Pediatric Nutrition

Fourth Edition

Edited by

Patricia Queen Samour, MMSc, RD

Director, Nutrition Services and Dietetic Internship Program
Beth Israel Deaconess Medical Center
Boston, Massachusetts

Kathy King, RD, LD

Private Practitioner
Publisher
Helm Publishing
Lake Dallas, Texas

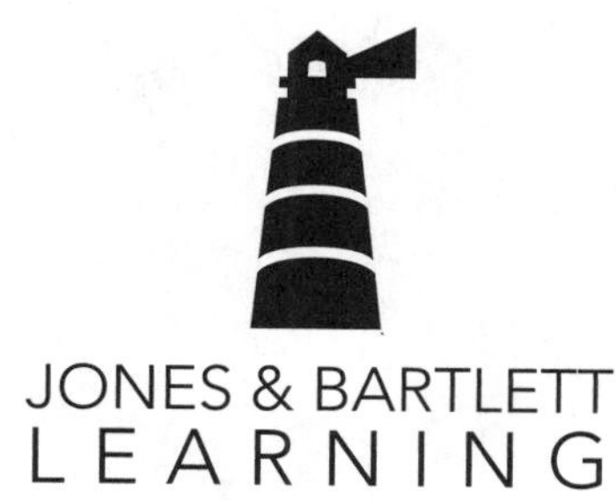

JONES & BARTLETT
LEARNING

World Headquarters
Jones & Bartlett Learning
40 Tall Pine Drive
Sudbury, MA 01776
978-443-5000
info@jblearning.com
www.jblearning.com

Jones & Bartlett Learning Canada
6339 Ormindale Way
Mississauga, Ontario L5V 1J2
Canada

Jones & Bartlett Learning International
Barb House, Barb Mews
London W6 7PA
United Kingdom

Jones & Bartlett Learning books and products are available through most bookstores and online booksellers. To contact Jones & Bartlett Learning directly, call 800-832-0034, fax 978-443-8000, or visit our website, www.jblearning.com.

Substantial discounts on bulk quantities of Jones & Bartlett Learning publications are available to corporations, professional associations, and other qualified organizations. For details and specific discount information, contact the special sales department at Jones & Bartlett Learning via the above contact information or send an email to specialsales@jblearning.com.

Production Credits
Publisher, Higher Education: Cathleen Sether
Senior Acquisitions Editor: Shoshanna Goldberg
Senior Associate Editor: Amy L. Bloom
Editorial Assistant: Prima Bartlett
Production Manager: Julie Champagne Bolduc
Production Editor: Jessica Steele Newfell
Associate Marketing Manager: Jody Sullivan
V.P., Manufacturing and Inventory Control: Therese Connell
Project Management: Thistle Hill Publishing Services, LLC
Composition: Dedicated Business Solutions, Inc.
Cover Design: Kristin E. Parker
Cover Images: (top left) © Bendao/Dreamstime.com; (top right) © Jperagine/Dreamstime.com; (bottom left) © Galina Barskaya/Dreamstime.com; (bottom right) © Jtphoto/Dreamstime.com
Printing and Binding: Malloy, Inc.
Cover Printing: Malloy, Inc.

Library of Congress Cataloging-in-Publication Data
Pediatric nutrition / [edited by] Patricia Queen Samour, Kathy King.—4th ed.
p. ; cm.
Rev. ed. of: Handbook of pediatric nutrition. 3rd ed. c2005.
Includes bibliographical references and index.
ISBN-13: 978-0-7637-8450-8 (pbk.)
ISBN-10: 0-7637-8450-8 (pbk.)
1. Children—Nutrition—Handbooks, manuals, etc. I. Samour, Patricia Queen. II. King, Kathy, RD. III. Handbook of pediatric nutrition.
[DNLM: 1. Child Nutritional Physiological Phenomena. 2. Child Nutrition Disorders. 3. Child. 4. Diet Therapy. 5. Infant Nutrition Disorders. 6. Infant. 7. Needs Assessment. WS 115]
RJ206.H23 2011
618.92—dc22
2010033533

6048

Printed in the United States of America
14 13 12 11 10 10 9 8 7 6 5 4 3 2 1

This edition of *Pediatric Nutrition* is dedicated to my dad, Joseph Emmett Queen, MD, who passed away in March 2010 at age 93. He was an internist and member of the Maryland State Medical Society who cared for many adult patients for over 60 years. His dad, my grandfather, was a pediatrician who cared for many infants and children. I thank them and my mom, who was a nurse, for their impact on my decision to be a registered dietitian.

—Patricia Queen Samour

This edition is dedicated to my parents, Iris Dean Nelson King and Walter Leroy King. Mother died in 1996, and I miss her dearly. She talked me into majoring in dietetics and was my business sounding board, manuscript copyeditor, and new product critic. She modeled high energy, jumping on new ideas and sticking with a job until it was at a standard I was proud of. My dad, Lee, was an instructor pilot in the Army Air Corps in WWII and then became an architect and engineer; he is now in a nursing home. He was always methodical and cautious—not an early adopter but always supportive and proud of my various new ventures. They are the flowers in my garden.

—Kathy King

Brief Contents

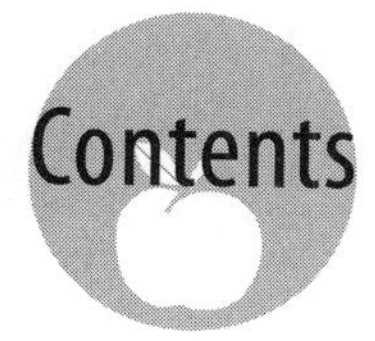

Contents

Preface

Commonly used by dietetic practitioners studying for their pediatric specialty exams, *Pediatric Nutrition, Fourth Edition*, is considered the most comprehensive textbook available on pediatric nutrition. Each chapter is written by experts in their practice area and contains detailed and comprehensive practical information. There are 21 chapters, with 13 returning chapter authors and 8 chapters with new authors. This book covers the latest clinical research, practical applications, alternative therapies, and study of the normal child from preconception through adolescence as well as children with special medical considerations.

This book is intended for use by all disciplines learning about pediatric nutrition and for practitioners managing the nutrition of pediatric groups and individuals. The goal for all infants and children is to grow and develop happily and in good health. As pediatric practitioners, we want to assess growth, evaluate nutrition status, and do everything possible to maximize health status. This goal is the same for all infants and children regardless of when they are born (full term or premature) and whether they have a disease condition or other health problem affecting their nutritional status. The growth charts, screening and assessment parameters, and routes of feeding may change, but the desired outcomes are the same.

Chapters of this text are written to help the reader identify and apply the key pediatric nutrition practices and principles. As is stated in many of the chapters, ongoing evidence-based research is needed in many of the conditions/diseases commonly seen in the pediatric population. New, emerging research and information (such as the use of botanicals) is addressed in this book. The appendixes, which contain the Centers for Disease Control and Prevention (CDC) growth charts, Tanner stages of sexual development, and other practical tables and figures, have now been expanded to include the World Health Organization (WHO) growth charts. Also included in the appendixes is the new Olsen and colleagues' intrauterine growth curves in Appendix A, an updated tool for growth assessment in U.S. neonatal intensive care units (NICUs).

For the first time, this book includes case studies with questions for the readers at the end of most chapters. We hope this will enhance the use and application of the chapter content. The *International Dietetics and Nutrition Terminology (IDNT), Third Edition*, published in 2009 and available online at http://www.eatright.org, is a resource used by registered dietitians (RDs) in learning about and documenting the nutrition care process. Additionally, this reference will help readers answer some of the case study questions. The nutrition care process consists of four steps: nutrition assessment, diagnosis, intervention, and monitoring and evaluation. The nutrition diagnosis (or problem [P]) is expressed using nutrition diagnostic terms and the etiologies (E), signs, and symptoms (S) that have been identified in the reference sheets describing each diagnosis. These result in a nutrition diagnostic statement or PES statement, as mentioned in many of the chapters' case studies.

Highlights of This Text

Chapter 1, Preconception and Prenatal Nutrition, includes the new guidelines for weight gain during pregnancy by the Institute of Medicine (IOM). It also includes the four goals from the CDC to improve health and pregnancy outcomes in the United States and addresses conditions such as polycystic ovary syndrome (PCOS).

Chapter 2, Physical Growth and Maturation, provides an overview of growth and maturation and their assessment, as illustrated by a case study and discussion about abnormal growth. Growth is assessed using the WHO and CDC growth charts in Appendix B.

Chapter 3, Nutritional Assessment, addresses the importance of nutrition screening and the components of a nutrition assessment, evaluation, and plan. Included are such topics as body mass index (BMI), the definitions of malnutrition, and failure to thrive.

Chapter 4, Nutrition for Premature Infants, addresses all aspects of nutrition management needed for the RD working with this high-risk population. Growth is assessed using special intrauterine and premature infant growth charts. Unique nutrient concerns and challenges for enteral and parenteral nutrition and common problems such as necrotizing enterocolitis (NEC) are detailed in this chapter.

Chapter 5, Normal Nutrition During Infancy, addresses the current recommended feeding practices for healthy full term infants and common feeding problems encountered during the first year of life. Information included in this chapter is applicable to all infants including those with diseases and/or conditions discussed in subsequent chapters.

Chapter 6, Normal Nutrition from Infancy Through Adolescence, focuses on the nutritional needs and issues of normal healthy children during their growth years. It also covers sports nutrition, pregnancy, and vegetarian diets. Developing sound nutrition and exercise habits is key to combating the problem of overweight children and obese adults.

Chapter 7, Food Hypersensitivities, deals with the pathophysiology, diagnosis, and treatment of infants and children with food hypersensitivities. This chapter is essential for the practitioner working with infants and/or children with true food hypersensitivities, and details such issues as food challenges, elimination diets, and the importance of label reading.

Chapter 8, Weight Management, addresses weight issues including the two extremes: obesity and eating disorders. Many factors that contribute to obesity and key issues such as prevalence trends, screening, assessment, and medical complications are discussed. The use of BMI, bariatric surgery, and intervention programs is detailed in the first section of this chapter. Eating disorders are discussed in the second part of the chapter because this is the third most common chronic illness in adolescents behind obesity and asthma. At-risk groups, such as female athletes and men, are discussed, as are key strategies to protect adolescents from developing an eating disorder.

Chapter 9, Genetic Screening and Nutrition Management, is a detailed resource for the practitioner having to manage the nutrition care of infants and children with inborn errors of metabolism (IEM). This chapter addresses newborn screening of IEMs and the principles and practical considerations in nutrition support of IEMs. Discussions cover the nutrition management of disorders of amino acid, nitrogen, carbohydrate, and fatty acid metabolism. Sample formula calculations for diet prescriptions are included which can help the RD less familiar with special medical foods determine accurate measurements on what to feed the infant or child with an IEM.

Chapter 10, Developmental Disabilities, addresses many of the more common types of disabilities, and their nutritional challenges and concerns. Topics such as performing a nutritional assessment on a child with cerebral palsy and managing a child with seizures on the ketogenic diet are addressed, along with nutritional considerations for children with attention deficit disorders.

Chapter 11, Pulmonary Diseases, includes the challenges of cystic fibrosis, bronchopulmonary dysplasia (BPD), and asthma. Some nutrition management issues discussed include cystic fibrosis during pregnancy, growth in infants with BPD, and the goals of asthma therapy. Family and caretakers learn their roles in the nutritional management of their child with pulmonary issues.

Chapter 12, Gastrointestinal Disorders, encompasses an array of common problems such as diarrhea and constipation, gastroesophageal reflux, and lactose intolerance as well as complex disorders such as celiac disease, liver transplant, and short gut syndrome. Properly handling the unique challenges of these conditions and their nutrition management is vital to health outcomes.

Chapter 13, Chronic Kidney Disease, addresses all nutrition care aspects of the infant or child before and during dialysis and after kidney transplant. The unique nutrients of concern in this disease and the challenges for normal growth are addressed. The frequent evaluation of food intake, growth, kidney function, and developmental stages is essential to adequately caring for these high risk infants and children.

Chapter 14, Cardiology, addresses the key concerns of infants and children with congenital heart disease and its inherent prevalence of malnutrition and growth disturbances. Issues such as extracorporeal membrane oxygenation (ECMO), cardiomyopathy, chylothorax, and hyerlipidemias are discussed here.

Chapter 15, Diabetes, stresses the challenge of the RD on the diabetes team to support the family's efforts of maintaining diabetes control of their infant or child and helping to promote healthy eating habits. Issues discussed include dysplipidemias, weight control, disordered eating, and use of the glycemic index. Diabetes is an area that continues to change rapidly with new research and technologies due to its high incidence in the U.S. population.

Chapter 16, HIV and AIDS, includes an in-depth description of the disease, and the goals and strategies of the nutrition management of infants and children with this disease. Use of highly active antiretroviral therapy (HAART) and other therapies and their impact on growth, body composition, and bone density are addressed.

Chapter 17, Hematology and Oncology, addresses the more common types of cancers in infants and children and their treatment challenges as well as other hematologic conditions such as sickle cell disease. Discussed are key aspects of nutrition support during cancer treatment, use of integrative medicine, and food safety.

Chapter 18, Nutrition for Burned Pediatric Patients, addresses the metabolic changes and physiologic challenges of providing adequate nutrition to the infant or child in this stressed state. Evaluation of energy requirements is emphasized, as is the use of nutrition support modalities used for rehabilitation post-burn.

Chapter 19, Enteral Nutrition, and Chapter 20, Parenteral Nutrition, contain the details needed to manage the nutritional status for all infants and children who cannot subsist and grow adequately on an oral diet. Use of enteral and/or parenteral nutrition may be short term or for longer periods of time and requires considerable knowledge of many factors by nutrition practitioners managing infants and children in the hospital, rehabilitation center, home, and other settings.

Chapter 21, Botanicals in Pediatrics, defines the nomenclature for herbs and phytomedicines. The use of herbs in pediatric practice and how to calculate the proper dose for medicinal herbs is included. This ever-growing consumer interest area requires the dietetics practitioner to be ever diligent in maintaining updated knowledge of research findings in this area.

The practice of pediatric nutrition with infants, young children, and adolescents in all settings, such as community, outpatient, and inpatient settings, continues to grow in complexity. It is balanced with an awareness of the importance of human contact and social development. It is hoped that readers of this fourth edition of *Pediatric Nutrition* will be challenged and reassured with the science and practice presented. Because infants and children have unique nutritional needs and physiology, advanced study in pediatric nutrition by health practitioners is vital for exemplary health care. This book contains the essential information that pediatric practitioners can use and apply in their individual setting for each infant or child.

Acknowledgments

Thank you to the staff at Jones & Bartlett Learning and our copyeditors for their fine work. Thank you also to all of our authors for being contributors to this book and for sharing your expertise with us. A special thanks to the nutrition volunteers, Aparna Kohli and Meg Schade, who worked with Patt to check references and tables and secure the necessary copyright permissions. And, a heartfelt thanks to all of our authors for the extra time and effort they spent finalizing their chapters for this new edition.

Contributors

Phyllis B. Acosta, MS, MPH, DrPH
Nutrition Consultant
Southeastern Region Genetics Group, Emory University
Atlanta, Georgia

Susan M. Akers, RD, LD
Pediatric Dietitian
MetroHealth Medical Center
Cleveland, Ohio

Diane M. Anderson, PhD, RD
Associate Professor of Pediatrics
Baylor College of Medicine
Houston, Texas

Jennifer Autodore, MA, RD, CSP, LDN
Pediatric Clinical Dietitian
Children's Hospital of Philadelphia
Philadelphia, Pennsylvania

Jenni Beary, MA, RD, CSP, LDN
Pediatric Clinical Dietitian
Children's Hospital of Philadelphia
Philadelphia, Pennsylvania

Susan Bessler, MS, RD, CSO
Clinical Pediatric Dietitian
Children's Hospital and Research Center Oakland
Oakland, California

Lynn Christie, MS, RD, LD
Research Project Manager Dietician
Department of Pediatric Allergy and Immunology
Arkansas Children's Hospital
Little Rock, Arkansas

Wm. Cameron Chumlea, PhD
Fels Professor
Lifespan Health Research Center
Departments of Community Health and Pediatrics
Boonshoft School of Medicine
Wright State University
Dayton, Ohio

Harriet Holt Cloud, MS, BS
Owner, Nutrition Matters
Birmingham, Alabama

Janice Hovasi Cox, MS, RD, CSP
Neonatal/Pediatric Dietitian
The Children's Hospital at Bronson
Kalamazoo, Michigan

Amanda L. Croll, RD, LDN
Pediatric Clinical Dietitian
Children's Hospital of Philadelphia
Philadelphia, Pennsylvania

Shannon Despino, RD, LDN
Clinical Dietitian Consultant
Scottsdale, Arizona

Maria Duarte-Gardea, PhD, RD
Chair, Department of Public Health Services
The University of Texas at El Paso
El Paso, Texas

Sharon Feucht, MS, RD, CSP
Nutritionist
Center on Human Development and Disability
University of Washington
Seattle, Washington

Michele Morath Gottschlich, PhD, RD, CNSD
Director, Nutrition Services
Shriners Hospital for Children
Cincinnati, Ohio

Sharon Groh-Wargo, PhD, RD, LD
Associate Professor and Senior Nutritionist
Case Western Reserve University
School of Medicine at Metro Health Medical Center
Cleveland, Ohio

Laurie Ann Higgins, MS, RD, LDN, CDE
Coordinator of Pediatric Nutrition Education and Research
Pediatric, Adolescent and Young Adult Section
Joslin Diabetes Center
Boston, Massachusetts

Laura Hudspeth, MS, RD
Infant and Pediatric Clinical Dietitian
University of Alabama at Birmingham
Birmingham, Alabama

Kathryn L. Hunt, BS, RD, CD
Clinical Pediatric Oncology Dietitian
Seattle Children's Hospital
Seattle, Washington

Susan Konek, MA, RD, CSP, CNSD, LDN
Director of Clinical Nutrition
The Children's Hospital of Philadelphia
Philadelphia, Pennsylvania

Haley W. Lacey, MD, RD, LD
Clinical Dietitian
Children's Health System of Alabama
Birmingham, Alabama

Michael J. LaMonte, PhD, MPH
Assistant Professor
Department of Social and Preventive Medicine
University of Buffalo–The State University of New York
Buffalo, New York

Betty Lucas, MPH, RD
Nutritionist
Center on Human Development and Disability
University of Washington
Seattle, Washington

Paula Charuhas Macris, MS, RD, FADA, CSO, CD
Nutrition Education Coordinator and Pediatric Nutrition Specialist
Seattle Cancer Care Alliance
Seattle, Washington

Theresa Mayes, RD
Clinical Dietitian
Shriners Hospital for Children
Cincinnati, Ohio

Ingrida Mara Melbardis, RD, CSP
Pediatric Dietitian
The Children's Hospital at Bronson
Kalamazoo, Michigan

Monica Nagle, RD, CNSD, LDN
Pediatric Clinical Dietitian
Children's Hospital of Philadelphia
Philadelphia, Pennsylvania

Beth Ogata, MS, RD, CSP
Nutritionist
Center on Human Development and Disability
University of Washington
Seattle, Washington

Linda A. Phelan, RD, CSR, LD
Pediatric Renal and NICU Dietitian
Oregon Health and Science University
Doernbecher Children's Hospital
Portland, Oregon

Erin Redding, RD, LDN
Nutrition Specialist
New England Dairy and Food Council
Boston, Massachusetts

Jill Rockwell, RD, CNSD
Clinical Dietitian
Children's Medical Center Dallas
Dallas, Texas

Melanie Savoca, MS, RD, LDN
Pediatric Clinical Dietitian
Children's Hospital of Philadelphia
Philadelphia, Pennsylvania

Lisa Simone Sharda, MA, RD
Children's Memorial Hospital
Chicago, Illinois

Bonnie A. Spear, PhD, RD
Professor of Pediatrics
University of Alabama at Birmingham
Birmingham, Alabama

Alyce Thomas, RD
Prenatal Nutrition Consultant
St. Joseph's Regional Medical Center
Paterson, New Jersey

John Westerdahl, PhD, MPH, RD, CNS
Director
Bragg Health Institute
Santa Barbara, California

Sarah C. Weston, RD, LDN
Clinical Dietitian for Gastroenterology
Children's Hospital of Philadelphia
Philadelphia, Pennsylvania

Preconception and Prenatal Nutrition

Alyce Thomas and María Duarte-Gardea

Infant care does not begin on the day a baby is born; it is a journey that takes place before conception. The health of the mother prior to and during pregnancy is one of the major determinants to a successful outcome. If a woman enters pregnancy in less than optimal health, the risk of adverse effects to her and her baby are increased. Preconception care, which includes nutrition, physical activity, and behavioral interventions, is an important adjunct to the health care of all women in their reproductive years. However, only a small percentage of women receive preconception care to follow healthy lifestyle recommendations.[1–3] As preconception care becomes the norm and not the exception to routine medical care, women will seek to enter prenatal care early in their pregnancy. Any delay in accessing prenatal care may result in an increase in negative outcomes. Important components of preconception and prenatal care are nutrition counseling for normal pregnancy with medical nutrition therapy (when needed), and they should be incorporated into the health care of all women.

Preconception

Despite having the highest per capita healthcare costs in the world, the United States ranks 29th in infant mortality rate.[4] The primary reason for the higher infant mortality rate is the number of preterm births when compared to other nations. One in eight infants in the United States is born preterm, which is defined as less than 37 weeks gestation.[4] In 2005, 8.2% of all U.S. infants were born at low birth weight or less than 2500 grams.[4] Although this includes an increase in the number of multiple births, the rates continue to rise for singleton births.

One of the contributing factors to the poor pregnancy outcome in the United States is the date when a woman enters prenatal care. If prenatal care does not begin until late in the first trimester or in the second or third trimester, the delay may result in serious health consequences for the mother and her infant. To reduce the risks associated with delayed prenatal care, the focus must be on improving the woman's health prior to pregnancy. Because more than half of all pregnancies are unplanned or unintended, preconception care should be incorporated into the routine primary medical care of every woman of childbearing age.[1,5] Ideally, the medical care for adolescent girls would transition from the pediatrician to the family physician. This would ensure continuous medical care.

Preconception care is defined as a set of interventions that aim to identify and modify biomedical, behavioral, and social risks to a woman's health or pregnancy outcome through prevention and management.[1] These interventions, when applied before conception, may decrease the risk of adverse health effects in the woman, fetus, and neonate. The goal of preconception care is for every woman to receive services that will enable her to achieve optimal health before pregnancy. This includes health care for women between pregnancies.[6]

The Centers for Disease Control and Prevention (CDC) has identified 4 goals and 10 recommendations to improve health and pregnancy outcomes in the United States (**Tables 1-1** and **1-2**). The American Academy of Pediatrics (AAP) and the American College of Obstetricians and Gynecologists (ACOG) have emphasized nutrition as one of the eight areas for risk screening.[7,8] Two of the CDC-selected preconception risk factors for adverse pregnancy outcomes that are directly affected by a woman's nutritional health are diabetes and obesity.

Two other conditions, hypertension and polycystic ovary syndrome, are not listed in the CDC's preconception health care recommendations, but they may also affect perinatal outcome.

Diabetes

Women with pregestational diabetes are at increased risk for poor perinatal outcomes. Maternal complications include retinopathy, neuropathy, nephropathy, and cardiovascular disease.[9,10] Congenital anomalies and increased risk of stillbirth and miscarriage are among the complications associated

TABLE 1-1 Goals to Improve Health and Pregnancy Outcomes in the United States

- **Goal 1.** To improve the knowledge, attitudes, and behaviors of men and women related to preconception health.
- **Goal 2.** To ensure that all U.S. women of childbearing age receive preconception care services (screening, health promotion, and interventions) that will enable them to enter pregnancy in optimal health.
- **Goal 3.** To reduce risks indicated by a prior adverse pregnancy outcome through interventions in the interconception (inter-pregnancy) period that can prevent or minimize health problems for a mother and her future children.
- **Goal 4.** To reduce the disparities in adverse pregnancy outcomes.

Source: From Centers for Disease Control and Prevention. Recommendations to improve preconception health and health care—United States. *MMWR.* 2006;55(RR06):1–23.

with hyperglycemia during pregnancy. Conception should be delayed until optimal glycemic levels are achieved. The risk of perinatal complications decreases in women with pregestational diabetes to a level comparable to pregnant women without diabetes if their glycosylated hemoglobin levels are as close to normal as possible without significant hypoglycemia.[9,11] The American Diabetes Association has recommended preconception counseling to all women with diabetes to reduce the risk of malformations associated with unplanned pregnancies and poor metabolic control.[9,10] Effective contraception methods should be used at all times until good metabolic control is achieved.[10]

Medical nutrition therapy (MNT) provided by registered dietitians has been shown to be effective in managing type 1 and type 2 diabetes.[11–13] The overall goals of MNT for women with preexisting diabetes are to achieve and maintain blood glucose levels in the normal range through dietary and lifestyle modifications to decrease the risk of perinatal complications.[9] Evidence-based nutrition recommendations for type 1 and type 2 diabetes can be found online at the American Dietetic Association's Evidence Analysis Library and the American Diabetes Association's position statement on nutrition recommendations.[12,13]

Women with previous gestational diabetes mellitus (GDM) are at risk of developing type 2 diabetes mellitus later in life or GDM in subsequent pregnancies.[11] Six to eight weeks after delivery, a 75-gram oral glucose tolerance test (OGTT) should be performed on all women with GDM. The American Diabetes Association also recommends GDM women be screened every year if the fasting glucose or 2-hour postprandial on the postpartum OGTT was elevated.[11] Nutrition recommendations for GDM are discussed in the pregnancy section of this chapter.

TABLE 1-2 Recommendations to Improve Preconception Health

- **Recommendation 1. Individual Responsibility Across the Lifespan.** Each woman, man, and couple should be encouraged to have a reproductive life plan.
- **Recommendation 2. Consumer Awareness.** Increase public awareness of the importance of preconception health behaviors and preconception care services by using information and tools appropriate across various ages; literacy, including health literacy; and cultural/linguistic contexts.
- **Recommendation 3. Preventive Visits.** As a part of primary care visits, provide risk assessment and educational and health promotion counseling to all women of childbearing age to reduce reproductive risks and improve pregnancy outcomes.
- **Recommendation 4. Interventions for Identified Risks.** Increase the proportion of women who receive interventions as follow-up to preconception risk screening, focusing on high priority intervention (i.e., those with evidence of effectiveness and greatest potential impact).
- **Recommendation 5. Interconception Care.** Use the interconception period to provide additional intensive interventions to women who have had a previous pregnancy that ended in an adverse outcome (i.e., infant death, fetal loss, birth defects, low birthweight, or preterm birth).
- **Recommendation 6. Prepregnancy Checkup.** Offer, as a component of maternity care, one prepregnancy visit for couples and persons planning pregnancy.
- **Recommendation 7. Health Insurance Coverage for Women with Low Incomes.** Increase public and private health insurance coverage for women with low incomes to improve access to preventive women's health and preconception and interconception care.
- **Recommendation 8. Public Health Programs and Strategies.** Integrate components of preconception health into existing local public health and related programs, including emphasis on interconception interventions for women with previous adverse outcomes.
- **Recommendation 9. Research.** Increase the evidence base and promote the use of the evidence to improve preconception health.
- **Recommendation 10. Monitoring Improvements.** Maximize public health surveillance and related research merchanisms to monitor preconception health.

Source: From Centers for Disease Control and Prevention. Recommendations to improve preconception health and health care—United States. *MMWR.* 2006;55(RR06):1–23.

Obesity

According to the Expert Panel from the National Heart, Lung and Blood Institute's (NHLBI) Obesity Education Initiative, overweight is defined as a body mass index (BMI) of 25 to 29.9 kg/m^2, and obesity is defined as a BMI >30 kg/m^2.[14,15]

The prevalence of overweight and obesity in women over 20 years of age has not increased over the past 4 years; it remains at 62% and 33.2%, respectively.[16]

Overweight and obesity continue to be the leading public health concerns in the United States.[16] Obesity is a risk factor for cardiovascular disease and diabetes, and substantially increases the risk of morbidity from hypertension, coronary artery disease, and certain types of cancers.[14,15] Obesity also affects the outcome of pregnancy in the mother and her fetus. A higher prevalence of gestational diabetes, impaired glucose tolerance, hypertension, thromboembolism, preeclampsia, sleep apnea, cesarean section, preterm delivery, and postpartum weight retention are associated with maternal obesity.[17,18] Fetal complications include macrosomia, congenital anomalies, shoulder dystocia, and childhood obesity.[17–19] Ideally, women should delay conception until they have achieved a normal weight to improve their pregnancy outcome.[17,19,20] Treatment of the overweight or obese woman consists of assessment and management.[15]

Assessment includes determining the degree of obesity and health status by evaluating the BMI, waist circumference, and overall medical risk. Body mass index is a better indicator than body weight alone because it provides a more accurate measure of total body fat.[17,21,22] Waist circumference is a useful indicator of abdominal fat mass.[15,21,22] The American Dietetic Association's Evidence Analysis Library Weight Management Guidelines recommends using BMI and waist circumference to classify overweight and obesity, estimate risk for disease, and identify treatment options.[23] BMI and waist circumference are highly correlated to obesity or fat mass and risk of other diseases.[21,23] Women are at increased relative risk for disease if their waist circumference is greater than 35 inches (89 cm). The classifications for BMI and waist circumference are found in **Table 1-3**.

Management involves weight loss, maintenance, and controlling other risk factors. The goals for weight loss and management include: (1) to reduce body weight, (2) to maintain lower body weight, and (3) to prevent further weight gain.

An initial weight loss of 10% of body weight within 6 months is considered achievable.[15,21] The weight loss should be at a rate of 1 to 2 pounds per week, based on a calorie reduction of 500–1000 kcal/day. Effective weight loss strategies include dietary therapy, physical activity, and behavioral therapy—or in certain cases, pharmacotherapy and surgery. Bariatric surgery is the most effective therapy for persons with BMI ≥ 40 or BMI ≥ 35 with comorbid conditions. This type of surgery could be considered warranted for adolescents under 18 years of age if they meet the following criteria: severely obese (BMI ≥ 40), attained skeletal maturity, and have comorbid conditions related to obesity.[24]

The BMI for girls under 20 years old is based on age. After the BMI is calculated, the number is plotted on the CDC BMI-for-age growth chart to obtain a percentile ranking. **Table 1-4** shows the weight status category and percentile range for adolescents.

Hypertension

Hypertensive disorders during pregnancy are a leading cause of maternal mortality and are associated with an increased risk of preterm birth and intrauterine growth retardation.[25] According to the Seventh Report of the Joint National Committee on Prevention, Detection, Evaluation, and Treatment of High Blood Pressure, a woman's blood pressure should be evaluated prior to conception in order to define its status, assess its severity, determine the presence of organ damage, and plan treatment strategies.[26] Certain medications, such as angiotensin II receptor blockers (ARBs)

TABLE 1-3 Classification of Overweight and Obesity in Women by BMI, Waist Circumference, and Associated Disease Risk

	BMI (kg/m²)	Obesity Class	Disease Risk (Relative to Normal Weight and Waist Circumference)	
			≤35 in (≤89 cm)	>35 in (89 cm)
Underweight	<18.5		—	—
Normal	18.5–24.9		—	—
Overweight	25.0–29.9		Increased	High
Obesity	30.0–34.9	I	High	Very High
	35.0–39.9	II	Very High	Very High
Extreme Obesity	≥40	III	Extremely High	Extremely High

Source: From National Heart, Lung and Blood Institute. *The Practical Guide. Identification, Evaluation, and Treatment of Overweight and Obesity in Adults*. Washington, DC: National Institutes of Health; 2000. NIH Publication No. 00–4084.

TABLE 1-4 BMI Categories for Adolescent Girls

Weight Status	Percentile
Underweight	Less than the 5th percentile
Healthy weight	5th percentile to less than the 85th percentile
Overweight	85th to less than the 95th percentile
Obese	Equal to or greater than the 95th percentile

Source: From Centers for Disease Control and Prevention. BMI children and teens. Available at: http://www.cdc.gov/healthyweight/assessing/bmi/childrens_bmi/about_childrens_bmi.html. Accessed September 3, 2010.

and angiotensin converting enzyme (ACE) inhibitors, are contraindicated in pregnancy and should be discontinued before the woman plans to conceive.[25] Methyldopa and beta blockers are safe to use during pregnancy.[25,26]

There is an increasing prevalence of hypertension in pregnant teenagers, which is related to higher rates of obesity among adolescents. Pregnant teenagers are more at risk of developing preeclampsia than women in the 20- to 30-year age group, and preeclampsia is most common among young primiparas.[27]

The American Dietetic Association's evidence-based nutrition practice guidelines for hypertension recommend a comprehensive program in the management of elevated blood pressure, which includes medical nutrition therapy, weight reduction, and physical activity.[28] Research indicates that a comprehensive program can prevent target organ damage and improve cardiovascular outcomes.[25,26,28,29] The DASH (Dietary Approaches to Stop Hypertension) dietary pattern has been shown to reduce systolic blood pressure by 8–14 mm Hg.[28–30] Lowering the daily sodium intake to less than 2300 mg also helps to lower blood pressure.[28–30]

Polycystic Ovary Syndrome

Polycystic ovary syndrome (PCOS) is an endocrine condition that affects about 1 in every 10 women.[31] It is associated with various metabolic dysfunctions, including menstrual irregularities, infertility, hyperandrogenism, hypertension, insulin resistance, and hyperinsulinemia.[31,32] Women with PCOS are at increased risk of developing cardiovascular disease, type 2 diabetes, and the metabolic syndrome.[31] Although most women with PCOS tend to be overweight, it is also seen in normal weight women with excessive abdominal fat distribution.[33]

Treatment for PCOS consists of dietary and lifestyle changes, including physical activity, weight management, behavior modification, and medication, if necessary. Insulin sensitivity has been shown to improve with weight loss.[34] Although there is no standardized food plan for PCOS, dietary patterns that emphasize unrefined carbohydrates with moderate protein and unsaturated fats have been recommended.[31–36] Dietary fats, especially saturated and trans fats, may play a role in insulin resistance by increasing inflammation. A prospective cohort study showed that a diet high in trans fats may increase the risk of ovulatory infertility.[37]

Metformin is commonly used in the treatment of PCOS to improve insulin resistance, reduce hyperandrogenism, and increase ovulation, and it may prevent the development of GDM.[31] Orlistat coupled with calorie restriction was shown to significantly decrease insulin resistance and weight in women with PCOS.[38]

Lifestyle Factors

Other modifiable risk factors have been identified that when addressed in the preconception period will help to improve pregnancy outcome. These risk factors include alcohol, folate deficiency, maternal phenylketonuria, and smoking.

Alcohol

Prenatal exposure to alcohol use during pregnancy is the leading cause of preventable birth defects and developmental disabilities.[39,40] Risks to the fetus include spontaneous abortions, intrauterine growth restriction, central nervous system and facial malformations, and mental retardation. Fetal alcohol spectrum disorders (FASD) is a term that describes a range of effects that can occur in persons exposed to alcohol in utero. Fetal alcohol syndrome (FAS) is the most commonly known of the disorders. In the United States, approximately 5000 babies are born each year with FAS. There is no safe level of alcohol consumption during pregnancy, so the U.S. Surgeon General's Advisory on Alcohol use in pregnancy urges women who are pregnant or who may become pregnant to abstain from alcohol use.[41]

Folate Deficiency

Each year in the United States, approximately 3000 pregnancies are affected by neural tube defects (NTDs), which include spina bifida and anencephaly.[42] Folate has been shown to protect against NTDs. All women of reproductive age are advised to take 400 mcg of folic acid daily, from fortified foods and/or supplements. Additional information on folate is found in the pregnancy section of this chapter.

Maternal Phenylketonuria

Phenylketonuria (PKU) is a metabolic disorder characterized by mental retardation, microcephaly, low birth weight, and congenital heart defects.[1,2,43,44] Women who were diagnosed with PKU as infants and enter pregnancy with elevated phenylalanine levels are at increased risk of delivering infants with congenital anomalies. Because the most critical period of pregnancy is in the first 10 weeks after conception, a phenylalanine-restricted diet is recommended for PKU women throughout their reproductive years.

Smoking

Cigarette smoking is the leading cause of preventable morbidity and mortality in the United States.[45,46] Women who smoke are at increased risk for heart disease, certain types of cancers, and lung disease.[45] Smoking during pregnancy has an adverse effect on both the woman and the fetus. Maternal effects include spontaneous abortion, premature rupture of the membranes, placenta previa, placenta abruption, and preterm delivery. Fetal effects associated with tobacco include intrauterine growth restriction, low birth weight, and sudden infant death syndrome. The CDC recommends cessation of smoking before pregnancy.[45] All women should be screened for tobacco use during their reproductive years and referred for counseling services.

Pregnancy

Pregnancy is a time of increased energy and nutrient needs for a woman to support fetal growth and development, as well as her own. As the length of gestation and the prepregnancy weight of the mother are two of the most influential factors affecting prenatal outcome, the mother's nutritional status is an important component to prenatal care.

Weight Issues in Pregnancy

Prepregnancy weight and weight gain are important aspects in pregnancy because both are associated with maternal outcomes, mode of delivery, preterm birth, birth weight, and postpartum weight retention.

BMI is the best available measure of prepregnancy weight; it serves as a baseline for weight gain recommendations. The World Health Organization (WHO) has established the following BMI categories to define weight status: underweight (<18.5), normal weight (18.5–24.9), overweight (25–29.9), and obese (>29.9).[47] The Institute of Medicine (IOM) provides guidelines for weight gain during pregnancy according to the prepregnancy BMI. These guidelines seek to improve maternal and infant outcomes.

Weight Gain Recommendations

Recommendations for weight gain during pregnancy should be individualized according to the prepregnancy BMI to improve pregnancy outcome, avoid excessive maternal postpartum weight retention, and reduce the risk of adult chronic disease in the child.[48]

After nearly two decades, the IOM reexamined the guidelines for weight gain during pregnancy, which took into consideration the recent increase in the prevalence of obese women of childbearing age. The new guidelines differ from the previous recommendations in two aspects: (1) they are based on the WHO BMI categories rather than the previous categories from the Metropolitan Life Insurance tables, and (2) they include a narrow range of weight gain for obese women. Recommendations of total and weekly weight gain for the second and third trimesters for each BMI are displayed in **Table 1-5**. The recommended total weight gain for the first trimester is 0.5–2 kg or 1.1–4.4 pounds, depending on the prepregnancy BMI.[49,50]

Overweight and Obesity

Obesity occurs in approximately 50% of non-Hispanic black women, followed by black Mexican American (38%), and non-Hispanic white (31%) women of childbearing age.[51] Numerous studies have reported an increased risk of gestational diabetes mellitus (GDM) among women who are overweight and obese. A meta-analysis of 20 studies determined the risk of developing gestational diabetes with maternal obesity. The unadjusted odds ratio (OR) of developing GDM were 2.14 (95% confidence of interval 1.82–2.53), 3.56 (3.05–4.21), and 8.56 (5.07–16.04) among overweight, obese, and severely obese women, respectively, compared with normal-weight

TABLE 1-5 Total and Mean Weight Gain Recommendations During Pregnancy

	Underweight (< 18.5)	Normal (18.5–24.9)	Overweight (25–29.9)	Obese (> 29.9)
Total				
Kg	12.5–18	11.5–16	7–11.5	5–9
Lb	28–40	25–35	15–25	11–20
Weekly Gain for Second and Third Trimesters				
Mean, Kg	0.51	0.4	0.28	0.22
Range, Kg	(0.44–0.58)	(0.35–0.50)	(0.23–0.33)	(0.17–0.27)
Mean, Lb	1	1	0.6	0.5
Range, Lb	(1–1.3)	(0.8–1)	(0.5–0.7)	(0.4–0.6)

Source: Adapted from Institute of Medicine. *Weight Gain During Pregnancy: Reexamining the Guidelines.* Report brief. Washington, DC: The National Academies Press; 2009. Reprinted with permission from the National Academies Press, Copyright 2009, National Academy of Sciences.

pregnant women. The authors concluded that high maternal weight is associated with a higher risk of GDM.[52] Other complications associated with maternal overweight and obesity are hypertension, preeclampsia, cesarean section, preterm delivery, labor induction, postpartum hemorrhage, macrosomia, and neonatal hypoglycemia.[53–59] Due to the multiple maternal and infant detrimental effects associated with maternal overweight and obesity, the American Dietetic Association and the American Society for Nutrition released the position statement that "all overweight and obese women of reproductive age should receive counseling on the roles of diet and physical activity in reproductive health prior to pregnancy, during pregnancy, and in the interconceptional period in order to ameliorate these adverse outcomes."[60]

Multiple Gestation

Multiple births have risen dramatically over the past 20 years in the United States, primarily due to the increasing use of assisted reproductive technologies (ART). Newborns conceived through ART are at higher risk for prematurity, low birth weight, and perinatal mortality. Women who conceive through ART are more likely to develop preeclampsia and gestational diabetes, and experience preterm birth or vacuum or forceps delivery. The most common antenatal complications include preterm premature rupture of membranes, hemorrhage, and anemia.[61–64] In a recent population study that included 316,696 twin, 12,193 triplet, and 778 quadruplet pregnancies from the 1995–2000 Matched Multiple Birth Data Set, triplet and quadruplet pregnancies had significantly higher risks than twin pregnancies for most maternal and neonatal complications. The study also showed that maternal anthropometric, nutritional, and previous reproductive factors may be particularly important in the reduction of these excess risks and improvement of outcomes in multiple births.[65] Most infants of multiple gestation are preterm births (37 weeks gestation) and are among the low birth weight (2500 g) and very low birth weight (1500 g) infant populations. Early preterm births (32 weeks gestation) occur in 35% of triplet and higher order births and 11% of twin births, compared with less than 2% of singleton births.[66] Weight gain recommendations for twin pregnancies from the IOM suggest a range of maternal weight gain of 37–54 pounds for the normal BMI category, 31–50 pounds for overweight women, and 25–42 pounds for obese women, with a suggested rate gain of 1.5 pounds per week during the second and third trimesters.[49] In a study by Luke and colleagues, optimal rates of fetal growth and birth weights in twins were achieved at rates of maternal weight gain that varied by period of gestation and maternal pregravid BMI status. For example, in normal weight women, the specific recommended rate of weight gain up to 20 weeks of gestation is 1–1.5 lb/wk (0.45–0.68 kg/wk), 1.25–1.75 lb/wk (0.57–0.79 kg/wk) between 20 and 28 weeks, and 1.0 lb/wk (0.45 kg/wk) from 28 weeks to delivery.[67]

Gastrointestinal Discomforts

Nausea and Vomiting

Symptoms of nausea and vomiting in pregnancy (NVP) constitute a frequent and often highly unpleasant syndrome during early gestation. Nausea and vomiting affect 70% of pregnant women during the first trimester and vomiting alone affects between 30% and 50% of pregnant women.[68] Commonly referred to as "morning sickness," nausea and vomiting may occur at any time during the day or night. Nausea, a frequent discomfort of early pregnancy, can last well into the second trimester and varies greatly in its severity. A prospective cohort study that included 2407 newly pregnant women in three U.S. cities found that 89% of women experienced NVP; in 99%, the symptoms started in the first trimester. NVP symptoms in multigravidas were more likely to last beyond the first trimester with each additional pregnancy.[69]

Management of nausea and vomiting depends on the severity of the symptoms. Dietary modifications may resolve mild cases. First trimester nausea may improve by consuming small amounts of liquid or food at frequent intervals, and avoiding fried, spicy, and high fat foods. Some pregnant women may tolerate foods high in carbohydrates such as crackers rather than high-protein or high-fat foods.[48] Some women respond by avoiding cooking odors, getting out of bed slowly in the morning, and drinking small amounts of liquid between meals.[70–72] Current dietary recommendations shown to have beneficial nausea-reducing effects and considered safe and effective include taking a multivitamin early in the pregnancy-planning process, supplementation with vitamin B_6, and eating ginger as a nonpharmacologic option.[73]

Hyperemesis gravidarum (HG), or severe nausea and vomiting, is a high-risk condition usually requiring hospital admission, antiemetic medications, rehydration, correction of electrolytes, and nutritional support. In a study of 819 women with HG, 214 (26.1%) experienced extreme weight loss, defined as a loss of greater than 15% of prepregnancy weight. Extreme weight loss ($p < 0.001$) was associated with indicators of the severity of HG, such as hospitalization, use of parenteral nutrition, gallbladder and liver dysfunction, renal failure, and retinal hemorrhage.[71] The interventions mentioned in the previous paragraph may help prevent excessive pregnancy weight loss and infants born with low birth weight.[72,73]

Heartburn

Heartburn is a common symptom in pregnancy, affecting up to 80% of women in the third trimester. The reasons for the increased symptoms during the latter stage of pregnancy are not well understood, but the effects of pregnancy hormones on the lower esophageal sphincter and gastric clearance are thought to play a part. A range of interventions has been used to relieve symptoms including advice on diet and lifestyle, antacids, antihistamines, and proton pump inhibitors.[74] In a systematic review of placebo controlled trials, three studies examined various medications to relieve heartburn (intramuscular prostigmine, an antacid preparation, and an antacid plus ranitidine). All three produced positive findings in favor of the intervention groups; however, the authors concluded that there was a paucity of information to draw conclusions on the overall effectiveness of interventions to relieve heartburn in pregnancy.[75]

Practical approaches that may ease heartburn in pregnancy include avoiding lying down immediately after eating; sleeping with the woman's head slightly elevated to avoid acid reflux; consuming small, frequent meals; and avoiding known irritants such as caffeine, chocolate, or highly seasoned foods.[48]

Ptyalism

Ptyalism is of unknown origin and is usually defined as an excessive secretion of saliva. It is common in women with nausea and vomiting who might have difficulty swallowing their saliva.[76] Dietary alterations to overcome ptyalism include the use of chewing gum or lozenges and restricting fluids.[77] In two case studies complicated by ptyalism during pregnancy, one case reported that ptyalism recovered spontaneously at 35–36 weeks gestation; in the other it did not resolve until after delivery.[75] Further research is needed to determine the physiologic origin of ptyalism and to identify treatment.[78]

Constipation

Constipation is common during pregnancy and occurs most frequently during the third trimester as the weight of the uterus puts pressure on the rectum, which may also result in hemorrhoids. Increased consumption of liquids in combination with high fiber foods and regular physical activity are recommended to alleviate constipation. It is recommended to drink from six to eight glasses of fluids daily. The dietary reference intake (DRI) for fiber during pregnancy is 28 g/day.[79] High fiber foods include whole grains, legumes, fruits, and vegetables.

Diarrhea

Diarrhea is characterized by several changes in the stool, including an increased frequency, looser consistency, and more volume. It is caused by an increase in water content in the stool. Diarrhea during pregnancy may be the result of foodborne infections, irritable bowel syndrome, or other causes. Acute diarrhea may lead to severe dehydration that can result in the loss of important electrolytes from the body. Symptoms of dehydration include excessive thirst, dry mouth, scant or no urine or dark yellow urine, decreased tears, severe weakness or lethargy, and dizziness. Fluids are the most effective treatment for preventing dehydration in pregnant women. Consumption of liquids, such as oral rehydration fluids, juice, or water, can help pregnant women reduce the risk of becoming dehydrated. Medical attention should be required when diarrhea is not resolved within 24 hours. Also diarrhea with bloody stools, fever, or severe abdominal pain requires immediate medical attention.

Eating Disorders

The eating disorders (EDs) anorexia nervosa, bulimia nervosa, and eating disorders not otherwise specified (EDNOS) have profound effects on the overall well-being of women and their children. Clinically, these disorders can present as menstrual dysfunction, low bone density, sexual dysfunction, miscarriage, preterm delivery, or low birth weight.[80] A recent study evaluated ED symptoms in pregnancy and reported that women with recent episodes of ED restricted their intake, used laxatives, self-induced vomiting, and exercised more than other groups during pregnancy. Their weight and body shape concern scores remained high during pregnancy. Women with past histories of ED were also more likely than controls to have some ED behaviors and/or concerns about weight gain during pregnancy.[81] Complications associated with eating disorders during pregnancy include miscarriage, premature labor, low birth weight, stillbirth or fetal death, and delayed fetal growth.

Physical Activity

The benefits of physical activity during pregnancy have been extensively documented. Physical activity is recommended by ACOG for most pregnant women without medical or obstetric risk. The recommendation for normal risk pregnant women in the absence of either medical or obstetric complications is 30 minutes or more of moderate-intensity physical activity on most, if not all, days of the week. According to the ACOG committee, in general, participation in a wide range of recreational activities appears to be safe during pregnancy. However, each sport should be reviewed individually for its potential risk, and activities with a high risk of abdominal trauma should be avoided. Physical activity is contraindicated if the following conditions are present: restrictive lung disease, incompetent cervix, multiple gestation, premature labor, rupture of membranes, preeclampsia/pregnancy-induced hypertension, persistent second and third trimester bleeding, and placenta previa.[82] A study of 44 healthy women in late pregnancy that compared active vs. inactive women reported that active women (those who engaged in more than 30 minutes of moderate-intensity physical activity per day) had significantly better cardiovascular fitness and lower sleeping heart rates without any negative effects on fetal condition or outcome of labor and delivery compared to the inactive women. The duration of the second stage of labor was 88 and 146 minutes, respectively, for the active vs. inactive women ($p = 0.05$).[83]

It is important to evaluate the overall health of pregnant women, including obstetric and medical risks, before prescribing an exercise program. Additional factors to take into consideration are prepregnancy BMI, weight gain goals, dietary intake, and history of physical activity.

Nutrient Recommendations

The quality of the diet during pregnancy has a profound impact on fetal and maternal outcomes. A well-balanced diet providing recommended calories and optimal nutrients throughout pregnancy should favor fetal normal growth and development and desired maternal outcomes. Conversely, maternal malnutrition, especially during the first trimester, a crucial period of fetal development, may predispose the infant to chronic diseases in adult years. Recent research suggests chronic diseases such as coronary heart disease, hypertension, and type 2 diabetes may originate in impaired intrauterine growth and development.[84,85]

The dietary reference intakes (DRIs) is a set of daily nutrient intake guidelines for different age groups and genders that encompasses several reference values such as the recommended dietary allowances (RDAs), adequate intake (AI), tolerable upper intake level (UL), and estimated average requirement (EAR). These values serve as a guide to prevent nutritional deficiencies and to promote optimal health benefits. Recommended levels of energy and nutrient intakes vary for adults, children, and women who are pregnant or breastfeeding.[79,86]

Energy

The energy allowance for pregnancy can be estimated by dividing the gross energy cost (80,000 kcal) by the approximate duration (250 days following the first month), yielding an average value of 300 kcal per day in addition to the allowance for nonpregnant females.[79,86] Caloric requirements for pregnant adolescents (14–18 years) and adult women (19–50 years) can be calculated by using the estimated energy requirements (EER) formula.[79] **Table 1-6** displays EER formulas to determine energy requirements for normal prepregnancy BMI for each trimester. The DRIs for total energy indicate that for healthful birth outcomes, pregnant women should consume an extra 340 kcal/day in the second trimester and 452 kcal/day in the third trimester.

The formulas displayed in Table 1-6 are not applicable to overweight and obese women. An estimate of the caloric requirement for overweight and obese women can be obtained by using an adjusted body weight in the Harris Benedict formula and adding 150–300 kcal for the second and third trimesters.[79,87] (See **Table 1-7**.)

A simple method to determine caloric needs during pregnancy for normal weight women is to estimate a daily need of 30 kcal per kilogram prepregnancy weight per day during the first trimester, and adding 300 kcal during the second and third trimesters. In underweight women, these caloric prescriptions would need to be increased.

Regardless of the method used to estimate caloric level, weight gain pattern, goals, and appetite are used by registered dietitians or other healthcare professionals to make the necessary caloric adjustments. Frequent monitoring ensures that pregnant women will consume adequate calories from nutrient-dense foods to sustain weight gain and provide appropriate nutrients.

Macronutrients

The main function of macronutrients in the diet is to provide energy. Besides providing the RDA or AI for carbohydrates, proteins, and fat, the DRIs for macronutrients also provide a range of daily macronutrient distribution. The Acceptable Macronutrient Distribution Range (AMDR) is the range of intake for a particular energy source that is associated with reduced risk of chronic disease while providing intakes of essential nutrients. If an individual consumes in excess of the AMDR, there is an increased risk of chronic

TABLE 1-6 Estimated Energy Requirements for Normal Prepregnancy BMI

First Trimester [EER + 0]	$EER = 354 - (6.91 \times A) + PA \times (9.36 \times Wt + 726 \times Ht)$
Second Trimester [EER + 340]	$EER = 354 - (6.91 \times A) + PA \times (9.36 \times Wt + 726 \times Ht) + 340$
Third Trimester [EER + 452]	$EER = 354 - (6.91 \times A) + PA \times (9.36 \times Wt + 726 \times Ht) + 452$

Abbreviations: A = age; PA = physical activity coefficient: sedentary (1.0), low activity (1.12), active (1.27), very active (1.45); Wt = weight in kilograms; Ht = height in meters.

Source: Data from Institute of Medicine. *Dietary Reference Intakes for Energy, Carbohydrates, Fiber, Fat, Fatty Acids, Cholesterol, Protein and Amino Acids (Macronutrients)*. Washington, DC: National Academies Press; 2002.

TABLE 1-7 Energy Requirements for Overweight and Obese Prepregnancy BMI

Energy = [655 + (9.6 × AdBWt kg) + (1.8 × Ht cm) − (4.7 × A)] × PA + (150 − 300) kcal

Abbreviations: AdBWt = Adjusted Body Weight: [(Actual Body Wt − Desirable Body Wt) × 0.25] + Desirable Body Wt.

diseases and/or insufficient intakes of essential nutrients. The AMDR for pregnancy is the same as for all healthy adults: 45–65% of kcal from carbohydrates, 10–35% of kcal from protein, and 20–35% of kcal from fat.[79]

Carbohydrates and Nutritive Sweeteners

The primary role of carbohydrates is to provide energy to cells. The major types of carbohydrates in the diet are starch, a complex carbohydrate, and simple sugars such as glucose, fructose, sucrose, and lactose. Sources of starch include grains and vegetables such as cereals and starchy vegetables. Natural sugars are found in foods such as fruits, vegetables, milk, and milk products. Added sugars include brown sugar, corn sweetener, corn syrup, dextrose, fructose, fruit juice concentrate, high-fructose corn syrup, and honey, and can be found in desserts, fruit drinks, soft drinks, and candy.[88]

The median intake of carbohydrates for women is approximately 180 to 230 g/day. To assure provision of glucose to the fetal brain (approximately 33 g/day), as well as to supply the glucose fuel requirement for the mother's brain independent of utilization of ketoacids, the RDA for pregnancy for ages 14 to 50 years is 175 g/day. There is no evidence to indicate that a certain portion of the carbohydrate must be consumed as starch or sugars.[86]

Carbohydrate-containing foods have been ranked according to their effect on blood glucose level response compared with a reference food (either glucose or white bread). This concept is known as the glycemic index (GI), and it classifies foods as low (< 55), medium (56–69), or high (> 70) GI foods. Foods with a low GI score contain slowly digested carbohydrates, which produce only small fluctuations in blood glucose and insulin levels. Examples of low GI foods include whole-wheat bread, old-fashioned oatmeal, bran cereal, legumes, vegetables, and fruits. Foods with high GI scores contain rapidly digested carbohydrates, which produce a rapid rise and fall in the blood glucose level. Examples of high GI foods are highly processed breakfast cereals, instant potatoes, instant noodles, sugar, honey, molasses, corn syrup, candy, and sweetened beverages.[89]

Several studies have evaluated the effects of glycemic index foods on pregnancy outcomes. For example, birth defects have been associated with poor glycemic control. One study reported that a diet high in sucrose and other high-glycemic foods increased the risk of neural tube defects by twofold in women among all weight groups, but the risk was fourfold among obese women (BMI > 29).[90] Another study reported that pregnant women who consumed diets with low-GI carbohydrates had reduced infant birth weight and an approximately twofold increased risk of a small-for-gestational-age baby.[91] Epidemiologic data from the Nurses' Health Study also showed that a low-glycemic, high-cereal-fiber diet reduced the risk for GDM by approximately one half.[92] A high-fiber and high-complex-carbohydrate diet may reduce the need for insulin after a meal, and theoretically decrease beta cell failure; however, efficacy data are limited.[60]

The concept of glycemic index foods is controversial and has not reached consensus among the scientific community. Additional studies are needed to determine if the glycemic index depends on food composition, cooking methods, or individual response. The IOM does not recommend the GI because of the lack of sufficient evidence in its use in the prevention of chronic diseases in generally healthy individuals.[79]

Fiber

Fiber is composed of complex carbohydrates and can be classified as insoluble or soluble fiber. Insoluble fiber such as cellulose, hemicellulose, and lignin increase water-holding capacity, thus increasing fecal volume and decreasing gastric transit time. Soluble fiber, such as gums and pectins, form gels, resulting in slowed gastrointestinal transit time and slowed or decreased nutrient absorption. Soluble fibers also bind other nutrients such as cholesterol and minerals to decrease their absorption. Foods high in insoluble fiber include wheat bran, whole grains, cereals, seeds, and the skin of fruits and vegetables. Foods containing high levels of soluble fiber are oats, legumes, barley, apples, strawberries, carrots, and citrus fruits. The DRI for fiber during pregnancy is 28 g/day.[86] Careful selection of fiber sources can help achieve the recommended level. Foods containing an average of 10–15 g of fiber per cup include baked beans, lentils, and chickpeas. Foods containing 5–10 g of fiber per cup include winter squash, spinach, mixed vegetables, peas, and cereals.[93]

Nonnutritive Sweeteners

The Food and Drug Administration (FDA) has approved five nonnutritive sweeteners: saccharin, aspartame, acesulfame potassium (or acesulfame K), sucralose, and most recently, neotame. The safety of these nonnutritive sweeteners has been determined with animal studies. The use of aspartame within FDA guidelines appears to be safe during pregnancy. Aspartame (Equal or Nutrasweet) is the methyl ester dipeptide of the natural amino acids L-aspartic acid and L-phenylalanine. Women with phenylketonuria (PKU) must restrict their phenylalanine intake. Because the amino acid phenylalanine is one of the metabolites of aspartame, women with PKU should avoid this sweetener. Maternal plasma levels of phenylalanine after ingestion of normal amounts of aspartame-containing foods are not higher than after the ingestion of protein-containing meals.[94]

Acesulfame potassium (Sweet One or Sunette) is considered safe for use during pregnancy. Sucralose (Splenda) is derived from sucrose and is safe for human consumption. The FDA concluded that sucralose does not pose carcinogenic, reproductive, or neurologic risk to human beings. Saccharin (Sweet'n Low) crosses the placenta and may remain in fetal tissue because of the slow fetal clearance. The American Medical Association and the American Dietetic Association suggest careful use of saccharin in pregnancy. Many practitioners suggest avoidance of saccharin during pregnancy. According to the American Dietetic Association position statement on the use of nonnutritive sweeteners during pregnancy, it is acceptable during pregnancy. Neotame® is a sweetener and flavor enhancer for beverages and foods. It is a derivative of the dipeptide composed of the amino acids aspartic acid and phenylalanine that is readily eliminated from the body. The FDA approved neotame as a general-purpose sweetener in 2002 after reviewing evidence of more than 100 scientific studies. It is considered safe for the general population, including pregnant and lactating women, children, and people with diabetes. Although no specific recommendations have been made regarding their use during pregnancy, moderation of ingestion of nonnutritive sweeteners may be appropriate.[95]

Dietary Fat

Dietary fat provides energy and is essential for the absorption and transport of fat-soluble vitamins. The main types of dietary fat are saturated, polyunsaturated, monounsaturated, and trans fats. Besides having an impact on weight gain, dietary fat also plays an important role in the modulation of lipid profile. Saturated fatty acids have been positively correlated with low-density lipoprotein (LDL) cholesterol levels, whereas monounsaturated and polyunsaturated fatty acids tend to decrease LDL cholesterol. Dietary trans-fatty acids are associated with increased LDL cholesterol levels. The main sources of trans-fatty acids in the diet are partially hydrogenated vegetable fats, baked goods, and commercial fried foods.

Essential fatty acids (EFA) are required in the human diet. Two closely related families of EFA are omega-3 and omega-6 fatty acids. The major fatty acids of the omega-6 series are linoleic (18:2n-6), γ-linolenic (18:3n-6), and arachidonic (20:4n-6) acids. The long-chain omega-3 fatty acids eicosapentaenoic acid (EPA) (20:5n-3) and docosahexaenoic acid (DHA) (22:66n-3) can be synthesized from α-linolenic acid.[96] Sources of omega-3 fatty acids include vegetable oils such as soybean, canola, and flaxseed oil; fish oils; and fatty fish, with smaller amounts found in meats and eggs. Sources of omega-6 fatty acids include nuts, seeds, and vegetable oils such as soybean, safflower, and corn oil. The AMDR of fat for pregnant women is 20–35% of total energy, the same as for nonpregnant women. Besides total fat recommendations, DRIs have been formulated for omega-3 and omega-6 fatty acids. The AI of omega-6 linoleic acid is 13 g/d and for omega-3, ∝-linolenic acid is 1.4 g/d.[86]

Protein

Pregnant women have additional protein requirements to support the expansion of maternal tissue and fetal growth. Protein intake has a significant effect on birth weight. In a study that increased the dietary protein intake by 1 g per day during preconception and in the 10th, 26th, and 38th weeks of gestation resulted in a significant increase of 7.8–11.4 g in birth weight.[97] A higher than average protein intake during pregnancy resulted in a significant depression of birth weight; in fact, a protein intake of more than 84 g/day on average was more detrimental than inadequate protein. It appears that moderate protein intake is optimal during pregnancy.[98]

Sources of protein providing all essential amino acids required for protein synthesis include meats, poultry, fish, milk, and eggs. Complementation of vegetable protein from a variety of cereals and legumes can also facilitate protein synthesis. The current RDA of 71 g of protein for pregnant women is 25 g more than the requirement for nonpregnant women. The additional 25 g is based on 1.1 g/kg/day using prepregnant weight.

Table 1-8 summarizes the DRIs for macronutrients for pregnant women ages <18–50 years of age.

Micronutrients

Certain vitamins and minerals are of particular significance during pregnancy. A deficiency of micronutrients during pregnancy has been associated with complications such as anemia and hypertension, as well as impaired fetal function, development, and growth. The main cause of multiple deficiencies is the quality of the diet. Women who avoid meat and/or milk in wealthier regions of the world are also at higher risk of micronutrient depletion during pregnancy and lactation. In certain dietary patterns high in unrefined grains and legumes, the amount of nutrients consumed may be adequate, but dietary constituents, such as phytates and polyphenols will limit micronutrient absorption.

TABLE 1-8 Dietary Reference Intakes (DRIs) of Macronutrients for Pregnant Women (grams/day)

	AMDR[a]	RDA[b]/AI[c] <18–50 years
Carbohydrates	45–65	175
Total fiber		28
Protein	10–35	71
Fat	20–35	ND[d]
Omega-6, linoleic acid	5–10	13
Omega-3, linolenic acid	0.6–1.2	1.4

Source: Adapted Institute of Medicine. Dietary reference intakes. National Academy of Sciences. www.nap.edu.

[a]Acceptable macronutrient distribution range (AMDR)

[b]Recommended dietary allowance (RDA)

[c]Adequate intake (AI)

[d]Not determinable (ND) due to lack of data of adverse effects in this age group and concern with regard to lack of ability to handle excess amounts. Source of intake should be from food only to prevent high levels of intake.

Several micronutrient deficiencies are well established as contributors to abnormal prenatal development and/or pregnancy outcome. These include magnesium, iron, folate, and vitamin D deficiencies. Less well recognized for their importance are deficiencies of B vitamins (and subsequently elevated plasma homocysteine concentrations).[99] See **Table 1-9** for the RDAs and adequate intakes for micronutrients for pregnant and nonpregnant adolescents and women.

Magnesium

Magnesium is an essential mineral for optimal metabolic functions, which include energy production, synthesis of essential molecules such as nucleic acids and proteins, bone structural integrity, ion transport across membranes, and cell signaling.[99] Research has shown that the mineral content of magnesium in food sources is declining, and magnesium depletion has been detected in persons with some chronic diseases. Magnesium may be effective in the management of eclampsia and preeclampsia, arrhythmia, severe asthma, and migraine.[100] Food sources of magnesium include green leafy vegetables, nuts, legumes, and whole grains. The RDA of 360 to 400 mg of magnesium in pregnancy is an increase of 40 mg over nonpregnant requirements.[86]

Iron

Iron is an essential component of multiple proteins and enzymes, and participates in oxygen transport and storage, electron transport and energy metabolism, and DNA synthesis. The requirement for iron is significantly increased during pregnancy due to increased iron utilization by the developing fetus and placenta, as well as blood volume expansion. Heme iron is readily absorbed and is present in meat, poultry, and fish. Non-heme iron sources, such as legumes, require the addition of vitamin C, organic acids, or meat, fish, or poultry to enhance its absorption. Inhibitors of non-heme iron absorption are phytates, polyphenols, and soy protein. Good sources of iron include beef, lentils, beans, bran cereal, and raisins.[99] Iron deficiency during pregnancy leads to maternal anemia, defined as a hematocrit less than 32% or a hemoglobin less than 11 g/dL. According to the Institute of Medicine, an appropriate time to begin iron supplementation at a dose of 30 mg/day is after 12 weeks of gestation, when iron requirements begin to increase.[101] The DRI for iron during pregnancy is 27 mg/day.[86]

Folate

Folate and folic acid participate in nucleic acid and amino acid metabolism and interact with vitamins B_6 and B_{12}. A deficiency of folate during the first days after conception may result in low birth weight, premature birth, and/or neural tube defects (NTDs) and elevated homocysteine levels, which may be a predictor of poor pregnancy outcomes.[99,102] Folate is naturally found in food; folic acid, the synthetic form of folate, is found in supplements and fortified foods. Folic acid is 100% absorbed when consumed whereas folate is only partially absorbed. Folic acid is added to breakfast cereals and many other foods with the purpose of preventing NTDs. Important sources of folate include asparagus, spinach, lentils, broccoli, and orange juice. The DRI for folate during pregnancy is 600 μg/day.[86]

Vitamin D

Vitamin D is essential for skeletal health, and a prolonged deficiency will result in infant rickets and adult osteomalacia. Besides being essential for the efficient utilization of calcium by the body, vitamin D also plays a role in cell differentiation, provides immunity, and participates in insulin secretion and blood pressure regulation. Serum 25(OH)D (25-hydroxyvitamin D) concentration is a useful indicator of vitamin D nutritional status.[100] A study of 180 pregnant women of various ethnic backgrounds evaluated the effects of daily and single-dose vitamin D supplementation at 27 weeks gestation. Study participants were randomly assigned to three treatment groups: a single oral dose of 200,000 IU vitamin D, a daily supplement of 800 IU vitamin D from 27 weeks until delivery, and a no treatment group. The women who received either the single or daily dose had significant improvement in their 25-hydroxyvitamin D levels.[103]

Common foods that are fortified with vitamin D include dairy products, cereals, and orange juice. The AI for

TABLE 1-9 Recommended Dietary Allowances and Adequate Intakes for Micronutrients

	Nonpregnant		Pregnant	
Micronutrient	Females 13–18 yr	Females 19–50 yr	Females 13–18 yr	Females 19–50 yr
Thiamin (mg/day)[a]	1.0	1.1	1.4	1.4
Riboflavin (mg/day)[a,c]	1.0	1.1	1.4	1.4
Niacin (mg/day)[a]	14	14	18	18
Biotin (μg/day)[b]	25	30	30	30
Pantothenic acid (mg/day)[b]	5	5	6	6
Vitamin B_6 (mg/day)[a]	1.2	1.3	1.9	1.9
Folate (μg/day)[a,d]	400	400	600	600
Vitamin B_{12} (μg/day)[a]	2.4	2.4	2.6	2.6
Choline (mg/day)[b]	400	425	450	450
Vitamin C (mg/day)[a]	65	75	80	85
Vitamin A (μg/day)[a,e]	700	700	750	770
Vitamin D (μg/day)[b,f]	5	5	5	5
Vitamin E (mg/day)[a,g]	15	15	15	15
Vitamin K (μg/day)[b]	75	90	75	90
Sodium (mg/day)[b]	1500	1500	1500	1500
Chloride (mg/day)[b]	2300	2300	2300	2300
Potassium (mg/day)[b]	4700	4700	4700	4700
Calcium (mg/day)[b]	1300	1000	1300	1000
Phosphorus (mg/day)[a]	1250	700	1250	700
Magnesium (mg/day)[a]	360	310	400	350
Iron (mg/day)[a]	15	18	27	27
Zinc (mg/day)[a]	9	8	12	11
Iodine (μg/day)[a]	150	150	220	220
Selenium (μg/day)[a]	55	55	60	60
Copper (μg/day)[a]	890	900	1000	1000
Manganese (mg/day)[b]	1.6	1.8	2.0	2.0
Fluoride (mg/day)[b]	3	3	3	3
Chromium (μg/day)[b]	24	25	29	30
Molybdenum (μg/day)[a]	43	45	50	50

[a]Recommended dietary allowance (RDA)

[b]Adequate intake (AI)

[c]Niacin recommendations are expressed as niacin equivalents (NE).

[d]Folate recommendations are expressed as dietary folate equivalents (DEF).

[e]Vitamin A recommendations are expressed as retinol activity equivalents (RAE).

[f]Vitamin D recommendations are expressed as cholecalciferol and assume absence of adequate exposure to sunlight.

[g]Vitamin E recommendations are expressed as α-tocoferol.

vitamin D recommended by the Institute of Medicine is 5 μg/day or 200 IU/day.

B Vitamins

B vitamins such as thiamin, riboflavin, niacin, biotin, pantothenic acid, vitamin B_6, folate, and vitamin B_{12} participate in many metabolic pathways, including those involved in energy metabolism. Poor maternal vitamin B status may be a major cause of homocysteinemia and poor pregnancy outcomes. It has not yet been established how homocysteinemia affects pregnancy outcome adversely, but proposed mechanisms include: (1) homocysteine increases free radical oxygen concentrations, which reduces nitrous oxide concentrations, leading to endothelial dysfunction; (2) homocysteine may cause oxidative stress and subsequent placental ischemia; (3) homocysteine may cause an inflammatory response that is cytotoxic to endothelial cells; (4) B-vitamin deficiencies lead to hypomethylation of DNA and altered gene expression; (5) homocysteine induces apoptosis of the endothelial cells; (6) birth defects may be caused by homocysteine interference with the N-methyl-D-aspartate receptor system; or (7) homocysteine is thrombogenic.[99]

Comorbidities During Pregnancy

There are certain conditions during pregnancy that require special dietary interventions. Pregnant women experiencing diabetes, hypertension, and pre-eclampsia require individualized dietary modification that will help to reduce the risks associated with these conditions.

Diabetes

The risk of developing gestational diabetes has increased in the last 10 years. Numerous studies have reported an increased risk of gestational diabetes mellitus (GDM) among women who are overweight or obese.[52] GDM is defined as glucose intolerance occurring during pregnancy.[104,105] Women at risk for GDM typically have a previous history of GDM, may exhibit obesity, have a strong family history of diabetes, or belong to an ethnic group with a high prevalence of diabetes. GDM is associated with fetal macrosomia, large-for-gestational-age infants, and an increased risk of a difficult labor and delivery.[106,107] Intensive treatment of hyperglycemia in women with GDM lessens the risk of adverse outcomes by reducing the risk of fetal macrosomia and providing the best outcome for normal or large-for-gestational-age infants.[108,109]

GDM nutrition management includes individualized nutrition counseling and medical nutrition therapy (MNT) by a registered dietitian. Nutrition management consists of specifying the appropriate amount of carbohydrates that will help the patient gain the recommended amount of weight, while achieving normoglycemia and preventing ketonuria. Carbohydrate intake affects postprandial blood glucose levels of women with GDM. The recommendation of a minimum of 175 g of carbohydrates per day is the same as for pregnant women without GDM.[110] Carbohydrates are less tolerated at breakfast than at other meals and should be adjusted based on monitoring weight, blood glucose, and ketones.[111] Food plans that contain 40% carbohydrates have been shown to reduce postprandial glucose levels.[112] For optimal glucose control, carbohydrates are usually distributed throughout the day in three meals and three snacks.

The amount of protein, fat, and vitamins and minerals should be based on DRI for pregnant women. Vitamin and mineral supplementation should be encouraged when DRIs are not met through dietary intake. Most women with GDM return to normal glucose levels in the postpartum period. Postpartum counseling should highlight the importance of attaining a normal BMI and regular physical activity in an effort to reduce the lifetime risk of GDM in subsequent pregnancies or type 2 diabetes.[113]

Hypertension and Preeclampsia

Gestational hypertension and preeclampsia are more common in overweight and obese pregnant women. Gestational hypertension, defined as a systolic blood pressure of at least 140 mm Hg or a diastolic blood pressure of at least 90 mm Hg, affects approximately 6% to 17% of nulliparous women and 2% to 4% of multiparous women.[60] Approximately 50% of women with gestational hypertension diagnosed before 30 weeks gestation develop preeclampsia. Risk factors include preeclampsia in a previous pregnancy, maternal age younger than 20 years or older than 40 years, obesity, insulin resistance, diabetes, and genetic factors.[48,114]

The cause of preeclampsia is unknown, but may be related to an inadequate placental blood supply, possibly due to maternal hypertension, which causes placental oxidative stress and the release of placental factors into maternal circulation that triggers an inflammatory response. Subclinical inflammation is more common in obese individuals, hence obese women may enter pregnancy with preexisting inflammation that enhances their risk for preeclampsia.[60,115]

The incidence of preeclampsia is greater in twins than in single births.[116] Preeclampsia is associated with preterm delivery, low birth weight infants, neonatal death, maternal morbidity and mortality, and an increased risk of developing cardiovascular disease later in life.[117–119] Theories abound concerning the management and prevention of preeclampsia. The role of diet and nutrient supplementation has not been adequately studied. Sodium restriction and calcium, zinc, and magnesium supplementation have not been proven effective.[120] A recent study of nulliparous pregnant Norwegian women at risk for preeclampsia suggests that a dietary pattern characterized by high intake of vegetables, plant foods, and vegetable oils decreases the risk of preeclampsia, whereas a dietary pattern characterized by high consumption of processed meat, sweet drinks, and salty snacks increases the risk.[115]

Food Safety

Seafood

Fish and shellfish are important additions to the diet, providing lean protein and essential nutrients such as omega-3 fatty acids. However, nearly all fish and shellfish contain traces of mercury. Mercury occurs naturally in the environment, but can also be released into the air through industrial pollution that may accumulate in oceans, thus exposing fish to this contaminant.[121] Microorganisms convert mercury into methylmercury, which the fish absorb as they feed in contaminated waters. Larger fish consuming smaller fish may contain additional methylmercury, although the contamination from methylmercury varies with fish age, size, diet, species, and water location.[122,123] Mercury contained in seafood products readily crosses the placental barrier and has the potential to damage the developing fetal nervous system.[121,122] To educate the public about the hazards of methylmercury, the FDA and the Environmental Protection Agency (EPA) issued a joint consumer advisory regarding mercury in fish and shellfish and recommended that pregnant women, women of childbearing age, and young children avoid eating shark, swordfish, mackerel, and tilefish.[124] The recommendation is to consume up to 12 ounces (two average meals) a week of a variety of fish and shellfish that are lower in mercury. Five of the most commonly eaten fish that are low in mercury are shrimp, canned light tuna, salmon, pollock, and catfish. Another recommendation is to check local advisories concerning the safety of fish caught by family and friends in local lakes, rivers, and coastal areas.

Listeriosis

Listeriosis is a serious infection caused by consuming food contaminated with the pathogen *Listeria monocytogenes*, a gram-positive anaerobe that grows at temperatures as low as 3°C (37°F) and can multiply in refrigerated foods.[125] Pregnant women, the elderly, and adults with weakened immune systems are susceptible to listeriosis.[126] Symptoms of listeriosis include influenza-like symptoms, persistent fever, and gastrointestinal symptoms such as nausea, vomiting, and diarrhea. The onset time to gastrointestinal symptoms is unknown but is probably greater than 12 hours; the onset time to the serious forms of listeriosis is unknown but may range from a few days to 3 weeks.

The manifestations of listeriosis include septicemia, meningitis (or meningoencephalitis), encephalitis, and intrauterine or cervical infections in pregnant women, which may result in spontaneous abortion or stillbirth.[127] Listeriosis is diagnosed by culturing the organism from blood, cerebrospinal fluid, or stool. The FDA recommends that all pregnant women avoid the following foods to prevent listeriosis:[125]

- Hot dogs or luncheon meats (including deli meats such as ham, turkey, salami, or bologna) unless reheated until steaming hot.
- Soft cheeses, such as feta, brie, Camembert, Roquefort, blue-veined, queso blanco, queso fresco, or Panela, unless the label clearly states the cheese is made with pasteurized milk. Hard cheeses, processed cheeses, cream cheese, and cottage cheese are safe.
- Refrigerated pâtés or meat spreads. Canned and shelf-stable versions are safe.
- Refrigerated smoked seafood unless cooked (as in a casserole). Canned and shelf-stable versions can be eaten safely.
- Unpasteurized milk, eggs, or juice, or foods made from these foods.

Post-Delivery Issues

Proper nutrition plays an important role not only before and during pregnancy but also after delivery. Obtaining the recommended types and amounts of nutrients after delivery can help women alleviate symptoms associated with postpartum depression.

Depression

Perinatal depression refers to major and minor episodes during pregnancy (antenatal) or within the first 12 months after delivery (postpartum or postnatal). The term *maternal depression* has been used interchangeably with perinatal depression. Signs and symptoms for perinatal depression are similar to those for the disease in the general population: depressed mood, loss of interest or pleasure, feelings of guilt or low self-worth, disturbed sleep or appetite, low energy, and poor concentration. Many factors have been associated with depression, including genetic predisposition and environmental factors, as well as a number of social, psychological, and biological factors. One biological factor given increasing consideration is inadequate nutrition. Women are particularly vulnerable to the adverse effects of poor nutrition on mood because pregnancy and lactation increase nutrient requirements. It has been suggested that depletion of nutrient reserves throughout pregnancy and a lack of recovery postpartum may increase a woman's risk for maternal depression.[128] Several studies have reported association between deficiency of some micronutrients such as folate, vitamin B_6, vitamin B_{12}, vitamin D, calcium, iron, zinc, and omega-3 fatty acids and postpartum depression.[128,129] Previous studies have shown that zinc levels are lower among patients with depression, and one study found that 25 mg zinc supplementation may improve depressive symptoms.[130]

Breastfeeding

The DRIs for lactation are similar to the dietary recommendations for pregnancy for macronutrients and most micronutrients. Nutrients required in greater amounts during lactation in women ages 19–50 years compared to pregnant women are: vitamin A (1300 μg/day), vitamin C (120 mg/day), riboflavin (1.6 mg/day), vitamin B_6 (2.0 mg/day), vitamin B_{12} (2.6 μg/day), choline (550 mg/day), copper (1300 mg/day), iodine (290 μg/day), selenium (70 μg/day), zinc (12 mg/day), and potassium (5100 mg/day).

The position of the American Dietetic Association on promoting and supporting breastfeeding states, "exclusive breastfeeding provides optimal nutrition and health protection for the first 6 months of life and breastfeeding with complementary foods from 6 months until at least 12 months of age is the ideal feeding pattern for infants. Breastfeeding is an important public health strategy for improving infant and child morbidity and mortality, and improving maternal morbidity and helping to control health care costs."[131] Breastfeeding provides multiple benefits to the infant and mother. Benefits for the infant include optimal nutrition, enhanced immune system, protection against allergies and intolerances, promotion of correct development of the jaw and teeth, and reduced risk for chronic disease. Advantages of breastfeeding for the mother include increased energy expenditure, which may lead to faster return to prepregnancy weight, and decreased risk for chronic diseases such as type 2 diabetes, breast and ovarian cancers, and postpartum depression.[131] Additional benefits of breastfeeding were reported from a 20-year prospective study that found the longer the duration of lactation, the lower the incidence of the metabolic syndrome among women with and without histories of GDM. Lactation may have persistent favorable effects on women's cardiometabolic health as well.[132] Currently there is no available evidence that any dietary factors significantly enhance breast milk production in healthy adult lactating women.[133] (See also Chapter 5, "Normal Nutrition During Infancy.")

Lifestyle Interventions

Lifestyle interventions aimed at the prevention of overweight and chronic disease in the perinatal and postpartum periods are important to prolong a state of optimal health. Nutrition education plays an important role in the modification of eating habits. A study of obese pregnant women evaluated two different nutrition education approaches. One group of women received nutritional advice from a brochure (passive group), the second group received the brochure and lifestyle education by a registered dietitian, and the third was a control group. Results indicated that energy intake did not change during pregnancy and was comparable in all groups. Fat intake, specifically saturated fat intake, decreased and protein intake increased from the first to the third trimester in the passive and active groups, as compared to an opposite change in the control group. Calcium intake and vegetable consumption increased during pregnancy in all groups. Physical activity decreased in all groups, especially in the third trimester. It was concluded that both lifestyle interventions improved the nutritional habits of obese women during pregnancy, although physical activity was not affected.[134] For women with GDM, dietary modifications including lowering fat and carbohydrate intake in combination with physical activity can reduce the risk of developing GDM in subsequent pregnancies.[135] In another study, a diagnosis of diabetes was prevented when diet and intense exercise were implemented for a 2-month period. This intervention was sufficient to reduce fasting glucose, normalize blood lipid profile, and achieve weight loss.[136] In addition to the implementation of dietary modifications and increased physical activity, the use of oral hypoglycemic agents was demonstrated to prevent or delay a diagnosis of type 2 diabetes.[137]

Case Study

Nutrition Assessment

Patient history: A 17-year-old female with history of irregular periods who has gained 20 pounds in the last 6 months. She also has noticed having heavy acne, and sprouting hair on her chest and face. She reports fatigue, depression, and alopecia. The pediatrician has diagnosed her as having PCOS. She is a senior in high school, and does not participate in gym classes. She usually does homework after school or is on the Internet or watches TV during the evening.

Family history: Mother has type 2 diabetes.

Food/nutrition-related history: Skips breakfast and occasionally eats lunch at the school cafeteria, but mostly eats a hamburger, French fries, and a soda at the fast food restaurant located two blocks from the school. Dinner is usually a large meal consisting of a meat, starch, and salad. Her average fiber intake is 16 g/day and sodium intake is 4000 mg/day.

Anthropometric Measurements

Weight: 190 pounds (86.2 kg)

Height: 64 in (1.63 m)

BMI: 32.5 kg/m^2

Estimated energy needs: Mifflin-St. Jeor's method BMR = 10 x weight (kg) + 6.25 x height (cm) – 5 x age (years) – 161

Estimated protein needs: 15–30% of total calories

Laboratory data: (normal values in parentheses)

Fasting insulin: 29 mIU/mL (1.8–24.6 mU/L)
Total testosterone: 58 ng/dL (20 ng/dL)
Luteinizing hormone (LH)/follicle stimulating hormone (FSH) ratio: 3.5:1 ↑ (1:1)
Prolactin, thyroid stimulating hormone (TSH), and liver function test: normal
Total cholesterol: 230 mg/dL (< 170 mg/dL)
LDL cholesterol: 150 mg/dL (< 110 mg/dL)
HDL cholesterol: 33 mg/dL (≥ 35 mg/dL)
Fasting glucose: 120 mg/dL (59–96 mg/dL)

Nutrition Diagnoses

1. Inappropriate eating choices related to (RT) lack of variety of foods and consumption of large meals
2. Excessive caloric intake from fat RT frequent consumption of high fat foods
3. Excessive caloric intake from high glycemic index carbohydrates RT frequent consumption of carbonated and sweetened beverages
4. Consumption of lower fiber and high sodium intake as evidenced by consumption of lower than recommended fiber intake and consumption of higher than recommended sodium intake
5. Inadequate meal pattern RT skipping breakfast
6. Continuous risk of weight gain RT lack of physical activity

Nutrition Interventions

Planning

1. Teach the basis of healthy eating including the following topics: importance of eating a variety of foods, meal planning, portion size, low-fat cooking methods, and food record keeping.
2. Plan consumption of three meals and three snacks a day to reduce body weight and improve hormone, lipid, and glucose profile.
3. Plan the following daily macronutrient distribution:
   - *Protein:* 15–30% of total calories (e.g., lean meats, egg substitute, low-fat dairy products, legumes, nuts, and soy products such as tofu, soymilk, and soynuts).
   - *Carbohydrates:* 35–40% calories from low GI carbohydrates (e.g., whole grains cereals, legumes).
   - *Fat:* 35–45% of total daily calories. Include sources of:

     Polyunsaturated fats (PUFAs): Corn, soybean, safflower, and cottonseed oils

     Monounsaturated fats (MUFAs): Olive oil, canola oil, peanuts, avocados, and olives

     Omega-3 fatty acids: Fatty types of fish, flaxseed, canola and olive oils, nuts

     Saturated fat: No more than 5% total calories from saturated fat

     Trans fats: Avoid consumption (fast foods, partially hydrogenated vegetable oil, commercial baked goods, chips, crackers, vegetable shortening)
   - *Fiber:* 25 g of insoluble fiber (wheat bran, whole grains, cabbage, carrots) and soluble fiber (oat bran, oatmeal, beans, peas, citrus fruits, vegetables). Increase fiber intake gradually and add 8 cups of water per day.
4. Plan to address the following micronutrients:
   - *Sodium:* Reduce sodium intake to 2300 mg/day (avoid canned soups, baked goods, soy sauce, seasoned salts, processed foods, and monosodium glutamate [MSG]).
   - *Magnesium:* Include dietary sources of magnesium (whole grains, legumes, vegetables, seeds and nuts, dairy products, and meats).
   - *Vitamin D:* Include dietary sources of vitamin D (salmon, tuna fish, orange juice, and dairy products fortified with vitamin D).
5. Recommend moderate to vigorous physical activity for 60–90 minutes daily. Initiate with 10 minutes, adding gradual increments of 5–10 minutes per day.

Implementation

1. Comprehensive nutrition education:
   - Instruct on healthy eating practices including variety and low-fat cooking methods.
   - Review cooking methods conducive to healthy meals.
   - Review portion size.
   - Review how to read food labels.
   - Instruct on meal planning to include three meals and three snacks, emphasizing the importance of eating breakfast.
   - Include low glycemic and high calcium foods.
   - Instruct on avoidance of high GI carbohydrates, sweetened beverages, unhealthy fats, and salty products.
   - Instruct on reducing fat, salt, and sodium when eating out.
   - Provide patient education related to lifestyle modification.
   - Provide patient education related to diabetes prevention.
2. Nutritional supplements:
   - Offer a chromium picolinate and biotin supplement as adjunctive therapy to improve glucose control and lipid profile.

Monitoring and Evaluation

- Evaluate meal patterns of three meals and three snacks a day and its effect on weight loss goals (nutrition-related behavioral and environmental outcomes and nutrition-related patient/client-centered outcome).

- Assess intake of low GI carbohydrates, fiber, protein, fat, sodium, and magnesium at follow-up clinic visits (food and nutrient intake outcomes).

Questions for the Reader

1. What is the patient's estimated energy needs based on her initial assessment?
2. What is the patient's estimated carbohydrate intake based on her initial assessment?
3. What is the purpose of including low glycemic index carbohydrates?
4. Why is it important to distribute total calories in three meals and three snacks throughout the day?
5. Write three possible Problem, Etiology, Signs/Symptoms (PES) statements.
6. What will you do during the follow-up visit 2 months later?
   a. If the patient has not lost any weight?
   b. If the patient has not changed her eating habits?
   c. If the patient has not engaged in physical activity?
   d. If the fasting glucose level continues to be elevated?
   e. If the total-cholesterol and LDL-cholesterol levels continue to be elevated?

REFERENCES

American Dietetic Association. Adult weight management evidence analysis project. Available at: http://www.adaevidencelibrary.com/topic.cfm?cat=1010. Accessed January 28, 2010.

American Dietetic Association. *International Dietetics and Nutrition Terminology (IDNT) Reference Manual: Standardized Language for the Nutrition Care Process*. Chicago, IL: 2009.

Grasso A. *The Dietitian's Guide to Polycystic Ovary Syndrome.* Haverford, PA: Luca Publishing; 2007.

Hoeger, KM. Obesity and lifestyle management in polycystic ovary syndrome. *Clin Obstet Gynecol.* 2007;50:277–294.

Moran LJ, Brinkworth GD, Norman RJ. Dietary therapy in polycystic ovary syndrome. *Semin Reprod Med.* 2008;26:85–92.

U.S. Department of Health and Human Services. Polycystic ovary syndrome. Available at: http://www.womenshealth.gov/faq/polycystic-ovary-syndrome.cfm#k. Accessed January 28, 2010.

Weight-control Information Network (WIN). Weight loss for life. Available at: http://win.niddk.nih.gov/publications/for_life.htm#yourplan. Accessed January 28, 2010.

Resources for Preconception and Prenatal Nutrition

Nutrition During Pregnancy Resource List, July 2008

http://www.nal.usda.gov/fnic/pubs/bibs/topics/pregnancy/pregcon.pdf

This publication is a collection of resources on the topic of nutrition during pregnancy. Resources include books, pamphlets, and audiovisuals, and are limited to those published in 2004 or later. Many of the pamphlets are available in single copies and some may also be purchased in bulk from the organization listed. (Web addresses are provided for materials available online.)

USDA. Lifecycle Nutrition: Pregnancy

http://fnic.nal.usda.gov/nal_display/index.php?info_center=4&tax_level=2&tax_subject=257&topic_id=1356

This site provides information on maintaining a healthy pregnancy, the nutritional needs of pregnancy, and breastfeeding. It also provides link to government agencies such as the National Center for Education in Maternal and Child Health and WIC, the Special Supplemental Program for Women, Infants, and Children. This site also provides a link to folic acid information and resources.

Interactive DRIs for Health Professionals

http://fnic.nal.usda.gov/interactiveDRI

Use this tool to calculate daily nutrient recommendations for dietary planning based on the dietary reference intakes (DRIs). Developed by the National Academy of Science's Institute of Medicine, these represent the most current scientific knowledge on nutrient needs. Individual requirements may be higher or lower than the DRIs.

USDA. MyPyramid for Mom

http://www.mypyramid.gov/mypyramidmoms/index.html

The MyPyramid Website is designed specifically for pregnant and breastfeeding mothers to provide interactive guidance. The site provides advice on healthy eating and on the importance of meeting nutrient recommendations. The site includes an interactive menu planner.

Dietary Supplement Fact Sheet: Folate

http://dietary-supplements.info.nih.gov/factsheets/folate.asp

A fact sheet of the Office of Dietary Supplements of the National Institutes of Health.

EPA. Fish Advisories. What You Need to Know about Mercury in Fish and Shellfish

http://www.epa.gov/fishadvisories/advice/

FDA toll-free food hotline: 1.800.SAFEFOOD

A fact sheet from the Environmental Protection Agency providing three essential recommendations for selecting and eating fish or shellfish to reduce exposure to the harmful effects of mercury.

REFERENCES

1. Centers for Disease Control and Prevention. *Proceedings of the Preconception Health and Health Care Clinical, Public Health, and Consumer Workgroup Meetings*. Atlanta, GA: CDC; 2006.
2. Centers for Disease Control and Prevention. Recommendations to improve preconception health and health care—United States. *MMWR*. 2006;55(RR06):1–23.
3. Inskip HM, Crozier SR, Godfrey KM, Borland SE, Cooper C, Robinson SM. Women's compliance with nutrition and lifestyle recommendations before pregnancy: general population cohort study. *BMJ*. 2009;388:b481.
4. MacDorman MF, Mathews TJ. Recent trends in infant mortality in the United States. *NCHS Data Brief*. 2008;9:1–8. Available at: http://www.cdc.gov/nchs/data/databriefs/db09.pdf. Accessed January 26, 2010.
5. Finer LB, Henshaw SK. Disparities in rates of unintended pregnancy in the United States, 1994–2001. *Perspect Sex Reprod Health*. 2006;38(2):90–96.
6. Lu MC, Kotelchuck M, Culhane JF, Hobel CJ, Klerman LV, Thorp JM. Preconception care between pregnancies: the content of internatal care. *Matern Child Health J*. 2006;10:S107–S122.
7. American Academy of Pediatrics, American College of Obstetricians and Gynecologists. *Guidelines for Perinatal Care*. 6th ed. Elk Grove, IL: American Academy of Pediatrics; 2007.
8. American College of Obstetricians and Gynecologists. ACOG Committee opinion no. 313. The importance of preconception care in the continuum of women's health care. *Obstet Gynecol*. 2005;106(3):665–666.
9. Kitzmiller JL, Block JM, Brown FM, et al. Managing preexisting diabetes for pregnancy: summary of evidence and consensus recommendations for care. *Diabetes Care*. 2008;31(5):1060–1079.
10. American Diabetes Association. Preconception care of women with diabetes. *Diabetes Care*. 2004;27(Suppl 1):S76–S78.
11. American Diabetes Association. Standards of medical care in diabetes—2010. *Diabetes Care*. 2010;33(Suppl 1):S11–S61.
12. American Dietetic Association. Diabetes 1 and 2 evidence analysis project. Evidence Analysis Library. Available at: http://www.adaevidencelibrary.com. Accessed December 18, 2009.
13. American Diabetes Association. Nutrition recommendations and interventions for diabetes. *Diabetes Care*. 2008;31(Suppl 1):S61–S78.
14. National Heart, Lung and Blood Institute. *Clinical Guidelines on the Identification, Evaluation and Treatment of Overweight and Obesity in Adults: Evidence Report*. Washington, DC: National Heart, Lung and Blood Institute. NIH Publication. No. 98-4083; 1998.
15. National Heart, Lung and Blood Institute. *The Practical Guide. Identification, Evaluation, and Treatment of Overweight and Obesity in Adults*. Washington, DC: National Institutes of Health. NIH Publication No. 00-4084; 2000.
16. Ogden CL, Carrol MD, Curtin LR, McDowell MA, Tabak CJ, Flegal KM. Prevalence of overweight and obesity in the United States, 1999–2004. *JAMA*. 2006;295(130):1549–1555.
17. Galtier F, Raingeard I, Renard E, Boulot P, Bringer J. Optimizing the outcome of pregnancy in obese women: from pregestational to long-term management. *Diabetes Metab*. 2008;34:19–25.
18. Zhong Y, Cahill AG, Macones GA, Zhu F, Odibo AO. The association between prepregnancy maternal body mass index and preterm delivery. *Am J Perinatol*. 2009. Available at: DOI 10.1055/s-0029-1241736. Accessed December 20, 2009.
19. Walters MR, Smith Taylor J. Maternal obesity: consequences and prevention strategies. *Nurs Womens Health*. 2009; 13(6):487–495.
20. Rasmussen KM, Catalano PM, Yaktine AL. New guidelines for weight gain during pregnancy: what obstetrician/gynecologists should know. *Curr Op Obstet Gynecol*. 2009;21:521–526.
21. American Dietetic Association. Position of the American Dietetic Association: weight management. *J Am Diet Assoc*. 2002;102(8):1146–1155.
22. Klein S, Allison DB, Heymsfield SB, et al. Waist circumference and cardiometabolic risk: a consensus statement from Shaping America's Health: Association for Weight Management and Obesity Prevention; NAASO, The Obesity Society; the American Society for Nutrition; and the American Diabetes Association. *Obesity*. 2007;15(5):1061–1067.
23. American Dietetic Association. Adult weight management evidence analysis project. Evidence Analysis Library. Available at: http://www.adaevidencelibrary.com. Accessed December, 20, 2009.
24. Inge TH, Krebs NF, Garcia VF, et al. Bariatric surgery for severely overweight adolescents: concerns and recommendations. *Pediatrics*. 2004;114:217–223.
25. Roberts JM, Pearson G, Cutler J, Lindheimer M. Summary of the NHLBI working group on research on hypertension during pregnancy. *Hypertens*. 2003;41:437–445.
26. National Heart, Lung and Blood Institute. *The Seventh Report of the Joint National Committee on Prevention, Detection, Evaluation, and Treatment of High Blood Pressure*. Washington, DC: NHLBI; 2004.
27. Alton I. Nutrition-related special concerns of adolescent pregnancy. In: Story M, Stang J, eds. *Nutrition and the Pregnant Adolescent: A Practical Reference Guide*. Minneapolis, MN: Center for Leadership, Education and Training in Maternal and Child Nutrition. University of Minnesota; 2000:89–112.
28. American Dietetic Association. Hypertension evidence analysis project. Evidence Analysis Library. Available at: http://www.adaevidencelibrary.com. Accessed December 21, 2009.
29. Sacks FM, Svetkey LP, Vollmer WM, et al. Effects on blood pressure of reduced dietary sodium and the Dietary Approaches to Stop Hypertension (DASH) diet. *N Engl J Med*. 2001;344:3–10.
30. Appel LJ, Moore TJ, Obarzanek E, et al. A clinical trial of the effects of dietary patterns on blood pressure. *N Engl J Med* 1997;336(16):1117–1124.
31. Glueck CJ, Pranikoff J, Aregawi D, Wang P. Prevention of gestational diabetes by metformin plus diet in patients with polycystic ovary syndrome. *Fertil Steri*. 2008;89(3):625–634.
32. Jeanes YM, Barr S, Smith K, Hart KH. Dietary management of women with polycystic ovary syndrome in the United Kingdom: the role of dietitians. *J Hum Nutr Diet*. 2009;22:551–558.
33. Moran LJ, Brinkworth GD, Norman RJ. Dietary therapy in polycystic ovary syndrome. *Semin Reprod Med*. 2008;26(1):85–92.
34. Franks S, Robinson S, Willis DS. Nutrition, insulin and polycystic syndrome. *J Reprod Fertil*. 1996;1:47–53.
35. American Dietetic Association. Case problem: dietary recommendations to combat obesity, insulin resistance, and other

concerns related to polycystic ovary syndrome. *J Am Diet Assoc.* 2000;100(8):955–960.

36. Marsh K, Brand-Miller J. The optimal diet for women with polycystic ovary syndrome. *Br J Nutr.* 2005;94:154–165.
37. Charvarro JE, Rich-Edwards JW, Rosner BA, Willett WC. Dietary fatty acids intakes and the risk of ovulatory infertility. *Am J Clin Nutr.* 2007;85:231–237.
38. Panidis D, Farmakiotis D, Rousso D, Kourtis A, Katsikis I, Krassas G. Obesity, weight loss, and the polycystic ovary syndrome: effect of treatment with diet and orlistat for 24 weeks on insulin resistance and androgen levels. *Am Soc Reprod Med.* 2008;89(4):899–906.
39. Centers for Disease Control and Prevention. Alcohol use among pregnant and nonpregnant women of childbearing age—United States, 1991–2005.*MMWR.* 2009;58(19):529–532.
40. Floyd RL, Jack BW, Cefalo R, et al. The clinical content of preconception care: alcohol, tobacco, and illicit drug exposure. *Am J Obstet Gynecol.* 2008;199(6 Suppl 2):S333–S339.
41. Office of the Surgeon General. U.S. Surgeon General releases advisory on alcohol use in pregnancy. News Release. February 2005. Available at: http://www.surgeongeneral.gov/pressreleases/sg02222005.html. Accessed March 13, 2010.
42. Gardiner PM, Nelson L, Shellhass CS, et al. The clinical content of preconception care: nutrition and dietary supplements. *Am J Obstet Gynecol.* 2008;199(6 Suppl 2):S345–S356.
43. Rouse B, Azen C. Effect of high maternal blood phenylalanine on offspring congenital anomalies and developmental outcome at ages 4 and 6 years: the importance of strict dietary control preconception and throughout pregnancy. *J Pediatr.* 2004;144:235–239.
44. Matalon KM, Acosta PB, Azen C. Role of nutrition in pregnancy with phenylketonuria and birth defects. *Pediatrics.* 2003;112(6):1534–1536.
45. Centers for Disease Control and Prevention. Smoking prevalence among women of reproductive age—United States, 2006. *MMWR.* 2008;57(31):849–852.
46. Ebrahim SH, Floyd RL, Merritt RK, Decoufle P, Holtzman D. Trends in pregnancy-related smoking rates in the United States, 1987–1996. *JAMA.* 2000;283(3):361–366.
47. World Health Organization. *Obesity: Preventing and Managing the Global Epidemic.* WHO Technical Report Series 894. Geneva: World Health Organization; 2000.
48. Kaiser LL, Allen L. Position of the American Dietetic Association: nutrition and lifestyle for healthy pregnancy outcome. *J Am Diet Assoc.* 2002;102:1479–1490.
49. Institute of Medicine. Weight gain during pregnancy: reexamining the guidelines. Available at: http://www.nap.edu/openbook.php?record_id=12584&page=254. Accessed December 1, 2009.
50. Institute of Medicine. *Weight Gain During Pregnancy: Reexamining the Guidelines.* Report brief. Washington, DC: The National Academies Press; 2009.
51. Krummel DA. Postpartum weight control. *J Am Diet Assoc.* 2007;107:37–40.
52. Chu SY, Callaghan WM, Kim C, et al. Maternal obesity and risk of gestational diabetes mellitus. *Diabetes Care.* 2007;30:2070–2076.
53. Baeten JM, Bukusi EA, Lambe M. Pregnancy complications and outcomes among overweight and obese nulliparous women. *Am J Public Health.* 2001;91:436–440.
54. Glazar NL, Hendrickson AF, Schellenbaum GD, Mueller BA. Weight change and the risk of gestational diabetes in obese women. *Epidemiol.* 2004;15:733–737.
55. Pirkola J, Puta A, Bloigu A, et al. Prepregnancy overweight and gestational diabetes as determinants of subsequent diabetes and hypertension after 20 years follow-up. *J Clin Endocrinol Metab.* 2009;94:2464–2470.
56. Doherty DA, Magann EF, Francis J, Morrison JC, Newnham JP. Prepregnancy body mass index and pregnancy outcomes. *Int J Gynaecol Obstet.* 2006;95:242–247.
57. Driul L, Cacciaguerra G, Citossi A, Della Martina A, Peressini L, Marchesoni D. Prepregnancy body mass index and adverse pregnancy outcomes. *Arch Gynecol Obstet.* 2008;278:23–26.
58. Cnattingius S, Bergstrom R, Lipworth L. Kramer MS. Prepregnancy weight and the risk of adverse pregnancy outcomes. *N Engl J Med.* 1998;338:147–152.
59. Edwards LE. Dickes WF, Alton IR, Hakanson EY. Pregnancy in the massively obese: course, outcome, and obesity prognosis of the infant. *Am J Obstet Gynecol.* 1978;131:479–483.
60. Position of the American Dietetic Association and American Society for Nutrition: obesity, reproduction, and pregnancy outcomes. *J Am Diet Assoc.* 2009;109:918–927.
61. Ellings JM, Newman RB, Hulsey TC, Bivins HA, Keenan A. Reduction in very low birth weight deliveries and perinatal mortality in a specialized, multidisciplinary twin clinic. *Obstet Gynecol.*1993;81:387–391.
62. Gardner MO, Goldenberg RL, Cliver SP, et al. The origin and outcome of preterm twin pregnancies. *Obstet Gynecol.* 1995;85:553–557.
63. Albrecht JL, Tomich PG. The maternal and neonatal outcome of triplet gestations. *Am J Obstet Gynecol.* 1996;174:1551–1556.
64. Peaceman AM, Dooley SL, Tamura RK. Antepartum management of triplet gestations. *Am J Obstet Gynecol.* 1992;167:1117–1120.
65. Luke B, Brown MB. Maternal morbidity and infant death in twin vs triplet and quadruplet pregnancies. *Am J Obstet Gynecol.* 2008;198:401.e1–e10.
66. Martin JA, MacDorman MF, Mathews TJ. Triplet births: trends and outcomes, 1971–94. *Vital Health Stat 21.* 1997;55:1–20.
67. Luke B, Hediger ML, Nugent C, et al. Body mass index-specific weight gains associated with optimal birth weights in twin pregnancies. *J Reprod Med.* 2003;48:217–224.
68. Kolasa KM, Weismiller DG. Nutrition during pregnancy. *Am Fam Physician.* 1997;56:205–212.
69. Chan RL, Olshan AF, Savitz DA, et al. Maternal influences on nausea and vomiting in early pregnancy. *Matern Child Health J.* 2009.
70. O'Brien B, Naber S. Nausea and vomiting during pregnancy: Effects on the quality of women's lives. *Birth.* 1992;19:138–143.
71. Chandra K, Magee L, Einarson A, Koren G. Nausea and vomiting in pregnancy: results of a survey that identified interventions used by women to alleviate their symptoms. *J Psychosom Obstet Gynaecol.* 2003;24:71–75.
72. Nelson-Piercy C. Treatment of nausea and vomiting in pregnancy: When should it be treated and what can be safely taken. *Drug Safety.* 1998;19(2):155–164.
73. American College of Obstetrics and Gynecology practice bulletin. Nausea and vomiting of pregnancy. *Obstet Gynecol.* 2004;103:803–814.

74. Feizo MS, Poursharif B, Korst LM, et al. Symptoms and pregnancy outcomes associated with extreme weight loss among women with hyperemesis gravidarum. *J Womens Health (Larchmt)*. 2009;18(12):1981–1987.
75. Dowswell T, Neilson JP. Interventions for heartburn in pregnancy. *Cochrane Database Syst Rev.* 2008 Oct 8;(4):CD007065
76. Erick M. Ptyalism gravidarum: an unpleasant reality [letter to the editors]. *J Am Diet Assoc.* 1998;98:129.
77. Van Dinter MC. Ptyalism in pregnant women. *J Obstet Gynecol Neonatal Nurs*. 1991;20:206–209.
78. Suzuki S, Igarashi M, Yamashita E, Satomi M. Ptyalism gravidarum. *North Am J Med Sci.* 2009;1:303–304.
79. Institute of Medicine. *Dietary Reference Intakes for Energy, Carbohydrates, Fiber, Fat, Fatty Acids, Cholesterol, Protein and Amino Acids (Macronutrients)*. Washington, DC: National Academies Press; 2002.
80. Andersen AE, Ryan GL. Eating disorders in the obstetric and gynecologic patient population. *Obstet Gynecol.* 2009;114:1353–1367.
81. Micali N, Treasure J, Simonoff E. Eating disorders symptoms in pregnancy: a longitudinal study of women with recent and past eating disorders and obesity. *J Psychosom Res.* 2007;63:297–303.
82. American College of Obstetricians and Gynecologists Committee. Opinion no. 267: exercise during pregnancy and the postpartum period. *Obstet Gynecol.* 2002;99:171–173.
83. Melzer K, Schutz Y, Soehnchen N, et al. Effects of recommended levels of physical activity on pregnancy outcomes. *Am J Obstet Gynecol.* 2009 Dec 18 (in press).
84. Godfrey KM, Barker DJ. Fetal nutrition and adult disease. *Am J Clin Nutr.* 2000;71(5 Suppl):1344S–1352S.
85. Godfrey KM, Barker DJ. Fetal programming and adult health. *Public Health Nutr.* 2001;4(2B):611–624.
86. Institute of Medicine, National Academy of Sciences. *Dietary Reference Intakes for Energy, Carbohydrate, Fiber, Fat, Fatty Acids, Cholesterol and Amino Acids*. Washington, DC: National Academies Press; 2005.
87. American Dietetic Association. *Medical Nutrition Therapy Evidence-Based Guide for Practice: Nutrition Practice Guidelines for Gestational Diabetes Mellitus* [CD-ROM]. Chicago, IL: American Dietetic Association; 2001.
88. U.S. Department of Agriculture. Dietary guidelines for Americans 2005. Available at: http://www.cnpp.usda.gov/Publications/DietaryGuidelines/2005/2005DGPolicyDocument.pdf. Accessed December 15, 2009.
89. Foster-Powell K, Holt SH, Brand-Miller JC. International table of glycemic index and glycemic load values. *Am J Clin Nutr.* 2002;76:55–56.
90. Shaw GM, Quach T, Nelson V, et al. Neural tube defects associated with maternal periconceptional dietary intake of simple sugars and glycemic index. *Am J Clin Nutr*. 2003;78:972–978.
91. Scholl TO, Chen X, Khoo CS, Lenders C. The dietary glycemic index during pregnancy: influence on infant birth weight, fetal growth, and biomarkers of carbohydrate metabolism. *Am J Epidemiol*. 2004;159:467–474.
92. Zhang C, Liu S, Solomon CG, Hu FB. Dietary fiber intake, dietary glycemic load, and the risk for gestational diabetes mellitus. *Diabetes Care*. 2006;29:2223–2230.
93. U.S. Department of Agriculture. National nutrient database for standard reference, release 22. Fiber, total dietary (g) content of selected foods per common measure, sorted by nutrient content. Available at: http://www.ars.usda.gov/SP2UserFiles/Place/12354500/Data/SR22/nutrlist/sr22w291.pdf. Accessed December 15, 2009.
94. Pitkin RM. Aspartame ingestion during pregnancy. In: Stegink LD, Filer JF, eds. *Aspartame: Physiology and Biochemistry*. New York: Marcel Dekker; 1984:555–564.
95. Position of the American Dietetic Association. Use of nutritive and nonnutritive sweeteners. *J Am Diet Assoc.* 2004;104:255–275.
96. Linus Pauling Institute Micronutrient Information Center. Essential fatty acids. Available at: http://lpi.oregonstate.edu/infocenter. Accessed July 28, 2010.
97. Cuco G, Arija V, Iranzo R, Vila J, Prieto MT, Fernandez-Ballart J. Association of maternal protein intake before conception and throughout pregnancy with birth weight. *Acta Obstet Gynecol Scand.* 2006;85:413–421.
98. Sloan NL, Lederman SA, Leighton J, Himes JH, Rush D. The effect of prenatal dietary protein intake on birth weight. *Nutr Res.* 2001;21:129–139.
99. Allen LH. Multiple micronutrients in pregnancy and lactation. *Am J Clin Nutr*. 2005;81:1206S–1212S.
100. Linus Pauling Institute Micronutrient Information Center. Magnesium. Available at: http://lpi.oregonstate.edu/infocenter. Accessed December 28, 2009.
101. Institute of Medicine. *Nutrition During Pregnancy. Weight Gain and Nutrient Supplements*. Washington, DC: National Academies Press; 1990.
102. Institute of Medicine. *Dietary Reference Intakes for Thiamin, Riboflavin, Niacin, Vitamin B_6, Folate, Vitamin B_{12}, Pantothenic Acid, Biotin, and Choline*. Washington, DC: National Academies Press; 2000.
103. Yu CK, Sykes L, Sethi M, Teoh TG, Robinson S. Vitamin D deficiency and supplementation during pregnancy. *Clin Endocrinol (Oxf)*. 2009;70:685–690.
104. Hadar E, Oats J, Hod M. Towards new diagnostic criteria for diagnosing GDM: the HAPO study. *Perinat Med.* 2009;37(5):447-9.
105. American Diabetes Association: Gestational diabetes mellitus position statement. *Diabetes Care*. 2004;27:S88–S90.
106. American College of Obstetricians and Gynecologists. Gestational diabetes. ACOG Practice Bulletin No. 30. *Obstet Gynecol.* 2001;98:525–538.
107. Casey BM, Lucas MJ, McIntire DD, Leveno KJ. Pregnancy outcomes in women with gestational diabetes compared with the general obstetric population. *Obstet Gynecol*. 1997;90:869–873.
108. Franz MJ, Bantle JP, Beebe CA, et al. Evidence-based nutrition principles and recommendations for the treatment and prevention of diabetes and related complications [technical review]. *Diabetes Care*. 2002;25:148–198.
109. Garcia-Patterson A, Corcoy R, Balsells M, et al. In pregnancies with gestational diabetes mellitus and intensive therapy, perinatal outcome is worse in small-for-gestational-age newborns. *Am J Obstet Gynecol*. 1998;179:481–485.
110. Thomas AM, Gutierrez YM. *American Dietetic Association Guide to Gestational Diabetes Mellitus*. Chicago IL: American Dietetic Association; 2005.

111. Peterson CH, Jovanovic-Peterson L. Percentage of carbohydrate and glycemic response to breakfast, lunch and dinner in women with gestational diabetes. *Diabetes*. 1991;40:S172–S174.
112. Major CA, Henry MJ, De Veciana M, Morgan MA. The effects of carbohydrate restriction in patients with diet-controlled gestational diabetes. *Obstet Gynecol.* 1998;91:600–604.
113. American Dietetic Association. Evidence analysis library. Gestational diabetes. Available at: http://www.adaevidencelibrary.com/topic.cfm?cat=1399. Accessed December 17, 2009.
114. Cedergren MI. Maternal morbid obesity and the pregnancy outcome. *Obstet Gynecol.* 2004;103:219–224.
115. Brantsæter AL, Haugen M, et al. A dietary pattern characterized by high intake of vegetables, fruits, and vegetable oils is associated with reduced risk of preeclampsia in nulliparous pregnant Norwegian women. *J Nutr.* 2009 June; 139: 1162–1168.
116. Kametras NA, McAuliffe F, Krampl E, Chambers J, Nicolaides, KH. Maternal cardiac function in twin pregnancy. *Obstet Gynecol.* 2003;102:806–815.
117. Sibai BM, Lindheimer M, Hauth J, et al. Risk factors for preeclampsia, abruption placentae and adverse neonatal outcomes among women with chronic hypertension. *N Eng J Med.* 1998;339:667–671.
118. Churchill D, Perry IJ, Beevers DG. Ambulatory blood pressure in pregnancy and fetal growth. *Lancet.* 1997;349:7–10.
119. Nijdam ME, Timmerman MR, Franx A, et al. Cardiovascular risk factor assessment after pre-eclampsia in primary care. *BMC Fam Pract.* 2009;8(10):77.
120. Dekker G, Sibai B. Primary, secondary and tertiary prevention of pre-eclampsia. *Lancet.* 2001;357:209–215.
121. Chan HM, Egeland GM. Fish consumption, mercury exposure and heart disease. *Nutrition Reviews*. 2004;62:68–72.
122. Dey PM, Gochfeld M, Reuhl KR. Developmental methylmercury administration alters cerebellar PSA-NCAM expression and Golgi sialytransferase activity. *Brain Res.* 1999;845:139–151.
123. Evans E. The FDA recommendations on fish intake during pregnancy. *J Obstet Gynecol Neonat Nurs.* 2002;31:541–546.
124. Environmental Protection Agency. Fish advisories. What you need to know about mercury in fish and shellfish. Available at: http://www.epa.gov/fishadvisories/advice. Accessed December 13, 2009.
125. Food and Drug Administration. Foodborne pathogenic microorganisms and natural toxins handbook. *Listeria monocytogenes.* Available at: http://www.fda.gov/Food/FoodSafety/FoodborneIllness/default.htm. Accessed December 17, 2009.
126. Lungu B, Ricke SC, Johnson MG. Growth, survival, proliferation and pathogenesis of *Listeria monocytogenes* under low oxygen or anaerobic conditions: a review. *Anaerobe.* 2009;15:7–17.
127. Posfay-Barbe KM, Wald ER. Listeriosis. *Semin Fetal Neonatal Med.* 2009;14:228–233.
128. Leung BM, Kaplan BJ. Perinatal depression: prevalence, risks, and the nutrition link—a review of the literature. *J Am Diet Assoc.* 2009;109(9):1566–1575.
129. Logan AC. Omega-3 fatty acids and major depression: a primer for the mental health professional. *Lipids Health Dis.* 2004;3:25.
130. Nowak G, Siwek M, Dudek D, Zieba A, Pilc A. Effect of zinc supplementation on antidepressant therapy in unipolar depression: a preliminary placebo-controlled study. *Pol J Pharmacol.* 2003;55:1143–1147.
131. James DC, Lessen R. Position of the American Dietetic Association. Promoting and supporting breastfeeding. *J Am Diet Assoc.* 2009;109:1926–1942.
132. Gunderson EP, Jacobs DR, Chiang V, et al. Duration of lactation and incidence of the metabolic syndrome in women of reproductive age according to gestational diabetes mellitus status: a 20-year prospective study in CARDIA—The Coronary Artery Risk Development in Young Adults Study. *Diabetes.* 2010;59(2):495–504.
133. American Dietetic Association. Evidence analysis library. Breastfeeding. Available at: http://www.adaevidencelibrary.com/topic.cfm?cat=4080. Accessed December 20, 2009.
134. Guelinckx I, Devlieger R, Mullie P, Vansant G. Effect of lifestyle intervention on dietary habits, physical activity, and gestational weight gain in obese pregnant women: a randomized controlled trial. *Am J Clin Nutr.* 2010;91(2):373–380.
135. Moses RG, Shand JL, Tapsell LC. The recurrence of gestational diabetes: could dietary differences in fat intake be an explanation? *Diabetes Care.* 1977;20:1647–1650.
136. Duarte-Gardea M. Case study: the prevention of diabetes through diet and intense exercise. *Clinical Diabetes.* 2004;22:45–46.
137. Knowler WC, Barret-Connor E, Fowler SE, et al. The diabetes prevention program research group. Reduction in the incidence of type 2 diabetes with lifestyle intervention or metformin. *N Engl J Med.* 2002;346:393–403.

Physical Growth and Maturation

Wm. Cameron Chumlea and Michael LaMonte

What Is Growth?

Physical growth is the increase in the mass of body tissues that occurs in genetically determined rates, patterns, and ages as a healthy infant grows into an adult. Good nutrition and exercise are necessary for optimal growth and maturation, and most normal, healthy children grow and mature with few, if any, problems. However, we are presently facing an obesity epidemic that affects and is interrelated with the growth and maturation of children and has potential consequences for both the current and future health of affected children.[1,2] This chapter provides an overview of growth and maturation and their assessment, and is illustrated by a case study and a brief discussion of abnormal growth.

How Is Growth Measured?

Accurate and reliable measures of body size present a broad description of a child's growth status. The most useful measures are recumbent length from birth to 3 years of age, stature after age 3 years, head circumference from birth to age 3 years (see **Figures 2-1**, **2-2**, and **2-3**, respectively), and weight at every age.[3] Descriptions and protocols for these measurements are available in video formats from the Centers for Disease Control and Prevention/National Center for Health Statistics,[4,5] and World Health Organization (http://www.cdc.gov/growthcharts and http://www.who.int/childgrowth/training/en).[6] These media demonstrate standardized measurement techniques similar to those in the *Anthropometric Standardization Reference Manual*.[3]

Recumbent length and stature describe linear growth, and weight is a measure of the mass of all body tissues. Weight indexed for stature can describe levels of overweight or obesity, but this measure of adiposity is most accurate when applied to groups rather than individuals. The body mass index (BMI) is the most common stature-standardized weight indicator of overweight or obesity in children.[7] BMI is computed as weight divided by stature squared, with all measures in the metric system ($kg/m^2 \times 10{,}000$). Additional measures related to body fatness are limb and trunk circumferences and skinfold thicknesses. Midarm circumference is an index of the underlying fat and muscle tissue; abdominal circumference is an indicator of abdominal fatness; and skinfolds measure subcutaneous adipose tissue thickness. Two common skinfold sites are the triceps on the back of the arm over the triceps muscle and the subscapular just below the scapula. Large values for BMI, midarm, and abdominal circumferences and triceps and subscapular skinfolds are positively correlated with total and percent body fat in children.[9,10]

It is important to assess a child's level of fatness because obesity is the most prevalent health problem of childhood. More children are obese today than in the past, and they are at greater levels of obesity than were children 10 to 20 years ago. Today, a big child, one who exceeds expected stature and weight standards for a given age, is likely overweight or obese rather than just healthy. Childhood obesity is frequently linked with type 2 diabetes, dyslipidemia, hypertension, and increased carotid intima-media thickness, measures of subclinical cardiovascular disease among children.[1] The childhood incidence of overweight, obesity, and cardiovascular disease track with high predictability into adulthood, which increases concern for future health.[1,7] It is also important to measure bone mineral content and bone mineral density in children in order to identify those with low levels (due to low calcium and protein intakes) who are at risk for osteopenia and osteoporosis in adulthood.[11,12] Measuring a child's body composition can identify risk factors for some chronic adult diseases at an early point in time when treatment may be most effective.

Periods and Patterns of Growth

A child's growth pattern can be divided into four periods: infancy from birth to 2 years of age, the preschool years from about 3 to 6 years of age, the middle childhood years

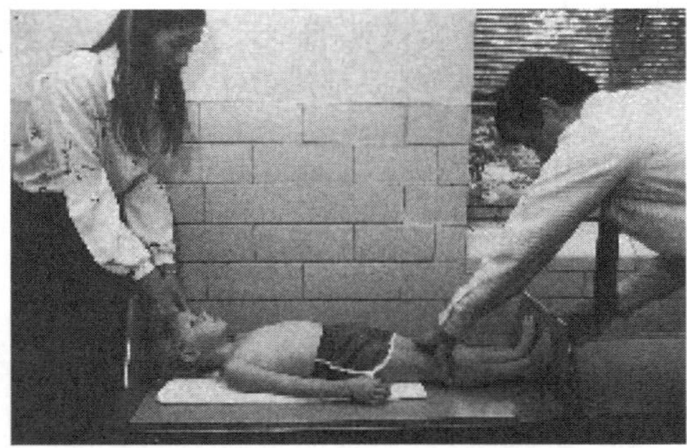

FIGURE 2-1 Measurement of Recumbent Length

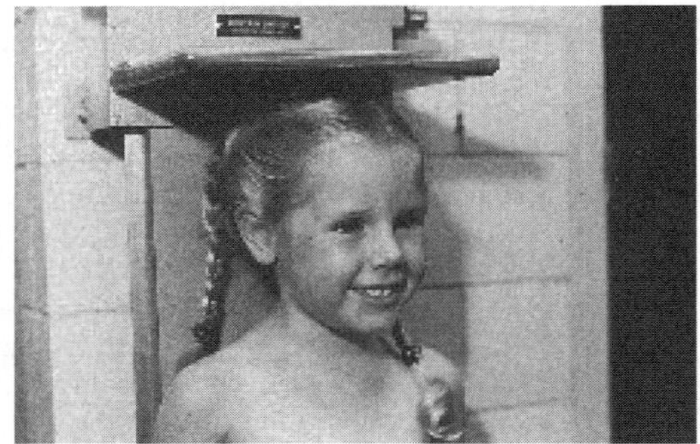

FIGURE 2-2 Measurement of Stature

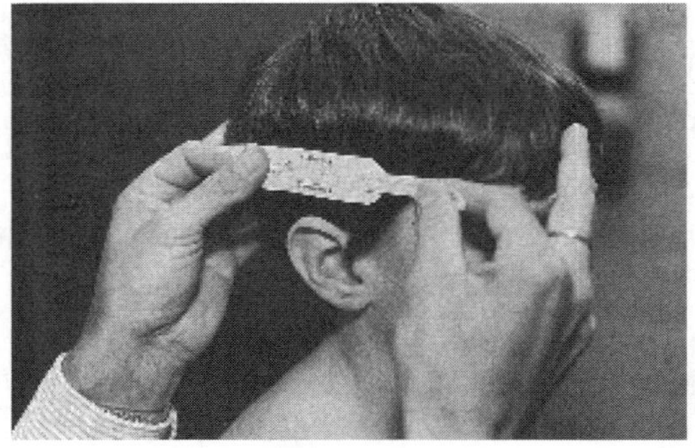

FIGURE 2-3 Measurement of Head Circumference

from about 7 to 10 years of age, and adolescence from about 11 to 18 years of age. Growth patterns and levels of maturation differ among children during these periods, and overlap occurs because of variation among children in the timing of their growth and maturation. A child's growth and size are related to his or her level of maturity and also reflect his or her genetic potential. At the same age, early-maturing children are taller and heavier than late-maturing children, and tall parents tend to have tall children and short parents tend to have short children. Weight has a strong genetic component that explains familial aspects of obesity, but epigenetic and environmental factors also affect the development of obesity.

Infancy: Birth to Age 2 Years

Infancy is distinguished by a very rapid growth period. Body size and dimensions increase faster than at any other time in postnatal life. Many healthy infants lose weight shortly after birth, but regain their birth weight after about a week.[13] Most normal infants double their birth weight by about 5 months and triple it by 1 year of age. During the first year of life, weight, on average, increases 200%, body length 55%, and head circumference 40%. Similar changes occur in the trunk, arms, and legs. Between 1 and 2 years of age, the average infant grows about 12 cm (4.7 inches) in length and gains about 2.5 kg (5.5 pounds) in weight.

An infant's head is disproportionately large compared with the dimensions of other body parts. At birth, its diameter exceeds that of the chest, and its length is about a quarter of the body's total length. Head circumference increases from an average of about 35–36 cm at birth to an average of about 45–46 cm at 1 year of age. Measures of head circumference reflect brain growth, and the brain doubles its birth weight by 1 year of age.

Preschool Years: 3 to 6 Years of Age

During the preschool years, the rate of growth slows, and it stabilizes by about 4 to 5 years of age. At 4 years of age, the average increase in stature and weight is about 6–8 cm (2.4–3.1 inches) and about 2–4 kg (4.4–8.8 pounds), respectively, per year. Head circumference remains an important measure during the preschool years because the brain more than triples its birth weight by 6 years of age. Sex differences in size and weight during the preschool years are slight, but the pattern of more adipose tissue in girls than boys appears by age 6 years. This is also a critical period for the development of overweight and onset of obesity in boys and girls, and the risk increases for subsequent obesity later in childhood and adulthood. During this period, overweight children should be monitored closely for increases in their BMI percentiles, patterns of dietary intake, and reduced physical activity.[7,14]

Middle Childhood: 7 to 10 Years of Age

During middle childhood, children grow at a steady rate. The average child at age 7 years grows about 5 to 6 cm (2–2.4 inches) per year in stature and about 2 kg (4.4 pounds) per year in weight, but the increase in weight is about 4 kg (8.8 pounds) per year by age 10 years. The legs grow at a greater rate than the trunk during middle childhood, so that although the trunk accounts for about 55% of total stature at age 7 years, it accounts for only about 45% by 10 years of age. During this period, the increasing maturity of the average girl causes her to grow more per year in stature and weight than the average boy, which contributes, in part, to the larger size of girls at the start of adolescence. At 7 years of age, boys are, on average, only about 2 cm (0.8 inch) taller than girls, but there is little difference in weight. By 10 years of age, the average girl is 1 cm (0.4 inch) taller, 1 kg (2.2 pounds) heavier, and the thickness of subcutaneous adipose tissue is about 25% greater than that of the average boy. Middle childhood is again a critical period of increased risk for the development of subsequent obesity. Based on their BMI percentiles, overweight and obese children during this period are at an increasing risk for being obese in adulthood.[7]

Adolescence: 11 to 18 Years of Age

Adolescence starts before puberty and spans the years until growth and maturation are mostly completed, which is around 16 to 18 years of age in girls and 18 to 20 years of age in boys. A final increase in body size, shape, and weight transforms a child into an adult. Most girls have their pubescent growth spurts between 11 and 14 years of age, and, on average, are taller than boys the same age. Boys, on average, enter their pubescent growth spurts about 2 years after girls, so they have an additional 2 years of prepubertal growth. In addition, the pubescent growth spurt lasts for a longer time in boys than girls, and the related amount of growth is larger in boys. The average peak height velocity (i.e., the maximum rate of growth in stature during the growth spurt) ranges in boys about 9.5–10.5 cm (3.7–4.1 inches) per year, while in girls the maximum velocity is about 8.5–9.0 cm (3.3–3.5 inches) per year. These sex differences result in the larger average body size in men than in women. During adolescence, girls add more total body fat than boys, but boys develop considerably more skeletal muscle tissue than girls. These differences result in the sex difference in adult body shape and, to a large extent, the increased physical ability and performance of the average boy.[15]

Assessing Growth Status

Recumbent length, stature, and weight along with head circumference and BMI are used to describe a child's growth status. These measures should be collected at regular intervals and plotted on growth charts (see Appendix B).[16] In the first year of life, the intervals for assessing growth are about every 3 months for well-baby visits and afterwards at annual physical examinations. Growth charts present an assessment or comparison of the stature or length, weight, head circumference, and BMI of an infant, child, or adolescent with the percentile distribution of other children at the same ages. The Centers for Disease Control and Prevention/National Center for Health Statistics (CDC/NCHS) and the World Health Organization (WHO) each produce growth charts, both of which are recommended for use with U.S. children.[3,5] Copies of these charts can be downloaded from the CDC (http://www.cdc.gov/growthcharts) and WHO (http://www.who.int/childgrowth) Websites.

CDC 2000 Growth Charts

In 2000, the CDC/NCHS revised the 1977 U.S. growth charts.[4] This revision combined national data from infants and children in the 1977 NCHS charts with additional data from the National Health and Nutrition Examination Survey (NHANES) II and III for a sample of over 64,000 U.S. children measured between 1960 and 1994. These charts are for infants and children from birth to 36 months of age and for children from 2 to 20 years of age (see Appendix B). The data represented on these revised charts include a greater proportion of non-Hispanic black and Hispanic children than the earlier 1977 national charts. The infants and children in this revised sample had feeding patterns common in the United States at the time the data were collected, and approximately 25% reportedly received some breastfeeding. The 2- to 20-year charts do not include any body weight data from the NHANES III conducted from 1988 to 1994 because the obesity epidemic affecting the United States' (and the rest of the world's) pediatric population would have resulted in spuriously higher weights of children in this sample.

WHO Growth Charts

Scientists in the Department of Nutrition for Health and Development at the WHO and their international collaborators[3,8] have created a new set of growth charts based on longitudinal and cross-sectional data from infants who were observed between 1997 and 2003. The healthy infants and children used to construct these WHO charts were recruited from nonsmoking families in urban, middle-class communities in Brazil, Ghana, Oman, Norway, India, and Davis, California. The more than 800 infants in the longitudinal sample were enrolled at birth and observed in their homes at 1, 2, 4, and 6 weeks, then monthly until 12 months, and then bimonthly until 24 months. These infants were exclusively or predominantly breastfed for the first 3 to 4 months of life with complete weaning occurring after the first birthday. These WHO charts come in two sets, one for infants from birth to 24 months of age, and the second for children from 2 to 5 years of age (see Appendix B).

The cross-sectional sample of almost 7000 children for the 2- to 5-year-old cross-sectional charts was from similar urban middle-class communities in these six countries. These children reportedly received some breastfeeding for at least 3 months. The infants and children in the longitudinal and cross-sectional groups comprised samples of convenience within their geographic locations. Recently, the WHO developed an additional set of growth charts for children and adolescents.[12] These WHO charts (see Appendix B) use a combination of data from the cross-sectional WHO 2- to 5-year-old growth charts and data for U.S. children from 2 to 19 years of age from the 1977 NCHS U.S. growth charts. These combined data were reanalyzed and statistically smoothed to provide a new WHO growth reference for older children and adolescents. These charts represent "healthy" weights and BMI values, and data from children who are directly part of the obesity epidemic are not included in the samples.

Using the CDC or the WHO Growth Charts

These CDC and WHO growth charts were created using large samples of children at all ages, and the data were statistically smoothed to minimize age-to-age variations,[17] but these charts are used clinically for a single infant or child. The primary clinical utility of growth charts is to help identify an infant or a child who is not growing normally (i.e., whose age- and sex-standardized percentile value for head circumference, recumbent length, weight, stature, or BMI indicates some possible clinical concern or health risk). To assist in screening for obesity and other growth disorders, the CDC and WHO charts are available in two percentile line versions at their Websites. The standard set for both has percentile lines on all charts from the 5th to the 95th percentiles (see Appendix B). The other set has percentile lines on all charts from the 3rd to the 97th percentiles, which improves discrimination of children at the extremes of the distributions for head circumference, recumbent length, weight, height, and BMI. The WHO infant and child growth charts are also available in several age groupings, resulting in differing widths between the lines from the 3rd to the 97th percentiles. This also facilitates the plotting of children at different ages or with possible growth disorders, in order to provide a clearer clinical interpretation.

Plotting a child's growth values on the CDC or WHO growth chart indicates that at this time and for this age, the child has a normal value (between the 15th and 85th percentiles), representing 70% of the population, or that additional information is needed to determine the validity of a possibly unusual value (below the 15th or above the 85th percentiles), representing 30% of the population. Additional health information is needed to determine the reason for a child's unusual percentile value location. For example, a child whose height is above the 85th or below the 15th percentile may have very tall or short parents, respectively, or may have a clinical growth deficiency or hormonal abnormality. The WHO charts are also available as z-score charts, where zero represents the mean and a positive or negative z-score is one standard deviation above or below the mean. These charts are not readily understandable to parents, but can be of greater clinical use than the percentile charts for some children.[3]

BMI Growth Charts

To help address the current pediatric obesity epidemic, the CDC and WHO sets of growth charts from 2 to 20 years of age now contain charts to plot a child's BMI (see Appendix B), a useful, recommended index of overweight and obesity.[6] The CDC classifies overweight in children as a BMI for age greater than the 95th percentile and obesity as greater than the 97th percentile. The WHO BMI charts are like the CDC charts, but the WHO defines overweight in children as a BMI for age between the 85th and 95th percentiles and obesity as above the 95th percentile.

Case Study

Demonstrating the Use of the CDC Growth Charts

In this example, a boy is observed for a regular checkup at 10, 11, and 12 years of age. At each visit, his weight and stature are measured and plotted on the CDC growth chart (**Figure 2-4**). His weight at 10 years was 37 kg, at 11 was 45 kg, and at 12 years was 54 kg. His stature was 143 cm at 10 years, 150 cm at 11 years, and 156 cm at 12 years. Plotting these values on his growth chart indicates that this boy had a weight at the 75th percentile at 10 years of age, but his weight has progressed to the 90th percentile by 12 years of age. His stature was at the 75th percentile at 10 years of age also, and it has risen slightly above the 75th percentile at 11 and 12 years of age. Based on these data, it is reasonable to assume that this boy, whose weight and stature were within normal values at age 10 years, is possibly entering his adolescent growth spurt early. However, no corresponding increase in stature accompanies his increase in weight, which limits this assumption.

To clarify these data, his BMI was calculated and plotted on the CDC BMI growth chart (**Figure 2-5**). At age 10 years, his BMI was 18 at the 75th percentile, which would be normal, but by age 12, his BMI had increased to 22 at the 90th percentile. The additional BMI plotted data lend support to the reasonable possibility that this boy has progressed from a normal weight to either a potential overweight category based on the CDC criteria or to an overweight category based on the WHO category. This change from a normal weight to overweight places this boy by 12 years of age at risk for obesity in adolescence and later in adulthood. Dietary intervention along with increased physical activity should be considered as possible treatments after further health information is obtained.

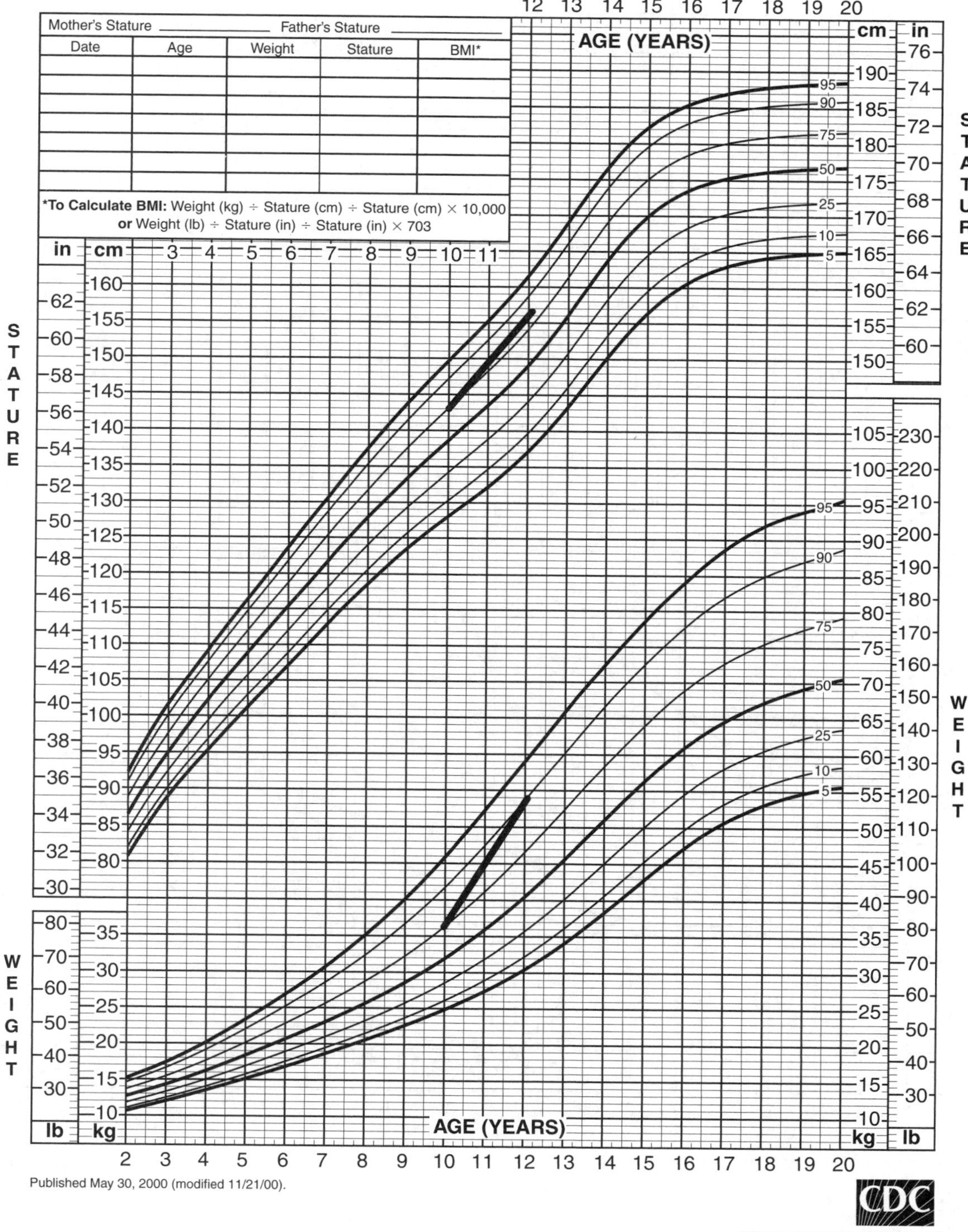

FIGURE 2-4 Stature-for-Age and Weight-for-Age Percentiles 2 to 20 Years: Boys

Source: Developed by the National Center for Health Statistics in collaboration with the National Center for Chronic Disease Prevention and Health Promotion (2000). Available at: http://www.cdc.gov/growthcharts.

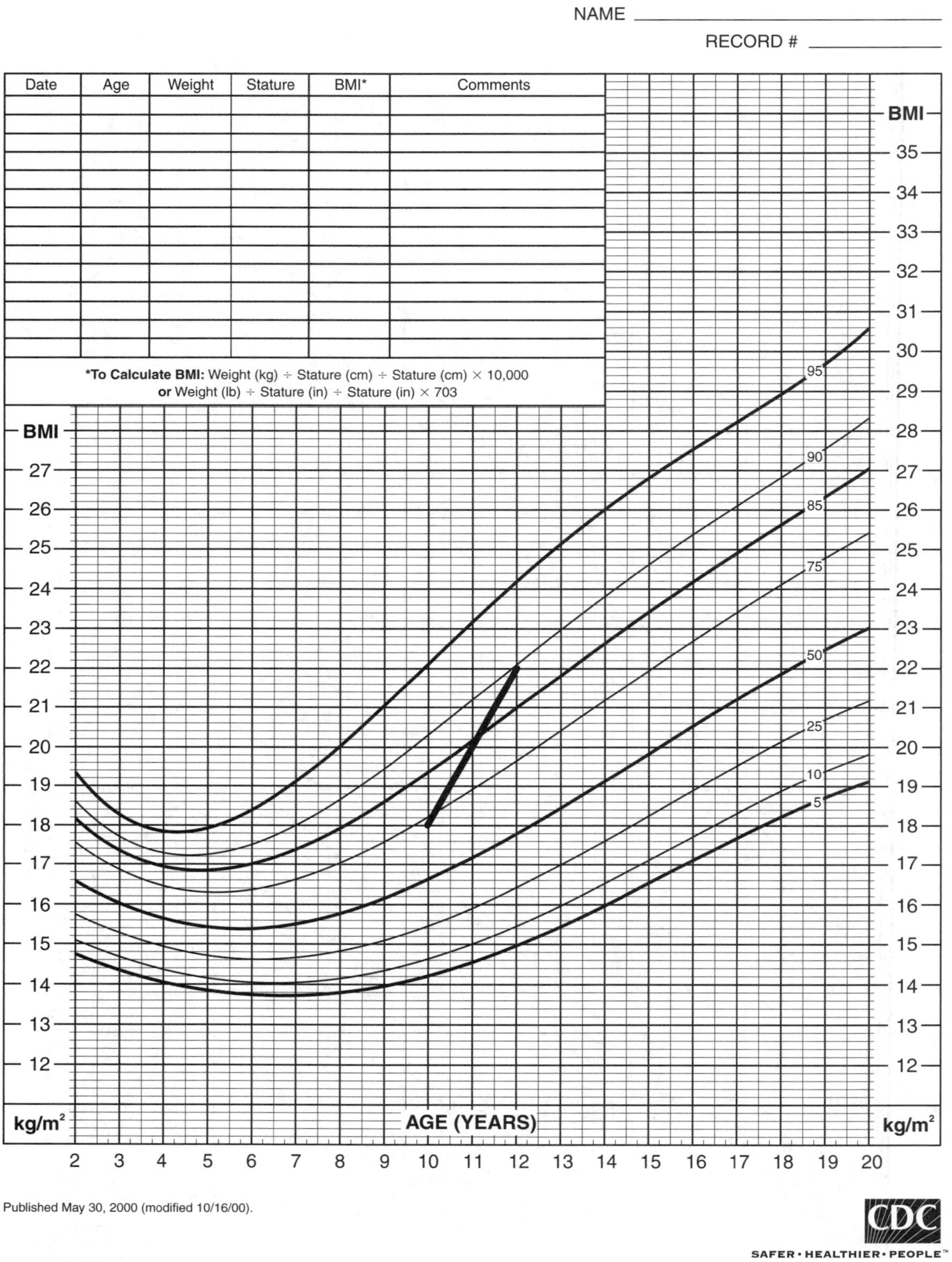
NAME
RECORD #
Date
Age
Weight
Stature
BMI*
Comments
*To Calculate BMI: Weight (kg) ÷ Stature (cm) ÷ Stature (cm) × 10,000
or Weight (lb) ÷ Stature (in) ÷ Stature (in) × 703
BMI
35 34 33 32 31 30 29 28 27 26 25 24 23 22 21 20 19 18 17 16 15 14 13 12
95
90
85
75
50
25
10
5
kg/m²
AGE (YEARS)
2 3 4 5 6 7 8 9 10 11 12 13 14 15 16 17 18 19 20
Published May 30, 2000 (modified 10/16/00).
CDC
SAFER • HEALTHIER • PEOPLE™

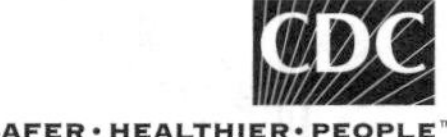

FIGURE 2-5 Body Mass Index-for-Age Percentiles 2 to 20 Years: Boys

Source: Developed by the National Center for Health Statistics in collaboration with the National Center for Chronic Disease Prevention and Health Promotion (2000). Available at: http://www.cdc.gov/growthcharts.

Race/Ethnicity

There are growth and maturational differences among black, white, and Mexican American children, but in most instances these differences, on average, are small.[4,13,14] There are also small differences in the growth and maturation of healthy Chinese American and Japanese American children or American children of other racial or ethnic groups compared with that of the white, black, and Mexican American children represented on the current CDC growth charts, and this is also the case for the WHO growth charts. Similar race/ethnicity differences are reported by clinicians in other countries who also use the CDC and WHO charts. In addition, when a child reaches puberty and progresses through his or her adolescent growth spurt, the individuality of that child creates large percentile differences during these adolescent years compared to earlier positions that usually dissipate with maturity. The percentile position on the growth chart of that infant or child is, in part, a function of the differences in his or her genetic background as compared to that of the children used to construct these growth charts, and these individual disparities occur regardless of the set of growth charts used.

Comparing the CDC and WHO Growth Charts

The 2000 CDC charts have flaws (as do all growth charts) because the combined data used to construct them were not collected in a single study over a defined period of time, the secular influences of the obesity epidemic limit the utility of the weight data from many of the NHANES samples, and there are differences and improvements in the statistical methods used to create and smooth the percentiles.[4] The majority of these cross-sectional data are from very large national probability samples of U.S. children, and these data were adjusted to reflect their complex national sampling structure. The 2000 CDC growth charts represent national data from the largest sample of U.S. children ever assembled for this purpose, and they are the best national data of their kind available today.

The WHO growth charts reflect the growth of breastfed infants for the first few months of life, and there are well-reported growth differences between breastfed and formula-fed infants and the potential subsequent health effects.[15,16] After infancy, the diet and nutrition of the children represented on the WHO charts, which may be above average in quality because they were selected from urban middle class families, may be similar to that of the U.S. children on the CDC growth charts. However, this information is either not known or unavailable. It is not possible in this brief discussion to cover the extensive literature on the growth differences between breastfed and formula-fed infants and subsequent health. However, if a mother plans to and can breastfeed her infant, it can be clinically helpful to plot the first few months of growth on both the CDC and the WHO charts. If that mother can successfully breastfeed her infant for a longer period of time (up to 6 months or more), then the WHO charts in most cases provide the best growth reference. Otherwise, it is difficult, on an individual basis, to provide an "ironclad" justification for the use of the CDC over the WHO growth charts for the majority of infants and children in the United States.

Premature Growth

It is important to account for the gestational age of premature infants or those small at birth when plotting their growth on the current CDC/NCHS growth charts.[13] The amount of prematurity is subtracted from an infant's chronologic age (e.g., for an infant with a gestational age of 28 weeks, this is a correction of 12 weeks or 3 months of chronological age). Current growth charts for preterm low-birth-weight infants include weight, recumbent length, and head circumference (see Appendix A).[18] However, an international study is under way to produce new fetal and premature growth charts for all children. This is the Intergrowth-21st Study (http://www.intergrowth21.org.uk), which is sponsored by the University of Oxford and the WHO with funding from the Bill and Melinda Gates Foundation. New fetal and premature growth charts should be available in the next few years. After about 2.5 years of age, it is frequently no longer necessary to make the adjustment for most healthy children who were premature.

Growth Velocity

When growth is measured at repeated visits, the amount of change in a measurement or the rate of growth per unit of time can be quantified. This provides additional information; for example, growth velocity can describe a child's response to nutritional intervention. Increment growth reference data supplement the status growth charts by indicating if a child's rate of growth is normal or unusual. The WHO has developed increment (or rate) charts with percentiles reflecting the tempo of growth for children between 1 and 5 years of age using the longitudinal data from the breastfed infants in their Multicentre Growth Reference Study (http://www.who.int/childgrowth). There are similar increment charts for U.S. children,[19,20] but these are almost 30 years old. Both assess the growth of children and monitor the results of nutritional therapy.

Maturation

The central nervous system integrates the activities of the endocrine system, coordinating growth and sexual maturation. Before puberty, the central nervous system inhibits hormone production, but this inhibition decreases near puberty when the sex hormones reach adult concentrations. Endocrine and adrenal androgens influence growth, sexual maturation, and the development of secondary sex characteristics.

The reproductive system matures at puberty, making sexual reproduction possible. Puberty is identified in girls by the onset of menstruation or menarche, but there is no similar marker in boys. The ages of individual children at the onset and completion of growth and sexual maturation are highly variable.

The progression of sexual maturation is assessed using Tanner stages as indicators of the development of breasts in girls, genitals in boys, and pubic hair in each sex (see Appendix F). Breast buds in girls (Tanner stage B-2) and genital enlargement in boys (Tanner stage G-2) indicate the onset of sexual maturation, which is followed by the appearance of pubic hair (Tanner stage PH-2) in both sexes. For girls, the 25th to 75th percentiles for the age at onset of sexual maturation, Tanner stage B-2, range from 8.5 to 10.5 years in non-Hispanic blacks, 8.6 to 11.2 years in Mexican Americans, and 9.5 to 11 years for non-Hispanic whites. The 25th to the 75th percentiles for the age at onset of sexual maturation, Tanner stage G-2 for boys, range from 7.5 to 10.9 years in non-Hispanic blacks, 8.9 to 11.7 years in Mexican Americans, and 8.6 to 11.4 years for non-Hispanic whites. The onset of sexual maturation is significantly earlier in non-Hispanic black girls and boys than in non-Hispanic white and Mexican American girls and boys.[21]

The sequence of Tanner stages between paired indicators is concordant for about 60% of healthy children. However, about 30% of healthy children are discordant (i.e., they enter or are in a stage for one indicator and at the same time enter or are in earlier or later stages for the other indicator), and this discordance affects their growth. Boys whose pubic hair stages are more advanced than their genital stages and girls whose breast development stages are more advanced than their pubic hair stages are heavier and have higher BMI percentiles than concordant children. Children with the opposite discordance have lesser weights and BMI percentiles than concordant children. This variation in weight and BMI among healthy concordant and discordant children is greater than that among early and late maturing children.

A girl attains menarche or starts to menstruate about 2 years after her breasts start to grow and about 12 to 18 months after her peak height velocity. Approximately 80% of non-Hispanic white girls start to menstruate between about 11.3 and 13.8 years of age, with a median age of 12.55 years, while 80% of non-Hispanic black girls start to menstruate between about 10.5 and 13.6 years of age, with a median age of 12.06 years, and 80% of Mexican American girls start to menstruate between about 10.8 and 13.7 years of age, with a median age of 12.25 years.[22] The ages at menarche for 50% of non-Hispanic black girls and 25% of Mexican American girls are significantly earlier than those of white girls, but there are no significant differences between the black girls and Mexican American girls in their ages at menarche. Girls who attain menarche before 10.5–11.0 years are relatively "early" and those who attain menarche after 13.75 years are relatively "late." Peak height velocity (age at most rapid growth in stature) occurs in girls about a year or two before it does in boys, but the sex difference in age between sexual maturity stages can be less than half a year.

Recently, it has been reported that the onset of puberty was possibly occurring earlier among U.S. children than in the past several decades[23] based on the prevalence of Tanner stage 2 breast and/or pubic hair development. Despite slight declines over the past two decades, there is currently no conclusive evidence of a significantly earlier age at menarche among non-Hispanic white girls and black girls. Analysis of U.S. national health survey data indicates that sexual maturation among U.S. children also has not become significantly earlier, but national survey data are needed to address this percentile trend and answer this important health concern.

Body Composition

Muscle, adipose tissue, and bone are the primary body tissues that change during growth. These tissues are frequently quantified using a model that divides the body into fat and fat-free components based upon assumptions that the densities of fat and lean tissues are constant.[24] The density of fat varies little at any age, but the density of lean tissue varies depending upon its hydration and the relative proportions of muscle and bone, which vary among children based on age, gender, race, level of maturation, exercise, and nutritional status.[25] Accurate body composition estimates are calculated from measures of body density, bone density, and the volume of total body water in a model that accounts for differences among growing children in their levels of fatness, muscle mass, age, ethnicity, and sex.[26] There are numerous methods for estimating body composition, but dual energy x-ray absorptiometry (DXA) is the most accurate, precise, and easiest method for children and even infants. There is a growing reference literature on the body composition of children and adolescents including fat-free mass (FFM), total body fat (TBF), and percent body fat (%BF),[27] but body composition references for infants and very young children remain limited. Reference averages for FFM and %BF estimates from bioelectrical impedance available from teenagers in the NHANES III are presented in **Figures 2-6** and **2-7**, respectively. There are differences in average values between non-Hispanic white and non-Hispanic black and Mexican American children for FFM and %BF. It is not possible to determine whether these differences are significant because of the limitations of the method used to produce these estimates. Shortly, NHANES national reference data for body composition from DXA will become available for U.S. children.

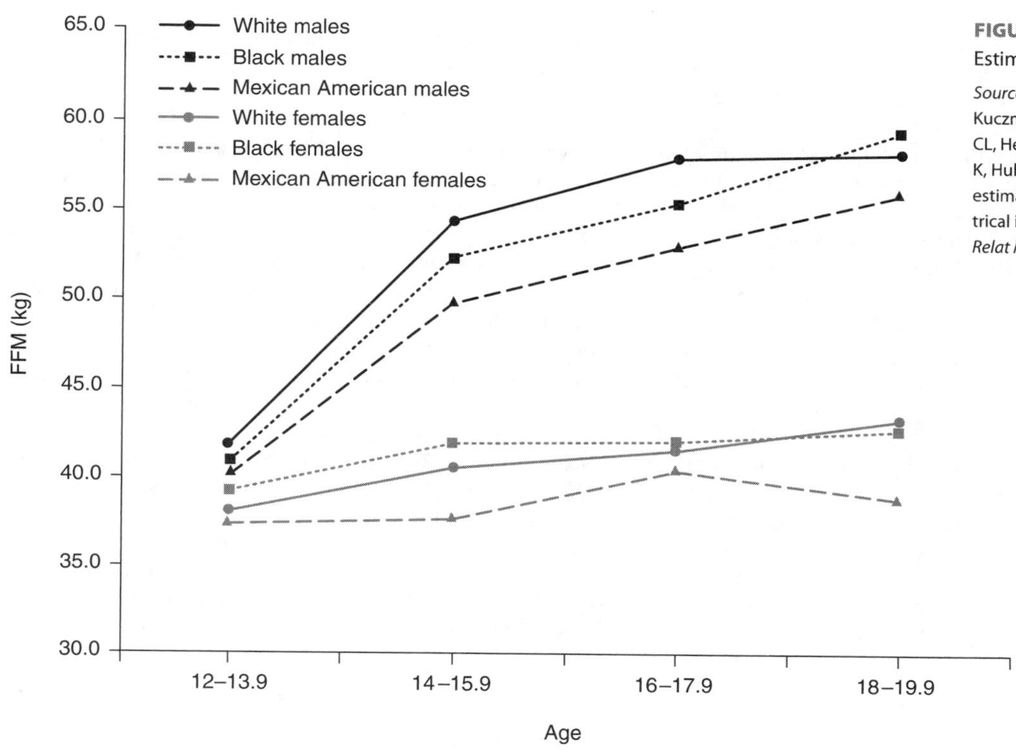

FIGURE 2-6 NHANES III FFM Estimates in Children

Source: From Chumlea WC, Guo SS, Kuczmarski RJ, Flegal KM, Johnson CL, Heymsfield SB, Lukaski H, Friedl K, Hubbard VS. Body composition estimates from NHANES III bioelectrical impedance data. *Int J Obes Relat Metab Disord*. 2002:1596–1609.

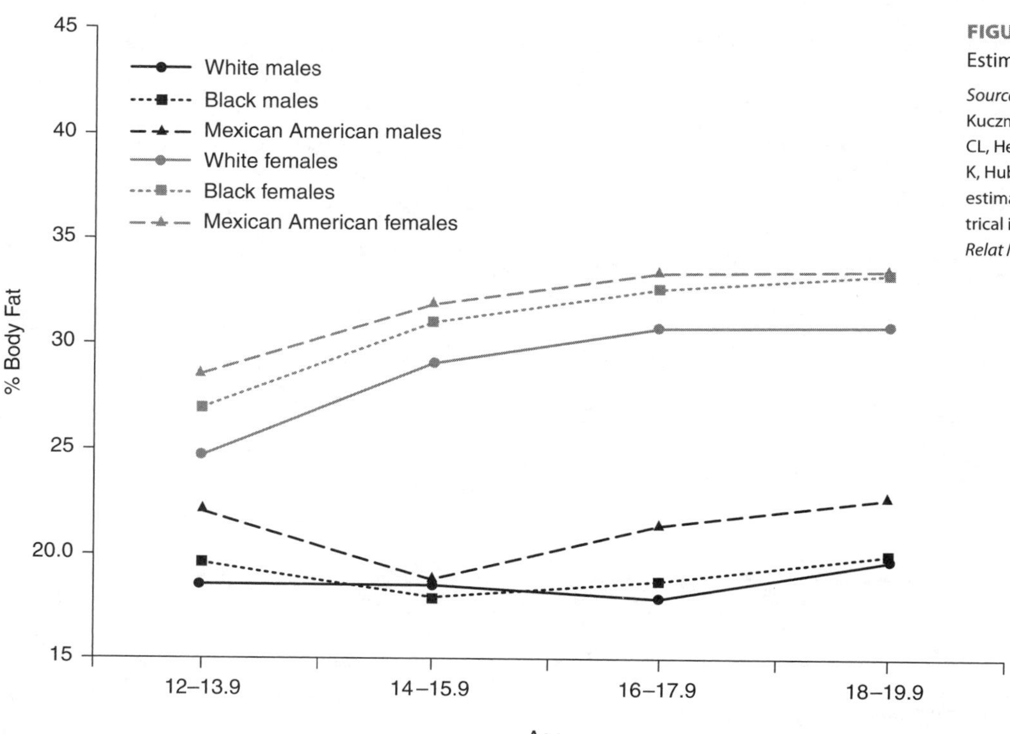

FIGURE 2-7 NHANES III %BF Estimates in Children

Source: From Chumlea WC, Guo SS, Kuczmarski RJ, Flegal KM, Johnson CL, Heymsfield SB, Lukaski H, Friedl K, Hubbard VS. Body composition estimates from NHANES III bioelectrical impedance data. *Int J Obes Relat Metab Disord*. 2002:1596–1609.

Growth of Muscle

Lean body mass (LBM) is metabolically active and is composed of muscle tissue, the internal organs, and the skeleton. Lean body mass contains a small amount of fat; in contrast, FFM is LBM without any fat. Growth in FFM and LBM is primarily due to an increase in skeletal muscle mass, which is the largest single tissue component of the body, the major constituent of which is body water. At birth, 25% of body weight is skeletal muscle, and this increases to about 50% of body weight at adulthood. FFM, LBM, and skeletal muscle mass are positively associated with stature (i.e., a tall child has a greater amount of these than a shorter child at the same level of maturity). Skeletal muscle mass increases in boys and girls during childhood and is roughly equal between them until about 13 to 14 years of age (**Figure 2-8**). In girls muscle continues to grow into adolescence, but stops around 16 years of age. In boys skeletal muscle grows rapidly after 13 years of age and well into late adolescence (Figure 2-8). This growth period in boys is about twice as long as in girls, and as a result, boys have several times as much skeletal muscle as girls, which is located primarily in the shoulders and arms. At maturity, boys have greater absolute amounts of FFM or LBM than girls, irrespective of stature.

Growth of Body Fat

Body fat stores energy. In children the majority of the body's fat is subcutaneous, but adipose tissue is also deposited in the visceral parts of the body. From infancy up to adolescence, the growth of body fat or adipose tissue is fairly steady in boys and girls. Adipose tissue thickness on the arms, legs, and trunk increases during childhood in both sexes but slightly more so in girls, so that by the onset of puberty, girls have about 25% more body fat than boys. Body fatness continues to increase during adolescence in girls, but in boys decreases after about 13 years of age because the underlying skeletal muscle and bone grow at a greater rate at this time. Boys and girls also differ in the deposition and patterning of adipose tissue during adolescence. Both sexes deposit adipose tissue on the torso, but adolescent girls add adipose tissue to breasts, buttocks, thighs, and across the back of the arms, which accentuates the adult sex differences in body shape. The majority of total body fat growth among obese children is subcutaneous, but

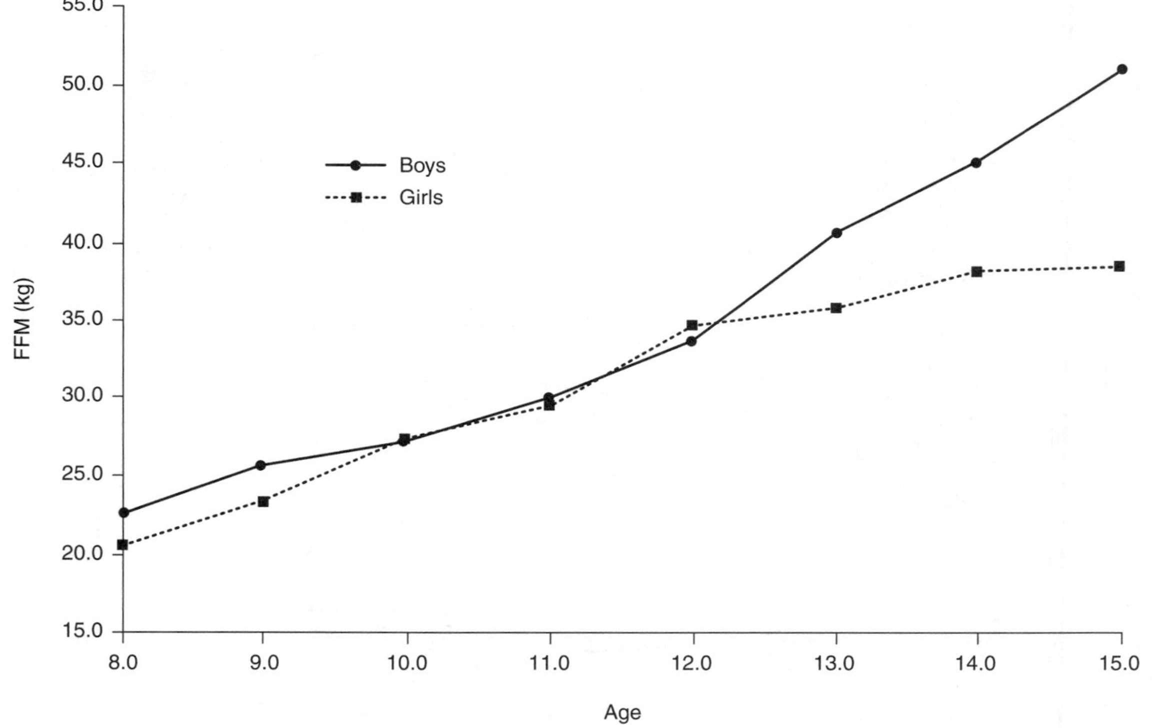

FIGURE 2-8 Fels Longitudinal Study

Source: Adapted from unpublished data. Used with permission of Dr. Cameron Chumlea.

recently, internal adipose tissue deposition similar to that of middle-aged adults is appearing in obese children.[28]

Skeletal Growth

Skeletal growth is a continuous process. The bones of the legs and the vertebrae are the major locations of growth in stature, which reflects growth in bone length. Bone growth is rather steady until the adolescent growth spurt, but slows afterward. By about 18 years of age for girls and around 20 to 22 years of age for boys, the epiphyses or growth plates at the ends of long bones have fused to the shaft or diaphysis and the skeleton is mature. Assessment of skeletal maturation from radiographs of the hand/wrist or knee is an index of a child's biological age known as *skeletal age*. Two children of the same chronological age may have different levels of skeletal maturation or skeletal ages, just as they may also have different levels of sexual maturation.

The skeleton is the body's reserve of calcium, and an important aspect of skeletal growth is the building of this calcium reserve. The importance of this reserve for children is that those who end growth with a low bone mass (i.e., a low calcium reserve) are at an increased risk for developing adult osteopenia and possible osteoporosis. Peak bone mass is the maximum mineral mass attained by the skeleton. This peak occurs in the late-middle part of the third decade of life, but by maturity, the majority of peak bone mass has been reached. With DXA, it is possible to measure the amount of calcium or bone mineral content and bone mineral density of the skeleton of children. Limited reference data for bone mineral content and density are now available for children at many ages,[29] and national data should be available in the future from the current National Health and Nutrition Survey. These data and the use of DXA along with calcium supplementation provide mechanisms for monitoring the growth of the skeleton and affecting its calcium content. This information can help children with low bone mass and density and low calcium intake attain their peak bone mass and reduce the prevalence of osteoporosis in their future.

Special Children

Assessing the growth status of children with Down's syndrome, cerebral palsy, contractures, braces, mental retardation, and the like is difficult. The heterogeneity of these conditions limits recommended standard methodology, and there is limited or no specific reference data.[30] If the child can stand, standard methods can be used. If the child is nonambulatory, then recumbent methods are recommended. Reference data from the NCHS need to be interpolated depending upon the condition of the child in question.

In a growth assessment of a handicapped child, one measurement is probably not sufficient. It may be necessary to take several measurements, especially with more difficult measurements or more uncooperative children. Several Websites provide useful information about measuring handicapped children. Accurate records are important, and the CDC/NCHS growth charts can be used. A child may be at the third percentile or less, but these growth charts can still provide information about a child's status, especially over time. For children with some specific conditions, such as Trisomy 21, growth charts are available[31] (see Appendix D). For other children, such as those with cerebral palsy, specific growth charts are being developed.

SUGGESTED READINGS

Malina RM, Bouchard C, Bar-Or O. *Growth, Maturation, and Physical Activity.* 2nd ed. Champaign, IL: Human Kinetics; 2004.

Roche AF, Sun SS. *Human Growth Assessment and Interpretation.* Cambridge, UK: Cambridge University Press; 2003.

World Health Organization. *WHO Child Growth Standards Length/Height-for-Age, Weight-for-Length, Weight-for-Height and Body Mass Index-for-Age, Methods and Development.* Geneva, Switzerland: World Health Organization; 2006.

REFERENCES

1. Dietz WH, Franks AL, Marks JS. The obesity problem. *N Engl J Med.* 1998;338(16):1157; author reply 1158.
2. Troiano RP, Flegal KM, Kuczmarski RJ, Campbell SM, Johnson CL. Overweight prevalence and trends for children and adolescents. The National Health and Nutrition Examination Surveys, 1963 to 1991. *Arch Pediatr Adolesc Med.* 1995;149(10):1085–1091.
3. Lohman TG, Roche AF, Martorell R. *Anthropometric Standardization Reference Manual.* Champaign, IL: Human Kinetics; 1988.
4. National Centers for Health Statistics, Centers for Disease Control and Prevention. *Analytic and Reporting Guidelines: The Third National Health and Nutrition Examination Survey (1988–1994)* [CD-ROM]. Washington, DC: National Centers for Health Statistics; 1997.
5. U.S. Department of Health and Human Services. *National Health and Nutrition Examination Survey III. Anthropometric Procedures* [videotape]. Washington, DC: U.S. Department of Health and Human Services, Public Health Services; 1996.
6. de Onis M, Onyangoa, AW, Van den Broeck J, Chumlea WC, Martorell R. Measurement and standardization protocols for anthropometry used in the construction of a new international growth reference. *Food Nutr Bull.* 2004;25(1):S27–S36.
7. Guo SS, Wu W, Chumlea WC, Roche AF. Predicting overweight and obesity in adulthood from body mass index values in childhood and adolescence. *Am J Clin Nutr.* 2002;76: 653–658.

8. Goran MI, Gower BA. Relation between visceral fat and disease risk in children and adolescents. *Am J Clin Nutr.* 1999;70(1 Part 2):149S–156S.
9. Roche AF, Siervogel RM, Chumlea WC, Webb P. Grading of body fatness from limited anthropometric data. *Am J Clin Nutr.* 1981;34:2831–2838.
10. Liem ET, De Lucia Rolfe E, L'Abee C, Sauer PJ, Ong KK, Stolk RP. Measuring abdominal adiposity in 6 to 7-year-old children. *Eur J Clin Nutr.* 2009;63(7):835–841.
11. Sakuragi S, Abhayaratna K, Gravenmaker KJ, et al. Influence of adiposity and physical activity on arterial stiffness in healthy children: the lifestyle of our kids study. *Hypertension.* 2009;53(4):611–616.
12. Matkovic V, Jelic T, Wardlaw GM, et al. Timing of peak bone mass in Caucasian females and its implication for the prevention of osteoporosis. Inference from a cross-sectional model. *J Clin Invest.* 1994;93(2):799–808.
13. Moore WM, Roche AF. *Pediatric Anthropometry*. 3rd ed. Columbus, OH: Ross Laboratories; 1987.
14. Whitaker RC, Wright JA, Pepe MS, Seidel KD, Dietz WH. Predicting obesity in young adulthood from childhood and parental obesity. *N Engl J Med.* 1997;337(13):869–873.
15. Beunen G. Muscular strength development in children and adolescents. In: Froberg K, Lammert O, Hansen H, Blimkie C, eds. *Exercise and Fitness—Benefits and Risks*. Denmark: Odense University Press; 1997:192–207.
16. Kuczmarski RJ, Ogden CL, Grummer-Strawn LM, et al. CDC growth charts: United States. *Adv Data.* 2000;314:1–27.
17. Chumlea WC. Which growth charts are the best for children today? *Nutr Today.* 2007;42(4):148.
18. Guo SS, Roche AF, Chumlea WC, Casey PH, Moore WM. Growth in weight, recumbent length, and head circumference for preterm low-birthweight infants during the first three years of life using gestation-adjusted ages. *Early Hum Dev.* 1997;47:305–325.
19. Baumgartner RN, Roche AF, Himes JH. Incremental growth tables: supplementary to previously published charts. *Am J Clin Nutr.* 1986;43:711–722.
20. Roche AF, Himes J. Incremental growth charts. *Am J Clin Nutr.* 1980;33:2041–2052.
21. Sun SS, Schubert CM, Chumlea WC, Roche AF, Kulin H, Lee PA, Himes J, Ryan AS. National estimates of the timing of sexual maturation and racial differences among U.S. children. *Pediatrics.* 2002;110:911–919.
22. Chumlea WC, Schubert CM, Roche AF, Kulin H, Lee PA, Himes JH, Sun SS. Age at menarche and racial comparisons in U.S. girls. *Pediatrics.* 2003;111(1):110–113.
23. Herman-Giddens ME, Slora EJ, Wasserman RC, Bourdony CJ, Bhapkar MV, Koch GG, Hasemeier CM. Secondary sexual characteristics and menses in young girls seen in office practice: a study from the Pediatric Research in Office Settings network. *Pediatrics.* 1997;99(4):505–512.
24. Siri W. Body composition from fluid spaces and density analysis of methods. In: Brozek J, Henschel A, eds. *Techniques for Measuring Body Composition*. Washington DC: National Academy Press; 1961:223–244.
25. Lohman TG. Applicability of body composition techniques and constants for children and youths. *Exerc Sport Sci Rev.* 1986;14:325–357.
26. Guo SS, Chumlea WC, Roche AF, Siervogel RM. Age- and maturity-related changes in body composition during adolescence into adulthood: the Fels Longitudinal Study. *Int J Obes Relat Metab Disord.* 1997;21:1167–1175.
27. Chumlea WC, Guo SS, Kuczmarski RJ, Flegal KM, Johnson CL, Heymsfield SB, Lukaski H, Friedl K, Hubbard VS. Body composition estimates from NHANES III bioelectrical impedance data. *Int J Obes Relat Metab Disord.* 2002:1596–1609.
28. Brambilla P, Bedogni G, Moreno LA, Goran MI, Gutin B, Fox KR, Peters DM, Barbeau P, De Simone M, Pietrobelli A. Crossvalidation of anthropometry against magnetic resonance imaging for the assessment of visceral and subcutaneous adipose tissue in children. *Int J Obes (Lond).* 2006;30(1):23–30.
29. Maynard LM, Guo SS, Chumlea WC, Roche AF, Wisemandle WA, Zeller CM, Towne B, Siervogel RM. Total body and regional bone mineral content and area bone mineral density in children aged 8 to18 years: the Fels Longitudinal Study. *Am J Clin Nutr.* 1998;68:1111–1117.
30. Stevenson RD, Hayes RP, Cater LV, Blackman JA. Clinical correlates of linear growth in children with cerebral palsy. *Dev Med Child Neurol.* 1994;36(2):135–142.
31. Cronk C, Crocker AC, Pueschel SM, Shea AM, Zackai E, Pickens G, Reed RB. Growth charts for children with Down syndrome: 1 month to 18 years of age. *Pediatrics.* 1988;81(1):102–110.

Nutritional Assessment

Susan Bessler

The assessment of nutritional status is an integral component of pediatric health care. It identifies nutritionally depleted or at-risk infants and children, provides essential information for developing achievable nutritional care plans, and serves as a mechanism for evaluating the effectiveness of nutritional care.

Screening

The completion of in-depth nutritional assessments on all children served by a healthcare system is neither practical nor essential for providing quality nutrition care. Well-designed nutritional screening performed by trained personnel is effective in identifying children who are at an elevated nutritional risk and therefore may require a more comprehensive nutritional assessment.[1–5] Nutritional screenings can also predict outcomes in specific diagnoses.[6] The information gathered for screening includes indices of nutritional status routinely collected during scheduled healthcare appointments or upon admission to a healthcare facility.[7,8]

Nutritional screening protocols must be adapted to the needs of the specific population served, staff and facility resources, and imposed credentialing requirements.[9] The participation of administration, medical staff, nursing staff, and often family members is essential in developing a nutritional screening program because the measurement and documentation of many of the parameters involve non-nutrition personnel and equipment. The success of the program depends upon the coordinated efforts of the multidisciplinary team in completing assigned responsibilities.[1,10]

Key issues to be resolved when planning a nutritional screening program include designation of team member responsibilities, selection of nutritional parameters to be screened, timing of the screening, determining how the data will be analyzed, and determining the intended action once the data have been evaluated. In the hospital setting, a dietetic technician may collect the selected data by interview and from the patient's medical record whereas a clinic or extended care facility may have a nurse complete the nutritional screening. Family-administered screening instruments that have the child's primary caretaker report data have been developed for use in the community setting.[11] Most pediatric nutrition screening tools routinely include age, weight, length or height, and head circumference. Information about the child's medical history as well as diet and feeding ability is also routinely requested. The routine collection of lab values depends on the needs of the population and the laboratory support available. Once the nutritional data have been obtained, the child is assessed for nutrition risk and the appropriate referral or action plan is made. **Exhibit 3-1** is an example of a hospital screening form that weighs the criteria and dictates the next appropriate step in the care plan. Ideally, the data selected for the nutrition screen are objective (reproducible regardless of who is completing the screen), specific (identifying patients truly at risk), and sensitive (identifying all at-risk patients).[12] The nutrition screening process generally takes place at or soon after a clinic visit or hospital admission. Additionally, extended care facilities and hospitals with long-term patients may perform periodic rescreening to monitor changes in nutritional risk status.[13]

Nutritional Assessment

The assessment of a child's nutritional status is based on pertinent information collected from the medical history, anthropometric data, laboratory data, physical findings, and dietary interview. These tools vary in time, invasiveness, and expense. Based on the patient and clinical setting, the practitioner needs to weigh the cost of the assessment tool against its potential benefit.

Medical History

Approximately 10–15% of children in the United States have special healthcare needs, defined as "having, or being at risk

EXHIBIT 3-1 Children's Hospital Oakland Nutrition Screening Profile

Admitting Diagnosis

[ ] Group 1 (8 points): New DM, CF, Inborn Errors of Metabolism, SBS, Iron Deficiency, Burns, Decubitus, IBD, FTT, Nutritional Rickets, Eating Disorder, Ketogenic Diet

[ ] Group 2 (4 points): CP, CHD, Liver Disease, Renal Disease, BPD, Bowel Surgery, Immunodeficiency, Obesity with Comorbidity, Chylothorax, Major Trauma

[ ] Group 3—Higher Risk Oncology (4 points): Relapsed ALL, AML, Bone Marrow Transplant, Solid Tumor Grade III or higher

[ ] Group 4 (0 points): All other diagnoses

Anthropometrics

wt: _______ kg: _______% ht: _______ cm: _______%

wt/ht: _______ % *or* BMI (kg/m^2): _________ %

[ ] Wt/ht or BMI <= 5% (8 points)

Diet Order

[ ] NPO (1 point) [ ] Modified/Special Diet (3 points)

[ ] Tube Feeding * (5 points) [ ] Food Allergies (1 point)

[ ] TPN * (5 points) [ ] Mechanical Feeding Problems (1 point)

[ ] Other (0 points)

Additional Information

[ ] Age <= 3 years old (1 point)

[ ] Admitted > 1 week ago (1 point)

Conclusion

[ ] Patient at high nutritional risk. Registered dietitian will provide further assessment and care planing within 48 hours of admission (8 or more points).

[ ] Patient at lower nutritional risk. Registered dietitian to monitor per standards and rescreen within the week. Contact registered dietitian for further assessment if status changes (less than 8 points).

* All patients receiving enteral or parenteral support will be assessed by the registered dietitian within 72 hours of initial nutrition support order.

Abbreviations: DM, diabetes mellitus; CF, cystic fibrosis; SBS, short bowel syndrome; IBD, irritable bowel syndrome; FTT, failure to thrive; CP, cerebral palsy; CHD, congenital heart defect; BPD, bronchopulmonary dysplasia; ALL, acute lymphocytic leukemia; AML, acute myelocytic leukemia; TPN, total parenteral nutrition.

Source: Courtesy of the Clinical Nutrition Service, Children's Hospital Oakland, Oakland, California.

for congenital or acquired conditions that affect physical and/or cognitive growth and development."[14] These children may be at risk for associated nutrition sequelae, as summarized in **Table 3-1**. A child's medical history should include a review of social history, growth, acute or chronic illnesses, history of preexisting nutrient deficiencies, history of surgical or diagnostic procedures, and history of relevant therapies such as chemotherapy or radiation.[15] Medications should be reviewed for possible drug–nutrient interactions.

Anthropometric Data

Age-appropriate growth is the hallmark of adequate nutrition. Although other factors play a role in growth, nutrition is the main determinant. Anthropometric data includes obtaining weight and measuring length/height and head circumference. Once this information is obtained, the BMI can be determined.

Weight, Height, and Head Circumference

Monitoring growth through measurement of weight, length/height, and head circumference (in children 3 years of age or less) is a routine practice in most pediatric healthcare systems. These data are plotted on growth charts according to age for comparison with growth of a reference population of healthy, normal infants/children. The most common charts used in the United States are the CDC 2000 growth charts as described in Chapter 2.[16,17] (See Appendix B.)

Upper Arm and Skinfold Measurements

Upper arm measurements and skinfold measurements (which include those on the triceps, biceps, subscapular area, and abdomen) are used to predict and monitor body fat and muscle stores, clarify other anthropometric findings, and in some settings, predict morbidity and mortality.[18] The upper arm measurements most commonly evaluated include triceps skinfold (TSF), midarm circumference (MAC), and midarm muscle circumference (MAMC). MAMC is calculated using the following equation. It can also be determined by using the nomogram for estimating surface area found in Appendix F.

$$\text{MAMC (cm)} = \text{MAC (cm)} - (0.314 \times \text{TSF [mm]})$$

The standards most commonly used for ages 1–75 are those revised by Frisancho et al.[19] based on data from the HANES survey.[17] Standards for children under 1 year of age have been published based on data from children in the United States[20] and England.[21,22] Oakly et al. created standards for children 37–42 weeks gestation that are based on both age and weight.[23] Mid-upper-arm-circumference (MUAC) standards have been developed by a World Health Organization (WHO) expert committee based on data from the NHANES I and II data (see Appendix D). The committee also developed MUAC standards for height when age is unknown.[24] Along with comparison to reference standards, skinfold measurements can be monitored using a child as his or her own control.

TABLE 3–1 Examples of Nutritional Risk Factors Associated with Selected Disorders

	Growth			Diet			Medical	
	Under-weight	Over-weight	Short Stature	Low Energy Needs	High Energy Needs	Feeding Problems	Constipation	Chronic Medications
Autism	✓[a]					✓		✓
Bronchopulmonary dysplasia	✓				✓			✓
Cerebral palsy	✓	✓	✓	✓	✓	✓	✓	✓
Cystic fibrosis	✓		✓		✓			
Down syndrome		✓		✓		✓		
Fetal alcohol syndrome	✓		✓					
Heart disease (congenital)	✓				✓			
HIV/AIDS[b]	✓				✓			✓
Prader-Willi syndrome		✓	✓	✓				
Premature birth	✓		✓		✓	✓		
Seizure disorder								✓
Spina bifida	✓	✓	✓	✓			✓	

[a]May be present

[b]HIV = human immunodeficiency virus; AIDS = acquired immunodeficiency syndrome

Source: Baer MT and Harris AB. Pediatric nutrition assessment: Identifying children at risk. Copyright The American Dietetic Association. Reprinted by permission from *Journal of the American Dietetic Association*, Vol. 97 (suppl 2): S107–S115, 1997.

Although useful, these measurements have limitations. Caution must be used in comparing a child to the reference data. The data published by Frisancho et al.[19] include measurements for a solely white population; therefore, use with other ethnic populations that may have different body compositions[25–28] may be erroneous. Even within the same reference population (i.e., ethnicity), mean body composition measurements can change over time.[21] Accurate skinfold measurements require both precise instruments that need to be checked and calibrated frequently and trained anthropometrists. Therefore, even under favorable conditions, varying compressibility of fat may make these measurements challenging to obtain and reproduce,[29] especially in an obese or active child.

Body Mass Index

The most widely used index to evaluate adiposity and proportionality is the body mass index (BMI). The BMI, also known as the Quetelet Index,[30] is derived by dividing weight in kilograms by height in meters squared (wt/ht^2). For example, the BMI of a 14-year-old female who is 5′1″ and 110 pounds is 50/(1.54)^2 or 21 kg/m^2. Standardized BMI curves are included on the most recent NCHS growth charts[16,31,32] (see Appendix B) and have been developed in other countries.[33–38] Based on the NHANES data,[17] mean BMI decreases from age 1 year to ages 4–6 years, at which point it increases. There is some evidence that children who rebound from this trough at earlier ages are at a higher risk for obesity later in life.[39] The American Academy of Pediatrics (AAP) considers a child greater than the 85th percentile overweight, and one at greater than the 95th percentile obese. Furthermore, it has been suggested that BMI be used to determine appropriate therapy to address the obesity.[40]

BMI doesn't consistently quantify adiposity in an individual, however. Two children with similar BMIs may have different proportions of fat and muscle mass.[41] Also, BMI may underpredict adiposity in some children with disease states.[42]

Other Considerations

Obtaining and interpreting anthropometric indices of premature infants and children with developmental disorders may require specialized equipment and standards. This is detailed further in Chapter 10.

The developmental maturity of the child needs to be considered when interpreting anthropometric data. Correction for gestational age at birth is essential in the assessment of infants born prematurely (refer to Chapter 4). Children evaluated for delayed or precocious growth often have bone age assessments based on radiographic studies, which should be considered. For the older child, data relating to the stage of sexual maturity can alter assessment findings.[43,44] See Appendix E for tables on progression of sexual development.

Laboratory Measurements

Some laboratory measurements of nutritional status are collected routinely as part of a normal healthcare evaluation. Others are performed when the diagnosis, medical history, or nutritional history indicates nutritional risk. Appendix G lists laboratory norms based on age categories for selected tests of nutritional status.[45] The interpretation of laboratory findings must take into consideration the present and past medical status of the child. Many biochemical indices of nutritional status for normal individuals are altered by acute or chronic disease.

Serum Proteins

Albumin is the serum protein most commonly measured for assessment of nutritional status because it is inexpensive and readily available. However, due to a relatively long half-life of approximately 2 weeks and reduced degradation during periods of low protein intake, diagnosis of nutritional depletion can be missed or delayed if based solely on serum albumin levels. Likewise, serum albumin level serves as a relatively late indicator of nutritional repletion. Serum albumin may be decreased during malnutrition due to inadequate availability of precursors.[46] However, independent of nutritional status, albumin can be depressed during infection, trauma, enteropathy, liver disease, or renal disease, and elevated in dehydration, third spacing, and after administration of exogenous albumin.[46,47] Serum proteins with shorter half-lives, including transferrin, retinal binding protein, and thyroxin-binding pre-albumin, more rapidly assess response to nutritional therapy though, like serum albumin, they may also be low during stress, sepsis, and acute illnesses secondary to fluid shifts and preferential synthesis of acute phase proteins.[46–49] Measurement of the acute phase protein C-reactive protein (CRP) may help determine whether a low serum protein level is caused by stress or nutritional deficiency.[50,51] Fibronectin and somatomedin have half-lives less than 1 day but may not be ideal indicators of nutritional repletion once adequate protein and caloric intake is attained. They are more useful in the research rather than the clinical setting.[51,52] **Table 3-2** lists half-life and normal reference values for serum proteins commonly used for nutritional assessment.

Iron Status

Iron deficiency anemia is a common pediatric nutritional problem in the United States[53–55] and is routinely assessed in the inpatient and community settings. Hemoglobin and/or hematocrit measurements are commonly used to assess iron nutrition. These are easily and relatively inexpensive to monitor; however, they are decreased only during later stages of iron deficiency and may be decreased for reasons other than iron deficiency including acute blood loss, acute or chronic infections, chronic inflammation, deficiencies of other micronutrients such as B_{12} or folate, or hereditary defects in red blood cell production (e.g., thalassemia major or sickle cell disease).[56,57] Serum ferritin level is highly correlated with total body stores of iron and is the most sensitive index of iron status among healthy individuals. An elevated free erythrocyte protoporphyrin level and a decreased serum iron/total iron-binding capacity ratio and transferrin saturation occur when iron stores are depleted. These biochemical findings are present before changes in hemoglobin and red blood cell morphology. With the exception of serum ferritin level, which rises, laboratory indicators for iron deficiency decrease during infection and chronic inflammation.[58–60] **Table 3-3** summarizes iron status and hematologic abnormalities in states of negative iron balance.

Immunologic Function

Protein-energy malnutrition as well as subclinical deficiencies of one or more nutrients can impair immune response

TABLE 3–2 Serum Proteins Used in Assessing Nutritional Status

Protein	Half-Life	Normal Value	Factors Known to Alter Concentration*
Albumin	18–20 days	Preterm: 2.5–4.5 g/dL Term: 2.5–5.0 g/dL 1–3 mo.: 3.0–4.2 g/dL 3–12 mo.: 2.7–5.0 g/dL > 1 year: 3.2–5.0 g/dL	↓inflammation, infection, trauma, liver disease, renal disease, protein-losing enteropathy; altered by fluid status
Transferrin†	8–9 days	180–260 mg/dL	↓inflammation, liver disease; ↑iron deficiency; altered by fluid status
Prealbumin	2–3 days	20–50 mg/dL	↓liver disease, cystic fibrosis, hyperthyroidism, infection, trauma
Retinol binding protein	12 hours	30–40 μg/mL	↓liver disease, zinc or vitamin A deficiency, infection; ↑renal disease

*Any condition that can alter a protein's rate of synthesis, degradation, or excretion has potential to alter the serum concentration.
†Transferrin may be calculated from total iron binding capacity (TIBC): (0.8 × TIBC) − 43.
Sources: Data from Dowliko J, Nomplegsi DJ. The role of albumin in human physiology and pathophysiology. Part III albumin and disease states. *J Parenter Enter Nutr.* 1991:15:477–487; Golden MHN. Transport proteins as indices of protein status. *Am J Clin Nutr.* 1982;35:1159–1165; and Yoder MC, Anderson DC, Gopalakrishna GS, Douglas SD, Polin RA. Comparison of serum fi bronectin, prealbumin and albumin concentrations during nutritional repletion in protein-calorie malnourished infants. *J Pediatr Gastroenterol Nutr.* 1987;6:84–88.

TABLE 3-3 Iron Status and Hematologic Abnormalities in States of Negative Iron Balance

	Normal	Iron Depletion	Iron Deficiency	Iron Deficiency Anemia: Early	Iron Deficiency Anemia: Advanced
Storage iron	NL	DECR	DECR	DECR	DECR
Erythron iron	NL	NL	DECR	DECR	DECR
Hemoglobin, Hematocrit, RBC count	NL	NL	NL	DECR	DECR
RBC indices	NL	NL	NL	NL	DECR

Abbreviations: NL, normal; DECR, decrease; RBC, red blood cell.

Source: Adapted with permission from Cecalupo AJ and Cohen HJ, Nutritional anemias, in *Pediatric Nutrition Theory and Practice*, R.J. Grand, J.L. Sutphen and W.H. Dietz, eds, p. 491, © 1987, Newton, MA: Butterworth Heinemann.

and increase risk for infection. The measurement of functional parameters of the immune system can therefore be useful to assess nutritional status. Among the immunologic indexes that are associated with nutritional status are levels of T-lymphocytes and leukocyte terminal deoxynucleotidyl transferase, appearance of delayed cutaneous hypersensitivity, opsonic function, salivary IgA, and total lymphocyte count. These tests vary in sensitivity for detecting nutritional depletion.[61] The total lymphocyte count (TLC) is the index of immune function most readily available for hospitalized patients. This value can be calculated from white blood cell (WBC) counts as follows:

$$\text{WBC/mm}^3 \times \%\ \text{lymphocytes} = \text{TLC/mm}^3$$

Values less than 1500 are associated with nutritional depletion. In infants less than 3 months of age, values of less than 2500 may be abnormal.[62] Independent of nutritional status, values of immunologic function may be altered during trauma, chemotherapy, immunosuppressant drug therapy, and lack of previous exposure to antigen (in the case of delayed cutaneous hypersensitivity).[61] Some studies find TLC to be a poor measure of nutrition status due to poor sensitivity and specificity.[63,64]

Clinical Evaluation

Examination and evaluation of general appearance and specific systems is an essential part of the nutritional assessment. In most cases, severe nutritional deprivation is easily detectable. Milder, nonspecific signs of malnutrition are more commonly observed but may be harder to detect. The presence of a suspected clinical deficiency is often reflected in the diet history and should be further supported by biochemical evaluation.[61,65] **Table 3-4** lists clinical signs associated with nutrient deficiencies and specifies laboratory findings recommended to substantiate the diagnosis.

Dietary Evaluation

The thorough collection of dietary data should include the quantity and quality of foods, psychosocial factors impacting food selection and intake, and clinical/physical factors related to nutritional status. Specific factors include:[65,66]

- Food-related factors
  - Chronological feeding history from birth or onset of nutritional problem
  - Current nutrient intake
  - Feeding skills
  - History of prescribed or self-imposed diets or outcome
  - Food allergies or intolerances
- Psychosocial factors
  - Family history and dynamics
  - Socioeconomic status including use of supplemental food programs
  - Patient's self-perception of nutritional status and/or caretaker's perception of child's nutritional status
  - Religious or cultural beliefs impacting food intake
- Clinical/physical factors
  - Vitamin supplements and medication
  - Stooling habits and characteristics
  - Activity
  - Sleep patterns

See **Exhibit 3-2** for a sample dietary interview worksheet.

Complementary and Alternative Medicine (CAM)

During the last 15 years the interest in and practice of CAM has increased.[67] Types of CAM may include, but are not limited to, homeopathic medicine, natural products, macrobiotics, megavitamins, and herbal medicine.[68] Families whose children have an acute or chronic condition may especially be seeking CAMs to augment routine medical

TABLE 3-4 Clinical Signs and Laboratory Findings in the Malnourished Child and Adult

Clinical Sign	Suspect Nutrient	Supportive Objective Findings
Epithelial		
Skin		
Xerosis, dry scaling	Essential fatty acids	Triene/tetraene ratio > 0.4
Hyperkeratosis, plaques around hair follicles	Vitamin A	↓Plasma retinol
Ecchymoses, petechiae	Vitamin K	Prolonged prothrombin time
	Vitamin C	↓Serum ascorbic acid
Hair		
Easily plucked, dyspigmented, lackluster	Protein-calorie	↓Total protein
		↓Albumin
Nails		↓Transferrin
Thin, spoon-shaped	Iron	↓Serum Fe
		↓TIBC
Mucosal		
Mouth, lips, and tongue	B vitamins	
Angular stomatitis (inflammation at corners of mouth)	B_2 (riboflavin)	↓RBC glutathione reductase
Cheilosis (reddened lips with fissures at angles)	B_2	See above
	B_6 (pyridoxine)	↓Plasma pyridoxal phosphate†
Glossitis (inflammation of tongue)	B_6	See above
	B_2	See above
	B_3 (niacin)	↓Plasma tryptophan
Magenta tongue	B_2	↓Urinary N-methyl nicotinamide†
Edema of tongue, tongue fissures	B_3	See above
Gums		See above
Spongy, bleeding	Vitamin C	↓Plasma ascorbic acid
Ocular		
Pale conjunctivae secondary to anemia	Iron	↓Serum Fe, ↑TIBC, ↓serum folic acid, or ↓RBC folic acid
	Folic acid	
	Vitamin B_{12}	↓Serum B_{12}
	Copper	↓Serum copper
Bitot's spots (grayish, yellow, or white foamy spots on the whites of the eye)	Vitamin A	↓Plasma retinol
Conjunctival or corneal xerosis, keratomalacia (softening of part or all of cornea)	Vitamin A	↓Plasma retinol
Musculoskeletal		
Craniotabes (thinning of the inner table of the skull); palpable enlargement of costochondral junctions ("rachitic rosary"); thickening of wrists and ankles	Vitamin D	↓25-OH-vit D ↓Alkaline phosphatase ± ↓Ca, ↓PO_4 Long bone films
Scurvy (tenderness of extremities, hemorrhages under periosteum of long bones; enlargement of costochondral junction; cessation of osteogenesis of long bones)	Vitamin C	↓Serum ascorbic acid Long bone films
Skeletal lesions	Copper	↓Serum copper X-ray film changes similar to scurvy because copper is also essential for normal collagen formation
Muscle wasting, prominence of body skeleton, poor muscle tone	Protein-calorie	↓Serum proteins ↓Arm muscle circumference

TABLE 3-4 *(Continued)*

Clinical Sign	Suspect Nutrient	Supportive Objective Findings
General		
Edema	Protein	↓Serum proteins
Pallor 2° to anemia	Vitamin E (in premature infants)	↓Serum vitamin E ↑Peroxide hemolysis Evidence of hemolysis on blood smear
	Iron	↓Serum Fe, ↑TIBC
	Folic acid	↓Serum folic acid Macrocytosis on RBC smear
	Vitamin B_{12}	↓Serum B_{12} Macrocytosis on RBC smear
	Copper	↓Serum copper
Internal systems		
Nervous		
Mental confusion	Protein	↓Total protein, ↓albumin, ↓transferrin
	Vitamin B_1 (thiamine)	↓RBC transketolase
Cardiovascular	Vitamin B_1	Same as above
Beriberi (enlarged heart, congestive heart failure, tachycardia)		
Tachycardia 2° to anemia	Iron Folic acid B_{12} Copper Vitamin E (in premature infants)	See above
Gastrointestinal		
Hepatomegaly	Protein-calorie	↓Total protein, ↓albumin, ↓transferrin
Glandular		
Thyroid enlargement	Iodine	↓Total serum iodine: inorganic, PBI*

*Bio Science Laboratories, 7600 Tyrone Avenue, Van Nuys, CA 91405

Abbreviations: Fe, iron; PBI, protein-bound iodine; RBC, red blood cells; TIBC, total iron-binding capacity.

Source: Reprinted with permission from Kerner A, *Manual of Pediatric Parenteral Nutrition*, pp. 22–23, © 1983, W.B. Saunders Company.

treatment. Information on a family's past or present use of a CAM is important; however, they may not readily volunteer this information. Specific questions, such as those outlined in **Exhibit 3-3**, may be useful to elicit this information. Any appearance of being judgmental may inhibit disclosure and discussion.[69] (See also Chapter 21 for more information about complementary and other alternative therapies.)

Collection of Current Intake Data

The diet history can be comprehensive, encompassing most of the aforementioned factors, or specific to support a suspected diagnosis. Several approaches to quantify nutrient intake data are available and include the following:

- A *diet history* is designed to determine the pattern of usual food intake. This type of history requires a detailed interview by a trained nutritionist.[70,71] An estimate of nutrient intake is calculated from the collected data. Studies indicate this method yields higher estimated values than the 24-hour recall and diet record.
- A *24-hour recall* provides an estimate of nutrient intake based on the individual's recollection of food consumed over the previous day. This method has been used successfully for groups of individuals; however, it is less valid in evaluating diet adequacy for an individual because the 24-hour period assessed may not be representative of the usual diet. Nutrient intakes calculated from 24-hour recalls are lower than those based on dietary histories or food records.[72–76]
- *Three-day to seven-day food records* provide prospective food intake data. These are recorded by the parent, child, or other caregiver (and therefore require literacy) and are returned to the nutritionist for analysis. Food records encompassing 7 days may provide more accurate information than one of shorter duration due to the inclusion of both weekend and

EXHIBIT 3-2 Dietary Interview Summary Portion of a Nutrition Clinic Evaluation

NUTRITION CLINIC EVALUATION

Date of Visit: ______________________ Age: ____________

Diagnosis: ______________________ Onset: ____________

Concomitant Conditions: ______________________

______________________ Ref. Phys. ____________

Problem: ______________________

Concerns of Parents or Patient: ______________________

Nutrition History: ______________________

Recent Nutrition History: ______________________

Formula: Kind ____________ Amount ____________ Cal. Density ____________

Food Intake: ______________________

Food Summary (no. of servings/day):

Meat ____________ Milk ____________ Fr/Veg ____________ Grains ____________

Fever/Vomiting: ____________ Elimination: ____________

Appetite: ______________________

Feeding Ability/Concerns: ______________________

Vitamin Mineral Supp: ______________________

Activity level 1–8, 8 high ______________________

Social Setting in Regard to Meal Prep: ______________________

Social History: ______________________

Pertinent Family Medical/Weight History: ______________________

EXHIBIT 3-3 Sample Questions to Elicit Information on Use of Complementary and Alternative Medicine

1. Is your child receiving any herbal preparations? If yes:
   - What is the name (if known)?
   - For what purpose is it given?
   - How is it administered (tea, tincture, fluid extract, tablet, or capsule)?
   - How much? How often?
   - Is it prescribed/recommended? Where is it purchased?
   - How is it tolerated? Any side effects noted?
2. Is your child receiving any additional vitamins or minerals? (If yes, the bulleted questions apply)
3. Are there any foods or vitamins you specifically avoid for your child?
4. Who are the people involved in your child's health care (caretakers and health providers)?
5. Do you have any questions regarding complementary or alternative health care?

weekday meal patterns; however, accuracy of diet recordkeeping often deteriorates over time. When a 7-day food record is not possible, use of shorter time periods including selected days of the week is an adequate alternative.[77]

- In inpatient facilities, *nutrient intake analyses (calorie counts)* are frequently ordered to assess a child's food intake. These are used to determine a child's ability to consume a sufficient amount of food for growth or to verify the achievement and adequacy of a prescribed feeding regimen. These records, however, do not provide data representative of intake within the home environment.
- *Food frequencies* estimate the frequency and amount of specific foods eaten. These often consist of questionnaires that can be self-administered and therefore reduce professional interview time. The questionnaire generally cannot retrieve unique details of an individual's diet unless designed to do so.[78] Over-reporting of food intake is common with this method.[72,73,79,80]

New methods of capturing dietary intake are being explored, using such technology as smart phone applications, laptop and other computers, and videoconferences [80–83]

Dietary Intake Evaluation

Estimated intakes of specific nutrients are calculated using values derived from food composition tables or computerized nutrient analysis programs. The calculated intake is evaluated for adequacy by comparing it with a reference intake. The *dietary reference intakes (DRIs)* are the most commonly used reference allowances in the United States.[84–90] DRIs are based on contemporary studies that address not only preventing classical nutritional deficiencies, but also reducing the risk of chronic diseases, promoting optimal health, and preventing nutrient toxicities.[90] The DRIs actually refer to at least six types of reference values: recommended dietary allowances (RDAs), adequate intakes (AIs), estimated average requirements (EARs), estimated energy requirements (EERs), acceptable macronutrient distribution range (AMDR), and tolerable upper limit (TUL). The RDA is the dietary intake level that is sufficient to meet the nutrient requirements of nearly all healthy persons, and is designed to include a wide margin of safety above amounts required to prevent deficiency.[91] Therefore, a healthy child whose estimated intake for a nutrient falls below the RDA may not have a nutritional deficiency or even a nutritional risk unless this intake is substantially below the RDA for a sufficient length of time. When assessing the adequacy of diets for infants and children with acute or chronic disease, potential alterations in nutrient requirements should be considered. In cases where sufficient scientific evidence is not available to estimate an average requirement, *AIs* have been set and should be used as a goal for intake where no RDAs exist. The *EAR* is the intake value that is estimated to meet the requirement defined by a specified indicator of adequacy in 50% of an age- and gender-specified group. The *EER* is the dietary energy intake predicted to allow for a level of physical activity consistent with normal health and development. The *AMDR* is the range of macronutrient intakes for a particular energy source that are associated with reduced risk of chronic disease while providing adequate intakes of essential nutrients. The *UL* is the maximum level of daily nutrient intake that is unlikely to pose risks of adverse health effects to almost all of the individuals in a life stage and/or gender group.

Calculation of Energy Requirements

Accurate prediction of energy requirements is important for the healthy child and is magnified in such clinical situations as treating the obese or failure-to-thrive child and implementing enteral or parenteral nutrition support in the acute or chronically ill child.[92] Energy needs can be estimated by using the DRIs[84] (see Appendix H); however, these are based on populations of normal healthy subjects and may not be applicable to the child with altered activity or with potential alterations in needs related to clinical status.

Many equations have been generated to predict basal or resting energy needs and to which the clinician can add factors accounting for activity and stress. In a subgroup of children with illnesses and concomitant malnutrition, energy expenditure may be most accurately predicted by the use of indirect calorimetry.[93]

Table 3-5 Equations for Predicting Energy Requirements of Children

Origin	Energy Determination	Gender	Age	Equation
Institute of Medicine[84]	Total energy requirement	Both Genders	0–3 mo	89 × wt + 75
			4–6 mo	89 × wt − 44
			7–12 mo	89 × wt − 78
			13–36 mo	89 × wt − 80
		Males	3–8 y	108.5 − 61.9 × age + PA × (26.7 × wt + 903 × ht [m])
			9–18 y	113.5 − 61.9 × age + PA × (26.7 × wt + 903 × ht [m])
				PA = 1.0 for sedentary 1.13 for low active 1.26 for active 1.42 for very active
		Females	3–8 y	155.3 − 30.8 × age + PA × (10 × w + 934 × ht [m])
			9–18 y	160.3 − 30.8 × age + PA × (10 × w + 934 × ht [m])
				PA = 1.0 for sedentary 1.16 for low active 1.31 for active 1.56 for very active
Harris-Benedict[97]	BMR	Male	Unspecified	66.47 + 13.75 W + 5.0 H − 6.76 A
		Female		655.1 + 9.56 W + 1.85 H − 4.68 A
World Health Organization (WHO)[98]	REE	Male	0–3 y	60.9 W − 54
			3–10 y	22.7 W + 495
		Female	0–3 y	61 W − 51
			3–10 y	22.5 W + 499
Schofield[99]	REE	Male	< 3 y	0.17 W + 15.17 H − 617.6
			3–10 y	19.6 W + 1.30 H + 414.9
			10–18 y	16.3 W + 1.37 H + 515.5
		Female	< 3 y	16.25 W + 10.23 H − 413.5
			3–10 y	16.97 W + 1.62 H + 371.2
			10–18 y	8.365 W + 4.65 H + 200.0
Altman and Dittmer[100]	REE	Male	3–16 y	19.56 W + 506.16
		Female		18.67 W + 578.64
Maffeis et al.[101]	REE	Male	6–10 y	1287 + 28.6 W + 23.6 H − 69.1 A
		Female		1552 + 35.8 W + 15.6 H − 36.3 A

Abbreviations: Unless otherwise specified, W = weight in kilograms; A = age in years; H = height in centimeters; REE, resting energy expenditure; BEE, basal energy expenditure.

Definition of Terms

Total energy expenditure (TEE) consists of the energy required to meet the basal metabolic rate (BMR), diet-induced thermogenesis, activity, and growth.[94] BMR assumes the following basal conditions:[95]

- Fasting (at least 10–12 hours after the last meal)
- Awake and resting in a lying position (measurements are taken shortly after awakening)
- Normal body and ambient temperature
- Absence of psychological or physical stress

Diet-induced thermogenesis, also referred to as the specific dynamic action of food, is the energy necessary for digestion, transport, and storage of nutrients. It accounts for 5–10% of daily energy expenditure.[96]

Resting energy expenditure (REE) is the energy expenditure of an individual at rest and in conditions of thermal neutrality. REE may include the thermal effect of a previous meal. BMR and REE usually differ by less than 10%.[95]

Standardized Equations

Equations have been developed to predict the BMR and REE of infants and children. A sampling of these equations are summarized in **Table 3-5**.[84,97–101] BMR and REE estimates using standard calculations are based on the assumption that the individual is free of pathology and fever that affect energy expenditure; therefore, applying these equations to the ill pediatric patient requires an additional stress factor. **Table 3-6** highlights a sampling of current findings regarding potential alterations in energy expenditure with different disease states.[102–118] Regular reevaluation of energy needs should be completed as clinical status changes. Caution must be taken not to overfeed a critically ill child because excess nutritional delivery can potentially increase pulmonary and hepatic pathophysiology.[119]

The final factor in determining energy needs is activity. A child's activity level can be established by determining the

TABLE 3-6 Potential Changes in Energy Expenditure Associated with Different Diagnoses

Diagnosis	Research	Population	Potential Stress Factor
Closed head injury Postinjury day 1–14	Phillips et al. (1987)[102]	2–17 years	Measured energy expenditure averaged 1.3 times Harris and Benedict's predicted value on postoperative days 1–14.
	Redmond et al. (2006)[103]	0–24 years	Caloric needs are ~ BEE × 1.0–1.2 (for paralyzed patients).
	Havalad et al. (2006)[104]	6–16 years	Energy expenditure in children with severe head injury cannot be estimated accurately by standard equations.
Sickle cell anemia	Williams et al. (2002)[105]	5–11 years	Measured REE was 15% greater than predicted REE.
Inflammatory bowel disease	Kushner et al. (1991)[106]	19–40 years	No significant increase in energy needs.
Cancer	Barale and Charuhas (1999)[107]	Unspecified	Supports adding 60–80% BEE to calculated BEE.
Allogeneic stem cell transplantation Week 3 post transplant	Duggan et al. (2003)[108]	3–15 years	Measured REE was 0.90–0.95 predicted REE.
End stage liver disease	Greer et al. (2003)[109]	0–2 years	Children with end stage liver disease had a 27% higher mean REE.
Extrahepatic biliary atresia	Pierro et al. (1989)[110]	2–73 months	Energy expenditure was 29% higher than normal.
Spastic quadriplegic cerebral palsy	Stallings et al. (1996)[111]	2–18 years	Nonbasal energy expenditure was minimal.
Burns	Mayes et al. (1996)[112]	0.5–10 years mean 30% BSA burns	Supports application of a factor 30% REE.
Postsurgery	Powis et al. (1998)[113]	0–3 years major abdominal surgery	No increase in metabolic rate after major abdominal operations.
	Jones et al. (1993)[114]	0–4 months various surgeries	Mean increase of 15% REE following surgery.
Congenital heart defects	Barton et al. (1994)[115]	Less than 6 months severe congenital heart disease	Needs 40% greater than RDA for age.
HIV	Alfaro et al. (1995)[116]	4 months–4 years	Perinatally infected children without secondary infections are not hypermetabolic.
	Henderson et al. (1998)[117]	2 years–11 years	Measured energy expenditure was ~ 120% predicted REE (WHO equation).
Fevers	Dubois (1954)[118]	NA	REE increases 13% for each degree Centigrade of fever (7.2% for each degree Fahrenheit).

Abbreviations: REE, resting energy expenditure; BEE, basal energy expenditure.

amounts of time spent performing various types of activities and calculating an activity factor based on a 24-hour time period. Activity factors of 1.3 are associated with sedentary lifestyles, whereas activity factors equal to or greater than 2.0 represent lifestyles high in physical activity. Children under normal unconstrained conditions are considered to be active if their activity factors range from 1.7 to 2.0 × REE. **Table 3-7** lists the approximate energy expenditure for various activities in relation to REE. **Table 3-8** demonstrates the method of calculating an activity factor and the total energy expenditure (TEE).

Individual variation in true energy expenditure may exist largely due to differences in lean body mass. The person with the higher lean body mass will have the higher energy expenditure.[120] In numerous studies, researchers have concluded that these standardized formulas may not be accurate in predicting individual energy needs for children with FTT, obesity, and some acute or chronic illnesses.[93,96,104,121,122]

Indirect Calorimetry

Indirect calorimetry is used to predict the energy needs for the subset of patients whose energy needs are elusive. This subset includes, but is not limited to, patients who are failing to thrive despite meeting predicted needs, obese patients, critically ill patients on nutrition support, and patients unable to be weaned from a ventilator. Indirect calorimetry measures oxygen consumption (VO_2) and carbon dioxide production (VCO_2). Most indirect calorimeters are open-circuit systems in which the patient breathes room air or air supplied from a mechanical ventilator and expires into a gas sampling system that eventually vents the expired air back into the room.[123] Indirect calorimetry provides two pieces of information: REE and a measure of substrate utilization as reflected in the respiratory quotient (RQ).[124]

The following abbreviated Weir equation calculates REE:[125]

$$\text{REE (kcal/min)} = 3.94 \times VO_2 + 1.11 \times VCO_2$$

Measured REE may need additional activity or stress added to accurately predict total energy needs. Also, measured REE does not account for anabolism or growth. In the adult or older child, this represents a fraction of total energy needs. In the very young infant, this potential energy has been measured to be 2.73 kcal/g tissue synthesized,[120] though in the very sick or traumatized child growth may be inhibited and applying growth factors may result in overfeeding.

Indirect calorimetry can also evaluate how the body is using fuel as reflected by the respiratory quotient (RQ). RQ is the ratio of carbon dioxide produced to oxygen consumed (VCO_2/VO_2). Glucose oxidation is associated with an RQ of 1.0, fat oxidation with an RQ of 0.7, and protein metabolism with an RQ of 0.8. Alcohol or ketone metabolism may reduce the RQ to 0.67, whereas overfeeding with lipogenesis may increase the RQ to 1.3. Knowledge of inefficient

TABLE 3-7 Approximate Energy Expenditure for Various Activities in Relation to Resting Needs for Males and Females of Average Size

Activity Category*	Representative Value for Activity Factor per Unit Time of Activity
Resting	REE × 1.0
Sleeping, reclining	
Very light	REE × 1.5
Seated and standing activities, painting trades, driving, laboratory work, typing, sewing, ironing, cooking, playing cards, playing a musical instrument	
Light	REE × 2.5
Walking on a level surface at 2.5 to 3 mph, garage work, electrical trades, carpentry, restaurant trades, house-cleaning, child care, golf, sailing, table tennis	
Moderate	REE × 5.0
Walking 3.5–4 mph, weeding and hoeing, carrying a load, cycling, skiing, tennis, dancing	
Heavy	REE × 7.0
Walking with load uphill, tree felling, heavy manual digging, basketball, climbing, football, soccer	

*When reported as multiples of basal needs, the expenditures of males and females are similar.

Source: Reprinted with permission from *Recommended Dietary Allowances*, 10th ed., © 1989 by the National Academy of Sciences. Published by National Academies Press.

TABLE 3-8 Example of Calculation for Total Energy Expenditure in an 11-Year-Old Boy*

Activity Type	REE Multiple	Duration (h)	Weighted REE Factor
Resting	1.0	9	9
Very light	1.5	8	12
Light	2.5	4	10
Moderate	5.0	2	10
Heavy	7.0	1	7
TOTALS		24	48

Activity factor = weighted REE ÷ hours
= 48 ÷ 24
= 2.0

Total energy expenditure:

Gender	Age (yr)	Wt (kg)	REE† (kcal/d)	×	Activity Factor	=	TEE (kcal/d)
Male	11	35	1190	×	2.0	=	2382

*Hypothetical activity pattern

†Calculated from Allman and Dittmer equation in Table 3-5

Source: Reprinted from Krug-Wispé S. Nutritional Assessment, in *Handbook of Pediatric Nutrition*, P. Queen and C.E. Lang, eds., p. 45, © 1993, Aspen Publishers, Inc., Gaithersburg, MD.

substrate utilization and subsequent reduction of RQ through alteration of energy substrates can be medically advantageous.[125–127]

Data Evaluation and Plan

The assessment of nutritional status is based on the careful evaluation of all gathered information. Interrelationships among the health status of the child, feeding abilities, eating habits, anthropometric data, and laboratory findings need to be considered.[128–130] The nutritional care plan is developed to correct nutritional problems or reduce nutritional risks identified through the assessment. Basic information included in the medical and dietary histories provides a foundation for designing a plan that is reasonable and achievable within a given setting. The effectiveness of the nutritional intervention is determined through periodic nutritional reassessment. The care plan is modified as needed for changes in nutritional status/risk. The following are examples of nutritional pathologies requiring a detailed assessment and care plan.

Protein-Energy Malnutrition

The identification of the presence and severity of protein-energy malnutrition (PEM) among children in hospitals and clinics is a valuable function of nutritional assessment. An estimated 20–40% of hospitalized pediatric patients may have PEM.[131] **Table 3-9** outlines anthropometric indices developed by Gomez and Waterlow to quantify the severity of chronic and acute PEM. Children may present with one or both forms of PEM. Acute, but not chronic, PEM may increase morbidity and increase length of hospital stay.[131]

Marasmus and Kwashiorkor

Marasmus and kwashiorkor are two classifications of severe, acute PEM. Marasmus develops over a period of weeks or months and is characterized by a wasted appearance due to diminished subcutaneous fat. Infants and children with marasmus have normal or low levels of serum albumin and other transport proteins and no evidence of edema. Liver size is normal.[128–131]

Conversely, kwashiorkor develops acutely, often in conjunction with an infection. Levels of serum albumin, other transport proteins, and lymphocytes are reduced. Edema is present over the trunk, extremities, and face. These infants and children often have subcutaneous fat stores that mask muscle wasting. Dermatitis and hair changes (flag sign) are usually present. In severe cases, fatty infiltration of the liver occurs.[128–131]

Marasmic kwashiorkor is the classification used to describe the presence of symptoms of kwashiorkor in a child with a weight for height less than 70% of standard or weight for age less than 60% of standard. This condition often develops following acute stress and is associated with high mortality.[131]

TABLE 3-9 Anthropometric Indexes Associated with Protein-Energy Malnutrition

		Degree of PEM			
Type of PEM	**Anthropometric Index**	**Normal**	**Mild**	**Moderate**	**Severe**
Chronic (stunting)	Height for age as % standard*	95	90–94	85–89	< 85
Acute (wasting)	Weight for age as % standard*	90	75–89	60–74	< 60
	Weight for height as % standard*	90	80–89	70–79	< 70
	Arm circumference/head circumference ratio†	> 0.31	0.28–0.31	0.25–0.28	< 0.25

*Original data for determining degree of PEM used the 50th percentile of Boston growth data as standard. The 50th percentile on CDC growth charts is now commonly used as the standard with these assessments.

†Ratio has been found to correlate with weight for age in children 3 months to 4 years of age.

Sources: Adapted with permission from Gomez F, Galvan R, Frenks, Munoz JC, Chavez R, Vasquez J. Mortality in second and third degree malnutrition. *J Trop Pediatr.* 1956;2:77; and Waterlow JC. Classification and definition of protein-calorie malnutrition. *Br Med J.* 1972;3:566–569.

Failure to Thrive

Failure to thrive (which is a symptom rather than a diagnosis) refers to the failure of weight gain and, in more severe cases, linear growth and head circumference.[132] It is identified in 1–5% of children under 2 years of age who are admitted to hospitals.[133,134] Traditionally, failure to thrive has been classified as organic or nonorganic depending on the presence or absence of a medical diagnosis. Most practitioners now recognize that most children may have mixed etiologies. Additionally, many cases of failure to thrive are idiopathic. Successful treatment of failure to thrive is dependent on a comprehensive work-up. A detailed growth chart with plots at several ages is useful in a number of ways. It identifies the age at which a child's growth began to deviate and therefore provides diagnostic clues as to the causes. It can support whether a child is truly decelerating in growth velocity (i.e., crossing growth percentiles) or is merely small for his or her age but gaining appropriately. It can pinpoint other sequelae associated with poor weight gain (e.g., microcephaly). Finally, a detailed growth curve can identify endocrine factors in the child's failure to thrive (i.e., a child who is gaining weight but not growing in height). The following criteria are commonly used to identify growth failure:

- Growth below a specified percentile on the growth chart
    - Weight for age plotting less than the third or fifth percentile on the Centers for Disease Control and Prevention (CDC) growth charts
    - Weight for length/height plotting less than the third or fifth percentile
- Poor growth velocity
    - Decreased growth velocity where weight falls more than two major percentiles over 3 to 6 months
    - Decrease of more than two standard deviations on the growth chart over a 3- to 6-month period

Standard Deviation

The standard deviation (SD) score, also called the Z score, is useful in expressing how far a child's weight and length/height fall from the median, or 50th percentile, on the reference growth charts for children of the same age and sex.[135] It is calculated as follows:

$$\text{Z score} = \frac{\begin{array}{c}\text{measurement value} - \text{median for age value}\\ \text{of reference population}\end{array}}{\begin{array}{c}\text{standard deviation for age}\\ \text{of reference population}\end{array}}$$

Categorizing growth according to progressive decrements in SD scores (22.0, 23.0, 24.0) can be used to describe the relative severity of undernutrition. Percentiles and equivalent SD scores for weight for age, length/height for age, and weight for length/height can be calculated easily using computer software developed by the CDC and the World Health Organization (WHO).[136] An SD of zero is equivalent to the 50th percentile; 21.65 SD corresponds to the 5th percentile cut-off used in the National Nutrition Surveillance System. The WHO recommends that a cut-off point of 22.0 SD below the 2000 CDC growth chart median weight for age, length/height for age, and weight for length/height be used to discriminate between well-nourished and poorly nourished children.[137] When compared over time, a positive change in SD indicates growth, whereas a negative change indicates a slowing of the growth rate.

Further work-up of failure to thrive is largely dependent on the age of the child. In the newborn period, the assessment will likely focus on the success of breastfeeding and bottle feeding including formula type, procurement, mixing, volume, and feeding tolerance. For a baby who is anorexic or who has significant vomiting or diarrhea, the nutrition assessment process will focus on identifying causes and treatment for these pathologies. Medical diagnoses associated with failure to thrive should be considered depending on the presence or absence of supporting factors. Some of these diagnoses include celiac disease, cystic fibrosis, cerebral palsy, food allergies, HIV, renal disease, and cardiac disease. A thorough diet history is paramount and should evaluate the type and quantity of food taken, meal patterns, family dynamics, family income, cultural beliefs, and relevant psychosocial information. Laboratory tests should be used to confirm the diagnosis or monitor treatment. Laboratory studies alone rarely identify the etiology of failure to thrive.[138]

Other nutritional diagnoses requiring therapeutic diet intervention will be further discussed in forthcoming chapters. Although most diagnoses share common components of the nutrition assessment process, each have unique foci.

Conclusion

The provision of quality nutritional services to children is dependent on identifying those who are nutritionally depleted or at nutritional risk. In-depth nutritional assessments include a medical history and clinical evaluation, evaluation of anthropometric indices, and dietary evaluation. Biochemical indices may be evaluated as part of a routine nutritional screen or to confirm a suspected nutritional aberration. Assessment data are used to identify specific nutritional problems and to develop workable care plans targeted to improve nutritional status.

REFERENCES

1. Shapiro LR. Streamlining and implementing nutritional assessment. The dietary approach. *J Am Diet Assoc.* 1979;75:230–237.
2. Hunt DR, Maslovitz A, Rowlands BJ, Brooks B. A simple nutrition screening procedure for hospital patients. *J Am Diet Assoc.* 1985;85:332–335.
3. Christensen KS, Gstundtner KM. Hospital-wide screening improves basis for nutrition intervention. *J Am Diet Assoc.* 1985;85:704–706.
4. DeHoog S. Identifying patients at nutritional risk and determining clinical productivity; essentials for an effective nutrition care program. *J Am Diet Assoc.* 1985;85:1620–1622.
5. Hedberg AM, Garcia N, Trejus IJ, Weinmann-Winkler S, Gabriel ML, Lutz AL. Nutrition risk screening: development of a standardized protocol using dietetic technicians. *J Am Diet Assoc.* 1988;88:1553–1556.
6. Mezoff A, Gamm L, Konek S, Beal KG, Hitch D. Validation of a nutritional screen in children with respiratory syncytial virus admitted to an intensive care complex. *Pediatrics.* 1996;97:543–546.
7. Fomon SJ. *Nutritional Disorders of Children.* Rockville, MD: U.S. Department of Health and Human Services, Education and Welfare; 1976. PHS publication no. (HAS) 75-5612.
8. Christakis G. Nutritional assessment in health programs. *Am J Public Health.* 1973;63(Suppl):1–56.
9. Joint Commission for the Accreditation of Healthcare Organizations. *Comprehensive Accreditation Manual for Hospitals. May Update.* Oakbrook Terrace, IL: TJC; 1998.
10. Kamath SK, Lawler M, Smith AE, Kalat T, Olson R. Hospital malnutrition: a 33 hospital screening study. *J Am Diet Assoc.* 1986;86:203–206.
11. Campbell MC, Kelsey KS. The PEACH survey: a nutrition screening tool for use in early intervention programs. *J Am Diet Assoc.* 1994;94:1156–1158.
12. Chima CS, Diet-Seher C, Kushner-Benson S. Nutrition risk screening in acute care: a survey of practice. *Nutr Clin Pract.* 2008;23:417–423.
13. Noel MB, Wojnarosk SM. Nutrition screening for long-term care patients. *J Am Diet Assoc.* 1987;87:1557–1558.
14. Baer MT, Farnan S, Mauer AM. Children with special health care needs. In: Shorbaugh CO, ed. *Call to Action: Better Nutrition for Mothers, Children, and Families.* Washington, DC: National Center for Education in Maternal and Child Health; 1991:191–208.
15. Klawittler BM. Nutrition assessment of infants and children. In: Williams CD, ed. *Pediatric Manual of Clinical Dietetics.* Chicago, IL: American Dietetic Assn.; 1998:19–34.
16. Centers for Disease Control and Prevention. 2000 CDC growth charts: United States. Available at: http://www.CDC.gov/growthcharts/. Accessed January 18, 2010.
17. National Center for Health Statistics. Plan and operation of the Health and Nutrition Examination Survey, United States, 1971–73. *Vital Health Stat.* 1973;1(10a and 10b):1–53.
18. Alam N, Wojtyniak B, Rahaman MM. Anthropometric indicators and risk of death. *Am J Clin Nutr.* 1989;49:884–888.
19. Frisancho AR. New norms of upper limb fat and muscle areas for assessment of nutritional status. *Am J Clin Nutr.* 1981;34:2540–2545.
20. Ryan AS, Martinez GA. Physical growth of infants 7–12 mos of age: results from a national survey. *Am J Phys Anthropol.* 1987;73:449–457.
21. Paul AA, Cole TJ, Ahmed EA, Whithead RG. The need for revised standards for skinfold thickness in infancy. *Arch Dis Child.* 1998;78:354–358.
22. Tanner JM, Whitehouse RH. Revised standards for triceps and subscapular skinfolds in British children. *Arch Dis Child.* 1975;50:142–145.
23. Oakley RR, Parsons RJ, Whitelaw AOC. Standards for skinfold thickness in British newborn infants. *Arch Dis Child.* 1977;52:287–290.
24. The development of MUAC-for-age reference data recommended by a WHO expert committee. *WHO Bull.* 1997;75:11–18.
25. Cronk CE, Roche AF. Race-and sex-specific reference data for triceps and subscapular skinfolds and weight/stature^2. *Am J Clin Nutr.* 1982;35:347–354.
26. Owen GM, Lubin AH. Anthropometric differences between black and white preschool children. *Am J Dis Child.* 1973;126:168–169.

27. Ryan AS, Martinez GA, Baumgartner RN, et al. Median skinfold thickness distributions and fat-wave patterns in Mexican-American children from the Hispanic Health and Nutrition Examination Survey (HHANES 1982–1984). *Am J Clin Nutr.* 1990;51:925S–935S.
28. Ryan AS, Martinez GA, Roche AF. An evaluation of the associations between socioeconomic status and the growth of Mexican-American children. Data from the Hispanic Health and Nutrition Examination Survey (HHANES 1982–1984). *Am J Clin Nutr.* 1990;51:944S–952S.
29. Bray GA, Greenway FL, Molitech ME. Use of anthropometric measures to assess weight loss. *Am J Clin Nutr.* 1978;31:769–773.
30. Quatelet LAJ. *Physique Sociale.* Vol. 2. Brussels: C Muquardt; 1869.
31. Hammer LD, Kraemer HC, Wilson DM, Ritter PL, Dornbusch SM. Standardized percentile curves of body-mass index for children and adolescents. *Am J Dis Child.* 1997;145:259–263.
32. Rosner B, Prineas R, Loggie J, Daniels SR. Percentiles for body mass index in US children 5 to 17 years of age. *J Pediatr.* 1998;132:211–222.
33. Leung SS, Cole TJ, Tse LY, Lau JT. Body mass index reference curves for Chinese children. *Ann Hum Bio.* 1998;25:169–174.
34. Cole TJ, Freeman JV, Preece MA. Body mass index reference curves for the UK 1990. *Arch Dis Child.* 1995;73:25–29.
35. Luciano A, Bressan F, Zoppi G. Body mass index reference curves for children ages 3–19 years from Verona, Italy. *Euro Clin Nutr.* 1997;51:6–10.
36. Bhalla AK, Walia BN. Percentile curves for body-mass index of Punjabi infants. *Indian Pediatr.* 1996;33:471–476.
37. Aurelius G, Khan NC, True DB, Ha TT, Lindren G. Height, weight and body mass index (BMI) of Vietnamese (Hanoi) schoolchildren aged 7–11 years related to parents' occupation and education. *Trop Pediatr.* 1996;42:21–26.
38. Lindgren G, Strandell A, Cole T, Healy M, Tanner J. Swedish population reference standards for height, weight and body mass index attained at 6–16 years (girls) or 19 years (boys). *Acta Paediatrica.* 1995;84:1019–1028.
39. Rolland-Cachera MF, Deheeger M, Bellisle F, Semp M, Guilloud-Bataillem, Patois E. Obesity rebound in children: a simple indicator for predicting obesity. *Am J Clin Nutr.* 1984;39:129–135.
40. Spear B, Barlow S, Ervin C, et al. Recommendations for treatment of child and adolescent overweight and obesity. *Pediatrics.* 2007;120:S254–S288.
41. Pietrobeloi A, Faith MS, Allison DB, Gallagher D, Chiumello G, Heymsfield SB. Body mass index as a measure of adiposity among children and adolescents: a validation study. *J Pediatr.* 1998;132:204–210.
42. Warner JT, Cowan FJ, Dunstan FDJ, Gregory JW. The validity of body mass index for the assessment of adiposity in children with disease states. *Ann Human Bio.* 1997;24:209–215.
43. Hannan WJ, Wrate RM, Cowen SJ, Freman CPL. Body mass index as an estimate of body fat. *Int J Eating Disord.* 1995;18:91–97.
44. Tanner JM. Issues and advances in adolescent growth and development. *J Adolesc Health Care.* 1987;8:470–478.
45. Behrman RE, Vaughan VC, eds. *Nelson Textbook of Medicine.* 13th ed. Philadelphia, PA: WB Saunders; 1987.
46. Russell MS. Serum proteins and nitrogen balance: evaluating response to nutrition support. *Dietetics in Nutrition Support Newsletter.* 1995;17:3–7.
47. Dowliko J, Nomplegsi DJ. The role of albumin in human physiology and pathophysiology. Part III albumin and disease states. *J Parenter Enter Nutr.* 1991:15:477–487.
48. Golden MHN. Transport proteins as indices of protein status. *Am J Clin Nutr.* 1982;35:1159–1165.
49. Yoder MC, Anderson DC, Gopalakrishna GS, Douglas SD, Polin RA. Comparison of serum fibronectin, prealbumin and albumin concentrations during nutritional repletion in protein-calorie malnourished infants. *J Pediatr Gastroenterol Nutr.* 1987;6:84–88.
50. Joyce DL, Waites KB. Clinical applications of C-reactive protein in pediatrics. *Pediatr Infect Dis J.* 1997;16:735–747.
51. Collier SB, Hendricks KM. Nutrition assessment. In: Baker RD, Baker SS, Daris AY, eds. *Pediatric Parenteral Nutrition.* New York: Wolters, Kluwer Law & Business; 1997:42–63.
52. Buopane EA, Brown RO, Boucher BA, Fabian TC, Luther RW. Use of fibronectin and somatomedin C as nutritional markers in the enteral support of traumatized patients. *Crit Care Med.* 1989;17:126–132.
53. Merritt RJ, Blackburn GL. Nutritional assessment and metabolic response to illness of the hospitalized child. In: Suskind R, ed. *Textbook of Pediatric Nutrition.* New York: Raven Press; 1981:296.
54. Cecalupo AJ, Cohen HJ. Nutritional anemias. In: Grand RJ, Sutphen JL, Dietz WH, eds. *Pediatric Nutrition.* Stonehaven, MA: Butterworth; 1987:489–499.
55. Expert Scientific Working Group. Summary of a report on assessment of the iron nutritional status of the United States population. *Am J Clin Nutr.* 1985;42:1318–1330.
56. Centers for Disease Control and Prevention. Recommendations to prevent and control iron deficiency in the United States. *MMWR.* 1983;47(RR-3):1–25.
57. Dallman RR, Yip R, Johnson C. Prevalence and causes of anemia in the United States, 1976–1980. *Am J Clin Nutr.* 1984;39:437–445.
58. Yip R, Johnson C, Dallman PR. Age-related changes in laboratory values used in the diagnosis of anemia and iron deficiency. *Am J Clin Nutr.* 1984;39:427–436.
59. Yip R, Dallman PR. The roles of inflammation and iron deficiency as causes of anemia. *Am J Clin Nutr.* 1988;48:1295–1300.
60. Cecalupo AJ, Cohen HJ. Nutritional anemias. In: Grand RJ, Sutphen JL, Dietz WH Jr, eds. *Pediatric Nutrition: Theory and Practice.* Boston, MA: Butterworth; 1987:489–491.
61. Puri S, Chandra RK. Nutritional regulation of host resistance and predictive value of immunologic tests in assessment of outcome. *Pediatr Clin North Am.* 1985;32:499–515.
62. Hattner JT, Kerner JA Jr. Nutritional assessment of the pediatric patient. In: Kerner JA Jr., ed. *Manual of Pediatric Parenteral Nutrition.* New York: John Wiley & Sons; 1983:19–60.
63. Forse RA, Rompre C, Crosilla P, O-Tuitt D, Rhode B, Shizgal HM. Reliability of the total lymphocyte count as a parameter of nutrition. *Can J Surg.* 1985;28(3):216–219.
64. Kuzuya M, Kanda S, Koike T, Suzuki Y, Iguchi A. Lack of correlation between total lymphocyte count and nutritional status in the elderly. *Clin Nutr.* 2005;24:427–432.
65. Christakis G. Nutritional assessment in health programs. *Am J Public Health.* 1973;63(Suppl):1–56.
66. Pipes PL, Bumbalo J, Glass RP. Collecting and assessing food intake information. In: Pipes P, ed. *Nutrition in Infancy and Childhood.* St. Louis, MO: Times Mirror Mosby; 1989:58–85.

67. Barrocas A. Complementary and alternative medicine: friend, foe or OWA. *J Am Diet Assoc.* 1997;97:1373–1376.
68. *Alternative Medicine: Expanding Medical Horizons.* Workshop on Alternative Medicine. Pittsburgh, PA: Government Printing Office; 1994. GPO No. 017-040-00537-7.
69. Eisenberg DM. Advising patients who seek alternative medical therapies. *Ann Intern Med.* 1997;127:61–69.
70. Burke BS. The dietary history as a tool in research. *J Am Diet Assoc.* 1947;23:1041.
71. Frank GC, Hollatz AT, Webber LS, Berenson GSS. Effect of interviewer recording practices on nutrient intake—Bogalusa Heart Study. *J Am Diet Assoc.* 1984;84:1432–1439.
72. Medlin C, Skinner JD. Individual dietary intake methodology; a 50-year review of progress. *J Am Diet Assoc.* 1988;88:1250–1257.
73. Block G. A review of validations of dietary assessment methods. *Am J Epidemiol.* 1982;114:492–504.
74. Persson LA, Carlgren G. Measuring children's diets: evaluation of dietary assessment techniques in infancy and childhood. *Int J Epidemiol.* 1984;113:506–517.
75. Carter RL, Sharbaugh CO, Stapell CA. Reliability and validity of the 24 hour recall. *J Am Diet Assoc.* 1981;79:542–547.
76. Emmons L, Hayes M. Accuracy of 24-hr recalls of young children. *J Am Diet Assoc.* 1973;62:409–415.
77. St Jeor SR, Guthrie HA, Jones MB. Variability in nutrient intake in a 28-day period. *J Am Diet Assoc.* 1983;3:155–162.
78. Rockett HRH, Colditz GA. Assessing diets of children and adolescents. *Am J Clin Nutr.* 1997;65:1116–1122.
79. Willett WC, Sampson L, Stampfer MJ, et al. Reproducibility and validity of a semiquantitative food frequency questionnaire. *Am J Epidemiol.* 1985;122:51–65.
80. Larkin FA, Metzner HL, Thompson FE, Flegal KM, Guire KE. Comparison of estimated nutrient intakes by food frequency and dietary records in adults. *J Am Diet Assoc.* 1989;89:215–223.
81. Fong AK, Kretsch MJ. Nutrition evaluation scale system reduces time and labor in recording quantitative dietary intake. *J Am Diet Assoc.* 1990;90:664–670.
82. Brown JE, Tharp TM, Dahlber-Luby EM, et al. Videotape dietary assessment: validity, reliability and comparison of results with 24-hour dietary recalls from elderly women in a retirement home. *J Am Diet Assoc.* 1990;90:1675–1679.
83. Ammerman AS, Kirkley BG, Dennis B, et al. A dietary assessment for individuals with low literacy skills using interactive touch-scan computer technology. *Am J Clin Nutr.* 1994;59:289S.
84. Institute of Medicine, Food and Nutrition Board. *Dietary Reference Intakes for Energy, Carbohydrate, Fiber, Fat, Fatty Acids, Cholesterol, Protein and Amino Acids.* Prepub ed. Washington, DC: National Academies Press; 2005.
85. Institute of Medicine, Food and Nutrition Board. *Dietary Reference Intakes: Dietary Reference Intakes for Vitamin A, Vitamin K, Arsenic, Boron, Chromium, Copper, Iodine, Iron, Manganese, Molybdenum, Nickel, Silicon, Vanadium, and Zinc.* Washington, DC: National Academies Press; 2002.
86. Institute of Medicine, Food and Nutrition Board. *Dietary Reference Intakes for Vitamin C, Vitamin E, Selenium, and Carotenoids.* Washington, DC: National Academies Press; 2000.
87. Institute of Medicine, Food and Nutrition Board. *Dietary Reference Intakes for Calcium, Phosphorus, Magnesium, Vitamin D and Fluoride.* Washington, DC: National Academies Press; 1997.
88. Institute of Medicine, Food and Nutrition Board. *Dietary Reference Intakes for Thiamin, Riboflavin, Niacin, Vitamin B_6, Folate, Vitamin B_{12}, Pantothenic Acid, Biotin and Choline.* Washington, DC: National Academies Press; 2000.
89. Institute of Medicine, Food and Nutrition Board. *Dietary Reference Intakes for Sodium, Potassium and Water.* Washington, DC: National Academies Press; 2004.
90. Yates AA, Schlicker SA, Suitor CW. Dietary reference intakes: the new basis for recommendations for calcium and related nutrients, B vitamins, and choline. *J Am Diet Assoc.* 1998:98:699–706.
91. Guthrie HA. The 1985 Dietary Allowance Committee; an overview. *J Am Diet Assoc.* 1985;85:1646–1648.
92. Garrel DR, Jobin N, De Jorge LHM. Should we still use the Harris and Benedict equations? *Nutr Clin Prac.* 1996;11:99–103.
93. Kaplan AS, Zemal BS, Neiswender KM, Stallings VA. Resting energy expenditure in clinical pediatrics: measured versus prediction equations. *J Pediatr.* 1995;127:200–205.
94. World Health Organization. *Energy and Protein Requirements.* Report of a joint FAO/WHO/UNU Expert Consultation. Geneva: World Health Organization; 1985. WHO Technical Report Series no. 724.
95. Bursztein S, Elwyn DH, Askanazi J, Kinney JM. The theoretical framework of indirect calorimetry and energy balance. *Energy Metabolism, Indirect Calorimetry and Nutrition.* Baltimore, MD: Williams & Wilkins; 1989:27–83.
96. Pencharz PB, Azcue MP. Measuring resting energy expenditure in clinical practice. *J Pediatr.* 1995;127:269–271.
97. Harris JA, Benedict FG. *A Biometric Study of Basal Metabolism in Men.* Washington, DC: Carnegie Institute of Washington; 1919. Publication no. 279.
98. World Health Organization. *Energy and Protein Requirements.* Geneva: WHO; 1985. WHO Technical Report Series no. 724.
99. Schofield WN. Predicting basal metabolic rate, new standards and review of previous work. *Hum Nutr Clin Nutr.* 1985;39c(1s):5–42.
100. Altman P, Dittmer D, eds. *Metabolism.* Bethesda, MD: Federation of American Societies for Experimental Biology; 1968.
101. Maffeis C, Schutz Y, Micciolo R, Zoccante L, Pinelli L. Resting metabolic rate in six- to ten-year-old obese and nonobese children. *J Pediatr.* 1993;122:556–562.
102. Phillips R, Ott K, Young B. Nutritional support and measured energy expenditure of the child and adolescent with head injury. *J Neuro Surg.* 1987;67:846–851.
103. Redmond C, Lipp J. Traumatic brain injury in the pediatric population. *Nutr Clin Pract.* 2006;21:450–461
104. Havalad S, Quaid MA, Sapiega V. Energy expenditure in children with severe head injury: lack of agreement between measured and estimated energy expenditure. *Nutr Clin Pract.* 2006;21:175–181.
105. Williams R, Olivi, S, Mackert P, Fletcher L, Tian, G, Wang W. Comparison of energy prediction equations with measured resting energy expenditure in children with sickle cell anemia. *J Am Diet Assoc.* 2002;102:956–961.
106. Kushner RF, Schoeller DA. Resting and total energy expenditure in patients with inflammatory bowel disease. *Am J Clin Nutr.* 1991;53:161–165.
107. Barale K, Charuhas P. Oncology and marrow transplantation. In: Samour PQ, King K, eds. *Handbook of Pediatric Nutrition.* Gaithersburg, MD: Aspen; 1999:480.

108. Duggan C, Bechard L, Donovan K, et al. Changes in resting energy expenditure among children undergoing allogeneic stem cell transplantation. *Am J Clin Nutr.* 2003;78(1):104–109.
109. Greer R, Lehnert M, Lewindon P, Cleghorn GJ, Shepherd RW. Body composition and components of energy expenditure in children with end-stage liver disease. *J Pediatr Gastroenterol Nutr.* 2003;36(3):358–361.
110. Pierro A, Koletzko B, Carnielli V, et al. Resting energy expenditure is increased in infants and children with extrahepatic biliary atresia. *J Ped Surg.* 1989;24:534–538.
111. Stallings VA, Zemol BS, Davies JC, Cronk CE, Charney EB. Energy expenditure of children and adolescents with severe disabilities; a cerebral palsy model. *Am J Clin Nutr.* 1996;64:627–634.
112. Mayes TM, Gottschlich MM, Khoury J, Warren GD. Evaluation of predicted and measured energy requirements in burned children. *J Amer Diet Assoc.* 1996;96:24–29.
113. Powis MR, Smith K, Renii M, Halliday D, Pierro A. Effect of major abdominal operations on energy and protein metabolism in infants and children. *J Ped Surg.* 1998;33:49–53.
114. Jones MO, Pierro P, Hammond P, Lloyd DA. The metabolic response to operative stress in infants. *J Ped Surg.*1993;28:1258–1262.
115. Barton JS, Hindmarsh PC, Scrimseour CM, Rennie MJ, Preece MH. Energy expenditure in congenital heart disease. *Arch Dis Child.* 1994;70:5–9.
116. Alfaro MP, Siegel RM, Baker RC, Heubi JE. Resting energy expenditure and body composition in pediatric HIV infection. *Pediatr AIDS HIV Infect.* 1995;6(6):276–280.
117. Henderson RA, Talusan K, Hutton N, Yoken R, Caballero B. Resting energy expenditure and body composition in children with HIV infection. *J Acquir Immune Defic Syndr Hum Retrovirol.* 1998;19:150–157.
118. Dubois EF. Energy metabolism. *Ann Rev Physiol.* 1954;16:125–134.
119. Chwals WJ. Overfeeding the critically ill child: fact or fantasy? *New Horizons.* 1994;2:147–155.
120. Subcommittee on the Tenth Edition of the RDAs, Food and Nutrition Board, National Research Council. *Recommended Dietary Allowances.* 10th ed. Washington, DC: National Academies Press; 1989.
121. Coss-Bu JA, Jefferson LS, Walding D, Yadin D, Smith EO, Klish W. Resting energy expenditure in children in a pediatric intensive care unit; comparison of Harris-Benedict and Talbot predictions with indirect calorimetry values. *Am J Clin Nutr.* 1998;67:74–80.
122. Bandini LG, Morelli JA, Must A, Dietz WH. Accuracy of standardized equations for predicting metabolic rate in premenarchal girls. *Am J Clin Nutr.* 1995;62:711–714.
123. Matarese LE. Indirect calorimetry: technical aspects. *J Am Diet Assoc.* 1997;97:s154–s160.
124. Porter C, Cohen NH. Indirect calorimetry in critically ill patients. Role of the clinical dietitian in interpreting results. *Am J Diet Assoc.* 1996;96:49–57.
125. Weir JB. New methods for calculating metabolic rate with special reference to protein metabolism. *J Physiol.* 1949;109:1–9.
126. Bursztein S, Elwyn DH, Askanazi J, Kinney JM. The theoretical framework of indirect calorimetry and energy balance. In: Elwyn DH, Askanazi J, Kinney JM, Bursztein S, eds. *Energy Metabolism, Indirect Calorimetry and Nutrition.* Baltimore, MD: Williams and Wilkins; 1989:27–83.
127. Ireton-Jones CS, Turner WW Jr. The use of respiratory quotient to determine the efficacy of nutrition support systems. *J Am Diet Assoc.* 1987;87:180–183.
128. Waterlow JC. Classification and definition of protein-calorie malnutrition. *Br Med J.* 1972;3:566–569.
129. Mclaren DS, Read WWC. Classification of nutritional status in early childhood. *Lancet.* 1972;2:146–148.
130. Waterlow JC. Note on the assessment and classification of protein-energy malnutrition in children. *Lancet.* 1973;2:87–89.
131. Pollack MM, Ruttimann UE, Wiley JS. Nutritional depletions in critically ill children; associations with physiologic instability and increased quantity of care. *J Parenter Enter Nutr.* 1985;9:309–313.
132. Leung AKC, Robson LM, Fagan JE. Assessment of the child with failure to thrive. *Am Fam Physician.* 1993;48(8):1432–1438.
133. Kirkland RT. Failure to thrive. In: Oski FA, DeAngelis CD, Feigin RD, Warshaw JB, eds. *Principles and Practice of Pediatrics.* Philadelphia: Lippincott; 1990:969–972.
134. Edwards AG, Halse PC, Parkin JM, Waterston AJ. Recognizing failure to thrive in early childhood. *Arch Dis Child.* 1990;65:1263–1265.
135. Waterlow JC, Buzina R, Keller W, Lane JM, Nichaman MZ, Tanner JM. The presentation and use of height and weight data for comparing the nutritional status of groups of children under the age of ten years. *Bull WHO.* 1977;55:486–498.
136. Centers for Disease Control and Prevention. *Epi Info, Version 3.5.1.* Available at: http://www.cdc.gov/epiinfo. Accessed January 18, 2010.
137. WHO Working Group. Use and interpretation of anthropometric indicators of nutritional status. *Bull WHO.* 1986;64:929–941.
138. Sills RH. Failure to thrive. The role of clinical and laboratory evaluation. *Am J Dis Child.* 1978;132:967–969.

Nutrition for Premature Infants

Diane M. Anderson

Introduction

Premature infants are defined as infants born before 37 weeks gestation, as compared to full-term infants born from 37 to 42 weeks.[1] The physiologic immaturity of premature infants renders them susceptible to a number of problems (see **Table 4-1**), many of which imperil their nutrition and growth (see **Table 4-2**). Low birth weight (LBW) refers to infants with a birth weight of less than 2500 g (5 pounds, 8 ounces); very low birth weight (VLBW) infants weigh less than 1500 g (3 pounds, 5 ounces), and extremely low birth weight (ELBW) infants weigh less than 1000 g (2 pounds, 3 ounces).[1] Infants can be LBW but yet be full term due to poor intrauterine growth.

Assessment of intrauterine growth is determined by plotting the infant's birth weight by gestational age on various charts. On the Lubchenco, Fenton, or Olsen growth chart, small-for-gestational-age (SGA) infants have a birth weight of less than the 10th percentile.[2–4] Large-for-gestational-age (LGA) infants have a birth weight greater than the 90th percentile.[2,3,5] Appropriate-for-gestational-age (AGA) infants are between the 10th and 90th percentiles (see Appendix A). On the Fenton and Olsen charts, SGA and LGA can also be defined as two standard deviations from the mean birth weight (approximately the 3rd and the 97th percentiles, respectively).[3,4,6] (See Appendix A. The Fenton chart also may be downloaded from http://members.shaw.ca/growthchart.) **Table 4-3** lists the etiologies for SGA, and **Table 4-4** lists the factors associated with LGA infants. These assessments are used to anticipate medical and nutritional problems and management needs of the infant (see **Table 4-5**). For example, consider an infant born at 34 weeks gestation whose birth weight is 1200 g. This infant is premature because the gestational age is less than 37 weeks. On these three intrauterine growth charts, the infant is SGA because birth weight is less than the 10th percentile or less than two standard deviations from the mean birth weight.[2–4]

SGA infants are further classified by their body length and head circumference as symmetrically or asymmetrically growth restricted.[6] The symmetrically SGA infant's birth weight, head circumference, and body length are all classified as small, whereas the asymmetrically SGA infant has a small body weight but an appropriate head circumference and body length. Infants who experience asymmetrical growth restriction usually stand a better chance for catch-up growth.[7] The potential for catch-up growth is determined by the etiology of the poor fetal growth.[7] Those infants who have the insult late in gestation due to placental insufficiency or uterine restrictions will grow when

TABLE 4-1 Potential Problems of the Premature Infant

• Undernutrition	• Apnea
• Poor growth	• Infection
• Glucose instability	• Hyperbilirubinemia
• Hypocalcemia	• Immature renal function
• Fat malabsorption	• Necrotizing enterocolitis
• Decreased gastric motility	• Osteopenia
• Uncoordinated sucking, swallowing, and breathing	• Intraventricular hemorrhage
• Perinatal depression	• Periventricular leukomalacia
• Respiratory distress syndrome	• Bronchopulmonary dysplasia
• Hypotension	• Retinopathy of prematurity
• Poor temperature control	• Anemia
• Patent ductus arteriosus	

Sources: Data from American Academy of Pediatrics Committee on Nutrition. Nutritional needs of preterm infants. In: Kleinman RE, ed. *Pediatric Nutrition Handbook*, 6th ed. Elk Grove Village, IL: American Academy of Pediatrics; 2009:79–112; and Lee KG. Identifying the high-risk newborn and evaluating gestational age, prematurity, postmaturity, large-for-gestational-age, and small-for-gestational age infants. In: Cloherty JP, Eichenwald EC, Stark AR, eds. *Manual of Neonatal Care*, 6th ed. Philadelphia: Wolters Kluwer/Lippincott Williams & Wilkins; 2008:41–58.

TABLE 4-2 Premature Infant's Risk Factors for Nutritional Deficiencies

1. Decreased nutrient stores
   - Premature infants are born before anticipated quantities of nutrients are deposited.
   - Low stores include glycogen, fat, protein, fat-soluble vitamins, calcium, phosphorus, magnesium, and trace minerals.
2. Rapid growth
   - Depletes small body nutrient stores.
   - With rapid growth, energy and nutrient needs will be increased.
3. Immature physiological systems
   - Digestion and absorption capabilities are decreased due to low concentrations of lactase, pancreatic lipase, and bile salts.
   - Gastrointestinal motility and stomach capacity are decreased, which limits gastric emptying and feeding volume.
   - A coordinated suck, swallow, and breathing is not developed until 32–34 weeks gestation.
   - Hepatic enzymes are deceased, which may make specific amino acids conditionally essential (cysteine) or toxic (phenylalanine), due to the inability to synthesize or degrade.
   - Immature renal function limits the infant's ability to control fluid, electrolytes, and acid/base status.
4. Cold stress results in energy expenditure for heat production instead of growth.
5. Illnesses
   - Respiratory distress syndrome will decrease gastrointestinal motility. Trophic feedings or small volume feedings will frequently be introduced.
   - Patent ductus arteriosus often requires fluid restriction, which limits caloric and nutrient intake. If the infant is treated with indomethacin, the infant will be made NPO.
   - Necrotizing enterocolitis forces nutrition management to parenteral nutrition for bowel rest. With refeeding, human milk is used but an elemental infant formula may be indicated. Some infants may develop short-gut syndrome as a complication and require extensive nutritional management for malabsorption.
   - Bronchopulmonary dysplasia can lead to an increased energy demand with fluid restriction. Nutrient-dense milks are often utilized. Chronic diuretic use will create electrolyte depletion.
   - Hyperbilirubinemia may be treated by phototherapy, which may increase the infant's insensible water loss and fluid requirement. If exchange transfusion is needed, introduction of enteral feedings will be delayed. Necrotizing enterocolitis has been reported as a complication of exchange transfusion therapy.
   - Sepsis may result in withholding all enteral fluids until it is established that the infant is stable.

Sources: Data from Schanler RJ, Anderson D. The low birth weight infant. Inpatient care. In: Duggan C, Watkins JB, Walker WA, eds. *Nutrition in Pediatrics: Basic Science Clinical Applications*, 4th ed. Hamilton, Ontario, Canada: BC Decker; 2008:377–394; Anderson DM. Nutritional assessment and therapeutic interventions for the preterm infant. *Clin Peri.* 2002;29:313–326; and Cloherty JP, Eichenwald EC, Stark AR. *Manual of Neonatal* Care, 6th ed. Philadelphia: Wolters Kluwer/Lippincott Williams & Wilkins; 2008.

provided appropriate nutrition.[7] Those infants who had an early perinatal insult related to congenital infection or genetic disorders remain small in physical size.[7]

Catch-up growth for premature infants continues until adulthood for weight and length.[8,9] Head circumference catch-up is limited to the first 6 to 12 months of life.[10,11] A suboptimal head circumference measurement at 8 months of age has been independently associated with decreased intellectual quotients, cognitive functioning skills, and behavior problems at school age.[12] Many premature infants remain smaller than infants born with normal birth weight or at term gestation.[9,10]

Premature infants represent a heterogeneous population for nutrition management. Intrauterine growth establishes nutritional status at birth, and gestational age determines nutrient need and feeding modality employed. As the infant matures, postnatal nutrient needs and feeding modality will vary. Finally, the infant's clinical condition can acutely change and alter nutrition care. Due to these factors, their nutrition management is a day-to-day decision-making process regarding what to feed, what volume and nutrient density to provide, and how to administer nourishment. The goal is to provide nutrition for optimal growth and development to take place. The intrauterine growth rate and weight gain composition without metabolic complications has been advocated as the goal for premature infant nutrition.[13]

AGA premature infants frequently become SGA before hospital discharge. The infants are growing at the intrauterine growth rate of 15 g/kg/day but their weight curve has fallen below the 10th percentile for their postmenstrual age.[14] Tsang and his group, in their Reasonable Nutrient Intakes, recommend providing more energy and protein

TABLE 4-3 Etiologic Factors for SGA Births

• Normal variation	• High altitude
• Pregnancy-induced hypertension	• Maternal age < 16 years or > 40 years
• Chronic hypertension	• Multiple gestation
• Chronic renal disease	• Congenital malformations
• Diabetes with vascular complications	• Chromosomal abnormalities
• Intrauterine infection	• Placental insufficiency
• Poor gestation weight gain	• Twin-to-twin transfusion
• Cigarette smoking	• Placental and cord defects
• Drug or alcohol abuse	• Short interpregnancy interval

Sources: Data from Lee KG. Identifying the high-risk newborn and evaluating gestational age, prematurity, postmaturity, large-for-gestational-age, and small-for-gestational age infants. In: Cloherty JP, Eichenwald EC, Stark AR, eds. *Manual of Neonatal Care*, 6th ed. Philadelphia: Wolters Kluwer/Lippincott Williams & Wilkins; 2008:41–58; Kliegman RM. Intrauterine growth restriction. In: Martin RJ, Fanaroff AA, Walsh MC, eds. *Fanaroff and Martin's Neonatal-Perinatal Medicine Diseases of the Fetus and Infant*, 8th ed. Philadelphia: Mosby Elsevier; 2006:271–306; and Institute of Medicine and National Research Council. *Weight Gain During Pregnancy: Reexamining the Guidelines*. Washington, DC: The National Academies Press; 2009.

TABLE 4-4 Factors Associated with LGA Births

• Infant of diabetic mother	• Genetic predisposition
• Beckwith's syndrome	• High gestation weight gain
• Some post-term infants	• Multiparity

Sources: Data from Lee KG. Identifying the high-risk newborn and evaluating gestational age, prematurity, postmaturity, large-for-gestational-age, and small-for-gestational age infants. In: Cloherty JP, Eichenwald EC, Stark AR, eds. *Manual of Neonatal Care*, 6th ed. Philadelphia: Wolters Kluwer/Lippincott Williams & Wilkins; 2008:41–58; and Institute of Medicine and National Research Council. *Weight Gain During Pregnancy: Reexamining the Guidelines*. Washington, DC: The National Academies Press; 2009.

than the American Academy of Pediatrics (AAP) has suggested as a means to prevent extrauterine growth restriction (EUGR)[15]; however, there are no studies to document that greater intakes would prevent this EUGR. The recent position of the Committee of Nutrition of the European Society for Paediatric Gastroenterology, Hepatology, and Nutrition is that the ELBW infant does not require more energy or nutrients except for protein.[16] Excess energy intake would lead to increased adipose tissue and not linear growth. In fact, just meeting the AAP guidelines may be effective for growth, and greater intakes are not indicated.[16] This increased protein of 4.6 g/kg would be only for those infants who had a history of not meeting the AAP guideline of 3.5–4 g/kg of enteral protein intake.[16]

TABLE 4-5 Anticipated Problems for SGA and LGA Infants

Problems	Issues
Small for Gestational Age	
Hypoglycemia	Caused by Low glycogen stores Decreased gluconeogenesis Decreased glycogenolysis Abnormal counter-regulatory hormones Hyperinsulinemia
Increased energy demand	Caused by Increased growth rate Increased energy cost of growth
Heat loss	Caused by Large surface area Decreased subcutaneous fat
Large for Gestational Age	
Birth trauma	Shoulder dystocia, fractured clavicle, depressed skull fracture, brachial plexus injury, facial paralysis
Hypoglycemia	Caused by hyperinsulinism

Sources: Data from Lee KG. Identifying the high-risk newborn and evaluating gestational age, prematurity, postmaturity, large-for-gestational-age, and small-for-gestational age infants. In: Cloherty JP, Eichenwald EC, Stark AR, eds. *Manual of Neonatal Care*, 6th ed. Philadelphia: Wolters Kluwer/Lippincott Williams & Wilkins; 2008:41–58; and Kliegman RM. Intrauterine growth restriction. In: Martin RJ, Fanaroff AA, Walsh MC, eds. *Fanaroff and Martin's Neonatal-Perinatal Medicine Diseases of the Fetus and Infant*, 8th ed. Philadelphia: Mosby Elsevier; 2006:271–306.

Parenteral Nutrition

Parenteral nutrition (PN) is often indicated and initiated in the first few days of life to allow the premature infant to adapt to the extrauterine environment and to supplement the small volume enteral feedings initiated. Enteral feedings are often slowly advanced, because premature infants have decreased enteral feeding tolerance and small gastric capacities, which limit volume intakes and advancements. Premature infants are at risk for necrotizing enterocolitis (NEC), and enteral feedings will be cautiously advanced.[13] For the VLBW infant, PN should be initiated within the first 24 hours of life to promote energy intake and glucose homeostasis, to establish nitrogen balance, and to prevent essential fatty acid deficiency.[17,18] The provision of amino acids as part of PN within the first 24 hours of life has been associated with nitrogen balance; improved glucose tolerance, which facilitates greater glucose administration; increased protein synthesis; and normal plasma amino acid levels.[17,18] **Tables 4-6** and **4-7** give suggested guidelines for parenteral administration of specific nutrients. **Table 4-8** briefly describes a protocol for parenteral nutrition management.

For the premature infant who is not fluid restricted, adequate nutrition can be provided by a peripheral line.[19] A central venous catheter is required for the infant who requires prolonged parenteral nutrition, has limited venous access, is fluid restricted, or has an increased nutrient demand that cannot be met by peripheral nutrition. Peripheral inserted central venous catheters (PICC) are frequently used with premature infants because the PICC line can be placed at an infant's bedside. A PICC line can reduce the stress to the infant caused by repeated insertion of peripheral lines, and facilitate the delivery of concentrated parenteral nutrients.[19] A tunneled, central venous catheter must be placed surgically under anesthesia and is used when a PICC line cannot be inserted.

TABLE 4-6 Parenteral Nutrition Guidelines: Energy, Protein, and Minerals per Day

Nutrient	Unit/kg
Energy (kcal)	90–100
Glucose (mg/kg/min)	6–12
Fat (g)	1–3
Protein (g)	2.7–3.5
Sodium (mEq)	2–4
Potassium (mEq)	1.5–2
Chloride (mEq)	2–4
Calcium (mg)	60–80
Phosphorus (mg)	39–67
Magnesium (mg)	4.3–7.2
Zinc (μg)	400
Copper (μg)	20
Chromium (μg)	0.2
Manganese (μg)	1
Selenium (μg)	2.0
Molybdenum (μg)	0.25
Iodide (μg)	1

Sources: Data from American Academy of Pediatrics Committee on Nutrition. Nutritional needs of preterm infants. In: Kleinman RE, ed. *Pediatric Nutrition Handbook*, 6th ed. Elk Grove Village, IL: American Academy of Pediatrics; 2009:79–112; and American Academy of Pediatrics, Committee on Nutrition. Parenteral Nutrition. In: Kleinman RE, ed. *Pediatric Nutrition Handbook*, 6th ed. Elk Grove Village, IL: American Academy of Pediatrics; 2009:519–540.

TABLE 4-7 Parenteral Vitamin Guidelines per Day

Vitamin	Dose/kg	Maximum Dose per Day*
Vitamin A (IU)	920	2300
Vitamin E (IU)	2.8	7
Vitamin K (μg)	80	200
Vitamin D (IU)	160	400
Vitamin C (mg)	32	80
Thiamin (mg)	0.48	1.2
Riboflavin (mg)	0.56	1.4
Niacin (mg)	6.8	17
Vitamin B_6 (mg)	0.4	1
Folate (μg)	56	140
Vitamin B_{12} (μg)	0.4	1
Biotin (μg)	8	20
Pantothenic acid (mg)	2	5

*Preterm infants receive 40% of the daily dose MVI Pediatric (INFUVITE Pediatric) per kg until the maximum daily dose is achieved at 2.5 kg.

Sources: Data from American Academy of Pediatrics Committee on Nutrition. Nutritional needs of preterm infants. In: Kleinman RE, ed. *Pediatric Nutrition Handbook*, 6th ed. Elk Grove Village, IL: American Academy of Pediatrics; 2009:79–112; and Greene HL, Hambidge KM, Schanler R, Tsang RC. Guidelines for the use of vitamins, trace elements, calcium, magnesium, and phosphorus in infants and children receiving total parenteral nutrition: report of the Subcommittee on Pediatric Parenteral Nutrient Requirements from the Committee on Clinical Practice Issues of the American Society for Clinical Nutrition. *Am J Clin Nutr.* 1988;48:1324–1342.

Management Concerns and Medical Problems

Fluid management is very individualized for the preterm infant. Insensible water losses will be high, and the infant's renal function and neuroendocrine control will be immature.[20] Fluid volume may be limited to prevent or treat patent ductus arteriosus (PDA) and bronchopulmonary dysplasia (BPD).[21,22] **Table 4-9** gives laboratory parameters that should be observed in guiding PN therapy.

Insensible fluid losses are high for many reasons.[20] First, the premature infant has a large surface area related to total weight, which facilitates easy heat and water losses. Second, the premature infant's skin offers little protection from evaporative losses. There is a high water content, and the epidermis is thin and highly permeable. Finally, environmental factors in the newborn intensive care unit, such

TABLE 4-8 Parenteral Nutrition Progression

	DOL to Begin	Beginning Quantity	Increase	Maximum or Goal	Considerations
Fluid (mL/kg/day)	1	80–100	10–20	140–160	• Fluid needs will vary by birth weight, gestational age, postnatal age, and environmental conditions. • The ELBW neonate may require 200 mL/kg/day to maintain normal hydration the first week of life. • Fluids should be provided to keep the infant in normal hydration status. Refer to Table 4-9 for monitoring guidelines.
Glucose (mg/kg/min)	1	4.5–6	1–2	11–12	• Begin on DOL 1 to prevent hypoglycemia. • Decrease glucose load for hyperglycemia. Glucose homeostasis will usually improve in 1–2 days. • Insulin infusions should be used with caution. Insulin usage may result in unstable blood glucose levels, hypoglycemia, and acidosis.
Protein (g/kg/day)	1	1–3	—	2.7–3.5	• Advance protein to meet needs. There is no documentation that gradual protein advancement is needed.
Lipids (g/kg/day)	1	1–2	1	3	• Provide over an 18–24 hour period. • The 20% intralipid is preferred over the 10% emulsion. Serum levels of cholesterol, triglycerides, and phospholipids are lower with use of the 20% emulsion.
Sodium chloride (mEq/kg/day)	2–3	1–3	—	2–4	• Allow diuresis to occur the first few days of life to decrease extracellular blood volume. • Start sodium to prevent hyponatremia.
Potassium (mEq/kg/day)	2	1.5–2	—	2–3	• Add potassium after urine flow is established and serum potassium level is normal. • Check for hyperkalemia because the ELBW infant has a decreased glomerular filtration rate, acidosis, and the release of nitrogen and potassium secondary to negative balance.
Magnesium (mg/kg/day)	1	4.3–7.2	—	4.3–7.2	• Remove from parenteral nutrition when mother has received magnesium.
Vitamins and trace minerals	1				

Abbreviations: DOL, day of life; ELBW, extremely low birth weight.

Parenteral nutrition progression may be slowed with fluid and electrolyte imbalance, glucose imbalance, renal failure, the anticipation of enteral feedings, or the initiation and tolerance of enteral feedings.

Sources: Data from American Academy of Pediatrics Committee on Nutrition. Nutritional needs of preterm infants. In: Kleinman RE, ed. *Pediatric Nutrition Handbook*, 6th ed. Elk Grove Village, IL: American Academy of Pediatrics; 2009:79–112; Schanler RJ, Anderson D. The low birth weight infant. Inpatient care. In: Duggan C, Watkins JB, Walker WA. eds. *Nutrition in Pediatrics: Basic Science Clinical Applications*, 4th ed. Hamilton, Ontario, Canada: BC Decker; 2008:377–394; Thureen PJ, Melara D, Fennessey PV, et al. Effect of low versus high intravenous amino acid intake on very low birth weight infants in the early neonatal period. *Pediatr Res*. 2003;53:24–32; and Doherty EG, Simmons CF. Fluid and electrolyte management. In: Cloherty JP, Eichenwald EC, Stark AR, eds. *Manual of Neonatal Care*, 6th ed. Philadelphia: Wolters Kluwer/Lippincott Williams & Wilkins; 2008:100–113.

as the use of radiant warmers, phototherapy, and high or low ambient temperature, increase insensible fluid losses.[21] These losses can be decreased by the use of humidified incubators, plastic shields, and plastic wraps or clothing.

Preterm infants have a limited ability to hydrolyze triglycerides. Elevated serum triglyceride levels are more frequently found with decreasing gestational age, infection, surgical stress, and malnutrition, and with the SGA infant.[13,23] It is recommended that serum triglyceride levels be kept under 200 mg/dL,[13] but there is a lack of data to support this level.[24] Although the free fatty acids from intralipid compete with indirect bilirubin for binding onto albumin,

TABLE 4-9 Fluid and Electrolyte Monitoring Parameters

Fluid intake	80–150 ml/kg*
Urine output	1–3 mL/kg/hour
Daily body weights	10–15% maximum total weight loss
Serum sodium	134–146 mmol/L
Serum potassium	3–7 mmol/L
Serum chloride	97–110 mmol/L
Serum creatinine	0.3–1 mg/dL
Blood urea nitrogen	3–25 mg/dL
Urine specific gravity	1.008–1.012

*The critically ill premature infant has highly variable fluid needs. This range represents the usual volume of fluid administered. To prevent over- or underhydration, fluids should be provided so as to keep the other monitoring parameters within normal levels.

Sources: Data from Pesce MA. Reference ranges for laboratory test and procedures. In: Kliegman RM, Behrman RE, Jenson HB, Stanton BF, eds. *Nelson Textbook of Pediatrics*, 18th ed. Philadelphia, PA: Saunders Elsevier; 2007:2943–2949; and Dell KM, Davis ID. Fluid, electrolyte, and acid base homeostasis. In: Martin RJ, Fanaroff AA, Walsh MC, eds. *Fanaroff and Martin's Neonatal-Perinatal Medicine Diseases of the Fetus and Infant*, 8th ed. Philadelphia: Mosby Elsevier; 2006:695–712.

intralipid may be provided during hyperbilirubinemia at the present recommended intakes. Intralipid should be administered at a maximum of 3 g/kg over a 24-hour infusion.[13,25] The concern is that free bilirubin may cross the blood–brain barrier and cause kernicterus. At this level of intake and rate of infusion, however, it appears to be safe.[25]

Several amino acid parenteral solutions are formulated for the pediatric patient.[26] These solutions contain a larger percentage of total nitrogen as essential amino acids and branch chain amino acids, and they have a balanced pattern of nonessential amino acids instead of a single amino acid concentration.[26] The use of a pediatric amino acid solution, as compared to an adult product, results in plasma amino acid levels that are similar to the breastfed infant and improve weight gain and nitrogen balance.[27] The addition of cystine to TrophAmine (Kendall McGraw Laboratories), one of the pediatric amino acid solutions, may improve nitrogen balance.[28] The addition of cysteine hydrochloride has not consistently improved nitrogen balance.[29] The addition of cysteine hydrochloride increases the pH of the solution, which allows greater levels of calcium and phosphorus to be added.[13,26]

Transition to Enteral Feedings

Weaning to enteral feedings is a slow process that is necessary to facilitate feeding tolerance and prevent the development of NEC.[13,30] Enteral feedings are gradually increased in volume and strength as parenteral fluids are decreased at a similar volume. The two fluid types are coordinated to keep stable the total fluids provided until enteral feedings provide adequate nutrition for growth. Parenteral fluids are discontinued at approximately 100 to 120 mL/kg/day of enteral feedings.

Enteral Nutrition

Premature infants are at risk for aspiration, NEC, and feeding intolerance, so enteral feedings are slowly introduced and advanced.[26] Infants with cardiovascular instability, which can present as severe acidosis, hypotension, or hypoxemia,[26] may not be fed. Trophic feedings have been advocated for the first week of life to facilitate gut development and have not been associated with increasing the incidence of NEC.[13,31] Trophic feedings are small volumes of feedings given to nourish the gut, but do not serve as a major source of nutrition. Volumes of 1 mL/kg to 25 mL/kg have been studied.[13] Benefits are listed in **Table 4-10**. These feedings can consist of human milk or premature infant formula provided at 10–20 mL/kg/day for 3 to 7 days.[26] The use of umbilical artery catheters should not be a contraindication for starting trophic feedings.[13,32] When the infant's condition stabilizes, feedings are advanced.[26] For the healthy premature infant, feedings can be initiated and advanced during the first week of life. Feeding advancement for the VLBW infant is often limited to 20 mL/kg/day or less because rapid feeding advancement has been associated with NEC.[33] In one study, the enteral feeding advancement of 35 mL/kg/day and 15 mL/kg/day were both tolerated.[34] The optimal volume of advancement needs to be further studied.[35] The use of a standardized feeding schedule, which includes time to initiate feeds, feed volume advancement, and milk strength, has been associated with a decreased incidence of NEC.[36]

The use of human milk has been linked to a decreased incidence of NEC.[37] Donor human milk is frequently used to supplement the mother's own milk for her infant to provide this protection.[38] A recent study demonstrated that the use of human milk and liquid donor milk fortifier decreased the incidence of NEC.[39] The type of milk selected depends on individual factors, and can sometimes involve complex decisions. **Table 4-11** lists factors that must be considered. Whatever milk is chosen, it should provide appropriate amounts of energy, protein, minerals, and vitamins (see **Table 4-12**). The goal is to promote growth and to prepare the infant for hospital discharge. In **Table 4-13**, selected nutrients are compared (at 150 mL of milk). This value represents the average volume intake for a premature infant on full enteral feedings. Fortified human milk or premature infant formulas will meet the needs of most premature infants.

TABLE 4-10 Benefits of Trophic Feedings

- Feeding
  - Improved feeding tolerance
  - Achieve full feedings sooner
  - Achieve full Per os PO sooner
- Gastrointestinal
  - Increased plasma gastrin
  - Decreased intestinal transit time
  - More mature intestinal motor pattern
  - Increased calcium, copper, and phosphorus retention
- Clinical
  - Decreased serum bilirubin and days of phototherapy
  - Decreased incidence of cholestasis
  - Lower serum alkaline phosphatase activity levels
- Decreased length of stay

Sources: Data from American Academy of Pediatrics Committee on Nutrition. Nutritional needs of preterm infants. In: Kleinman RE, ed. *Pediatric Nutrition Handbook*, 6th ed. Elk Grove Village, IL: American Academy of Pediatrics; 2009:79–112; Schanler RJ, Anderson D. The low birth weight infant. Inpatient care. In: Duggan C, Watkins JB, Walker WA, eds. *Nutrition in Pediatrics: Basic Science Clinical Applications*, 4th ed. Hamilton, Ontario, Canada: BC Decker; 2008:377–394; Dunn L, Hulman S, Weiner J, Kliegman R. Beneficial effects of early hypocaloric enteral feeding on neonatal gastrointestinal function: preliminary report of a randomized trial. *J Pediatr*. 1988;112:622–629; Ziegler EE, Thureen PJ, Carlson SJ. Aggressive nutrition of the very low birthweight infant. *Clin Peri*. 2002;29:225–244; and Schanler RJ, Shulman RJ, Lau C, et al. Feeding strategies for premature infants: randomized trial of gastrointestinal priming and tube-feeding method. *Pediatrics*. 1999;103:434–439.

The premature infant's vitamin needs will be met by the use of powdered bovine-fortified human milk or premature infant formula; no additional supplementation is indicated.[13] Commercial donor milk fortifiers are not vitamin fortified, so multiple vitamin supplementation is recommended. Iron needs will be met by the consumption of 120 kcal/kg of an iron-fortified premature infant formula, because this will provide 2 mg/kg of iron, which is the goal.[13] For the infant receiving human milk, iron supplementation can be initiated at 2 to 4 mg/kg/day once full-volume feedings have been achieved or after 2 weeks of age.[13] The fortifiers vary in their iron content, and extra iron supplements should be limited to those that have low iron content. When erythropoietin therapy is employed, iron supplementation at 6 mg/kg/day to facilitate red cell production is recommended.[13]

Pharmacological dosage of vitamin E (50 to 100 mg/kg/day) for premature infants to prevent retinopathy of prematurity, BPD, or intraventricular hemorrhage is not recommended.[13] Although vitamin E is an antioxidant, it has not consistently prevented these illnesses; complications associated with its pharmacological dosing include NEC, sepsis, intraventricular hemorrhage, and death.[40]

To prevent BPD in the ELBW infant, vitamin A supplementation has been suggested due to its role in cell differentiation and tissue repair.[41] Providing 5000 IU of vitamin A intramuscularly (IM) three times per week for the first month of life will lower oxygen requirements at 36 weeks gestation.[41] Developmental follow-up scores at 18 months corrected age demonstrated no difference from premature infants who had not received extra vitamin A.[42] It is recommended that physicians decide whether to use vitamin A supplementation in their nurseries.[13] Considerations include the variation in the incidence of BPD among nurseries, the lack of additional benefits of vitamin A supplementation, and the acceptance of IM therapy.[13,43] Additional factors associated with the occurrence of BPD are antenatal steroids, exogenous surfactant, mode of ventilation, and postnatal steroids. The criteria used to prescribe oxygen varies among NICU practices which will alter the incidence of BPD by the definition of BPD being the oxygen requirement at 36 weeks postmenstrual age (PMA).[43]

Osteopenia or poor bone mineralization is commonly reported for premature infants when the intake of calcium and phosphorus is inadequate, and this is in addition to their poor nutrient stores at birth.[44] Risk factors include prolonged PN and/or diets of unfortified human milk. A diet of fortified human milk or premature infant formula will meet the infant's needs.[45] Vitamin D intake at 200 to 400 IU per day with the calcium- and phosphorus-enriched premature formula is adequate.[46] Chronic diuretic use can increase urinary calcium losses.[44]

Premature infants are at risk for trace mineral deficiency due to their poor nutrient stores at birth, rapid growth, and the dependence on adequate intake. With use of today's PN guidelines, premature infant formula, or fortified human milk, deficiencies should be uncommon.[47] Infants who have excessive losses via an ileostomy drainage or high urine output related to renal failure could need two to three times the recommended guidelines for zinc.[26,48] Additional case reports of zinc deficiency have been reported when the mother's milk had an extremely low zinc content or the infant had been provided with copper and/or iron supplements that compete with zinc for absorption.[49]

The two long chain polyunsaturated fatty acids, docosahexaenoic acid, and arachidonic acid, are present in human milk and have been added to infant formulas. However, study results on the addition of these two fatty acids to the premature infant's diet have been mixed for physical growth, visual function, and neurodevelopment.[50]

The feeding method employed will depend on the infant's gestational age, clinical condition, and nursery staff experience.[13] **Table 4-14** describes methods in use, and **Table 4-15** gives guidelines for amounts and rates of feedings. Due to the

TABLE 4-11 Milk and Formula Selection Indications and Concerns

Milk	Indications	Concerns
Human milk	• Nutrients are readily absorbed. • Anti-infective factors are present. • Decreased incidence of NEC and sepsis. • Nutrient composition is unique. • Maternal–infant attachment enhanced. • Maternal emotional support by family and healthcare team is indicated to facilitate lactation. • Quicker achievement of full enteral feedings versus premature infant formula. • Slower weight gain, but earlier discharge has been demonstrated on fortified human milk feedings versus premature infant formula.	• Milk from mothers who deliver prematurely will often contain a higher protein concentration than that found in the milk from mothers who deliver at term. This elevated protein concentration decreased by 28 days of lactation and may not meet the protein needs of the rapidly growing premature infant. • The concentration of protein, calcium, phosphorous, and sodium is too low to meet the needs of many premature infants. To increase nutrient density, human milk fortifiers should be added to the milk. • Iron supplementation at 2–4 mg/kg is needed for those infants receiving the low iron–containing fortifier. For those who are provided the fortifier with iron, no iron supplementation is needed. • Milk volume production may be inadequate to nourish the infant.
Formulas for premature infants	• Glucose polymers comprise 50–60% of the carbohydrate calories, which decreases the lactose load presented to the premature infant for digestion. Glucose polymers also decrease the osmolality of the formula. • Lactose comprises 40–50% of the carbohydrate calories. • Medium chain triglycerides (MCTs) are 40–50% of the fat calories. MCTs do not require pancreatic lipase or bile salts for digestion and absorption. • Protein is at a higher concentration than that incorporated into standard infant formula to meet the increased protein needs of the preterm infant. • The protein is a 60/40 or 100/0 whey/casein ratio as compared with the 18/82 ratio found in bovine milk. This whey predominance prevents the elevation of plasma phenylalanine and tyrosine levels. • Calcium and phosphorous are two to three times the concentration found in standard infant formulas. These levels will maintain normal serum calcium and phosphorous levels, prevent osteopenia, and promote calcium and phosphorous accretion at the fetal rate. • Sodium, potassium, and chloride concentrations are greater than in standard infant formulas to meet the increased electrolyte needs of the premature infant. • Vitamins, trace minerals, and additional minerals are incorporated into these formulas at high concentration to meet the infant's increased nutrient need while facilitating a limited volume intake. • Iron-fortified formulas are available, which eliminates the need for iron supplementation. • Formula osmolality is within the physiologic range at 235–300 mOsm/kg water for the 20–24 kcal/ounce, which facilitates formula tolerances and decreases the risk of NEC. • A 30 kcal/ounce formula is available for the infant who needs fluid restriction to support growth, such as the infant with BPD. The osmolality is 325 mOsm/kg water. • Premature formulas can be used until the infant reaches 2.5–3.6 kg, depending on the formula vitamin concentration and volume intake.	• Feeding volumes should be advanced slowly with the very-low-birth weight infant. • Vitamin and iron supplements are not indicated for the infant receiving iron-fortified premature infant formula.

Premature discharge formulas (transition formulas)	• Designed for the premature infant at discharge. The infant should weigh at least 1.8 kg when this formula is provided. • Formula should be initiated at least 3 days prior to discharge to document formula tolerance and weight gain. • Formulas have a nutrient composition between the concentrated premature formulas and the standard infant formulas. • Glucose polymers comprise 50–60% of the carbohydrate calories, and lactose comprises 40–50%. • Medium Chain Triglycerides (MCTs) are 20–25% of the fat calories. • The protein is either a 60/40 or 50/50 whey/casein ratio. • Improved bone mineral concentration and greater weight and length gains were documented with premature infants fed a transition formula for the first 9 months of life.	• Indications for this formula are not clearly defined. There is no consensus as to which premature infants should receive this formula nor the length of time they should remain on this formula. One suggestion is that the premature infant should remain on this formula until weight for length is between the 25th and 50th percentiles. • Transitional formulas can be provided up to 1 year of corrected age if needed. The greatest effect is during the first 3 to 6 months of corrected age. • Formulas are iron fortified and vitamin dense such that nutrient supplementation may not be needed. To meet the term infant guideline of 400 IU/day for vitamin D, a vitamin D supplement may be needed. • Formulas are available as a powder and can be concentrated to meet the needs of the infant with bronchopulmonary dysplasia. This formula can be provided in the nursery and in the home setting.
Standard infant formulas	• Can be used at discharge for larger premature infants who can gain 20–30 g/day while consuming at least 180 mL/kg/day of this formula.	• Nutrient content is inadequate for the premature infant during the neonatal period. • During the early neonatal period, these formulas may not be tolerated well. Lactose is the sole carbohydrate source, and only long chain fatty acids are incorporated into these formulas.
Elemental infant formula	• Infants who are recovering or suffering from gastrointestinal disorders can benefit from elemental infant formula. • Casein hydrolysates and amino acid formulas are available. • MCTs are a component of some of these formulas. • Glucose or glucose and sucrose are the carbohydrate sources.	• Nutrient content is inadequate for the premature infant, with special reference to calcium and phosphorus levels. • The time to switch to a premature formula must always be considered to improve nutrient intake. Depending on the infant's feeding history, the formulas can be switched or the premature infant formula can be provided as one feed per day and advanced by one additional feed per day as tolerated.
Soy formulas		• These formulas are not indicated for premature infants. • The premature infant is at risk for osteopenia. The phytates in the formula bind phosphorous and make it unavailable for absorption. The aluminum content may also interfere with appropriate bone growth. • The amino acid profile may be inappropriate for the premature infant. • Decreased weight gain and length growth have been reported when soy formulas were fed to premature infants.

Sources: Data from American Academy of Pediatrics Committee on Nutrition. Nutritional needs of preterm infants. In: Kleinman RE, ed. *Pediatric Nutrition Handbook*, 6th ed. Elk Grove Village, IL: American Academy of Pediatrics; 2009:79–112; Schanler RJ, Anderson D. The low birth weight infant. Inpatient care. In: Duggan C, Watkins JB, Walker WA, ed. *Nutrition in Pediatrics: Basic Science Clinical Applications*, 4th ed. Hamilton, Ontario, Canada: BC Decker; 2008:377–394; American Academy of Pediatrics Committee on Nutrition. Failure to thrive. In: Kleinman RE, ed. *Pediatric Nutrition Handbook*, 6th ed. Elk Grove Village, IL: American Academy of Pediatrics; 2009:601–636; Abbott Nutrition. Our products. Available at: www.abbottnutrition.com/Our-Products/Our-Products.aspx. Accessed March 15, 2010; MeadJohnson Nutrition. Healthcare Professional Resource Center Product Information. Available at: http://www.mjn.com/app/iwp/hcp2/content2.do?dm=mj&id=/HCP_Home2/ProductInformation&iwpst=MJN&ls=0&csred=1&r=3456090752. Accessed March 15, 2010; and American Academy of Pediatrics, Bhatia J, Greer F, Committee on Nutrition. Use of soy protein-based formulas in infant feeding. *Pediatrics*. 2008;121:1062–1068.

TABLE 4-12 Enteral Nutrient Guidelines per kg/day

Nutrient	Amount	Nutrient	Amount
Energy (kcal)	105–130	Molybdenum (μg)	0.3
Protein (g)	3.5–4	Iodine (μg)	10–60
Carbohydrate (g)	10– 14	Vitamin A (IU)	700–1500
Fat (g)	5–7	Vitamin D (IU)	150–400*
Sodium (mEq)	2–3	Vitamin E (IU)	6–12
Potassium (mEq)	2–3	Vitamin K (μg)	8–10
Chloride (mEq)	2–3	Vitamin C (mg)	18–24
Calcium (mg)	100–220	Thiamin (μg)	180–240
Phosphorus (mg)	60–140	Riboflavin (μg)	250–360
Magnesium (mg)	7.9–15	Niacin (mg)	3.6–4.8
Iron (mg)	2–4	Vitamin B_6 (μg)	150–210
Zinc (μg)	1000–3000	Folate (μg)	25–50
Copper (μg)	120–150	Vitamin B_{12} (μg)	0.3
Chromium (μg)	0.1–2.25	Biotin (μg)	3.6–6
Manganese (μg)	0.7–7.5	Pantothenic acid (mg)	1.2–1.7
Selenium (μg)	1.3–4.5		

*Maximum of 400 IU/day

Source: Data from American Academy of Pediatrics Committee on Nutrition. Nutritional needs of preterm infants. In: Kleinman RE, ed. *Pediatric Nutrition Handbook*, 6th ed. Elk Grove Village, IL: American Academy of Pediatrics; 2009:79–112.

TABLE 4-13 Milk Comparison for the Premature Infant at 150 mL/kg

Guideline (per kg)	EBM + HMF 24 kcal/oz (powder bovine)	EBM + HMF 24 kcal/oz (liquid donor milk)	Premature Infant Formula 24 kcal/oz	Premature Discharge Formula 22 kcal/oz
105–130 kcal	120	120	120	110
3.5–4 g protein	2.9–3	2.9	3.6–4	3.1–3.2
100–220 mg calcium	169–209	203	197–219	117–132
2–4 mg iron	0.5–2.3	0.2	2.2	2
1–3 mg zinc	1.38–1.8	0.99	1.56–1.8	1.33–1.38
150–400 IU vitamin D	180–225	39	183–288	77–88

Abbreviations: EBM, expressed breast milk; HMF, human milk fortifier; term human milk nutrient concentrations used for calculations.

Sources: Data from American Academy of Pediatrics Committee on Nutrition. Nutritional needs of preterm infants. In: Kleinman RE, ed. *Pediatric Nutrition Handbook*, 6th ed. Elk Grove Village, IL: American Academy of Pediatrics; 2009:79–112; Abbott Nutrition. Our products. Available at: www.abbottnutrition.com/Our-Products/Our-Products.aspx. Accessed March 15, 2010; MeadJohnson Nutrition. Healthcare Professional Resource Center Product Information. Available at: http://www.mjn.com/app/iwp/hcp2/content2.do?dm=mj&id=/HCP_Home2/ProductInformation&iwpst=MJN&ls=0&csred=1&r=3456090752. Accessed March 15, 2010; Gerber. Start healthy stay healthy resource center. Gerber infant nutritional products. Available at: http://medical.gerber.com/products. Accessed March 15, 2010; and Prolact + H^2MF^{TM} *Nutrient Values*. Prolacta Bioscience MKT-0164 Rev-1. 2009.

TABLE 4-14 Methods of Feeding

Type	Considerations
Breast/bottle	Most physiological methods. Infant at least 32 to 34 weeks gestation. Infant medically stable. Infant's respiratory rate less than 60 breaths per minute.
Gavage	Supplement to breast/bottle feedings. Suggested for infants less than 32 weeks gestation. Use for intubated infant. Use for neurologically impaired neonate.
Transpyloric	Employ when gavage feedings not tolerated. Use when the infant is at risk for milk aspiration. Use for the infant with decreased gut motility. Use for the infant with anatomic abnormality of the gastrointestinal tract. Infant intubated. Tube is placed under guided fluoroscopy. Complications include dumping syndrome, nutrient malabsorption, and perforation of intestine. Continuous infusions indicated.
Gastrostomy	Gastrointestinal malformation. Infant neurologically impaired.

Sources: Data from American Academy of Pediatrics Committee on Nutrition. Nutritional needs of preterm infants. In: Kleinman RE, ed. *Pediatric Nutrition Handbook*, 6th ed. Elk Grove Village, IL: American Academy of Pediatrics; 2009:79–112; Schanler RJ, Anderson D. The low birth weight infant. Inpatient care. In: Duggan C, Watkins JB, Walker WA, eds. *Nutrition in Pediatrics: Basic Science Clinical Applications*, 4th ed. Hamilton, Ontario, Canada: BC Decker; 2008:377–394; Sapsford A. Enteral nutrition. In: Pediatric Nutrition Practice Group, Groh-Wargo S, Thompson M, Cox JH, eds. *ADA Pocket Guide to Neonatal Nutrition*. Chicago: American Dietetic Association; 2009:64–103; and Ellard D, Anderson DM. Nutrition. In: Cloherty JP, Eichenwald EC, Stark AR, eds. *Manual of Neonatal Care*, 6th ed. Philadelphia: Wolters Kluwer/Lippincott Williams & Wilkins; 2008:114–136.

TABLE 4-15 Feeding Guidelines

Trophic feedings*	Provide to infants < 1250 g BW Give for 3 days 10–20 mL/kg/day Human milk or 20 kcal/oz premature infant formula Bolus feedings
Feeds initiation and advancement	< 1250 g BW 10–20 mL/kg/day 1250–1500 g BW 20 mL/kg/day 1500–2000 g BW Initiate at 20 mL/kg/day and advance by 20–40 ml/kg/day 2000–2500 g BW Initiate at 20–30 mL/kg/day and advance by 20–40 mL/kg/day to ab libitum (ab lib) depending on clinical status of infant > 2500 g BW Start at 50 mL/kg/day or ab lib with minimum and advance by 20–40 mL/kg/day
Milk selection	< 1800–2000 g BW or < 34 weeks PMA • Human milk; fortify with four packs human milk fortifier/100 mL milk when 100 mL/kg feeds achieved. • Liquid donor milk fortifier added at 40–100 mL/kg/day of human milk • Premature infant formula ≥ 2000 g BW or ≥ 34 weeks PMA • Human milk • Standard infant formula

* Trophic feedings should begin on day 1 or 2 for the medically stable infant. The infant should have a physiologic range blood pressure while receiving 5 μg/kg/min or less of dopamine.

Abbreviations: BW, birthweight; PMA, postmenstrual age.

Source: Data from Clinical Review Committee Nutriton, Metabolic Management Nutrition. In: Anderson DM, Eichenwald EC, Chan SW, et al., eds. *Guidelines for Acute Care of the Neonate*, 17th ed. Houston, TX: Section of Neonatology Department of Pediatrics, Baylor College of Medicine; 2009:97–108.

infant's constantly changing clinical condition and development, several methods will be used. Both continuous and bolus infusions are used with gavage feedings.[13] A recent study demonstrated improved weight gain and feeding tolerance with the use of bolus versus continuous infusion.[51] The use of transpyloric feedings dictates the use of continuous infusion to prevent an osmotic load presented to the intestine and dumping from occurring.[26] The delivery of nutrients to the infant is decreased with continuous infusions.[13,52] Specifically, human milk fat and fat additives and minerals in the human milk fortifier adhere to or precipitate in the delivery system.[52] A bolus feeding or a feeding given over 30 to 120 minutes on a pump can decrease the nutrient loss.[26,52]

Breastfeeding

Mothers who want to breastfeed their premature infant must usually express their milk. During the infant's prolonged hospitalization, it will be difficult for the mother to be available for 24-hour breastfeeding. Further, their infants are too little and/or sick to nurse. Family members, friends, and nursery staff must provide support for these women to enable them to be successful in providing milk during this stressful period (see **Table 4-16**). Kangaroo care (skin-to-skin contact between the parent and the infant) will facilitate parent–infant bonding and has been linked to a longer period of lactation by the mother who delivers prematurely.[53]

TABLE 4-16 Steps to Support Lactating Women

1. Instruction
   - Methods of milk expression
   - Sterilization of expression equipment
   - Storage and transport of milk
   - Diet for lactation
   - Tips for relaxation
2. Tips to help with let down prior to expression
   - Showering
   - Hand massaging of the breasts
   - Applying warm washcloths to the breasts
   - Consuming warm beverages
   - Visiting the infant
   - Talking to the infant's nurse by phone
   - Placing the infant's picture on the pump
3. Nursery staff and nursery support
   - Availability of lactation consultant for mothers and staff
   - Education of nursery staff on milk expression and breastfeeding
   - Electric pump and pumping room conveniently available to the nursery
   - Electric pumps available for rental and hand pumps for purchase
   - Mother's milk used to feed the infant whenever it is available
   - Help mother with the initiation of nursing
   - Promote kangaroo care for skin-to-skin contact
4. Initiation of breastfeeding
   - Wake baby up
   - Express a little milk prior to nursing so nipple is easier to grasp by the small infant
   - Position infant so mother and infant are stomach to stomach
   - Allow mother to room in with baby prior to discharge to establish breastfeeding pattern

Sources: Data from American Academy of Pediatrics Committee on Nutrition. Nutritional needs of preterm infants. In: Kleinman RE, ed. *Pediatric Nutrition Handbook*, 6th ed. Elk Grove Village, IL: American Academy of Pediatrics; 2009:79–112; Hurst NM, Valentine CJ, Renfro L, Burns P, et al. Skin-to-skin holding in the neonatal intensive care unit influences maternal milk volume. *J Peri.* 1997;17:213–217; and Hurst NM, Myatt A, Schanler RJ. Growth and development of a hospital-based lactation program and mother's own milk bank. *JOGNN.* 1998;27:503–510.

Nutritional Assessment

Nutrition assessment is a continual process for the premature infant to ensure optimal nutritional intakes. Dietary considerations, anthropometric measurements, feeding tolerance and laboratory indices will need to be monitored.

Dietary Considerations

Daily assessment is necessary to determine the need for changing feeding volume, solution strength, or feeding method. Intake is evaluated against nutrient guidelines. Finally, feeding technique needs to be advanced to the most physiological method possible for the infant. Breast or bottle feedings are introduced as the infant's coordination of sucking, swallowing, and breathing is developed at 32 to 34 weeks gestation.[13] The number of oral feedings should be increased per day as the infant demonstrates the ability to effectively feed. Feedings are frequently limited to 20 minutes per feeding period to prevent fatigue and excessive energy expenditure.[54] Enteral feedings may be limited to once a day until the infant demonstrates successful feeding.

Anthropometric Measurements

Anthropometric measurements are difficult to perform on premature infants, principally due to an infant's small size and clinical condition. Medical equipment can interfere with the measurement or can add to the recorded weight. Also, the infant is at risk for cold stress during these procedures, which diverts energy from growth to heat production. The new high humidity hybrid incubators contain bed scales that enable infants to be weighed without removing them from their humidity- and temperature-controlled environment.[22]

Weekly weights, lengths, and head circumferences are plotted on intrauterine growth charts to track longitudinal growth and to assess whether the infant is growing at the intrauterine growth rate. Most premature infants will parallel their birth curve and demonstrate catch-up growth later in life. Initial weight loss that reflects the loss of extracellular fluid ranges from 10% to 15% of birth weight during the first week of life.[55] After regaining birth weight, the weight gain goal is 15–20 g/kg/day for infants who weigh less than 2000 g.[26,56] When the infant weighs 2 kg or more, a weight gain of 20 to 30 g/day is appropriate.[26,56] Head circumferences and length measurements should increase by 0.7–1.0 cm/wk.[26]

Daily weights and weekly lengths and head circumferences can be plotted on postnatal premature infant growth charts.[14] (See Appendix A.) These charts reflect the growth of a population of premature infants after birth. The infant's growth is assessed against a group of their peer premature infants and demonstrates how the infant is growing as compared to other premature infants. These charts profile the initial weight loss seen with infants at week 1 of life. The goal is for the infant to stay on his or her growth curve or demonstrate greater growth. Intrauterine growth cannot be assessed by these postnatal growth charts.

Weights will be influenced by the medical equipment attached to the infant, the use of different scales, the infant's hydration status, and total nutrient intake. Weights taken at the same time each day will avoid recording diurnal variations. Alterations in the head circumference measurement will occur from birth to week 1 of life due to head molding or edema. Length board measurements should be used to obtain accurate length measurements.

Skinfolds and mid-arm circumference measurements do not change rapidly enough to be more helpful than weight measurements for diet changes. These measurements are generally not employed for routine clinical care, but are indicated for growth studies. There are limited standards.[14,57,58]

Assessing Inadequate Weight Gain

When a series of daily or weekly measurements indicates inadequate growth, a search must be made for the cause. **Table 4-17** outlines areas to check.

Assessment of Feeding Tolerance

Feeding intolerance and clinical compromise are common for the premature infant, so constant surveillance is required to detect early signs of feeding intolerance, sepsis, or NEC.[56] Depending on the findings, feedings may be held, decreased, diluted, discontinued, or their frequency may be changed. Feedings will often be held due to signs of illness, including persistent apnea and bradycardia, temperature instability, or

TABLE 4-17 Possible Etiologies for Inadequate Weight Gain

1. Nutrient calculations are incorrect.
2. Parenteral nutrition is not optimized.
3. Infant just achieved full enteral feedings meeting guidelines.
4. Infant is not receiving ordered diet.
   - Intravenous fluid administration has been interrupted to give blood or drugs, or the intravenous line has become infiltrated.
   - Infant is unable to consume what is ordered by bottle, and no gavage supplements were provided.
   - Feedings were held because the infant's respiratory rate increased or body temperature instability developed.
   - Feedings were held for clinical tests.
5. Infant does not tolerate given formula.
6. Calculated nutrient guidelines are inadequate for the infant due to illness.
7. Infant is cold stressed.
8. Infant has outgrown previous diet order.
9. Nutrition solution was not prepared correctly.
10. Incorrect formula was provided to infant.
11. Human milk issues
    - Continuous infusion will lead to fat separation in feeding syringe. Switch to bolus feedings or put over a pump for 30 to 90 minutes.
    - Ensure correct number of fortifier packets were added to milk.
    - Ensure infant is not receiving only the foremilk, which is low in fat.
12. Metabolic issues
    - Acidosis
    - Electrolyte abnormality
13. Low hemoglobin
14. Ostomy output

Sources: Data from Anderson DM. Nutritional assessment and therapeutic interventions for the preterm infant. *Clin Peri.* 2002;29:313–326; and Anderson DM. Nutrition for premature infants. In: Samour PQ, King K, eds. *Handbook of Pediatric Nutrition*, 3rd ed. Boston, MA: Jones and Bartlett Publishers; 2005:53–74.

lethargy. There are no universally agreed upon criteria for feeding assessment.[26]

Gastric residuals are often present, but what exactly constitutes an unacceptable volume is difficult to define. Residuals may be due to immature intestinal motor activity, because they are seen prior to feeds initiation.[56] Often during trophic feedings, residuals are acceptable if the infant is clinically stable.[59] Some infants have small aspirates no matter what the feeding volume, and yet are tolerating feedings.[60] With bolus feedings, a residual up to 50% of the feeding volume or 1.5 times the hourly rate for continuous feeding is often accepted.[26] A fixed volume of 2–3 mL/kg/feed has also been used.[26] Mucus residuals are not a concern and are present in the infant recovering from lung disease. Undigested formula may indicate that the feeding volume is too large, that the infant does not tolerate this formula, that the infant has poor gastrointestinal motility, or that the infant has NEC or intestinal obstruction. Residuals containing bile may indicate feeding tubes have moved into the intestine, and are not uncommon when the infant is fed transpylorically.[56] Bile also may indicate intestinal obstruction.[56] Residuals are not a consistent marker of feeding intolerance or NEC, but should be noted in relation to other clinical parameters.[26]

The tonicity of the abdomen should be observed. Increases will occur with air swallowing, feeding intolerance, infrequent stooling, or NEC. When the abdomen is distended and/or tender, an evaluation to rule out bowel obstruction is done.[61] A workup for sepsis and NEC may be considered with other signs of feeding intolerance or when an increase in abdominal tone is noted. Visible loops of bowel may indicate illness.

Blood in the stool or residual is a concern and should be evaluated. Blood may be a sign of illness, feeding-tube irritation of the intestine, anal fissure, or swallowed blood during delivery.

Assessing Nutrient Adequacy and Tolerance

Both the specific clinical signs of nutrient deficiency/toxicity and the associated laboratory values should be assessed regularly. Vitamin and trace mineral assays should be performed when a deficiency is suspected.[62] Serial plasma trace mineral levels may be more helpful than one plasma level when assessing a trace mineral deficiency.[26] There are several reviews on clinical signs.[47,63] Acceptable standards for laboratory values are difficult to establish because premature infants differ by their physical maturity, clinical condition, and nutrient stores; for example, serum proteins will vary by the infant's hepatic maturity, energy and protein intake, vitamin and mineral nutritional status, and clinical condition. Blood urea nitrogen does not correlate to parenteral protein intake the first week of life, but may be helpful for the premature infant fed human milk to determine protein supplementation needs.[64,65]

During the first week of life, serum electrolytes, glucose, creatinine, and urea nitrogen are monitored daily, or more frequently when values are abnormal. As these blood parameters stabilize, they can be examined as clinically indicated.[26] Serum electrolytes are assessed for those infants receiving diuretics or those with a history of abnormal values until values are normal. Additional parameters monitored when PN is being administered include serum triglycerides to check lipid tolerance, direct bilirubin to detect cholestasis, and serum alanine aminotransferase (ALT, serum glutamic-pyruvic transaminase) to evaluate hepatic function.[26] Serum calcium, phosphorus, and alkaline phosphatase levels may be monitored to detect osteopenia in the premature infant.[26] Hematocrit and hemoglobin levels are checked as needed.[26]

Discharge Concerns

The premature infant is ready for discharge from the hospital when body temperature can be maintained, breastfeeding or bottle feeding supports growth, and cardiorespiratory function is mature and stable.[66] Most important, the caretaker must be ready to care for this high-risk infant. Twenty-four-hour visitation allows the parents to become active in caring for their infant. Rooming in with the infant will help to facilitate care and give confidence to the parent.[67]

The infant should be evaluated for participation in the Special Supplemental Nutrition Program for Women, Infants, and Children (WIC), early intervention programs, and a developmental follow-up program for premature infants. The follow-up program should monitor the infant's growth and development, offer aid with chronic illness management, provide early detection of problems, make referrals to specialized services as indicated, and give the parents support and guidance in caring for their prematurely born infant.[11] These clinics not only aid with early detection of problems, but also evaluate the care that newborn intensive care units provide. A primary care physician must be identified to provide well-baby and sick care, and an appointment should be established prior to discharge to home.[66] Most infants will be discharged home on human milk, standard infant formula, or preterm discharge (transition) formula. The breastfed infant should receive a daily multiple vitamin containing 400 IU of vitamin D and a 2 mg/kg iron supplement.[13,68] Breastfed premature infants may need additional nutrients to grow well. Two to three feedings may be given as the discharge formula in place of breastfeeding to enrich their intake of protein and other nutrients. The infant formula-fed with iron will not require additional iron supplementation. Infants receiving the premature discharge formula may require extra vitamins, and the premature infant receiving term formula should receive a multivitamin until 3 kg of body weight is achieved.[13] There is no consensus on which infants should be provided with the discharge formula and how long they should be given it.[13] In Carver's group study, infants provided discharge formula were < 1800 g birth weight. Infants with a birth weight < 1250 g had improved growth for 6 to 12 months of corrected age; the larger infants had improved growth for 1 to 3 months.[69] Lucas and group reported infants < 1750 g birth weight had improved growth for 9 months of corrected age,[70] whereas Koo and Hockman found no growth advantage for premature infants fed premature discharge formula versus a standard, term formula.[71] Infants with a birth weight < 1800 grams should be evaluated for use of preterm discharge formula. The AAP has suggested that the infants remain on the discharge formula until weight for length is at the 25th percentile or greater.[7] Infants suffering from BPD may need a nutrient-dense formula. The premature discharge formulas can be concentrated easily to 24 or 27 kcal/oz.

Conclusion

Although premature infants begin life in a compromised nutritional state, nutrition and medical therapies continue to evolve that enhance the infant's potential for optimal growth and development.[13] Daily nutrition evaluation of the premature infant is necessary to ensure that appropriate nutrition therapy can be provided.

Case Study

Nutrition Assessment

Patient history: A 980-gram female infant was born at 27 weeks gestation and classified as an appropriate for gestational age premature infant on the Fenton growth chart. Length was 36 cm and head circumference was 25 cm. Today the patient is 21 days old or 30 weeks postmenstrual age (PMA). Patient had respiratory distress syndrome, which required intubation and surfactant therapy. Patient is now on room air.

Nutrition history: Patient was on parenteral nutrition, but is now on total enteral feedings of human milk from her mother at 160 mL/kg.

Anthropometric Measurements

Weight: 1085 g

Length: 38 cm

Head circumference: 27 cm

Nutrition Problem

Nutrient intake is inadequate for the premature infant.

Nutrition Interventions

As discussed on team rounds, human milk fortifier will be added to human milk to provide 24 kcal/oz milk. At 160 mL/kg the infant will receive 128 kcal/kg and 3 g protein/kg. The fortifier will bring the nutrient content up to meet the guidelines for prematurity.

Monitoring and Evaluation

The infant's weekly rate of weight, head circumference and length will be calculated and measurements recorded on the Fenton Growth Chart.

Questions for the Reader

1. How did weight, length, and head circumference plot at birth and at 3 weeks or 30 weeks gestation on the Fenton growth chart?
2. What are the kilocalorie and protein goals per kg for this infant?
3. What milk is recommended for the premature infant?
4. What would the feed volume be per feed for feeding every 3 hours at 160 mL/kg?
5. Write one PES.
6. Calculate energy and protein intakes on fortified human milk with powdered bovine fortifier at 160 mL/kg.
7. What should be monitored on a weekly basis in this infant before discharge?

REFERENCES

1. American Academy of Pediatrics, American College of Obstetricians and Gynecologists. *Guidelines for Perinatal Care*, 6th ed. Elk Grove, IL: American Academy of Pediatrics; 2007.
2. Battaglia FC, Lubchenco LO. A practical classification of newborn infants by weight and gestational age. *J Pediatr*. 1967;71:159–163.
3. Fenton TR. A new growth chart for preterm babies: Babson and Benda's chart updated with recent data and a new format. *BMC Pediatrics*. 2003;3:13.
4. Olsen IE, Groveman SA, Lawson ML, et al. New intrauterine growth curves based on United States data. *Pediatrics*. 2010;125:e214–e224.

5. Cloherty JP, Eichenwald EC, Stark A, eds. *Manual of Neonatal Care*, 6th ed. Philadelphia: Wolters Kluwer/Lippincott Williams & Wilkins; 2008.
6. Lee KG. Identifying the high-risk newborn and evaluating gestational age, prematurity, postmaturity, large-for-gestational-age, and small-for-gestational-age infants. In: Cloherty JP, Eichenwald EC, Stark AR, eds. *Manual of Neonatal Care*, 6th ed. Philadelphia: Wolters Kluwer/Lippincott Williams & Wilkins; 2008:41–58.
7. American Academy of Pediatrics Committee on Nutrition. Failure to thrive. In: Kleinman RE, ed. *Pediatric Nutrition Handbook*, 6th ed. Elk Grove Village, IL: American Academy of Pediatrics; 2009:601–636.
8. Hack M, Schluchter M, Cartar L, et al. Growth of very low birth weight infants to age 20 years. *Pediatrics*. 2003;112:e30–e38. Available at: http://www.pediatrics.org/cgi/content/full/112/1/e30. Accessed August 8, 2010.
9. Hack M. Young adult outcomes of very-low-birth-weight children. *Semin Fetal Neonat Med*. 2006;11:127–137.
10. Farooqi A, Hagglof B, Sedin G, Gothefors L, Serenius F. Growth in 10- to 12-year-old children born at 23 to 25 weeks' gestation in the 1990s: a Swedish national prospective follow-up study. *Pediatrics*. 2006;118:e1452–e1465.
11. Wilson-Costello DE, Hack M. Follow-up for high risk neonates. In: Martin RJ, Fanaroff AA, Walsh MC, eds. *Fanaroff and Martin's Neonatal-Perinatal Medicine Diseases of the Fetus and Infant*, 8th ed. Philadelphia: Mosby Elsevier; 2006:1035–1044.
12. Hack M, Breslau N, Weissman B, et al. Effect of very low birth weight and subnormal head size on cognitive abilities at school age. *N Engl J Med*. 991;325:231–237.
13. American Academy of Pediatrics Committee on Nutrition. Nutritional needs of preterm infants. In: Kleinman RE, ed. *Pediatric Nutrition Handbook*, 6th ed. Elk Grove Village, IL: American Academy of Pediatrics; 2009:79–112.
14. Ehrenkranz RA, Younes N, Lemons JA, et al. Longitudinal growth of hospitalized very low birth weight infants. *Pediatrics*. 1999;104:280–289.
15. Tsang RC, Uauy R, Koletzko B, Zlotkin SH, eds. *Nutrition of the Preterm Infant. Scientific Basis and Practical Guidelines*, 2nd ed. Cincinnati, OH: Digital Educational Publishing; 2005.
16. Agostoni C, Buonocoe G, Carnielli VP, et al. Enteral nutrient supply for preterm infants: commentary from the European Society of Paediatric Gastroenterology, Hepatology and Nutrition Committee on Nutrition. *J Pediatr Gastroenterol Nutr*. 2010;50:85–91.
17. Thureen PJ, Melara D, Fennessey PV, et al. Effect of low versus high intravenous amino acid intake on very low birth weight infants in the early neonatal period. *Pediatr Res*. 2003;53:24–32.
18. Te Braake FWJ, Van Den Akker CHP, Wattimena DJL, et al. Amino acid administration to premature infants directly after birth. *J Pediatr*. 2005;147:457–461.
19. Carlson SJ. Parenteral nutrition. In: Pediatric Nutrition Practice Group, Groh-Wargo S, Thompson M, Cox JH, eds. *ADA Pocket Guide to Neonatal Nutrition*. Chicago, IL: American Dietetic Association; 2009:29–63.
20. Doherty EG, Simmons CF. Fluid and electrolyte management. In: Cloherty JP, Eichenwald EC, Stark AR, eds. *Manual of Neonatal Care*, 6th ed. Philadelphia: Wolters Kluwer/Lippincott Williams & Wilkins; 2008:100–113.
21. Stephens BE, Gargus RA, Walden RV, et al. Fluid regimens in the first week of life may increase risk of patent ductus arteriosus in extremely low birth weight infants. *J Perinatol*. 2008;28:123–128.
22. Kim SM, Lee EY, Chen J, et al. Improved care and growth outcomes by using hybrid humidified incubators in very preterm infants. *Pediatrics*. 2010;125:e137–e145.
23. Shulman RJ, Phillips S. Parenteral nutrition in infants and children. *J Pediatr Gastroenterol Nutr*. 2003;36:587–607.
24. Neu J. Is it time to stop starving premature infants? *J Perinatol*. 2009;29:399–400.
25. Putet G. Lipid metabolism of the micropremie. *Clin Perinatol*. 2000;27:57–69.
26. Schanler RJ, Anderson D. The low birth weight infant. Inpatient care. In: Duggan C, Watkins JB, Walker WA, eds. *Nutrition in Pediatrics: Basic Science Clinical Applications*, 4th ed. Hamilton, Ontario, Canada: BC Decker; 2008:377–394.
27. Helms RA, Christensen ML, Mauer EC, et al. Comparison of pediatric versus standard amino acid formulation in preterm neonates requiring parenteral nutrition. *J Pediatr*. 1987;110:466–472.
28. Rivera A, Bell EF, Stegink LD, Ziegler EE. Plasma amino acid profiles during the first three days of life in infants with respiratory distress syndrome: effect of parenteral amino acid supplementation. *J Pediatr*. 1989;115:464–468.
29. Zlotkin SH, Bryan MH, Anderson GH. Cysteine supplementation to cysteine-free intravenous feeding regimens in newborn infants. *Am J Clin Nutr*. 1981;34:914–923.
30. American Academy of Pediatrics Committee on Nutrition. Parenteral nutrition. In: Kleinman RE, ed. *Pediatric Nutrition Handbook*, 6th ed. Elk Grove Village, IL: American Academy of Pediatrics; 2009:519–540.
31. Dunn L, Hulman S, Weiner J, Kliegman R. Beneficial effects of early hypocaloric enteral feeding on neonatal gastrointestinal function: preliminary report of a randomized trial. *J Pediatr*. 1988;112:622–629.
32. Davey AM, Wagner CL, Cox C, et al. Feeding premature infants while low umbilical artery catheters are in place: a prospective, randomized trial. *J Pediatr*. 1994;124:795–799.
33. Jesse N, New J. Necrotizing enterocolitis: relationship to innate immunity, clinical features, and strategies for prevention. *NeoReviews*. 2006;7:e143–e150.
34. Rayyis SF, Ambalavanan N, Wright L, et al. Randomized trial of "slow" versus "fast" feed advancements on the incidence of necrotizing enterocolitis in very low birth weight infants. *J Pediatr*. 1999;134:293–297.
35. Kennedy KA, Tyson JE. Rapid versus slow rate of advancement of feedings for promoting growth and preventing necrotizing enterocolitis in parenterally fed low-birth-weight infants (Cochrane Review). *The Cochrane Library*. 2005. Available at: http://www.nichd.nih.gov/cochrane/Kennedy/KENNEDY.HTM. Accessed August 8, 2010.
36. Patole SK, de Klerk N. Impact of standardized feeding regimens on incidence of neonatal necrotising enterocolitis: a systematic review and meta-analysis of observational studies. *Arch Dis Child Fetal Neonatal Ed*. 2005;90:F147–F151.
37. Schanler RJ, Shulman RJ, Lau C. Feeding strategies for premature infants: beneficial outcomes of feeding fortified human milk versus preterm formula. *Pediatrics*. 1999;103:1150–1157.

38. Morales Y, Schanler RJ. Human milk and clinical outcomes in VLBW infants: how compelling is the evidence of benefit? *Sem Perinatol*. 2007;31:83–88.
39. Sullivan S, Schanler RJ, Kim JH, et al. An exclusively human milk-based diet is associated with a lower rate of necrotizing enterocolitis than a diet of human milk and bovine milk-based products. *J Pediatr*. 2010;156:562–574.
40. Institute of Medicine. *Dietary Reference Intakes for Vitamin C, Vitamin E, Selenium and Carotenoids*. Washington, DC: National Academies Press; 2000.
41. Tyson JE, Wright LL, Oh W, et al. Vitamin A supplementation for extremely-low-birth-weight infants. *N Eng J Med*. 1999;340:1962–1968.
42. Ambalavanan N, Tyson JE, Kennedy KA, et al. Vitamin A supplementation for extremely low birth weight infants: outcome at 18 to 22 months. *Pediatrics*. 2005;115:e249–e254.
43. Darlow BA, Graham PJ. Vitamin A supplementation for preventing morbidity and mortality in very low birthweight infants (Cochrane Review).*The Cochrane Library*. 2008. Available at: http://www.nichd.nih.gov/cochrane/ Darlow/Darlow.htm. Accessed March 15, 2010.
44. Mitchell SM, Rogers S, Hicks PD, et al. High frequencies of elevated alkaline phosphatase activity and rickets exist in extremely low birth weight infants despite current nutritional support. *BMC Pediatr*. 2009;9:47. doi:10.1186/1471-2431-9-47.
45. Kliegman RM.. Intrauterine growth restriction. In: Martin RJ, Fanaroff AA, Walsh MC, eds. *Fanaroff and Martin's Neonatal-Perinatal Medicine Diseases of the Fetus and Infant*, 8th ed. Philadelphia: Mosby Elsevier; 2006:271–306.
46. Koo WWK, Krug-Wispe S, Neylan M, et al. Effect of three levels of vitamin D intake in preterm infants receiving high mineral containing milk. *J Pediatr Gastroenterol Nutr*. 1995;21:182–189.
47. Rao R, Geoergieff M. Microminerals. In: Tsang RC, Uauy R, Koletzlo B, Zlotkin SH, eds. *Nutrition of the Preterm Infant: Scientific Basis and Practical Guidelines*. Cincinnati, OH: Digital Educational Publishing; 2005:277–310.
48. Shulman RJ. Zinc and copper balance studies in infants receiving total parenteral nutrition. *Am J Clin Nutr*. 1989;49:879–883.
49. Atkinson SA, Zlotkin S. Recognizing deficiencies and excesses of zinc, copper, and other trace elements. In: Tsang RC, Zlotkin SH, Nichols BL, Hansen JW, eds. *Nutrition During Infancy: Principles and Practice*, 2nd ed. Cincinnati, OH: Digital Educational Publishing; 1997:209–232.
50. Heird WC, Lapillonne A. The role of essential fatty acids in development. *Annu Rev Nutr*. 2005;25:549–571.
51. Schanler RJ, Shulman RJ, Lau C, et al. Feeding strategies for premature infants: randomized trial of gastrointestinal priming and tube-feeding method. *Pediatrics*. 1999;103:434–439.
52. Rogers S, Hicks PD, Hamzo M, et al. Continuous feedings of fortified human milk lead to nutrient losses of fat, calcium and phosphorous. *Nutrients*. 2010;2:230–240. doi:10.3390/nu2030240.
53. Hurst NM, Valentine CJ, Renfro L, et al. Skin-to-skin holding in the neonatal intensive care unit influences maternal milk volume. *J Perinatol*. 1997;17:213–217.
54. Kalhan SC, Price PT. Nutrition and selected disorders of the gastrointestinal tract. In: Klaus MH, Fanaroff AA, eds. *Care of the High-Risk Neonate*, 5th ed. Philadelphia: W.B. Saunders; 2001:147–194.
55. Dell KM, Davis ID. Fluid, electrolyte, and acid base homeostasis. In: Martin RJ, Fanaroff AA, Walsh MC, eds. *Fanaroff and Martin's Neonatal-Perinatal Medicine Diseases of the Fetus and Infant*, 8th ed. Philadelphia: Mosby Elsevier; 2006:695–712.
56. Anderson DM. Nutritional assessment and therapeutic interventions for the preterm infant. *Clin Peri*. 2002;29:313–326.
57. Vaucher YE, Harrison GG, Udall JN, Morrow G. Skinfold thickness in North American infants 24–41 weeks gestation. *Hum Biol*. 1984;56:713–731.
58. Sasanow SR, Georgieff MK, Pereira GR. Mid-arm circumference and mid-arm/head circumference ratios: standard curves for anthropometric assessment of the neonatal nutritional status. *J Pediatr*. 1986;109:311–315.
59. Metabolic Management Committee. Nutrition. In: Anderson DM, Eichenwald EC, Chan SW, et al., eds. *Guidelines for Acute Care of the Neonate*, 17th ed. Houston, TX: Section of Neonatology Department of Pediatrics, Baylor College of Medicine; 2009:97–108.
60. Rickard K, Gresham E. Nutritional considerations for the newborn requiring intensive care. *J Am Diet Assoc*. 1975;66:592–600.
61. Premji SS, Paes B, Jacobson K, et al. Evidence-based feeding guidelines for very low-birth-weight infants. *Adv Neonat Care*. 2002;2:5–18.
62. Moyer-Mileur LJ. Anthropometric and laboratory assessment of very low birth weight infants: the most helpful measurements and why. *Sem Perinatol*. 2007;31:96–103.
63. Greer FR. Vitamins A, E, and K. In: Tsang RC, Uauy R, Koletzlo B, Zlotkin SH, eds. *Nutrition of the Preterm Infant: Scientific Basis and Practical Guidelines*. Cincinnati, OH: Digital Educational Publishing; 2005:141–172.
64. Ridout E, Melara D, Rottinghaus S, et al. Blood urea nitrogen concentration as a marker of amino-acid intolerance in neonates with birthweight less than 1250 g. *J Perinatol*. 2005;25:130–133.
65. Arslanoglu S, Moro GE, Ziegler EE. Preterm infants fed fortified human milk receive less protein than they need. *J Perinatol*. 2009;29:489–492.
66. American Academy of Pediatrics Committee on Fetus and Newborn. Hospital discharge of the high-risk neonate. *Pediatrics*. 2008;122:1119–1126.
67. American Academy of Pediatrics Committee on Hospital Care. Family-centered care and the pediatrician's role. *Pediatrics*. 2003;112:691–696.
68. American Academy of Pediatrics, Wagner CL, Greer FR, Section on Breastfeeding and Committee on Nutrition. Prevention of rickets and vitamin D deficiency in infants, children, and adolescents. *Pediatrics*. 2008;122:1142–1152.
69. Carver JD, Wu PYK, Hall R, et al. Growth of preterm infants fed nutrient-enriched or term formula after hospital discharge. *Pediatrics*. 2001;107:683–689.
70. Lucas A, Fewtrell MS, Morley R, et al. Randomized trial of nutrient-enriched formula versus standard formula for postdischarge preterm infants. *Pediatrics*. 2001;108:703–711.
71. Koo WWK, Hockman EM. Post hospital discharge feeding for preterm infants: effects of standard compared with enriched milk formula on growth, bone mass, and body composition. *Am J Clin Nutr*. 2006;84:1357–1364.

Normal Nutrition During Infancy

Susan Akers and Sharon Groh-Wargo

At no other time in the lifecycle is nutrition delivery more important for health, growth, and development than during infancy. Ideal feeding experiences are those that meet nutrient demands while focusing on the individual developmental readiness of the infant. The objectives of this chapter are to cover current recommended feeding practices for healthy, full-term infants and to discuss common feeding problems encountered during the first year.

Nutrition Issues at Birth

Newborn infants are born with a relatively poor vitamin K status due to low placental transfer of vitamin K, decreased gastrointestinal vitamin K synthesis, and the low content of vitamin K in breast milk. Therefore, newborns are at risk for vitamin K deficiency bleeding including gastrointestinal bleeding as well as bleeding at the umbilicus and the site of circumcision. A one-time intramuscular injection of 0.5–1 mg vitamin K is recommended for all newborn infants at birth.[1]

All states in the United States are now encouraging parents to have their newborn infants tested for congenital disorders within 48 hours of life. Each year, over 4.1 million infants are screened. Approximately 4000 of these infants will be diagnosed with having a congenital disorder. The test is performed by taking small droplets of blood and placing them onto a screening card. State laboratories then analyze them using tandem mass spectrometry. Actual test procedures and the various disorders screened are state specific. Most states are screening for a core panel of 29 disorders, with an additional potential for 25 other disorders. Some states include more than 50 congenital disorders on their newborn screen test at birth.[2]

The goal of newborn screening is to identify congenital disorders such as in-born errors in metabolism, endocrine disorders, hemoglobinopathies, and perinatally acquired infectious diseases before symptoms occur. Some of these disorders, such as phenylketonuria and maple syrup urine disease, are treatable with alterations in nutrition. It is the responsibility of the primary care physician to make sure newborn screening is done in the appropriate time frame. The dietitian's role is to help determine the appropriate method of feeding when a congenital disease is diagnosed. (See Chapter 9.)

Links to state-specific education and support can be accessed through the National Newborn Screening and Genetics Resources Center (http://genes-r-us.uthscsa.edu/resources/consumer/statemap.htm), the American Academy of Pediatrics (http://www.aap.org), or the American College of Medical Genetics (www.acmg.net/resources/policies/ACT/condition-analyte-links.htm).

The American Academy of Pediatrics Committee on Genetics has developed Newborn Screening Fact Sheets to be used as a reference for providers performing or evaluating newborn screening tests or treating infants with positive tests. Fact sheets are available at http://www.pediatrics.org/cgi/content/full/118/3/e934.[3]

Nutrient Needs

Most newborns can obtain all necessary nutrient requirements from human milk or infant formula alone. Vitamin D is the most likely exception. As the infant reaches 4 to 6 months, nutrient needs become greater than human milk or formula alone can provide. Solid foods become necessary for adequate satiety. Supplemental iron and fluoride also may become necessary. During infancy, distribution of calories is generally recommended to be 40% to 50% fat and 7% to 11% protein, with the remaining calories from carbohydrates.[4] Adding solid foods to the diet may alter the distribution of nutrients. This is a significant factor when deciding on the type and amount of solids to add to the diet. (See "Supplementation" and "Weaning and Feeding Progression" later in this chapter.)

Dietary reference intakes (DRIs) for infants are available as adequate intakes (AI) from the Institute of Medicine. Fluid needs are estimated at 700 mL per day for 0- to 6-month-old infants and 800 mL per day for 7- to 12-month-old infants.[5] Average estimated daily energy requirements (kcal/kg) based on reference body weights for 0–6 months (6 kg) and 7–12 months (9 kg) of age are 90 kcal/kg and 80 kcal/kg, respectively, with a range of 80–110 kcal/kg. Specific energy needs can be estimated with the equations in **Exhibit 5-1**.[4] Mean daily protein needs are estimated at 1.5 g protein/kg and 1.2 g protein/kg for 0- to 6-month-old and 7- to 12-month-old infants, respectively. DRIs are available online at http://www.nap.edu. A complete listing of AIs for infants is in Appendix H.

Breastfeeding

Breastfeeding is the recommended method of feeding for virtually all infants.[1,6] Both the American Academy of Pediatrics (AAP)[7] and the American Dietetic Association (ADA)[8] promote breastfeeding as the best source of infant nutrition. The distribution of women who choose to breastfeed varies among different cultures, ethnic backgrounds, education levels, and ages. Statistically, those with the lowest initiation rates for breastfeeding are African Americans, the poor, the less educated, those younger than 20 years of age, and those women participating in the Special Supplemental Nutrition Program for Women, Infants, and Children (WIC).[8] The greatest increases in initiation rates since the 1990s were observed in African American women and mothers younger than 20 years old.[9] Recent data suggest that we are approaching the goal established in 2010 Healthy People that 75% of newborns receive breast milk during the early postpartum period.[8,10] The average rates of infants being exclusively breastfed at 6 and 12 months are 43% and 21%, respectively, and are lower than the Healthy People 2010 goals of 50% and 25%, respectively.[8] Women returning to work and those participating in WIC are the most likely to wean from the breast before these ages.[8,9] Education and support can help these groups make informed choices. Health professionals need to be knowledgeable about both the science and art of breastfeeding, as well as understand the general nutrition needs of their patients.[11]

EXHIBIT 5-1 Equations for Calculating Energy Needs of Infants

0–3 months: (89 × weight [kg] − 100) + 175 kcal
4–6 months: (89 × weight [kg] − 100) + 56 kcal
7–12 months: (89 × weight [kg] − 100) + 22 kcal

Source: Data from Institute of Medicine. *Dietary Reference Intakes for Energy, Carbohydrate, Fiber, Fat, Fatty Acids, Cholesterol, Protein, and Amino Acids (Macronutrients).* Washington, DC: National Academies Press; 2005.

Informed Choice

In order to make an informed decision, each mother, together with the baby's father or other significant family member, needs to weigh the implications of feeding choices. This process is ideally completed early in the pregnancy. Studies have shown that women's attitudes regarding breastfeeding are influenced more by familial and social opinions than by sociodemographic factors.[12] Nutritional and health advantages commonly listed for human milk and breastfeeding include:

- Superior nutritional composition[6–8,13]
- Provision of immunologic and enzymatic components[6,7]
- Health benefits for mothers[6,7]
- Lower cost and increased convenience[7]
- Enhanced maternal–infant bonding[6]
- Decreased incidence of respiratory and gastrointestinal infections[7,14]
- Leaner body composition for infants at 1 year of age[15]
- Decreased incidence of atopic dermatitis[16]
- Controversial benefits of decreased risk for obesity in adulthood[17,18] and improved cognitive development[13]

Human Milk Composition

Human milk is not a uniform body of fluids but a secretion of the mammary gland with changing composition.[6] The composition of human milk varies from individual to individual, and also with stage of lactation, time of day, time into feeding, and maternal diet.[19] Laboratory techniques continue to improve, allowing the over 200 constituents of maternal milk to be analyzed and identified.[6] (See **Table 5-1**.) The four stages of human milk expression are colostrum, transitional milk, mature milk, and extended lactation, each containing its own significant biochemical components and properties.

- Colostrum is the milk produced during the first several days following delivery. It is lower in fat and energy than mature milk but higher in protein, fat-soluble vitamins, minerals, and electrolytes.[6] This early stage of lactation also provides a rich source of antibodies.[6] Human milk has a ratio of about 80:20 casein-to-whey ratio[6] in colostrum, which decreases to about 55:45 in mature human milk.
- Transition milk begins approximately 7 to 14 days postpartum, when the concentration of immunoglobulins and total proteins decreases and the amount of lactose, fat, and total calories increases.[6]
- The third phase, beginning at about 2 weeks postpartum, referred to as mature milk and described above, continues throughout lactation until about 7 to 8 months.[6]

- Extended lactation (7 months to 2 years) results in milk different from colostrum, transitional, and mature human milk. Its carbohydrate, protein, and fat content remains relatively stable, but concentrations of vitamins and minerals continue to decrease gradually over time until weaning off breast milk. Some of these declining nutrients include calcium, zinc, and lactose.[6,20]

Maternal Diet During Breastfeeding

Throughout pregnancy, the maternal body is preparing for lactation by increasing the development of breast tissue and storing additional nutrients and energy.[6] The nutritional requirements during lactation are high, exceeding those in both pregnancy and the nonpregnant state, and are designed to meet the additional demands of lactation without compromising the nutrient stores of the mother.[19] The DRIs for the lactation period can be found online at http://www.nap.edu and in Appendix H. In general, the recommendations for breastfeeding women during lactation include a well-balanced diet, with an additional 300–400 calories and 25 grams of protein per day for milk production. For those mothers not motivated to eat a well-balanced diet or for those avoiding primary food groups, continuation of a prenatal vitamin and possibly calcium supplementation are recommended. Lactation will not produce a net drain on the mother if the amount of energy available and the requirements of any given nutrient are replaced in the diet.[6,19] Energy requirements are greater if weight gain during the pregnancy was low, weight during lactation falls below standards for height and age, and/or more than one infant is being nursed. There is some evidence that successful lactation can be maintained at energy intakes somewhat lower than the DRIs, without adversely affecting lactation performance or infant growth.[6,19,21] It is suggested that iron supplementation of the mother be continued postpartum whether breastfeeding or not, in order to replenish iron stores depleted by pregnancy.[22]

Most breastfeeding women experience increased thirst. This should naturally result in additional intake of fluids. There is no evidence that forcing fluids will increase, or restricting fluids will decrease, milk production.[6,23] Regular exercise and weight loss up to 2 kg per month should not affect milk production,[23] but both should be kept within moderate levels to help conserve the mother's energy to care for the infant.

In summary, the composition of breast milk remains stable even with significant variability in women's diets. Except in cases of chronic deficiency, the quantity and quality of breast milk can support growth and promote the health of infants even when the mother's supply of nutrients is

TABLE 5-1 Composition of Mature Human Milk and Cow Milk

Nutrient (per liter)	Human Milk	Cow Milk
Macronutrients		
Energy (kcal)	650–700	627
Protein (g)	9	32
Carbohydrate (g)	67–70	46
Fat (g)	35	35
Vitamins		
Retinol (mg)	0.3–0.6	Variable
Carotenoids (mg)	0.2–0.6	N/A
Vitamin D (μg)	0.33	—*
Vitamin E (mg)	3–8	0.4
Vitamin K (μg)	2–3	1–4
Vitamin C (mg)	100	30
Thiamine (μg)	200	388
Riboflavin (μg)	400–600	914
Vitamin B_6 (μg)	90–310	554
Vitamin B_{12} (μg)	0.5–1	4.3
Nicotinic acid (μg)	1800–6000	1667
Folic acid (μg)	80–140	60
Pantothenic acid (μg)	2000–2500	3251
Biotin (μg)	5–9	47
Minerals		
Calcium (mg)	200–250	1150
Phosphorus (mg)	120–140	910
Magnesium (mg)	30–35	96
Iron (mg)	0.3–0.9	0.5
Zinc (μg)	1000–3000	4
Manganese (μg)	3	40
Copper (μg)	200–400	30
Chromium (μg)	0.5	<5
Selenium (μg)	7–33	Variable
Fluoride (μg)	4–15	45
Sodium (mg)	120–250	515
Potassium (mg)	400–550	1400
Chloride (mg)	400–450	970
Other Composition Data		
Protein source	60–70% whey; 30–40% casein	18% whey; 82% casein
% calories protein	6–7	20
Carbohydrate source	Lactose	Lactose
% calories carbohydrate	43	30
Fat source	Human	Butterfat
% calories fat	50	50
Potential renal solute load (mOsm/L)	93	308
Osmolality (mOsm/kg H_2O)	290–300	275

*Vitamin D added.

Abbreviation: N/A, not available.

Sources: Data from Lawrence RA, Lawrence RM. *Breastfeeding: A Guide for the Medical Profession*, 6th ed. St. Louis, MO: Mosby; 2005; American Academy of Pediatrics, American College of Obstetricians and Gynecologists. *Breastfeeding Handbook for Physicians.* 2006; Fomon SJ. *Nutrition of Normal Infants*. St. Louis, MO: Mosby; 1993; and Jensen RG. *Handbook of Milk Composition*. New York: Academic Press; 1995.

somewhat limited.[16] However, maternal diet can affect milk composition in the following ways:

- Fatty acid composition mirrors maternal intake.[13,19]
- Vitamin content is reduced in maternal deficiency and increases with supplementation; pharmacological doses of vitamin D (4000–6000 IU per day) can increase vitamin D content of milk, but current recommendations are for supplementing the infant rather than the breastfeeding mother.[6,24,25]
- Mineral content is generally unaffected by maternal intake with two notable exceptions: selenium and iodine.[6]
- Colic symptoms may appear in babies whose mothers drink a lot of cow milk, due to transmission of allergens in the milk.[26]
- Caffeine, nicotine, and alcohol will pass into milk, possibly causing adverse affects in the baby when maternal consumption is high.[6,27,28]
- Medications, both prescription and over-the-counter, and environmental contaminants may pass into milk.[1,6,7]

Management of Lactation

Successful lactation is greatly influenced by the motivation and confidence of the mother, and by support from family and friends, especially the father, and medical professionals. The ability to lactate is a natural characteristic of all mammals, and infants have the capability to suckle even in utero. Infant suckling stimulates release of the hormones prolactin, responsible for milk production, and oxytocin, responsible for milk release, from the pituitary.[29] In order to establish and sustain lactation, therefore, it is necessary to allow the baby access to the breast on demand. The more a mother nurses, the more milk she will produce. The following list offers some tips for ensuring breastfeeding success:

- *Initial breastfeeding:* This should take place as soon after delivery as possible, ideally within the first hour of life.
- *Positioning:* The mother should find a comfortable position either lying down or sitting up. Pillows can support the baby's body and the mother's back and arms. She should change the position of the baby with every feeding during the first few weeks so that pressure on the mother's nipple is rotated, allowing complete emptying of all milk ducts. The mother should use one hand to support and guide her breast and the other hand around the baby's back, cupping the infant's bottom to support and move the baby.
- *Latching on:* The mother can stimulate the rooting reflex by touching the baby's closest cheek. When the mouth is open wide, she pulls the baby close. Be sure that most of the mother's areola is in the baby's mouth, the baby's lower lip is turned out, and the tongue is under the mother's nipple. Rapid sucking, followed by slower, rhythmic sucking and swallowing, will stimulate the milk ejection reflex (MER), or the actual release of milk. Signs that let-down has occurred include rapid swallowing by the infant, tingling in the breast, tightening in the uterus, milk around the baby's mouth, or milk dripping from the other breast. The mother can insert her finger in the side of the baby's mouth to break the suction before moving the baby off the breast.
- *Timing:* During the first few weeks, the baby should be nursed 8 to 12 times a day, or about every 2 to 3 hours. The feedings will become less frequent after breastfeeding is established. It is more important to completely empty the first breast and get adequate hind milk than it is to breastfeed from both sides. Alternating breasts from feeding to feeding establishes good milk supply on both sides. The baby should dictate the duration of feeding.
- *Assessing adequacy (or "How do I know if my baby is getting enough?"):* A newborn who is receiving adequate fluid and calories will (1) have at least six to eight thoroughly wet diapers a day (maybe only four to five heavy wet diapers if they are disposable); (2) have a bowel movement with most feedings; (3) nurse 8 to 12 times a day; (4) seem satisfied after nursing; and (5) gain approximately 1 oz a day in the first 3 months of life.[6,29,30]

A number of situations arise during the early weeks of breastfeeding that, if unanticipated and poorly managed, can jeopardize a successful nursing experience. **Table 5-2** points out the most frequent complaints from breastfeeding mothers and possible treatments. Many new mothers return to work or school after their babies are born. They can continue to breastfeed by

- Arranging to go to the baby or having the baby brought to them
- Pumping and saving the milk in a refrigerator for use within 48 hours or a freezer for up to 3 months
- Discontinuing the feeding(s) when they are away but continuing to nurse at other times

There are several good sources that discuss these alternatives, as well as issues related to milk storage.[6,29,30,31,32]

Bottle-Feeding

Breast milk composition continues to be the gold standard by which infant formulas are modeled. However, when breastfeeding is not chosen, is unsuccessful, or is stopped before 1 year of age, bottle-feeding with a commercially

TABLE 5-2 Most Frequent Complaints from Breastfeeding Mothers

Problem	Description	Treatment
Sore nipples	These are most often the result of improper positioning.	Involves nursing on the least sore nipple first and changing the position of the baby's mouth on the mother's nipple.
Engorgement	This painful swelling of the breast can occur as mature milk production begins and is accompanied by an increase in blood flow and fluid accumulation.	Frequent nursing may help to minimize the discomfort until the breast adjusts. Expressing more milk than is necessary to relieve the pressure will only result in increased milk production and should be discouraged.
Jaundice	In the newborn, this is associated with an elevated bilirubin level and is often the result of inadequate feeding.[2]	Early and frequent feedings will facilitate a good milk supply and stimulate increased gut motility, thus decreasing the absorption of bilirubin.
Poor milk supply	This is probably more a theoretical concern than an actual problem because many mothers are insecure with their ability to successfully provide adequate nutrition without tangible evidence of consumption. Overuse of pacifiers may deter the mother from offering the breast as comfort.	Information about assessing adequacy should be presented in a positive and supportive manner. Frequent feedings and adequate rest will do more to promote milk production than forcing fluids or increasing calories in the mother, unless the diet is severely restricted.

Sources: American Academy of Pediatrics, American College of Obstetricians and Gynecologists. *Breastfeeding Handbook for Physicians*. Elk Grove Village, IL: American Academy of Pediatrics; 2006; and Meek JY, ed. *New Mother's Guide to Breastfeeding*. New York: Bantam Books; 2002.

prepared iron-fortified infant formula is the recommended alternative.[1] The infant formula market continues to expand and offers a wide variety of products.

Infant Formula Composition

The AAP[4] and the Food and Drug Administration (FDA)[33] have identified the importance of regulating the composition and safety of infant formulas. The Infant Formula Act of 1980 was reviewed and updated by an expert panel within the Life Science Research Office (LSRO) and focused on the minimums and maximums of nutrients present in infant formulas.[1,33] These desirable ranges for each nutrient must remain at optimal bioavailable levels throughout the shelf life of each product and provide complete nutrition for the first 4 to 6 months of life.[1] Formulas are grouped by the following categories: standard, soy, protein hydrolysate, elemental or amino acid, and follow-up formulas. A recent review is available.[34] This chapter discusses formulas indicated for term infants. See **Table 5-3** for an overview of infant formula products and **Tables 5-4 through 5-8** for detailed nutritional information of selected products. Updated product information is available at company Websites including:

- http://abbottnutrition.com (Abbott Nutrition/Similac products)
- http://www.gerber.com (Gerber/Nestle Good Start products)
- http://www.mjn.com (Mead Johnson/Enfamil products)
- http://www.nutriciahealthcare.com (Nutricia/Neocate products)
- http://www.pbmproducts.com (store brand); detailed nutritional information on Wal-Mart store brand at http://www.parentschoicemedical.com

Formulas for premature infants or babies older than 1 year old are discussed in Chapters 4 and 6.

Standard Formulas

The most common human milk substitute is standard infant formula. These formulas are made from cow's milk by removing the butterfat, adding vegetable oils, and decreasing the protein. Standard formulas vary in their ratio of casein to whey. Although the addition of demineralized whey appears to result in a product that more closely mimics human milk, there is a lack of scientific data to support superior performance over other standard formulas when fed to babies.[1,35]

Approximately 40–50% of energy provided by standard infant formula comes from fat.[1] The addition of arachidonic acid (ARA) and docosahexaenoic acid (DHA) to infant formulas is recognized as safe, but clinical trials reporting effects on cognitive, social, and motor development have been inconsistent.[34,36] Significant benefits are still controversial.[36] The use of palm olein oils as a source of fat in infant formulas has been found to decrease the absorption of calcium, negatively affecting bone mineralization.[37]

Although the incidence of primary lactose intolerance remains rare in infancy, the infant formula market has

TABLE 5-3 Summary of Formula Products for Infants and Young Toddlers

Product Names	Manufacturer	Comments on Composition[#]	Forms Available[§]				
			P	LC	RTF	H	ALL
Milk-Based: For healthy full term infants when breast milk not available							
Enfamil Premium Triple Health Guard	Mead Johnson	Prebiotic; Nucleotides					✓
Nestle Good Start Gentle Plus	Gerber		✓	✓	✓		
Nestle Good Start Protect Plus	Gerber	Probiotic	✓				
Nestle Good Start Nourish Plus	Gerber	No DHA/ARA	✓				
Similac Advance Early Shield	Abbott Nutrition	Prebiotic; carotenoids; nucleotides					✓
Similac Organic	Abbott Nutrition	Certified USDA organic; nucleotides	✓		✓	✓	
Store Brand Standard	PBM Products*	Nucleotides	✓				
Store Brand Organic	PBM Products*	Certified USDA organic; nucleotides	✓				
Store Brand Prebiotic	PBM Products*	Prebiotic; nucleotides	✓				
Store Brand Probiotic	PBM Products*	Probiotic	✓				
Milk-Based Low/No Lactose: Perceived sensitivity to lactose; fussiness; gas							
Enfamil Gentlease	Mead Johnson	Partially hydrolyzed protein; reduced lactose	✓				
Similac Sensitive	Abbott Nutrition	Lactose free; nucleotides					✓
Store Brand Sensitivity	PBM Products*	Lactose free; nucleotides	✓				
Store Brand Gentle	PBM Products*	Partially hydrolyzed protein; reduced lactose	✓				
Milk-Based Added Rice Starch: Frequent spit-up							
Enfamil A.R	Mead Johnson		✓		✓	✓	
Similac Sensitive RS	Abbott Nutrition	Lactose free	✓		✓		
Store Brand Added Rice Starch	PBM Products*		✓				
Soy-Based: Galactosemia; lactose free for primary or secondary lactose intolerance; vegetarian family							
Good Start Soy Plus	Gerber		✓	✓	✓		
Isomil Advance	Abbott Nutrition						✓
Isomil DF	Abbott Nutrition	Added dietary fiber to firm loose/watery stools			✓		
Prosobee	Mead Johnson						✓
Store Brand Soy	PBM Products*		✓				
Store Brand Organic Soy	PBM Products*	Certified USDA organic	✓				
Protein Hydrolysate: hypoallergenic; extensively hydrolyted protein for allergy to cow milk							
Alimentum	Abbott Nutrition		✓		✓	✓	
Nutramigen	Mead Johnson						✓
Nutramigen with Enflora LGG	Mead Johnson	Probiotic	✓				
Pregestimil	Mead Johnson		✓			✓	
Amino Acid–Based: nonallergenic; elemental formula for severe cow milk protein allergy							
EleCare	Abbott Nutrition	33% MCT	✓				
Neocate Infant	Nutricia	5% MCT; No DNA or ARA	✓				
Neocate Infant with DNA and ARA	Nutricia	33% MCT	✓				
Nutramigen AA	Mead Johnson	0% MCT	✓				

TABLE 5-3 *(Continued)*

Product Names	Manufacturer	Comments on Composition#	Forms Available§				
			P	LC	RTF	H	ALL
Follow-up: complete nutrition for older infants and toddlers							
Enfagrow Premium Next Step	Mead Johnson	10–36 months	✓		✓		
Enfagrow Premium Next Step Soy	Mead Johnson	10–36 months	✓				
Go and Grow Milk-Based	Abbott Nutrition	9–24 months	✓				
Go and Grow Soy-Based	Abbott Nutrition	9–24 months	✓				
Good Start Gentle Plus 2	Gerber	9–24 months	✓				
Good Start Protect Plus 2	Gerber	9–24 months; Probiotic added	✓				
Good Start Soy Plus 2	Gerber	9–24 months	✓				
Store Brand Follow-up	PBM Products*	9 months and older	✓				

#Products contain DHA and ARA unless otherwise noted

*Store brands include: CVS/pharmacy; Walgreens; Wegmans; AAFES; Publix; Target; PathMark; Sam's Club; NEX; VyVee; Shopko; Walmart; RiteAid; Topco; ToysRus; Safeway; Giant Eagle; Weis; Food Lion; Price Chopper; Meijer; BJ's; Winn Dixie; Western Family; Drug Mart; Kroger; Ralphs; Fry's; QFC; Dillons; Smith's; King Soopers; FredMeyer; Food4Less; Roundy's; SuperValu; Albertsons; Jewel-Osco; Cub Foods; ACME; Bigg's; Shaw's Star; Amway

§P = powder; LC = liquid concentrate; RTF = ready to feed; H = ready to feed for hospital use.

Sources: Table data retrieved from manufacturers' websites (accessed January 10, 2010): Abbott Nutrition, http://abbottnutrition.com; Gerber, http://www.gerber.com; Mead Johnson, http://www.mjn.com; Nutricia, http://www.nutriciahealthcare.com; WalMart Store Brand, http://www.pbmproducts.com (detailed nutritional information on WalMart Store Brand at http://www.parentschoicemedical.com).

expanded standard formulas to include lactose-free products. The only indications for using a lactose-free formula are galactosemia, primary lactase deficiency, and relief of temporary or secondary lactose intolerance following gastroenteritis.[34]

Prebiotics, probiotics, and mixtures of pre- and probiotics are now being added to infant formulas. Oligosaccharides function as prebiotics that selectively target the growth of "friendly" bacteria in the colon and are the third most abundant component of human milk.[38] Most, but not all, studies suggest that infants fed formulas supplemented with galacto-oligosaccharides and/or other prebiotics may have more bifidobacteria and lactobacillus in the colon, which results in softer stools, and may benefit from protection against the development of allergies and infections.[39–42] Limited experience with probiotic-supplemented infant formula is promising regarding safety, tolerance, and gastrointestinal benefit.[43,44] There are fewer concerns about potential adverse effects of probiotic-supplemented products when they are fed to infants older than 5 months because these infants have a more mature immune response, an established intestinal colonization, and a history of exposure to a variety of organisms from the environment.[45]

Cow's milk–based formulas thickened with added rice starch are available for infants for gastroesophageal reflux (GER).[34] Anti-reflux formulas appear safe, are nutritionally adequate, and have been shown to decrease episodes of regurgitation and emesis.[46,47] It is not known if they improve growth or development. An added rice starch formula intended to help babies sleep longer is also available (http://www.mjn.com). See also Chapter 12.

Standard formulas are marketed as iron fortified (12 mg/quart) and low iron (1 mg/quart). Only the iron-fortified formulas meet the iron requirements of infancy; the AAP has discouraged the use of low-iron formulas.[48]

Soy Formulas

In the 1960s, soy formulas were developed for infants who could not tolerate cow's milk protein or lactose. Soy formulas can also be useful for infants with galactosemia, with congenital lactase deficiency, or who are born to families practicing vegetarianism.[34] Despite limited indications, soy formulas currently represent about 25% of the infant formula market in the United States.[49] Recent studies have discouraged the use of soy formulas for infants with cow's milk protein (CMP) allergy. About 10–14% of infants with CMP allergy will also have a soy allergy.[50,51] For example, an infant who cannot tolerate a standard milk-based formula such as Similac also may not tolerate a soy formula such as Isomil. Infants with CMP allergy, or infants with CMP-induced enteropathy or enterocolitis, should be fed protein hydrolysates or amino acid–based formulas. The routine use of soy formula has no proven value in the prevention or management of infantile colic or fussiness.[49]

Soy formulas contain methionine-, carnitine-, and taurine-fortified soy protein isolate. The protein content of soy

TABLE 5-4 Standard Infant Formulas (Composition per 100 kcal)

	Enfamil Premium Triple Health Guard (3)	Nestle Good Start Gentle Plus (2)*	Similac Advance Early Shield (1)	Store Brand Standard (5)**
Macronutrients				
Energy (kcal)	100	100	100	100
Volume (ml)	150	150	150	150
Protein				
g	2.1	2.2	2.1	2.1
% kcal	8.5	9	8	8.5
Source	Whey and nonfat milk	Whey protein concentrate	Nonfat milk; whey protein concentrate	Nonfat milk; whey protein concentrate
Carbohydrate				
g	11	11.2	11.2	10.9
% kcal	43.5	45	43	43.5
Source	Lactose; GOS	Lactose	Lactose; GOS	Lactose
Fat				
g	5.3	5.1	5.4	5.3
% kcal	48	46	49	48
Source	Palm olein, soy, coconut and high oleic sunflower oils	Palm olein, soy, coconut and high oleic sunflower (or safflower) oils	High oleic safflower, soy and coconut oils	Palm olein, coconut, soy and high oleic sunflower (or safflower) oils
Linoleic acid (mg)	860	900	1000	N/A
Vitamins				
Vitamin A (IU)	300	300	300	300
Vitamin D (IU)	60	60	60	60
Vitamin E (IU)	2	2	1.5	2
Vitamin K (mcg)	9	8	8	8
Vitamin C (mg)	12	10	9	12
Thiamine B_1 (mcg)	80	100	100	80
Riboflavin B_2 (mcg)	140	140	150	140
Vitamin B_6 (mcg)	60	75	60	60
Vitamin B_{12} (mcg)	0.3	0.33	0.25	0.3
Niacin (mcg)	1000	1050	1050	1000
Folic acid (mcg)	16	15	15	16
Pantothenic acid (mcg)	500	450	450	500
Biotin (mcg)	3	4.4	4.4	3
Minerals				
Calcium (mg)	78	67	78	78
Phosphorus (mg)	43	38	42	43
Magnesium (mg)	8	7	6	8
Iron (mg)	1.8	1.5	1.8	1.8

TABLE 5-4 *(Continued)*

	Enfamil Premium Triple Health Guard (3)	Nestle Good Start Gentle Plus (2)*	Similac Advance Early Shield (1)	Store Brand Standard (5)**
Zinc (mg)	1	0.8	0.75	1
Manganese (mcg)	15	15	5	15
Copper (mcg)	75	80	90	75
Iodine (mcg)	15	12	6	10
Selenium (mcg)	2.8	3	1.8	2.8
Sodium (mg)	27	27	24	27
Potassium (mg)	108	108	105	108
Chloride (mg)	63	65	65	63
Other data				
kcal/oz (usual dilution)	20	20	20	20
DHA/ARA added?	yes	Yes; product without DHA/ARA also available	yes	yes

Abbreviation: GOS, galactooligosaccharide.
*Similar product with probiotics also available
**Similar product with GOS available
(1) Abbott Nutrition
(2) Gerber
(3) Mead Johnson
(4) Nutricia
(5) PBM

TABLE 5-5 Soy Protein-Based Infant Formulas (Composition per 100 kcal)

	Good Start Soy Plus (2)	Isomil Advance (1)#	Prosobee (3)	Store Brand Soy (5)
Macronutrients				
Energy (kcal)	100	100	100	100
Volume (ml)	150	150	150	150
Protein				
g	2.5	2.4	2.5	2.5
% kcal	10	10	10	10
Source	Soy protein isolate, L-methionine	Soy protein isolate, L-methionine	Soy protein isolate, L-methionine	Soy protein isolate, L-methionine
Carbohydrate				
g	11.1	10.3	10.6	10.6
% kcal	44	41	42	42
Source	Corn maltodextrine and sugar	Corn syrup solids and sugar	Corn syrup solids	Corn syrup
Fat				
g	5.1	5.5	5.3	5.3
% kcal	46	49	48	48
Source	Palm olein, soy, coconut and high oleic sunflower (or safflower) oils	High oleic safflower, soy and coconut oils	Palm olein, soy, coconut and high oleic sunflower oils	Palm olein, coconut, soy and high oleic sunflower (or safflower) oils

(continued)

TABLE 5-5 *(Continued)*

	Good Start Soy Plus (2)	Isomil Advance (1)*	Prosobee (3)	Store Brand Soy (5)
Linoleic acid (mg)	920	1000	860	N/A
Vitamins				
Vitamin A (IU)	300	300	300	300
Vitamin D (IU)	60	60	60	60
Vitamin E (SU)	3	1.5	2	2
Vitamin K (mcg)	9	11	8	8
Vitamin C (mg)	12	9	12	12
Thiamine B_1 (mcg)	60	60	80	80
Riboflavin B_2 (mcg)	94	90	90	90
Vitamin B_6 (mcg)	60	60	60	60
Vitamin B_{12} (mcg)	0.3	0.45	0.3	0.3
Niacin (mcg)	1050	1350	1000	1000
Folic acid (mcg)	16	15	16	16
Pantothenic acid (mcg)	500	750	500	500
Biotin (mcg)	5	4.5	3	3
Minerals				
Calcium (mg)	105	105	105	105
Phosphorus (mg)	63	75	69	69
Magnesium (mg)	11	7.5	11	11
Iron (mg)	1.8	1.8	1.8	1.8
Zinc (mg)	0.9	0.75	1.2	1.2
Manganese (mcg)	25	25	25	25
Copper (mcg)	80	75	75	75
Iodine (mcg)	15	15	15	15
Selenium (mcg)	3	1.8	2.8	2.8
Sodium (mg)	40	44	36	36
Potassium (mg)	116	108	120	120
Chloride (mg)	71	62	80	80
Other data				
kcal/oz (usual dilution)	20	20	20	20
DHA/ARA added?	yes	yes	yes	yes

*Similar product with added fiber available

(1) Abbott Nutrition

(2) Gerber

(3) Mead Johnson

(4) Nutricia

(5) PBM

TABLE 5-6 Protein Hydrolysate[#] Infant Formulas (Composition per 100 kcal)

	Alimentum (1)	Nutramigen (3)*	Pregestimil (3)
Macronutrients			
Energy (kcal)	100	100	100
Volume (m1)	150	150	150
Protein			
g	2.8	2.8	2.8
% kcal	11	11	11
Source	Casein hydrolysate; L-amino acids	Casein hydrolysate; L-amino acids	Casein hydrolysate; L-amino acids
Carbohydrate			
g	10.2	10.3	10.2
% kcal	41	41	41
Source	Sugar, modified tapioca starch	Corn syrup solids and modified corn starch**	Corn syrup solids, dextrose and modified corn starch**
Fat			
g	5.5	5.3	5.6
% kcal	48	48	48
Source	Safflower and soy oils, medium chain triglycerides	Palm olein, soy, coconut and high oleic sunflower oils	Soy, corn and high oleic oils, medium chain triglycerides
Linoleic acid (mg)	1900	860	940
Vitamins			
Vitamin A (IU)	300	300	350
Vitamin D (IU)	45	50	50
Vitamin E (1U)	3	2	4
Vitamin K (mcg)	15	8	12
Vitamin C (mg)	9	12	12
Thiamine B_1 (mcg)	60	80	80
Riboflavin B_2 (mcg)	90	90	90
Vitamin B_6 (mcg)	60	60	60
Vitamin B_{12} (mcg)	0.45	0.3	0.3
Niacin (mcg)	1350	1000	1000
Folic acid (mcg)	15	16	16
Pantothenic acid (mcg)	750	500	500
Biotin (mcg)	4.5	3	3
Minerals			
Calcium (mg)	105	94	94
Phosphorus (mg)	75	52	52
Magnesium (mg)	7.5	11	8
Iron (mg)	1.8	1.8	1.8
Zinc (mg)	0.75	1	1
Manganese (mcg)	8	25	25

(continued)

TABLE 5-6 *(Continued)*

	Alimentum (1)	Nutramigen (3)*	Pregestimil (3)
Copper (mcg)	75	75	75
Iodine (mcg)	15	15	15
Selenium (mcg)	1.8	2.8	2.8
Sodium (mg)	44	47	47
Potassium (mg)	118	110	110
Chloride (mg)	80	86	86
Other data			
kcal/oz (usual dilution)	20	20	20
DHA/ARA added?	Yes	Yes	Yes

#Extensively hydrolyzed
*Similar product with probiotics also available
**Ready to feed has slightly different carbohydrate blend
(1) Abbott Nutrition
(2) Gerber
(3) Mead Johnson
(4) Nutricia
(5) PBM

TABLE 5-7 Amino Acid-Based Infant Formulas (Composition per 100 kcal)

	EleCare (1)	Neocate Infant with DHA and ARA (4)	Nutramigen AA (3)
Macronutrients			
Energy (kcal)	100	100	100
Volume (m1)	150	150	150
Protein			
g	3.1	3.1	2.8
% kcal	15	12	11
Source	Free L-amino acids	Free L-amino acids	Free L-amino acids
Carbohydrate			
g	10.7	11.7	10.3
% kcal	43	47	41
Source	Corn syrup solids	Corn syrup solids	Corn syrup solids and modified tapioca starch
Fat			
g	4.8	4.5	5.3
% kcal	42	41	48
Source	High oleic safflower and soy oils, medium chain triglycerides	High oleic sunflower and soy oils, medium chain triglycerides	Palm olein, soy, coconut and high oleic sunflower oils
Linoleic acid (mg)	840	677	860

TABLE 5-7 *(Continued)*

	EleCare (1)	Neocate Infant with DHA and ARA (4)	Nutramigen AA (3)
Vitamins			
Vitamin A (IU)	273	409	300
Vitamin D (IU)	42	60	50
Vitamin E (1U)	2.1	1.1	2
Vitamin K (mcg)	6	9	8
Vitamin C (mg)	9	9	12
Thiamine B_1 (mcg)	210	93	80
Riboflavin B_2 (mcg)	105	138	90
Vitamin B_6 (mcg)	84	124	60
Vitamin B_{12} (mcg)	0.4	0.3	0.3
Niacin (mcg)	1680	1544	1000
Folic acid (mcg)	29.5	10	16
Pantothenic acid (mcg)	421	620	500
Biotin (mcg)	4.2	3.1	3
Minerals			
Calcium (mg)	116	124	94
Phosphorus (mg)	84.2	93	52
Magnesium (mg)	8.4	12.4	11
Iron (mg)	1.5	1.8	1.8
Zinc (mg)	0.8	1.7	1
Manganese (mcg)	84	90	60
Copper (mcg)	105	124	75
Iodine (mcg)	8.4	15.4	15
Selenium (mcg)	2.3	3.7	2.8
Sodium (mg)	45	37	47
Potassium (mg)	150	155	110
Chloride (mg)	60	77	86
Other data			
kcal/oz (usual dilution)	20	20	20
DHA/ARA added?	Available with and without	Yes; product without DHA/ARA and with less MCT is available	Yes

(1) Abbott Nutrition
(2) Gerber
(3) Mead Johnson
(4) Nutricia
(5) PBM

TABLE 5-8 Follow-Up Formulas (Composition per 100 kcal)

	Enfagrow Premium Next Step (3)[#]	Go and Grow Milk-Based (1)[#]	Good Start Gentle Plus 2 (2)[#*]	Store Brand Follow-up (5)
Macronutrients				
Energy (kcal)	100	100	100	100
Volume (m1)	150	150	150	150
Protein				
g	2.6	2.1	2.2	2.6
% kcal	10	8	9	10
Source	Nonfat milk	Nonfat milk and whey protein concentrate	Whey protein concentrate	Nonfat milk
Carbohydrate				
g	10.5	10.6	11.2	10.5
% kcal	42	43	45	42
Source	Lactose and corn syrup solids	Lactose	Lactose and corn maltodextrine	Corn syrup and lactose
Fat				
g	5.3	5.5	5.1	5.3
% kcal	48	49	46	48
Source	Palm olein, soy, coconut and high oleic sunflower oils	High oleic safflower, soy and coconut oils	Palm olein, soy, coconut and high oleic sunflower (or safflower) oils	Palm olein, soy, coconut and high oleic sunflower (or safflower) oils
Linoleic acid (mg)	860	1000	900	N/A
Vitamins				
Vitamin A (IU)	300	300	300	300
Vitamin D (IU)	60	60	60	60
Vitamin E (1U)	2	3	2	2
Vitamin K (mcg)	8	8	8	8
Vitamin C (mg)	12	12	12	12
Thiamine B_1 (mcg)	80	100	100	80
Riboflavin B_2 (mcg)	140	150	140	140
Vitamin B_6 (mcg)	60	60	75	60
Vitamin B_{12} (mcg)	0.3	0.25	0.33	0.3
Niacin (mcg)	1000	1050	1050	1000
Folic acid (mcg)	16	15	15	16
Pantothenic acid (mcg)	500	450	450	500
Biotin (mcg)	3	4.4	4.4	3
Minerals				
Calcium (mg)	195	150	190	195
Phosphorus (mg)	130	81	106	130
Magnesium (mg)	8	6	7	8
Iron (mg)	2	2	2	2

TABLE 5-8 *(Continued)*

	Enfagrow Premium Next Step (3)#	Go and Grow Milk-Based (1)#	Good Start Gentle Plus 2 (2)#*	Store Brand Follow-up (5)
Zinc (mg)	1	0.75	0.8	1
Manganese (mcg)	15	5	15	15
Copper (mcg)	75	90	80	75
Iodine (mcg)	10	6	12	10
Selenium (mcg)	2.8	1.8	3	2.8
Sodium (mg)	36	24	27	36
Potassium (mg)	130	105	108	130
Chloride (mg)	80	65	65	80
Other data				
kcal/oz (usual dilution)	20	20	20	20
DHA/ARA added?	Yes	Yes	Yes	Yes

#Also available as a soy-based protein, lactose-free product
*Similar product with probiotics also available
(1) Abbott Nutrition
(2) Gerber
(3) Mead Johnson
(4) Nutricia
(5) PBM

formula is higher than that of standard formula because the biologic value of soy protein is lower than cow's milk protein. Soy formulas contain a blend of vegetable oils and most are supplemented with ARA and DHA. Though all soy formulas are lactose free, some are also sucrose free or corn free. Soy phytates and fiber oligosaccharides contained in soy formulas have been found to interfere with the absorption of calcium, phosphorous, zinc, and iron. For this reason, calcium and phosphorous levels in soy formulas have been increased by 20% over those of cow's milk–based formulas and are fortified with zinc and iron.[48,49] These formulas then meet the requirements for vitamins and minerals established by the AAP and FDA.[49]

Overall, studies have confirmed that soy formulas are adequate for promoting normal growth and development when fed to full-term, healthy infants. Soy formulas are not recommended for premature infants.[49]

Protein Hydrolysates

Indications for using hydrolyzed protein formulas include CMP allergy, soy allergy, or significant nutritional challenges related to a variety of gastrointestinal or liver diseases.[34,51] CMP allergy is usually diagnosed in infants with a strong family history of allergy and can present with any combination of cutaneous (e.g., atopic dermatitis), respiratory (e.g., asthma), and gastrointestinal complaints; blood in the stool is a classic symptom.[34,51] Both partially hydrolyzed and extensively hydrolyzed formulas are available. Extensively hydrolyzed formulas contain only peptides that have a molecular weight of less than 3000 D and are considered truly hypoallergenic.[51] Data support the use of extensively hydrolyzed formulas during the first year of life for infants who are at risk for atopic disease when exclusive breastfeeding for 4–6 months is not possible or for infants who are formula fed.[51] Sources of carbohydrate and fat vary among the protein hydrolysate formulas and should be considered when they are fed for indications other than protein allergy or hypersensitivity. The AAP takes no position on the use of hypoallergenic formulas for the treatment of colic or irritability. Initial experience with a hydrolyzed formula supplemented with probiotics suggests it is well-tolerated in healthy infants[52] (http://www.mjn.com). Extensively hydrolyzed formulas are significantly more expensive than milk- or soy-based formulas.

Amino Acid–Based Formulas

Infants with severe protein hypersensitivity and persistence of symptoms on other formulas can be switched to nonallergenic, amino acid–based formulas.[34] The use of amino acid–based formulas for the prevention of atopic disease has not been studied.[51] Amino acid–based formulas are extremely expensive and difficult for families to obtain. WIC participants in some states can obtain these formulas; other families must pay out of pocket or fight for insurance coverage, often with limited success.

Follow-Up Formulas

"Follow-up formulas" are designed for older infants and toddlers who are taking solid foods but not enough to meet all essential nutrients needed for optimal growth and development.[34] The AAP has stated that although nutritionally adequate, these formulas offer no clearly established superiority over traditional formulas or breast milk for infants. They may be appropriate as a beverage for a toddler whose diet is consistently poor.[1] In general, follow-up formulas cost less than standard infant formula but more than cow's milk, and are higher in iron than cow's milk. There is no evidence of a growth or developmental advantage over whole milk.[34]

Other Products Fed to Infants

The AAP does not support the use of evaporated milk preparations for infants because of their inadequate nutrient composition.[1] Although not recommended, a home-prepared formula from evaporated milk is probably preferable to using unmodified cow's milk when commercial formula or breast milk is temporarily unavailable. The usual recipe is one can of evaporated whole milk (13 oz), 19.5 oz of water, and 3 tablespoons of sugar or corn syrup.[53] The evaporation process denatures the protein, rendering it softer and more digestible, and adding the sugar or corn syrup improves the protein:fat:carbohydrate ratio. Evaporated milk formula has all of the same disadvantages as unmodified cow's milk: poorly digested fat; low concentration of essential fatty acids, iron, zinc, and vitamins E and C; and excessive amounts of protein, sodium, potassium, chloride, and phosphorous. A multivitamin supplement is recommended, and additional iron is needed unless the infant takes sufficient quantities of appropriate solid foods. After 6 months of age supplemental fluoride is prescribed unless the water used in formula preparation is fluoridated.[1]

Goat's milk is not recommended. If fed to infants, goat's milk must be supplemented with folic acid.[1] Cow's milk is not recommended until 1 year of age.[1] Soy (e.g., Silk), rice (e.g., Rice Dream), and almond (e.g., Blue Diamond Almond Breeze) "milks" are not nutritionally adequate for infants and should not be fed during the first year of life.[1]

Management of Formula Feedings

Pediatric professionals should not assume that caregivers are familiar with how to purchase or prepare infant formulas. The Infant Formula Act requires packaging to provide instructions for preparation, including pictorials.[1] Bottle-feeding parents need assistance from their healthcare professionals on appropriate volumes required to meet nutrient needs and the addition of age-appropriate solids.

Infant formulas come packaged in three ways: ready-to-feed, concentrated liquid, and powder. Ready-to-feed formulas provide sterile feedings of known caloric concentration for those who like the convenience or do not have the capability of preparing formulas at the time of a feeding (e.g., while traveling). Ready-to-feed formulas do not contain fluoride. They are generally the most expensive form of formula. Concentrated liquid formulas are readily available and mix easily by combining with water in a 1:1 ratio. Powder is ideal if only a small amount of formula is desired, and it may be the cheapest form of formula. Powder formula is popular among breastfeeding mothers who may want to occasionally offer a bottle feeding. Powder formula is generally prepared by mixing one level scoop of powder with 2 ounces of water. It is important to use the scoop provided in the can of powder because scoop sizes vary across different formula powders.

The source of water is important to consider. Both powder and concentrated liquid formula can be the source of fluoride for the infant if reconstituted with fluoridated water. This is especially important when the infant reaches 6 months of life and needs a source of dietary fluoride. Sterile water is used for formula preparation. The U.S. Food and Drug Administration recommends mixing infant formula "using ordinary cold tap water that's brought to a boil and then boiled for 1 minute and cooled."[54] Boiling longer than 1 minute may concentrate the minerals in the water to an undesirable degree.[1] For most infants older than 3 months of age, water no longer needs to be boiled, and formula prepared with water directly from the tap is satisfactory.[55] Bottled waters, including distilled and spring water, cannot be assumed to be sterile unless specifically labeled as such.[56] Bottled "nursery" water is sold near infant formula in many stores and is often labeled as sterile.

Hands should be washed thoroughly before mixing and feeding formula. All equipment used in preparing and storing formula should be clean and formula should be fed from clean bottles and clean nipples. Items should be thoroughly washed in hot soapy water, rinsed well with clean water, and air dried or dried with a clean towel.[55] The use of a dishwasher for cleaning equipment is acceptable. Bottles made of polycarbonate plastic contain bisphenol A, an environmental toxin. Infants may experience low-dose exposure to bisphenol A due to leaching from the bottle, especially if the plastic is scratched or worn. Long-term consequences from bisphenol A exposure are uncertain.[57,58]

Most prepared formulas can be kept in the refrigerator for 24 to 48 hours; however, it is safest to consume formula within 24 hours. Open cans of powder have a 30-day shelf life. Powder formulas are not sterile and may contain the bacterium *Enterobacter sakazakii*.[59] Safe handling practices are especially important for reconstituting powders for very young infants. Mixing the smallest batch of formula practical and limiting storage periods decreases the time a potential pathogen has to proliferate.

There is currently no evidence that babies prefer warmed milk; however, most caregivers do not feed cold bottles from the refrigerator. Warming is best done by putting the unopened bottle in a bowl of warm water for 5–10 minutes prior to feeding.[1] Microwave heating is not advised because it is difficult to monitor the actual temperature of formula in the center of the bottle. In addition, steam building within the bottle can result in an explosion and spraying of hot liquid. Reports have associated facial and palatal burns of babies with the heating of bottles in a microwave.[60,61]

An update on infant formula for consumers entitled "FDA 101: Infant Formula" is available at http://www.fda.gov/ForConsumers/ConsumerUpdates/ucm048694.htm.

Feeding Techniques and Schedules

Good bottle-feeding technique includes holding the infant, so that face-to-face contact is maximized, and tilting the bottle so that the nipple is filled with milk. Interaction between caregiver and infant can be just as intimate during bottle-feeding as with breastfeeding. Bottles should never be propped. This practice removes the socialization aspect of feeding and can lead to dental caries.[55] Breast- or bottle-feeding in the supine position is associated with an increased risk of ear infections.[62] Infants should be fed in a semi-upright position. The addition of sugar to the formula or sucrose-containing fluids to the bottle is not recommended because it increases the risk of dental caries.[1,55] Adding solids, such as cereal, to the bottle also is not recommended.[55]

Most infants can finish a bottle in 15 to 30 minutes. If most feedings exceed this time frame, it is recommended that a pediatric feeding specialist evaluate the infant to rule out any severe oral or motor delay or dysfunction. Other possible reasons for slow feeding include a nipple with a hole that is too small or clogged or a collapsed nipple. Burping is usually done midway through the feeding and at the end of the feeding. Partially used bottles should be discarded after the feeding and not saved for the next feeding time. **Table 5-9** gives a suggested bottle-feeding schedule for infants.[63]

Supplementation

The human race has evolved over the centuries on an infant diet of human milk alone, raising the argument that no routine supplementation should be necessary. There are several nutrients, however, for which this may not be entirely true. **Table 5-10** summarizes the most up-to-date vitamin and mineral supplementation recommendations for vitamin K, vitamin D, iron, and fluoride.[1] **Table 5-11** gives the composition of selected infant vitamin and mineral drops.

TABLE 5-9 Suggested Number and Volume of Bottle Feedings for a Healthy Infant

Age	Feedings/Day	Ounces/Feeding
Birth–4 months	8–12	2–6
4–6 months	5–8	6–7
6–8 months	3–5	7–8
8–12 months	3–4	7–8

Source: Misra M, Pacaud D, Petryk A, et al. Vitamin D deficiency in children and its management: review of current knowledge and recommendations. *Pediatrics*. 2008;122:398–417.

A one-time intramuscular dose of vitamin K at birth (0.5–1.0 mg) is effective protection against hemorrhagic disease of the newborn and is recommended for both breast- and bottle-fed newborns.[1]

Rickets continues to occur in infants.[64] In addition, vitamin D is now known to have important extraskeletal effects, including protection against infection.[65,66] The AAP recommends supplementing all newborn infants with 400 IU vitamin D per day within the first few days of life.[64] Supplementation should continue until at least 1 liter per day of vitamin D–fortified milk is consumed. Infants particularly at risk for vitamin D deficiency are those who live at higher latitudes (particularly above 40°), especially during the winter, and are dark skinned. Consideration should be given to supplementing these high-risk infants with up to 800 IU vitamin D per day.[65] One mL per day of a tri-vitamin drop or D-Vi-Sol (Mead Johnson) provides 400 IU vitamin D.

Term infants usually have adequate iron stores for the first 4 to 6 months of life.[1] Although the amount of iron in human milk is minimal, its bioavailability is quite high, approximately five times greater than bovine milk.[1] However, by 6 months of age, exclusively breastfed infants require additional iron (1 mg/kg/day) either as a supplement or through the introduction of sufficient iron-fortified infant cereal and/or meat.[1,67,68] For example, an average of two servings (1/2 oz or 15 g of dry cereal per serving) is needed to meet the daily iron requirement. The AAP supports the use of iron-fortified formulas (12 mg iron/quart) as the preferred alternative to feeding infants if breastfeeding is not chosen.[1] Iron-fortified formula provides approximately 2 mg/kg per day of iron when fed at about 120 kcal/kg per day. Several well-designed studies have shown that iron-fortified formulas are as well tolerated as low-iron formulas.[1] These interventions to maintain iron status will decrease the risk of iron-deficiency anemia and its irreversible association with cognitive and motor impairments.[1]

A source of dietary fluoride is recommended for infants after 6 months of age. Commercial formulas do not contain fluoride, but if they are mixed with fluoridated water, no supplement is needed. The AAP recommends daily supplements of 0.25 mg fluoride for those infants over 6 months of age living in areas where tap or well water supplies contain less than 0.3 ppm of fluoride, who consume ready-to-feed formula or formula reconstituted with nonfluoridated bottled water, or who continue to be exclusively breastfed.[1] Fluoride supplements, with dosages changing over time,

TABLE 5-10 Suggested Vitamin and Mineral Supplementation for Full-Term Infants (0–12 Months)

Product	Initiated at	Infants Fed Human Milk	Infants Fed Infant Formula
Vitamin K	Birth	Single dose 0.5–1 mg IM	
Vitamin D	First few days of life	400 IU/day until 1 L/day of vitamin D–fortified milk is consumed	
Iron	4–6 months	1 mg/kg/day as two servings per day of 15 g infant cereal each, or iron supplement	At least 11 mg/day as iron-fortified formula (12 mg/qt)
Fluoride	6 months	If exclusively breastfed OR is partially breastfed AND local water has < 0.3 ppm fluoride; 0.25 mg/day	If using ready-to-feed formula OR local water has < 0.3 ppm fluoride; 0.25 mg/day

Abbreviations: IM, intramuscular; ppm, parts per million.
Source: Data from Kleinman R. *Pediatric Nutrition Handbook*, 6th ed. Elk Grove Village, IL: American Academy of Pediatrics; 2009.

TABLE 5-11 Composition of Selected Infant Vitamin and Mineral Drops (1 mL)

Product	Brand Name and Manufacturer	Vitamin D (IU)	Vitamin C (mg)	Vitamin A (IU)	Iron (mg)	Fluoride (mg)
Tri-Vitamin	Tri-Vi-Sol (Mead Johnson)	400	35	1500		
Tri-Vitamin with Iron	Tri-Vi-Sol with Iron (Mead Johnson)	400	35	1500	10	
Vitamin D	D-Vi-Sol (Mead Johnson)	400				
Iron	Fer-In-Sol (Mead Johnson)				15	
Fluoride	Luride* (Colgate)					0.5

*Prescription required
Sources: Table data retrieved from manufacturers' websites (accessed January 10, 2010): Mead Johnson, http://www.mjncom; Colgate, http:// www.colgate.com.

are recommended until 16 years of age in children who do not have access to fluoridated water.[1]

Diets of breastfeeding mothers should be assessed for adequacy of vitamin B_{12} if the mother is following an animal protein–restricted diet, especially those who comply with vegan guidelines.[1] When the mother takes a limited diet in any nutrient, supplementation is indicated for both the mother and infant.

Weaning and Feeding Progression

During infancy, the most important source of nutrition for growth and development is breast milk or iron-fortified infant formulas. During the second half of infancy, the addition of infant cereal and solid foods benefits the infant nutritionally as well as developmentally. Complementary feedings allow caregivers the opportunity to expose infants to an array of flavors and food textures that can initiate lifelong healthy eating habits. The optimal timing and kinds of "complementary" foods introduced has been questioned for decades. Currently, the AAP, the World Health Organization (WHO), and the United Nations Children's Fund (UNICEF) all believe there is no nutritional benefit to adding solids to an infant's diet until at least the fourth month of life. The latest recommendations from these organizations encourage waiting until closer to 6 months of age before complementary foods are initiated.[1]

Studies looking at the timing of food introduction have not been able to prove or disprove any significant consequences to when or how the various complementary foods are initiated. However, infants who are exclusively breastfed are at the greatest risk of deficiencies and may benefit from the addition of complementary foods earlier than those who are formula fed.[1] Around 6 months of age, breastfed infants may be at risk for iron deficiency anemia and can benefit from an additional iron source such as iron-fortified cereals or meats. When considering the introduction of complementary foods, caregivers should consider the individual readiness of the infant along with the following potential concerns:

- Energy requirements and growth of the infant
- Iron and zinc status of the infant and foods being introduced
- Risk of infectious morbidity for the infant (mainly in underdeveloped countries where sanitation is a concern)
- Potential risk of atopic disease if there is a personal or family history of intolerance
- Long-term impact on neurocognitive development and behavior

Readiness to start solid foods generally occurs during the first 4 to 6 months of life. Observations of individual physical and psychological developments are better determinants of readiness for starting complementary foods than age alone. All infants develop at different rates, and caregivers should respect this unique trait and level of comfort with initiating spoon feeding and new textures. Awareness of the infant's hunger and satiety cues with spoon feeding are just as important as feeding cues during breast- and bottle-feeding. Infants who turn away during a feeding are usually indicating they are satisfied and want the feeding to stop. "Infants have the innate ability to self regulate their energy intake."[69] This self-regulating instinct can be affected by factors such as coercive feeding, overly restrictive feeding, or the feeding environment in general. Encouraging infants to establish a healthy self-confidence in regard to satiety and hunger is one of the most important aspects of infant feeding. New studies are looking at the significance of infant feeding practices and the impact they have on eating behaviors and risk of obesity later in life. The main goal of solid food introduction during infancy is to balance nutrient needs with a variety of foods and textures while encouraging development of independent feeding skills. Feedings transition from exclusive liquids at birth, with breast milk or iron-fortified formulas, to a well-balanced diet of table foods shared by the family at 1 year of age.

Physical Readiness for Solids

Physical readiness includes gross motor development as well as oral motor development. Prior to about 4 months of age, infants have poor head control and are uncoordinated with lip closure. In addition, infants possess an extrusion reflex that permits them to swallow only liquid foods easily.[70] During this phase there is limited or no interest in oral feeding other than breast- or bottle-feeding. Around 4 to 6 months of age, infants learn oral and gross motor skills that aid in accepting solid foods. At this age, oral motor skills evolve from the reflexive suck to the ability to swallow nonliquid foods and transfer contents from the front of the tongue to the back of the mouth. Gross motor development includes sitting independently and maintaining balance while using hands to reach and grasp for objects.[67] Head control is improved at this stage, and infants are ready to sit in a high chair and grasp pieces of food. Infants will begin to turn toward food or watch others eating, but still lack the hand-to-mouth coordination necessary to feed themselves and need assistance from caregivers.[71] At this stage of development, infants should be encouraged to sit in high chairs by themselves. It is important that they begin to start developing more independence with feeding and join the family around a table setting.

Psychological Readiness for Solids

Independent eating behaviors are encouraged as infants advance from reflexive and imitative behaviors to more independent and exploratory behaviors. This transitional milestone occurs sometime during the fourth month of life.[72] By 6 months, infants are able to indicate a desire for food by opening their mouth, leaning forward to indicate hunger, and leaning back and turning away to show disinterest or satiety. Until an infant can express these feelings, feeding of solids will probably represent a type of forced feeding, potentially leading to overfeeding and risk of obesity or general anxiety around eating for the infant.

In addition to determining the quantity of feedings, infants should be encouraged to develop more independence with feeding in the following ways:

- Self-feeding of soft finger foods
- Sipping from a cup by 6 to 8 months of age[72]
- Holding the bottle or cup independently
- Controlling the timing of feeds in an effort to promote self-regulation of hunger and satiety[73]

A variety of foods should be experienced throughout infancy. The introduction of unfamiliar foods is noteworthy because it allows the infant to gain experience with various tastes and textures, promoting successful weaning to the family diet. The importance of diversifying the diet at specific intervals during the infant's psychological development can be observed in deprived environments in which the eating pattern is unvaried and monotonous, or where weaning is delayed. Both of these situations fail to stimulate interest in solid foods[73,74] or self-feeding. Caregivers who find it difficult to give freedom or control to infants with self-feeding often promote frustration and insecurity around eating for infants. Food refusal and failure to thrive often result from this negative feeding environment.

Complementary Foods

As the complementary foods begin to displace breast milk or formula in the diet, vitamin and mineral intake are also affected. Foods selected for the infant feeding should be nutrient-dense items. Some studies have encouraged the introduction of meats between 4 and 6 months to help prevent deficiency of either iron or zinc,[1] especially for exclusively breastfed infants. Introduction of solids should not mislead caregivers into thinking consumption of breast milk or infant formula is any less significant. Optimal volumes of breast milk and/or iron-fortified infant formula are still essential to meet the majority of the infant's nutrient needs. The Feeding Infants and Toddlers Study (FITS) from 2002 reported dramatic decreases in energy intake from breast milk and/or formula with the introduction of solid foods. The most significant decrease in breast milk or formula volume occurs from about 4 to 5 months of age to 6 to 8 months of age, with a total energy decrease from 88% to 66% of total intake.[75]

Review breast milk and infant formula composition in Table 5-1, Tables 5-3 through 5-8, and Table 5-13 to identify nutrient delivery of select infant feedings. For more information on infant foods and infant feeding, go to http://www.gerber.com, http://www.heinzbaby.com, http://www.beechnut.com, http://www.healthychildren.org (an AAP-sponsored site), or http://www.pediatrics.about.com/od/startingsolidfoods/startingsolid_foods.htm.

First Foods

Commercial infant rice cereal thinned to a semi-liquid consistency with breast milk or infant formula is generally recommended as an infant's first food. This has become customary because allergy to rice is unlikely in infancy.[67] The cereal is traditionally introduced on a small spoon. Resistance to the initial spoon-feeding is common because infants are not familiar with the spoon as a dispenser of nutrition. Holding the infant in one's arms, rather than sitting him or her in a high chair, may relieve some of the initial apprehension the infant may experience. Each new food item introduced in the infant's diet should be fed for 2 to 3 days while examining the infant for symptoms of intolerance. Signs of potential intolerance may include skin rashes, vomiting, diarrhea, or wheezing. In the absence of such symptoms, the quantity, frequency, and consistency of the food item can be increased, and a second food can be presented. Refer to **Table 5-12** for further recommendations regarding the progression of solid foods. Once a variety of single ingredients have been introduced and tolerated, a combination of these ingredients can be offered.

TABLE 5-12 Guidelines for Progression of Solid Foods

Age in Months	Feeding Skills	Oral Motor Skills	Types of Food	Suggested Activities
Birth–4		Rooting reflex Sucking reflex Swallowing reflex Extrusion reflex	Breast milk Infant formula	Breast-feeding Bottle-feeding
5	Able to grasp objects voluntarily Learning to reach mouth with hands	Disappearance of extrusion reflex		Possible introduction of thinned cereal
6	Sits with balance while using hands Ready for high chair	Transfers food from front of tongue to back Closes lips around spoon	Infant cereal Strained fruit Strained vegetables	Prepare cereal with formula or breast milk to a semi-liquid texture Use spoon Feed from a dish Advance to ⅓–½ cup cereal before adding fruits and vegetables
7	Improved grasp Drinks from cup with help	Mashes food with lateral movements of jaw Learns side-to-side or "rotary" chewing	Infant cereal Strained to junior texture of fruits, vegetables, and meats	Thicken texture to lumpier texture Sit child in high chair with feet supported Introduce cup
8–10	Holds bottle without help Drinks from cup without spilling Decreases fluid intake and increases solids Coordinates hand-to-mouth movement	Swallows with closed mouth	Soft, mashed, or minced table foods	Begin finger foods Do not add salt, sugar, or fats to foods Present soft foods in chunks ready for finger feeding
10–12	Feeds self with fingers and spoon Holds cup without help	Tooth eruption Improved ability to bite and chew	Soft, chopped table foods	Provide meals in pattern similar to rest of family Use cup at meals

Sources: Data from Fomon SJ. *Nutrition of Normal Infants*. St. Louis, MO: Mosby; 1993; Butte N, Cobb K, Duyer J, Graney L, Heird W, Rickard K. The start healthy feeding guidelines for infants and toddlers. *J Amer Diet Assoc*. 2004;104:442–484; and Hinton S, Kerwin D. *Maternal and Child Nutrition*. Chapel Hill, NC: Health Sciences Consortium Corporation; 1981.

A gag reflex of varying degrees is apparent until about the age of 7 to 9 months. At this time, most infants are beginning to chew and tolerate smooth to chunky foods, and a normal gag reflex is developing. Choking, however, indicates that, despite the infant's chronologic age, he or she is not ready for the transition to solid foods. It is not unusual for caregivers to be overly cautious about this natural gag reflex and mistake it for choking. Providers must be attentive to situations where infant feeding and solid texture progression is being delayed due to caregiver anxiety. Infants will pick up on this anxiety around feeding and begin to develop insecurity around the feeding environment. Parental support, encouragement, and even a feeding demonstration while at a medical visit can reduce some of this anxiety early on. Moms can be very influential with eating and role modeling. Repeat introduction of foods and supportive encouragement will open opportunity for more flexibility with eating.[76]

Many commercial baby food products are available on the market today. Virtually all are prepared without added sodium and many without added sugar. Juices are generally enriched with vitamin C, and cereals are enriched with iron, thiamine, riboflavin, niacin, calcium, and phosphorus. Those advertised as "first foods" are single-ingredient foods, in contrast to "dinners," baked goods, desserts, "graduates," "junior foods," and some cereals, which contain a combination of ingredients. Textures from strained to chunky are available, along with foods designed for teething. Baby food manufacturers use various descriptors to identify the different textures. Words such as "stage," "first," "second," or "graduate" can tell a parent or caregiver approximately when in infancy the baby might be ready to handle the texture of the food. Commercial baby foods are a time-efficient means of providing an infant with solids, and if chosen wisely, can supply a nutrient-dense diet. Certain items will provide more nutrients than seemingly comparable choices. For example, plain meats contain from 220% to 250% of the protein and up to 200% of the iron of "meat dinners." The nutrient contents of selected commercial baby foods are listed in **Table 5-13**. Providers and caregivers can use the Nutrient Data Laboratory Website to view a nutrient analysis of commercial baby foods. The

TABLE 5-13 Nutrient Composition of Selected Commercial Baby Food Products

Food		Amount	Calories	Protein	Carbohydrates	Fat	Sodium	Sugar	Fiber
Instant Cereal	Single grain rice	¼ cup	60	1	12	0.5	0	17	0
Stage 1 Vegetable	Carrots G	1 pack	25	< 1	5	0	80	4	1
	Carrots H	1 jar	50	1	9	1	25	6	3
Stage 1 Fruit	Bananas G	1 pack	60	< 1	15	0	5	12	1
	Bananas H	½ bowl	65	1	15	0	1.5	11	1
Stage 2 Vegetable	Garden Vegetable G	1 pack	40	2	7	0.5	35	3	2
	Mixed Vegetable H	1 jar	50	3	10	0.3	22	1	2
Stage 2 Fruit	Apple Berry G	1 pack	50	0	12	0	0	10	1
	Apple Berry H	1 jar	90	0	23	0	6	19	2
Stage 2 Dinner	Sweet Potato Turkey G	1 jar	80	2	16	1	50	9	2
	Sweet Potato Turkey H	1 jar	90	4	20	0.3	35	4	2
Graduate	Chicken and Pasta G	1 tray	110	9	16			3	3
Stage 3 Dinner	Chicken Cass. Veg w/Rice H	1 tray	180	8	35	6	40	5	3

Abbreviations: G, Gerber; H, Heinz.

Note: Mean values derived from http://www.gerber.com and http://www.heinzbaby.com.

site is at http://www.nal.usda.gov/fnic/foodcomp/search/. Analysis includes macro and micronutrients as well as amino acid profiles of various serving sizes.

Home Preparation of Baby Foods

Home-prepared baby foods are an alternative to commercially prepared foods. They are more economical and allow greater flexibility in altering food consistency. Preparation can be time consuming, but many families feel it's important for the child. Families should not be encouraged to prepare baby foods from their own meals if they lack variety in their diet, lack refrigeration and freezing, or have poor sanitation in their homes.[77] Infants from developing countries are at a greater risk of food contamination or foodborne illness related to poor sanitation and unsafe water supplies. Homegrown foods should not be prepared for infants if the lead concentration of soil in residential areas is excessive.[78] These precautions are to ensure a varied diet and to prevent nutrient deficiencies, foodborne illness, and lead toxicity.

Infants can experience different tastes from maternal diets via amniotic fluid and breast milk.[79] For this reason, it is reasonable to consider that infants can handle a little spice in their foods. Families should start with single ingredients and then progress to multiple ingredient foods and spices after the infant has shown tolerance without adverse reaction. It is more important to avoid excessive sodium, sugar, and additives commonly found in some table foods. **Table 5-14** provides detailed instructions for the home preparation of baby foods.

Home-prepared foods should focus on providing safe and adequate nutrition. Diets for infants should have variety and include foods that are nutrient dense. Foods should be easy to hold, vary in texture and temperature, and contain a balance of all the food groups. The FITS data showed that 18% to 33% of infants and toddlers over 6 months of age consumed no fruits and vegetables.[80] This low level of produce intake continues into childhood and adolescence. The primary influence of this reduction in produce consumption may be the poor example from parents, caregivers, and other children in the home.

The diets of family members and caregivers play a significant role in influencing the types of foods infants are eating. The final phase of infant feeding, between the 10th and 12th months, is a combination of mimicry and increasing independence with self-feeding. The caregiver and child interactions around eating are significant at this point to help establish healthy eating relationships that will extend into childhood and adulthood. See the following Websites for suggestions on making baby foods and recipes:

- http://www.homecooking.about.com/library/archive/blbabyfood.htm
- http://www.pediatrics.about.com/od/startingsolidfoods/starting_solid_foods.htm

TABLE 5-14 Steps in the Home Preparation of Baby Foods

1. Choosing appropriate foods:
    - Use fresh or unsalted frozen foods. Do not use canned foods because they may contribute excessive sodium to the infant diet.
    - Spinach, carrots, broccoli, and beets should not be pureed at home because they may contain sufficient nitrite to cause methemoglobinemia in young infants.
2. Preparing fruits and vegetables:
    - Thaw frozen vegetables; wash fresh produce.
    - Remove peels, cores, and seeds.
    - Steam or boil.
    - Puree in blender or food processor to desired consistency. Use liquid from cooking to preserve nutrients otherwise lost in cooking. Do not over-blend because this may cause excessive oxidation of nutrients.
3. Preparing meats:
    - Bake, broil, or stew meat.
    - Remove all skins.
    - Chop into small pieces.
    - Puree in blender to desired consistency.
4. Storing prepared foods:
    - Keep refrigerated in a covered container. Use refrigerated foods within 48 hours.
    - Freeze in 2-tablespoon portions by pouring pureed food into an ice cube tray. Thaw desired portions in refrigerator before using.

Sources: Data from Kleinman R. *Pediatric Nutrition Handbook*, 6th ed. American Academy of Pediatrics; 2009; Hinton S, Kerwin D. *Maternal and Child Nutrition.* Chapel Hill, NC: Health Sciences Consortium Corporation; 1981; American Academy of Pediatrics, Committee on Nutrition. Infant methemoglobinemia: the role of dietary nitrate. *Pediatrics.* 1970;46:475–478; and Kerr C, Reisinger K, Plankey F. Sodium concentration of homemade baby foods. *Pediatrics.* 1978;62:331–335.

Risk for Obesity

The epidemic and global rise in childhood obesity remains a concern as the numbers of infants and children affected continues to increase. Currently, one out of every three children is at risk of being overweight or becoming obese during childhood.[1] The National Health and Nutrition Examination Survey (NHANES) reports from 2003 to 2004 revealed that the number of infants and children less than 2 years old who were clinically overweight had increased from 7.2% (1976–1980) to 11.5%.[81] As the incidence of overweight and obesity rises, research has started focusing on when the initial risk for childhood overweight or obesity begins and who is at greatest risk.

Initial risk factors for infants and children becoming overweight or obese appear to develop sooner than anticipated. Prior to conception, mothers can already have risk factors for unhealthy weight gain in their children. Mothers who are overweight themselves, smoke, or gain excessive weight during pregnancy have a greater risk of having an infant and/or child who will be overweight at some point during childhood.[82] From birth, studies have looked at the possible influence of various infant feeding methods on risk of childhood overweight and obesity. Researchers initially comparing breastfeeding and formula-feeding believed that breastfeeding had a protective effect against infants and children becoming overweight. Comparison studies revealed that formula-fed infants started to outgrow the breastfed infants by as early as 2–3 months of age.[81] However, the many confounding variables common with choosing whether to breastfeed make it difficult to declare breastfeeding as more protective against overweight and obesity. The nutritional differences between breast milk and infant formulas may not be as significant as the method of feeding itself. Infants put to breast learn very early on how to self-regulate their intake of nutrition to meet individual satiety. Formula-fed infants are often given standard amounts of formula, and parents and caregivers are not as attentive to feeding cues. This subtle difference in feeding environment may be enough to teach self-regulation with eating for years to come.

Research has found that being breastfed and the duration of breastfeeding appears to be inversely related to fat mass at 4 years of age.[83] Infants who are fed more fruits, vegetables, and home-prepared foods were also leaner at 4 years.[83] The greatest risk factor for overweight or obesity in infancy or childhood was having an overweight parent. The earlier an infant or child is identified as overweight, the better predictability of life-long overweight.

The following goals have been established for infant feeding to prevent childhood overweight or obesity:[76]

- Breastfeed exclusively for 6 months.
- Avoid sweet beverages.
- Respect infant self-regulation during feeding (breast-, formula-, or solid food feedings).
- Avoid using food for comfort.

Dental Caries in Infancy

It has been said that tooth decay is the most common chronic disease of childhood.[1] Baby bottle tooth decay (BBTD) is an oral health disorder characterized by rampant dental caries associated with inappropriate infant feeding practices (see **Figure 5-1**). The disorder affects the primary teeth of infants and young children, particularly those who are permitted to fall asleep with a bottle filled with juice or other fermentable liquid.[1] Nursing caries, similar to tooth decay caused by BBTD from formulas, can also occur with prolonged or inappropriate breastfeeding at naptime or too frequently throughout the day. Recent studies have found that children have a 32 times greater chance of having caries by 3 years of age if they come from a low socioeconomic background, eat sugary foods, and have a mother with a low education level.[1]

Certain feeding practices can be altered to prevent BBTD. The American Academy of Pediatric Dentistry (AAPD) recommends the cessation of ad lib breast- or bottle-feeding with the initial eruption of teeth. Providing liquids concentrated in mono- and disaccharides, such as juice and sweetened beverages, are the leading cause of BBTD. While sleeping with a bottle in his or her mouth, an infant's swallowing and salivary flow decrease. This creates a pooling of liquid around the teeth. Sweet fluid contacting the teeth for a prolonged period of time provides plaque-forming bacteria, particularly *Streptococcus mutans*, with energy.[1,84] The outcome is dental plaque. Another contributing factor for tooth decay is the early introduction of juice. By the age of 1 year, nearly 90% of all infants in the United States have been introduced to juice; 25% before the age of 6 months.[1] Infants who refuse cold foods or grimace when chewing

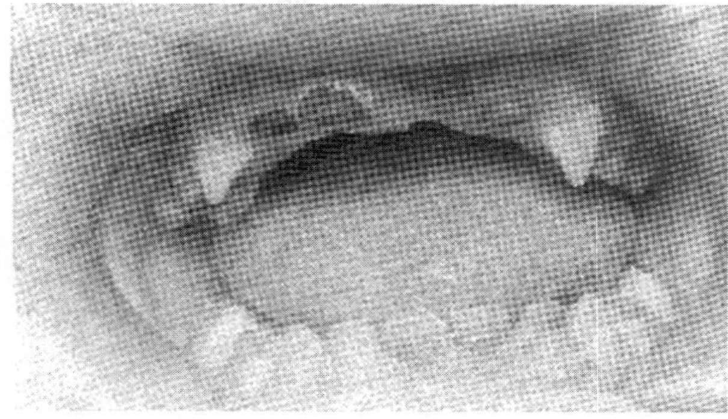

FIGURE 5-1 Baby Bottle Tooth Decay

Source: S.L. Groh and K. Antonelli, Normal Nutrition During Infancy, in *Handbook of Pediatric Nutrition*, P.M. Queen and C.E. Lang, eds., © 1993, Aspen Publishers, Inc. Gaithersburg, MD.

should be examined for BBTD. Those afflicted will have tooth discoloration varying from yellow to black. Preventive measures include the following:

- Feeding only infant formula or water from a bottle.
- Cleaning the infant's teeth and gums with a damp washcloth or gauze pad after each feeding.
- Avoiding juices in the first year; if given offer them in a cup rather than a bottle.
- Filling bedtime bottles with water, if necessary.

In other words, the greater the exposure to sugary rich foods and beverages, the more likely an infant is to develop tooth decay.

Whole Cow's Milk

During the first 12 months of life, The AAP Committee on Nutrition recommends that in order to maintain optimal nutrition status, infants should be provided breast milk, with the only alternative being iron-fortified formulas.[1] As mentioned earlier, potential detrimental effects of early introduction of whole cow's milk in the diet of infants include increased risks of milk protein allergy, excessive renal solute load, gastrointestinal blood loss, poor iron delivery, and overall poor nutritional status of the infant.[1] More current studies have expanded this list of medical concerns to include chronic constipation, and possibly an increased risk for type 1 diabetes.[1]

The incidence of cow's milk protein allergy remains about 2% during the first 2 years of life.[85] Very early introduction of cow's milk increases the risk of developing allergy to milk protein and potentially other foods as well. Resistance to allergy increases with gastrointestinal maturity,[1,86] so that at 6 months of age, small amounts of foods containing cow's milk protein can be introduced into the infant's diet with a reduced risk of developing allergy.

Risks of iron deficiency anemia[87] and other micronutrient deficiencies remain a problem when cow's milk replaces breast milk or formula before 12 months of age. Occult loss of blood from the gastrointestinal tract is associated with the introduction of cow's milk in both early and later infancy. Blood loss, along with the lower concentration and bioavailability of iron in cow's milk, predisposes the infant to iron deficiency anemia.[88] Cow's milk is also a poor source of vitamin C, vitamin E, and essential fatty acids (EFAs).

Lastly, the additional protein and electrolytes in cow's milk increases the renal solute load and places the infant at risk for dehydration during periods of vomiting, diarrhea, or exposure to dry heat in winter or to the sun in the summer. For all of these reasons, it is best to delay the introduction of cow's milk until the infant is 1 year old. When the infant's diet is changed to cow's milk after the first year, it should be whole cow's milk, as opposed to 2% or skim milk, to provide essential fat and calories. Despite these recommendations and negative medical consequences, the FITS study found that nearly one third of all infants were introduced to cow's milk and were consuming it daily within the first year of life.[80]

Water in First Year

Additional water is not necessary during the first year if infants are receiving adequate amounts of breast milk or formula to sustain adequate weight gain. Even in hot months, infants can obtain adequate amounts of free water from breast milk or iron-fortified formula. Caregivers often feel thirsty or hot themselves and offer water to infants. Unfortunately, the free water usually displaces nutrient- and calorie-dense breast milk or infant formula, putting the infant at increased risk for electrolyte imbalance and weight loss. The only exception to this rule is if the caregiver observes the infant having a reduction in urine output or urine appears to be dark in color.[1]

Juice Consumption During Infancy

There has been debate in the past among healthcare providers regarding the benefit of consuming fruit juices during infancy. Juice had been suggested in the second half of infancy as a treatment for hard stools; however, too often infants were consuming excessive amounts, leading to inappropriate growth and malabsorption during infancy. Today, the American Academy of Pediatrics strongly encourages the avoidance of juices in the first 6 months of life. There is concern that any amount of juice intake will put the infant at risk of displacing nutrient-dense breast milk or formula with high-sugar and low-nutrient juices.

If an infant is experiencing harder stools, small amounts of juice can be tried on an as-needed basis only. The carbohydrate source in fruit juice is primarily from a combination of fructose, glucose, and sorbitol. See **Table 5-15** for the carbohydrate sources in various fruit juices.[89] Studies

TABLE 5-15 Carbohydrate Sources in Select Juices (g/100 g of food) (mOsm/kg H_2O)

Juice	Fructose	Glucose	Sucrose	Sorbitol	Osmolality
Apple	6.0	2.4	2.5	0.5	638
Pear	6.6	2.0	3.7	2.2	764
White grape	7.5	7.1	0.6		1030

Values may vary depending on the dilution of the juice and type of fruit used.
Sources: Data from Fomon SJ. *Nutrition of Normal Infants*. St. Louis, MO: Mosby; 1993; Smith MM, Davis M, Chasalow FI, et al. Carbohydrate absorption from fruit juice in young children. *Pediatrics*. 1995;95:340–344; and Hyams JS, Etienne NL, Leichtner AM, et al. Carbohydrate malabsorption following fruit juice ingestion in young children. *Pediatrics*. 1988;82:64–68.

summarized by Fomon suggest that infants better absorb and have greater tolerance to juices containing fructose when found in combination with sucrose and glucose.[89,90] Fruit juices containing these sugars appear to have beneficial effects similar to those of fiber for infants suffering from constipation. Juices containing the greatest amounts of fructose and sorbitol include apple and pear juice.[91,92]

Excessive juice intake puts infants and children at risk for dental caries, failure to thrive, short stature, and obesity later in the preschool years.[93] If an infant has poor weight gain, it is very important to obtain a thorough diet history with specific inquiry into juice or water consumption. The FITS Study revealed that more than 20% of infants ages 4–6 months were already having small amounts of juice in their diets daily.[80,94] When juice is included, only 100% juice should be used, and volumes should not exceed 4–6 ounces a day for children up to 6 years old.[1]

Feeding Problems

Formula intolerance, constipation, acute diarrhea, and food refusal are common feeding problems encountered during infancy. These problems can usually be resolved through simple measures. If ignored, the problems may become exacerbated and cause detrimental effects to an infant's nutritional status and growth.

Food Allergy in Infancy

The concern around food allergies has become apparent in all age groups. Food labels have altered how ingredients are listed and now highlight the most common allergens: milk, soy, egg, wheat, nut, and fish. Airlines have become more cautious about serving peanuts on flights, and physicians suggest restriction of potential food allergens in pregnancy and early infancy to help avoid or delay onset of allergic reactions. After years of potentially over-restricting diets, researchers now wonder whether there is any way to prevent allergies or if current techniques merely delay the onset to later ages.

Incidence of allergy in infants and children appears to range between 1% and 8%, depending upon the patient's age and the specific allergen.[1] Most infants and children appear to outgrow their food allergy as they go through the toddler years; however, some reactions can be severe or even life threatening and never outgrown. Media stories and fear of potentially life-threatening reactions with true allergy have caused some caregivers and parents to be overly sensitive to infant behaviors. It is not unusual to interview caregivers who have changed their infant's formula more than a few times because of perceived intolerances. A true intolerance may be present, but if formulas are changed too quickly, it is difficult to assess the true problem. Intolerance to lactose must not be confused with milk protein allergy. Lactose intolerance is not common in infancy and has an enzymatic etiology, whereas milk allergy is based on immunologic mechanisms. Gastrointestinal disturbance is common to both disorders. Diarrhea is frequently observed in both, but vomiting is exclusive to milk allergy. In addition to gastrointestinal symptoms, dermatologic, respiratory, and possibly systemic reactions, such as anaphylactic shock (although this is rare), may occur in milk allergy.[95]

Milk allergy is usually identified in the first 4 months of infancy. This onset is due to the immaturity of both the gastrointestinal tract and the immune system. In early infancy, the gastrointestinal tract adapts to the extrauterine environment, protecting against the penetration of harmful substances such as bacteria, toxins, and antigens within the intestinal lumen.[96] Mechanisms act to control and maintain the epithelium as an impermeable barrier to the uptake of such antigens as β-lactoglobulin and α-lactalbumin found in cow's milk.

Much research has been done to find the best way to prevent development of allergy. Studies have looked at maternal avoidance during pregnancy and lactation. Other studies evaluated the development of allergy with late introduction of solids or specific allergens during infancy. Unfortunately, there has not been a clear benefit to any of these interventions; in fact, other potential risk factors have been identified, including exposure to tobacco smoke, alcohol, and medications.[97] At best, allergic reactions may be delayed to later in infancy or childhood. Presence of milk protein allergy may correlate with allergies to other foods. Withholding the more allergenic foods from the diet for the first 6 to 12 months of life can be a prophylactic measure; however, the benefit of potential allergen avoidance should be weighed against the risk of over-restriction for the infant. Restricting these allergenic foods until the milk allergy has resolved may be indicated for only the more severe cases. (See Chapter 7 on food sensitivities.) Infants at "high risk" are those with at least one parent with food allergies or siblings with allergies. Recommendations suggest exclusive breastfeeding for at least 4 if not 6 months. If supplementation is needed, consider hypoallergenic or less allergenic formulas to supplement breastfeeding.[98]

Constipation and Stool Characteristics

Constipation is defined by timing and consistency of the stool compared with the usual number of bowel movements. By definition, infants have constipation if they do not have a bowel movement for several days or defecation is extremely dry, hard, or painful.[99] Caregivers may fail to understand that different types of infant feedings are expected to produce variations in stool patterns. "Normal" stooling patterns vary from infant to infant and with differences in dietary intake.

After passing meconium, hopefully within the first 24 hours of life, the number of stools gradually decreases from over four times a day to one to two a day by the end of the first year.[100] Infants being breastfed or receiving hydrolyzed protein formulas typically experience between 1 and 12 bowel movements a day.[100] This can be at least twice as many stools as infants consuming cow's-milk-based or soy-based formulas.[101] Infants fed soy-based formulas tend to have more stools, which are hard and firm.[101]

Stool color also varies with protein source in milk or formula. Breast milk–fed infants typically have stools that look loose to pasty and are yellowish in color. Constipation is rare in breastfed infants; however, infants may have days when they do not have a bowel movement due to enhanced absorption of nutrients from breast milk. Formulas with soy, whey, or casein hydrolyzed protein sources may produce stools that range from yellow to green or brownish in color.[100] Behaviors characteristic during infant stooling that might alarm parents or caregivers include flushing, grunting, and change in stool color with change in diet.[99] These behaviors are actually normal and should decrease over time.

Treating nonanatomic constipation requires dietary intervention. Five measures can be taken in the following sequence:

1. Verify constipation through family interview.
2. Ensure the proper diet, including free fluid intake versus fluid losses.
3. Ensure accurate preparation of formula if infant is bottle-fed.
4. Feed two additional ounces of water after each feeding.
5. Provide two ounces of pear or apple juice per day.

If there is no relief from these recommendations and the infant appears to be in pain or cramping, a physician should be notified.

As discussed earlier, the most recent change in the infant formula market is the addition of prebiotics, attempting to mimic the complex mixture of oligosaccharides present in human breast milk. Initial studies have found potential benefits when prebiotics were added, including softer stools, increased stool frequency, and reduction in infection rates and atopic dermatitis. Ongoing research is being conducted to look at potential benefits in other areas such as improved bone mineral density and calcium absorption.[102]

Regardless of which formula infants are being fed, parents should be discouraged from "formula jumping." This only causes confusion for the infant and the professional attempting to distinguish between a "fussy" infant and a true intolerance or allergic finding.

Acute Diarrhea

Acute infantile diarrhea is defined as the sudden onset of increased stool frequency, volume, and water content with greater than three stools in a 24-hour period.[103] There may be many causes for acute diarrhea (e.g., viral infection, excessive juice intake, antibiotic-associated diarrhea), but most occur in rural areas of developing countries where there is poor sanitation and limited availability of clean water supplies. Persistent diarrhea is defined as lasting greater than 14 days. Infants with persistent diarrhea are usually malnourished and have repetitive cycles of infection and malabsorption.

Diarrhea lasting more than 4 days or resulting in greater than 10% dehydration may require intravenous fluid therapy. However, bottle-fed infants suffering from mild to moderate diarrhea can be rehydrated with an oral rehydration solution for 4 to 6 hours (refer to **Table 5-16**).

After dehydration status is assessed and resolved, reintroduction of age-appropriate foods and liquids should occur as soon as possible. Studies revealed that this approach did not worsen stool output and helped maintain nutritional status.[103] Beverages such as juice, broth, carbonated beverages, or sport drinks should not be provided because their high osmolality may induce osmotic diarrhea, exacerbating the initial problem.[100] Continued breastfeeding is beneficial, despite controversial concerns related to secondary lactose intolerance during acute diarrhea. Lactose-free formulas could be considered in infants who are malnourished or have severe dehydration with persistent diarrhea.[103]

Gastroesophageal Reflux

Gastroesophageal reflux (GER), or chalasia, affects many infants. GER is otherwise referred to as regurgitation or spitting up. A clinical definition is the presence of gastric contents in the esophagus. When complications arise from recurrent reflux, the condition is called GERD, or gastroesophageal reflux disease.[104] All infants experience some degree of GER. Most infants have no significant complications associated with it, whereas others may develop irritability, poor weight gain, failure to thrive, or pulmonary aspiration with pneumonia.[104] Mild GER may be treated with modifications in feeding positions and dietary regimens. More severe GERD may require pharmaceutical or surgical interventions.

An upright position during feeding may prevent GER. In this position, gravity aids in gastric emptying. When an infant is placed in the semi-upright position of an infant seat, however, reduced truncal tone, common in early infancy, may result in slumping.[105] Slumping submerges the infant's posterior gastroesophageal junction into the stomach, increasing abdominal pressure and GER. A truly upright position is most reliable in preventing GER.[106] Regardless of the presence of GER, infants should sleep in supine position in order to reduce the risk of sudden infant death syndrome (SIDS).[104]

Thickening formula with cereal has been routine practice in preventing GER. There has been documentation of

TABLE 5-16 Nutrient Comparisons of Clear Liquids and Rehydration Solutions

Product	Na (mEq/L)	K (mEq/L)	Cl (mEq/L)	Sugar (g/L)	Starch (g/L)	Osmolality (mOsm/L)
Cola	1.7	0.1–0.6	—	53–58.5	—	750
Apple Juice	4.6	26	1.1	39.5	—	747
Gatorade	20–23	2.5–3	23	25–28	—	330–365
Chicken Broth	250	8	—	—	—	500
Enfalyte	50	25	45	25	—	167
Pedialyte	45	20	35	25	—	270

Sources: Data from Swedberg J, Steiner J. Oral rehydration therapy in diarrhea: not just for Third World children. *Postgrad Med.* 1983;74:335–341; and Synder J. Oral rehydration therapy for acute diarrhea. *Semin Pediatr Gastroenterol Nutr.* 1990;1:8; and from product information provided by Abbott Nutrition and Mead Johnson Nutritionals.

anecdotal responses to this treatment, including decreased emesis and crying time, and increased sleeping time in the postprandial period. Some believe a trial of a commercially prepared formula with added rice starch may be beneficial to reduce visible regurgitation; however, it does not decrease the number of esophageal reflux episodes. The clinician must also be aware that cereal increases the caloric concentration of formula, altering the protein:carbohydrate:fat ratio, interfering with breastfeeding, and possibly delaying gastric emptying.

Milk protein intolerance can be a cause of reflux or vomiting in infants. If the feeding regimens suggested above do not improve symptoms, switching to an alternate protein source may be warranted.

Food Refusal

The two important feeding milestones during infancy are self-feeding and developing a positive relationship with food and eating. If these do not occur, a spiral effect of food refusal and poor nutrient intake can ensue. It is currently estimated that feeding problems may occur in up to 25–35% of infants and children.[107] Food refusal can occur in infancy because of physical or emotional stress. This is more typically classified as organic, indicating a medical or functional etiology, caused by environmental influences. Illness and an unfavorable atmosphere for feeding are typical contributors to food refusal. The consequence of this problem is failure to thrive.

During illness, infants become irritable due to fever, congestion, or lack of sleep. At these times, food refusal is inevitable. The encouragement of oral fluid intake, and in severe cases administration of parenteral fluids, is necessary to prevent or treat dehydration. Although food refusal of this nature can still cause significant weight loss and deplete nutrient stores, if identified early, it is usually self-limited.

Food refusal originating from excessive or deficient stimulation is more difficult to discern. Commotion and overly aggressive or restrictive caregivers can cause development of negative associations with feeding. Routine negative interactions at mealtime can keep an infant from wanting to explore and advance with the normal self-feeding progression. As the stages of eating advance from liquid and dependence as a newborn to table foods as a toddler, parents need to be attuned to their child's developmental transition with eating.[108] The caregiver may restrict the infant's exploration of food and/or rush through a meal, disrupting the feeding pace. Under these circumstances, it is not uncommon for an infant to begin to refuse food entirely. Concerned that the infant is feeding poorly or losing weight, caregivers become tense. This tension only exacerbates the reluctance to feed.

The most effective means of treating feeding disorders after identification is to increase appropriate behavior and decrease maladaptive behavior between the infant and caregiver and between the infant and the feeding experience. As infants get closer to their first birthday, their interest in self-feeding and encouragement of self-regulation with food intake should be promoted. Most literature related to feeding disorders promotes a calm, interactive, and supportive environment, and encourages the most positive relationship with infant feeding.

Suggested Websites

http://www.mypyramid.gov
http://www.aap.org
http://www.eatright.org
http://www.babycenter.com
http://www.keepkidshealthy.com
http://www.healthychildren.org
http://www.gerber.com
http://www.heinzbaby.com

Conclusion

Issues related to breastfeeding, bottle-feeding, vitamin and mineral supplementation, the introduction and progression of solids, and common feeding problems have all been discussed in this chapter. Translating this scientific information into practical suggestions for parents and caregivers is necessary. Infancy is a time for developing healthy eating habits and family relationships around mealtimes. As early as infancy, pediatric healthcare professions have a responsibility for identifying those at greatest risk for developing feeding and nutrition problems and providing appropriate education and intervention as soon as possible.

Case Study

Patient history: BA is a 6-month-old girl born at term to a healthy, 26-year-old mother with no family history of allergy. The baby is being seen today for WIC recertification. BA's anthropometric measurements are 7.1 kg (weight), 65 cm (length), and 42.25 cm (head circumference). Mother puts the baby to breast five to six times per day using one breast at each feeding. Each feeding lasts about 15 minutes. BA is this mother's first baby, and the mother reports that the baby "is a good breastfeeder"—she latches well with audible sucking and visible swallowing—and she burps easily with minimal spitting up. The baby has three or more very soft, yellow stools each day. In the last few weeks, the mother has noticed that the baby seems less satisfied after feeding. The baby had been sleeping through the night but now occasionally wakes early for a feeding. The baby gets a daily 1 mL dose of Tri-vi-sol, an infant vitamin drop. The WIC dietitian notices that BA has good head control and puts her hands in her mouth.

Anticipatory guidance is offered so that the parents know what to expect. This includes:

- Obtain a high chair if one is not currently available.
- Provide opportunities for the infant to eat with others.
- Add more solid food variety in the next 1–2 months starting with Stage One meats followed by fruits and vegetables.
- Advance texture as tolerated. Wait 2–3 days between new foods to assess for a possible allergic reaction.
- Offer finger foods (dry cereal or toast; small tender pieces of meat, vegetables, or fruits; noodles; etc.) as tolerated around 8–9 months.
- Assess for anemia at 9–15 months.
- Offer cup feeding as tolerated at 9–12 months.
- Delay juice and cow's milk until 12 months.
- Continue the vitamin D supplement until the baby consumes 1 liter or quart per day of vitamin D–fortified milk.

Questions for the Reader

1. Plot BA's length, weight, head circumference, and weight-for-length on a CDC growth chart. What percentiles is she in?
2. Using the Nutrition Care process, does BA have a nutritional diagnosis?
3. What interventions are needed at this WIC visit (what food and/or nutrient supplements would you recommend for BA)?

REFERENCES

1. Kleinman R. *Pediatric Nutrition Handbook*, 6th ed. Elk Grove Village, IL: American Academy of Pediatrics; 2009.
2. Newborn Screening Authoring Committee. Newborn screening expands: recommendations for pediatricians and medical homes—implications for the system. *Pediatrics*. 2008;121:192–217. (doi:10.1542/peds.2007-3021)
3. Kaye CI, Committee on Genetics. Introduction to the newborn screening fact sheets. *Pediatrics*. 2006;118(3):1304–1312.
4. Institute of Medicine. *Dietary Reference Intakes for Energy, Carbohydrate, Fiber, Fat, Fatty Acids, Cholesterol, Protein, and Amino Acids (Macronutrients)*. Washington, DC: National Academies Press; 2005.
5. Institute of Medicine. *Dietary Reference Intakes for Water, Potassium, Sodium, Chloride, and Sulfate*. Washington, DC: National Academies Press; 2005.
6. Lawrence RA, Lawrence RM. *Breastfeeding: A Guide for the Medical Profession*, 6th ed. St. Louis, MO: Mosby; 2005.
7. American Academy of Pediatrics. Breastfeeding and the use of human milk. *Pediatrics*. 2005;115:496–506.
8. Position of the American Dietetic Association: promoting and supporting breast-feeding. *J Am Diet Assoc*. 2009;109:1926–1942.
9. Ahluwalia I, Morrow B, Hsia J, Grummer-Strawn L. Who is breast-feeding? Recent trends from the pregnancy risk assessment and monitoring system. *J Pediatrics*. 2003;142:486–491.
10. Grummer-Strawn LM, Scanlon KS, Fein SB. Infant feeding and feeding transitions during the first year of life. *Pediatrics*. 2008;122:S36–S42.
11. American Academy of Pediatrics, Committee on Practice and Ambulatory Medicine. Pediatrics' responsibility for infant nutrition. *Pediatrics*. 1997;99:749–750.
12. Scott JA, Binns CW, Aroni RA. The influence of reported paternal attitudes on the decision to breast-feed. *J Pediatr Child Health*. 1997;33:305–307.

13. Heird W. The role of polyunsaturated fatty acids in term and preterm infants and breast-feeding mothers. *Pediatr Clin North Am.* 2001;48:173–188.
14. Scariati PD, Grummer-Strawn LM, Fein SB. A longitudinal analysis of infant morbidity and the extent of breast-feeding in the United States [Abstract]. *Pediatrics.* 1997;99(6):5.
15. Dewey KG, Heinig MJ, Nommsen LA, et al. Breast-fed infants are leaner than formula-fed infants at 1 year of age: the DARLING study. *Am J Clin Nutr.* 1993;57:140–145.
16. Gdalevich M, Mimouni D, David M, Mimouni M. Breast-feeding and the onset of atopic dermatitis in childhood: a systemic review and meta-analysis of prospective studies. *J Am Acad Dermatol.* 2001;45:520–527.
17. Gillman M. Breast-feeding and obesity. *J Pediatr.* 2002;141:749–750.
18. American Academy of Pediatrics, Committee on Nutrition. Prevention of pediatric overweight and obesity. *Pediatrics.* 2003;112:424–430.
19. Picciano MF. Representative values for constituents of human milk. *Pediatr Clin North Am.* 2001;48:263–264.
20. Karra MV, Udipi SA, Kirksey A, Roepke JLB. Changes in specific nutrients in breast milk during extended lactation. *Am J Clin Nutr.* 1986;43:495–503.
21. Lourdes B, Butte NF, Villalpando S, et al. Maternal energy balance and lactation performance of Mesoamerindians as a function of body mass index. *Am J Clin Nutr.* 1997;66:575–583.
22. Institute of Medicine. *Nutrition During Lactation.* Washington, DC: National Academy of Sciences; 1991.
23. Jensen RG. *Handbook of Milk Composition.* San Diego, CA: Academic Press; 1995.
24. Misra M, Pacaud D, Petryk A, et al. Vitamin D deficiency in children and its management: review of current knowledge and recommendations. *Pediatrics.* 2008;122:398–417.
25. Wagner CL, Greer FR, Section on Breastfeeding and Committee on Nutrition. Prevention of rickets and vitamin D deficiency in infants, children, and adolescents. *Pediatrics.* 2008;122:1142–1152.
26. Hill DJ, Roy N, Heine RG, et al. Effect of a low-allergen maternal diet on colic among breastfed infants: a randomized, controlled trial. *Pediatrics.* 2005;116:e709–e715.
27. Berlin CM, Denson HM, Daniel CH, Ward RM. Deposition of dietary caffeine in milk, saliva, and plasma of lactating women. *Pediatrics.* 1984;73:59–63.
28. Luck W, Nau H. Nicotine and cotinine concentrations in serum and urine of infants exposed via passive smoking or milk from smoking mothers. *J Pediatr.* 1985;107:816–820.
29. American Academy of Pediatrics, American College of Obstetricians and Gynecologists. *Breastfeeding Handbook for Physicians. Elk Grove Village, IL:American Academy of Pediatrics:* 2006.
30. Meek JY, ed. *New Mother's Guide to Breastfeeding.* New York: Bantam Books; 2002.
31. Fomon SJ. *Nutrition of Normal Infants.* St. Louis, MO: Mosby; 1993.
32. Jensen RG. *Handbook of Milk Composition.* New York: Academic Press; 1995.
33. Life Science Research Office. LSRO report: assessment of nutrient requirements for infant formulas. *J Nutr.* 1998;128:2059–2078.
34. O'Connor NR. Infant formula. *Am Fam Physician.* 2009;79(7): 565–570.
35. Ziegler EE. Milk and formulas for older infants. *J Pediatr.* 1990;117:76.
36. Simmer K, Patole SK, Rao SC. Longchain polyunsaturated fatty acid supplementation in infants born at term. *Cochrane Database Syst Rev.* 2008;(1):CD000376.
37. Koo W, Hammami M, Margeson D, et al. Reduced bone mineralization in infants fed palm olein-containing formula: a randomized, double-blinded, prospective trial. *Pediatrics.* 2003;111:1017–1023.
38. Boehm G, Stahl B. Oligosaccharides from milk. *J Nutr.* 2007;137:847S–849S.
39. Fanaro S, Marten B, Bagna R, et al. Galacto-oligosaccharides are bifidogenic and safe at weaning: a double-blind randomized multicenter study. *J Pediatr Gastroenterol Nutr.* 2008;48:82–88.
40. Ziegler E, Vanderhoof JA, Petschow B, et al. Term infants fed formula supplemented with selected blends of prebiotics grow normally and have soft stools similar to those reported for breast-fed infants. *J Pediatr Gastroenterol Nutr.* 2007;44:359–364.
41. Moro G, Minoli I, Mosca M, et al. Dosage-related bifidogenic effects of galacto- and fructooligosaccharides in formula-fed term infants. *J Pediatr Gastroenterol Nutr.* 2002;34:291–295.
42. Arslanoglu S, Moro GE, Schmitt J, et al. Early dietary intervention with a mixture of prebiotic oligosaccharides reduces the incidence of allergic manifestations and infections during the first two years of life. *J Nutr.* 2008;138:1091–1095.
43. Saavedra JM, Abi-Hanna A, Moore N, Yolken RH. Long-term consumption of infant formula containing live probiotic bacteria: tolerance and safety. *Am J Clin Nutr.* 2004;79:261–267.
44. Langhendries JP, Detry J, Van Hees J, et al. Effect of a fermented infant formula containing viable bifidobacteria on the fecal flora composition and pH of healthy full-term infants. *J Pediatr Gastroenterol Nutr.* 1996;21:177–181.
45. Agostoni C, Axelsson I, Braegger, C, et al. Probiotic bacteria in dietetic products for infants: a commentary by the ESPGHAN Committee on Nutrition. *J Pediatr Gastroenterol Nutr.* 2004;38:365–374.
46. Craig WR, Hanlo-Dearman A, Sinclair C, et al. Metoclopramide, thickened feedings, and positioning for gastro-oesophageal reflux in children under two years. *Cochrane Database Syst Rev.* 2004;(4):CD003502.
47. Moukarzel AA, Abdelnour H, Akatcherian C. Effects of a prethickened formula on esophageal pH and gastric emptying of infants with GER. *J Clin Gastroenterol.* 2007;41(9):823–829.
48. American Academy of Pediatrics, Committee on Nutrition. Iron fortification of infant formulas. *Pediatrics.* 1999;104:119–123.
49. Bhatia J, Greer F, Committee on Nutrition. Use of soy protein-based formulas in infant feeding. *Pediatrics.* 2008;121:1062–1068.
50. Zeiger RS, Sampson HA, Bock SA, et al. Soy allergy in infants and children with IgE-associated cow's milk allergy. *J Pediatr.* 1999;134:614–622.
51. Greer FR, Sicherer SH, Burks AW, Committee on Nutrition and Section on Allergy and Immunology. Effects of early nutritional interventions on the development of atopic disease in infants and children: the role of maternal dietary restriction, breastfeeding, timing of introduction of complementary foods, and hydrolyzed formulas. *Pediatrics.* 2008;121:183–191.
52. Scalabrin DM, Johnston WH, Hoffman DR, et al. Growth and tolerance of healthy term infants receiving hydrolyzed

infant formulas supplemented with *Lactobacillus rhamnosus* GG: randomized, double-blind, controlled trial. *Clin Pediatr.* 2009;48(7):734–744.
53. Fomon SJ, Filer LJ, Anderson TA, Ziegler EE. Recommendations for feeding normal infants. *Pediatrics*. 1979;63:52–59.
54. U.S. Food and Drug Administration. FDA 101: infant formula. Available at: http://www.fda.gov/ForConsumers/ConsumerUpdates/ucm048694.htm. Accessed December 29, 2009.
55. Dietz WH, Stern L, eds. *American Academy of Pediatrics Guide to Your Child's Nutrition*. New York: Villard; 1999.
56. Teske S, Robbins S. Formula preparation and handling. In: Robbins ST, Beker LT, Pediatric Nutrition Practice Group, eds. *Infant Feedings: Guidelines for Preparation of Formula and Breastmilk in Health Care Facilities*. Chicago, IL: American Dietetic Association; 2004:31–67.
57. Kang J, Kondo F, Katayama Y. Human exposure to bisphenol A. *Toxicology.* 2006;226:79–89.
58. Gillman MW, Barker D, Bier D, et al. Meeting report on the 3rd International Congress on Developmental Origins of Health and Disease (DOHaD). *Pediatr Res.* 2007;61:625–629.
59. Centers for Disease Control and Prevention. *Enterobacter sakazakii* infections associated with the use of powdered infant formula. *MMWR*. 2002;51:297–300.
60. Hibbard RA, Blevins R. Palatal burn due to bottle warming in a microwave oven. *Pediatrics*. 1988;82:382–384.
61. Puczynski M, Rademaker D, Gatson RL. Burn injury related to the improper use of a microwave oven. *Pediatrics*. 1983;72:714–715.
62. Tully SB, Bar-Halm Y, Bradley RL. Abnormal tympanography after supine bottle-feeding. *J Pediatr*. 1995;126:S105–S111.
63. Nevin-Folino NL, ed. *Pediatric Manual of Clinical Dietetics*, 2nd ed. Chicago: American Dietetic Association; 2003.
64. Wagner CL, Greer FR, Section on Breastfeeding and Committee on Nutrition. Prevention of rickets and vitamin D deficiency in infants, children, and adolescents. *Pediatrics*. 2008;122:1142–1152.
65. Misra M, Pacaud D, Petryk A, et al. Vitamin D deficiency in children and its management: review of current knowledge and recommendations. *Pediatrics.* 2008;122:398–417.
66. Holick MF. Vitamin D deficiency. *N Engl J Med.* 2007;357:266–281.
67. Fomon S. Feeding normal infants: rationale for recommendations. *J Am Diet Assoc*. 2001;101:1002–1005.
68. Butte N, Cobb K, Duyer J, Graney L, Heird W, Rickard K. The start healthy feeding guidelines for infants and toddlers. *J Amer Diet Assoc*. 2004;104:442–484.
69. Fox MK, Devaney B, Reidy K, Razafindrakoto C, Ziegler P. Relationship between portion size and energy intake among infants and toddlers: evidence of self-regulations. *J Am Diet Assoc.* 2006;106:S77–S83.
70. Lipsitt L, Crook C, Booth C. The transitional infant: behavioral development and feeding. *Am J Clin Nutr.* 1985;41:485–496.
71. Cloud H, Feeding problems of the child with special health care needs. In: Ekvall SW,ed. *Pediatric Nutrition in Chronic Diseases and Developmental Disorders: Prevention, Assessment, and Treatment*. New York: Oxford University Press; 1993:203–218.
72. Chatoor I, Hirsch R, Persinger M. Facilitating internal regulation of eating: a treatment model of infantile anorexia. *Infants Young Child.* 1997;9(4):12–22.
73. Underwood B. Weaning practices in deprived environments: the weaning dilemma. *Pediatrics*. 1985;75(Suppl):194–198.
74. Pipes P, Trahms CM. *Nutrition in Infancy and Childhood*, 5th ed. St. Louis, MO: Mosby; 1993.
75. Fox MK, Reidy K, Novak T, Ziegler P. Sources of energy and nutrients in the diets of infants and toddlers. *J Am Diet Assoc.* 2006;106:S28–S42.
76. Murray R, Battista M. Managing the risk of childhood overweight and obesity in primary care practice. *Curr Probl Pediatr Adolesc Health Care*. 2009;39:145–166.
77. Oskarsson A. Exposure of Infants and Children to Lead: Working Document for the 30th meeting of the Joint FAO/WHO Expert Committee on Food Additives . Renouf Publishing Co. Rome Italy,1989.
78. Shils ME, Olson JA, Shike M. *Modern Nutrition in Health and Disease*, 8th ed. Philadelphia, PA: Lea & Febiger; 1994.
79. Blumberg S. Infant feeding: can we spice it up a bit? *J Am Diet Assoc.* 2006;106:504–505.
80. Fox MK, Pac S, Devaney B, Jankowski L. Feeding infants and toddlers study: what foods are infants and toddlers eating? *J Am Diet Assoc.* 2004;104(Suppl 1):S22–S30.
81. Worobey J, Lopez MI, Hoffman D. Maternal behavior and infant weight gain in first year. *J Nutr Educ Behav.* 2009;41:169–175.
82. Owen, CG, Martin RM, Whincup PH, et al. Effect of infant feeding on risk of obesity across the life course: a quantitative review of published evidence. *Pediatrics.* 2005;115:1367–1377.
83. Robinson SM, Marriott LD, Crozier SR, et al. Variations in infant feeding practice are associated with body composition in childhood: a prospective cohort study. *J Clin Endocrinol Metab.* 2009;94:2799–2805.
84. Nowak A. What pediatricians can do to promote oral health. *Contemp Pediatr*. 1993;10:90–106.
85. Sampson HA. Update on food allergy. *J Allergy Clin Immunol.* 2004;113:805–819.
86. Tunnessen WW, Oski FA. Consequences of starting whole cow milk at 6 months of age. *J Pediatr*. 1987;111:813–816.
87. Walter T, DeAndraca I, Chadud P, et al. Iron deficiency anemia: adverse effects on infant psychomotor development. *Pediatrics.* 1989;84:7–17.
88. Ziegler EE, Fomon SJ, Nelson SE, et al. Cow milk feeding in infancy: further observations on blood loss from the gastrointestinal tract. *J Pediatr.* 1990;116:11–18.
89. Fomon SJ. *Nutrition of Normal Infants.* St. Louis, MO: Mosby; 1993.
90. Hoekstra JH, van Kempen AA, Kneepkens CM. Apple juice malabsorption: fructose or sorbitol? *J Pediatr Gastroenterol Nutr.* 1993;16:39–42.
91. Smith MM, Davis M, Chasalow FI, et al. Carbohydrate absorption from fruit juice in young children. *Pediatrics.* 1995;95:340–344.
92. Lifschitz CH. Fruit juice [Letter to the editor]. *Pediatrics*. 1995;96:376.
93. Levine AA. Excessive fruit juice consumption: how can something that causes failure to thrive be associated with obesity? [Selected summary]. *J Pediatr Gastroenterol Nutr*. 1997;25:554–555.
94. Skinner JD, Ziegler P, Ponza M. Transitions in infants' and toddlers' beverage patterns. *J Am Diet Assoc.* 2004;104:S45–S50.

95. Wyllie R, Hyams JS. *Pediatric Gastrointestinal Diseases*. Philadelphia, PA: WB Saunders; 1993.
96. Walker A. Absorption of protein and protein fragments in the developing intestine: role in immunologic/allergic reactions. *Pediatrics*. 1985;75(Suppl):167.
97. Pali-Scholl I, Renz H, Jensen-Jarolim E. Update on allergies in pregnancy, lactation, and early childhood. *J Allergy Clin Immunol*. 2009;123:1012–1021.
98. Sicherer SH, Burks AW. Maternal and infant diets for prevention of allergic diseases: understanding menu changes in 2008. *J Allergy Clin Immunol* 2008;122:29
99. Montgomery DF, Navarro F. Management of constipation and encopresis in children. *J Pediatr Health Care*. 2008;22:199–204.
100. Hyams J, Treem WR, Etienne NL, et al. Effects of infant formula on stool characteristics of young infants. *Pediatrics*. 1995;95:50–54.
101. Hillemier C. Gastroesophageal reflux. *Pediatr Clin North Am*. 1996;43(1):197–212.
102. Sherman PM, Cabana M, Gibson GR et al. Potential roles and clinical utility of prebiotics in newborns, infants, and children: proceedings from a global prebiotic summit meeting, New York City, June 27–28, 2008. *J Ped*. 2009;155:S61–S70.
103. Grimwood K, Forbes D. Acute and persistent diarrhea. *Pediatr Clin N Am*. 2009;56:1343–1361.
104. Vandenplas Y, Rudolph C, Lorenzo CD, et al. Pediatric gastroesophageal reflux clinical practice guidelines: joint recommendations of the North American Society of Pediatric Gastroenterology, Hepatology, and Nutrition and the European Society of Pediatric Gastroenterology, Hepatology, and Nutrition. *J Pediatr Gastroenterol Nutr*. 2009;49:498–547.
105. Herbst J. Gastroesophageal reflux. *J Pediatr*. 1981;98:859–870.
106. Orenstein S, Whitington P. Positioning for prevention of infant gastroesophageal reflux. *J Pediatr*. 1983;103:534–537.
107. Rudolph C, Link D. Feeding disorders in infants and children. *Pediatr Clin N Am*. 2002;49:97–112.
108. Couch SC, Falciglia GA. Improving the diets of the young: considerations for intervention design. *J Am Diet Assoc*. 2006; 106:S10–S11.
109. Hinton S, Kerwin D. *Maternal and Child Nutrition*. Chapel Hill, NC: Health Sciences Consortium Corporation; 1981.
110. American Academy of Pediatrics, Committee on Nutrition. Infant methemoglobinemia: the role of dietary nitrate. *Pediatrics*. 1970;46:475–478.
111. Kerr C, Reisinger K, Plankey F. Sodium concentration of homemade baby foods. *Pediatrics*. 1978;62:331–335.
112. Hyams JS, Etienne NL, Leichtner AM, et al. Carbohydrate malabsorption following fruit juice ingestion in young children. *Pediatrics*. 1988;82:64–68.
113. Snyder J. Oral rehydration therapy for acute diarrhea. *Semin Pediatr Gastroenterol Nutr*. 1990;1:8.
114. Swedberg J, Steiner J. Oral rehydration therapy in diarrhea: not just for Third World children. *Postgrad Med*. 1983;74:335–341.

Normal Nutrition from Infancy Through Adolescence

Betty Lucas, Beth Ogata, and Sharon Feucht

From 1 year of age through adolescence, children experience the most changes in physical, cognitive, and social-emotional growth. The 1-year-old toddler is taking his or her first steps into the bigger world, becoming more independent in self-help skills, and rapidly learning to communicate. At the other end of the spectrum, the 18-year-old is also taking steps into the world, becoming more independent and self-sufficient in many areas, and planning for the future. This chapter will focus on the nutritional needs and issues of normal, healthy children during these growing years.

Progress in Growth and Development

After the rapid growth of infancy, there is considerable slowing in physical growth during the preschool and school years. The elementary school years are often referred to as the *latent period* prior to the pubertal growth spurt of adolescence. Children will have individual growth patterns, which may be erratic at times, with spurts in height and weight followed by periods of little or no growth. These patterns usually correspond to similar changes in appetite and food intake in healthy children and teenagers. Parents and other caregivers need to realize that these changes are normal so they can avoid struggles over food and eating.

Developmental progress during the growing years influences many aspects of food and eating. The very young child prefers food that can be picked up or doesn't have to be chased across the plate. Food jags may be more an expression of independence than of actual likes and dislikes. In older children, the influence of peers and of the media will affect snack choices. Teenagers want foods that fit into their lifestyles, are quick and easy to fix, and are inexpensive. Understanding the developmental characteristics and milestones at any particular age will help parents and professionals to set realistic expectations, support eating behavior and food decisions that are developmentally appropriate, and avoid unnecessary conflicts. Satter[1] has described well the feeding relationship between parents and children of all ages, which incorporates these developmental aspects.

Nutrient Needs

The primary factor in determining nutrient needs is usually a child's rate and stage of growth. Other factors include physical activity, body size, basal energy expenditure, and state of health. There is a wide range of actual needs based on individual characteristics. The dietary reference intakes (DRIs), which include the recommended dietary allowances (RDAs) and adequate intake (AI), serve as a guide to prevent deficiency and/or to provide positive health benefits.[2] Many of the data for children and adolescents, however, are extrapolated values. Because these guidelines provide a margin of safety greater than the physiologic requirements for most children in the United States, they are not meant to be marker goals for individual children. Intakes less than these guidelines do not presume inadequacies or adverse effects (see Appendix H-1 and H-2).

Energy

Energy needs are the most variable, due to individual differences in basal metabolism, growth, physical activity, onset of puberty, and body size. The DRIs include equations for estimated energy requirements (EERs) for children who are not overweight, and weight maintenance total energy expenditure (TEE) for children who are overweight. Unlike previous guidelines for energy intake, the DRIs incorporate direct measures of energy expenditure using doubly labeled water studies. EER equations through age 2 years include allowances for age and weight. EER and TEE equations for children 3 years and older include allowances for age, sex, weight, height, and level of physical activity.[3] These references for energy intake in children and adolescents provide tools to both assess energy intake and develop nutrition care plans that incorporate the individual child's size, activity, and state of health.

Protein

Adequate protein intake is needed to provide for optimal growth in children and adolescents. National surveys have reported actual protein intakes to be in the range of 10–15% of energy for these ages.[4] This level assumes that enough energy is provided so that protein is spared for growth. Protein needs decrease as the growth rate slows after infancy, then increase again at puberty. Total protein intake increases steadily until about 12 years of age in girls and 16 years of age in boys.

In the United States, protein intakes usually exceed recommended allowances. Some children and adolescents, however, may be at risk for protein malnutrition if energy is inadequate so that protein is used for energy. Examples include those with inadequate energy intakes (extreme use of low-fat diets, limited access to food, dieting to lose weight, and athletes in training who limit food), those who are strict vegetarians, and some with food allergies. Dietary evaluation of protein intake should include the growth rate, energy intake, and quality of the protein sources.

Minerals and Vitamins

Although clinical signs of vitamin or mineral deficiency are rare in the United States, dietary intake studies have reported that the nutrients most likely to be low or deficient in the diets of children and adolescents are calcium, vitamin D, magnesium, vitamin A, vitamin E, and vitamin C.[5–9] Certain populations of children, such as low-income, Native American, and other groups with limited food and health resources (e.g., the homeless), are more at risk for poor diet and nutrient deficiencies. Most of the recommended allowances for children and adolescents have been extrapolated from studies on infants and adults.

Calcium

Primarily needed for bone mineralization, calcium needs are determined by growth velocity, rates of absorption, and other nutrients, such as phosphorus, vitamin D, and protein. Because of individual variability, a child receiving less than the recommended allowance of calcium is not necessarily at risk. Approximately 100 mg of calcium per day is retained as bone in the preschool years. This doubles or triples for adolescents during peak growth periods.[10] Adolescence is a critical period for optimal calcium retention to achieve peak bone mass, especially for females who are at risk for osteoporosis in later years. Calcium intake, however, often decreases during the teen years. Balance studies indicate that young adolescent girls (younger than 16 years of age) may need to consume as much as 1600 mg per day to achieve maximum calcium intake and calcium balance.[10] Even prepubertal children have demonstrated increased bone mineral density when their diets have been supplemented with calcium.[11] The Food and Nutrition Board recommends an AI of 1300 mg of calcium per day for ages 9 to 18 years to support optimal bone mineralization.[2]

Those who consume none or only limited amounts of dairy products—the major source of calcium—are at risk for calcium deficiency. Some adolescents may also receive less calcium than needed because of rapid growth, dieting practices, and substituting carbonated beverages for milk. In assessing calcium status, vitamin D intake should be considered because of its major role in calcium metabolism. For children with limited sunshine exposure, dietary intake is critical. Vitamin D–fortified milk is the primary food source of this nutrient; other dairy products are not usually made with fortified milk. A child may be receiving adequate calcium from cheese and yogurt but taking very little fluid milk and, thus, receiving minimal dietary vitamin D. **Table 6-1** contains a list of calcium food sources. Levels of physical activity also affect an individual's calcium needs for optimal bone development.[12]

Iron

Requirements for iron are determined by the rate of growth, iron stores, increasing blood volumes, and rate of absorption from food sources. Menstrual losses, as well as rapid growth, increase the need in adolescent females. To reach adulthood with an adequate storage of iron, recommended daily intakes are 7 mg for children ages 1 to 3 years, 10 mg for 4- to 8-year-olds, 11 mg for pubertal males, and 15 mg

TABLE 6-1 Calcium Equivalents

1 cup milk* = approx. 300 mg calcium	1 cup (8 oz) yogurt†
	1 cup calcium-fortified orange juice
	1 cup calcium-fortified soy milk‡
	1 cup calcium-fortified rice milk or almond milk‡,§
¾ cup milk =	1 oz cheddar, jack, or Swiss cheese
⅔ cup milk =	1 oz mozzarella or American cheese
	2 oz canned sardines (with bones)
½ cup milk =	2 oz canned salmon (with bones)
	½ cup custard or milk pudding
	½ cup cooked greens (mustard, collards, kale)
¼ cup milk =	½ cup cottage cheese
	½ cup ice cream
	¾ cup dried beans, cooked or canned

*Some low-fat or skim milks and some low-fat yogurts have additional nonfat dry milk (NFDM) solids added. Some labels will read "fortified." Such products will contain more calcium than indicated here.

†Most commercially prepared yogurt does not contain vitamin D.

‡The amount of calcium varies; not all milks are fortified with calcium and/or vitamin D.

§Rice and almond milks (and other nut milks) have significantly less protein than cow's milk and soy milk.

for pubertal females.[13] (See the iron deficiency anemia discussion later in this chapter.)

Vitamin D

Vitamin D is increasingly recognized as an important nutrient for its role in bone health, and for other potential roles, including prevention of cancer, autoimmune disorders, cardiovascular disease, and infectious diseases. The American Academy of Pediatrics has increased recommendations for intake to 400 IU per day for all infants, children, and adolescents, beginning in the first few days of life.[14] Serum 25-hydroxyvitamin D (25[OH]D) levels are used to measure deficiency and insufficiency; however, there is some controversy about the cut-off levels to indicate insufficiency; many experts feel the levels have been too low in the past. An analysis of National Health and Nutrition Examination Survey (NHANES) data indicated vitamin D deficiency in about 9% of children, and insufficiency in 61%.[15]

The recent recommendations to increase vitamin D intake will require a careful evaluation of a child's intake to determine if a supplement is needed to reach these goals, especially in young children.[14]

Vitamin–Mineral Supplements

The use of supplements is a common practice in the United States. Almost 40% of preschool children take supplements, typically a multivitamin–mineral preparation. Supplement use declines among older children—29% for children ages 9–13 years and 26% among 14- to 18-year-olds.[16] Children taking supplements do not necessarily represent those who need them. Higher rates of use are found in families with higher incomes. However, the supplements may not be providing the marginal or deficient nutrients either; for example, a child may be taking a children's vitamin but may actually need extra calcium, not always provided in a supplement.

Except for fluoride supplementation in nonfluoridated areas, the American Academy of Pediatrics does not support routine supplementation for normal, healthy children.[17] It does, however, identify six groups at nutritional risk who might benefit from supplementation. These include children and adolescents:

1. With anorexia, inadequate appetite, or who consume fad diets
2. With chronic disease (e.g., cystic fibrosis, inflammatory bowel disease, hepatic disease)
3. From deprived families or those who are abused or neglected
4. Using a dietary program to manage obesity
5. Who do not consume adequate amounts of dairy products
6. With failure to thrive

Both the American Dietetic Association and the American Medical Association also have recommended that nutrients for healthy children should come from food, not supplements.[18,19]

Children with food allergies, those who omit entire food groups, and those with limited food acceptances will be likely candidates for supplementation. No risk is involved if parents wish to give their children a standard pediatric multivitamin. Megadose levels of nutrients should be discouraged and parents counseled regarding the dangers of toxicity, especially of fat-soluble vitamins. The DRIs include tolerable upper intake levels (UL), which can be used to determine excessive levels of vitamins and minerals from supplemental sources.[2] Because many children's vitamins look and taste like candy, parents should be educated to keep them out of reach of children.

Use of other dietary supplements, including herbal preparations, is becoming more widespread. Although many supplements are harmless and may be beneficial, others may be dangerous and/or affect nutritional status. Evaluation of dietary intake should include questions about the use of supplements.[20] This topic is covered in Chapter 21.

Food Intake Patterns and Guidelines

Because appetite usually follows the rate of growth, food intake is not always smooth and consistent. After observing a good appetite in infancy, parents frequently describe their preschool children as having fair to poor appetites, a response to a slower growth rate. There is a wide variability in nutrient intake in healthy children. Daily energy intake of preschool children is surprisingly constant, despite a high variability from meal to meal. One classic longitudinal study found that the maximum intake of energy, carbohydrate, fat, and protein was two to three times the minimum intake. For ascorbic acid and carotene, the maximum/minimum ratios were 10:1 and 20:1, all in healthy children.[21] With such variability (especially in micronutrient intake) being the norm for children, nutrition professionals need to use dietary assessment tools that include intake over time.

Just as there are changing trends of dietary patterns in the general public, similar patterns are seen in children. National dietary studies have shown decreased intake of whole milk and eggs, greater use of low-fat and nonfat milk, more snacking, and more eating away from home among children and adolescents.[5,8] These shifts in intake, however, still do not meet national recommendations such as the U.S. Dietary Guidelines or the USDA Food Guide (see Appendix I). Using national data, one study reported an average of 35% of energy intake from fat, and only about one-third of the group met recommendations for fruit, vegetable, grain, and meat intake.[22]

Factors Influencing Food Intake

Food intake and habits are determined by numerous factors. Major influences for children include the family, peers, media, and body image.

Family

Family food choices and eating-related behaviors influence the types of foods children will accept.[23] Eating habits and food likes and dislikes are formed in the early years and often continue into adulthood. Parents and siblings are primary models for young children to imitate behavior. Mealtime atmosphere, both positive and negative, can influence how a child approaches and handles family meals. The positive effects of regular family meals can last into adulthood.[24]

With more women employed outside the home, there may be less time available for food preparation and more use of fast food, prepared foods, and restaurant meals. Mothers' employment, however, is not associated with poorer dietary intakes for their children.[25] There is also a larger percentage of single-parent families, usually headed by women. This usually translates into lower income, with less money available for food.

Quality of dietary intake has been linked to family meals. School-aged children and adolescents who ate dinner with their families most often had higher consumptions of fruits and vegetables and nutrients including fiber, folate, calcium, iron, and vitamins B_6, B_{12}, C, and E. Intakes of saturated fat, soda, and fried foods were lower among individuals who ate with their families more often than among children with less frequent family meals.[24,26]

Media

Television is the primary media influence on children of all ages. It has been estimated that by the time the average child in the United States graduates from high school, he or she will have watched about 15,000 hours of television, compared with spending 11,000 hours in the classroom. The average child views more than 500 food references per week on television, and 20% of commercials during children's programming are for food.[27,28] In addition, food products are marketed through cross-promotions with programs and characters and through fast-food restaurant promotions. The food items generally advertised to young audiences are sweetened cereals, fast food, snack foods, and candy—foods high in sugar, fat, and salt.[29]

The commercial messages are not based on nutrition but on an emotional/psychological appeal—fun, gives you energy, yummy taste. Younger children generally cannot discriminate between the regular program and commercial messages, frequently giving more attention to the latter because of their fast, attention-getting pace. Television viewing and other types of "screen time" have been suggested as factors in the rising rate of obesity among children and teenagers in the U.S. screen time and low physical activity levels are related to overweight and obesity,[28] and television viewing has been inversely associated with fruit and vegetable intake.[28,30–32] In addition to encouraging inactivity, there is the steady presentation of food and eating cues.

Peers

As children move into the world, others influence their food choices. In preschool, the group snack time may encourage a child to try a new food. During school years, friends rather than the menu may decide participation in the school lunch program. Peer influence is particularly strong in adolescence as teenagers strive for more independence and eating becomes a more social activity outside the home. A chronic illness or disorder that requires diet modification, such as diabetes, phenylketonuria, or food allergies, can be a problem for children and teenagers when they want to be part of the group. These individuals need education regarding diet rationale appropriate to their developmental level, as well as problem-solving methods to explain it to their peers.

Body Image

Puberty is the period of greatest awareness of body image. It is normal for teens to be uncomfortable and dissatisfied with their changing bodies. The media and popular idols offer a standard that adolescents compare themselves with, no matter how unrealistic it may be (e.g., store mannequins are usually size 7 or 8, magazine models weigh about 23% less than the average female). Even prepubertal school-age girls have been increasingly preoccupied with body image and "dieting." To change their body image, they may try restrictive diets, purchase weight loss products, or in the case of males, try supplements or diets in the hope of increasing their muscles. Some of these dietary measures may put them at risk for poor nutritional status. The increasing prevalence of childhood overweight has also impacted the positive body image of growing children and adolescents.

Feeding the Toddler and Preschool Child

Parents often become concerned when their toddler refuses some favorite foods and appears to be disinterested in eating. These periods (food jags) vary in intensity from child to child and may last a few days or years. At the same time, the child is practicing self-feeding skills, with frequent spills, and is often resorting to the use of fingers. These changes and behaviors during the preschool years are a normal part of the development and maturation of young children.[33] When parents understand this, they are more likely to avoid struggles, issues of control, and negative feedback around food and eating.

Portion sizes for young children are small by adult standards. **Table 6-2** provides a guide for foods and portion sizes. A long-standing rule of thumb is to initially offer 1 tablespoon of each food for every year of age for preschool children, with more provided according to appetite.

Because of smaller capacities and fluctuating appetites, most children eat four to six times a day. Snacks contribute significantly to the total day's nutrient intake and should be planned accordingly. Foods that make nutritious snacks are listed in **Table 6-3**. Foods chosen for snacks should be those least likely to promote dental caries.

Parents of young children frequently become concerned about the adequacy of their children's intakes; plain meats are often refused because they are more difficult to chew, very little or too much milk may be consumed, and cooked vegetables are pushed away. **Table 6-4** offers nutrition solutions to these common, normal variations in eating behaviors.

Just as important as providing adequate nutrients to young children is supporting a positive feeding environment—both physically and emotionally—so that, as they grow, they acquire skills, develop positive attitudes, and have control over food decisions as appropriate for their developmental level. General guidance in this area is listed in **Table 6-5**.

Children under age 4 are at greatest risk for choking on food. In some cases, this can lead to death from asphyxiation.[34] Foods most likely to cause choking are those that are round, hard, and do not readily dissolve in saliva, such as hot dogs, grapes, raw vegetables, popcorn, peanut butter, nuts, and hard candy. Other foods can also cause choking problems if too much is stuffed into the mouth, if the child is running while eating, or if the child is unsupervised. Choking episodes can be prevented by common-sense management of foods and the eating environment. **Table 6-6** outlines preventive approaches.

TABLE 6-2 Feeding Guide for Children

The following is a guide to a basic diet. Fats, sauces, desserts, and snack foods will provide additional energy to meet the growing child's needs. Foods can be selected from this pattern for both meals and snacks.

Food	2- to 3-Year-Olds Portion Size	Servings	4- to 6-Year-Olds Portion Size	Servings	7- to 12-Year-Olds Portion Size	Servings	Comments
Milk and dairy products	½ cup (4 oz.)	4	½–¾ cup (4–6 oz.)	3–4	¾–1 cup (6–8 oz.)	3–4	The following may be substituted for ½ cup liquid milk: ½–¾ oz. cheese, ½ cup yogurt, 2 ½ Tbsp. nonfat dry milk.
Meat, fish, poultry, or equivalent	1–2 oz.	2	1–2 oz.	2	2 oz.	3–4	The following may be substituted for 1 oz. meat, fish, or poultry: 1 egg, 2 Tbsp. peanut butter, 4–5 Tbsp. cooked legumes.
Fruits and vegetables							
Vegetables						5	Include one green leafy or yellow vegetable for vitamin A, such as carrots, spinach, broccoli, or winter squash.
Cooked	2–3 Tbsp.	4–5	3–4 Tbsp.	4–5	¼–½ cup		
Raw*	Few pieces		Few pieces		Several pieces		
Fruit							Include one vitamin C–rich fruit, vegetable, or juice, such as citrus juices, orange, grapefruit, strawberries, melon, tomato, or broccoli.
Raw	½–1 small		½–1 small		1 medium		
Canned	2–4 Tbsp.		4–6 Tbsp.		¼–½ cup		
Juice	3–4 oz.		4 oz.		4 oz.		
Bread and grain products							The following may be substituted for 1 slice of bread: ½ cup spaghetti, macaroni, noodles, or rice; 5 saltines; ½ English muffin or bagel; 1 tortilla
Whole-grain or enriched bread	½–1 slice	3–4	1 slice	4–5	1 slice	5–6	
Cooked cereal	¼–½ cup		½ cup		½–1 cup		
Dry cereal	½–1 cup		1 cup		1 cup		

*Do not give to young children until they can chew well.

Source: Adapted from Lowenberg ME, Development of food patterns in young children, in *Nutrition Infancy and Childhood,* ed 4 (pp. 146–147) by PL Pipes (ed) with permission of Times Mirror/Mosby College Publishing, © 1989 with permission of W.B. Saunders Company.

TABLE 6-3 Foods that Make Nutritious Snacks

Protein Foods	Fruits#	Breads and Cereals#	Vegetables
Natural cheese	Apple wedges*	Whole-grain breads	Carrot sticks*
Milk	Bananas	Whole-grain, low-fat crackers	Celery*
Plain yogurt	Pears	Rice crackers	Green pepper strips*
Cooked turkey or beef	Berries	English muffins	Cucumber slices*
Unsalted nuts and seeds*	Melon	Bagels	Cabbage wedges*
Peanut butter*	Oranges and other citrus fruits	Tortillas	Tomatoes
Hard-cooked eggs	Grapes*	Pita bread	Jicama*
Cottage cheese	Unsweetened canned fruit	Popcorn*	Vegetable juices
Tuna	Unsweetened fruit juices		Cooked green beans
			Broccoli and cauliflower florets

*Foods that are hard, round, and do not easily dissolve can cause choking. Do not give to children under 3 years of age. (Peanut butter is more dangerous when eaten in chunks or spread thickly rather than thinly on crackers or bread.)

#Fruits, juices, and most cereal/bread products contain fermentable carbohydrate, which is a factor in the development of dental caries.

TABLE 6-4 Common Feeding Concerns in Young Children

Common Concerns	Possible Solutions
Refuses meats	• Offer small, bite-size pieces of moist, tender meat or poultry. • Incorporate into meatloaf, spaghetti sauce, stews, casseroles, burritos, or pizza. • Include legumes, eggs, and cheese. • Offer boneless fish (including canned tuna and salmon).
Drinks too little milk	• Offer cheeses and yogurt, including cheese in cooking (e.g., macaroni and cheese, cheese sauce, pizza). Use milk to cook hot cereals. Offer cream soups and milk-based puddings and custards. • Allow child to pour milk from a pitcher and use a straw. • Include powdered milk in cooking and baking (e.g., biscuits, muffins, pancakes, meatloaf, casseroles)
Drinks too much milk	• Offer water if thirsty between meals. • Limit milk to one serving with meals or offer at end of meal; offer water for seconds. • If bottle is still used, wean to cup.
Refuses vegetables and fruits	• If child refuses vegetables, offer more fruits, and vice versa. • Prepare vegetables that are tender but not overcooked. • Steam vegetable strips (or offer raw if appropriate) and allow child to eat with fingers. • Offer sauces and dips (e.g., cheese sauce for cooked vegetables, dip for raw vegetables, yogurt to dip fruit). • Include vegetables in soups and casseroles. • Add fresh or dried fruit to cereals. • Prepare fruit in a variety of ways (e.g., fresh, cooked, juice, in gelatin, as a salad). • Continue to offer a variety of fruits and vegetables.
Eats too many sweets	• Limit purchase and preparation of sweet foods in the home. • Avoid using as a bribe or reward. • Incorporate into meals instead of snacks for better dental health. • Reduce sugar by half in recipes for cookies, muffins, quick breads, and the like. • Work with staff of day care, preschools, and others to reduce use of sweets.

Fruit juice is a common beverage for young children, usually replacing water and sometimes milk. Excessive fruit juice consumption has been linked to chronic diarrhea and failure to thrive, with improvement when juice is limited.[35] Although excess juice consumption has been suggested as a factor in short stature and obesity, studies have not shown associations between fruit juice intake and growth parameters.[36,37] Frequent juice intake could dull the

TABLE 6-5 Tips for a Happy Mealtime

Physical Setting

- Schedule meals at regular times.
- Avoid having a child get too hungry or too tired before mealtime.
- Snacks should be at least 1½ to 2 hours before meals.
- Child should be able to sit up to the table comfortably without reaching.
- Provide support for the legs and feet, such as a booster seat or stool.
- Use nonbreakable, sturdy dishes with sides to push food against.
- Spoons and forks should be blunt with broad, short handles.
- Use cups that are nonbreakable, broad based, and small.

Social-Emotional

- Serve a new food with familiar ones—don't be surprised by an initial rejection.
- Offer at least one food at a meal that you know your child will eat, but do not cater to his or her likes and dislikes.
- Avoid coaxing, nagging, bribing, or any other pressure to get your child to eat.
- Serve dessert (if any) with the meal—it becomes less important and cannot be used as a reward.
- Let children determine when they are full; amounts eaten will vary from child to child and day to day.
- Use the child's developmental stage to determine expectations for neatness and manners, but set limits on inappropriate behaviors (e.g., throwing food, playing).
- Attempt to have family meals be as pleasant as possible; avoid arguments and criticism.
- Allow children to help set the table or do part of the meal preparation.

appetite and result in less food consumed, or, for some children, the extra energy from juice (instead of water) could cause excess weight gain. The AAP suggests that fruit juice intake be limited to 4–6 ounces per day for children 1 to 6 years of age and 8–12 ounces for children 7 to 18 years of age. The AAP recommends that fruit juice provide up to half of the suggested fruit servings, and whole fruit should be encouraged to provide dietary fiber.[38] Intake of 100% fruit juice at levels recommended by the AAP (about 4 ounces per day) did not have a negative effect on weight status, but was associated with higher intakes of some vitamins and minerals and total whole fruit.[39] A recent study compared intakes of fruit juice, milk, and sweetened beverages and adiposity. Intake of sweetened beverages (but not milk or 100% fruit juice) at age 5 years was predictive of adiposity between ages 5 and 15 years.[40]

TABLE 6-6 Guidelines for Feeding Safety: Preschool Children

- Have children sit while eating. It lets them concentrate on chewing and swallowing. While preschool-age children do have molars, they are still learning to chew effectively. Eating while walking or running may cause choking.
- An adult should supervise children at all times while they are eating.
- Children can be easily distracted, so meals and snacks should be presented in a calm atmosphere; overexcitement may cause choking.
- Offer well-cooked foods, modified if needed, so that the child can chew and swallow without difficulty.
- For children under age 3, avoid offering foods that can cause choking (e.g., hard candy, mini-marshmallows, popcorn, pretzels, chips, spoonfuls of peanut butter, nuts, seeds, large chunks of meat, hot dogs, raw carrots, raisins and other dried fruits, and whole grapes). For children between the ages of 3 and 5, modify these foods to make them safer (e.g., cut hot dogs in quarters lengthwise and into small pieces, cut whole grapes in half lengthwise, chop nuts finely, slice carrots into thin strips, spread peanut butter thinly on crackers or bread).
- Avoid eating in the car. If the child starts choking, it may be difficult to get to the side of the road safely and help the child.

Sources: American Academy of Pediatrics Committee on Injury, Violence, and Poison Prevention. Prevention of choking among children. *Pediatrics.* 2010;125:601–607; Harris CS, Baker SP, Smith GA. Childhood asphyxiation by food: a national analysis and overlook. *JAMA.* 1984;251:2231–2235; and Story M, Holt K, Sofka D, eds. *Bright Futures in Practice: Nutrition,* 2nd ed. Arlington, VA: National Center for Education in Maternal and Child Health; 2002:69.

Feeding the School-Age Child

The years from 6 to 12 are a period of slow but steady growth, with increases in food intake as a result of appetite (see Table 6-2). Most food behavior problems from early childhood have been resolved except for extreme cases, but food dislikes may persist, especially if attention is given to them.

Because children are in school, they may eat fewer times in the day, but after-school snacks usually are a routine. Skipping breakfast may begin in these years, with contributing factors such as time constraints, children left to get themselves off to school, and early school starts. With participation in organized sports, music programs, and other activities, sitting down to a family meal may be less frequent.

An emerging trend in the United States is the increased responsibility of children not yet in their teens to do family shopping and cooking. Some children are frequently responsible for their own breakfasts, lunches, snacks, and even the dinner meal. They also do food shopping on a regular basis and influence the family food purchases. Several factors contribute to this trend, including working parents, increased use of microwave ovens, more money available to spend on prepared foods, and less emphasis on family meals. Along with this trend, increasingly sophisticated advertising is being aimed at these children.

Feeding the Adolescent

Adolescents in their rapid-growth period seem to eat all the time. Their appetites usually guide their intakes. As teenagers achieve more independence and spend a greater amount of time away from home, they have additional variable intakes and irregular eating patterns. Skipping meals is greatest in this age group, particularly for breakfast and lunch. On the other hand, snacking tends to be a common practice. Whether they are called snacks or meals, adolescents who eat less than three times a day have poorer diets than do those eating more often.

Although fast foods are popular with all segments of the population, they appeal most to teenagers. The food is inexpensive, well-accepted, and can be eaten informally without utensils or plates. Fast food restaurants are also socially acceptable and a common employer of adolescents. Generally, the menu items tend to be energy-dense, high in fat (some items provide more than 50% of energy as fat), high in sodium, and low in fiber, vitamin A, ascorbic acid, calcium, and folate. Although these establishments now offer more salads and lower-fat sandwiches, these foods are not necessarily chosen by teens. Negative impacts of fast foods on the diets of adolescents will depend on how frequently they are eaten and the choices made. During a 2-day survey, the majority of adolescents consumed at least one fast food item on at least 1 day.[41] Increased fast food consumption was associated with decreased intake of milk, fruits, and vegetables.

School Nutrition

Children and teens spend much time in school and many participate in events outside the academic school day but in the school setting. Most children eat at least one meal daily in the school environment; others may consume 2 meals and a snack. School lunches, school wellness policies, and food sources outside the cafeteria all have received attention with the goal to maximize health.

School Lunch Programs

Children usually participate in the school lunch program or bring a packed lunch from home. The National School Lunch Program is administered by the U.S. Department of Agriculture (USDA) and supported by means of reimbursements and supplemental commodity foods. Federal guidelines are established for food groups and portion sizes so that the lunch provides approximately one-third of the RDAs or AIs for students. About 85% of schools also participate in the School Breakfast Program. Free and reduced-price meals are available for low-income children.

Problems with the school lunch program have included plate waste, poor menu acceptance by students, competition from vending machines, and concerns regarding the amount of fat, sugar, and salt in the food. These problems have been addressed by including the students in menu planning, offering popular items more frequently (e.g., pizza, tacos, hamburgers, salad bars), and allowing students to refuse one or two items from the menu. Incorporating the U.S. Dietary Guidelines into child nutrition programs has also encouraged menus with a lower fat content, and more fresh fruits, vegetables, and whole-grain products.[42] A sack lunch prepared at home will likely provide more calcium, iron, and fruit than a school lunch; however, school lunches tend to be lower in sugar, sodium, and fat and have more vegetables than packed lunches.[43] The same favorite foods tend to be packed with less variety, and foods are limited to those that don't require heating or refrigeration. Children who participate in the school lunch program are more likely to consume milk, fruit, and vegetables and less likely to consume desserts and snack items than children who did not participate.[44]

Vending Machines and Other Competing Foods

Vending machines, especially those that sell soft drinks, may be available to children and adolescents during the school day. This issue is complex as educators and healthcare providers weigh the health risks associated with excessive intake of these foods and beverages (including 100% fruit juice) with the school program funding that is often provided by vending machine profits. Problems associated with increased soda consumption include risk of obesity, deficits in bone mass (because of decreased intake of calcium and other nutrients when soft drinks replace milk), and increased dental caries. The AAP encourages healthcare providers to work to eliminate sweetened drinks in schools.[45] Other approaches to promoting better choices from vending machines include price reductions on lower fat options. In one study, this approach did not affect profits,[46] and other studies have demonstrated positive effects on overall nutrient intake.[47]

School Wellness Policies

Since 2006–2007, school wellness policies have been required in institutions that participate in school meal programs. School districts set goals for nutrition education, physical activity, campus food provision, and other school-based activities to promote student wellness. Ideally, efforts are collaborative and include input and action from administrators, teachers, students, food service personnel, families, and the community.

A joint position statement of the American Dietetic Association, the Society for Nutrition Education, and the

American School Food Service Association calls for the integration of school nutrition services with a coordinated, comprehensive school health program and school nutrition policy.[48]

Other Nutrition Issues

As children grow and develop, various nutrition-related issues or problems arise. These are not uncommon in otherwise healthy children, and they can be prevented or managed with minimal intervention. Other specific problems—obesity, allergies, and chronic diseases—are discussed in other chapters.

Diet and Oral Health

Despite successful efforts in the past few decades, dental caries remain a common oral health disease in the pediatric population. National Health and Nutrition Examination Survey III (NHANES III) data indicate for 2- to 11-year-olds, the prevalence of dental caries in primary teeth is 42% (28% for 2- to 5-year-olds, and 51% for 6- to 11-year-olds). For 6- to 8-year-olds, the prevalence of caries in permanent teeth is about 10%, and for 9- to 11-year-olds is about 31%. Adolescent caries rates are about 59%. Increased use of dental sealants have led to improved caries rates; however, oral health remains a significant problem in the United States.[49]

Nutrition and oral health are closely related. Inadequate intake of energy and protein can delay tooth eruption, affect tooth size, and cause salivary gland dysfunction. Micronutrients (e.g., calcium and vitamin D for mineralization, fluoride for enamel formation) are also critical to the development and maintenance of oral structures.[50,51] A comparison of dietary quality and caries found lower rates of caries among young children who scored highest on the Healthy Eating Index (a measure of diet quality compared to federal dietary guidance).[52]

Poor oral health can negatively affect a child's nutritional status and has implications for overall health as well. Missing or decayed teeth may increase the risk of nutrient deficiency by preventing a child from eating certain foods. Pain or malformed teeth can contribute to problems with speech and communication, interfere with sleep, and negatively affect an individual's self-image, psychological status, and overall social function.

Dental caries develop in the presence of carbohydrate, bacteria, and a susceptible tooth. The process of decay begins with the interaction of bacteria (*Streptococcus mutans*) and fermentable carbohydrate on the tooth surface. When the bacteria within the dental plaque (the gelatinous substance on the tooth surface) metabolize the carbohydrate, organic acids are produced. When the acid reduces the pH to 5.5 or less, demineralization of the tooth enamel occurs.[53] Some individuals seem to be more susceptible to caries than others, suggesting a hereditary influence. About 80% of the caries in 5- to 17-year-olds are found in only 25% of the children and adolescents.[54] Individual salivary counts of *S. mutans* that are high appear to be a risk for caries.[55]

Sucrose is the most common carbohydrate recognized in the caries process. Although starch is considered less cariogenic than sucrose, it can easily be broken down into fermentable carbohydrate by salivary amylase. Also, many foods high in starch often contain sucrose or other sugars, which may make the food more cariogenic than sugar alone because starch is retained longer in the mouth. Honey is just as cariogenic as sucrose.

The cariogenicity of specific foods depends not only on the type and amount of fermentable carbohydrate, but also on the retentiveness of foods to the tooth surface and the frequency of eating. Dental researchers believe that all of these factors influence the length of time the teeth are exposed to an acidic environment, which leads to tooth decay.[53]

Some protein foods (e.g., nuts, hard cheeses, eggs, meats) do not decrease plaque pH and are thought to have a protective effect against caries.[56] Eating these foods at the same time as high-sugar foods prevents a reduction in plaque pH. Why these foods are protective is not known, but theories include the presence of protein and lipids in these foods, the presence of calcium and phosphorus, and the stimulation of alkaline saliva. Chewing gum sweetened with xylitol or sorbitol after a sugar-containing snack may also counteract the decrease in pH and reduce caries.[57]

Prevention of Caries

Because children of all ages eat frequently, snacks should emphasize foods that are low in sucrose, are not sticky, and stimulate saliva flow, thereby limiting acid production in the mouth (Table 6-3). Including protein foods such as cheese and nuts may provide nutritional as well as dental benefits. Desserts, when consumed, should be eaten with meals. School-age children and adolescents may benefit from chewing sugarless gum after snacks containing fermentable carbohydrate.

Good oral hygiene complements dietary efforts. In infancy, parents can clean the gums and teeth with a clean cloth. The toothbrush should be introduced in the toddler period. The key is to incorporate brushing and flossing as a regular, consistent routine, with parental supervision in the early years. If the water supply is not fluoridated, use of a fluoride supplement is recommended into the teen years. Topical fluoride applications are recommended, based on assessment of caries risk. Varnishes, rinses, gels, and foams are also available to prevent caries and are often incorporated into local public health activities (e.g., partnership with the public health department, schools, and early intervention program).

The AAP and American Academy of Pediatric Dentistry (AAPD) suggest establishing a dental home (a primary dental care provider that provides or coordinates comprehensive care, including preventive oral health supervision and emergency care) with regular visits beginning in early childhood. The AAPD recommends a visit by 12 months of age or 6 months after the first tooth erupts.[58,59]

The U.S. Surgeon General's Report on Oral Health identifies assessment and action by nondental providers as critical to improving oral health. Screening (and appropriate referral) and anticipatory guidance are included in these actions.[60]

Early Childhood Caries

Children under 3 years of age are most likely to have early childhood caries (ECC). ECC is also known as baby bottle tooth decay, nursing caries, and nursing bottle caries. ECC affects 28% of all U.S. toddlers and preschoolers.[49] Rampant caries develops on the primary upper front teeth (incisors) and often on the cheek surface of primary upper first molars. Children from poor families are at highest risk for ECC. A history of ECC seems to increase the risk for future caries in permanent teeth.[58]

The primary cause of ECC is prolonged exposure of the teeth to a sweetened liquid (formula, milk, juice, soda pop, or sweetened drinks). This occurs most often when the child is routinely given a nursing bottle at bedtime or during naps. During sleep, the liquid pools around the teeth, saliva flow decreases, and the child may continue to suck liquid over an extended period of time. Although ECC has been documented in ad libitum breastfeeding, the occurrence is believed to be less than with bottle-feeding.[61] Toddlers who hold their own bottles and have access to bottles or sippy cups with sweetened liquids anytime throughout the day are also at high risk. Dental treatment of ECC is expensive, often requires a general anesthetic, and may be traumatic for the child and family.

Education is the primary strategy to prevent ECC. Parents should be counseled about the disorder early in infancy and encouraged to avoid putting a baby to sleep with a bottle, as previously addressed in Chapter 5. Juices and liquids other than milk or formula should be offered in a cup. In typically developing infants, weaning from the bottle should begin at about 1 year of age. Day care providers and other caregivers should also be informed of the threat to oral health posed by use of the nursing bottle as a pacifier. For this educational approach to be successful, families often need help with positive parenting strategies and behavioral counseling.

Iron Deficiency Anemia

Iron deficiency anemia is most common in children between 1 and 2 years of age, with a prevalence of about 7%. Other high-risk groups are adolescent females, with deficiency noted among 9% of 12- to 15-year-olds and 16% of 16- to 19-year-olds.[62] Over the past three decades, there has been an overall decrease in the prevalence of iron deficiency anemia, both in low-income and middle-class pediatric populations. Factors influencing this positive trend include increased and prolonged use of iron-fortified infant formulas, more breastfeeding, increased iron intake from other food sources, and the Women, Infants, and Children (WIC) food program. Despite the encouraging trends, some young children, especially those in low-income households, are at high risk for iron deficiency. Although the relationship between iron deficiency and cognitive/behavioral function has been debated for a long time, poorer cognitive performance and delayed psychomotor development have been reported in infants and preschool children with iron deficiency, compared with children without iron deficiency. Iron deficiency in infancy may have long-term consequences, as demonstrated by poorer performance on developmental tests in late childhood and early adolescence.[63,64] Children who are iron deficient are also at risk for increased lead absorption when exposed to sources of lead.

Dietary factors, as well as growth and physiologic needs, play a role in development of anemia. Some toddlers consume a large volume of milk to the exclusion of solids; plain meats are often not well-accepted by preschool children because they require more chewing. For many of these children, most dietary iron comes from nonheme sources such as vegetables, grains, and cereals. Because the typical U.S. diet contains approximately 6 mg iron per 1000 calories, adolescents dieting to lose weight will have minimal iron intake.

Absorption of iron from food depends on several factors. One is the iron status of the individual; those with low iron stores will have a higher absorption rate. There is a higher rate of absorption from heme iron (in meat, fish, and poultry) than from nonheme iron (in vegetables and grains). Absorption of nonheme iron can be increased by two enhancing factors: (1) ascorbic acid and (2) meat, fish, or poultry (MFP).[65] The presence of an ascorbic acid–rich food and/or MFP in a meal will increase the rate of nonheme-iron absorption. Other foods or compounds inhibit iron absorption. **Table 6-7** identifies good iron sources as well as absorption enhancers and inhibitors. Simple but conscientious menu planning can help improve iron availability to children and teenagers.

Universal screening up to 2 years of age is recommended for communities and populations with significant levels of iron deficiency anemia or for infants whose diets put them at risk. Screening should be performed at approximately 12 months of age and again at approximately 18 months of age. Selective screening would be based on individual risk factors such as prematurity, low-birth-weight infants, and dietary intake in communities with a 5% or less rate of anemia. Routine screening is not recommended after age

TABLE 6-7 Food Sources of Iron

Food	Iron (mg)
Meat, Fish, and Poultry (1 oz)*	
Chicken liver	2.8
Beef liver	2.2
Turkey, roasted	1.7
Beef pot roast	1.3
Hamburger	1.1
Fresh pork, roasted	1.1
Ham	0.7
Chicken	0.6
Tuna, canned	0.5
Hot dog	0.3
Salmon	0.3
Fish stick	0.1
Cereals, Grains, Vegetables, and Fruits#	
Cooked cereals (½ cup)	0.7–1.3
Ready-to-eat cereals (¾ cup)	0.3–9.0
Whole-wheat bread, enriched	0.6–0.8
bread (1 slice)	1.3–3.0
Legumes, cooked (½ cup)	1.5–2.0
Greens (spinach, mustard,	1.3
beet), cooked (½ cup)	1.0–1.5
Green peas, cooked (½ cup)	1.0
Dried fruit (¼ cup)	0.5
Nuts, most kinds (2 Tbsp.)	0.9
Wheat germ (1 Tbsp.)	
Molasses, light (1 Tbsp.)	

Dietary Enhancers of Nonheme Iron Absorption	Dietary Inhibitors of Noneheme Iron Absorption
Meat, fish, poultry	Tea (tannic acid)
Ascorbic acid	Sequestering additives (such as EDTA used in fats and soft drinks to clarify and prevent rancidity)
Antacids	

*Heme iron sources (approximately 40% of the iron in these foods); well-absorbed.

#Nonheme sources; lower level of absorption; enhancers eaten at the same time will increase absorption.

2 except for risk factors such as poor diet, poverty/limited access to food, and special healthcare needs. Guidelines for treatment and follow-up of iron deficiency anemia have been developed.[62]

A heme profile (hemoglobin or hematocrit) is usually used to screen for anemia; however, other tests are more sensitive, and can provide more information about an individual's iron status. The AAP currently suggests using hemoglobin, serum ferritin, and C-reactive protein to screen for iron deficiency, based on risk. The combination of hemoglobin and serum transferrin receptor tests is also suggested, once standards for the latter are developed. [66]

Effect of Diet on Learning and Behavior

What impact does a child's diet have on his or her school performance and behavior? For decades people have debated whether skipping breakfast affects classroom learning. Food additives, sugar, and allergies have been suggested as causes of hyperactivity in children. Although these are controversial issues, some scientific studies have examined them.

Diet and Learning Behavior

Although severe malnutrition early in life is known to negatively affect intellectual development, the impact of marginal malnutrition, skipping meals, or hunger has been more difficult to document. Experimental studies have used standardized tests to measure cognitive functions (e.g., problem solving, attention, and memory) in healthy school-age children who were given either breakfast or no breakfast. The "fasted" children had slower memory recall, increased errors, and slower stimulus discrimination.[67] Similar studies comparing healthy children to those stunted, those who suffered severe malnutrition early in life, and those currently wasted (low weight for height) showed even poorer results for the malnourished/undernourished children when they missed breakfast.[67,68]

In a community study, standardized achievement test scores were compared before and after implementation of the School Breakfast Program in six schools in a predominantly low-income community.[69] Children participating in the breakfast program demonstrated improved academic performance compared with those qualified but not participating. The findings also noted decreased tardiness and absenteeism among the children in the breakfast program. These results and those of other similar studies indicate that efforts of nutrition education and feeding programs should be targeted to children at risk so they might be better able to achieve in school.[70]

The impact of diet and nutrition on a child's behavior has been a controversial topic for some time. Although malnourished children and those experiencing iron deficiency anemia often demonstrate decreased attention and responsiveness, less interest in their environment, and reduced problem-solving ability, the effects of periodic hunger or "food insecurity" is less clear. A report of families from a large Community Childhood Hunger Identification Project (CCHIP) found that the "hungry" children were three times more likely than "at-risk for hunger" children, and seven times more likely than "not hungry" children to have scores indicating irritability, anxiety, aggression, and oppositional behavior.[71] Data from NHANES III showed negative academic and psychosocial outcomes associated with food insufficiency. Children who were classified as food-insufficient had lower math scores and were more likely to have repeated a grade, to have seen a psychologist, and to have difficulty getting along with other children. Adolescents with food insufficiency were also more likely to have been suspended from school.[72] Although other unstudied factors could also be related to these negative behaviors, they could be tied to the family's food insecurity. With federal welfare reform legislation and state budget limitations, more low-income families are likely to be at risk for limited food resources. Without broad policies to ensure children their basic needs, these children may suffer worsening behavioral and academic functioning.

Attention Deficit Hyperactivity Disorder

Commonly known as hyperactivity, attention deficit hyperactivity disorder (ADHD) is a developmental disorder with specific criteria: inattention, impulsivity, hyperactivity, onset before 7 years of age, and duration of at least 6 months. The etiology of ADHD is not clear; however, some nutritional factors have been proposed as causes, including food additives, sugar, and food allergies. Although treatment usually includes behavioral management, medication, and/or special education, various dietary treatments have been proposed.

The Feingold diet, popularized in the 1970s, theorized that artificial colorings and flavorings in the food supply caused hyperactivity. Treatment was to remove from the child's diet those substances, natural salicylates (found mostly in fruits), and some preservatives (BHA, BHT). Controlled double-blind challenge studies have not supported the Feingold hypothesis,[73] although it is generally accepted that a small percentage (no more than 5–10%) of children with ADHD (usually preschoolers) may benefit from the diet. Another report, using the Feingold diet plus elimination of foods that the family thought were bothersome to their child (e.g., chocolate, sugar, or caffeine) found that almost 50% of the preschool hyperactive boys showed some improvement in behavior, using accepted rating scales.[74] The modified Feingold diet, including fruits, has been evaluated favorably according to nutrient content and thus poses little risk for the child.[75] Families using the diet should receive nutritional counseling and should not disregard other helpful treatment for their child's ADHD.

Sugar (sucrose) is popularly believed to cause hyperactivity in children or behavior problems and delinquency in adolescents. Controlled challenge studies, however, have failed to show any negative behavioral effects from sucrose.[76] In one study, children receiving the sugar were less active and quieter afterward than were those receiving the placebo.[77] A double-blind challenge study with juvenile delinquents did not show impaired behavioral performance after a sucrose load.[78] There are many reasons for reducing sugar consumption, including improved oral health and diets that are more nutrient dense. This can be reinforced with families, while helping them remain objective about a sugar–behavior relationship. There is always the rare possibility that a child may have an individual intolerance to sugar.

Stimulant medications, such as methylphenidate (e.g., Ritalin, Concerta, Metadate, and Focalin), dextroamphetamine (e.g., Dexedrine or Dextrostate), and mixed salts of a single entity amphetamine (e.g., Adderall), are commonly used to treat ADHD.[79] These medications are available in short- and long-acting preparations. They usually result in improvement of motor restlessness, short attention span, and irritability.

Anorexia is a side effect of stimulant medications, and this has been shown to cause suppression of physical growth. Data suggest there is a direct relationship between dosage of the medication and the degree of reduced growth.[80] Over time, there seems to be more tolerance for a medication's negative effect on growth, but the response is individual. The effects of stimulant medications on height gain, however, seem to be temporary, with no differences in heights-for-age by late adolescence.[80] Nonstimulant medications, including atomoxetine (Strattera), are sometimes prescribed for ADHD.

Although the mechanisms involved are not clear, decreased energy intake is a factor in decreased growth rates for those receiving stimulant medication. Individuals who take stimulant medications should have regular monitoring of growth, and the efficacy of the drug effect should be reassessed routinely. Because the effect of the medication will be noted shortly after being ingested, food should be offered to take advantage of the child's optimal appetite; in other words, the medication should be given with or after meals and healthy snacks should be offered when the effects of the short-action preparations are wearing off. The long-acting preparations appear to suppress appetite less dramatically. Overall, children are less hungry but as the medication effects lessen toward the end of the day they express hunger and will eat.

Megavitamin therapy has been promoted for many disorders, including ADHD and behavior problems. Of the controlled studies done, none have supported the use of megavitamins, and there is the potential for vitamin toxicity or other negative effects.[81] The use of fatty acid supplements, specifically polyunsaturated fatty acids such as docosahexaenoic acid (DHA) and evening primrose oil, has been suggested because of observed differences in plasma and erythrocyte phospholipid levels in children with ADHD. One double-blind, placebo-controlled study indicated no significant clinical improvements with DHA supplementation after 4 months. The authors suggest future supplementation studies with different doses and other fatty acids.[82]

Food allergies and intolerances as a factor in ADHD or behavioral difficulties in children are unclear. Many reports are subjective and the validity and interpretation of allergy tests can be controversial. It is certainly possible that children with allergies may manifest behaviors (irritability, poor attention) seen in children with ADHD, but whether or not elimination diets alleviate these symptoms is not clear. Children suspected of having food allergies should be seen by an allergist for diagnosis. Periodic nutrition evaluations are warranted for any child using an atypical dietary regimen.

Vegetarian Nutrition

Well-planned vegetarian diets are appropriate throughout the life cycle including childhood and adolescence.[83] Children, adolescents, and/or their families may practice vegetarian diet patterns for a variety of reasons including health benefits, economic issues, environmental concerns, religious beliefs, and animal rights. By definition, a vegetarian diet does not contain meat, fish, or fowl or products containing these foods.[83] However, vegetarian diet patterns cover a wide range, from lacto-ovo vegetarians (consume grains, vegetables, fruits, legumes, seeds, nuts, dairy products, and eggs), lacto vegetarians (no eggs consumed), ovo vegetarians (no dairy consumed), and vegans (exclude all products of animal origin) to food patterns that include only raw food or other specific food types. The more restrictive vegetarian food diets will most likely not meet the needs of growing children and adolescents.[84] Therefore, if a vegetarian lifestyle is reported a careful nutrition assessment will determine the actual intake and pattern used by the family or individual.

In 2005, 3% of 8- to 18-year-olds said they never ate meat, poultry, fish, or seafood. Previous polls indicated 2% of this population reported the same information. This 3% equates to approximately 1.4 million 8- to 18-year-olds in the United States.[85]

Evidence indicates that those following a vegetarian pattern have a lower risk of death from ischemic heart disease. It appears that a vegetarian lifestyle can result in lower low-density lipoprotein cholesterol levels, lower blood pressure, lower rates of hypertension and type 2 diabetes, and lower overall cancer rates, and can contribute to a tendency for a lower body mass index.[83] However, vegans and other vegetarians may have lower intakes of vitamin B_{12}, calcium, vitamin D, zinc, and long chain omega-3 fatty acids. Key nutrients to assess include the previous list plus iron and riboflavin.[83] Health benefits and risks of vegetarian food patterns were examined among 15- to 23-year-olds as part of the Project EAT (Eating Among Teens)-II study. Benefits of vegetarian patterns included increased intake of fruits and vegetables. Current vegetarians were at increased risk for binge eating with loss of control, and former vegetarians were at increased risk for unhealthful weight control behaviors.[86]

Families may choose to implement vegetarian food patterns throughout their child's development. Infants can be breastfed or receive soy formula (vegan) or cow's milk formula (lacto-). Infants born prematurely should not receive soy formula, because of increased osteopenia with soy-based formulas, compared to milk-based formulas. (See Chapter 4.) Solid foods should be introduced following recommended guidelines, based on developmental readiness. Depending on the type of vegetarian diet followed by the family, anticipatory guidance may include explanations of the need for offering foods with appropriate textures, and foods that are energy- and nutrient-dense. Children consuming a well-planned and not overly restrictive diet grow and develop as their peers.[84] Adolescents with vegetarian food patterns may need guidance to ensure they consume a variety of foods to meet their needs. This guidance may also include use of vitamin and/or mineral supplements at appropriate levels.

A vegetarian food guide was published in 2003, and includes practical recommendations for ensuring that vegetarian food patterns are nutritionally adequate.[87]

Adolescent Pregnancy

Although pregnancy is a normal physiologic state, there are more risks and complications for pregnant teens compared to any other age group. They have higher rates of low-birth-weight infants, especially among those younger than 15 years old. Birth rates among adolescents declined between 1990 and 2005, but rose in 2006 from 40.5 births per 1000 females to 41.9 births.[88]

The nutritional status of the pregnant adolescent is influenced by both physiologic and environmental/social factors. There is evidence that young pregnant teenage girls are still growing, creating a maternal–fetal competition for nutrients, and thus indicating increased nutrient needs in addition to pregnancy.[89,90] Other risk factors include a low prepregnancy weight and minimal nutrient stores at the time of conception. Many social factors can also affect the health and nutritional status of the teen, including late or no prenatal care, little financial support, limited food resources, poor eating habits, family difficulties, and various other emotional stresses.

For a positive outcome of pregnancy, weight gain for the pregnant adolescent may need to be more than the usual 25 to 35 pounds. The Committee to Reexamine Institute of Medicine (IOM) Pregnancy Weight Guidelines of the Food and Nutrition Board released new recommendations for weight gain, based on BMI. The 2009 report recommends that pregnant teens follow the adult BMI cutoff points, recognizing that many adolescents will be categorized in a lighter group and advised to gain more weight. The committee also notes that younger adolescents often need to gain more to improve birth outcomes[91] (see Appendix H), and it may be more prudent to use pediatric cut-off ranges to estimate energy needs. The pattern of weight gain is important, with weight gain in the first and early second trimesters being related to improved birth weights.[92] Studies document that weight gain in adolescent pregnancy includes maternal weight gain and nutrient accretion (i.e., continued growth), in addition to the typical maternal weight and fetal weight gain that is expected during pregnancy in an adult.[93]

Dietary guides for pregnant teens have usually added the pregnancy DRIs to the DRIs for 15- to 18-year-old females (see Appendix H-1 and H-2). Energy needs can vary greatly, depending on pubertal maturation and physical activity. An adequate weight gain is the best indicator of an appropriate energy intake. The pregnancy RDA for protein is 1.1 grams protein per kilogram body weight per day, which is slightly more than the RDA for 14- to 18-year-old females.[3] Higher protein intakes may be needed, depending on body build and growth needs. A sufficient energy intake will protect the protein to be used for growth. Individualized nutrition assessments will help identify the nutrition and diet concerns to be prioritized for ongoing nutrition counseling and education.

Many adolescents do not have adequate intakes of calcium, folic acid, and/or iron and may, in fact, have iron deficiency anemia before pregnancy. These nutrients are of special concern, both to maintain good nutritional status of the mother and because of potential long-term effects on their children. A study of adolescent mothers found long-term effects of iron deficiency. At age 3, children of iron-deficient mothers were less active than children whose mothers had adequate iron status.[94] A U.K. study documented increased risk of small-for-gestational-age (SGA) births among adolescents with poor micronutrient (folate, iron, and vitamin D) intake and status.[93] Supplementation of iron, folate, and other micronutrients is often necessary.[95]

Education and counseling are needed for the teen to accept the needed weight gain, plus the likelihood of a higher postpartum weight as part of a healthy pregnancy. An interdisciplinary healthcare team can best help pregnant teenagers to deal with their multiple health, psychosocial, and economic issues. This is most effective when provided as accessible prenatal care targeted to the teenage population in their own communities.[96] Education and resource referrals are also needed regarding infant care and feeding, continued schooling of the mother, parenting, and financial services (also see Chapter 3).

Substance Abuse

Alcohol, tobacco, and marijuana are the most widely used substances among teenagers. Inhalants and nonmedical use of prescription medications are also common.[97] Alcoholism in adolescence is a significant public health problem. A survey (1999–2004) of 12- to 17-year-olds indicates that 16% of teens have had some exposure to alcohol before age 13 years; 39% have had at least one drink by age 17 years. Binge drinking (five or more drinks in a few hours) is reported by 10% of 12- to 17-year-olds.[98] Any negative effect on nutritional status will depend on the frequency and amount of drinking as well as usual food habits. A survey of teenage males who were alcohol and marijuana abusers did not show significant differences in biochemical measures, but decreased intakes of milk, fruits, and vegetables were reported, as well as more snack food consumption and more symptoms of poor nutrition (tiredness, bleeding gums, muscle weakness).[99] For the female who consumes alcohol and becomes pregnant, there is risk of fetal alcohol syndrome in her infant.

Despite a decrease in cigarette smoking among adults in recent years, smoking remains relatively popular among teenagers. There may be increased need for some nutrients such as ascorbic acid, and smoking during pregnancy can reduce infant birth weight. Smokeless (chewing) tobacco and water-pipe tobacco smoking have also become popular with both school-age children and adolescents.[100,101] Not a benign substance, regular use is related to periodontal disease, oral cancer, dependence, and hypertension.

The negative nutritional consequences of a substance user's habit will depend on factors such as lifestyle, available food, and money to buy food. During a nutrition evaluation, the areas of alcohol consumption, tobacco use, and illegal drug use should be explored. Information will most likely be shared if a matter-of-fact, nonthreatening approach is used. Depending on the individual's situation, nutrition education and counseling can focus on improving health and nutrition. Other teenagers will need comprehensive treatment programs, which include a nutrition component.

Nutrition and Physical Activity

A child and adolescent's food intake contributes to growth, development, and overall health. In addition to nutrition, regular physical activity throughout life is important for maintaining a healthy body, enhancing psychological well-being, and preventing premature death.[102]

Physical Activity in Children and Teens

A youth surveillance survey of those in 9th to 12th grades in 2007 indicated about one-third of students met recommended levels of physical activity. The survey standard was activity that increased the student's heart rate and made them breathe hard some of the time for a total of at least 60 minutes per day on 5 or more days. No changes in this level of activity occurred between the 2005 and 2009 data; however, an increase did occur over the same time period in the amount of time this teen population played video or computer games unrelated to schoolwork.

Television watching time decreased slightly during the same time period.[103]

Others have found that for children 4 to 11 years of age, just over one-third have low levels of active play. Two-thirds of the sample had high screen time, and approximately 25% of these children had both low activity levels of play and high screen time.[104]

Preschoolers' activity has also been examined; more research is needed to understand physical activity behavior in this age group. A review indicated that boys were more active than girls, children with active parents tended to be more active, and children who spent more time outdoors were more active than those spending less time outdoors.[105]

Physical activity should be encouraged for all children and adolescents. Through physical activity, an individual's endurance, flexibility, and strength are improved.[106] For those 6–17 years of age, strong evidence for benefits from physical activity include improved cardiorespiratory endurance, improved muscular fitness, favorable body composition, improved bone health, and improved cardiovascular and metabolic health biomarkers. Moderate evidence suggests that activity may reduce symptoms of anxiety and depression in this age group.[106] In addition, physical activity can help children and adolescents have fun, make new friends, and/or spend quality time with their families.[107]

Current physical activity recommendations for those ages 6 through 17 years of age are:[106]

- Children and adolescents should do 1 hour or more of physical activity every day.
- Most of the 1 hour or more a day should be either moderate- or vigorous-intensity aerobic physical activity.
- As part of their daily physical activity, children and adolescents should do vigorous-intensity activity on at least 3 days per week. They also should do muscle-strengthening and bone-strengthening activity on at least 3 days per week.

The 2008 Physical Activity Guidelines for Americans contain information regarding activities that will meet these recommendations and are appropriate for children.[106]

Sports Nutrition

Many children and adolescents participate in competitive sports, and they (or their parents and/or coaches) are interested in the effects of nutrition on athletic performance. It is important to ensure that an individual's energy and fluid intake is adequate to support growth and to meet the increased demands of physical activity. See **Table 6-8** for exercise levels with age, nutrition, fluid, and health assessment guidelines.[108–115] Children and adolescents who participate in sports may need to adjust their intakes pre-event, during long events, and/or post-event (for example, pregame snacks of foods with complex carbohydrates). Children with some medical conditions (e.g., diabetes) may require additional adjustments to food patterns and/or medications.

A large market exists for sports-focused nutritional supplements, and children and adolescents as well as parents and coaches are targeted by marketers. Evidence is not available to suggest that healthy athletes have increased needs beyond the recommended nutrition requirements for active individuals.[116] Little evidence is available to support the use of dietary sports supplements in young athletes to enhance performance, lean muscle mass, or endurance. The AAP policy states that performance-enhancing substances for athletic or other purposes should be strongly discouraged.[117] Parents, coaches, and other youth sports organizations should encourage the young athlete to consume whole, nutritious foods for a balanced diet in addition to participating in appropriate physical training.[117]

Health Promotion

Americans have been gradually altering their eating habits as a result of increased interest in their health and their concern about preventing heart disease, cancer, obesity, and hypertension. The federal government and nonprofit organizations have provided recommendations, such as the dietary guidelines, to promote healthy eating. To what degree, if any, should this advice be applied to growing children and adolescents?

For overall health promotion, moderation and common sense continue to be the best policy. Although prevention of obesity and other chronic conditions is a worthy goal, there is no conclusive data to support a massive change in the diets of growing children. For healthy, growing children, the use of low-fat dairy products and fewer high-fat foods is appropriate for those over 2 years of age. Limiting the intake of fermentable carbohydrate will enhance dental health. Increasing the intake of fruits, vegetables, whole-grain products, and legumes above the usual reported levels can have several benefits, including reducing the percentage of fat in the diet, increasing the fiber content, increasing the amount of beta-carotene and other dietary factors that may help prevent cancer, and making the total diet more nutrient dense. The more varied the diet, the more likely the child's nutrient needs will be met.

Heart Health

Recommendations for lipid screening and cardiovascular health in children have been published by the AAP, and are very similar to guidelines recommended by the National Cholesterol Education Program (NCEP) and the American Heart Association.[118–121] These groups recommend that everyone over 2 years of age follow a diet that includes no more than 30% of energy as fat (10% or less from saturated fat) and no more than 200–300 mg cholesterol per day. Population-based recommendations also include a balanced energy intake;

TABLE 6-8 Exercise Levels with Age, Nutrition, Fluid, and Health Assessment Guidelines

Definitions	Examples (not inclusive)	Recommended Age	Nutrition Comments	Fluid Intake	Recommended Health Assessment
1. ROUTINE: The duration of the activity is less than 20 min, and it may or may not reach 60% of maximum heartbeat rate.	Recess play, casual walking, recreational noncontinual sport (i.e., T-ball, volleyball)	Minimum activity level for any age	Normal nutrition for age from MyPyramid.	Normal for age.	Yearly routine exam from a pediatrician or physician for all ages of children.
2. HEALTH FITNESS: 60—80% of maximum heartbeat rate is achieved for greater than 20 min at least three times per week for a minimum of 6 months. The activity should involve muscular strength and flexibility.	Brisk walking, jogging, running, cycling, hiking, swimming, dancing	Preferred level for any age	Normal nutrition for age from the Food Guide Pyramid. If desired weight for height, possibly more calories.	Good hydration, especially in adverse weather. Normal requirements for age and replacement of lost fluid from activity.	Yearly routine exam from a pediatrician or physician for all ages of children. Education from a physician or health professional on healthy practices (diet, fluid, injury prevention, warm-up and cool-down techniques, etc.). Immediate attention from an appropriate health professional for an injury or insult.
3. COMPETITIVE SPORTS: An activity less than or equal to 6 months that consists of team involvement, preseason training, and competing either as a team member or individually at an intramural or interschool level.	Swimming, gymnastics, diving, volleyball, wrestling, sprinting, relay, football, soccer, basketball, tennis, field hockey, crosscountry	Junior high age and above	Nutrition assessment, recommendations, and education, preferably from a registered dietitian, for an individual's season intake to achieve weight and body composition for the sport. Recommendations will be dependent on type of activity, duration, and intensity.	Pre-event, event, and postevent (or prepractice and postpractice) hydration. Good hydration at other times. Electrolyte replacement may be needed if heavy sweating occurs or in adverse weather conditions.	Preparticipation assessment by a health team consisting of a physician, dietitian, nurse or nurse practitioner, and possibly a physical therapist. Examination as well as education should be given to students at this time. Immediate attention from an appropriate health professional for any injury or insult during the sports season.
3a. Competitive under 6 months: Short endurance—intense activity that lasts for 20 min or less.	Same as 3.	Junior high age and above	2 g pro/kg for growing athletes ≥1 g pro/kg for mature athletes.		
3b. Competitive under 6 months: Long endurance—activity, intense or nonintense, that lasts for longer than 20 min.	Same as 3.	High school age and above	May need refueling with carbohydrate during the event if long in duration (more than 4 h).	Electrolyte replacement needs assessed and replacement given if necessary.	
4. COMPETITIVE SPORTS: Longer than 6 months. Same as Competitive, but usually involved at a personal level other than school.	Same as 3, but may include state or national competition	High school age and above	Same as 3.	Same as 3.	Same as 3. It is very important that a physician determine that the maturation age of the participant is appropriate for the sport.

4a. Competitive at least 6 months: Short endurance—same as 4.	Same as 3.				
4b. Competitive at least 6 months: Long endurance—same as 4.	Same as 3.				
5. PERFORMING: An activity that requires dedicated practice (several times a week) to perform with a group or individually a routine lasting anywhere from 5 min to 1 hr (or longer) in competition or performance.	Ballet, dance, or gymnastics	Junior high age and above as determined by a physician	Nutrition assessment, recommendations, and education provided, preferably by a registered dietitian due to the usually restricted intake to achieve desired weight for performance.	Normal hydration and replacement of lost fluids from practice or performance	Preparticipation assessment by a physician, dietitian, and possibly an orthopedist or physical therapist. Injury attention as in competitive sports.
6. MARCHING BAND: Involvement with a band that competes or performs in marching or choreographed performance. Includes preseason training as well as competition or performance.	High school marching or competing bands	Junior high age and above	Nutrition assessment, recommendations, and education, preferably from a registered dietitian, in a group setting, or individually if necessary.	Same as in 3a and 3b.	Same as in 2 or 3a and 3b. Nutrition attention by a registered dietitian if the participant is less than 85% or greater than 120% of desired weight for height.
7. SEASONAL: Intramural involvement with a team or individual activity, not based heavily on winning but just participation. Practice required. May or may not last longer than 20 min three or more times a week, but activity is not sustained longer than 2 or 3 months.	Soccer, softball, swimming lessons	All ages	Same as in 2.	Same as in 3a and 3b.	Preparticipation assessment by a pediatrician or physician, as in 2. Nutrition attention by a registered dietitian if the participant is less than 85% or greater than 120% of desired weight for height.

Sources: Luckstead SR. Cardiac risk factors and participation guidelines for youth sports. *Ped Clin North Am.* 2002;49:4; National Academy of Sciences. Institute of Medicine. Food and Nutrition Board. Dietary reference intakes: recommended intakes for individuals. Available at: http://iom.edu/en/Global/News%20Announcements/~/media/Files/Activity%20Files/Nutrition/DRIs/DRISummaryListing2.ashx. Accessed March 28, 2010; U.S. Department of Agriculture. MyPyramid.gov. Available at: http://www.mypyramid.gov. Accessed March 28, 2010; Story M, Holt K, Sofka D, eds. *Bright Futures in Practice: Nutrition*, 2nd ed. Arlington, VA: National Center for Education in Maternal and Child Health; 2002: 203–211; American Academy of Pediatrics Committee on Sports Medicine and Fitness. Medical concerns in the female athlete. *Pediatrics*. 2000;106(3):610–613; Rogoi A. Effects of endurance training on maturation. *Consultant*. 1985;25:68–83; Bar-Or O, Barr S, Bergeron M, et al. Youth in sport: nutritional needs. Gatorade Sports Science Institute. 1997;RT30(8):4. Available at: http://www.gssiweb.com. Accessed August 9, 2010.

sufficient physical activity to maintain a healthy weight; increased intake of fruits, vegetables, fish, whole grains; and use of low-fat dairy products. Low-fat milk is suggested for children 12–24 months of age who are obese or who have a family history of obesity, dyslipidemia, or cardiovascular disease (CVD).[118] The AAP also recommends cholesterol screening for children (ages 2 years and above) at risk: those with a positive family history of dyslipidemia or premature ($\leq$ 55 years of age for men and $\leq$ 65 for women) CVD. Other risk factors that might indicate a need for screening include family history of overweight, hypertension, cigarette smoking, or diabetes mellitus. Although controversy exists regarding universal versus selective cholesterol screening,[122] screening in childhood appears to be a sensitive predictor of adult lipid levels.[123]

For children identified by screening, the NCEP intervention is dependent on low-density lipoprotein (LDL) cholesterol categories.[119] For those with an acceptable level (less than 110 mg/dL), the recommended dietary pattern (step-one diet) is suggested, with a repeat lipoprotein analysis in 5 years. Children with a borderline level of LDL cholesterol (110–129 mg/dL) would be provided with a step-one diet prescribed and individualized for them and a reevaluation in 1 year. Those with high LDL cholesterol levels (greater than 130 mg/dL) would initially be given the step-one diet, and if necessary the step-two diet (further reduction to less than 7% saturated fat and less than 200 mg cholesterol per day). These guidelines were included in the 2005 AAP and AHA Consensus Statement.[121]

Some experts believe that these recommendations are not appropriate, especially for the young child.[124] Growth failure has been seen in some infants and toddlers whose parents, well intentioned but misguided, restricted their children's diet to prevent atherosclerosis, obesity, and poor eating habits.[125] Although there is little evidence that dietary intervention in the growing years will decrease serum cholesterol levels or modify other risk factors later in life, young children appear to be able to consume low-fat diets (less than 30% of energy as fat) without negatively influencing the level of energy or micronutrients consumed or affecting growth.[126,128] It seems appropriate to recommend a gradual transition to a diet meeting the NCEP guidelines for children over 2 years of age.

A 10-year study of 2379 girls showed that a significant number of adolescents are exceeding NCEP recommendations for total and saturated fat and cholesterol intakes. A higher percentage of black girls than white girls are not meeting recommendations.[129] Another large national study indicated that children in low-income families with food insufficiency had higher cholesterol intakes than their peers from higher income, food-sufficient households. They were more likely to be overweight, consumed less fruit, and watched more television than peers from low-income, food-sufficient families.[130]

Bone Health

Prevention of osteoporosis begins with optimal calcium and vitamin D intake and maximal bone density in the growing years. However, many young people, especially adolescents, do not receive the recommended AI of 1300 mg calcium. Those who consume limited amounts of dairy products are at risk for calcium deficiency. Some adolescents may also receive less calcium than needed because of rapid growth, dieting practices, and substituting carbonated beverages for milk. Nutrition education public media campaigns are being used to improve these diet trends.

Fiber

National diet intake data have shown that children and adolescents consume a less-than desirable intake of fiber and whole-grain foods, similar to the adult population.[131] An AI for fiber has been established as part of the DRIs. This new recommendation is significantly higher for children and adolescents than previous guidelines[3] (see Appendix H). Increasing dietary fiber can help prevent constipation, protect against coronary heart disease, and often results in greater intake of fruits and vegetables.

Nutrition Education

Children first learn about food and nutrition from their families in their own homes. This begins in an informal manner, with parental attitudes, foods commonly served (e.g., potatoes or tortillas may be served daily; okra or bok choy may never be served), and family opinions about what foods are good nutritionally. Later, more formal nutrition education occurs in preschools, Head Start programs, day care, schools, and clubs such as 4-H. Information is also assimilated from the media, advertising, written materials, the Internet, and peers.

A child's developmental level should be taken into account when teaching nutrition concepts. For example, Piaget's learning theory can be used to correlate developmental periods and cognitive characteristics with progress in feeding and nutrition.[132] Younger children definitely do best with hands-on personal experience with food, not abstract nutrition concepts. A personal approach works well with children and adolescents, such as the use of computer software to examine their own dietary profiles. Social marketing strategies including television, print, radio, and Internet media have been used to communicate health messages to "tweens" (9- to 13-year-olds).[133] Using theoretical concepts to design nutrition education programs and evaluating the effectiveness of these programs is necessary to have an impact on the target population.[134,135] The use of an ecological model has been suggested to increase understanding of eating behaviors, especially among adolescents. The ecological model examines the influences of individual (e.g., biologic), social environmental (e.g., peers), physical environmental (e.g., school), and macrosystem or societal (e.g., marketing) factors on behaviors.[136] Lastly, nutrition education efforts for children should not overlook parents and the family as a whole.

Case Study

Nutrition Assessment

Patient history: A 6.5-year-old male (Ryan) was referred to the nutritionist due to lack of weight gain and slowed growth over the past year. At age 6 years Ryan was diagnosed with attention deficit hyperactivity disorder (ADHD). Concerta (methylphenidate HCI) was prescribed. Current dose is 36 mg daily, but it has varied based on a balance between medication effectiveness and reduced appetite.

Food/Nutrition-Related History

Typical intake: 3 meals and 2 snacks—estimated energy intake 1500 kcal/day

Early morning: Ryan wakes at 5:45 am. He prepares for school, takes his medication, and watches television for ½ hour before the family leaves. Prior to starting before-school care 5 months earlier, Ryan ate breakfast at home: 3 packets instant oatmeal or 1.5 cups Cheerios or 2 eggs. Drank 10 ounces 2% milk and ate ½ cup fruit.

Breakfast: 7:30 am offered at before-school care, but Ryan is not hungry at this time—he may eat a few bites.

Lunch: Parents send lunch. Ryan consumes ½ peanut butter and jelly sandwich, perhaps ½ a small bag of chips; he may eat a 4-ounce cup of applesauce, and drinks water. Family sends a juice box but Ryan usually does not drink it. He prefers milk but does not like school milk.

Snack: Offered at after-school program; they report Ryan always eats the snack and drinks water.

5 pm: Family picks up from after-school program. Ryan is hungry and will finish some of his lunch (chips and applesauce).

6:30 pm: Eats 1½ cups casserole, chili, or stew or 3 ounces chicken and 1 cup rice. Eats ¼ cup vegetables; if green beans can eat 2 cups. Drinks 10 ounces milk.

7 pm: 4–5 times each week Ryan asks for a snack after dinner and will eat applesauce, cheese, or 1 piece of bologna.

A pediatric chewable vitamin, Flintstones Complete, is offered daily. For the past 4 months the family has offered L'il Critters Immune C plus Zinc and Echinacea daily.

Ryan is described as active by family.

Anthropometric Measurements

Weight: 21 kg

Height: 125 cm

BMI: 13.4

Previous growth: According to records from Ryan's primary care provider, for the previous 3 years height has been following the 95th percentile, weight plotted between the 50th and 75th percentiles, and BMI plotted between the 10th and 25th percentiles.

Estimated energy needs: Calculate EER (estimated energy requirement).

EER (boys 3 through 8 years) = $88.5 - 61.9 \times$ age [years] + PA ($26.7 \times$ wt [kg] + $903 \times$ ht [m]) + 20 = $88.5 - 61.9(6.5) + 1.26(26.7 \times 21 + 903 \times 1.25) + 20 = 1835$

Calculate estimated protein needs, based on the DRI: $0.95 \times$ wt [kg] = 21 grams

Medical tests: None indicated

Nutrition Diagnoses

Inadequate energy intake related to decreased appetite from use of Concerta, as evidenced by reported intake below EER and lack of weight gain during the past year.

Intervention Goals

1. Increase energy intake to initially meet EER.
2. Gain weight at a rate appropriate for age.

Nutrition Interventions

Energy intake (NI-1.4):

- Offer breakfast at home before giving medication dose.

Monitoring and Evaluation

- Evaluate growth and weight gain in 3 months.
- Evaluate diet for energy intake in 3 months.

Questions for the Reader

1. What are the nutrition-related side effects, if any, from this medication?
2. What are Ryan's BMI, height, and weight percentiles on the growth chart?
3. How do current BMI, height, and weight compare to previous percentiles?
4. How does Ryan's actual energy intake compare to the calculated EER?

RESOURCES

Knowledge Path on Child and Adolescent Nutrition

http://www.mchlibrary.info/KnowledgePaths/kp_childnutr.html

This extensive resource has information for professionals and families, with strategies for improving nutrition and eating behaviors within families, schools, and communities. There are resources on child care/early childhood, food safety, food marketing to children, food security and assistance programs, and school-based food and nutrition programs. Also included are many related nutrition Websites, electronic publications and newsletters, and many databases.

Bright Futures in Practice: Nutrition, 2nd edition

http://www.brightfutures.org/nutrition

This nutrition guide emphasizes prevention and early recognition of nutrition concerns and provides developmentally appropriate nutrition supervision guidelines for infancy through adolescence. The publication is out of print, but PDFs of the materials can be downloaded. Additional resources, educational materials, and a pocket guide are also available.

Additional Bright Futures resources are listed on the Bright Futures at Georgetown University Website (http://www.brightfutures.org/georgetown.html). Links to educational materials, training materials, and other tools are listed, including those related to social and emotional development, mental health, oral health, and physical activity.

American Academy of Pediatrics

http://www.aap.org

The American Academy of Pediatrics (AAP) Website features resources for professionals (e.g., policy statements, clinical practice guidelines, technical reports) and for families (e.g., educational materials, Health Topics, and Parenting Corner).

Food and Nutrition Information Center (FNIC) Resource Lists

http://www.nal.usda.gov/fnic/resource_lists.shtml

This site includes resource lists related to child nutrition and health, food allergies, food and nutrition education, food safety, and nutrition and food assistance.

Physical Activity and Children and Adolescents Knowledge Path

http://www.mchlibrary.info/knowledgepaths/kp_phys_activity.html

This knowledge path offers a selection of recent, high-quality resources that analyze data, describe public health campaigns and other promotion programs, and report on research aimed at identifying promising strategies for improving physical activity levels within families, schools, and communities.

REFERENCES

1. Satter E. *How to Get Your Kid to Eat . . . But Not Too Much*. Palo Alto, CA: Bull Publishing; 1987.
2. Food and Nutrition Board, Institute of Medicine. *Dietary Reference Intakes: The essential guide to nutrient requirements*. Washington, DC: National Academies Press; 2006.
3. Food and Nutrition Board, Institute of Medicine, National Academy of Sciences. *Dietary Reference Intakes for Energy, Carbohydrate, Fiber, Fat, Fatty Acids, Cholesterol, Protein, and Amino Acids*. Washington, DC: National Academies Press; 2005.
4. Wright JD, Wang CY, Kennedy-Stephenson JK, Ervin RB. Dietary intake of ten key nutrients for public health, United States: 1999–2000. *Adv Data Vital Health Stat*. 2003;334.
5. U.S. Department of Agriculture, Agricultural Research Service. Food and nutrient intakes by children 1994–96, 1998. ARS Food Surveys Research Group. Available at: www.ars.usda.gov/SP2UserFiles/Place/12355000/pdf/scs_all.pdf. Accessed February 10, 2004.
6. Alaimo K, McDowell MA, Briefel RR, et al. Dietary intake of vitamins, minerals, and fiber of persons ages 2 months and over in the United States: third National Health and Nutrition Examination Survey, Phase I, 1988–1991. *Adv Data Vital Stat*. 1994;258. PHS 95–1250.
7. Suitor CW, Gleason PM. Using dietary reference intake–based methods to estimate the prevalence of inadequate nutrient intake among school-aged children. *J Am Diet Assoc*. 2002;102(4):530–536.
8. Moshfegh A, Goldman J, Cleveland L. *What We Eat in America, NHANES 2001–2002: Usual Nutrient Intakes from Food Compared to Dietary Reference Intakes*. Washington, DC: U.S. Department of Agriculture, Agricultural Research Service; 2005.
9. Moshfegh A, Goldman J, Ahuja J, Rhodes D, LaComb R. *What We Eat in America, NHANES 2005–2006: Usual Nutrient Intakes from Food and Water Compared to 1997 Dietary Reference Intakes for Vitamin D, Calcium, Phosphorus, and Magnesium*. Washington, DC: U.S. Department of Agriculture, Agricultural Research Service; 2009.
10. Matkovic V, Fontana D, Tominac C. Factors that influence peak bone mass formation: a study of calcium balance and the inheritance of bone mass in adolescent females. *Am J Clin Nutr*. 1990;52:878–888.
11. Johnston CC, Miller JZ, Slemenda CW, et al. Calcium supplementation and increases in bone mineral density in children. *N Engl J Med*. 1992;327:82–87.
12. Anderson JJ. Calcium requirements during adolescence to maximize bone health. *Pediatrics*. 2001;20(2 Suppl):186S–191S.
13. Food and Nutrition Board, Institute of Medicine, National Academy of Sciences. *Dietary Reference Intakes: Vitamin A, Vitamin K, Arsenic, Boron, Chromium, Copper, Iodine, Iron, Manganese, Molybdenum, Nickel, Silicon, Vanadium, and Zinc*. Washington, DC: National Academies Press; 2001.
14. Wagner CL, Greer FR. Prevention of rickets and vitamin D deficiency in infants, children, and adolescents. *Pediatrics*. 2008; 122:1142–1152.
15. Kumar J, Muntner P, Kaskel F, Hailpern SM, Melamed ML. Prevalence and associations of 25-hydroxyvitamin D deficiency in US children: NHANES 2001–2004. *Pediatrics*. 2009;124(3):e362–e370.

16. Picciano MF, Dwyer JT, Radimer KL, et al. Dietary supplement use among infants, children, and adolescents in the United States, 1999–2002. *Arch Pediatr Adolesc Med.* 2007;161(10):978–985.
17. Feeding the child. In: Kleinman RE, ed. American Academy of Pediatrics, Committee on Nutrition. *Pediatric Nutrition Handbook*, 6th ed. Elk Grove Village, IL: American Academy of Pediatrics; 2009:155–156.
18. American Dietetic Association. Position of the American Dietetic Association: nutrient supplementation. *J Am Diet Assoc.* 2009;109:2073–2085.
19. American Medical Association, Council on Scientific Affairs. Vitamin preparations as dietary supplements and as therapeutic agents. *JAMA.* 1987;257:1929.
20. Lanski SL, Greenwald M, Perkins A, Simon HK. Herbal therapy use in a pediatric emergency department population: expect the unexpected. *Pediatrics.* 2003;111(5):981–985.
21. Beal VA. Dietary intake of individuals followed through infancy and childhood. *Am J Public Health.* 1961;51:1107–1117.
22. Munoz KA, Krebs-Smith SM, Ballard-Barbash R, et al. Food intakes of U.S. children and adolescents compared with recommendations. *Pediatrics.* 1997;100:323–329.
23. Galloway AT, Lee Y, Birch LL. Predictors and consequences of food neophobia and pickiness in young girls. *J Am Diet Assoc.* 2003;103(6):692–698.
24. Larson NI, Neumark-Sztainer D, Hannan PJ, Story M. Family meals during adolescence are associated with higher diet quality and healthful meal patterns during young adulthood. *J Am Diet Assoc.* 2007;107(9):1502–1510.
25. Johnson RK, Crouter AC, Smiciklas-Wright H. Effects of maternal employment on family food consumption patterns and children's diets. *J Nutr Educ.* 1993;25:130–133.
26. Gillman MW, Rifas-Shiman SL, Frazier AL, et al. Family dinner and diet quality among older children and adolescents. *Arch Fam Med.* 2000;9:235–240.
27. Borzekowski D. Watching what they eat: a content analysis of televised food references reaching preschool children. Unpublished manuscript; 2001 [as cited in Kaiser Family Foundation. *The Role of Media in Childhood Obesity*]. Menlo Park, CA: Kaiser Foundation; 2004.
28. Laurson KR, Eisenmann JC, Welk GJ, Wickel EE, Gentile DA, Walsh DA. Combined influence of physical activity and screen time recommendations on childhood overweight. *Pediatrics.* 2008;153(2):209–214.
29. Bell RA, Cassady D, Culp J, Alcalay R. Frequency and types of foods advertised on Saturday morning and weekday afternoon English- and Spanish-language American television programs. *J Nutr Educ Behav.* 2009;41(6):406–413.
30. American Public Health Association. Policy statement 2003-17. Food marketing and advertising directed at children and adolescents: implications for overweight. Available at: http://www.apha.org/advocacy/policy/policysearch/default.htm?id=1255 Accessed August 9, 2010.
31. Boynton-Jarrett R, Thomas TN, Peterson KE, et al. Impact of television viewing patterns on fruit and vegetable consumption among adolescents. *Pediatrics.* 2003;112(6 Pt 1):1321–1326.
32. Harris JL, Bargh JA, Brownell KD. Priming effects of television food advertising on eating behavior. *Health Psychology.* 2009;28(4):404–413.
33. Wright CM, Parkinson KN, Shipton D, Drewett RF. How do toddler eating problems relate to their eating behavior, food preferences and growth? *Pediatrics.* 2007;120:e1069–e1075.
34. Harris CS, Baker SP, Smith GA. Childhood asphyxiation by food: a national analysis and overlook. *JAMA.* 1984;251:2231–2235.
35. Smith MM, Lifshitz F. Excess fruit juice consumption as a contributing factor in nonorganic failure to thrive. *Pediatrics.* 1994;93:438–443.
36. Skinner JD, Carruth BR, Moran J, et al. Fruit juice intake is not related to children's growth. *Pediatrics.* 1999;103(1):58–64.
37. Alexy U, Sicher-Hellert W, Kersting M, et al. Fruit juice consumption and the prevalence of obesity and short stature in German preschool children: results of the DONALD study. *J Pediatric Gastroenterol Nutr.* 1999;29(3):343–349.
38. Committee on Nutrition, American Academy of Pediatrics. The use and misuse of fruit juice in pediatrics. *Pediatrics.* 2001;107(5):1210–1213. [Policy statement reaffirmed October 2006.]
39. Nicklaus TA, O'Neil CE, Kleinman R. Association between 200% juice consumption and nutrient intake and weight of children aged 2 to 11 years. *Arch Pediatr Adolesc Med.* 2008;162(6):557–565.
40. Fiorito LM, Marini M, Francis LA, Smiciklas-Wright H, Birch LL. Beverage intake of girls at age 5 y predicts adiposity and weight status in childhood and adolescence. *Am J Clin Nutr.* 2009;90:935–942.
41. Sebastian RS, Wilkinson C, Goldman JD. US adolescents and MyPyramid: associations between fast-food consumption and lower likelihood of meeting recommendations. *J Am Diet Assoc.* 2009;109:226–235.
42. U.S. Department of Agriculture, Food and Nutrition Service, Office of Analysis, Nutrition and Evaluation. School Nutrition Dietary Assessment Study-II Summary of Findings. Alexandria, VA: USDA; 2001:1-44.
43. Rees GA, Richards CJ, Gregory J. Food and nutrient intakes of primary school children: a comparison of school meals and packed lunches. *J Hum Nutr Diet.* 2008;21(5):420-427.
44. Condon EM, Crepinsek MK, Fox MK. School meals: types of foods offered to and consumed by children at lunch and breakfast. *J Am Diet Assoc.* 2009;109:S67–S78.
45. Committee on Nutrition, American Academy of Pediatrics. Soft drinks in schools. *Pediatrics.* 2004;113(1):152–154. [Policy statement reaffirmed January 2009.]
46. French SA, Jeffery RW, Story M, et al. Pricing and promotion effects on low-fat vending snack purchases: the CHIPS study. *Am J Public Health.* 2001;91(1):112–117.
47. Schwartz MB, Novak SA, Fiore SS. The impact of removing snacks of low nutritional value from middle schools. *Health Educ Behav.* 2009;36(6):999–1011.
48. Briggs M, Safaii S, Beall D. Position of the American Dietetic Association, Society for Nutrition Education, and American School Food Service Association—nutrition services: an essential component of comprehensive school health programs. *J Am Diet Assoc.* 2003;103:505–514.
49. Dye BA, Tan S, Smith V, et al. Trends in oral health status: United States, 1988–1994 and 1999–2004. *Vital Health Stat.* 2007;11(248):1–92.
50. Faine MP. Nutrition issues and oral health. In: *Proceedings from Promoting Oral Health of Children with Neurodevelopmental*

Disabilities and Other Special Health Care Needs. May 4-5, 2001. Center on Human Development and Disability, University of Washington, Seattle, WA. Available at: http://www.mchoral health.org/PDFs/LEND2001.pdf. Accessed February 10, 2004.

51. Palmer CA. *Diet and Nutrition in Oral Health*. Upper Saddle River, NJ: Prentice Hall; 2003.
52. Nunn ME, Braunstein NS, Krall Kaye EA, Dietrich T, Garcia RI, Henshaw MM. Healthy eating index is a predictor of early childhood caries. *J Dent Res* 2009;88(4):361–366.
53. White-Graves MV, Schiller MR. History of foods in the caries process. *J Am Diet Assoc*. 1986;86:241–245.
54. Kaste LM, Selwitz RH, Oldakowski RJ, et al. Coronal caries in the primary and permanent dentition of children and adolescents 1–17 years of age: United States, 1988–1991. *J Dent Res*. 1996;75:631–641.
55. Garcia-Closas R, Garcia-Closas M, Sera-Majem L. A cross-sectional study of dental caries, intake of confectionery and foods rich in starch and sugars, and salivary counts of *Steptococcus mutans* in children in Spain. *Am J Clin Nutr*. 1997;66:1257–1263.
56. Navia JM. Carbohydrates and dental health. Am *J Clin Nutr*. 1994;59(Suppl):719S–727S.
57. Makinen KK, Hujoel PP, Bennett CA, et al. A descriptive report of the effects of a 16-month xylitol chewing gum programme subsequent to a 40-month sucrose gum programme. *Caries Res*. 1998;32:107–112.
58. American Academy of Pediatric Dentistry. Policy on early childhood caries (ECC): classifications, consequences, and preventive strategies. 2003, revised 2008. Available at: http://www.aapd .org/media/Policies_Guidelines/P_ECCClassifications.pdf. Accessed November 1, 2009.
59. American Academy of Pediatrics, Section on Pediatric Dentistry. Oral health risk assessment timing and establishment of the dental home. *Pediatrics*. 2003;111(5):1113–1116. [Policy statement reaffirmed May 2009.]
60. U.S. Department of Health and Human Services. *Oral Health in America: A Report of the Surgeon General—Executive Summary*. Rockville, MD: U.S. Department of Health and Human Services, National Institute of Dental and Craniofacial Research, National Institutes of Health; 2000. Available at: http://www.nidcr.nih .gov/DataStatistics/SurgeonGeneral/Report/ExecutiveSummary .htm. Accessed August 9, 2010.
61. Caplan LS, Erwin K, Lense E, Hicks J. The potential role of breast-feeding and other factors in helping to reduce early childhood caries. *J Public Health Dent*. 2008;68(4):238–241.
62. Centers for Disease Control and Prevention. Iron deficiency—United States, 1999–2000. *MMWR*. 2002;51(40):897–899.
63. Lozoff B, Beard J, Connor J, Felt B, Georgieff M, Schallert T. Long-lasting neural and behavioral effects of iron deficiency in infants. *Nutr Rev*. 2006;64(5):S34–S43.
64. Lozoff B, Corapci F, Burden MJ, et al. Preschool-aged children with iron deficiency anemia show altered affect and behavior. *J Nutr*. 2007;137:683–689.
65. Monsen ER, Hallberg L, Layrisse M, et al. Estimation of available dietary iron. *Am J Clin Nutr*. 1978;31:134–141.
66. Iron. In: Kleinman RE, ed. American Academy of Pediatrics, Committee on Nutrition, ed. *Pediatric Nutrition Handbook*, 6th ed. Elk Grove Village, IL: American Academy of Pediatrics; 2004:402–422.
67. Pollit E, Cueto S, Jacoby ER. Fasting and cognition in well- and undernourished school children: a review of three experimental studies. *Am J Clin Nutr*. 1998;67(Suppl):779S–784S.
68. Simeon DT, Grantham-McGregor S. Effects of missing breakfast on the cognitive functions of school children of differing nutritional status. *Am J Clin Nutr*. 1989;49:646–653.
69. Meyers AF, Sampson A, Weitzman M, et al. School breakfast program and school performance. *Am J Dis Child*. 1989;143:1234–1239.
70. Powell CA, Walker SP, Chang SM, Grantham-McGregor SM. Nutrition and education: a randomized trial of the effects of breakfast in rural primary school children. *Am J Clin Nutr*. 1998;68:873–879.
71. Kleinman RE, Murphy J, Little M, et al. Hunger in children in the United States: potential behavioral and emotional correlates. *Pediatrics*. 1998;101:e3.
72. Alaimo K, Olsom CM, Frongillo EA. Food insufficiency and American school-aged children's cognitive, academic, and psychosocial development. *Pediatrics*. 2001;108(1):44–51.
73. Lipton MA, Mayo JP. Diet and hyperkinesis: an update. *J Am Diet Assoc*. 1983;83:132–134.
74. Kaplan BJ, McNicol J, Conte RA, et al. Dietary replacement in preschool-aged hyperactive boys. *Pediatrics*. 1989;83:7–17.
75. Harper PH, Goyette CH, Conners CK. Nutrient intakes of children on the hyperkinesis diet. *J Am Diet Assoc*. 1978;73:515–519.
76. Wolraich ML, Wilson DB, White JW. The effect of sugar on behavior or cognition in children: a metaanalysis. *JAMA*. 1995;274:1617–1621.
77. Behar D, Rapoport JL, Adams AJ, et al. Sugar challenge testing with children considered behaviorally sugar reactive. *Nutr Behav*. 1984;1:277–288.
78. Bachorowski J, Newman JP, Nichols SL, et al. Sucrose and delinquency: behavioral assessment. *Pediatrics*. 1990;86:244–253.
79. American Academy of Pediatrics Subcommittee on Attention-Deficit/Hyperactivity Disorder. Clinical practice guideline: treatment of the school-aged child with attention-deficit/hyperactivity disorder. *Pediatrics*. 2001;108(4):1033–1044.
80. Spencer T, Biederman J, Wilens T. Growth deficits in children with attention deficit hyperactivity disorder. *Pediatrics*. 1998;102:501–506.
81. Haslam RHA, Dalby JT, Rademaker AW. Effects of megavitamin therapy on children with attention deficit disorders. *Pediatrics*. 1984;74:103–111.
82. Voigt RG, Llorente AM, Jensen CL, et al. A randomized, double-blind, placebo-controlled trial of docosahexaenoic acid supplementation in children with attention-deficit/hyperactivity disorder. *J Pediatr*. 2001;139:189–196.
83. Craig WJ, Mangels AR, American Dietetic Association. Position of the American Dietetic Association: vegetarian diets. *J Am Diet Assoc*. 2009;109(7):1266–1282.
84. Kleinman RJ. Nutritional aspects of vegetarian nutrition. In: American Academy of Pediatrics, Committee on Nutrition, ed. *Pediatric Nutrition Handbook*, 6th ed. Elk Grove Village, IL: American Academy of Pediatrics; 2009:201–224.
85. Vegetarian Resource Group. How many youth are vegetarian? Available at: http://www.vrg.org/journal/vj2005issue4/vj2005 issue4youth.htm. Accessed October 30, 2009.

86. Robinson-O'Brien R, Perry CL, Wall MM, Story M, Neumark-Sztainer D. Adolescent and young adult vegetarianism: better dietary intake and weight outcomes but increased risk of disordered eating behaviors. *J Am Diet Assoc.* 2009;109:648–655.
87. Messina V, Melina V, Mangels AR. A new food guide for North American vegetarians. *J Am Diet Assoc.* 2003;103(6):771–775.
88. Centers for Disease Control and Prevention, National Center for Health Statistics. NCHS data on adolescent health. December 2008. Available at: http://www.cdc.gov/nchs/data/infosheets/infosheet_adoleshealth.pdf. Accessed August 9, 2010.
89. Hediger ML, Scholl TO, Schall JI. Implications of the Camden study of adolescent pregnancy: interactions among maternal growth, nutritional status, and body composition. *Ann N Y Acad Sci.* 1997;817:281–291.
90. Rees JM, Lederman SA. Kiely JL. Birth weight associated with lowest neonatal mortality: infants of adolescent and adult mothers. *Pediatrics.* 1996;98:1161–1166.
91. Institute of Medicine. *Weight Gain During Pregnancy: Reexamining the Guidelines.* Washington, DC: National Academies Press; 2009.
92. Hediger ML, Scholl TO, Belsky DH, Ances IG, Salmon RW. Patterns of weight gain in adolescent pregnancy: effect on birth weight and preterm delivery. *Obstet Gynecol.* 1989;74:6–12.
93. Scholl TO, Hediger ML, Schall JI. Maternal growth and fetal growth: pregnancy course and outcome in the Camden study. *Ann N Y Acad Sci.* 1997;817:292–301.
94. Lozoff B, Georgieff MK. Iron deficiency and brain development. *Semin Pediatr Neurol.* 2006;13(3):158–165.
95. Baker PN, Wheeler SJ, Sanders TA, et al. A prospective study of micronutrient status in adolescent pregnancy. *Am J Clin Nutr.* 2009;89:1114–1124.
96. Story M. Promoting healthy eating and ensuring adequate weight gain in pregnant adolescents: issues and strategies. *Ann N Y Acad Sci.* 1997;817:321–333.
97. Substance Abuse and Mental Health Services Administration, Office of Applied Studies. *The NSDUH Report: Trends in Substance Use, Dependence or Abuse, and Treatment among Adolescents: 2002 to 2007.* Rockville, MD: SAMHSA; 2008.
98. Fryar CD, Merino MC, Hirsch R, Porter KS. Smoking, alcohol use, and illicit drug use reported by adolescents aged 12–17 years: United States, 1991–2004. *Nat Health Stat Rep.* 2009;15:1–23.
99. Farrow JA, Rees JM, Worthington-Roberts B. Health, developmental and nutritional status of adolescent alcohol and marijuana abusers. *Pediatrics.* 1987;79:218–223.
100. Centers for Disease Control and Prevention. Tobacco use among middle and high school students—United States, 2002. *MMWR.* 2003;52(45):1096–1098.
101. Primack BA, Walsh M, Bruce C, Eissenberg T. Water-pipe tobacco smoking among middle and high school students in Arizona. *Pediatrics.* 2009;123(2):e282–e288.
102. U.S. Department of Health and Human Services. Physical activity and fitness health indicators. *Healthy People 2010: Understanding and Improving Health,* 2nd ed. Washington, DC: U.S. Government Printing Office; 2000. Available at: http://www.healthypeople.gov/pdf/Volume2/22Physical.pdf. Accessed August 10, 2010.
103. Centers for Disease Control and Prevention. Youth risk behavior surveillance – United States, 2009. *MMWR Surveill Summ,* 2010;59(5):1–142.
104. Anderson SE, Economos CD, Must A. Active play and screen time in US children aged 4 to 11 years in relation to sociodemographic and weight status characteristics: a nationally representative cross-sectional analysis. *BMC Public Health.* 2008;8:366.
105. Hinkley T, Crawford D, Salmon J, Okely AD, Hesketh K. Preschool children and physical activity: a review of correlates. *Am J Prev Med.* 2008;34(5):435–441.
106. U.S. Department of Health and Human Services. 2008 physical activity guidelines for Americans. Available at: http://www.health.gov/paguidelines/guidelines/default.aspx. Accessed August 9, 2010.
107. President's Council on Physical Fitness and Sports. The president's challenge. Available at: http://www.presidentschallenge.org. Accessed November 25, 2009.
108. Goldberg B, Saraniti A, Witman P, Gavin M, Nicholas JA. Pre-participation sports assessment: an objective evaluation. *Pediatrics.* 1980;66:736–745.
109. Luckstead SR. Cardiac risk factors and participation guidelines for youth sports. *Ped Clin North Am.* 2002;49:4.
110. National Academy of Sciences. Institute of Medicine. Food and Nutrition Board. Dietary reference intakes: recommended intakes for individuals. Available at: http://iom.edu/en/Global/News%20Announcements/~/media/Files/Activity%20Files/Nutrition/DRIs/DRISummaryListing2.ashx. Accessed March 28, 2010.
111. U.S. Department of Agriculture. MyPyramid.gov. Available at: http://www.mypyramid.gov. Accessed March 28, 2010.
112. Story M, Holt K, Sofka D, eds. *Bright Futures in Practice: Nutrition,* 2nd ed. Arlington, VA: National Center for Education in Maternal and Child Health; 2002: 203–211.
113. American Academy of Pediatrics Committee on Sports Medicine and Fitness. Medical concerns in the female athlete. *Pediatrics.* 2000;106(3):610–613.
114. Rogoi A. Effects of endurance training on maturation. *Consultant.* 1985;25:68–83.
115. Bar-Or O, Barr S, Bergeron M, et al. Youth in sport: nutritional needs. Gatorade Sports Science Institute. 1997;RT30(8):4. Available at: http://www.gssiweb.com. Accessed August 9, 2010.
116. Spear BA. Sports nutrition for adolescents. *Building Block Life.* 2008;31(1):1–8.
117. American Academy of Pediatrics. Use of performance-enhancing substances. *Pediatrics.* 2005;115(4):1103–1106. [Policy statement reaffirmed August 2008.]
118. Daniels SR, Greer FR, Committee on Nutrition. Lipid screening and cardiovascular health in childhood. *Pediatrics.* 2008;122:198–208.
119. National Heart, Lung, and Blood Institute, National Cholesterol Education Program. *Report of the Expert Panel on Blood Cholesterol Levels in Children and Adolescents.* Bethesda, MD: National Heart, Lung, and Blood Institute; 1991.
120. Lichtenstein AH, Appel LJ, Brands M, et al. Diet and lifestyle recommendations revision 2006: a scientific statement from the American Heart Association Nutrition Committee. *Circulation.* 2006;114(1):82–96. [Published corrections appear in *Circulation.* 2006;114(23):e629 and *Circulation.* 2006;114(1):e27.]
121. Gidding SS, Dennison BA, Birch LL, et al. Dietary recommendations for children and adolescents: a guide for practitioners:

consensus statement from the American Heart Association. *Circulation*. 2005;112(13):2061–2075.

122. Steiner NJ, Neinstein LS, Pennbridge J. Hypercholesterolemia in adolescents: effectiveness of screening strategies based on selected risk factors. *Pediatrics*. 1991;88:269–275.
123. Stuhldreher WL, Orchard TJ, Donahue RP, et al. Cholesterol screening in childhood: sixteen-year Beaver County Lipid Study experience. *J Pediatr*. 1991;119:551–556.
124. Olson RE. The folly of restricting fat in the diet of children. *Nutr Today*. 1995;30(6):234–245.
125. Pugliese MT, Weyman-Daum M, Moses N, et al. Parental health beliefs as a cause of nonorganic failure to thrive. *Pediatrics*. 1987;80:175–182.
126. Luepker RV, Perry CL, McKinlay SM, et al. Outcomes of a field trial to improve children's dietary patterns and physical activity. The Child and Adolescent Trial for Cardiovascular Health (CATCH). *JAMA*. 1996;275:768–776.
127. Dixon LB, McKenzie J, Shannon BM, et al. The effect of changes in dietary fat on the food group and nutrient intake of 4- to 10-year-old children. *Pediatrics*. 1997;100:863–872.
128. Obarzanek E, Kimm SYS, Barton BA, et al. Long-term safety and efficacy of a cholesterol-lowering diet in children with elevated low-density lipoprotein cholesterol: seven-year results of the Dietary Intervention Study in Children (DISC). *Pediatrics*. 2001;107(2):256–264.
129. Kronsberg SS, Obarzanek E, Affenito SG, et al. Macronutrient intake of black and white adolescent girls over 10 years: the NHLBI Growth and Health Study. *J Am Diet Assoc*. 2003;103(7):852–860.
130. Casey PH, Szeto K, Lansing S, et al. Children in food-insufficient, low-income families: prevalence, health, and nutrition status. *Arch Pediatr Adolesc Med*. 2001;155(4):508–514.
131. Harnack L, Walters SH, Jacobs DR. Dietary intake and food sources of whole grains among US children and adolescents: data from the 1994–1996 Continuing Survey of Food Intakes by Individuals. *J Am Diet Assoc*. 2003;103(8):1015–1019.
132. Lucas B, Feucht S. Nutrition in childhood. In: Mahan LK, King K, eds. *Krause's Food, Nutrition, & Diet Therapy*, 12th ed. Philadelphia, PA: Saunders, Elsevier; 2008:22–245.
133. Huhman M, Bauman A, Bowles HR. Initial outcomes of the VERB campaign: tweens' awareness and understanding of campaign messages. *Am J Prev Med*. 2008;34(6 Suppl):S241–S248.
134. Contento I, Balch GI, Bronner YL, et al. The effectiveness of nutrition education and implications for nutrition education and policy, programs, and research: a review of research. *J Nutr Educ*. 1995;27:298–311.
135. Sigman-Grant M. Strategies for counseling adolescents. *J Am Diet Assoc*. 2002;102(3 Suppl):S32–S39.
136. Story M, Neumark-Sztainer D, French S. Individual and environmental influences on adolescent eating behaviors. *J Am Diet Assoc*. 2002;102(3 Suppl):S40–S51.

Food Hypersensitivities

Lynn Christie

Identifying health problems associated with foods, the mechanisms of the problems, and appropriate treatments have plagued medicine for centuries. Hippocrates was one of the first to report an adverse food reaction to milk over 2000 years ago.[1] The National Institutes of Allergy and Infectious Diseases and the American Academy of Allergy, Asthma, and Immunology established a common language describing adverse food reactions. An adverse food reaction is a clinically abnormal response to an ingested food or food additive. Adverse food reactions (food sensitivities) are categorized either as hypersensitivities (food allergy) or as intolerances. Food hypersensitivity is caused by an immunologic reaction resulting from the ingestion of a food or food additive. Food intolerance is an abnormal physiological response to an ingested food or a food additive that has not been proven to be immunologic in nature.

Food hypersensitivity involves either immunoglobulin E (IgE)-mediated or non-IgE-mediated immune mechanisms. IgE-mediated reactions occur after ingestion of a specific food, occur usually within 1 hour, and can be followed by a late-phase reaction. Non-IgE-mediated reactions such as food protein–induced enterocolitis, proctocolitis, allergic eosinophilic diseases, and gluten-sensitive enteropathy are cell-mediated reactions. Food hypersensitivities are further described in **Table 7-1** by their clinical manifestations and whether the disorder is IgE mediated.

Food intolerances that are proven not to be immunologic in nature are secondary to factors that include toxic contaminants, pharmacological properties of foods, metabolic disorders, and idiosyncratic responses. **Table 7-2** provides a differential diagnosis for adverse food reactions.

Eggs, milk, peanuts, soybeans, wheat, tree nuts, fish, and shellfish cause approximately 90% of food hypersensitivities in children in the United States.[2] Milk, egg, peanut, soybean, and wheat are the primary foods responsible for hypersensitivity in children 3 years of age and younger.

Clinical Manifestations

Contact with an allergen is necessary before an IgE immunological response can occur. The dermal, gastrointestinal tract, and respiratory tract are involved with an allergic reaction. More severe, life-threatening reactions involve the cardiovascular system. IgE mediated food allergy is responsible for oral allergy syndrome, exercise-induced anaphylaxis, and possibly colic in infants with milk allergy. Non-IgE mediated food allergies involve the gastrointestinal tract. No matter what the mechanism is, elimination of the allergen is the basis of the medical management.

Pathophysiology

The allergic immune response begins with sensitization to a particular antigen, a glycoprotein in a food. Therefore, the susceptible individual must come in contact with a food before becoming allergic. The plasma cells (mature B-cells) begin producing IgE to a particular food antigen. The food-specific IgE becomes bound to mast cells and basophils, and then recurrent antigen exposure leads to a cross-linking of the food-specific IgE molecules, activating the mast cells and basophils. This activation causes the release of histamine, leukotrienes, and other mediators. These mediators produce the vasodilation, smooth muscle contraction, and mucous secretion resulting in the clinical symptoms detected in the skin, respiratory system, and gastrointestinal system. The immediate allergic reaction can occur within seconds and up to 2 hours after contact with the food allergen. This cross-linking can lead to the synthesis of proinflammatory cytokines and chemokines that are responsible for a late-phase reaction that might occur within 4 to 48 hours after the initial exposure. A chronic inflammatory response seen primarily with the skin and respiratory systems is thought to be due to the repetitive ingestion of a food allergen.[3]

TABLE 7-1 Food Hypersensitivity Disorders

	IgE Mediated	Mixed (May Involve Both IgE-Mediated and Cell-Mediated Mechanisms)	Non-IgE Mediated
Gastrointestinal	Oral allergy syndrome (oral and perioral pruritis and angioedema, throat tightness) Gastrointestinal anaphylaxis (nausea, cramping, emesis, diarrhea) Infantile colic (~15% of infants with colic)	Allergic eosinophilic esophagitis (subset) Allergic eosinophilic gastroenteritis (postprandial nausea, emesis, weight loss)	Food-induced enterocolitis (1 to 3 hours postingestion: emesis, diarrhea, failure to thrive, and rarely, hypotension) Food-induced proctocolitis (2 to 12 hours postingestion; blood in stools) Food-induced malabsorption syndrome ("celiac-like"; nausea, steatorrhea, weight loss) Celiac disease
Cutaneous	Acute (common) and chronic (rare) urticaria Generalized flushing	Atopic dermatitis (pruritic morbilliform rash leading to eczematous lesion)	Dermatitis herpetiformis Contact hypersensitivity Contact irritation (especially with acid fruits and vegetables)
Respiratory	Rhinoconjunctivitis Laryngeal edema	Asthma (both acute wheezing and increased bronchial hyperreactivity)	Heiner's syndrome (rare form of pulmonary hemosiderosis)
Other: Mechanism Unknown	Migraine (rare)		

Source: Adapted with permission from Sampson HA. Diagnosing food allergies in children. In: Lichtenstein LM, Busse WW, Raif SG, eds. *Current Therapy in Allergy, Immunology, and Rheumatology*, 6th ed. St. Louis, MO: Mosby; 2004:147–153.

IgE-Mediated Food Hypersensitivities

The organ systems generally related to IgE-mediated allergic reactions are the skin, gastrointestinal (GI) tract, and respiratory tract. Once foods are ingested, there may be immediate oral symptoms such as itching mouth and swelling of the lips, palate, tongue, or throat. In the gastrointestinal tract, nausea, cramping, gas, distention, vomiting, abdominal pain, or diarrhea may be experienced. Once the antigen spreads through the bloodstream and lymphatics, degranulation of mast cells may occur in the skin, causing urticaria, angioedema, pruritis, or an erythematous macular rash. Respiratory symptoms include coughing, wheezing, profuse nasal rhinorrhea, sneezing, or laryngeal edema. The eyes may experience edema, tearing, excess mucus, itching, or burning. The relationship of food hypersensitivities to migraine headaches, epilepsy, rheumatoid arthritis, enuresis, or attention deficit hyperactivity remains controversial.[4] Physical findings associated with gluten sensitivity can be found in Chapter 12.

Systemic anaphylaxis is an acute and potentially fatal reaction. Anaphylaxis can begin with any of the symptoms just mentioned plus cardiovascular symptoms including chest tightness, tachycardia, hypotension, and shock. A fatal reaction may begin with mild symptoms and progress to cardiorespiratory arrest and shock rapidly within 1 to 3 hours. Risk factors for fatal or near-fatal hypersensitivity reactions include: (1) children with asthma; (2) allergies to peanuts, tree nuts, fish, and/or shellfish; (3) individuals who do not receive epinephrine immediately after the reaction begins; and (4) patients who had a previous allergic reaction to a food.[5] Milk, egg, and soy are less likely than the previously listed items to produce fatal reactions in children.[6]

Exercise-induced anaphylaxis is associated with the ingestion of a specific food prior to exercise. Then, during or shortly after exercise, the individual experiences allergic symptoms that may progress to anaphylaxis.[7] The individual can usually exercise without any reaction as long as the specific food has not been ingested within the past 8 to 12 hours. Individuals with exercise-induced anaphylaxis typically have a positive skin prick test to foods that provoke symptoms. A skin prick test is a diagnostic test defined in the "Diagnosing Food Hypersensitivity" section of this chapter. Management requires identifying the food through a food challenge that includes strenuous exercise after food ingestion and avoiding the food at least 8 to 12 hours prior to any expected exercise.

TABLE 7-2 Differential Diagnosis for Adverse Food Reactions

I. Food additives
  A. Food colors: Azo dye F, D, and C, yellow no. 5 (tartrazine)
  B. Preservatives
    1. Sulfiting agents
    2. Nitrate/nitrite
    3. BHA/BHT
  C. Flavor enhancers: l-monosodium glutamate (MSG)
  D. Sweeteners: aspartame, sorbitol, sucrose
  E. Miscellaneous: antibiotics (penicillin)

II. Unintentional food contaminants
  A. Plant toxins
    1. Cyanogenic compounds: glycosides in fruit pits and cassava
    2. Oxalates: spinach
    3. Solanine alkaloids: potatoes
  B. Microbial toxins
    1. Bacterial
      a. *Staphylococcus aureus*, *Clostridium botulinum*, etc.
      b. Scromboid poisoning: tuna, mackerel
    2. Fungal (mycotoxins): aflatoxins, ergot
    3. Algal (dinoflagellates)
      a. Ciguatera poisoning: grouper, snapper, barracuda
      b. Saxitoxin: shellfish
  C. Foodborne infectious agents
    1. Bacterial: salmonellosis, *Campylobacter jejuni*, *Clostridium perfringens*, etc.
    2. Parasitic: *Giardia lamblia*, *Trichinella spiralis*, flukes, etc.
    3. Viral: hepatitis

III. Naturally occurring pharmacologic agents
  A. Methylxanthines: caffeine, theobromine
  B. Biologically active amines: tyramine, phenylethylamine, serotonin, histamine

IV. Gastrointestinal diseases
  A. Structural abnormalities
    1. Gastroesophageal reflux
    2. Hiatal hernia
    3. Pyloric stenosis
    4. Intestinal obstruction
  B. Carbohydrate intolerance
    1. Congenital carbohydrate deficiency: lactase, sucrase, isomaltase, galactose-4-epimerase
    2. Acquired carbohydrate intolerance: lactase, sucrase, isomaltase
  C. Malignancy
  D. Other conditions
    1. Gastroenteritis
    2. Gastric/duodenal ulcer disease
    3. Cholelithiasis
    4. Pancreatic insufficiency
    5. Irritable bowel syndrome
    6. Inflammatory bowel disease
    7. Mucosal damage secondary to drug therapy

V. Other conditions
  A. Malnutrition
  B. Endocrine disorders: hypothyroidism, hyperthyroidism
  C. Eating disorders

Source: Adapted with permission from Olejer V. Food hypersensitivities. In: Queen PM, Lang CE, eds., *Handbook of Pediatric Nutrition*. Gaithersburg, MD: Aspen Publishers. 1993:206–231.

Oral allergy syndrome (OAS), also referred to as pollen-food allergy syndrome, is another form of IgE-mediated food allergy.[8] OAS occurs mainly in patients allergic to pollens. The proteins in the pollens that cause allergic rhinitis immunologically cross-react to the allergens in related raw fruits and vegetables.[9] The reaction is limited to the lips, tongue, palate, and throat, followed by a rapid resolution of symptoms. In rare instances, systemic anaphylaxis can occur. People allergic to birch tree pollen may have OAS symptoms when they eat raw carrots, celery, apples, pears, cherries, apricots, and kiwis. Those allergic to ragweed may react when they eat watermelon, cantaloupe, honeydew, and bananas. Generally, cooking fruits and vegetables denatures the relevant proteins, allowing symptom-free consumption.

Infants with cow's milk allergy have a high rate (44%)[10] of colic that improves with extensively hydrolyzed formulas. All causes of colic need to be considered, but if there are additional symptoms of cow's milk allergy or a poor response to other measures (for example, medicines), a trial elimination diet may be reasonable. Studies[11,12] have suggested that infantile colic may represent an early manifestation of food allergy.

Non-IgE–Mediated Food Hypersensitivity

Food protein–induced enterocolitis syndrome, food protein–induced enteropathy, allergic proctocolitis, and celiac disease (gluten-sensitive enteropathy) are immunologically mediated food hypersensitivity disorders, but are not IgE mediated.[10] Food protein–induced enterocolitis, enteropathy, and protocolitis tend to be outgrown by 12 to 36 months of age. Diagnosis is usually made through clinical history and response to an elimination diet. (Skin prick test to foods will be negative.) Management is dietary elimination of the offending foods. Up to half of all cases of cow's milk allergy in childhood may manifest with symptoms limited to the GI tract.

Food protein–induced enterocolitis syndrome (FPIES) presents with projectile emesis and excessive diarrhea that can lead to dehydration, hypotension, and lethargy within 2–3 hours after exposure. FPIES usually occurs in formula-fed infants. Most infants present with this classic history of severe reactions and become asymptomatic when the suspected food is eliminated. Oral food challenges of the suspected food are required prior to reintroducing the food back into the diet. Cow's milk, soybeans, grains, vegetables, and/or poultry are often the offending foods.[13]

Dietary protein enteropathy presents within the first 1–2 months of life and can be seen as late as 9 months of age in the cow's milk formula–fed infant. The onset of symptoms mimics acute enteritis with transient emesis, anorexia, and protracted diarrhea that leads to failure to thrive. Diagnosis through an intestinal biopsy reveals patchy, subtotal villus injury. The foods commonly associated with food-sensitive enteropathy are cow's milk, soy, egg, rice, chicken, and/or fish.

Allergic proctocolitis presents with rectal bleeding within the first few weeks to months of life in well-nourished infants. These children do not have growth delay or poor weight gain. Biopsy of the large intestine reveals eosinophils in the lamina propria. Cow's milk and soy proteins are the usual offending foods.

Allergic eosinophilic gastroenteropathy is inflammation in the gastrointestinal tissues caused by eosinophilic inflammation. When eosinophils are found in the esophagus the disease is labeled allergic eosinophilic esophagitis (AEE). If eosinophils are located in the stomach and intestines, the diagnosis is allergic eosinophilic gastroenteritis (AEG). Symptoms are pain, nausea, poor appetite, vomiting, and diarrhea. Strictures and dysmotility also occur. Endoscopic biopsies are required to establish the diagnosis. Fifty percent are atopic and benefit from removal of identified foods, reducing the need for corticosteroids or repeated esophageal dilations.[14] Medical management is controversial.

Celiac disease is an intolerance to gliadin, which is found in wheat, spelt, kamut, rye, and barley. Oats do not contain gliadin and are safe for those with celiac disease; however, oats may be contaminated during processing with other grains that do contain gliadin.[15] Refer to Chapter 12 on gastrointestinal disorders for more information on celiac disease.

Diagnosing Food Hypersensitivity

The evaluation of a suspected adverse food reaction requires a thorough medical history, physical examination, possibly a diet diary, and various laboratory studies. If food hypersensitivity is suspected, an elimination diet is indicated and food challenges may need to be performed. Incomplete food hypersensitivity work-ups and unorthodox procedures can erroneously label one with food allergies, resulting in incorrect diagnoses, nutrient deficiencies (e.g., calcium or vitamin D), and delay in treating treatable disease.[16–21]

History

The medical history is useful in diagnosing food allergy in acute events (e.g., systemic anaphylaxis following the ingestion of peanuts). Historically, reported adverse food reactions have been confirmed less than 50% of the time using double-blind, placebo-controlled food challenge (DBPCFC).[22–24] The history may be helpful in distinguishing IgE-mediated food reactions from other forms of adverse food reactions. The history should include:

- Food suspected to have provoked the reaction
- Quantity of the food ingested
- Length of time between ingestion and development of symptoms
- Description of the symptoms provoked
- What similar symptoms developed on other occasions when the food was eaten
- If other factors (e.g., exercise) are necessary for the reaction to occur
- Length of time since the last reaction

If reactions occur within minutes to 1–2 hours of ingesting a specific food and the symptoms are consistent with those previously mentioned, one should suspect a food hypersensitivity.

Adverse food reactions or intolerances and disorders that mimic food allergic reactions are listed in Table 7-2. Lactose intolerance produces symptoms similar to cow's milk allergy. Lactose intolerance is frequently seen after a bacterial or viral gastroenteritis. Toddler's diarrhea or chronic nonspecific diarrhea is aggravated by consumption of simple sugars, especially sorbitol found in fruits (e.g., apple and pear juice), some sugar-free candies, and chewing gums. Unintentional consumption of food contaminants (infectious organisms and toxins) may result in symptoms similar to an allergic reaction.

Physical Exam

No specific features of the physical examination will suggest IgE-mediated food hypersensitivity. The physical exam can identify other atopic diseases that increase the chance that the symptoms are related to food hypersensitivity. Atopic diseases are food and environmental allergy, asthma, allergic rhinitis, and atopic dermatitis; they share allergic mechanisms. Thirty-five percent of young children with atopic dermatitis have food allergies as a trigger for the condition.[25] Anthropometrics, assessment of growth and development, and nutritional status should be performed. (Refer to Chapters 2 and 3.) Abnormal physical findings and a patient's behavior may suggest a diagnosis other than adverse reactions to foods.

Skin Testing and In Vitro Assays

If IgE-mediated food sensitivity is suspected, skin prick testing (SPT) with food extracts will help screen for the responsible food allergens. SPT is the first test used because of the ease of use, low cost, and immediate results. Glycerated food extracts, and positive (histamine) and negative (saline) controls are applied by a prick technique.[26,27] After 15–20 minutes, the diameter of the wheal is measured. If the wheal, defined as a localized area of edema not including erythema, is at least 3 mm greater than the negative control, it is considered positive; anything else is considered negative. A positive SPT indicates the presence of food-specific IgE, not necessarily that the child will have a clinical reaction to the food. Individuals may or may not be hypersensitive to a specific food because the positive predictive accuracy of a SPT is less than 50%. A good history is critical when evaluating SPT results. If the SPT is negative, there is no detected food-specific IgE. With a negative history, it is highly unlikely that an IgE allergic reaction would occur to the tested food. The negative predictive value is greater than 95%, but severe reactions may occur in patients with negative test results.[28]

The mean diameter of the wheal can be used to predict whether an oral food challenge is indicated. **Table 7-3** provides guidelines that can be used to determine the likelihood of a positive reaction with ingestion of milk, egg, or peanut.[29] If the SPT is ≤ 3 mm in response to egg or peanut, there is a 50% likelihood of a negative food challenge.

To diagnose OAS, a skin prick test is recommended with the prick to prick technique. This involves pricking the fresh food first and then the patient's skin with the same lancet.[30] This induces a minor reaction that does not require a challenge to confirm. It is important to distinguish the OAS from oropharyngeal symptoms that may precede systemic symptoms, including urticaria, GI symptoms, rhinitis, and anaphylactic shock.

There are a few exceptions to the clinical findings to consider when interpreting the SPT results. A child less than 1 year of age may have an IgE-mediated food allergy without a positive SPT because of the lower concentration of IgE present in the skin; a child less than 2 years of age may have smaller wheals when tested by the SPT method.[31] Therefore, do not discount histories of strongly suspected foods for which the SPT is negative. Patients may have a positive SPT long after they have outgrown the food allergy. Another exception is when a SPT is positive to a food; if that food had been ingested in isolation causing a serious systemic anaphylactic reaction, this scenario is considered diagnostic. A SPT is not indicated in patients with extensive skin disease, dermatographism, those who cannot be taken off antihistamines, or if prior exposure to minute amounts resulted in near-fatal anaphylaxis. In vitro tests for specific IgE would be indicated in these patients. Intradermal skin tests are not recommended because of the increased risk of inducing a systemic reaction.[26]

In vitro assays are available to detect and quantify food-specific serum IgE antibodies. The Phadia ImmunoCAP (Pharmacia-Upjohn Diagnostics, Uppland, Sweden) system has been validated with double-blind, placebo-controlled food challenges to show that there are food-specific serum levels of IgE that indicate a ≥ 95% probability of a reaction if that individual undergoes a food challenge to the specific food[29] (see Table 7-3). The ImmunoCAP positive values for milk and egg are lower for younger children because of the less developed immune system.[32,33] The ImmunoCAP is helpful in quantifying the amount of food-specific serum IgE for other foods, but it has not been validated to predict reactivity to those foods. Like SPT, the ImmunoCAP test for other foods has a false positive rate of less than 50%.

TABLE 7-3 Tests to Assess the Likelihood of Obtaining a Positive or Negative OFC in Children

	Serum Food-IgE (kIU/L)*		SPT Wheal (mm)*	
Food	**~95% Positive**	**~50% Negative†**	**~95% Positive**	**~50% Negative†**
Cow's milk	≥15 ≥5 if younger than 1 year	≤2	≥8	
Egg white	≥7 ≥2 if younger than 2 years	≤2	≥7	≤3
Peanut	≥14	≤2 with and ≤5 without history of peanut reaction	≥8[1]	≤3
Fish	≥20			

A subset of patients with undetectable serum food-specific IgE antibody and negative SPT has been reported to have objective reactions confirmed by OFC.

*Phadia ImmunoCAP; SPT with commercial food extracts.

†In the authors' experience, children with about 50% chance of experiencing a negative challenge are the optimal candidates for an office-based OFC. However, serum levels of food-specific IgE antibodies and SPT wheal sizes are not absolute indications or contraindications to performing an OFC. Laboratory test results always have to be interpreted in the context of clinical history. For example, if a child had a recent anaphylactic reaction (past 6 mo) to a food, it is more prudent to defer an office OFC even if the test values are at 50% pass rate. In contrast, a child with peanut IgE of 20 kUA/L who recently tolerated an accidental ingestion of a product containing peanut butter may be a candidate for an OFC.

Source: Adapted with permission from Nowak-Wegrzyn A, Assa'ad AH, Bahna SL, et al. Work Group report: Oral food challenge testing. *J Allergy Clin Immunol.* 2009;123:S365–383.

Monitoring food-specific serum IgE levels is clinically important in the follow-up of patients with food hypersensitivity. Pediatric food allergy is a dynamic process, with the majority of children developing oral tolerance. Patients destined to "outgrow" their allergies to milk or egg protein will demonstrate lowering levels of IgE antibodies to the food.[34] Food-specific serum IgE test results indicate an approximately 50% or better chance of tolerance with egg, milk, and peanut IgE[35] (Table 7-3). A diagnostic food challenge would be indicated when food-specific serum IgE values drop below these levels and if there is no known reaction to that food over the past 6 months. Again, these tests are to be viewed as guidelines rather than set diagnostic points. The food-specific serum IgE levels give no indication of the dose the patient may react to or predict the severity of the reaction.

Cross-reactivity occurs when an individual is allergic to more than one food in a food family. Clinical reactivity to more than one member of an animal species or botanical family is more common with fish, shellfish, tree nuts, and OAS, as previously mentioned.[36,37] A significant amount of cross-reactivity is demonstrated through the food-specific positive SPTs and food-specific serum IgE because of the shared homologous proteins. SPT and food-specific serum IgE cannot determine the clinical relevance of cross-reactivity between foods because of the high rate of false-positive results. An example of test cross-reactivity is when the SPT or food-specific serum IgE is positive to environmental grasses and dietary wheat and the child suffers from allergic rhinitis. The child has always consumed and tolerated wheat products. The tests identified the common proteins found in grasses; wheat is part of this family. The positive wheat test was false positive. With a negative dietary history and a diagnosis of allergic rhinitis, dietary wheat should not be avoided. Several alternative tests for food hypersensitivity have been evaluated, but the results are no better than chance at diagnosing food hypersensitivity.[38,39] These alternatives are vega testing (electrodiagnostic devices),[40] applied kinesiology, hair analysis, pulse test, sublingual or subcutaneous provocative challenge, ELISA/ACT, IgG or IgG4 antibody food test, lymphocyte activation, and food antigen-antibody complexes.

Diet Diary

A diet diary may be helpful in identifying a relationship between the foods ingested and the symptoms experienced. Families are asked to keep a timed, chronological record of the amount of formula and/or food (including condiments) ingested for each meal or snack over a specified period of time. Brand names (with ingredient labels), methods of preparation, and recipes are important. The families and other caregivers should record any prescription or over-the-counter medications, including vitamin and mineral supplements or herbal preparations, along with the duration and severity of any symptoms experienced during this time. This experience helps the family pay greater attention to what the child is actually eating. The registered dietitian can evaluate the diet for nutritional adequacy. If a food intolerance is responsible for the symptoms, minor dietary changes may be adequate as opposed to elimination diets.

Elimination Diets

Food elimination followed by selected food challenges is important to determine whether a food is responsible for the reported symptoms. The food(s) to be eliminated and tested by oral food challenge are based on patient history, food diary, skin prick test, and/or food-specific serum IgE results. The elimination diet used in diagnosing a food allergy may be the same as one needed in treatment of the diagnosed food hypersensitivity. If used as part of the diagnostic process, it should be for a specified trial period to avoid iatrogenic malnutrition. There are several types of elimination diets.

A single food elimination diet is used when a child has a history of a sudden acute reaction and positive test for IgE to the food (e.g., egg). If an infant is breastfed, the mother will need to eliminate the food(s) in question from her diet.[41,42]

A multiple food elimination diet removes a number of foods from the diet based on history and positive tests. Children with chronic disease (e.g., asthma or atopic dermatitis) may not have noticeable reactions to a specific food but will have a positive test. A trial elimination diet for 2–6 weeks of the identified foods will determine whether the foods play a role in the child's chronic disease when accompanied by medical management for asthma and/or atopic dermatitis. An example of this would be a child with atopic dermatitis and a positive food-specific IgE test to egg, milk, peanuts, and tree nuts. The child's atopic dermatitis improves immensely over a 3-week period once these foods are eliminated from the diet. The purpose of the multiple food elimination diet is to provide a clean baseline. Food challenges then would begin with the patient's favorite nutrient-dense foods, if appropriate. A few-foods diet, also called an "eat-only" or "oligoantigenic" diet, eliminates a large number of food allergens suspected of playing a role in severe chronic diseases such as atopic dermatitis and eosinophilic gastroenteropathies. This diet includes foods that cannot be related to symptoms or were negative on testing. To begin, select one meat, one grain, three cooked vegetables, three fruits, and all condiments from the following list:

- *Meats:* Chicken, turkey, or lamb
- *Grain:* Rice or corn
- *Vegetables (cooked):* Carrots, broccoli, cauliflower, sweet potato, squash, spinach, or cucumber

- *Fruits:* Apple, pear, peach, plum, canned pineapple, or grapes
- *Condiments:* Salt, pepper, canola and/or olive oil, white vinegar, or sugar

An extensively hydrolyzed or amino acid formula may be needed to provide adequate nutrients for growth and development. Once symptoms resolve on the few-foods diet, slowly expand the diet using additional fruits and vegetables, then meats and grains based on testing and history. Individual condiments may be expanded to help increase palatability of the safe foods. The time frame used to introduce new foods, including condiments to flavor foods, is based on the disease (e.g., every 5–7 days with severe atopic dermatitis). Several foods are slowly introduced with eosinophilic gastroenteropathies followed by endoscopic biopsies. Biopsies used with eosinophilic gastroenteropathies occur every 3–6 months to determine tolerance of new foods. This is a very slow process that requires patience and cooperation between the allergist and gastroenterologist.

Individualization of allowed foods improves compliance. Educate the family on the different forms of the food available to help with variety and advancement of the child's developmental feeding skills. For example, if rice is the selected grain, white rice, brown rice, rice bread, rice cereals, rice cakes, rice pasta, and rice milk can be used. Fresh, frozen, or canned corn; corn cereals; corn chips; corn pasta; polenta; and homemade popcorn can be used when corn is an allowed grain.

An elemental diet requires the use of amino acid–based formulas as the sole source of nutrition. This eliminates all foods to help establish whether food consumption plays a role in the symptoms. Once the patient is symptom-free, foods cited in the previous list may be added slowly to the diet.

Resolution of symptoms during the elimination phase suggests that the symptoms were triggered by one or more of the eliminated foods. An oral food challenge is recommended to reintroduce foods that are not responsible for the clinical reactions. In order to diagnose the allergy or intolerance appropriately, the symptoms must be documented after oral ingestion of the suspected food. If improvement of symptoms is not detected within 2 weeks on the elimination diet either:

- A food sensitivity is not responsible for the symptoms.
- There is poor dietary compliance.
- The unrecognized offending food continues to be present in the diet.
- Other chronic conditions are causing the flair of symptoms (e.g., asthma, atopic dermatitis).

Oral Food Challenges

Oral food challenges (OFCs) determine whether an individual is, in fact, reactive to a food. There are three types of OFCs: (1) open, (2) single-blind, and (3) double-blind, placebo-controlled. The double-blind, placebo-controlled food challenge (DBPCFC) is considered the "gold standard" for accurately diagnosing food allergies and for examining a wide variety of food-related complaints.[29,43,44] Open or single-blind food challenges are useful in the medical practice setting to determine whether symptoms can be reproduced when a food is ingested. Challenges are labor intensive and require equipment to treat an anaphylactic reaction. Any challenge should be supervised by personnel appropriately trained to recognize and manage any severe food reaction.[45]

Open Food Challenge

During an open food challenge, the patient eats a serving of the food in its traditional form (e.g., a cup of milk, a scrambled egg). Examples of good candidates for an open food challenge are patients who have had negative skin tests and doubtful histories and/or patients who have been "avoiding the food" yet ingest foods that contain the allergen (e.g., someone who eats cookies symptom free that contain milk and eggs). Open challenges also are performed following a single-blind or double-blind OFC. A negative open challenge—no reaction within 2 hours after ingestion—will convince the individual that the food does not cause any symptoms.

Single-Blind Food Challenge

A single-blind OFC is where the patient and parent do not know what food is being challenged; therefore, it eliminates the bias of the subject and family. It is easily performed in an office setting to confirm objective symptoms. This challenge would be performed under the same conditions as a double-blind, placebo-controlled food challenge (outlined in the next section) except the nurse, dietitian, or doctor performing the challenge would know which food is being challenged.

Double-Blind, Placebo-Controlled Food Challenge

The DBPCFC has the patient, parent, and medical personnel performing the challenge "blinded" to what substance is being administered. During the DBPCFC there are two servings of a food (vehicle)—one contains the food allergen (active arm) and the other contains a safe similar food (placebo arm). The active and placebo containing vehicles are randomized and fed to the patient in that order. The DBPCFC may be performed on one or two days. The DBPCFC is the most objective of the three tests and provides the most accurate information.

For an OFC to be accurate, suspected foods should be totally eliminated for at least 10 to 14 days, or up to 12 weeks in some gastrointestinal disorders, prior to the challenge. The subject should be symptom-free during the elimination diet. It might be assumed that once symptoms resolve and the skin tests are positive, a diagnosis could be made; however, less than 50% of positive histories will be confirmed by DBPCFC.[23] Certain medications (e.g., antihistamines and oral or injected steroids) may inhibit food hypersensitivity reactions. Recommended avoidance of medication prior to food challenge may range from 36 hours to 1 month.[44] Children with atopic dermatitis may require aggressive skin care prior to food challenges.

Note of caution: If there is a clear history of severe anaphylaxis following an isolated ingestion of a specific food and there is a positive skin test, this patient should *not* be challenged.

Foods to be used in OFCs can be found locally. Powdered milk, individually packed flours, powdered egg, and baby foods are found in grocery and health food stores. Challenge substance and placebo material should be well mixed in a carrier food (vehicle). The vehicle should mask the smell, flavor, and texture of the food to be tested. Vehicles to use in food challenges include baby food fruits, hot cereals, applesauce, ice cream, mashed potatoes, fruit smoothies, and ground chicken or beef patties. Placebos can be safe foods not under suspicion, such as dextrose, cornstarch, another grain, or baby food meat.

The OFC is administered in a fasting state, starting with a dose unlikely to cause symptoms (10 to 100 mg of dry powder food, 0.1–1% of the total amount to be consumed). The dose is doubled every 10 to 60 minutes, depending on the type of reaction that might occur based on the history. Clinical reactivity is generally ruled out once the patient has tolerated 10 grams of a dried food, 100 mL of a wet food, or 30–60 g of meat/fish without symptoms. Following completion of the challenge, the individual should be observed for 2 hours for food allergic reactions and 4 to 8 hours for food intolerances, based upon the child's history. If the immediate onset of symptoms is suspected, the DBPCFC can be performed in a day. One series of challenges (active or placebo) is given in the morning. In the afternoon, a second series of challenges (the opposite of the earlier challenge) is performed. If the blinded challenge is negative, the food must be given openly in usual quantities, under observation, to rule out a rare false-negative challenge. Overall, this method works well except for delayed or late onset reactions. The Food Allergy and Anaphylaxis Network (FAAN) has published a book titled *A Health Professional's Guide to Food Challenges* that is more detailed, for those interested in performing food challenges.[46]

Summation of Diagnosing Food Allergies and Food Challenges

In summary, the medical history identifies possible food hypersensitivity reactions. If IgE-mediated food hypersensitivity is suspected, perform skin prick tests for suspected and common food allergens (e.g., milk, egg, wheat, soy, peanut, fish). If positive, perform food-specific serum IgE to those foods. If negative, either stop or consider other possible non-IgE immunological disorders (see Tables 7-1 and 7-2). If the tests are positive and there is a convincing history of anaphylaxis, restrict the food(s) and stop the workup. Otherwise, place the child on an elimination diet for the suspected food allergens for 2 to 4 weeks. If there is no improvement, food hypersensitivity may not be the cause. If there is improvement, and considering the SPT and ImmunoCAP results, begin the food-challenge process.

To determine what kind of OFC to perform, ask whether there is concern about the child's bias, whether the child has had a positive OFC in the past, and whether symptoms will be difficult to interpret. If yes, a blinded OFC is indicated; otherwise, an open OFC is appropriate. If there are no symptoms during the OFC, the child is not or is no longer reactive to the food. If there are subjective symptoms, a blinded OFC is needed. If there are objective symptoms, the individual has a food allergy to that food.

If a food protein–induced enteropathy is suspected, the OFC needs to be done in a hospital setting with placement of an IV to treat a reaction. Offer 0.15–0.3 g protein per kg weight for milk or soy, or 8–10 g dried food (e.g., dry baby rice cereal mixed with a safe liquid).[29] Divide into three servings and give it to the patient over 30 minutes. Observe for 6–8 hours.

If food intolerance is suspected, eliminate the suspected offending food(s) from the diet. If symptoms persist, add the foods back and look for other causes. If symptoms improve, add the food(s) back to the diet after an OFC.

Diet Therapy

Education

Once a diagnosis has been made, management of food hypersensitivities is strict avoidance of the offending allergen(s) supported by pharmacological treatment during an allergic reaction, such as injection of epinephrine in the event of anaphylaxis. Education is the cornerstone for good compliance and a nutritionally adequate diet. This requires extensive education for the patient and family regarding all forms of the food to be avoided, how to read food labels, where the food may be hidden, and alternative food sources for the nutrients that may be affected. This is overwhelming to the family and impacts most aspects of their life. Follow-up for newly diagnosed individuals is best 1 to 2 months after diagnosis to reinforce education and address issues that have come up with the family. If a child is allergic to a single food, such as peanuts or fish, the nutritional adequacy of the diet may not be compromised; however, the elimination of milk, eggs, soybeans, or wheat can have a major impact on the quality of a diet. These foods are found in the food supply in many forms, making complete elimination difficult. Milk, soy, wheat, and egg food hypersensitivities traditionally can be outgrown. Therefore, long-term follow-up involves repeated testing to determine if a child is still reactive to a food and to prevent unnecessary food avoidance.

In a published study,[47] children with two or more food hypersensitivities were shorter in length and height stature than those with only one food hypersensitivity. Twenty-five percent of the children with food hypersensitivities consumed inadequate amounts of calcium, vitamin D, and vitamin E. Children with two or more food hypersensitivities and those hypersensitive to milk were at greatest risk. The Food Guide Pyramid (FGP) can be used to quickly assess one's diet for nutrient deficiencies by comparing the diet to a personalized FGP and other tools in the preschooler and kids section available on http://www.mypyramid.gov. The original Food Guide Pyramid for Young Children[48] provides a list of foods in each food group that helps to explain what the child can eat. Alternative foods based on the allergens to avoid can be worked into the pyramid to demonstrate a balanced diet.

Labels

Label reading is critical to successfully avoiding a food allergen. The patient and family should read all product labels every time they shop because ingredients change without warning. This is the only way food manufacturers communicate that the ingredients have changed. One brand may be allergen free but another brand of the same food may not.

The Food Allergen Labeling and Consumer Protection Act of 2004 (http://www.fda.gov/food/labelingnutrition), effective January 2006, has made label reading much easier for families. This act requires that major allergens (milk, egg, wheat, soy, peanuts, tree nuts, fish, and seafood) be identified in plain English on packaged foods. Specific tree nut, fish species, or crustacean shellfish must be identified. Mollusks are not considered major allergens and will not be fully disclosed on the food label like crustacean shellfish. The allergen can be listed on the label in the following ways:

- Included in the ingredient list (e.g., milk, wheat)
- Parenthetically following a scientific term (e.g., whey, milk)
- Below the ingredient list in a "contains" statement (e.g., Contains: egg)

If a child is allergic to other foods (e.g., chicken or sesame), the family must contact manufacturers to determine if the food is allergen-free, especially if terms like *flavors* or *spices* are listed. Only intentional ingredients, not contaminants, are listed on the food product label. Other household products, including pet food, cosmetics, bath products, lotions, sunscreens, and so forth, are known to contain food allergens and may use creative terms for the ingredients on the label. It is advantageous for families to know specific terms for the allergens, such as casein or whey for milk. **Table 7-4** contains information from FAAN on how to read a label for the major allergens. This also can be found on their Website: http://www.foodallergy.org under education.

Advisory labeling declares potential cross-contact. This is completely voluntary and unregulated. Advisory labeling uses phrases such as "may contain (*allergen*)" or "produced in a facility that also produces (*allergen*)." Risk is not less with one phrase over another; in addition, absence of advisory labeling does not mean there is no risk.[49,50] A *D* (dairy) or *DE* (dairy equipment) next to Rabbinical agency symbols (such as a *U* in a circle) is a form of advisory labeling indicating the possible presence of milk protein, which may or may not be found in the ingredient statement.

Avoidance of products with advisory labeling is suggested, and contacting the company for more information is recommended. Families must be specific when they contact the company. Ask "Does this product contain these allergens?" not "What is in brand *X* sauce?" Ask about potential cross-contamination by asking whether production lines are shared with allergen-containing foods; if so, ask how the production lines are cleaned between runs. Most large manufacturers have this information. If a company cannot provide appropriate information, it is best to avoid the product. Imported foods are required to follow U.S. labeling regulations, but U.S. distributors often do not track down ingredient information from foreign sources.

Cross-Contact

Cross-contact occurs when an allergen-containing food comes in contact with a "safe" food. As a result, each food now contains a small and usually hidden amount of the other food. Cross-contact happens during the manufacturing, preparation, and serving of a food throughout the food industry and at home.

Packaged and processed foods are at risk for cross-contact because equipment for related products is shared. Failure to clean the equipment satisfactorily between processing different products can leave allergenic food residues. Guidelines for the cleaning and care of equipment for manufactured foods ("good manufacturing practice") do not eliminate all the sources of cross-contact. This may occur with any food, such as egg-containing and egg-free pastas, or breakfast cereals/cereal bars with or without nuts, dark chocolate, and milk chocolate. Formulation errors and packaging or labeling mistakes may also occur. There may or may not be advisory labeling. Families can contact manufacturers to clarify how a product was produced.

At the grocery store, cross-contact occurs in the deli, where meats and cheeses are sliced on the same equipment; in the

TABLE 7-4 How to Read Food Labels for the Major Allergens

How to Read a Label for a Milk-Free Diet

All FDA-regulated manufactured food products that contain milk as an ingredient are required by U.S. law to list the word "milk" on the product label.

Avoid foods that contain milk or any of these ingredients:

butter, butter fat, butter oil, butter acid, butter ester(s)	lactose
buttermilk	lactulose
casein	milk *(in all forms, including condensed, derivative, dry, evaporated, goat's milk and milk from other animals, low-fat, malted, milkfat, nonfat, powder, protein, skimmed, solids, whole)*
casein hydrolysate	milk protein hydrolysate
caseinates *(in all forms)*	pudding
cheese	Recaldent®
cottage cheese	rennet casein
cream	sour cream, sour cream solids
curds	sour milk solids
custard	tagatose
diacetyl	whey *(in all forms)*
ghee	whey protein hydrolysate
half-and-half	yogurt
lactalbumin, lactalbumin phosphate	
lactoferrin	

Milk is sometimes found in the following:

artificial butter flavor	luncheon meat, hot dogs, sausages
baked goods	margarine
caramel candies	nisin
chocolate	nondairy products
lactic acid starter culture and other bacterial cultures	nougat

How to Read a Label for a Soy-Free Diet

All FDA-regulated manufactured food products that contain soy as an ingredient are required by U.S. law to list the word "soy" on the product label.

Avoid foods that contain soy or any of these ingredients:

edamame	soybean *(curd, granules)*
miso	soy protein *(concentrate, hydrolyzed, isolate)*
natto	soy sauce
shoyu	tamari
soy *(soy albumin, soy cheese, soy fiber, soy flour, soy grits, soy ice cream, soy milk, soy nuts, soy sprouts, soy yogurt)*	tempeh
soya	textured vegetable protein *(TVP)*
	tofu

Soy is sometimes found in the following:

Asian cuisine	vegetable gum
vegetable broth	vegetable starch

Keep the following in mind:

- **The FDA exempts highly refined soybean oil from being labeled as an allergen.** Studies show most allergic individuals can safely eat soy oil that has been highly refined (*not* cold pressed, expeller pressed, or extruded soybean oil).
- Most individuals allergic to soy can safely eat soy lecithin.
- Follow your doctor's advice regarding these ingredients.

How to Read a Label for a Peanut-Free Diet

All FDA-regulated manufactured food products that contain peanut as an ingredient are required by U.S. law to list the word "peanut" on the product label.

Avoid foods that contain peanuts or any of these ingredients:

artificial nuts	goobers	monkey nuts	peanut butter
beer nuts	ground nuts	nut pieces	peanut flour
cold pressed, expeller pressed, or extruded peanut oil	mixed nuts	nutmeat	peanut protein hydrolysate

Peanut is sometimes found in the following:

African, Asian *(especially Chinese, Indian, Indonesian, Thai, and Vietnamese)*, and Mexican dishes	baked goods *(e.g., pastries, cookies)*	chili	marzipan
	candy *(including chocolate candy)*	egg rolls	mole sauce
		enchilada sauce	nougat

Keep the following in mind:

- Mandelonas are peanuts soaked in almond flavoring.
- **The FDA exempts highly refined peanut oil from being labeled as an allergen.** Studies show that most allergic individuals can safely eat peanut oil that has been highly refined (not cold pressed, expeller pressed, or extruded peanut oil). Follow your doctor's advice.
- A study showed that unlike other legumes, there is a strong possibility of cross-reaction between peanuts and lupine.
- Arachis oil is peanut oil.
- Many experts advise patients allergic to peanuts to avoid tree nuts as well.
- Sunflower seeds are often produced on equipment shared with peanuts.

How to Read a Label for a Wheat-Free Diet

All FDA-regulated manufactured food products that contain wheat as an ingredient are required by U.S. law to list the word "wheat" on the product label. The law defines any species in the genus Triticum as wheat.

Avoid foods that contain wheat or any of these ingredients:

bread crumbs	matzoh, matzoh meal *(also spelled as matzo, matzah, or matza)*
bulgur	pasta
cereal extract	seitan
club wheat	semolina
couscous	spelt
cracker meal	sprouted wheat
durum	triticale
einkorn	vital wheat gluten
emmer	wheat *(bran, durum, germ, gluten, grass, malt, sprouts, starch)*
farina	wheat bran hydrolysate
flour *(all purpose, bread, cake, durum, enriched, graham, high gluten, high protein, instant, pastry, self-rising, soft wheat, steel ground, stone ground, whole wheat)*	wheat germ oil
hydrolyzed wheat proteins	wheat grass
kamut	wheat protein isolate
	whole wheat berries

Wheat is sometimes found in the following:

glucose syrup	starch *(gelatinized starch, modified starch, modified food starch, vegetable starch)*
soy sauce	surimi

How to Read a Label for a Shellfish-Free Diet

All FDA-regulated manufactured food products that contain a crustacean shellfish as an ingredient are required by U.S. law to list the specific crustacean shellfish on the product label.

Avoid foods that contain shellfish or any of these ingredients:

crab	*Mollusks are not considered major allergens* under food labeling laws and may not be fully disclosed on a product label.
crawfish *(crayfish, ecrevisse)*	
lobster *(langouste, langoustine, scampo, coral, tomalley)*	
prawn	
shrimp *(crevette)*	

Your doctor may advise you to avoid mollusks or these ingredients:

abalone	octopus
clams *(cherrystone, littleneck, pismo, quahog)*	oysters
cockle *(periwinkle, sea urchin)*	snails *(escargot)*
mussels	squid *(calamari)*

Shellfish are sometimes found in the following:

bouillabaisse	seafood flavoring *(e.g., crab or clam extract)*
cuttlefish ink	surimi
fish stock	

Keep the following in mind:

- Any food served in a seafood restaurant may contain shellfish protein due to cross-contact.
- For some individuals, a reaction may occur from inhaling cooking vapors or from handling fish or shellfish.

How to Read a Label for an Egg-Free Diet

All FDA-regulated manufactured food products that contain egg as an ingredient are required by U.S. law to list the word "egg" on the product label.

Avoid foods that contain eggs or any of these ingredients:

albumin *(also spelled albumen)*	eggnog	mayonnaise	ovalbumin
egg *(dried, powdered, solids, white, yolk)*	lysozyme	meringue *(meringue powder)*	surimi

Egg is sometimes found in the following:

baked goods	lecithin	marzipan	nougat
egg substitutes	macaroni	marshmallows	pasta

Keep the following in mind:

- Individuals with egg allergy should also avoid eggs from duck, turkey, goose, quail, etc., as these are known to be cross-reactive with chicken egg.

(continued)

TABLE 7-4 *(Continued)*

How to Read a Label for a Tree Nut–Free Diet			
All FDA-regulated manufactured food products that contain a tree nut as an ingredient are required by U.S. law to list the specific tree nut on the product label.			
Avoid foods that contain nuts or any of these ingredients:			
almonds	filberts/hazelnuts	natural nut extract *(e.g., almond, walnut)*	pili nut
artificial nuts	gianduja *(a chocolate-nut mixture)*	nut butters *(e.g., cashew butter)*	pine nuts *(also referred to as Indian, pignoli, pigñolia, pignon, piñon, and pinyon nuts)*
beechnut	ginkgo nut	nut meal	pistachios
Brazil nuts	hickory nuts	nut paste *(e.g., almond paste)*	praline
butternut	litchi/lichee/lychee nut	nut pieces	shea nut
cashews	macadamia nuts	nutmeat	walnuts
chestnuts	marzipan/almond paste	pecans	
chinquapin	Nangai nuts	pesto	
coconut			
Tree nuts are sometimes found in the following:			
black walnut hull extract *(flavoring)*	natural nut extract nut distillates/alcoholic extracts	nut oils *(e.g., walnut oil, almond oil)*	walnut hull extract *(flavoring)*
Keep the following in mind:			
• Mortadella may contain pistachios. • There is no evidence that coconut oil and shea nut oil/butter are allergenic. • Many experts advise patients allergic to tree nuts to avoid peanuts as well. • Talk to your doctor if you find other nuts not listed here.			

Source:

bakery, where pastries with and without nuts are side by side, and in bins where bulk foods are accidentally mixed. Advise families to purchase sealed packages with ingredient labels.

Food service industry practices can lead to cross-contact. Cooking utensils, serving utensils, and containers may be shared on buffets, salad bars, and cafeteria lines, and in ice cream stores. The same frying oil may be used for all of the foods (e.g., potatoes, fish, foods dipped in egg or milk and battered in wheat). Seafood and steaks or eggs and bacon may be prepared on the same grill.

At home, cooking utensils may be used to stir an allergen-containing food and then a safe food, contaminating the safe food. An allergen-containing food may spill or splatter into safe foods. All cooking equipment must be cleaned with soap and water prior to preparing allergen-free foods.

Elimination Diets

All forms of a food to be eliminated must be completely removed from an individual's diet once diagnosed with food hypersensitivity. Labels must be read to identify words that are terms for the offending foods (Table 7-4).

Milk Hypersensitivity

If cow's milk protein hypersensitivity is suspected in infancy, an extensively hydrolyzed protein-based formula (Alimentum, Nutramigen, or Pregestimil) rather than a soy-based formula is recommended until the child is 1 year of age or has had a negative test to soy.[51]

The breastfed infant with any food allergy would benefit from maternal avoidance of the identified allergen from the diet. Partially hydrolyzed milk-based formulas (Good Start, Enfamil, Gentlease, Lipil) contain whole cow's milk allergens and will continue to cause allergic reactions in the milk-allergic child. In children with IgE-associated hypersensitivity to milk, 14% cannot tolerate soy formulas:[52] 30–50% of those with non-IgE–mediated enterocolitis and enteropathy syndromes are reactive to soy protein. Ten percent of infants or toddlers fail to tolerate an extensively hydrolyzed milk protein–based formula; therefore, an amino acid–based formula (Neocate, Elecare, Nutramigen AA) would be required.[53,54] Health professionals also need to contact these companies to ensure the product is free of milk or soy contamination. Goat's milk is not an alternative to cow's milk because of the potential cross-reactivity with the beta-lactoglobulins in cow's milk.[55] The vitamin and mineral–fortified infant formulas will provide the calcium, phosphorus, vitamin D, vitamin B_{12}, riboflavin, and pantothenic acid that would be provided by the milk products. Encourage parents to continue milk-free formulas as long as the milk-hypersensitive child will consume them; age is not a factor.

Alternative enriched beverages can be considered if the child begins to refuse formula and is able to consume at least two-thirds of the total daily nutrient requirement from a wide variety of solid foods. Cow milk substitutes have their strengths and weaknesses based on the product's fortification. Enriched soy milk provides dietary calcium, vitamin D, and protein, almost equivalent to milk. If the child is allergic to soy and cow's milk, rice milk may provide dietary calcium and vitamin D but it is very low in protein, fat, and other nutrients. Hemp and oat enriched products may be fortified with calcium and vitamin D. Stress the need for appropriate amounts of high biological proteins during counseling if the child refuses or consumes very little formula or milk alternative.

The Daily Value of calcium on food labels is a helpful tool. Teach families how to calculate whether their child is consuming adequate calcium from fortified ready-to-eat cereals, breads, and beverages. A calcium and vitamin D supplement may still be needed. Some ready-to-eat cereals, breads, and fruit juices are calcium fortified but may not be fortified with vitamin D. Vitamin D deficiency has been the culprit for rickets in children with milk allergy.[56,57] The adequate intake for vitamin D established by the Food and Nutrition Board in 1997 is now under review. If a low intake is suspected, it may be appropriate to check serum levels of 25(OH) vitamin D in infants and children with milk allergy.[58,59]

When cooking from scratch at home, fruit juice, water, rice milk, or soy milk are appropriate substitutes for milk in recipes. Whole grains, legumes, meats, and nuts can provide alternative sources of other nutrients such as phosphorus, riboflavin, and pantothenic acid that are found in milk.

Egg Hypersensitivity

Nutrients in eggs are easily replaced by other high-protein foods and whole grains. However, eggs are incorporated into breads, pastas, baking mixes, breaded or processed meats, custards, fat substitutes, salad dressings, sauces, candies, and other commercially prepared foods. It is the elimination of all of these other foods containing egg that causes problems in providing a nutritionally balanced diet. For instance, eggs are used for a shiny glaze on products in bakeries. Beware of fried foods because eggs are frequently used in batters, and consequently the oil may be contaminated with egg protein.

Families can be taught how to modify recipes at home to provide substitutes for the binding and leavening properties of eggs. Not all egg substitutes are alike; egg whites are commonly used in most egg substitutes, for example, Egg Beaters. Ener-g Foods, Inc. has an egg-free powder called Egg Replacer. For other substitutes for eggs in a recipe, try one of the following for each egg:

- 1 tsp. of baking powder, 1 Tbsp. of water, 1 Tbsp. of vinegar (add vinegar separately at end)
- 1 tsp. baking soda, 1 Tbsp. oil, 2 Tbsp. baking powder, 1 Tbsp. vinegar (add vinegar separately at end)
- 1 tsp. of yeast dissolved in ¼ cup of warm water
- 1½ Tbsp. of water, 1½ Tbsp. of oil, 1 tsp. of baking powder
- 1 Tbsp. of apricot (or other fruit) puree (binder)
- 1 packet of plain gelatin mixed with 1 cup boiling water (binder). Substitute 3 Tbsp. of this liquid for each egg. Refrigerate remainder for 1 week; microwave to liquefy.

Soybean Hypersensitivity

Soybean flour and soybean protein are major ingredients used by food manufacturers. Soy can be found in processed grains (crackers, cereals, baked goods), processed meats, frozen dinners, salad dressings, sauces, Asian foods, and soups. A balanced diet may be a challenge in this population, and cooking from scratch with basic ingredients may be a necessity. Soybean oil and soy lecithin are considered safe for most soy allergic individuals because the processing of the oil removes the protein portion.[60,61] The highly refined soybean oil is exempt from allergen labeling, but not soy lecithin. Products that contain soy lecithin may have a "contains soy" statement. To ensure that a product is safe, call the manufacturer to determine if any soy protein ingredients are included in the product.

Wheat Hypersensitivity

Wheat and wheat products are the foundation of the U.S. diet and are difficult to eliminate from the diet. Wheat is found in baked products, pastas, cereals, crackers, snacks, sauces, soups, and breaded and processed meats. Wheat flours are fortified with niacin, riboflavin, thiamin, and iron. A child's diet composed of very few whole grain products may be deficient in these and other nutrients. Encourage the use of fortified or 100% whole grains. Products made with the flours of amaranth, arrowroot, barley, buckwheat, corn, oats, potato, quinoa, rice, rye, soybean, and tapioca are suitable wheat alternatives. These foods and grains can be found in grocery stores, health food stores, and mail-order companies. Gluten-free products used by individuals with celiac disease or gluten sensitivity may be good alternatives but often contain milk or egg products. Packaged gluten-free mixes or home baked recipes can be prepared with egg replacement and cow's milk substitute.

Peanut Hypersensitivity

Peanuts are legumes, but an allergy to peanuts does not automatically make one allergic to other legumes (soybeans, peas, beans, green beans, and lentils). However, there is a strong possibility of cross-reaction between peanuts and lupine,[62] a legume used predominantly in Europe but that may be found in high-protein and baked products manufactured in the United States. Individuals allergic to peanuts are advised to avoid tree nuts (such as pecans, almonds, and walnuts) for several reasons. Roughly a third of the people who are allergic to peanuts are also allergic to one type of tree nut.[63,64] Peanuts are often substituted for tree nuts in recipes or flavored as tree nuts. Tree nuts are commonly processed on equipment shared with peanuts. Peanuts, especially peanut flour, are found in pastries, candies, fruit nut breads, salads, sauces, cereals, crackers, soups, and ethnic foods, particularly those of Africa, China, and Thailand. Peanut oil is considered safe for most individuals with peanut allergies,[61,65] but not crude peanut oil that has been cold pressed, expressed, extruded, or expelled. Nutrients such as vitamin E, niacin, magnesium, manganese, and chromium found in peanuts can also be found in legumes, whole grains, meats, and vegetable oils.

Tree Nut Hypersensitivity

Tree nut hypersensitivity is more common in adults than children and has a reputation of causing anaphylactic reactions. Almond, Brazil nut, cashew, chestnut, filbert/hazelnut, macadamia, pecan, pine nut, pistachio, and walnut are considered tree nuts. Tree nuts are used in cereals, crackers, ice cream, marinades, and sauces, making avoidance more difficult. Nut paste and nut butters are often made on shared equipment. Pure tree nut extracts, such as almond and walnut, may contain allergens.

Individuals hypersensitive to any tree nut are advised to avoid all tree nuts because of potential cross-reactivity.[63,64] Nuts are frequently processed on the same equipment and substituted for each other in recipes. But, if a specific tree nut has previously been eaten and tolerated, that nut is OK to include in the diet if it is shelled at home, not commercially shelled (e.g., pecans).

Fish and Shellfish Hypersensitivity

An individual may be hypersensitive to one fish and tolerate others,[36] but in the marketplace, substituting one fish for another is a common occurrence and is dangerous for the fish-allergic individual. In addition, there is a 50% rate of cross-reactivity with fish allergies.[37] Cross-contamination occurs in restaurants because of shared equipment (frying oil, grill, and spatula). Those allergic to fish but not shellfish need to be aware of Surimi, an imitation shellfish made with fish. Nutrients in fish such as vitamin B_6, vitamin B_{12}, vitamin E, niacin, phosphorus, and selenium are also found in meats, grains, and oils.

If one is allergic to shellfish, all shellfish need to be avoided. The risk of cross-reactivity is 75% with shellfish.[37] Crustacean shellfish (crab, crawfish, shrimp, and lobster) are considered major allergens and listed on product labels. Mollusks (clams, mussels, oysters, scallops, and squid) are not considered major allergens under the food labeling laws. Therefore, the food company will need to be called to determine whether clams, for example, are used in a seafood flavoring. Shellfish are traditionally not hidden in foods, but beware of cross-contamination in seafood restaurants. Asian dishes use a number of fish and shellfish and should also be avoided. Imitation seafood may not be safe because the flavoring used may be made from shellfish.

Other Principles of Management and Treatment

The registered dietitian can play a critical role in working with children who have food hypersensitivities and their families. The key is avoiding all of the necessary foods, suggesting alternatives to the avoided foods, providing recipes and meal plans where necessary, evaluating compliance, and ensuring adequacy and enjoyment of the diet. Families need to be educated about new cooking techniques, how to eat away from home and at social events, and dealing with other family members and schools where food is served. This section builds upon basic information previously provided to enhance families' education.

Ideally, everyone in the family follows the allergen-free diet at home so the home can be a safe place for the child. Preparing the same food for everyone minimizes the amount of cooking needed. It also reduces the chance for cross-contact between allergen-containing foods and allergen-free foods. Cooking that begins with fresh, unprocessed foods or single ingredients is an excellent way to protect the allergic child from accidental ingestions. However, families may need to be educated on basics of cooking, how to adapt recipes, and how to make appropriate safe substitutions. Recommend food allergen–free cookbooks located at the local library and through inter-library loan. Cooking lessons with recipes can alleviate anxiety and help with the time management of cooking.

If the allergen is brought into the home, extra care should be taken. Wash hands and cooking utensils. The allergen-free meal should be prepared first and protected from cross-contact before mealtime. The allergen-containing foods can be prepared afterwards. In a household with an allergy, it is helpful for everyone to always eat at a table and not in other rooms throughout the home; hands are washed after eating to avoid the spread of the allergen throughout the home. It may be helpful to have designated areas in the pantry and refrigerator for allergen-free "safe" foods. Each family should decide what strategy works best for its household.

Parents of infants must be warned that they may cause developmental and behavioral feeding issues by continuing to feed jarred baby foods and not preparing allergen-free food, or by not feeding the family meal to the older infant.

Parents also may rely on "safe" fast foods to avoid allergen-free food preparation that may lead to potentially nutritionally deficient diets.

Eating out creates a high risk situation for the food-allergic individual. Factors that put one at risk include not telling the staff about a child's food allergy, cross-contact between foods (caused by shared cooking surfaces or utensils), and restaurant errors. Creative or ethnic recipes lead to allergens found in unexpected places. Desserts are responsible for 43% of allergic reactions when eating out, followed by entrées (35%), appetizers (13%), and others (9%).[66] Avoiding Asian-type restaurants would be best if one is allergic to peanuts or tree nuts. Seafood restaurants should be avoided if one is allergic to fish or shellfish. The food-allergic individual or parent may want to contact the manager or chef to decide if the restaurant would be able to provide safe foods. It is best to avoid buffet service, sauces, combination foods, fried foods, and desserts. Select simple, single food items. For clearer communication, written information about one's food allergy can be shared with the manager or chef. "Chef Cards" can be created at the FAAN Website (found in the site's education section). In the restaurant, state that the child has a food allergy. Families can ask that food be prepared with cleaned equipment. Have the same person responsible for preparing the safe meal and delivering it directly to the table. If there is a restaurant that the family prefers, get to know the manager or owner so the child's special requests can be met. Avoid the restaurant's busiest time. Always bring safe foods in case there are problems.

Social events can be stressful because there is food everywhere and the parent has no idea how most of the foods were prepared. Other individuals may try to feed the allergic child without knowing of the child's food hypersensitivity. Children need to be taught not to accept any food or candy from anyone without their guardian's approval. Eating before events may help curb the child's hunger. Grandparents and other close friends need to be educated on a child's food hypersensitivity. The parent must be firm about avoiding allergens with those who do not understand that even a little amount can hurt the child.

Schools and day cares need aggressive education for those caring for children with food allergies. Families need to work closely with the school to ensure that all of the school personnel are educated on avoidance of the allergen(s), strategies to prevent allergen contact, and treatment of an allergic reaction. Thanks to Public Law 93-112, the Rehabilitation Act of 1973, Section 504, and the U.S. Department of Agriculture's 7 CFR 15b, federally funded day cares and schools are required to modify their health services, which includes making available menu information, providing substitutions for the foods to be omitted (identified by a doctor's signed statement), and administering medications at school. FAAN has developed a program to assist in managing food allergy at school and day cares; it can be found on its Website under schools.

Accidental ingestions do occur in spite of the best avoidance efforts, and the family will need to be educated on how to manage an allergic reaction. This information is provided on a Food Allergy Action Plan available through the child's physician. Most accidental ingestions that lead to severe systemic anaphylaxis occur when foods are eaten away from home and are disguised. If the allergic reaction is mild (only urticaria or rhinitis), the treatment may be a quick-acting antihistamine. Antihistamines or albuterol (for those with asthma), however, are never a substitute for epinephrine when an allergic reaction becomes more severe. Individuals with food hypersensitivities must be taught how to self-inject epinephrine once an allergic reaction is recognized. Epinephrine is available by prescription for emergency use in premeasured doses. These include EpiPen Jr. and the EpiPen, Twinject and Twinject Jr, or generic epinephrine, Adrenaclick. Because accidental ingestions commonly occur away from the home, it should be stressed to carry emergency medicine at all times. Epinephrine provides valuable time for transport to the hospital emergency room for observation. Once epinephrine is used, the individual must go to a hospital emergency room. The medically supervised observation period is critical for immediate treatment of an unexpected late phase reaction. No one can predict how a reaction will progress; guidelines are available on medical treatment.[67] Emergency medical identification systems (such as MedicAlert; Turlock, California) may also be indicated.

A family's quality of life is impacted when a child is diagnosed with a food allergy.[68] Parents may be fearful of a life-threatening allergic reaction, giving rise to anxiety on their part. These families may feel that a situation is beyond their ability to manage, and feel out of control, vulnerable, and helpless. This can be picked up by the child, leading to food fears. The more informed the family is about living with a food allergy, the more control they have, and the less stress they will experience.[69]

At this time, the only proven treatment is strict elimination of the offending allergen and pharmacological and/or medical intervention if there is an allergic reaction. The effectiveness of subcutaneous neutralization or provocation has not been demonstrated. Untested herbal remedies and nutrition supplements do not affect the outcome of a food hypersensitivity reaction. Atopic individuals should be warned of rare but potential adverse reactions after ingesting some nutrition supplements. Case reports have documented anaphylaxis to bee pollen,[70,71] royal jelly,[72,73] and echinacea.[74]

Research efforts[75] are directed at identifying the molecular and immunologic mechanisms involved in food allergen–receptor recognition and the cascade of events that lead to allergic reactions through anti-IgE, probiotics,

Chinese herbal medicine, and vaccines. Immunotherapy methods are under investigation and appear to help prevent serious food allergic reactions in the future.

Natural History and Prevention

Several studies[76–81] evaluating the development of food hypersensitivity emphasize that approximately a quarter of all parents report one or more adverse food reactions that can be confirmed in 5–10% of young children. The peak prevalence is around 1 year of age, and then it progressively falls until late childhood. Then the prevalence remains stable at about 3.5%.[2] A child with one IgE-mediated food hypersensitivity has an increased chance of developing additional food allergies and atopic diseases.

The general understanding is that most children "outgrow" food hypersensitivities by school age. The allergens responsible for the sensitivities will affect whether one will outgrow the allergic response. Two studies suggest that tolerance is occurring at a slower rate. A retrospective chart review of children with cow's milk allergy at Johns Hopkins found that the allergy resolved in 19% by age 4 years, 42% by age 8 years, 64% by age 12 years, and 79% by age 16 years.[82] A similar study at the same facility focused on egg allergy and found the resolution rates were 11% by age 4 years, 41% by age 8 years, 65% by age 12 years, and 82% by age 16 years.[83] Both studies found that the presence of additional atopic diseases and higher concentrations of food-specific IgE were associated with a reduced chance of outgrowing their food allergy. Children with peanut, tree nut, fish, or shellfish hypersensitivity rarely will lose their allergic reactivity. The exception is that roughly 20% of children with peanut hypersensitivity do lose their clinical reactivity.[84,85,86] If the child has not had a clinical reaction to peanut for 1 to 2 years and the peanut ImmunoCAP is low (under 2 kU/L), this child may have lost clinical reactivity. Consider a food challenge to peanut. Nine percent of children allergic to tree nuts outgrow their nut allergy.[87] Infants with non-IgE–mediated food hypersensitivities also appear to outgrow their food reactivity by 3 years of age.[88]

In 2000, the AAP published guidelines for the primary prevention of food allergy in high-risk children.[51] Avoidance of foods in infants, young children, and pregnant nursing women was recommended, though based on limited evidence. In 2008 the AAP Committee on Nutrition and Section of Allergy and Immunology[89] published revised recommendations that were evidence-based. In summary, the committee stressed the lack of appropriate studies designed to draw conclusions about primary prevention of food allergy through dietary intervention. The documented benefits of nutritional intervention that may prevent or delay the onset of atopic disease are largely limited to infants at high risk of developing allergy (i.e., infants with at least one parent or sibling with allergic/atopic disease [food and/or environmental allergy, asthma, allergic rhinitis, and atopic dermatitis]). This is not a universal guide for the general population. For the at-risk infant, the current evidence suggests:[89]

- Maternal dietary restrictions during pregnancy or lactation do not play a significant role in preventing atopic disease in infants.
- Exclusively breastfeeding the high-risk infant for at least 4 months compared to feeding intact cow's milk protein formula (CMF) decreases the incidence of atopic dermatitis and milk allergy during the first 2 years of life.
- Extensively hydrolyzed formulas and, less effectively, partially hydrolyzed formulas may prevent atopic disease compared to CMF.
- Soy-based formula plays no role in allergy prevention.
- Delaying the introduction of solids until after 4 to 6 months of age does not provide a protective effect, whether the infant is breastfed or CMF fed; this includes potentially allergenic foods such as eggs, peanuts, and fish.
- Data are lacking to support a protective effect of any dietary intervention in infants after 4 to 6 months of age for prevention of atopic disease.
- If a child develops a food allergy or other atopic disease triggered by foods, the food allergen must be identified and restricted.

If an infant is diagnosed with food hypersensitivity and is breastfed, the mother will need to completely remove the allergen from her diet.[42,90] This may place the lactating mother at nutritional risk. She will need to be counseled on alternative sources of the nutrients that are lost through the avoidance diet. This can be difficult, may impact her nutritional status, and can have an impact on the infant's growth.[90] If the mother cannot follow a strict avoidance diet, an extensively hydrolyzed formula is appropriate.

For the food-allergic infant/child, in 2000 the AAP[51] recommended delaying the introduction of milk or soy until after 1 year of age; eggs until 2 years of age; and peanuts, tree nuts, fish, and shellfish until after 3 years of age to prevent the development of those food allergies. Postponing the introduction of food allergens does not prevent this disorder, but does delay the development of food hypersensitivity and other atopic diseases in high-risk infants.[91,92] Food allergy testing and longer periods of avoidance may need to be considered; more research on prevention and treatment is needed.

Conclusion

In summary, it is important to make an accurate diagnosis of food hypersensitivity. Nutrition assessment and education for avoidance diets is complex. Without appropriate education, the child is at risk of accidental reactions, persistent food allergies, growth problems, and social stigmas.

Case Study

Nutrition Assessment

Patient history: 16-month-old female was a term newborn with no perinatal complications. At 2 months of age she developed atopic dermatitis that keeps getting worse, not better, with medically directed skin care.

Family history: There is a family history of seasonal allergies in the child's mother.

Food/nutrition-related history: Infant was breastfed and had mild reflux that worsened when supplemented with a milk-based formula around 5 months of age. The child's physician placed the child on an extensively hydrolyzed formula at 6 months; reflux improved. Mom took child off formula at 12 months and tried whole milk; 15 minutes later the child vomited and broke out in hives. The physician told mom to avoid milk, measured food-specific serum IgE, and referred the child to an allergy and immunology clinic. Mom has been avoiding milk and cheese in the child's diet. The child is eating table food; eats a wide variety of fruits, vegetables, grains, and meats; and drinks juice, no milk alternative. She has not been offered peanuts or tree nuts, but eats salmon and catfish and has had shrimp without any problems. She takes no vitamin or mineral supplement.

Anthropometric Measurements

Weight: 9.8 kg (25th percentile)

Height: 78 cm (50th percentile)

Weight for length: (25th–50th percentile)

Estimated energy needs: 792 kcal [(89 × wt (kg) – 100) + 20]

Estimated protein needs: 11 grams [1.1 × wt (kg)]

Medical test: ImmunoCAP (kU/L): milk—13, egg—0.9, soy—0.35, wheat—0.35, peanut—1.1, walnut—0.35, cod—0.35 (Note: 0.35 is considered negative.)

Diet order: Avoidance diet for milk, egg, peanuts, and tree nuts

Nutrition Diagnoses

1. Food and nutrition-related knowledge deficit related to newly diagnosed food allergy as evidenced by allergy test
2. Inadequate mineral (calcium) intake and inadequate vitamin intake (vitamin D) related to food allergy as evidenced by current diet restrictions requiring the avoidance of dairy foods

Intervention Goals

1. Remove all forms of milk, egg, peanut, and tree nuts from diet.
2. Increase consumption of calcium and vitamin D to meet AI.

Nutrition Interventions

1. Comprehensive nutrition education:
   - Instructed on strict avoidance of milk, egg, peanut, and tree nuts
   - Reviewed how to read labels
   - Discussed sources of cross-contact
   - Explained how to eat out
   - Instructed how to prepare safe foods at home
   - Provided sources of information on food allergies and day cares for the future
2. Vitamin/mineral supplement:
   - Offer a fortified soy beverage instead of juice at meals (minimum of 16 ounces/day to provide > 500 mg of calcium/day to meet AI).
   - Begin a multiple vitamin for vitamin D (to provide a minimum of 200 IU of vitamin D/day to meet AI).

Monitoring and Evaluation

- Evaluate for accidental ingestions associated with allergens at follow-up clinic visits.
- Assess intake of calcium and vitamin D (goal of 16 oz of fortified soy beverage and a multiple vitamin) at follow-up clinic visits.
- Monitor atopic dermatitis improvement with elimination of food allergy triggers.
- Educate parents regarding possible food challenge to egg in future.

Questions for the Reader

What will you do during the follow-up visit 2 months later:

1. If the child only has the fortified soy beverage on her cereal in the morning, and refuses to drink it?
2. If the child's atopic dermatitis has not improved?
3. If the child has not gained any weight since her last visit?

Resources for Food Hypersensitivities

American Academy of Allergy, Asthma, and Immunology
To locate a board-certified allergist
http://www.aaaai.org

American Partnership for Eosinophilic Disorders
http://www.apfed.org

The Food Allergy and Anaphylaxis Network
http://www.foodallergy.org

Kids with Food Allergies
http://www.kidswithfoodallergies.org

Medline Plus: Food Allergy
http://www.nlm.nih.gov/medlineplus/foodallergy.html

REFERENCES

1. Anderson JA, Song DD, eds. *Adverse Reactions to Foods*. American Academy Allergy and Immunology/NIAID; 1984:1–6. NIH Publ. #84-2442.
2. Sicherer SH, Sampson. Food allergy. *J Allergy Clin Immunol.* 2006;117:S470–S475.
3. Sellge G, Bischoff SC. The immunological basis of IgE-mediated reactions. In: Metcalfe DD, Sampson HA, Simon RA, eds. *Food Allergy: Adverse Reactions to Foods and Food Additives*, 4th ed. Malden, MA: Blackwell Science; 2008:15–28.
4. Metcalfe DD, Sampson HA, Simon RA. *Food Allergy: Adverse Reactions to Foods and Food Additives*, 4th ed. Malden, MA: Blackwell Science; 2008.
5. Sampson HA. Anaphylaxis and food allergy. In: Metcalfe DD, Sampson HA, Simon RA, eds. *Food Allergy: Adverse Reactions to Foods and Food Additives*, 4th ed. Malden, MA: Blackwell Science; 2008;157–170.
6. Munoz-Furlong A, Weiss CC. Characteristics of food-allergic patients placing them at risk for a fatal anaphylactic episode. *Curr Allergy Asthma Rep*. 2009;9:57–63.
7. Castells MC, Horan RF, Sheffer AL. Exercise-induced anaphylaxis. *Curr Allergy Asthma Rep*. 2003;3:15–21.
8. Tatachar P, Kumar S. Food-induced anaphylaxis and oral allergy syndrome. *Pediatr Rev.* 2008;29:23–27
9. Ortolani C, Ispano M, Pastorello EA, et al. Comparison of results of skin prick test (with fresh foods and commercial food extracts) and RAST in 100 patients with oral allergy syndrome. *J Allergy Clin Immunol.* 1989;83:683–690.
10. Sicherer SH. Clinical aspects of gastrointestinal food allergy in childhood. *Pediatrics*. 2003;111:1609–1616.
11. Iacono G, Carroccio A, Montalto G, et al. Severe infantile colic and food intolerance: a long-term prospective study. *J Pediatr Gastroenterol Nutr.* 1991;12:332–335.
12. Lothe L, Lindberg T, Jakobsson I. Cow's milk formula as a cause of infantile colic: a double-blind study. *Pediatrics*. 1982;70:7–10.
13. Norwak-Wegrzyn A, Sampson HA, Wood RA, et al. Food protein-induced entercolitis syndrome caused by solid food proteins. *Pediatrics*. 2003;111:829–835.
14. Liaciuras CA, Spergel JM, Ruchelli E, et al. Eosinophilic esophagitis: a 10-year experience in 381children. *Clin Gastroenterol Hepatol*. 2005;95:336–343.
15. Janetuinen EK, Kemppainen TA, Julkunen RJ, et al. No harm from five-year ingestion of oats in celiac disease. *Gut*. 2002;50:332–335.
16. Lloyd-Still JD. Chronic diarrhea of childhood and the misuse of elimination diets. *J Pediatr.* 1979;95:10–13.
17. Libib M, Gama R, Wright J, et al. Dietary maladvice as a cause of hypothyroidism and short stature. *Br Med J.* 1989;298:232–233.
18. Robertson DAF, Ayres RCS, Smith CL, Wright R. Adverse consequences arising from misdiagnosis of food allergy. *Br Med Jr.* 1988;297:719–720.
19. Roesler TA, Barry PC, Bock SA. Factitious food allergy and failure to thrive. *Arch Pediatr Adolesc Med.* 1994;148:1150–1155.
20. Noimark L, Cox HE. Nutritional problems related to food allergy in childhood. *Pediatr Allergy Immunol.* 2008;19:188–195.
21. Fortunato JE, Scheimann AO. Protein-energy malnutrition and feeding refusal secondary to food allergies. *Clin Pediatr.* 2008;47:496–499.
22. Bock SA, Lee WY, Remigio LK, et al. Studies of hypersensitivity reactions to foods in infants and children. *J Allergy Clin Immunol.* 1978;62:327–334.
23. Sampson HA, Albergo R. Comparison of results of skin test, RAST and double-blind, placebo-controlled food challenge in children with atopic dermatitis. *J Allergy Clin Immunol.* 1984;74:26–33.
24. Venter C, Pereira B, Voigt K, et al. Prevalence and cumulative incidence of food hypersensitivity in the first 3 years of life. *Allergy.* 2008;63:354–359.
25. Burks AW, James JM, Hiegel A, et al. Atopic dermatitis and food hypersensitivity reactions. *J Pediatr.* 1998;132:132–136.
26. Bock SA, Buckley J, Houst A, May CD. Proper use of skin test with food extracts in diagnosis of food hypersensitivity. *Clin Allergy.* 1978;8:559–564.
27. American Academy of Allergy, Asthma and Immunology. The use of standardized allergen extracts. *J Allergy Clin Immunol.* 1997;99:583–586.
28. Sampson HA. Utility of food specific IgE concentration in predicting symptomatic food allergy. *J Allergy Clin Immunol.* 2001;107:891–896.
29. Nowak-Wegrzyn A, Assa'ad AH, Bahna SL, et al. Work Group report: Oral food challenge testing. *J Allergy Clin Immunol* 2009;123:S365–S383.
30. Ortoloni C, Ispano M, Partorella EA, et al. Comparison of results of skin prick test (with fresh foods and commercial food extracts) and RAST in 100 patients with oral allergy syndrome. *J Allergy Clin Immunol.* 1989;83:683–689.
31. Menurdo JL, Bousquet J, Rodiere M, et al. Skin test reactivity in infancy. *J Allergy Clin Immunol.* 1985;74:646–651.
32. Garcia-Ara C, Boyano-Martinez T, Diaz-Pena JM, et al. Specific IgE levels in the diagnosis of immediate hypersensitivity

of cows' milk protein in the infant. *J Allergy Clin Immunol.* 2001;107:185–190.

33. Boyano-Martinez T, Garcia-Ara C, Diaz-Pena JM, et al. Validity of specific IgE antibodies in children with egg allergy. *Clin Exp Allergy*. 2001;31:1464–1469.
34. Shek LP, Soderstrom L, Ahlstedt S, et al. Determination of food specific IgE levels over time can predict the development of tolerance in cow's milk and hen's egg allergy. *J Allergy Clin Immunol.* 2004;114:385–391.
35. Perry TT, Matsui EC, Conover-Walker MK, et al. The relationship of allergen-specific IgE levels and oral food challenge outcome. *J Allergy Clin Immunol.* 2004;114:144–149.
36. Bernhisel-Broadbent J, Scanlon SM, Sampson HA. Fish hypersensitivity. I. In vitro and oral challenge results in fish allergic patients. *J Allergy Clin Immunol.* 1992;89:730–737.
37. Sicherer SH. Clinical implications of cross-reactive food allergens. *J Allergy Clin Immunol.* 2001;108:881–890.
38. Niggemann B, Gruber C. Unproven diagnostic procedures in IgE-mediated allergic diseases. *Allergy.* 2004;59:806–808.
39. Teuber SS, Beyer K. IgG to foods: a test not ready for prime time. *Curr Opin Allergy Clin Immunol.* 2007;7:257–258.
40. Krop J, Lewith GT, Gziut W, et al. A double blind, randomized controlled investigation of electrodermal testing in the diagnosis of allergies. *J Altern Complement Med.* 1997;3:241–248.
41. Jarvinen KM, Makinen-Kiljunen S, Suomalainen H. Cow's milk challenge through human milk evokes immune responses in infants with cow's milk allergy. *J Pediatr.* 1999;135:506–512.
42. Vadas P, Wai Y, Burks AW, et al. Detection of peanut allergens in breast milk of lactating women. *JAMA.* 2001;106:346–349.
43. Sicherer SH. Food allergy: when and how to perform oral food challenges. *Pediatr Allergy Immunol.* 1999;10:226–234.
44. Reibel S, Rohr C, Zeigert M, et al. What safety measures need to be taken in oral food challenges in children? *Allergy.* 2000;55:940–944.
45. Executive Committee of the Academy of Allergy and Immunology: Reactions caused by immunotherapy with allergic extracts (position statement). *J Allergy Clin Immunol.* 1986;77:271–273.
46. Mofidi S, Bock SA. *A Health Professional's Guide to Food Challenges*. Fairfax, VA: Food Allergy and Anaphylaxis Network; 2004.
47. Christie L, Hine RJ, Parker JG, et al. Food allergies in children affect nutrient intake and growth. *J Am Diet Assoc.* 2002;102:1648–1651.
48. U.S. Department of Agriculture, Center for Nutrition Policy and Promotion. Food guide pyramid for young children 2 to 6 years of age. Washington, DC: U.S. Department of Agriculture, Center for Nutrition Policy and Promotion; 1999.
49. Hefle, SL, Furlong TJ, Niemann L, Lemon-Mule H, Sicherer SH, Taylor SL. Consumer attitudes and risks associated with packaged foods having advisory labeling regarding the presence of peanuts. *J Allergy Clin Immunol.* 2007;120:171–176.
50. Pieretti MM, Chung D, Pacenza R, Slotkin T, Sicherer SH. Audit of manufactured products: use of allergy advisory labels and identification of labeling ambiguities. *J Allergy Clin Immunol.* 2009:124:337–341.
51. American Academy of Pediatrics, Committee on Nutrition. Hypoallergenic infant formulas. *Pediatrics.* 2000;106:346–349.
52. Zeiger RS, Sampson HA, Bock SA, et al. Soy allergy in infants and children with IgE-associated cow's milk allergy. *J Pediatr.* 1999;134:614–622.
53. Niggemann B, Christaine B, Dupont C, et al. Prospective, controlled, multi-center study on the effect of an amino acid-based formula in infants with cow's milk allergy/intolerance and atopic dermatitis. *Pediatr Allergy Immunol.* 2001;12:78–82.
54. Sicherer SH, Noone SA, Koerner CB, et al. Hypoallergenicity and efficacy of an amino acid–based formula in children with cow's milk and multiple food hypersensitivities. *J Pediatr.* 2001;138:688–693.
55. Bellioni-Businco B, Paganelli R, Lucenti P, et al. Allergenicity of goat's milk in children with cow's milk allergy. *J Allergy Clin Immunol.* 1999;103:1191–1194.
56. Fox AT, Du Toit G, Lang A, Lack G. Food allergy as a risk factor for nutritional rickets. *Pediatr Allergy Immunol.* 2004;15:566–569.
57. Yu JW, Pekeles G, Legault L, McCusker CT. Milk allergy and vitamin D deficiency rickets: a common disorder associated with an uncommon disease. *Ann Allergy Asthma Immunol.* 2006;96:615–619.
58. Holick MF. Vitamin D deficiency. *N Engl J Med.* 2007;357:266–281.
59. Holick MF, Chen TC. Vitamin D deficiency: a worldwide problem with health consequences. *Am J Clin Nutr.* 2008;87:1080S–1086S.
60. Bush RK, Taylor CL, Nordlee JA, Busse WW. Soybean oil is not allergenic to soybean-sensitive individuals. *J Allergy Clin Immunol.* 1985;76:242–245.
61. Crevel RWR, Kerhoff MAT, Konig MMG. Allergenicity of refined vegetable oils. *Food Chem Toxicol.* 2000;109:385–293.
62. Moneret-Vuatrin DA, Guerin L, Kanny G, et al. Cross-allergenicity of peanut and lupine: the risk of lupine allergy in patients allergic to peanuts. *J Allergy Clin Immunol.* 1999;104:883–888.
63. Sicherer S, Burks AW, Sampson H. Clinical features of acute allergic reactions to peanut and tree nuts in children. *Pediatrics.* 1998;102:6.
64. Sampson HA. Update on food allergy. *J Allergy Clin Immunol.* 2004;113:805–819.
65. Taylor SL, Busse WW, Sachs MI, Parker JL, et al. Peanut oil is not allergenic to peanut-sensitive individuals. *J Allergy Clin Immunol.* 1981;68:372–375.
66. Furlong TJ, Desimone J, Sicherer SH. Peanut and tree nut allergic reactions in restaurants and other food establishments. *J Allergy Clin Immunol.* 2001;18:867–870.
67. Sampson HA. Anaphylaxis and emergency treatment. *Pediatrics.* 2003;111:1601–1608.
68. Sicherer SH, Noone SA, Munoz-Furlong A. The impact of childhood food allergy on quality of life. *Ann Allergy Asthma Immunol.* 2001;87:461–464.
69. Munoz-Furlong A. Daily coping strategies for patients and their families. *Pediatrics.* 2003;111:S1654–S1661.
70. Mansfield LE, Goldstein GB. Anaphylactic reaction after ingestion of local bee pollen. *Ann Allergy*. 1981;47:154–156.
71. Cohen SH, Yunginger JW, Rosenberg N, Fink JN. Acute allergic reaction after composite pollen ingestion. *J Allergy Clin Immunol.* 1979;64:270–274.
72. Leung R, Ho A, Chan J, et al. Royal jelly consumption and hypersensitivity in the community. *Clin Exp Allergy*. 1997;27:333–336.
73. Thien FC, Leung R, Baldo BA, Weiner JA, et al. Asthma and anaphylaxis induced by royal jelly. *Clin Exp Allergy*. 1996;26:216–222.

74. Mullins RJ. Echinacea-associated anaphylaxis. *Med J Australia.* 1998;168:170–171.
75. Sicherer SH, Sampson HA. Food allergy: recent advances in pathophysiology and treatment. *Annu Rev Med.* 2009;60:261–277.
76. Bock SA. Prospective appraisal of complaints of adverse reactions to foods in children during the first 3 years of life. *Pediatrics.* 1987;79:683–688.
77. Kajosaari M. Food allergy in Finnish children aged 1 to 6 years. *Acta Paediatr Can.* 1982;71:815–819.
78. Eggelsbo M, Kalvorsen R, Tambs K, et al. Prevalence of parentally perceived adverse reactions to food in young children. *Pediatr Allergy Immunol.* 1999;10:122–132.
79. Eggelsbo M, Botten G, Halvorsen R, et al. The prevalence of allergy to egg: a population-based study in young children. *Allergy.* 2001;56:403–411.
80. Host A, Halken S. A prospective study of cow milk allergy in Danish infants during the first 3 years of life. Clinical course in relation to clinical and immunologic type of hypersensitivity reaction. *Allergy.* 1990;45:587–596.
81. Tariq SM, Stevens M, Matthews S, et al. Cohort study of peanut and tree nut sensitization by the age of 4 years. *BJM.* 1996;313:514–517.
82. Skripak JM, Matsui EC, Mudd K, Wood RA. The natural history of IgE-mediated cow's milk allergy. *J Allergy Clin Immunol.* 2007;120:1172–1177.
83. Savage JH, Matsui EC, Skripak JM, Wood RA. The natural history of egg allergy. *J Allergy Clin Immunol.* 2007;120:1413–1417.
84. Hourihane JO, Roberts SA, Warner JO. Resolution of peanut allergy: case-control study. *BMJ.* 1998;316:1271–1275.
85. Skolnick HS, Conover-Walter MK, Barnes-Koerner C, et al. The natural history of peanut allergy. *J Allergy Clin Immunol.* 2001;107:265–274.
86. Fleischer DM, Conover-Walker MK, Christie L, et al. The natural progression of peanut allergy: resolution and the possibility of recurrence. *J Allergy Clin Immunol.* 2003;112:183–189.
87. Fleischer DM, Conover-Walker MK, Matsui EC, Wood RA. The natural history of tree nut allergy. *J Allergy Clin Immunol.* 2005;116:1087–1093.
88. Host A, Halken S, Jacobsen HP, et al. The natural course of cow's milk allergy in Danish infants during the first 3 years of life. Clinical course in relation to clinical and immunological type of hypersensitivity reaction. *Allergy.* 1990;45:587–596.
89. Greer FR, Sicherer SH, Burks AW, Committee on Nutrition and Section on Allergy and Immunology. Effects of early nutritional interventions on the development of atopic disease in infants and children: the role of maternal dietary restriction, breastfeeding, timing of introduction of complementary foods, and hydrolyzed formulas. *Pediatrics.* 2008;121:183–191.
90. Isolauri E, Tahvanainen A, Peltola T, et al. Breast-feeding of allergic infants. *J Pediatr.* 1999;134:27–32.
91. Kjellman MIM. Atopic disease in seven-year-old children. Incidence in relation to family history. *Acta Paediatr Scand.* 1977;66:465–471.
92. Zeiger RS, Heller S. The development and prediction of atopy in high-risk children: follow-up at age 7 years in a prospective randomized study of combined maternal and infant food allergen avoidance. *J Allergy Clin Immunol.* 1995;95:1179–1190.

Weight Management: Obesity to Eating Disorders

Laura V. Hudspeth, Bonnie A. Spear, and Haley W. Lacey

Introduction

It has been well documented that the growing epidemic of childhood overweight and obesity is one of the most significant public health concerns facing the United States today. The number of obese and overweight children and adolescents continues to climb despite efforts by the weight loss industry, local and state governments, the media, and nutrition and medical communities to reverse the trend. Current medical and scientific evidence suggest that excessive weight gain is a result of several factors including genetic predisposition and biological issues related to weight regulation, environmental and behavioral influences such as dietary and exercise habits, and sociocultural influences.

But, in a culture that glorifies being thin, many youth become overly preoccupied with their physical appearance and, in an effort to achieve or maintain a thin body, begin to diet obsessively. A minority of these youth eventually develops an eating disorder such as anorexia nervosa, bulimia nervosa, or eating disorders not otherwise specified.

Symptoms of eating disorders usually first become evident early in adolescence. Factors that appear to place girls at increased risk include low self-esteem, poor coping skills, and perfectionism. Additionally, adolescents who have mothers, aunts, or siblings with eating disorders are at particular risk for developing an eating disorder themselves.

Adults and health professionals should take it seriously when children or adolescents express concerns about their body weight. Health professionals can help children and their parents understand the importance of physical activity and appropriate nutrition for maintaining health. In doing so, it is important to keep in mind the family's resources and their cultural background, both of which may influence the family's ability to make changes.

This chapter provides a review of literature about obesity and eating disorders and also provides the reader with clinical and community interventions that can help providers to address and treat these medical issues and concerns.

Overweight/Obesity

Childhood obesity has become the most prevalent pediatric nutritional problem in the United States. The most recent data from the National Health and Nutrition Examination Study (NHANES, 2007–2008) show that over the past 25 years, the prevalence of obesity in children and adolescents has tripled, reaching 19.6% in children 6–11 years of age and 18.1% in children 12–19 years of age.[1,2] Children are also becoming obese at younger ages. This increased prevalence is problematic because obesity that occurs early in life and persists throughout childhood is more difficult to treat.

Prevalence and Trends

The NHANES 2007–2008 data also show that 9.5% of infants and toddlers were at or above the 95th percentile of the weight for recumbent length growth charts. According to the findings, 19.6% of children 6–11 and 18.1% of adolescents ages 12 through 19 were at or above the 95th percentile of body mass index (BMI)-for-age. The increases are occurring in both boys and girls, across all states and socioeconomic lines as well as among all racial and ethnic groups; however, African American and Hispanic children and adolescents are disproportionately affected.[1] **Table 8-1** shows changes in obesity rates over time.

Concerns for children and adolescents experiencing rapid weight gain are enhanced by the research indicating that children are likely to carry obesity into adulthood and thus experience significant health problems related to obesity. Researchers have documented the persistence of obesity from childhood into adolescence and on into adulthood. The probability that obese school-age children will become obese adults is estimated at 50%,

TABLE 8-1 Obesity Prevalence/Trends

Age	NHANES 1988–1994	NHANES 1999–2000	NHANES 2003–2006	NHANES 2007–2008
2- to 5-year-olds	7.2%	10.4%	12.4%	10.4%
6- to 11-year-olds	11.3%	15.3%	17.0%	19.6%
12- to 19-year-olds	10.5%	15.5%	17.6%	18.1%

Sources: Ogden CL, Carroll MD, Curtin LR, Lamb MM, Flegal KM. Prevalence of high body mass index in US children and adolescents, 2007–2008. *JAMA*. 2010;303(3):242–249; and Ogden CL, Carroll MD, Flegal KM. High body mass index for age among US children and adolescents, 2003–2006. *JAMA* 2008;299(20):2401–2405.

and the likelihood that obese adolescents will become obese adults is between 70% and 80%.[3]

Medical Complications of Obesity in Children and Adolescents

Obesity is associated with significant health problems in the pediatric age group and is an important early risk factor for much of adult morbidity and mortality. Medical problems are common in obese children and adolescents and can affect cardiovascular health, the pulmonary system, the musculoskeletal system, the endocrine system, gastrointestinal system and mental health.[4]

Cardiovascular Concerns

The cardiovascular complications associated with obesity include hypertension, dyslipidemia, left ventricular hypertrophy, and pulmonary hypertension. Cardiovascular risk factors tend to cluster in obese and overweight children. Data from the Bogalusa Heart Study showed that children who were obese (BMI ≥ 95th percentile) had a greater risk for cardiovascular risk factors than their peers,[5] increasing from 27% (nonobese) to 61% (obese). Obese children also had increased risks for elevated cholesterol (2.4% increased risk), elevated triglycerides (7.1% increased risk), and low high-density lipoprotein cholesterol (HDL-C; 3.4% increased risk).

Rises in the rate of hypertension in childhood are now found to be more commonly associated with obesity than with renal disease. Blood pressure tends to track with BMI; as BMI increases, so does blood pressure. It has been shown that the risk for elevated blood pressure in children is three times greater in obese children compared to nonobese children. The correlation of BMI and hypertension has been reported independently of race, gender, or age.

Pulmonary Concerns

Childhood obesity has been shown to be related to increases in childhood pulmonary complications, such as sleep apnea, exercise intolerance, and asthma. Elamin showed that there were significantly more children with asthma (30.6%) who were obese (≥ 95th BMI percentile) compared with only 11.6% of the nonobese.[6] The difference in asthma rates between the obese and nonobese was significant for both sexes and across all age groups, although the severity of asthma was not related to obesity. In many children, asthma is triggered by exercise (exercise-induced asthma); if left untreated, it limits the child's ability to be active, which may increase the risk for obesity. However, weight loss improves lung function in individuals who have asthma and obesity.

Obstructive sleep apnea (OSA) is a common condition in children characterized by episodes of stopped breathing during sleep. Loud snoring, mouth breathing, daytime sleepiness, depression, and hyperactive behavior in children are all indicators of possible OSA. Consequences of untreated OSA include delayed growth, bedwetting, behavior problems, poor academic performance, and cardiopulmonary disease. Although obesity is not the only cause of obstructive sleep apnea, Rosen found that children who had high BMIs had obstructive sleep apnea 28% more frequently than their peers.[7] Daytime sleepiness and fatigue secondary to obstructive sleep apnea may impair the ability of a child to get adequate physical activity, which in turn may worsen the obesity. The diagnosis of obstructive sleep apnea should be confirmed by polysomnography (sleep study).

Musculoskeletal Concerns

Overweight has been found to be associated with increased incidence of slipped capital femoral epiphysis, the most common hip disorder among young teenagers. Slipped capital femoral epiphysis happens when the cartilage plate (epiphysis) at the top of the thighbone (femur) slips out of place. The classic patient is an obese, early pubertal boy with delayed bone age. Symptoms include a limp, and hip or knee pain. This can only happen during growth, before the epiphysis plates fuse.

Blount's disease, also known as tibia vera, presents as a bowing of the tibia and femur, affecting one or both knees. Patients usually present with a limp with or without pain. Obesity has been reported in two-thirds of the patients with Blount disease. It is unclear whether this abnormality is caused by excess weight placed on the joint at a critical stage in development or whether it is an underlying condition aggravated by excessive weight.[10]

Endocrine Concerns

In 1988, the metabolic syndrome was first described in adults. It is defined as a link between insulin resistance and hypertension, dyslipidemia, type 2 diabetes, and other metabolic abnormities and is associated with an increased risk of atherosclerotic cardiovascular disease. Obesity is the most common cause of insulin resistance in children and is associated with dyslipidemia, type 2 diabetes, and long-term vascular complications. Weiss and others modified the adult criteria for metabolic syndrome to apply to children and adolescents.[11] Because body proportions normally change during pubertal development and may vary among persons of different races and ethnic groups, waist-to-hip ratios (used as criteria in adults) are difficult to interpret and not appropriate to use in children at this time due to lack of national reference standards. The authors classified children and adolescents as having metabolic syndrome if they met three or more of the following criteria:

- BMI for age and gender above the 97th percentile
- A triglyceride level above the 95th percentile
- An HDL cholesterol level below the 5th percentile
- Systolic or diastolic blood pressure above the 95th percentile (for age, gender, and height)
- Impaired glucose tolerance

Results of this study suggested that the metabolic syndrome was more common among children and adolescents than previously reported and that its prevalence increased directly with the degree of obesity. Insulin resistance in obese children was found to be strongly associated with specific adverse metabolic factors. Preliminary follow-up of the subjects suggested that the metabolic syndrome persists over time and tends to progress clinically. Many of the children diagnosed with metabolic syndrome developed type 2 diabetes in a very short period of time.[11]

The American Diabetes Association reported that type 2 diabetes now accounts for up to 45–50% of newly diagnosed cases of diabetes in children and adolescents, especially minority youth.[12] This increase in adolescent diabetes is almost completely attributable to childhood obesity. Family history is strongly associated with type 2 diabetes in children. The frequency of a history of type 2 diabetes in a first- or second-degree relative of obese youth ranges from 74% to 100%.

Acanthosis nigricans is often associated with insulin resistance and type 2 diabetes. It is seen in 85–90% of individuals with insulin resistance. This condition is characterized by hyperpigmentation and velvety thickening that occurs in the skin of the neck, axillae, and groin. Skin tags are seen in more severe cases. Many patients present with complaints of a dirty neck that they cannot get clean with soap and water.

Polycystic ovarian syndrome is one of the most common endocrine problems in females.[13] Patients usually present with menstrual irregularities. It is characterized by insulin resistance in the presence of elevated androgens. Patients present with irregular menstrual periods or amenorrhea, hirsutism, acne, polycystic ovaries, and obesity. Hair usually forms mid-line with hair on face, chest, abdomen, and back. Weight loss will improve symptoms, but treatment with hormones will often help in the short-term. Because of the significant increase in diagnosis in adolescents there is a new diagnosis called teen polycystic ovarian syndrome, which has the following symptoms: elevated BMI (however, one-third of individuals have normal BMI), hyperinsulinemia, abnormal lipid profile, anovulatory/polycystic ovaries, and early development of auxiliary (underarm) hair.

Gastrointestinal Concerns

Obesity is a major risk factor for the development of cholelithiasis (gallstones) and cholecystitis. Symptoms include right upper quadrant abdominal pain and tenderness. It is mostly seen in females (70%), and 50% of adolescents presenting with cholelithiasis are obese. Gallstones are three times more common in obese individuals than nonobese subjects.

Nonalcoholic fatty liver disease (NAFLD) has increased with the increased rate of childhood obesity. As many as 75% of pediatric obesity patients may have evidence of NAFLD. NAFLD is the early stages of hepatic steatosis and is associated with the degree of obesity, elevated triglycerides, and insulin resistance. Patients with NAFLD usually have no symptoms, although some may present with right upper quadrant abdominal pain or tenderness. Serum alanine aminotransferase (ALT) and aspartate aminotransferase (AST) levels are usually elevated and can be used as good screening tests for NAFLD. ALT or AST levels two times normal levels should prompt a consult with a hepatologist.[14]

Neurological Concerns

Obesity occurs in 30–80% of children diagnosed with pseudotumor cerebri. This is often diagnosed due to an elevated intracranial pressure, but no tumor or other abnormalities are seen. Pseudotumor cerebri presents with headache, dizziness, diplopia, and mild unsteadiness, and generally has a gradual onset. Neck, shoulder, and back pain have also been reported. Weight loss is recognized as the best treatment.[14]

Psychological Concerns

Children and adolescents are at risk of developing psychosocial problems related to being obese in a society that values thinness. The likelihood of a severely obese child or adolescent having impaired health-related quality of life was 5.5 times greater than a healthy child or adolescent, and similar to a child diagnosed as having cancer.[15] Overweight children and youth with decreased levels of self-esteem reported increased rates of loneliness, sadness, and nervousness.[15] Overweight adolescents also are more likely to be socially isolated than normal weight adolescents. Additionally, obese children and adolescents are four times more likely than healthy children to report impaired school function. Psychological effects may also contribute to worsening obesity.[15]

Assessment and Diagnosis

The assessment of an obese child or adolescent is critical in the treatment of childhood obesity. The assessment is based on a wide variety of factors, including age, sex, family history, developmental stage, ethnicity, and social environment. Each of these factors will influence the treatment goal, the selection of type of treatment, and the course of therapy. Obesity is a complex disease, and even with excellent adherence to treatment recommendations, progress may be slow. Because of the extended time that children may need to be in treatment, the assessment must include a careful review of family lifestyle patterns and the child's social environment.

Growth Assessment

In 2007, 14 professional organizations met to develop a set of evidence-based recommendations for the prevention, assessment, and management of pediatric overweight and obesity. All recommendations were endorsed by these professional organizations.[14] The Expert Committee on Assessment recommended that BMI be used as the preferred measure for evaluating obesity in children and adolescents 2 to 19 years of age. Weight-for-length is still recommended to assess children less than 2 years of age. BMI expresses the weight-for-height relationship as a ratio: weight (kg)/height (m^2). BMI is recommended because it is easily obtained, is highly correlated with body fat percentage, and can correctly identify the fattest individuals (BMI $>$ 95th percentile) with acceptable accuracy (e.g., greater than 95th percentile).[13] For children and teens, age- and sex-specific percentiles are used to interpret the BMI because the amount of body fat changes with age and differs between girls and boys. The Centers for Disease Control and Prevention (CDC) growth charts take into account these differences and allow the BMI number to be translated into a percentile for a child's sex and age. A BMI in the 85th to 94th percentile defines overweight. Children and adolescents with BMI in this range often have excess body fat and health risks, although for some, the BMI category will reflect high lean body mass rather than fat. A BMI $\geq$ 95th percentile defines obesity. Almost all children and adolescents with BMI in this range are likely to have excess body fat and associated health risks.[4]

Work by Freedman and colleagues showed that children with extreme obesity were increasing in prevalence, and that these children were at higher risk for cardiovascular diseases.[5] Although the Expert Committee on the Prevention, Assessment and Treatment of Childhood Obesity suggested the use of the 99th percentile defined by Freedman using NHANES data, the sample of children and adolescents with BMI at this level was small.[14] Children and adolescents with BMI at or above the 99th percentile have a higher health risk, and therefore intervention is more urgent. The 97th percentile, which is the highest curve available on the growth charts, may be used to determine the highest risk children and adolescents and can be used to implement a higher degree of assessment and treatment.[14]

BMI Rebound

BMI changes substantially with age. After about 1 year of age, BMI-for-age begins to decline, and it continues falling during the preschool years until it reaches a minimum around 4 to 6 years of age. After 4 to 6 years of age, BMI-for-age begins a gradual increase through adolescence and most of adulthood. The rebound or increase in BMI that occurs after it reaches its lowest point is referred to as *BMI rebound*. This is a normal pattern of growth that occurs in all children. The age when the BMI rebound occurs may be a critical period in childhood for the development of obesity as an adolescent or adult. An early BMI rebound, occurring before ages 4 to 6, has been cited as a risk factor for the development of obesity.[13] However, studies have yet to determine whether the higher BMI in childhood is truly adipose tissue versus lean body mass or bone. Additional research is needed to further understand the impact of early BMI rebound on adult obesity.

Other Anthropometric Measures

Many clinicians and researchers use other measures of body composition including skinfold measures and waist circumferences to assess children. The Expert Committee on Assessment[13] reviewed the use of these measures to determine whether they provide important clinical information beyond just using the BMI. Although skinfold measurements are predictive of total body fat in children and adolescents, the expert committee did not recommend their use in routine clinical assessment because they are often difficult to measure, require expertise in assessment techniques, and therefore are not feasible in routine medical care. Waist circumference measures assess visceral adiposity and can track with cardiovascular disease and metabolic risk factors. They are easier to assess than skinfold measurements. They are used when assessing obesity in adults; however, reference values for children and adolescents are not available. It was the opinion of the expert committee that waist circumference measurements do not provide additional information for identifying risk that is not identified by BMI percentiles. In the future, once reference values become available for children and adolescents, waist circumference values may be useful in providing an adjunct to identify children who are at increased risk for metabolic co-morbidities.

Screening

Screening for obesity risk is an ongoing process. It starts with BMI evaluation, and then incorporates evaluation of medical conditions and risks, current behaviors, family attitudes, and psychosocial situations. Based on this information, clinicians can provide obesity prevention or obesity treatment. In general, children with BMI below the 85th percentile will benefit from prevention counseling, which will guide them toward healthier behaviors or reinforce current healthy behaviors. This counseling should be framed as growing healthy bodies rather than achieving a specific weight.

Children whose BMI is in the overweight category (85th–95th percentile), but just above the 85th percentile category, are unlikely to have excess body fat; however, they should receive standard obesity prevention counseling without necessarily a goal of a lower BMI percentile. These children and adolescents should be seen more frequently to ensure that the BMI is remaining stable and not increasing. If BMI begins to increase, these children would need more in-depth intervention.

Steps in nutrition screening/assessment include:

1. *BMI assessment:* BMI calculation and plotting at least once a year to identify current category. See the previous sections for how to assess BMI.
2. *Screening:* Screening includes:
   a. *Parental obesity:* Parental obesity is one of the strongest risk factors in childhood obesity that persists into adulthood.
   b. *Family medical history:* A positive family history includes history of early cardiovascular disease, parental hypercholesterolemia, parental hypertension, or a first- or second-generation relative with type 2 diabetes (siblings, parents, aunts, uncles, and grandparents). Providers should regularly review and update family history, especially for at-risk children.
   c. *Blood pressure:* Elevated systolic blood pressure is seen in 13% of obese children. Blood pressure should be checked at all health supervision visits. Children's and adolescents' blood pressure evaluation should be based on age, gender, and height. Blood pressure greater than the 90th percentile for age/gender/height is considered at risk; blood pressure greater than the 95th percentile for age/gender/height is considered high if elevated on three or more occasions.[13]
3. *Assessment of weight-related problems:* A review of systems through a detailed family and patient history as well as a physical examination for current obesity-related conditions should be performed. The provider should be aware that even with a thorough history, some of the co-morbidities have no symptoms or signs.[14] Laboratory assessment may be necessary to complete the assessment.
4. *Laboratory assessment/testing:* History and physical examination cannot effectively screen for abnormal cholesterol, NAFLD, and type 2 diabetes mellitus; therefore, these conditions must be identified by laboratory tests. The expert committee recommended that children with BMI between the 85th and 94th percentiles have a lipid panel performed. If risk factors are present, then a fasting glucose and ALT and AST should also be measured every 2 years for individuals age 10 years or older. When the BMI is ≥ 95th percentile, the expert committee suggests a fasting glucose and ALT and AST every 2 years starting at age 10 years, regardless of other risk factors. Elevation of ALT or AST on two occasions may indicate the need for further evaluation, probably with guidance from a pediatric gastroenterology/hepatology expert.[14]
5. *Behavior assessment:* Providers often find it helpful for parents and/or the child (depending on age) to complete a quick screening form in the waiting room prior to being seen for their first visit. This allows the provider to target the assessment and counseling to potential problem areas.

   Behavior assessment includes:
   a. *Dietary:* A brief assessment of foods and beverages typically consumed and the pattern of consumption can uncover modifiable behaviors associated with excess caloric intake. Not all areas can be assessed or addressed at one visit. The following questions are areas that should be assessed during subsequent visits:
      - Frequency of eating food prepared outside the home, including restaurants, school and work cafeterias, fast food establishments, and food purchased for take-out
      - Amount of sugar-sweetened beverages consumed each day
      - Amount of 100% juice consumed each day
      - Frequency and quality of breakfast
      - Energy density in the diet, such as high-fat foods
      - Number of fruit and vegetable servings each day
      - Number of meals and snacks each day, including frequency and quality of snacks
      - Number of meals eaten together as a family
      - Portion sizes
      - Number of calcium sources
      - Number of fiber sources

- History of breastfeeding, especially if the child was breastfed to age 6 months and if breastfeeding was continued after introduction of solids to age 12 months and beyond

b. *Physical activity:* It is important to assess age-appropriate vigorous activity, both structured and unstructured, and routine activity. Areas to be addressed include the following:
   - Time spent in moderate to vigorous physical activity each day, to estimate whether the goal of 60 minutes of activity daily is met. One hour or more should be vigorous intensity at least 3 days per week.[16]
   - Frequency of participating in muscle- and bone-strengthening activities. This should be occurring at least 3 days per week. These include climbing, jumping, running, and hanging/climbing on playground equipment.
   - Barriers to physical activity.

c. *Physical inactivity:* Asking about hours of television viewing and other "screen time" will uncover a very important opportunity to modify behavior for improved energy balance. A large number of hours of television watched each day has been associated with increased risk of obesity. A reduction in the number of hours can improve weight. Therefore, hours of television, video/DVD, and video game viewing, and non-homework computer use should be limited to less than 2 hours per day, with no television for children less than 2 years of age.[17] It is also important to ask about sleep habits. Counseling to ensure adequate amounts of sleep may be helpful in prevention and treatment of obesity.

d. *Sleep and obesity:* Many pediatric practitioners are also looking at whether poor sleep increases the risk of children becoming obese. Acute sleep deprivation leads to increased food intake, increased norepinephrine levels, and decreased body temperature. Assessment of sleeping habits and sleep time need to be part of an initial nutritional assessment. Studies in the United States, Japan, and Spain have shown a significant association between short sleep time and obesity in adults, with other studies showing an increase in BMI with shorter sleep duration. Sleep loss has been associated with altered glucose metabolism. Poor quality and insufficient quantity of sleep are common problems in children. In fact, Mamun and colleagues found that in young adults, BMIs and the prevalence of obesity were greater in those who had sleeping problems at 2–4 years of age.[8] Landhuis, Poulton, Welch, and Hancox also found that shorter childhood sleep times were significantly associated with higher adult BMI values.[9] It is estimated that 80% of adolescents get less than the recommended sleep on school nights. Recommended sleep time for adolescents is 9 to 9½ hours of sleep per night, but they average only 7 hours per night. Many factors impact teens' sleep time, including school, jobs, sports, friends, TV, phones, and computers.

6. *Attitude assessment:* The complexity of obesity prevention and intervention lies less in the identification of target health behaviors and much more in the process of influencing families to change behaviors when habits, culture, and environment promote less physical activity and more energy intake. Prior to providing counseling about new behaviors, clinicians should assess attitude, capacity, and motivation for change of the parents and child.

Nutritional Factors in Prevention and Treatment of Obesity

Although there is limited evidence of nutritional factors in the prevention and treatment of childhood obesity, the following sections review current information about nutritional intakes and behaviors.

Fruits and Vegetables

Fruits and vegetables have been promoted for the prevention of childhood obesity due to their low energy density, high fiber content, and satiety value. Many studies have shown that when children have higher intakes of fruits and vegetables they have lower risk of obesity and a lower BMI. Unfortunately, these are the foods that are less likely to be consumed by children. The National Youth Risk Behavior Survey (YRBS) is conducted every 2 years and surveys students in grades 7–12.[18] The YRBS provides data on dietary intakes, physical activity, and nutrition behaviors. Nationwide, only 21.4% of high school students eat at least 5 servings fruits and vegetables per day.

Sweetened Beverages

Intake of nondiet soft drinks and sweetened fruit drinks has increased dramatically among children in the United States in recent decades, particularly among adolescents. According to a national survey, soft drinks were the sixth leading food source of energy among children, comprising more than 50% of total beverage consumption. Soft drinks represent the number one source of calorie intake in the diets of U.S. adolescents.[19] Soft drinks are becoming substitutes for healthier options such as low-fat milk, water, or 100% fruit juices. According to the YRBS, 33.8% of students drank a can, bottle, or glass of soda or pop (not including diet) at least one time per day. The Growing up Today Study[20] assessed intakes of 2- to 19-year-olds and found soft drink intake was higher among overweight than nonoverweight youth in all age groups. Consuming excessive quantities of low-nutrient, energy-dense foods such as sugar-sweetened beverages are a risk factor for obesity.

Dairy

Recent research from some observational studies suggests that lower intakes of dairy products and/or calcium are associated with obesity in children. Research studies' findings are mixed, with half finding no associations with obesity and half finding that children who have low calcium intake have increased obesity.[21] However, none of the studies showed increased obesity with intake of dairy products. Additionally, an increased intake of calcium and dairy foods may play a role in the prevention of weight gain in youth.

Fiber

Higher fiber foods induce greater satiation. The recommendation for children's fiber intake is an "age + 5" rule; for example, a 5-year-old should consume at least 10 grams of fiber per day. Unfortunately, dietary fiber intake throughout childhood and adolescence averages approximately 12 grams per day, an amount that has not changed over time.[22] There is reason to conclude that fiber-rich diets containing nonstarchy vegetables, fruits, whole grains, legumes, and nuts may be effective in the prevention and treatment of obesity in children.

Breakfast

Obese children are more likely to skip breakfast or eat smaller breakfasts than leaner children. The evidence seems to suggest that breakfast skipping may be a risk factor for increased obesity, particularly among older children or adolescents. Population-based surveys have revealed that many children, particularly adolescents, skip breakfast and other meals, but consume more food later in the day, and that this pattern has increased in recent years. In addition to having a poorer nutritional intake, children who skip breakfast have been shown to have a decrease in academic performance.

Eating Out

Eating out can negatively impact the diets of children, and consumption of foods away from home has increased considerably in recent years. This increase may be associated with obesity, especially among adolescents.[21] The proportion of foods that children consume from restaurants (including fast food restaurants) has increased by nearly 300% over the past 2 decades. The frequency of eating foods away from home has been associated with greater intakes of total energy, sugar-sweetened beverages, and trans fats as well as lower consumption of low-fat dairy foods and fruits and vegetables.[23] Adding to this, portion sizes have increased in restaurants. Portion sizes can significantly influence energy intake. Diliberti and colleagues found that customers who purchased the larger portion of an entrée served at a fast food outlet increased their energy intake by 43%.[24] (Also see the following section on portion size.) Additionally, children and adolescents who consumed fast food more frequently had higher energy intakes, poorer diet quality, and higher BMIs.[13] The currently available evidence suggests that frequent eating at fast food restaurants may be a risk factor for obesity in children, and fast food ingestion year after year may accumulate to larger weight gains that can be clinically significant.[14]

Portion Size

Research indicates that portion size may contribute to the increasing prevalence of overweight among children by promoting excessive energy intake.[25] A study of preschool children 4 to 6 years of age found that the most powerful determinant of the amount of food consumed at meals was the amount served. Reducing food portion sizes may be an effective strategy for decreasing energy intake[13] when eating out or in the home.

Snacks

The majority of research shows that snacking frequency or snack food intake is not likely to be a major risk factor associated with obesity in children.[21] According to national surveys, although the average size of snacks and the energy content of snacks have remained relatively constant, only when the frequency of snacking increases (greater than two or three per day) does snacking become a risk factor among children of all age groups. Reportedly, between one-fourth and one-third of the energy intake of adolescents is derived from snacks.[17] Snack foods tend to have higher energy density and fat content than meals, and frequent snacking has been associated with high intakes of fat, sugar, and calories. The primary snacks selected by teens include potato chips, ice cream, candy, cookies, breakfast cereal, popcorn, crackers, soup, cake, and carbonated beverages. It is important not to eliminate snacks, but to help children choose healthy snacks and watch portion sizes.

Physical Activity

Along with diet, physical activity is the other key factor in the maintenance of energy balance. In addition to helping to control weight, physical activity provides numerous mental and physical benefits to health including reduction in the risk of cardiovascular disease, hypertension, diabetes, depression, and cancer. The greatest benefits of physical activity are gained from regular participation. The 2008 Physical Activity Recommendations for Americans[16] state that children and adolescents should participate in 60 minutes or more of physical activity every day. Unfortunately, the trend is for children to spend less and less time engaging in physical activity, with U.S. children spending approximately 75% of their waking hours being inactive. Physically active children are also more likely to remain physically active throughout adolescence and possibly into adulthood. However, measuring physical activity in children is challenging because children often have difficulty understanding the concepts of time, duration, and intensity of activity. The nature, context, and practice of physical activity vary with age.[26]

Particular individuals are at increased risk of having low levels of physical activity, including children from ethnic minorities, those living in poverty, children with disabilities, those residing in apartments or public housing, and children living in neighborhoods where outdoor physical activity is restricted by climate or safety concerns. Many barriers exist that may prevent children and youth from getting the recommended 60 minutes of daily physical activity. Communities and neighborhoods where inadequate after-school programs exist, lack of community recreation facilities, inadequate access to quality daily physical activity, and lack of discretionary income may contribute to the high obesity rates in these populations. Additionally, safety concerns such as heavy traffic, high crime rate, lack of equipment, lack of space, and urban development that favors cars are significant barriers to outside play. Walking or biking to and from school can help students meet their physical activity needs. However, heavy traffic, lack of bicycle lanes, unmarked intersections, and other obstacles have reduced the number of children who transport themselves to school today compared to previous generations.[17]

Motivational Interviewing

Most healthcare professionals, such as nurses, dietitians, and physicians, have not been adequately trained in behavioral counseling and have even less experience in counseling children and adolescents with obesity. In order to successfully treat obesity, providers must address not only diet and exercise, but also behavior change. Often healthcare professionals provide information they think the patient needs to know without finding out what the person wants to know or what changes the client thinks would be most helpful to them. Understanding of behavioral interviewing and counseling is critical to successfully working with overweight and obese children and adolescents.

Motivational interviewing (MI) can be defined as a directive, client-centered counseling style for eliciting behavioral change by helping clients explore and resolve ambivalence.[27] The resolution of ambivalence is one of the central purposes of MI and is particularly effective for individuals who are initially not ready to make changes. The tone of MI is nonjudgmental, empathetic, and encouraging. It provides a supportive environment where clients feel comfortable expressing both positive and negative aspects of their current behaviors.[28] Traditional models of counseling for nutrition rely on information exchange and counselor insight on what should be done. In contrast, the MI approach has the patient do much of the psychological work. In other words, the client is responsible for making the change. MI encourages clients to make fully informed and contemplated life choices, even if the decision is not to change.

MI operates under the premise that behavior change is affected more by motivation than information. There are specific techniques and strategies that, when used effectively, help ensure that the spirit of MI is evoked.[28] MI counselors rely heavily on reflective listening and positive affirmations. Clients make changes when they assign value to the change. In other words, clients are motivated to change what they value as important. Other core MI techniques include setting an agenda, rolling with resistance, building discrepancy, and eliciting self-motivation statements.

Prevention

Intervention programs are few and program cost may prevent many from being able to participate in or integrate into school curriculums. As we continue to intervene with already-at-risk children and adolescents, we also need to increase our preventative measures. Prevention is the responsibility of the provider, the family, the child, the school, and the community as well as the insurer and government agencies.[29] The following provides an overview of prevention activities for each segment.

Primary Care Provider

- Early recognition of overweight/obesity. Plot BMI routinely, and if the BMI percentile increases, address this prior to reaching more than 95%.
- Identify those at risk. Risk factors can include:
  - Parents are overweight.
  - Sibling is overweight.
  - Lower socioeconomic status.
  - Children with less cognitive stimulation.
- Provide anticipatory guidance in nutrition and physical activity. Anticipatory guidance is information and counseling that helps patients and families understand what to expect during a child or adolescent's current and/or approaching stage of development (e.g., growth spurts, increased/decreased energy needs, ways to prevent obesity through exercise and nutrition). Healthcare professionals can provide anticipatory guidance on nutrition and physical activity to help with obesity and eating disorder prevention as well as provide information to families.
  - Promote water and milk consumption over juice and soda.
  - Eat as a family.
  - Encourage nonsedentary family activities.
  - Do not use food as a reward.
  - Limit TV/computer/video games to 1–2 hours per day.
  - Do not eat in front of the TV.
  - Do not put a TV in the child's room.

Family

- Parents act as a role model.
  - Nutrition
  - Physical activity
- Limit eating out.
- Eat family meals.
- "Special times" do not have to involve food or sedentary activities.

School

- Promote physical activity.
- Provide nutritious meals.
- Have recess prior to lunch when possible.
- Control vending machines/healthy vending.
- Have nutrition and activity education integrated into school curriculum.
- Encourage children to walk or bike to school when safe.

Community

- Have safe playgrounds.
- Provide safe places for bike riding and walking.
- Promote physical activity outside of school.

Insurance and Government

- Acknowledge obesity as a medical condition for which one can be reimbursed.
- Provide reimbursement for anticipatory guidance on nutrition and physical activity.

Treatment

Treatment for children who are overweight or obese seems easy—just counsel children and their families to eat less and exercise more. In practice, however, treatment of childhood obesity is often time-consuming, frustrating, difficult, and expensive. Choosing the most effective methods for treating overweight and obesity in children is complex, especially for healthcare providers who have limited resources to offer interventions. It's also complicated by the lack of third-party reimbursement for healthcare services related to obesity.[17]

To date, no clinical trials have determined whether specific dietary modifications alone (i.e., without behavioral interventions and increased physical activity) are effective in reducing childhood overweight and obesity. Comprehensive interventions that include behavioral therapy along with changes in nutrition and physical activity are the most closely studied and appear to be the most successful approaches to improving long-term weight and health status.[21] Ultimately, children and adolescents (and adults, for that matter) become overweight or obese because of an imbalance between energy intake and expenditure. Dietary patterns, television viewing and other sedentary activities, and an overall lack of physical activity play key roles in creating this imbalance, and therefore represent opportunities for intervention. Interventions should focus on improving these eating and activity behaviors. Components of a successful weight management program include the following:

- Nutrition/dietary
- Increasing physical activity
- Reducing physical inactivity
- Behavioral modification

Nutrition/Dietary Component

It is often difficult to determine which part of nutritional intervention is responsible for the greatest behavioral change in treating obesity. In fact, the majority of studies that show a positive effect are comprehensive and include physical activity and behavioral counseling. Although comprehensive approaches that provide intervention in diet, physical activity, family behavior, and the social and physical environment are undoubtedly needed, studies involving multiple modalities cannot assess the efficacy of any specific component (e.g., diet).[17] The following dietary interventions have been components of most obesity treatment programs:

- *Fruits and vegetables:* Five or more a day
- *Fruit juice:* The American Academy of Pediatrics recommends that 100% fruit juice consumption be limited to 4 oz. per day for children 1–6 years of age and 8 to 12 oz. per day for children 7–18 years of age.[30] Unfortunately, many patients and families cannot distinguish between 100% fruit juice and fruit drinks, which are high in sugar and low in nutrients. It is often helpful for interventions to provide education about the difference between fruit drinks and 100% fruit juice and ways to limit 100% juice in children who drink excessive amounts.
- *Sweetened beverages:* Reducing the intake of these type of beverages may be one of the easiest and most effective ways to reduce energy intake and thereby decease weight.[17]
- *Dairy foods and calcium:* Increasing fat-free or low-fat dairy products to three to four servings a day while consuming a lower calorie diet may assist with weight loss. However, more research in this area is needed.[17]
- *Dietary fiber:* Dietary fiber may be related to regulation of body weight in children. Increasing fiber increases satiety, causing the child to eat less. Additionally, high fiber foods such as vegetables, fruits, and whole grains tend to be lower calorie foods and high in nutrients (high nutrient density), which also contributes to weight loss.[17]
- *Breakfast:* Incorporating breakfast as one of the key elements in an intervention program may assist with weight reduction.

- *Snacking:* Choosing healthy snacks should be encouraged in any intervention program.
- *Eating out:* Interventions should target education in eating out and increases in family meals.

Increasing Physical Activity

The 2008 Physical Activity Guidelines for Americans recommends the following for children and adolescents ages 6–17.[16]

- Aerobic activity should make up most of the child's 60 or more minutes of physical activity each day. This can include either moderate-intensity aerobic activity, such as brisk walking, or vigorous-intensity activity, such as running. Include vigorous-intensity aerobic activity on at least 3 days per week
- Muscle strengthening activities should be included at least 3 days per week.
- Bone strengthening activities, such as jumping rope or running, should be included at least 3 days per week as part of the 60 minute activity per day.

Reducing Physical Inactivity

Reducing television viewing and sedentary behaviors may be of more importance in obesity reduction than increasing physical activity.

Behavioral Modification

Behavior intervention for pediatric obesity uses a number of techniques that modify and control children's food and activity environment to bring about weight loss. These interventions include removing unhealthy foods from the home, monitoring behavior by asking children or parents to keep logs of behavioral components (e.g., food consumed, TV time, physical activity amounts), setting goals for nutrient intake and physical activity, and rewarding children's and sometimes parents' successful changes in diet and physical activity.

Staged Approach to Treating Childhood Obesity

Because limited studies have been conducted on obesity treatment, especially in the primary care setting, the Expert Committee on Childhood Obesity Treatment provides guidance for providers. The Expert Committee used available evidence to propose a comprehensive staged approach to treatment. The recommendations suggest that providers should counsel patients on healthy behaviors, utilize MI techniques to motivate patients and families, establish office systems that help providers monitor and care for these children, and implement a staged approach to intervention that is tailored to the individual child and family.[14,17] Stages 1 and 2 occur in the primary care setting, stage 3 in the community, and stage 4 in tertiary care centers. **Table 8-2** provides an overview of the staged approach.

Stage 1: Prevention Plus

All children should receive prevention counseling in the form of healthy lifestyle eating and activity habit. It is estimated that 40% of children with BMIs in the 50th to 85th percentile become overweight during adolescence. For children ages 2 to 18 years who are above the 85th percentile, stage 1 (Prevention Plus) should be implemented. This differs from basic prevention counseling by recommending that providers spend more time and intensity while providing closer follow-up every 3–6 months.

All intervention in this stage should be based on the family's and/or child's readiness to change. Intervention should focus on basic prevention behavior strategies. The outcome goal for this stage is based on the age of the child and improving the BMI status of the child or adolescent. Positive outcomes can be maintaining weight until BMI is less than the 85th percentile or gradual weight loss until BMI is less than the 85th percentile. Specific behavioral components to address in this stage include:

Eating behaviors:

- Minimize or eliminate sugar-sweetened beverages, such as soda, sports drinks, and punches. If sweetened beverages cannot be eliminated, children who consume large amounts will benefit from reduction to one serving a day.
- Consume at least five servings of fruits and vegetables daily. Families may subsequently increase to nine servings a day, as recommended by the USDA dietary guidelines.
- Limit eating out and purchasing restaurant food.
- Eat at the table as a family (family meals).
- Consume a healthy breakfast daily.
- Involve the whole family in lifestyle changes.

Physical activity behaviors:

- Decrease television viewing as well as other forms of nonhomework screen time to 2 or fewer hours a day. If the child is less than 2 years of age the committee recommends no television viewing. Removing the television from the bedroom will help reduce TV viewing time.
- Engage in 1 hour or more of physical activity per day. It is important to gradually increase physical activity for sedentary children. Initially, children may be unable to achieve 1 hour per day, but can gradually increase activity to reach 1 hour or more per day. Unstructured play is most appropriate for young children; older children may enjoy sports, dance, martial arts, bike riding, and walking. Physical activity can be done all at one time or in several shorter periods of activity over an entire day.

TABLE 8-2 Staged Approach for Treatment of Childhood and Adolescent Obesity

Stage	Stage Recommendations	Setting and Staff	Frequency of Visits
Stage 1: Prevention Plus	• 5+ fruits and vegetables a day • < 2 hours/day screen time • ≥ 1 hour/day physical activity • Reduce/eliminate sugar-sweetened beverages • Modify eating behaviors (e.g., three meals a day, family meals, limit eating out) • Family-based change	Primary care office–based Ensure scheduled follow-up visits	Frequency of visits based on readiness to change/ behavioral counseling. Reevaluate in 3 to 6 months. Advance to next level if no improvement.
Stage 2: Structured Weight Management	Develop a plan for the family and/or adolescent to include: • More structure (timing and content) of daily meals and snacks • Balanced macronutrient diet • Reduced screen time (< 1 hour/day) • Increased time spent in physical activity • Monitoring to improve success (e.g., logs of screen time, physical activity, dietary intake, or dietary patterns)	Office-based (dietitian, physician, nurse) trained in motivational interviewing/ behavioral counseling	Monthly visits tailored to child/adolescent and family. Advance if needed or if no improvement after 3 to 6 months.
Stage 3: Comprehensive Multidisciplinary Intervention	• Structured behavioral program (e.g., food monitoring, goal setting, contingency management) • Improved home food environment • Structured dietary and physical activity interventions designed to result in negative energy balance • Strong parental/family involvement, especially for children under 12 years of age	Multidisciplinary team (includes dietitian and counselor or behavioralist, with medical oversight)	Weekly for 8–12 weeks, then monthly for 6–12 months. Consider stage 4 if no improvement for children ages 12–18.
Stage 4: Tertiary Care Intervention	Continued diet and activity behavioral counseling plus consider more aggressive approaches, such as medication, surgery, or meal replacement	Pediatric weight management center operating under established protocols Multidisciplinary team	According to protocol.

Sources: Adapted from Barlow SE. Expert committee recommendations regarding the prevention, assessment and treatment of child and adolescent overweight and obesity: summary report. *Pediatrics.* 2007;120:S164–S192; and Spear BA, Barlow SE, Ervin C, et al. Recommendations for treatment of child and adolescent overweight and obesity. *Pediatrics.* 2007;120:S254–S288.

Follow-up visit frequency will be tailored to the individual family, and MI techniques may be useful to set the frequency. After 3 to 6 months, if the child has not made appropriate improvement, the provider can offer the next level of obesity care, Structured Weight Management.

Stage 2: Structured Weight Management

This stage targets the same behaviors as the Prevention Plus stage (food consumption, activity, and screen time), and offers additional support and structure to help the child and family achieve healthy behaviors in eating and physical activity. This stage requires the primary provider to have additional training in behavioral counseling. The eating plan requires a dietitian or a clinician who has received additional training in creating this kind of eating plan for children. Additionally, this stage requires the ability to add monitoring to the recommendations. Patients who monitor behavior change through such things as behavior logs, food diaries, or exercise logs have greater success in weight changes. This stage is characterized by closer follow-up, more structure, and monitoring of activities. The outcome goal for this stage is based on the age of the child and improving the BMI status of the child or adolescent. Positive outcomes can be maintaining weight until BMI is less than the 85th percentile or gradual weight loss until BMI is less than the 85th percentile. Specific behavioral components to address in this stage include:

Eating behaviors:

- Planned and structured daily meals and snacks (breakfast, lunch, dinner, with one or two snacks) with the following characteristics:
  - Balanced macronutrients based on the U.S. Dietary Guidelines
  - Emphasis on foods low in energy density, such as those with high fiber or water content
  - Mild energy (caloric) deficit
- Behavioral monitoring such as the use of food, activity, and screen time logs
- Planned reinforcement for achieving targeted behavior goals

Physical activity behaviors:

- Planned and supervised physical activity or active play for 60 minutes daily
- Reduction in screen time for leisure to 60 minutes or less each day (not including time dedicated to schoolwork). For example, the patient or family can record the minutes spent watching television, and they can keep a 3-day recording of foods and beverages consumed.

Ideally, monthly office visits are most effective at this level. After 3 to 6 months, if the child has not made significant improvement based on age and BMI level, the provider can offer the next level of obesity care, Comprehensive Multidisciplinary Intervention.

Stage 3: Comprehensive Multidisciplinary Intervention

The eating and activity goals associated with the Comprehensive Multidisciplinary Intervention stage are generally the same as those of the other treatment stages. The distinguishing characteristics of this stage are an increased intensity of behavioral change strategies, greater frequency of patient–provider contact, and an increase in the number of disciplines/specialists involved. The need for formalized behavioral therapy and a multidisciplinary treatment team exceeds the capacity of services that most primary care offices can provide. Specific behavioral components to address in this stage include:

Eating behaviors:

- Negative energy balance achieved through structured diet and physical activity (e.g., lower calorie diets that will help with weight reduction, decreasing high intake of sugar-sweetened beverages in children who have excessive consumption, or decreased TV viewing in children who watch greater than 2 hours per day).
- Planned and structured daily meals and snacks (breakfast, lunch, dinner, and one or two snacks) with the following characteristics:
  - Balanced macronutrients based on U.S. Dietary Guidelines
  - Emphasis on foods low in energy density, such as those with high fiber or water content
- Behavioral monitoring such as the use of food, activity, and screen time logs. For example, the patient or family can record the minutes spent watching television, and they can keep a 3-day recording of foods and beverages consumed.
- Planned reinforcement for achieving targeted behavior goals.
- Education for parents to improve home environment.

Physical activity behaviors:

- Planned and supervised physical activity or active play for at least 60 minutes daily
- Planned and supervised muscle-strengthening and bone-strengthening activity at least 3 days per week[16]
- Reduction in screen time for leisure to 60 minutes or less each day

Frequent office visits, weekly for a minimum of 8–12 weeks, appears most efficacious. Subsequently, monthly visits will help maintain new behaviors. Patients ages 6 to 18 years old who do not show improvement in weight after participating in stage 3 for 3 to 6 months may benefit from a referral to a tertiary care center. However, when these centers are not available or if families are motivated they may achieve success with longer implementation of components in Stage 3 with closer follow-up by healthcare providers.

Stage 4: Tertiary Care Intervention

The intensive interventions in this category have been used only to a limited extent in the pediatric population but may be an option for some severely obese youth who have significant co-morbidities. These interventions are more intensive and need more supervision than recommendations in the other stages. Candidates being considered for this stage should have attempted weight loss at the level of stage 3, Comprehensive Multidisciplinary Intervention; have the maturity to understand possible risks associated with stage 4 interventions; and be willing to maintain physical activity, follow a prescribed diet, and participate in behavior monitoring. However, lack of success with stage 3 is not by itself a qualification for stage 4 treatment. It is recommended that programs that provide these intensive treatments operate under established protocols to evaluate patients, implement the program, and monitor patients.

Although the interventions included in this stage have been used in adolescents, careful consideration should be made in implementing the components of this stage. The appropriateness of each of these interventions depends on the patient, family resources, age, and the geographic area's resources. Interventions to consider include the following:

- *Very-low-calorie diet/meal replacement:* There are few reports on the use of highly restrictive diets in children or adolescents. A restrictive diet has been employed as the first step in a childhood weight management program, followed by a mildly restrictive diet.[10] Long-term outcome data have not been reported.
- *Pharmacotherapy/medication:* Only two medications have been approved for use in adolescents: sibutramine (for those over 16 years of age) and orlistat (for those over 12 years of age). Both have significant side effects, and individuals on these medications should be followed closely. Studies showed positive long-term results when the medication was used in conjunction with nutrition, physical activity, and behavioral counseling.
- *Weight control surgery:* Because of the increasing number of youth with severe obesity who are not responsive to behavioral intervention, a few centers offer bariatric surgery. (See the "Bariatric Surgery" section below.)

Recommended Weight Change Goals

The general goal for all ages is for the BMI to deflect downwards until it is less than the 85th percentile. This may be done by maintaining weight while height increases. In other cases, a gradual weight loss may be needed to reach a BMI less than the 85th percentile. However, realizing that some children will be healthy between the 85th and 95th percentiles, clinical judgment will play a critical role in weight recommendations. Although monitoring BMI over the long term is ideal, in the short term (< 3 months), weight changes may be an easier parameter to measure.

Bariatric Surgery

Often, severe obesity is persistent even when treated through diet and lifestyle change and weight management medications. The increased use of bariatric surgery to treat morbid obesity and associated co-morbidities in adults has generated interest in using this therapy in adolescents. However, there is a limited amount of research regarding the safety, efficacy, and long-term outcomes of bariatric surgery in adolescents. For some very obese adolescents, however, bariatric surgery may be a justifiable treatment option. An expert panel made up of pediatricians and pediatric surgeons have developed stringent guidelines for the use of bariatric surgery in physically mature adolescents.[31] These guidelines include strict qualification criteria for the patients and the centers performing the surgery, and take into account the noncompliant nature of adolescents. They cover the specific nutritional and developmental needs for adolescents. As a further precaution, the expert committee felt it was critical that only experienced surgeons in a pediatric center with a multi-disciplinary team capable of long-term follow-up should perform adolescent bariatric surgery. **Table 8-3** shows criteria for bariatric surgery in adolescents.

Unfortunately, no data are available to assess the impact of bariatric surgery on bone mineral density and brittle bone or fractures in later life. Ongoing assessments of skeletal health should be performed in patients who have had bariatric surgery. Bariatric surgery results in consistent initial weight loss in approximately 90% of patients. Patients are expected to lose about 20–30 pounds in the first month following surgery and an additional 10 pounds per month until weight loss plateaus after about 12–18 months. Preliminary data from adolescents show a decrease in BMI from 59 kg/m^2 to 38 kg/m^2 in the first year following surgery. Persistent and long-lasting weight loss occurs in many adolescents following surgery; however, it is possible to regain excess body weight.[32]

TABLE 8-3 Criteria for Adolescents Receiving Bariatric Surgery

To be eligible for bariatric surgery, the patient must:

- Have reached physical maturity. (Adolescents who have achieved 95% of adult stature on skeletal exam and Tanner stage 4 can be cleared for surgery.)
- Have a BMI $\geq$ 50 or a BMI $\geq$ 40 with significant co-morbidities.
- Have failed a formal 6-month weight loss program.
- Be capable of adhering to the long-term lifestyle changes that are required postoperatively.
- Understand that the surgery is not a cure for obesity, but instead is an effective weight loss tool when used in conjunction with recommended dietary and physical activity regimens.
- Be aware of the known risks and possible side effects of the surgery.
- Undergo preoperative testing focusing on identifying co-morbidities associated with obesity and routine lab screenings including:
  - Fasting insulin and glucose
  - Oral glucose tolerance test
  - Lipid profile
  - Liver profile
  - Complete blood count
  - Vitamin B_1, B_{12}, and folate levels

Sources: Adapted from Inge TH, Krebs NF, Garcia VF, et al. Bariatric surgery for severely overweight adolescents: concerns and recommendations. *Pediatrics.* 2004;114:217–223; and Helmrath MA, Brandt ML, Inge TH. Adolescent obesity and bariatric surgery. *Surg Clin North Am.* 2006;86(2):441–454.

Success in maintaining weight loss long term depends on the patient's ability to adhere to behavior changes and a reduced calorie diet. Taking into account the developmental behaviors of adolescents and their propensity to rebel against strict regimens, it is important to provide consistent support and follow-up postoperatively. Meticulous, lifelong medical supervision of patients who undergo bariatric procedures during adolescence is essential to ensure optimal postoperative weight loss, eventual weight maintenance, and overall health. This is particularly important for adolescents, given the fact that the long-term effects of bariatric surgery in younger, reproductively active populations have not been well characterized.[31,33] Postoperative vitamin and mineral supplementation is critical in a reduced calorie diet, and usually consists of a chewable adult multivitamin, calcium supplement, B-complex vitamins, and folic acid in females.[32]

Weight regain and nutritional complications can be avoided by the patient's adherence to five basic rules: (1) Eat low-fat, high-protein foods first at mealtimes; (2) drink at least 64 ounces of low-calorie liquids per day; (3) do not snack between meals; (4) get at least 30 minutes of exercise daily; and (5) take vitamin and mineral supplements as instructed.[32]

Resources

There are many weight-loss programs available for individuals, families, schools, and communities. Unfortunately, many do not have long-term outcomes. The following are programs that are nationally available and provide nutrition and physical activity programming/resources or obesity prevention/treatment in a variety of settings.

Clinical Intervention Programs

The use of formal weight loss programs in healthcare settings has increased in recent years. Several academic institutions, in conjunction with their associated medical school or health systems, have implemented and evaluated child and adolescent weight management programs. The advantages of clinical weight loss interventions delivered in the healthcare setting are the ability to utilize a team of experts from different disciplines (e.g., nutrition, mental health, exercise, medicine) for the treatment programs and the ability of researchers to follow patients over an extended period of time. Disadvantages have tended to be associated with higher costs and dropout rates. The range of weight loss demonstrated in studies varies greatly among individual patients and programs. Programs that utilize behavior modification (as opposed to education alone) resulted in a greater change in weight status.

Committed 2 Kids
Individual and family-based; team approach; clinically based for ages 5–14
http://www.kazabee.com/html/committed_to_kids.html

Fit Kids
Family-based for overweight kids and their caregivers
http://www.choa.org/default.aspx?id=3226

HealthWorks!
Family-based; team approach; hospital- and community-based program for ages 5–19
http://www.cincinnatichildrens.org/svc/alpha/h/heart/clinical/healthworks/default.htm

KidShape
Family-based; team approach for children 6–14 years of age
http://kidshape.com

L.E.S.T.E.R. (Let's Eat Smart Then Exercise Right)
Individual- and group-based; hospital-based for children (6–11 years)
http://weight.chsys.org/

On Target
Medical; individual; hospital-based for pre-teens and teens
http://www.schneiderchildrenshospital.org/sch_ado_obesity.html

Shapedown
Family-based; team approach; clinical-based for children and teens (6–18 years)
http://www.Shapedown.com

School-Based Prevention and Intervention Programs

The school environment provides an ideal setting in which to intervene in improving children's nutrition and physical activity habits. Much has been written in the media and scientific literature about the need for modification of the school environment, including policy changes to promote healthier dietary intake and more opportunities for physical activity. Past research has demonstrated the link between a child's health and his or her ability to learn.[34]

Few school-based studies have targeted specifically overweight children because it may increase sensitivity to the stigma associated with participation in such programs at school. More recent programs have provided for school-wide interventions addressing healthy eating, increasing physical activity, and behavior change. Many have also focused on changing the school environment.

A number of evaluated school intervention programs are available that address the topics of childhood obesity prevention and physical activity and nutrition behaviors. These may provide nutrition professionals the opportunity to reach out to local schools to serve as partners in education to promote a healthy school environment. A selected few school and government programs include the following:

Animal Trackers
School-based for children (3–5 years)
http://www.healthy-start.com/prog_anim.html

Balance First Elementary School and Middle School
Children (grades 1–5 and 6–8)
http://school.discoveryeducation.com/balancefirst/learnMore.html

CATCH (Coordinated Approach to Child Health)
Formerly known as Child and Adolescent Trial for Cardiovascular Health Children (grades K–5)
http://www.sph.uth.tmc.edu/catch/

CATCH Kids Club
After-school/summer program for children (grades K–5)
http://www.sph.uth.tmc.edu/catch/KidsClub.htm

Eat Well & Keep Moving
Students (grades 4 and 5)
http://www.eatwellandkeepmoving.org

Generation FIT
Students (grades 3–12)
http://www.generation-fit.com/index.asp

Healthy Hearts for Kids
School-based (utilizes the Internet) for children (grades 5 and 6)
http:/healthyhearts4kids.org

Healthy Start
Children (3–5 years)
http://www.healthy-start.com

Pathways
American Indian children (grades 3–5)
http://hsc.unm.edu/pathways

Planet Health
Teens (grades 6 and 7)
http://www.planet-health.org

Stanford S.M.A.R.T (Student Media Awareness to Reduce Television)
Students (grades 3 and 4)
http://notv.stanford.edu/

SPARK (Sports, Play and Active Recreation in Kids)
School-based PE curriculum for students (Pre-K to 8th grade)
http://www.sparkpe.org

Take 10!
School-based for students (grades K–5)
http://www.take10.net

WAY (Wellness Academics & You Program)
School-based classroom-based curriculum for students (grades 4 and 5)
http://www.i4learning.com

We Can! (Ways to Enhance Children's Activity and Nutrition)
Children (8–13 years)
http://www.nhlbi.nih.gov/health/public/heart/obesity/wecan/

Community-Based Prevention and Intervention Programs

There are few community intervention programs, and many programs that are offered are often not evaluated. The following provides an overview of community programs that could be incorporated into other communities or offer resources for community programs:

Action For Healthy Kids
Family-, school-, and community-based for youth
http://www.actionforhealthykids.org

Body Works
Community- and family-based for females (9–13 years) and moms
http://www.womenshealth.gov/bodyworks

CANFit (California Adolescent Nutrition and Fitness)
Community-based for students (10–14 years) who are African American, Latino, and Pacific Islander youth
http://www.canfit.org/index.html

CHIP (Cardiovascular Health in Children)
Individual- and school-based (grades 3, 4, and 6–8)
http://www.epi.umn.edu/cyhp/r_catch.htm

Girls on the Run International
After-school or recreation center: Girls on the Run (grades 3–5) and Girls on Track (grades 6–8)
http://www.girlsontherun.org/default.html

Hearts N' Parks
Community-based for everyone
http://www.nhlbi.nih.gov/health/prof/heart/obesity/hrt_n_pk/index.htm

Materials to Develop Programs

Bright Futures
Resources for families, schools, and healthcare professionals
http://www.brightfutures.aap.org

Center for Weight and Health
Provides resources on nutrition, physical activity, and obesity, some free and some for sale
http://cwh.berkeley.edu/

Eat Smart. Move More North Carolina
Provides school, communities, families, churches with resources
http://www.eatsmartmovemorenc.com/index.html

Fit, Healthy and Ready to Learn: A School Health Policy Guide
Aids state and local decision makers in the creation of effective policies that allow for academic success and the development of lifelong healthy habits
http://nasbe.org/index.php/shs/53-shs-resources/396-fit-healthy-and-ready-to-learn-a-school-health-policy-guide

FitSource: Physical Activity & Nutrition in Child Care Setting
Resource database for parents, child care providers, and afterschool providers; provides tools that can be used to increase physical activity and improve nutrition in children
http://fitsource.nccic.acf.hhs.gov/fitsource/

Kidnetic.com
Interactive Website for children that promotes good health
http://www.kidnetic.com

Make It Happen! School Success Stories
Provides success stories from 32 schools and districts about improving nutrition in schools
http://www.fns.usda.gov/TN/Resources/makingithappen.html

A Parent's Guide to Healthy Eating and Physical Activity
Promotes healthy eating and an active lifestyle for the entire family
http://www.healthychildrenhealthyfutures.org

Project LEAN (Leaders Encouraging Activity and Nutrition)
Promotes healthy eating and physical activity to reduce chronic diseases
http://www.californiaprojectlean.org

School Health Index
An assessment tool for schools to assess the health of their school. It includes modules on nutrition, physical activity, school food service, health education, and school wellness. It is designed for the school to assess itself. A great tool for the PTA to utilize for assessment and to help plan school intervention.
http://apps.nccd.cdc.gov/ski/default.aspx

Shape Up America! (Healthy Weight for Life)
Increases awareness of obesity as a major public health problem
www.shapeup.org/

Team Nutrition
Educational materials for schools to provide meals that follow the dietary guidelines and MyPyramid. Most of the materials are free to health professionals.
http://www.fns.usda.gov/tn/

Eating Disorders

Eating disorders are the third most common chronic illness in adolescents behind obesity and asthma. They remain a serious cause of morbidity in children, adolescents, and young adults.[35] Eating disorders are considered medical illnesses with diagnostic criteria based on psychological, behavioral, and physiologic characteristics.[36] As a general rule, these illnesses are characterized by abnormal eating patterns and cognitive distortions related to food and weight, which in turn result in adverse effects on nutrition status, medical complications, and impaired health status and mental function.[37–40] The major characteristics of eating disorders are a disturbed body image in which the person perceives his or her body as being fat (even at normal or low weight), an intense fear of weight gain or becoming fat, and a relentless obsession to become thinner. Primary prevention combined with early recognition and treatment help decrease the rate of morbidity and mortality in adolescents suffering from these illnesses.[41]

Diagnostic Criteria

Diagnostic criteria for anorexia nervosa, bulimia nervosa, and eating disorders not otherwise specified (EDNOS) are identified in the fourth edition of the *Diagnostic and Statistical Manual of Mental Disorders* (DSM-IV) and shown in **Table 8-4**.[42] These clinical diagnoses are based on psychological, behavioral, and physiologic characteristics. It is important to note that patients cannot be diagnosed with both anorexia nervosa (AN) and bulimia nervosa (BN) at the same time. AN can develop from about 8 years of age, reaching a peak around 15–18 years old, while bulimia nervosa is rare below the age of 13 but becomes more common than anorexia by young adulthood. Atypical forms occur at higher rates than full syndrome disorders.[43] Patients with EDNOS do not fall into the diagnostic criteria for either AN or BN, but account for about 50% of the population with eating disorders and up to 70% of children and adolescents with eating disorders. Binge eating disorder is currently classified within the EDNOS grouping.

In a medical setting, the psychiatric diagnoses of AN and BN often are not used because medical providers often are not covered for psychiatric diagnoses. Because they are treating medical problems, their diagnoses are related to medical problems/symptoms such as severe malnutrition, bradycardia, hypotension, amenorrhea, vomiting, and esophageal pain.

Because of the complex biopsychosocial aspects of eating disorders, the optimal assessment and ongoing management of these conditions are under the direction of an interdisciplinary team consisting of professionals from medical, nursing, nutrition, and mental health disciplines.[39–40] Medical nutrition therapy (MNT) provided by a registered dietitian (RD) trained in the area of eating disorders and pediatrics is an integral component of treatment of children and adolescents with eating disorders. The RD's role should be to provide nutritional counseling, recognize clinical signs related to eating disorders, and assist with medical monitoring while remaining cognizant of psychotherapy that is the cornerstone of eating disorder treatment. The main objective of MNT should be to normalize the eating patterns and nutritional status of the patient.[36]

Children and Adolescents

The prevalence of eating disorders in children and adolescents has increased dramatically over the past three decades, especially in females, with an incidence of up to 5%.

TABLE 8-4 Diagnostic Criteria for Eating Disorders

Anorexia Nervosa (Diagnostic Code 307.10)

A. Refusal to maintain body weight at or above a minimally normal weight for age and height, e.g., weight loss leading to maintenance of body weight less than 85% of that expected; or failure to make expected weight gain during period of growth, leading to body weight less than 85% of that expected.

B. Intense fear of gaining weight or becoming fat, even though underweight.

C. Disturbance in the way in which one's body weight, size, or shape is experienced, undue influence of body weight or shape on self-evaluation, or denial of the seriousness of the current low body weight.

D. In postmenarcheal females, amenorrhea, i.e., the absence of at least three consecutive menstrual cycles. (A woman is considered to have amenorrhea if her periods occur only following hormone, e.g., estrogen, administration.)

Specific type:

Restricting Type: during the current episode of Anorexia Nervosa, the person has not regularly engaged in binge-eating or purging behavior (i.e., self-induced vomiting or the misuse of laxatives, diuretics, or enemas)

Binge-Eating/Purging Type: during the current episode of Anorexia Nervosa, the person has regularly engaged in binge-eating or purging behavior (i.e., self-induced vomiting or the misuse of laxatives, diuretics, or enemas)

Bulimia Nervosa (Diagnostic Code 307.51)

A. Recurrent episodes of binge eating. An episode of binge eating is characterized by both of the following:

1. eating, in a discrete period of time (e.g., within any 2-hour period), an amount of food that is definitely larger than most people would eat in a similar period of time under similar circumstances
2. a sense of lack of control over eating during the episode (e.g., a feeling that one cannot stop eating or control what or how much one is eating)

B. Recurrent inappropriate compensatory behavior in order to prevent weight gain, such as self-induced vomiting; misuse of laxatives, diuretics, enemas, or other medications; fasting or excessive exercise.

C. The binge eating and inappropriate compensatory behaviors both occur, on average, at least twice a week for three months.

D. Self-evaluation is unduly influenced by body shape and weight

E. The disturbance does not occur exclusively during episodes of Anorexia Nervosa.

Specific Type:

Purging Type: during the current episode of Bulimia Nervosa, the person has regularly engaged in self-induced vomiting or the misuse of laxatives, diuretics or enemas

Nonpurging Type: during the current episode of Bulimia Nervosa, the person has used other inappropriate compensatory behaviors, such as fasting or excessive exercise, but has not regularly engaged in self-induced vomiting or the misuse of laxatives, diuretics or enemas.

Eating Disorder Not Otherwise Specified (EDNOS) (Diagnostic Code 307.5)

The Eating Disorder Not Otherwise Specified category is for disorders of eating that do not meet the criteria for any specific Eating Disorders. Examples include:

1. For females, all of the criteria for Anorexia Nervosa are met except that the individual has regular menses.
2. All of the criteria for Anorexia Nervosa are met except that despite significant weight loss, the individual's current weight is in the normal range.
3. All of the criteria for Bulimia Nervosa are met except that the binge eating and inappropriate compensatory mechanism occurs at a frequency of less than twice a week or for a duration of less than 3 months.
4. The regular use of inappropriate compensatory behavior by an individual of normal body weight after eating small amounts of food (e.g., self-induced vomiting after the consumption of two cookies).
5. Repeatedly chewing and spitting out, but not swallowing large amounts of food.
6. Binge-eating disorder: recurrent episodes of binge eating in the absence of the regular use of inappropriate compensatory behaviors characteristic of Bulimia Nervosa.

Binge Eating Disorder (Research Criteria of Eating Disorders Not Otherwise Specified EDNOS)

A. Recurrent episodes of binge eating. An episode of binge eating is characterized by both of the following:

1. eating, in a discrete period of time[1] (e.g., within any 2-hour period), an amount of food that is definitely larger than most people would eat in a similar period of time under similar circumstances
2. a sense of lack of control over eating during the episode (e.g., a feeling that one cannot stop eating or control what or how much one is eating)

B. The binge-eating episodes are associated with three (or more) of the following:

1. eating much more rapidly than normal
2. eating until feeling uncomfortably full
3. eating large amounts of food when not feeling physically hungry
4. eating alone because of being embarrassed by how much one is eating
5. feeling disgusted with oneself, depressed, or very guilty after overeating

C. Marked distress regarding binge eating is present.

D. The binge eating occurs, on average, at least 2 days a week for 6 months.

E. The binge eating is not associated with the regular use of inappropriate compensatory behaviors (e.g., purging, fasting, excessive exercise) and does not occur exclusively during the course of Anorexia Nervosa or Bulimia Nervosa.

Source: Reprinted with permission from the American Psychiatric Association: *Diagnostic and Statistical Manual of Mental Disorders*, Fourth Edition, Text Revised, Washington, DC: American Psychiatric Association; 2000.

More specifically, 10% of 13-year-old females report the use of self-induced vomiting in an attempt to lose weight, and atypical eating disorders are estimated to occur in 3–6% of middle-school-age females and 2–13% of high-school-age females.[41,44–46] Large numbers of adolescents who have disordered eating do not meet the strict DSM-IV criteria for either AN or BN but can be classified as EDNOS. Diagnostic criteria for eating disorders, such as those in the DSM-IV, may not be entirely applicable to children and adolescents. The wide variability in the rate, timing, and magnitude of both height and weight gain during normal puberty, the absence of menstrual periods in early puberty along with the unpredictability of menses within the first year after menarche, and the lack of abstract concept limit the application of diagnostic criteria to adolescents. A thorough screening process can help prevent delays in diagnosis.[30,47–48]

Because of the potentially irreversible effects of an eating disorder on physical and emotional growth and development in adolescents, the onset and intensity of the intervention in adolescents should be more aggressive than with adults. Medical complications in adolescents that are potentially irreversible include growth retardation if the disorder occurs before closure of the epiphyses, pubertal delay or arrest, impaired acquisition of peak bone mass during the second decade of life, increased risk of osteoporosis in adulthood, and structural brain changes.[47,49]

Healthcare Team

Adolescents with eating disorders require evaluation and treatment focused on biological, psychological, family, and social features of these complex, chronic health conditions. The expertise and dedication of the members of a treatment team who work specifically with adolescents and their families are more important than the particular treatment setting. In fact, traditional settings such as a general psychiatric ward/clinic may be less appropriate than an adolescent medical clinic/unit. Smooth transition from inpatient to outpatient care can be facilitated by an interdisciplinary team that provides continuity of care in a comprehensive, coordinated, developmentally oriented manner.

The healthcare team needs to be familiar with working not only with the patient, but also with the family, school, coaches, and other agencies or individuals who are important influences on healthy adolescent development.[46,50] Many patients with eating disorders have a fear of eating in front of others. Often it can be difficult for the patient to achieve adequate intake from meals at school. Because school is a major element in the life of adolescents, treatment team members need to be able to help adolescents and their families work within the system to achieve a healthy and varied nutrition intake. In working with the family of an adolescent, it is important to remember that the adolescent is the patient and that all nutritional therapy should be planned on an individual basis. It is often helpful to have the dietitian meet with adolescent patients and their parents separately to provide nutrition education and to clarify and answer questions. Parents are often frightened and want a quick fix. Educating the parents regarding the stages of the nutrition plan may be helpful.

Prognosis

There is limited research on the long-term outcomes of adolescents with eating disorders. There appears to be limited prognostic indicators to predict outcome.[20,39–41] Generally, poor prognosis has been reported when adolescent patients have been treated almost exclusively by mental health professionals.[44,51] Data from treatment programs based in adolescent medicine show more favorable outcomes. Reviews by both Kriepe and Durkarm and Becker et al. showed a 71–86% satisfactory outcome when patients are treated in adolescent-based programs.[38,47] Strober, Freeman, and Morrell conducted a long-term prospective follow-up of adolescents with severe AN admitted to the hospital.[52] At follow-up, results showed that nearly 76% of the cohort met criteria for full recovery. In this study, approximately 30% of patients had relapses following hospital discharge. The authors also noted that the time to recovery ranged from 57 to 79 months.

Adolescents who recover medically and are able to maintain a healthy weight usually have no long-term medical side effects of the malnutrition. The only exception may be that total peak bone mass density may not reach the genetic potential. This is especially critical to individuals who suffer from malnutrition during peak growth phases. Bone density may be in the normal range, but may not be as high as it would have been without the eating disorder. This may be linked to high cortisol levels and growth hormone resistance in adolescents with AN, which can contribute to decreased bone turnover and bone mass density leading to suppressed bone formation.[53,54]

Nutrition Assessment

The initial interview/visit provides the dietitian with the first opportunity to develop a therapeutic alliance with the patient while gathering information critical to the assessment. Developing an alliance with the patient is important in building a trusting relationship. Ensuring an atmosphere of acceptance during the interview allows the patient to feel comfortable and to share openly. **Table 8-5** lists the topics to cover during the initial interview. In addition to the information gathered from the initial interview, a nutrition assessment should include the data listed in **Table 8-6**. These topics will be covered in more detail in the following sections.

Medical Consequences and Intervention in Eating Disorders

Nutritional factors and dieting behaviors may influence the development and course of eating disorders.[40,47,50,55] Higher

TABLE 8-5 Important Topics for Initial Interviews

1. Background information
   - Diagnosis
   - Current age and age of onset
   - Treatment history: previous treatment plans, time in treatment
   - Weight: premorbid and current
   - Height
   - Menstruation history: last menstrual period, typical cycle
2. Food/dieting
   - "Usual" intake prior to diagnosis
   - Typical day's intake or food frequency or 24-hour recall
   - Safe and forbidden foods
   - Food likes and dislikes
   - Weight loss techniques employed
3. Exercise history
   - Exercise and activity level: current and premorbid, including
     - Type of exercise (e.g., running, weight training, riding bike)
     - Intensity (e.g., how long to run 1 mile, how many miles)
     - Setting (e.g., alone in room, at gym)
4. Weight history
   - History of weight conflicts
   - Weight high/low
   - Patient's goal/desired weight
   - Total weight loss
5. Binge/purge activity
   - Frequency of binges
   - Method of purging
   - Frequency of purging
   - Subjective report on severity of bingeing/purging
6. Family history
   - Family members at home
   - Food/dieting/exercise/weight conflicts among other members
   - History of psychiatric illness, especially affective illness
   - Mother or sibling with eating disorder
7. Social history
   - School and grade
   - Overall school performance: current and premorbid
   - Peer interactions: current and premorbid
8. Physical status
   - General observations: hair loss; dry, flaking skin; swollen parotid glands; calluses on knuckles (Russell sign)
   - Reported clinical effects of starvation: decreased tolerance to cold, poor sleep habits, lightheadedness, dizziness, symptoms of hypoglycemia, increased moodiness
9. Medication and substance use
   - Prescription medication
   - Over-the-counter medication, including laxatives, diuretics, and vomiting agents, such as ipecac
   - Alcohol use
   - Other substance use

TABLE 8-6 Data Needed for the Initial Nutritional Assessment

1. Growth data
   - Height
   - Weight
   - BMI percentile
   - Expected weight range for height (using Hamwi method)
   - Percent of expected weight for height
2. Energy
   - Basal energy expenditure (BEE) for ideal body weight for height
   - Requirement for weight gain (BEE $\times$ 1.5)
3. Body composition data (if appropriate)
   - Skinfolds: tricep, bicep, subscapular, suprailiac
   - Calculate percent body fat
4. Physical assessment
   - Subjective muscle wasting (e.g., glutial wasting)
   - Symptoms of gastroesophageal reflux (GER) or *H. pylori*
   - Symptoms of hypoglycemia (lightheadedness, dizziness)
   - Calluses on knuckles
   - Dental erosions
5. Biochemical data (labs are based on symptoms; not all will be needed)
   - CBC
   - Electrolytes
   - Glucose
   - Bone density (only recommended if $>$ 6 months amenorrheic)
   - Lipid status (cholesterol level)
   - Phosphorus status
   - Urine specific gravity
   - Amylase
   - Stool antigen for *H. pylori*
   - T4, TSH

prevalence rates among specific groups, such as athletes and patients with diabetes mellitus,[56] support the concept that increased risk occurs with conditions in which dietary restraint or control of body weight assumes great importance. However, only a small proportion of individuals who diet or restrict intake develop an eating disorder. In many cases, psychological and cultural pressures must exist along with physical, emotional, and societal pressures for an individual to develop an eating disorder.

Anorexia Nervosa

Medical Symptoms

Essential to the diagnosis of AN is that patients weigh less than 85% of that expected (Table 8-4). There are several ways to determine whether a patient is less than the 85th percentile. For postmenarchal adolescents and young adults, the Hamwi method can be used to determine expected weight for height.[57] This method allows 100 pounds for

5 feet of height plus 5 pounds for each inch over 5 feet tall, ± 10% to determine 90–110% expected weight for height, which is a normal healthy range. The 85th percentile of expected weight for height can be diagnostic of AN.[39,58–60] Additionally, for children and younger adolescents the percentage of expected weight for height can be calculated by using CDC growth charts or the CDC BMI charts. (See Appendix B.)[28] Individuals with BMIs less than the 10th percentile are considered at risk for underweight, and BMIs less than the 5th percentile are at risk for AN.[40,61] In all cases, the patient's body build, weight history, and stage of sexual development should be considered.

Physical characteristics of anorexia include lanugo hair on face and trunk, brittle listless hair, cyanosis of hands and feet, and dry skin. Cardiovascular changes include bradycardia (HR < 60 beats/min), hypotension (systolic < 90 mm Hg), and orthostatic changes in pulse and blood pressure.[37,40,47] Many patients, as well as some healthcare providers, attribute the low heart rate and low blood pressure to these patients' physical fitness and exercise regimen; however, Nudel and colleagues showed these lower vital signs actually altered cardiovascular responses to exercise in patients with AN.[62] A reduced heart mass also has been associated with the reduced blood pressure and pulse rate.[58,59,63] Cardiovascular complications have been associated with death in AN patients.

AN can also significantly affect the gastrointestinal tract and brain mass of these individuals. Self-induced starvation can lead to delayed gastric emptying, decreased gut motility, and severe constipation. Long-term rehabilitation, as opposed to short-term refeeding, has been shown to improve these symptoms.[64] There is also evidence of structural brain abnormalities (tissue loss) with prolonged starvation, which appears early in the disease process and may be of substantial magnitude. Although it is clear that some reversal of brain changes occurs with weight recovery, it is uncertain whether complete reversal is possible. Studies have shown abnormal cognitive function and brain structure in female subjects with adolescent-onset AN compared to healthy individuals, despite an extended period since diagnosis.[65] To minimize the potential long-term physical complications of AN, early recognition and aggressive treatment are essential for young people who develop this illness.[49,66,67]

Amenorrhea is a primary characteristic of AN. Amenorrhea is associated with a combination of hypothalamic dysfunction, weight loss, decreased body fat, stress, and excessive exercise. The amenorrhea appears to be caused by an alteration in the regulation of gonadotropin-releasing hormone. In AN, gonadotropins revert to prepubertal levels and patterns of secretion.[40,47] Complications of amenorrhea, often seen in athletes, include impaired endothelium-dependent arterial vasodilation, which reduces the perfusion of the working muscle; impaired skeletal muscle oxidative metabolism; and elevated low-density lipoprotein cholesterol levels.[68]

Low bone mineral density (BMD) is an established risk in AN. Fifty percent of anorexics develop osteopenia within 20 months of experiencing amenorrhea. Thirty-eight percent subsequently develop osteoporosis after having amenorrhea for less than 24 months. BMD declines as the number of missed menstrual cycles increases. Osteopenia and osteoporosis, like brain changes, are serious and possibly irreversible medical complications of AN. This may be serious enough to result in vertebrae compression and stress fractures. Stress fracture occurrence is estimated to be two to four times more common in physically active women with amenorrhea and/or low BMD.[60,69,70] Optimal intervention is to promote weight restoration early, before bone mineral loss has occurred.[71] Study results indicate that some recovery of bone may be possible with weight restoration and recovery, but compromised bone density has been evident 11 years after weight restoration and recovery.[72,73] In younger adolescents, more bone recovery may be possible. Providing exogenous estrogen (e.g., oral contraceptives) has not been shown to preserve or restore bone mass in the AN patient.[74] Calcium supplementation alone (1500 mg/day) or in combination with estrogen has not been observed to promote increased bone density;[37] however, adequate calcium intake may help to lessen bone loss.[47] Only weight restoration to > 90% expected weight for height has been shown to increase bone density.

In patients with AN, laboratory values usually remain in normal ranges until the illness is far advanced; however, true laboratory values may be masked by chronic dehydration. Some of the earliest lab abnormalities include bone marrow hypoplasia, including varying degrees of leukopenia and thrombocytopenia.[75] Despite low-fat and low-cholesterol diets, patients with AN often have elevated cholesterol and abnormal lipid profiles. Reasons for this include mild hepatic dysfunction, decreased bile acid secretion, abnormal eating patterns, and increased cholesterol metabolism.[76] Additionally, serum glucose tends to be low, secondary to a deficit of precursors for gluconeogenesis and glucose production.[77] Patients with AN may have repeated episodes of hypoglycemia.

Despite dietary inadequacies, vitamin and mineral deficiencies are rarely seen in AN. This has been attributed to a decreased metabolic need for micronutrients in a catabolic state. Additionally, many patients take vitamin and mineral supplements, which may mask true deficiencies. Despite low iron intakes, iron deficiency anemia is rare. This may be due to decreased needs due to amenorrhea, decreased needs in a catabolic state, and altered states of hydration.[78] Prolonged malnutrition, however, may lead to low levels of zinc, vitamin B_{12}, and folate. Any low nutrient levels should be treated appropriately with food and supplements as needed.

Medical and Nutritional Management

Treatment for AN may be inpatient- or outpatient-based, depending upon the severity and chronicity of both the medical and behavioral components of the disorder. No single professional or professional discipline is able to provide the necessary broad medical, nutritional, and psychiatric care necessary for patients to recover. An interdisciplinary team approach is necessary whether the individual is undergoing inpatient or outpatient treatment.

Outpatient Treatment

In AN, the goals of outpatient treatment are to focus on nutritional rehabilitation, weight restoration, cessation of weight reduction behaviors, improvement in eating behaviors, and improvement in psychological and emotional state. Clearly, weight restoration alone does not indicate recovery, and forcing weight gain without psychological support and counseling is contraindicated. Typically, the patient is terrified of weight gain and may be struggling with hunger and urges to binge, but the "safe" foods he or she allows him- or herself are too limited to enable sufficient energy intake.[40] Individualized guidance and a meal plan that provides a framework for meals and snacks and food choices (but not a rigid diet) is helpful for most patients.

The registered dietitian determines the individual caloric needs and with the patient develops a nutrition plan that allows the patient to meet these nutrition needs. In the early treatment of AN, this may be done on a gradual basis by increasing the caloric prescription in increments to reach the necessary caloric intake. The dietitian helps the patient to select foods that the patient feels he or she can accept, thereby starting the process of relearning how to eat normally. A critical balance exists between allowing gradual, small changes in a patient with very restricted eating patterns and ensuring adequate nutrition and weight gain. Reminding the patient that the treatment team does not want the patient's weight gain to be out of control but reflective of physiologic changes may soothe fears about adding new foods and increasing the amount of calories consumed. Guidelines for nutritional intervention for AN are shown in **Table 8-7.**

MNT should be targeted at helping the patient understand nutritional needs as well as helping the patient begin to make wise food choices by increasing variety in diet and practicing appropriate food behaviors.[37] One effective counseling technique is cognitive behavioral therapy, which involves challenging erroneous beliefs and thought patterns with more accurate perceptions and interpretations regarding dieting, nutrition, and the relationship between starvation and physical symptoms.[78,79]

TABLE 8-7 Nutrition Intervention in Anorexia Nervosa

A. General guidelines
   1. Provide a nutritionally balanced diet with some individual preferences included (e.g., vegetarian).
   2. Provide multivitamin/mineral supplements at recommended dietary allowance (RDA) levels.
   3. Provide dietary fiber from grain sources to enhance elimination.
   4. Whenever possible, permit small, frequent feedings to reduce sensation of bloating.
   5. Use liquid supplements only when the patient cannot achieve goal intake via foods.
   6. Provide cold or room-temperature food to reduce satiety sensations.
   7. Reduce caffeine intake, if appropriate.
   8. Provide parenteral nutrition only in severe cases.
   9. Provide interactive nutritional counseling on an ongoing basis.

B. Energy recommendations
   1. Initial nutrition counseling (outpatient)
      a. Determine average kcal intake.
      b. Develop nutrition plan with patient that
         i. Contains three meals and one or two snacks a day.
         ii. Provides increasing energy levels (50–75% of DRI for energy or approximately 1000–1500 kcal/day). This depends on the current intake. It may take several visits to reach this level of kcal intake because of fears of food and weight gain.
      c. Continue to assess for refeeding syndrome.
   2. Follow-up counseling
      a. Increase diet prescription in small, progressive increments to provide for:
         i. 0.5–1 lb gain/week—outpatient
         ii. 2–4 lb gain/week—inpatient
      b. Maintain kcal level as long as appropriate weight gain continues.
      c. Increase kcal level if weight gain stops or weight loss occurs.
      d. Because of increased energy demands for repair and growth, patients may require higher than expected energy intake (½ to 2 times DRI for energy).
      e. If patient continues to lose or fails to gain on adequate kcal level evaluate for vomiting, discarding food, increased exercise, or increased activity.

C. Micronutrients
   1. Protein
      a. RDA in g/kg ideal body weight
      b. 15–20% of calories
      c. High biological value
   2. Carbohydrates
      a. 50–60% of calories
      b. High fiber for treatment of constipation

(continued)

TABLE 8-7 (Continued)

3. Fat
   a. 20–25% of calories
   b. Encourage small increases in fat intake until goal attained

D. Micronutrients
   1. 100% of RDA for micronutrients with supplements as needed.
   2. 1300–1500 mg of calcium from food and supplements may help to prevent rapid bone loss.
   3. Iron supplement may aggravate constipation.

E. Physical activity
   1. Monitor physical activity levels; increases in physical activity will affect kcal recommendations.
   2. Increase physical activity levels as weight restoration occurs.
      a. Begin with flexibility exercises (~80% expected weight for height).
      b. Next add strength exercises (e.g., free weights, pushups, crunches) (~85% expected weight for height)
      c. Last add aerobic activities. Begin with 10 minutes and increase time as long as weight restoration continues (~88–90% expected weight for height).

In many cases, monitoring skinfold measurements can be helpful in determining composition of weight gain as well as being useful as an educational tool to show the patient the composition of any weight gain (lean body mass vs. fat mass). The percentage of body fat can be estimated from the sum of four skinfold measurements (triceps, biceps, subscapular, and suprailiac crest) using the calculations of Durnin.[80] The results of skinfold measurements have been found to be significantly correlated with dual energy x-ray absorptiometry (DEXA) measurements of body fat percentage.[77,81] This method also has been validated against underwater weighing in adolescent girls with AN. Bioelectrical impedance analysis has been shown to be unreliable in patients with AN secondary to changes in intracellular and extracellular fluid and chronic dehydration.[82,83]

Dietary supplements may be recommended as needed to meet nutritional needs. Physical activity recommendations need to be based on medical status, psychological status, and nutritional intake. Physical activity may need to be limited or initially eliminated with the compulsive exerciser who has AN, so that weight restoration can be achieved. The counseling effort needs to focus on the message that exercise is an activity undertaken for enjoyment and fitness rather than a way to expend energy and promote weight loss. Supervised strength training using a low level of weights is less likely to impede weight gain than other forms of activity and may be psychologically helpful for patients.[51] Nutrition therapy must be ongoing to allow the patient to understand his or her nutritional needs as well as to adjust and adapt the nutrition plan to meet the patient's medical and nutritional requirements.

Inpatient Treatment

Although many patients may respond to outpatient therapy, others do not. Low weight is only one index of malnutrition; weight should never be used as the only criterion for hospital admission. Most patients with AN are knowledgeable enough to falsify weights through such strategies as excessive water/fluid intake. If body weight alone is used for hospital admission criteria, these behaviors (e.g., excessive water intake) may result in acute hyponutremia or dangerous degrees of unrecognized weight loss. All criteria for admission (shown in **Table 8-8**) should be considered.[47]

The goals of inpatient therapy are the same as for outpatient management except more intense. If admitted for medical instability, medical and nutrition stabilization is the first and most important goal of inpatient treatment. This is often necessary before psychological therapy can be optimally effective. Often, the first phase of inpatient treatment is on a medical unit.

A medical malnutrition protocol is used to stabilize a patient with AN from both a medical and nutritional standpoint. The goals of this protocol are to establish adequate energy intake, maintain hydration status, maintain medical stability, and prevent purging activity through supervision.[61] The dietitian team member should guide the nutrition plan. The nutrition plan should help the patient, as quickly as possible, to consume a diet that is adequate in energy intake and nutritionally well-balanced. The energy intake as well as body composition should be monitored to ensure that appropriate weight gain is achieved. As with outpatient therapy, MNT should be targeted at helping the patient understand nutritional needs as well as helping them to begin to make wise food choices by increasing variety in diet and practicing appropriate food behaviors. In very rare instances, enteral or parenteral feeding may be necessary; however, risks associated with aggressive nutrition support in these patients are substantial, including hypophosphatemia, edema, cardiac failure, seizures, aspiration of enteral formula, and death.[37] Reliance on foods (rather than enteral or parenteral nutrition support) as the primary method of weight restoration contributes significantly to successful long-term recovery. The overall goal is to help the patient normalize eating patterns and learn that behavior must involve planning and practicing with real food.

Refeeding Syndrome

During the refeeding phase (especially early in the refeeding process), the patient needs to be monitored closely for signs of refeeding syndrome. Refeeding syndrome is characterized by sudden and sometimes severe hypophosphatemia, sudden

TABLE 8-8 Indications for Hospitalization in an Adolescent with an Eating Disorder

- Severe malnutrition (weight < 75% expected weight for height)
- Dehydration
- Electrolyte disturbances (hypokalemia, hyponatremia, hypophosphatemia)
- Cardiac dysrhythmia (including prolonged QT)
- Physiological instability
  - Severe bradycardia (heart rate < 50 beats/min)
  - Hypotension (< 80/50 mm Hg)
  - Hypothermia (body temperature < 96°F)
    - Orthostatic changes in pulse (> 20 beats per minute) or blood pressure (>10 mm Hg)
- Arrested growth and development
- Failure of outpatient treatment
- Acute food refusal
- Uncontrollable bingeing and purging
- Acute medical complication of malnutrition (e.g., syncope, seizures, cardiac failure, pancreatitis, etc.)
- Acute psychiatric emergencies (e.g., suicidal ideation, acute psychoses)
- Co-morbid diagnosis that interferes with the treatment of the eating disorder (e.g., severe depression, obsessive-compulsive disorder, severe family dysfunction)

Sources: Sturdevant MS, Spear BA. Eating disorders and obesity. In: Burg F, Ingelfinger J, Polin R, Gershon A. *Current Pediatric Therapy*. Philadelphia, PA: Saunders; 2006:334–336; Position of the American Dietetic Association: Nutrition intervention in the treatment of anorexia nervosa, bulimia nervosa and eating disorders not otherwise specified (EDNOS). *J. Am Diet Assoc.* 2001;101:810–819.

drops in potassium and magnesium, glucose intolerance, hypokalemia, gastrointestinal dysfunction, and cardiac arrhythmias (a prolonged QT interval is a contributing cause of the rhythm disturbances).[58] Refeeding syndrome can follow sudden increases in nutritional intake after a period of starvation.[43] Water retention during refeeding should be anticipated and discussed with the patient. Guidance with food choices to promote normal bowel function should be provided as well. A weight gain goal of 1–2 pounds per week for outpatients and 2–3 pounds for inpatients is recommended. In the beginning of therapy, the dietitian will need to see the patient on a frequent basis. If the patient responds to medical, nutritional, and psychiatric therapy, nutrition visits may be less frequent. After a normal, safe weight is achieved, caloric intake should be adjusted for weight maintenance.[43] Refeeding syndrome can be seen in both the outpatient and inpatient setting, and the patient should be monitored closely during the early refeeding process. Because more aggressive and rapid refeeding is initiated on the inpatient units, refeeding syndrome is more common, especially when being fed parenterally.[43]

Bulimia Nervosa

Bulimia nervosa (BN) occurs in approximately 2–5% of the population. Most patients with BN tend to be of normal weight or moderately overweight and therefore are often undetectable by appearance alone. However, they place a strong emphasis on physical appearance and are often frustrated because they cannot maintain underweight status. The average onset of BN occurs between mid-adolescence and the late 20s, with a great diversity of socioeconomic status.[61] The individual at risk for the disorder may also have a risk for depression that may be exacerbated by a chaotic or conflicting family as well as the stress of social expectations.[84,85] A subgroup of BN patients began bingeing before dieting. This group tends to be of a higher body weight.[85]

The patient with BN has an eating pattern that is typically chaotic, with self-imposed rules of what should be eaten, how much, and what constitutes good and bad foods. These thoughts occupy the thought process for the majority of the patient's day. Although the amount of food consumed that is labeled a binge episode is subjective, the criteria for BN requires other measures such as the feeling of being out of control during the binge (see Table 8-4).

The diagnostic criteria for this disorder focuses on the binge/purge behavior; however, much of the time, the person with BN is restricting her or his diet. The dietary restriction can be the physiological or psychological trigger to subsequent binge eating. Also, the trauma of breaking "the rules" by eating something other than what was intended or more than what was intended may lead to self-destructive binge/purge eating behavior. Any sensation of stomach fullness may trigger the person to purge. Common purging methods consist of self-induced vomiting (with or without the use of syrup of ipecac) and other compensatory behaviors including laxative use, diuretic use, and excessive exercise.[87] After purging, the patient may feel some initial relief, which is often followed by feelings of guilt and shame. However, resuming normal eating commonly leads to gastrointestinal complaints such as bloating, constipation, and flatulence. This physical discomfort, as well as the guilt from bingeing, often results in the patient trying to get back on track by restricting once again. The binge/purge behavior is often a means for the person to regulate and manage emotions and to medicate psychological pain.

Medical Symptoms

In the initial assessment, it is important to assess and evaluate for medical conditions that may play a role in the purging behavior. Conditions such as gastroesophageal reflux (GER) and *Helicobacter pylori* may increase the pain and the need for the patient to vomit. Medical interventions for these conditions may help in reducing the vomiting and allow the treatment for BN to be more focused. Nutritional abnormalities for patients with BN depend on the amount of restriction during the nonbinge episodes. It is important to note that purging behaviors do not completely prevent the utilization of calories from the binge; an average retention of 1200 calories occurs from binges of various sizes and contents.[36]

Muscle weakness, fatigue, cardiac arrhythmias, dehydration, and electrolyte imbalance can be caused by purging, especially self-induced vomiting and laxative abuse. It is common to see hypokalemia and hypochloremic alkalosis as well as gastrointestinal problems involving the stomach and esophagus. Some patients may have calluses on one or both hands around the knuckles (Russell signs). This is caused from the teeth hitting the hand when patients use their fingers to induce vomiting. Dental erosion from self-induced vomiting can be quite serious. Although laxatives are used to purge calories, they are quite ineffective. Chronic ipecac use has been shown to cause skeletal myopathy, electrocardiographic changes, and cardiomyopathy with consequent congestive heart failure, arrhythmia, and sudden death.[37,50]

Medical and Nutritional Management of Bulimia Nervosa

As with AN, interdisciplinary team management is essential to care for BN. The majority of patients with BN are treated in an outpatient setting. Indications for inpatient hospitalization include severe disabling symptoms that are unresponsive to outpatient treatment or additional medical problems such as uncontrolled vomiting, severe laxative abuse withdrawal, metabolic abnormalities or vital sign changes, or suicidal ideations.[61]

The primary goal of nutrition therapy intervention is to normalize eating patterns and eliminate chaotic eating habits by recommending three meals a day with snacks as needed. Any weight loss that is achieved would occur as a result of a normalized eating plan and the elimination of bingeing. Helping patients combat food myths often requires specialized nutrition knowledge.[36] Bulimic patients of normal or excess body weight often present with a history of attempts to control weight through severe caloric restriction. Foods become categorized as "good" and "bad" or "safe" and "forbidden." Low-fat foods (e.g., fruits, vegetables, rice cakes, nonfat yogurt) become the staples at meals, leading to decreased satiety at meals and an increased vulnerability to bingeing. Food intake patterns are usually quite rigid, and the patient often believes that this seemingly controlled intake is healthy and is the only way to eat to lose or maintain weight. These unrealistic diet restrictions need to be met with clear guidelines that promote satiety, thereby reducing the risk of bingeing. Specific recommendations for nutrition intervention in BN are shown in **Table 8-9**.

TABLE 8-9 Nutrition Intervention with Bulimia Nervosa

A. General guidelines
  1. Eat regularly planned, nutritionally balanced meals and snacks.
  2. Adequate but not excessive energy intake.
  3. Include warm foods rather than cold or room-temperature foods to increase meal satiety.
  4. Avoid dieting behavior.
  5. Minimize food avoidance.
  6. Increase the variety of foods consumed.
  7. Increase dietary fiber for meal satiety and to aid elimination.
  8. Develop control strategies for high risk situations.

B. Energy intake
  1. 75–100% DRI for age/height/weight at physical activity level (PAL) 1 (sedentary).
  2. Monitor anthropometric status and adjust caloric intake to ensure weight maintenance.
  3. Depending on beginning entry weight, adjust kcal to help patient achieve healthy weight.
  4. Initial plans are around 1500 kcal/day.

C. Macronutrients
  1. Protein
     a. RDA in g/kg/ideal body weight
     b. 15–20% of total kcal
  2. Carbohydrate
     a. 50–55% of total kcal
     b. Fiber to help with constipation
  3. Fat
     a. 20–30% of total kcal

D. Micronutrients
  1. 100% of RDA through food or supplements.

Cognitive-behavioral therapy (CBT) is now a well-established treatment modality for BN. A key component of the CBT process is nutrition education and dietary guidance. Meal planning, assistance with a regular pattern of eating, and rationale for and discouragement of dieting are all included in CBT. Nutrition education consists of teaching about body weight regulation, energy balance, effects of starvation, misconceptions about dieting and weight control, and the physical consequences of purging behavior. Meal planning consists of three meals a day with one to three snacks per day prescribed in a structured fashion to help break the chaotic eating pattern that continues the cycle of bingeing and purging. Caloric intake should initially be based on the maintenance of weight to help prevent hunger because hunger has been shown to substantially increase the susceptibility to bingeing. One of the hardest challenges of normalizing the eating pattern of a person with BN is to expand the diet to include the patient's self-imposed "forbidden" or "feared" foods. CBT provides a structure to plan for and expose patients to these foods from least feared to most feared, while in a safe, structured, supportive environment. This step is critical in breaking the all or none behavior that goes along with the deprive–binge cycle.

Discontinuing purging and normalizing eating patterns are a key focus of treatment. A common symptom of stopping purging is fluid retention. The patient needs education and understanding of this temporary, yet disturbing phenomenon. Education should consist of information about the length of time to expect the fluid retention. It is helpful to provide evidence that the weight gain is not causing body fat mass gain. In some cases, utilization of skinfold measurements to determine body fat percentage may be helpful in determining body composition changes. The patient must also be taught that continual purging or other methods of dehydration such as restricting sodium or using diuretics or laxatives will prolong the fluid retention. If the patient is laxative dependent, a protocol for laxative withdrawal should be implemented to prevent bowel obstruction. The patient should be instructed on a high fiber diet with adequate fluids while the physician monitors the slow withdrawal of laxatives.

Self-monitoring tools can be helpful in revealing to the patient his or her food beliefs and eating patterns. Through recognition of certain harmful or self-defeating thoughts and behaviors, choices can be made to find alternatives. Records or journals should include facts, state of mind, and some reflection about his or her emotional world, for example:

- Type and amount of food eaten
- Time of day
- Degree of hunger (low, medium, high) and fullness (low, medium, high)
- Binge/purge activity

Medication management is more effective in treating BN than AN, especially with patients who present with co-morbid conditions.[57,88] Current evidence cites combined medication management and CBT as most effective in treating BN,[89] although research continues looking at the effectiveness of other methods and combinations of methods of treatment.

Eating Disorders Not Otherwise Specified

The majority of adolescents seeking treatment for an eating disorder do not classify as having AN or BN, and therefore are considered to have EDNOS.[90] The nature and intensity of the medical and nutritional problems and the most effective treatment modality will depend on the severity of impairment and the symptoms. These patients may have met all criteria for anorexia except that they have not missed three consecutive menstrual periods. Or, they may be of normal weight and purge without bingeing. Although the patient may not present with medical complications, they do often present with medical concerns.

EDNOS also includes binge eating disorder (BED) (see Table 8-4), in which the patient has bingeing behavior without the compensatory purging seen in BN. It is estimated that prevalence of this disorder is 1–2% of the population. Binge episodes must occur at least twice a week and have occurred for at least 6 months. Most patients diagnosed with BED are overweight and suffer the same medical problems faced by the nonbingeing obese population, such as diabetes, high blood pressure, high blood cholesterol levels, gallbladder disease, heart disease, and certain types of cancer.

The patient with BED often presents with weight management concerns rather than eating disorder concerns. Although researchers are still trying to find the treatment that is most helpful in controlling binge eating disorder, many treatment manuals exist utilizing the CBT model shown effective for BN.[91–93]

Populations at High Risk

Specific population groups who focus on food or thinness, such as athletes, models, culinary professionals, and young people who may be required to limit their food intake because of a disease state, are at risk for developing an eating disorder. Additionally, risks for developing an eating disorder may stem from predisposing factors such as a family history of mood, anxiety, or substance abuse disorders. A family history of an eating disorder or obesity, and precipitating factors such as the dynamic interactions among family members and societal pressures to be thin, are additional risk factors.[94] Eating disorders are becoming increasingly common in athletes in particular due to increased physiologic demands imposed by high-intensity and high-volume sports training. Thirty-three percent of males and 62% of females are estimated to have experienced some type of eating disorder.[95]

Female Athlete Triad

The female athlete triad summarizes the symptoms that many female athletes experience (**Table 8-10**). It can impact all physically active females, not just elite competitors.[96] However, numerous studies have shown a higher rate of food restriction, vomiting, diuretic use, and other purging methods among female athletes involved in weight-sensitive sports such as gymnastics, swimming, figure skating, rowing, and long-distance running. This type of weight control behavior may be practiced during the particular sport's season or year round.[68,97,98] The three components of the triad are energy availability, menstrual function, and BMD. Clinical manifestations of the triad can be eating disorders, amenorrhea, and/or osteoporosis. It is important for

TABLE 8-10 Common Signs and Symptoms of Female Athlete Triad

- Irregular or absent menstrual cycles
- Chronic fatigue
- Difficulty sleeping
- Frequent or recurrent stress fractures or injuries
- Restriction of food intake
- Eating less than needed in an effort to improve performance or physical appearance
- Constant effort to be thin
- Cold hands and feet
- Electrolyte abnormalities

Source: Gable KA. Special Nutrition Concerns for the Female Athlete. *Current Med Reports*. 2006;5:187–191.

athletes to maintain a positive energy balance. Energy balance compares the amount of calories a patient consumes to the amount he or she expends during physical activity.

Early intervention is the key to preventing female athletes from developing the triad. In order to prevent eating disorders in the athlete population it is important to educate parents, athletes, coaches, and trainers on adequate nutrition. Proper screening for eating disorders should be done annually during preperformance physicals.[99,100] Even if an athlete is experiencing only one or two of the three symptoms upon examination, she may still be at risk for other long-term health problems. A multidisciplinary approach is generally the most effective form of treatment. It is important to stress to the athlete that the eating disorder can impair athletic performance, increase injury risk, and lead to other serious medical complications.[68,101–103]

Eating Disorders in the Male Population

The prevalence of formally diagnosable AN and BN in males is accepted to be from 5% to 10% of all patients with an eating disorder. Young men who develop AN are usually members of subgroups that emphasize weight loss. Sport-specific eating behaviors are more common in men. The male anorexic is more likely to have been obese before the onset of symptoms. Dieting may have been in response to past teasing or criticisms about his weight. Additionally, the association between dieting and sports activity is stronger among males. Both a dietary and activity history should be taken, with special emphasis on body image, performance, and sports participation on the part of the male patient. These same young men should be screened for androgenic steroid use. The DSM-IV diagnostic criterion for AN of < 85th percentile of ideal body weight is less useful in males. A focus on the BMI, nonlean body mass (body fat percentage), and the height–weight ratio are far more useful in assessing a male with an eating disorder. Adolescent males below the 25th percentile for BMI, upper arm circumference, and subscapular and triceps skinfold thicknesses should be considered to be in an unhealthy, malnourished state.[104–107]

Conclusion

Although more research is needed in the treatment of eating disorders, some general strategies to protect adolescents from developing an eating disorder or an obsession with weight include the following:

- Promote the acceptance of a broad range of appearances.
- Promote positive self-image and body image.
- Educate adolescents and their families about the detrimental consequences of a negative focus on weight.
- Educate school personnel, including coaches, on risk factors and symptoms for early identification of eating disorders.
- Promote a positive focus on sources of self-esteem other than physical appearance, such as academic, artistic, or athletic accomplishments.
- Promote healthy eating and normal food patterns and behaviors.
- Promote adequate (not excessive) physical activity.

Case Study

Nutrition Assessment

Patient and family history: Adam is a 12-year-old white male who presents in clinic today with complaints of stomach pain for > 6 months. Family history reveals that his parents have been divorced for approximately 1 year and he is not able to see his father as often as he would like. Because of the divorce, mom and Adam have moved to a new neighborhood and mom often works late and is unable to prepare home-cooked meals on a regular basis. Adam is not allowed to cook when mom is not at home. Mother has just recently been diagnosed with diabetes and his father is overweight and has hypertension. His mother is concerned about Adam's rapid weight gain but feels the new neighborhood is not safe and does not allow Adam to be outdoors unsupervised. He watches TV or plays video games after school. Adam's main concern is stomach pain, although he does identify concerns about his weight gain.

Food/nutrition-related history: Diet history shows an average intake of 3100 kcal (range 2900–3400). Average protein intake is 90 g/day (range 60–120 g/day). Fat intake is approximately 37% of total kcal. Fiber intake is approximately 14 g/day. Average intake of calcium is approximately 1000 mg/day, iron 14 mg/day, and sodium 3800 mg/day from food. Estimated beverage intake is ~ 40 oz/day of sweetened beverages. Physical activity history reveals TV viewing/computer games 3–4 hours/day.

Anthropometric Measurements

Height: 64.5 inches (156 cm)

Weight: 130 lbs (59 kg)

BMI: 21.9 (85th–90th percentile)

One year ago, Adam was 62″ (157.5 cm) and 100 lbs (45.45 kg). His BMI was 18.2 (50th–75th percentile). Patient has had a 30-pound weight gain over the past year. Sexual Maturity Rating or Tanner State 2. Blood pressure and heart rate are normal for age and height. Bowel history shows two bowel movements per week.

Nutrition Diagnoses

There could be many nutrition diagnoses which may include lack of physical activity, high level of physical inactivity, unhealthy snacking, high intake of sugar sweetened beverages.

Intervention Goals

The overall goal of treatment is to decrease overall caloric intake and increase activity to maintain current weight until appropriate height for weight is achieved. Increasing fluid and fiber intake will address the patient's concern of constipation.

Monitoring and Evaluation

The expert committee recommends monthly follow-up for children in stage 2 treatment. The patient and his mother should be encouraged to monitor suggestions and return for weight checks and nutrition counseling to ensure BMI maintenance or BMI trending downward during growth spurt. Weight loss is not necessarily recommended.

Questions for the Reader

1. What does Adam's BMI percentile mean? Where was he 1 year ago?
2. What are Adam's energy needs and protein needs?
3. What factors are affecting nutrient and physical activity requirements?
4. Write at least one PES statement for this patient.
5. Identify interventions in at least two domains of nutrition intervention to use in counseling Adam and his mother.

Nutrition Documentation Form

ASSESSMENT: Summary of subjective and objective data from chart review and interview.

Age: 12	**Sex:** Male	**Family health hx:** Mother has diabetes, father overweight and hypertensive
Ht: 64.5″ (156 cm)	**Wt:** 130 lb (59 kg)	**BMI:** 85th to 90th percentile—overweight; 1 year ago in normal weight range
Estimated nutritional needs: Energy: 2200–2500 kcal/day; protein: ~45–55 g/day; calcium: 1300 mg/day; fiber: 20–30 g/day. SMR level of 2 indicates that growth spurt has not yet started; opportune time to affect BMI as height changes.		
Intake: Average of 3100 kcal per day, 90 g protein, 37% of calories from fat, 14 g fiber, 1000 mg calcium, 14 mg iron, 3800 mg sodium. Fast food two times/week; sweetened beverages (~40 oz per day) and two or less servings of fruit and vegetables/day; no whole grain servings/day. Access to fresh fruits and vegetables and ability to prepare foods is minimal during after school hours before mother arrives home, limited availability of home-prepared meals. Symptoms of constipation may be affected by fiber intake and lack of physical activity.		
Physical activity: PE at school; greater than 3 hours TV/video games per day; after-school activities limited by mother's perception of lack of safety in neighborhood.		
Food allergies or intolerances: None		**Medications/supplements:** None

Nutrition Diagnosis	Signs and Symptoms (As Evidenced By)	Etiology (Related to)	Goals	Planned Interventions
Excessive energy intake	Weight gain of 30 pounds over past year, 500–700 kcal/day above EER	Undesirable food choices and physical inactivity	Decrease daily calorie intake approximately 400–500 kcal/day; BMI maintenance or trending downward.	Provide meal plan to include healthier snacks and lower caloric beverages, and increase fruits and vegetables to five a day.
Physical inactivity	Greater than 3 hours/day of TV/video game use	Unsafe neighborhood and mother's increased work hours	Decrease physical inactivity.	Limit television viewing/computer games to 1–2 hours per day.
Undesirable food choices	Consuming greater than 40 oz sweetened beverages/day	Limited intake of foods consistent with Dietary Guidelines	Limit sweetened beverages to 6–8 oz juice/day.	Work with patient and mom to provide sugar-free drinks and water.
Inadequate fiber intake	Constipation (bowel movements two times per week)	Limited intake of fruits and vegetables and whole grain foods	Increase intake of fiber-rich foods: fruits, vegetables, and whole grains.	Develop with patient a meal plan that includes at least five fruits and vegetables per day, increase high fiber foods, whole grain foods, and healthy snacks.

Follow-up in one month

Date:__________________ **Dietitian**________________________ **Nutrition Provider #**___________________________

REFERENCES

1. Ogden CL, Carroll MD, Curtin LR, Lamb MM, Flegal KM. Prevalence of high body mass index in US children and adolescents, 2007–2008. *JAMA*. 2010;303(3):242–249.
2. Centers for Disease Control and Prevention. Healthy weight. 2008. Available at: http://www.cdc.gov/nccdphp/dnpa/healthy weight. Accessed November 5, 2008.
3. Whitaker RC, Wright JA, Pepe MS, Seidel KD, Dietz WH. Predicting obesity in young adulthood from childhood and prenatal obesity. *New Engl J Med.* 1997;337:869–873.
4. American Academy of Pediatrics. Policy statement: prevention of pediatric overweight and obesity. *Pediatrics.* 2003;112(2):424–430.
5. Freedman DS, Zuguo M, Berenson GS, Srinivasan S, Dietz WH. Risk factors and excess adiposity in very overweight children and adolescents: the Bogalusa Heart Study. *J Pediatr.* 2007;150:12–17.
6. Elamin EM. Asthma and obesity: a real connection or a casual association? *Chest.* 2004;125:1972–1974.
7. Rosen C, Storfer-Isser A, Taylor HG, Kirchner HL, Emancipator J, Redline S. Increased behavioral morbidity in school aged children with sleep-disordered breathing. *Pediatrics.* 2004;114:1640–1648.
8. Mamun A, Lawlor DA, Cramb S, O'Callaghan M, Williams G, Najman J. Do childhood sleeping problems predict obesity in young adulthood? Evidence from a prospective birth cohort study. *Am J Epidemiol.* 2007;166(12):1366–1373.
9. Landhuis CE, Poulton R, Welch D, Hancox RJ. Childhood sleep time and long-term risk for obesity: a 32-year prospective birth cohort study. *Pediatrics.* 2008;122(5):955–960.
10. Sothern MS, Gordon ST, von Almen TK. *Handbook of Pediatric Obesity.* Boca Raton, FL: Taylor and Francis; 2006:38.
11. Weiss R, Dziura J, Burget TS, et al. Obesity and the metabolic syndrome in children and adolescents. *N Engl J Med.* 2004;350:2362–2374.
12. American Diabetes Association. Type 2 diabetes in children and adolescents. *Diabetes Care.* 2000;286:1427–1430.
13. Krebs NF, Himes JH, Jacobson D, Nicklas TA, Guilday P, Styne D. Assessment of child and adolescent overweight and obesity. *Pediatrics*. 2007;120:S193–S288.
14. Barlow SE. Expert committee recommendations regarding the prevention, assessment and treatment of child and adolescent overweight and obesity: summary report. *Pediatrics.* 2007;120:S164–S192.

15. Feld LG, Hyams JS. Childhood obesity. *Consensus Pediatr.* 2007;1(4):1–36.
16. U.S. Department of Health and Human Services. Physical activity guidelines for Americans. Office of Disease Prevention and Health Promotion. 2008. Available at: http://www.health.gov/PAGuidelines/default.aspx. Accessed October 12, 2008.
17. Spear BA, Barlow SE, Ervin C, et al. Recommendations for treatment of child and adolescent overweight and obesity. *Pediatrics.* 2007;120:S254–S288.
18. Centers for Disease Control and Prevention. Youth risk behavior surveillance (YRBS), United States, 2007. *MMWR.* 2008;57:SS-4.
19. Murphy M, Douglass J, Latulippe M, Barr S, Johnson RK, Frye C. Beverages as a source of energy and nutrients in diets of children and adolescents. *FASEBJ.* 2005;19 (3) 434:275.
20. Ebbeling CB, Feldman HA, Osganian SK, Chomitz VR, Ellenbogen SJ, Ludwig DS. Effects of decreasing sugar-sweetened beverage consumption on body weight in adolescents: a randomized controlled pilot study. *Pediatrics.* 2006;117:673–680.
21. American Dietetic Association. What we know about childhood overweight. Evidence Analysis Library. 2009. Available at: http://www.adaevidencelibrary.com. Accessed December 15, 2009.
22. Pereira MA, Ludwig DS. Dietary fiber and body weight regulation: observations and mechanisms. *Pediatr Clin North Am.* 2001;48:969–980.
23. Guthrie JF, Lin BH, Frazao E. Role of food prepared away from home in the American diet, 1977–78 versus 1994–96: changes and consequences. *J Nutr Educ Behav.* 2002;34(3):140–150.
24. Diliberti N, Bordi PL, Conklin MT, Roe LS, Rolls BJ. Increased portion size leads to increased energy intake in a restaurant meal. *Obes Res.* 2004;12(3):562–568.
25. McConahy KL, Smiciklas-Wright H, Mitchell DC, Picciano MF. Portion size of common foods predicts energy intake among preschool-aged children. *J Am Diet Assoc.* 2004;104(6):975–979.
25. Resnicow K, Davis R, Rollnick S. Motivation interviewing for pediatric obesity: conceptual issues and evidence review. *J Am Diet Assoc.* 2006;106:2024–2033.
26. Davis MM, Gance-Cleveland B, Hassink S, Johnson R, Paradis G, Resincow K. Recommendations for prevention of childhood obesity. *Pediatrics.* 2007;120(4):S229–S253.
27. Rollnick S, Miller WR. What is motivational interviewing? *Behav Cogn Psychother.* 1995;23:325–334.
29. Society for Nutrition Education, Weight Realities Division. Guidelines for childhood obesity prevention programs: promoting healthy weight in children. *J Nutr Educ Behav.* 2003;35:1–5.
30. American Academy of Pediatrics. Policy statement. Identifying and treating eating disorders. *Pediatrics.* 2003;111:204–211.
31. Inge TH, Krebs NF, Garcia VF, et al. Bariatric surgery for severely overweight adolescents: concerns and recommendations. *Pediatrics.* 2004;114:217–223.
32. Helmrath MA, Brandt ML, Inge TH. Adolescent obesity and bariatric surgery. *Surg Clin North Am.* 2006;86(2):441–454.
33. Apovian CM, Baker C, Ludwig DS, et al. Best practice guidelines in pediatric/adolescent weight loss surgery. *Obes Res.* 2005;13:274–282.
34. Story M. School-based approaches for preventing and treating obesity. *Int J Obes Relat Metab Disord.* 1999;23:S43–S51.
35. Gonzalez A, Kohn MR, Clarke SD. Eating disorders in adolescents. *Aust Fam Physician.* 2007;36(8):614–619.
36. American Dietetic Association. Position of the American Dietetic Association: nutrition intervention in the treatment of anorexia nervosa, bulimia nervosa, and other eating disorders. *J Am Diet Assoc.* 2006;106(12):2073.
37. Rock CL. Nutritional and medical assessment and management of eating disorders. *Nutr Clin Care.* 1999;2:332–343.
38. Kreipe RE, Durkarm CP. Outcome of anorexia nervosa related to treatment utilizing an adolescent medicine approach. *J Youth Adolesc.* 1996;25:483–497.
39. Gralen SJ, Levin MP, Smolak L. Dieting and disordered eating during early and middle adolescence: do the influences remain the same? *Int J Eating Disord.* 1990;9:501–512.
40. Kreipe RE, Birndorf DO. Eating disorders in adolescents and young adults. *Medical Clin North Am.* 2000;84(4):1027–1049.
41. Rome ES. Children and adolescents with eating disorders: the state of the art. *Pediatrics.* 2003;111(1):e98.
42. American Psychiatric Association. Practice guidelines for the treatment of patients with eating disorders. *Am J Psychol.* 2000;157(Suppl):1–39.
43. Gowers SG. Management of eating disorders in children and adolescents. *Arch Dis Child.* 2008;93(4):331.
44. Bryant-Waugh R, Markham L, Kreipe RE, Walsh BT. Feeding and eating disorders in childhood. *Int J Eat Disord.* 2010;43(2): 98–111.
45. Patrick LL. Eating disorders: a review of the literature with emphasis on medical complications and clinical nutrition. *Alt Med Rev.* 2002;7(3):184.
46. Fisher M, Golden NH, Datzman KD, et al. Eating disorders in adolescents: a background paper. *J Adolesc Health Care.* 1995;16:420–437.
47. Becker AE, Grinspoon SK, Klibanski A, Herzog DB. Current concepts: eating disorders. *N Engl J Med.* 1999;340(14):1092–1098.
48. Rosen DS. Eating disorders in children and young adolescents: etiology, classification, clinical features, and treatment. *Adolesc Med.* 2003;14(1):49.
49. Katzman DK, Zipursky RB. Adolescents with anorexia nervosa: the impact of the disorder on bones and brains. *Ann N Y Acad Sci.* 1997;817:127–137.
50. Harris JP, Kriepe RE, Rossback CN. QT prolongation by isoproterenol in anorexia nervosa. *J Adolesc Health.* 1993;14:390–393.
51. Szabo CP. Hospitalized anorexics and resistance training: impact on body composition and psychological well-being. A preliminary study. *Eating Weight Disord.* 2002;7(4):293.
52. Strober M, Freeman R, Morrell W. The long-term course of severe anorexia nervosa in adolescents: survival analysis of recovery, relapse and outcome predictors over 10–15 years in a prospective study. *Int J Eating Disord.* 1997;22:339–369.
53. Misra MM. Alterations in growth hormone secretory dynamics in adolescent girls with anorexia nervosa and effects on bone metabolism. *J Clin Endocrinol Metab.* 2003;88(12):5615.
54. Misra MM. Alterations in cortisol secretory dynamics in adolescent girls with anorexia nervosa and effects on bone metabolism. *J Clin Endocrinol Metab.* 2004;89(10):4972.
55. Ressler A. A body to die for: eating disorders and body-image distortion in women. *Int J Fertil Womens Med.* 1998;43(3):133–138.

56. Rodin GG. Eating disorders in young women with type 1 diabetes mellitus. *J Psychosom Res.* 2002;53(4):943.
57. Hammond KA. Dietary and clinical assessment. In: Mahan K, Escott-Stump S, eds. *Krause's Food, Nutrition and Diet Therapy,* 11th ed. Philadelphia: Saunders; 2004: 407–435.
58. Swenne I. Heart risk associated with weight loss in anorexia nervosa and eating disorders: electrocardiographic changes during the early phase of refeeding. *Acta Paediatr.* 2000;89:447–452.
60. Jayasinghe Y. Current concepts in bone and reproductive health in adolescents with anorexia nervosa. *Br J Obstet Gynaecol.* 2008;115(3):304.
61. Sturdevant MS, Spear BA. Eating disorders and obesity. In: Burg F, Ingelfinger J, Polin R, Gershon A. *Current Pediatric Therapy.* Philadelphia, PA: Saunders; 2006:334–336.
62. Nudel DB, Gootman N, Nussbaum MP, Shenker IR. Altered exercise performance in patients with anorexia nervosa. *J Pediatr.* 1984;105:34–42.
63. Schebendach J, Reichert-Anderson P. Nutrition in eating disorders. In: Mahan K, Escott-Stump S, eds. *Kraus's Nutrition and Diet Therapy.* New York: McGraw-Hill; 2000:594-615.
64. Benini LL. Gastric emptying in patients with restricting and binge/purging subtypes of anorexia nervosa. *Am J Gastroenterol.* 2004;99(8):1448.
65. Chui HT. Cognitive function and brain structure in females with a history of adolescent-onset anorexia nervosa. *Pediatrics.* 2008;122(2):e426.
66. Cooke RA, Chambers JB. Anorexia nervosa and the heart. *Br J Hosp Med.* 1995;54:313–317.
67. Lantzouni E, Frank GR, Golden NH, Shenker RI. Reversibility of growth stunting in early onset anorexia nervosa: a prospective study. *J Adolesc Health.* 2002;31:162–165.
68. American College of Sports Medicine. American College of Sports Medicine position stand. The female athlete triad. *Med Sci Sports Exerc.* 2007;39(10):1867.
69. Bachrach LK, Guido D, Datzman C. Decreased bone density in adolescent girls with anorexia nervosa. *Pediatrics.* 1990;86:440–447.
70. Biller BMK, Saxe V, Herzog DB. Mechanisms of osteoporosis in adult and adolescent women with anorexia nervosa. *J Clin Endocrinol Metab.* 1989;68:548–554.
71. Mehler PS. Treatment of osteopenia and osteoporosis in anorexia nervosa: a systematic review of the literature. *Int J Eating Disord.* 2009;42(3):195.
72. Bachrach LK, Katzman DK, Litt JF, Buido D, Marcus R. Recovery from osteopenia in adolescent girls with anorexia nervosa. *J Clin Endocrinol Metab.* 1991;72:602–606.
73. Carmichael KA, Carmichael DI. Bone metabolism and osteopenia in eating disorders. *Medicine.* 1995;74:254–267.
74. Robinson E, Bachrach KL, Katzman DK. Use of hormone replacement therapy to reduce the risk of osteopenia in adolescent girls with anorexia nervosa. *J Adolesc Health.* 2000;26:343–348.
75. Hütter G. The hematology of anorexia nervosa. *Int J Eating Disord.* 2009;42(4):293.
76. Ohwada R, Hotta M, Oikawa S, Takano K. Etiology of hypercholesterolemia in patients with anorexia nervosa. *Int J Eat Disord.* 2006;39(7):598–601.
77. Probst M. Body composition in female anorexia nervosa patients. *Br J Nutr.* 1996;76:639–644.
78. Kennedy A. Iron status and haematological changes in adolescent female inpatients with anorexia nervosa. *J Paediatr Child Health.* 2004;40(8):430.
79. Wilson GT. Cognitive behavior therapy for eating disorder: progress and problems. *Behavior Research Ther.* 1999;37(Suppl 1): S79–S95.
80. Durnin JVGA, Rahaman MM. The assessment of the amount of body fat in the human body from measurements of skinfold thickness. *Br J Nutr.* 1967;21:681–685.
81. Kerruish KP. Body composition in adolescents with anorexia nervosa. *Am J Clin Nutr.* 2002;75(1):31.
82. Birmingham CL. The reliability of bioelectrical impedance analysis for measuring changes in the body composition of patients with anorexia nervosa. *Int J Eating Disord.* 1996;19: 311–313.
83. Scalfi L. Bioimpedance and resting energy expenditure in undernourished and refed anorectic patients. *Eur J Clin Nutr.* 1993;47:61–68.
84. Kirkley BG. Bulimia: clinical characteristics, development and etiology. *J Am Diet Assoc.* 1986;86:468–475.
85. Haiman C, Devlin MJ. Binge eating before the onset of dieting: a distinct subgroup of bulimia nervosa. *Int J Eating Disord.* 1999;25:151–157.
85. Heatherington MM, Altemus M, Nelson ML. Eating behavior in bulimia nervosa: multiple meal analyses. *Am J Clin Nutr.* 1994;60:864–873.
87. Shapiro JR. Bulimia nervosa treatment: a systematic review of randomized controlled trials. *Int J Eating Disord.2007* 40(4): 321.
50. Society for Adolescent Medicine. Eating disorders in adolescents: a position paper of the Society of Adolescent Medicine. *J Adolesc Health.* 200333:496–503.
88. Boardley D. The treatment of eating disorders: role of the dietitian. *Academy for Eating Disorders Newsletter.* Winter 2000;1-4.
89. Sysko R, Hildebrandt T. Cognitive-behavioural therapy for individuals with bulimia nervosa and a co-occurring substance use disorder. *Eur Eat Disord Rev.* 2009;17(2):89–100.
90. Eddy J, Kamryn TK. Eating disorder not otherwise specified in adolescents. *J Am Acad Child Adolesc Psychiatry.* 2008;47(2):156.
91. Grilo CM. The assessment and treatment of binge eating disorder. *J Practical Psychiatry Behav Health.* 1998;4:191–201.
92. Williamson DA, Martin CK. Binge eating disorder: a review of the literature after publication of the DSM-IV. *Eating Weight Disord Stud Anorexia Bulimia Obes.* 1999;4(3):103–114.
93. Goldfein JA, Devlin JH, Spitzer RL. Cognitive behavioral therapy for the treatment of binge eating disorder: what constitutes success? *Int J Eating Disord* 2000;157(7):1051–1056.
94. Woodside DB, Field LL, Garfinkel PE, Heinman M. Specificity of eating disorders diagnoses in families of probands with anorexia nervosa and bulimia nervosa. *Compr Psychiatry.* 1998;39(5):261–264.
95. Bonci CM. National athletic trainers' association position statement: preventing, detecting, and managing disordered eating in athletes. *J Athletic Train.* 2008;43(1):80.
96. Hobart JA, Smucker DR. The female athlete triad. American Academy of Family Physicians. Available at: http://www.aafp.org/afp/20000601/3357.html. Accessed October 11, 2007.

97. Sanborn CF, Horea M, Simers BJ, Dieringer KL. Disordered eating and the female athlete triad. *Clin Sports Med Athletic Woman*. 2000;19:199–213.
98. Otis C. *The Athletic Women's Survival Guide*. Indianapolis, IN: Human Kinetics; 2000.
99. American Academy of Pediatrics Committee on Sports Medicine and Fitness. Promotion of healthy weight-control practices in young athletes. *Pediatrics*. 2005;116:1557–1564.
100. Gable KA. Special nutritional concerns for the female athlete. *Curr Sports Med Reports*. 2006;5:187–191.
101. International Olympic Committee Medical Commission. Working group on women in sport: position stand on the female athlete triad. Available at: http://multimedia.olympic.org/pdf/en_report_917.pdf. Accessed January 4, 2010.
102. Cabera D. *Eating Disorders across the Lifespan*. Remuda Ranch Program for Eating Disorders; Wickenburg, AZ, 2007.
103. Hoch AZ. Prevalence of the female athlete triad in high school athletes and sedentary students. *Clin J Sport Med*. 2009;19(5):421.
104. Farrow JA. The adolescent male with an eating disorder. *Pedia Ann*. 1992;21:769–773.
105. Carlat DJ, Camargo CA, Herzog DB. Eating disorders in males: a report on 135 patients. *Am J Psychiatry*. 1997;154(8):1127–1132.
106. Braun D., Sunday SR, Huang A, Halmi KA. More males seek treatment for eating disorders. *Int J Eating Disord*. 1999;25(4):415–424.
107. Ogden CL, Carroll MD, Flegal KM. High body mass index for age among US children and adolescents, 2003–2006. *JAMA*. 2008;299(20):2401–2405.

Genetic Screening and Nutrition Management

Phyllis B. Acosta

Introduction

Nutrition support of infants and children with inborn errors of metabolism (IEMs) requires in-depth knowledge of metabolic processes; the science and application of nutrition, growth, and development; and food science. When providing nutrition support for patients with inborn errors, the specific nutrient needs of each patient, based on individual genetic and biochemical constitution, must be considered. Nutrient requirements established for normal populations[1] may not apply to individuals with IEMs.[2] Some chemical compounds, normally not considered essential because they can be synthesized de novo, may not be synthesized in patients with a metabolic defect. Consequently, dependent on the inborn error, the subsequent organ damage that accrues, and the rate of loss of specific chemicals from the body, several compounds become conditionally essential. Among these are the amino acids arginine,[3] carnitine,[4] cystine,[5] and tyrosine[6] and the "vitamin" tetrahydrobiopterin (BH_4).[7] Failure to adapt nutrient intakes to the needs of each patient can result in mental retardation, metabolic crises, neurological crises, growth failure, and with some inborn errors, death. Quality care is best achieved by an experienced team of specialists in a genetic/metabolic center.[8]

This chapter addresses newborn screening for IEMs; principles and practical considerations in nutrition support of IEMs first suspected by newborn screening[9,10] and later diagnosed by appropriate methods; nutrition support of these disorders of amino acid, nitrogen, carbohydrate, and fatty acid metabolism; selected areas needing further research; and roles and functions of the dietitian in nutrition support of IEMs. For a detailed guide to nutrition support, see the *Nutrition Management of Patients with Inherited Metabolic Disorders*.[11]

Newborn Screening

The American College of Medical Genetics recommends the core panel for screening newborns and includes tests for 24 inherited metabolic disorders in which nutrition management is important (see **Table 9-1**). Twenty-four metabolic disorders that are secondary targets include some for which it is as yet unknown whether diet therapy will be beneficial (see Table 9-1). Disorders in the core panel were chosen based on (1) availability and sensitivity of a specific screening test that can be carried out within 24 to 48 hours after birth, (2) efficacious therapy, and (3) adequate knowledge of the natural history of the disease.[9,10] Diseases in the secondary target are conditions essential in the differential diagnosis of a disorder in the core panel. Differential diagnosis by other analytes, enzymes, or mutation analysis is necessary for appropriate therapy, including nutrition management, to prevent the disastrous effects of many IEMs. Marker analytes for disorders recommended for newborn screening by mass spectrometry (MS/MS) are noted in Table 9-1.[10]

Many other IEMs are known for which newborn screening does not occur. These may be diagnosed at a later age by clinical symptoms, and diet therapy may be used to ameliorate or prevent worsening of symptoms.[11] However, early identification, diagnosis, and treatment are essential to prevent the disastrous effects of IEMs.

Principles and Practical Considerations in Nutrition Support

Principles of Nutrition Support

This section discusses a number of approaches to nutrition support of IEMs. The appropriate approach is dependent on the biochemistry and pathophysiology of disease expression. Several therapeutic strategies may be used simultaneously:[2]

- *Enhancing anabolism and depressing catabolism:* This involves the use of high-energy feeds; appropriate amounts of amino acid mixtures, carbohydrates, and fats; and administration of insulin, if needed. Fasting

TABLE 9-1 Core and Secondary Targets of Inborn Errors of Metabolism Recommended for Newborn Screening and Marker Analytes Used with MS/MS Screening

Inborn Error	Marker Analyte
Core Targets	
Amino Acid Disorders	
Argininosuccinic acidemia (ASA)	Citrulline (CIT)
Citrullinemia (CIT)	CIT
Homocystinuria (HCY)	Methionine (MET)
Maple syrup urine disease (MSUD)	Leucine (LEU) ± Valine (VAL)
Phenylketonuria (PKU)	Phenylalanine (PHE), PHE/Tyrosine (TYR)
Tyrosinemia type I (TYR I)	TYR
Fatty Acid Oxidation Disorders	
Carnitine uptake deficiency (CUD)	C[a]O[b]
Long-chain-hydroxy-acyl-CoA dehydrogenase deficiency (LCHAD)	C16-OH[c]; C[a]18:1[d]-OH
Medium-chain acyl-CoA dehydrogenase deficiency (MCAD)	C[a]8/C[a]10 ± C[a]6, C[a]10:1, C8[a]
Trifunctional protein deficiency (TFP)	C[a]16-OH, C[a]18:1-OH
Very-long-chain acyl-CoA dehydrogenase deficiency (VLCAD)	C14:1, C14:1/C12:1 (± C14, C16, C18:1)
Organic Acid Disorders	
β-ketothiolase deficiency (BKT)[e]	C[a]5:1, ± C[a]5OH[c]
β-methylcrotonyl-CoA carboxylase deficiency (3MCC)[e]	C[a]5-OH[c], ± [a]C5:1
Cobalamin A and B defects (Cbl A, B)[e]	C[a]3, C[a]3/C[a]2
Glutaric acidemia type I (GA I)[e]	C[a]5-DC[f]
HMG-CoA lyase deficiency (HMG)[e]	C[a]5-OH, ± C[a]6-DC[f]
Isovaleric acidemia (IVA)[e]	C[a]5
Methylmalonic acidemia (MUT)[e]	C[a]3, C[a]3/C[a]2
Multiple carboxylase deficiency (MCT)[e]	C[a]5-OH, ± C[a]3
Propionic acidemia (PROP)[e]	C[a]3, C[a]3/C[a]2
Other Disorders	
Biotinidase deficiency (BIOT)[e]	± C[c]5-OH[c], C[a]5:1
Cystic fibrosis (CF)	
Galactose-1-phosphate uridyltransferase deficiency (GALT)[g]	
Secondary Targets	
Amino Acid Disorders	
Argininemia (ARG)	ARG
Biopterin regeneration deficiency (Biopt REG)	PHE, PHE/TYR
Biopterin synthesis defect (BS)	PHE, PHE/TYR
Citrin deficiency (CIT II)	CIT
Hypermethioninemia (MET)	MET
Hyperphenylalaninemia (Hyper-PHE)	PHE
Tyrosinemia type II (TYR II)	TYR
Tyrosinemia type III (TYR III)	TYR
Fatty Acid Oxidation Disorders	
Carnitine acylcarnitine transporter defect (CACT)	C[a]16:1; C[a]18:1
Carnitine palmitoyltransferase I defect (CPT IA)	Carnitine
Carnitine palmitoyltransferase II defect (CPT II)	C[a]16:1, C[a]18:1
Dienoyl-CoA reductase deficiency (DE RED)	
Glutaric acidemia type II (GA2)[e]	C[a]4, C[a]5, C[a]5-DC[d], C[a]6, 8, 12, 14, 16
Medium-chain ketoacyl-CoA thiolase deficiency (MCKAT)	C[a]8, C[a]8/C[a]10, ± C[a]6, C[a]10:1
Medium-/short-chain hydroxy-acyl-CoA dehydrogenase deficiency (M/SCHAD)	C[a]4-OH[c]
Short-chain acyl-CoA dehydrogenase deficiency (SCAD)	C[a]4

Organic Acid Disorders	
α-methyl-β-hydroxy-butyric acidemia (2M3HBA)[e]	C^a5, $C^a5:1$, C^a5-OH[c]
α-methylbutyryl-CoA dehydrogenase deficiency[e] (2MBG)	C^a5
β-methylglutaconyl hydratase deficiency (3MGA)[e]	C^a5-OH[c]
Cobalamin C and D defects (Cbl C, D)[e]	C^a3/C^a2
Isobutyryl-CoA dehydrogenase deficiency (IBG)[e]	C^a4
Malonic acidemia (MAL)	C^a3
Other Disorders	
Galactokinase deficiency (GALK)[g]	
Galactose epimerase deficiency (GALE)[g]	

a. C = acyl group or carbon chain.

b. O = number of carbons: 0 to 18.

c. OH = hydroxy.

d. Colon (:) followed by number represents double bonds.

e. One or more amino acids involved in disorder.

f. DC = dicarboxyl.

g. Screened for by measuring blood galactose.

Sources: American College of Medical Genetics. Newborn screening: toward a uniform screening panel and system. *Genet Med.* 2006;8(Suppl 1):1S–252S; Chace DH, Lim T, Hansen CR, Adam BW, Hannon WH. Quantification of malonylcarnitine in dried blood spots by use of MS/MS varies by stable isotope internal standard composition. *Clin Chim Acta.* 2009;402(1–2):14–18; Frazier DM. Newborn screening by mass spectrometry. In Acosta PB, ed. *Nutrition Management of Patients with Inherited Metabolic Disorders.* Sudbury, MA: Jones and Bartlett Publishers; 2010:21–67; Gillingham MB. Nutrition management of patients with inherited disorders of mitochondrial fatty acid oxidation. In Acosta PB, ed. *Nutrition Management of Patients with Inherited Metabolic Disorders*. Sudbury, MA: Jones and Bartlett Publishers; 2010:369–403; Korman SH. Inborn errors of isoleucine degradation. *Mol Genet Metab.* 2006;89:289–299; Matalon KM. Introduction to genetics and genetics of inherited metabolic disorders. In Acosta PB, ed. *Nutrition Management of Patients with Inherited Metabolic Disorders*. Sudbury, MA: Jones and Bartlett Publishers; 2010:1–19; Miinalainen IJ, Schmitz W, Huotari A, et al. Mitochondrial 2, 4-dienoyl-CoA reductase deficiency in mice results in severe hypoglycemia with stress intolerance and unimpaired ketogenesis. *PLoS Genet.* 2009;5:e1000543; Molven A, Matre GE, Duran M, et al. Familial hyperinsulinemia and hypoglycemia caused by a defect in the SCHAD enzyme of mitochondrial fatty acid oxidation. *Diabetes.* 2004;53:221–227; and Sim KG, Wiley V, Carpenter K, et al. Carnitine palmitoyltransferase I deficiency in neonate identified by dried blood spot free carnitine and acylcarnitine profile. *J Inherit Metab Dis*. 2001;24:51–59.

should be prevented. This therapeutic maneuver is important to the management of all inborn errors involving catabolic pathways.

- *Correcting the primary imbalance in metabolic relationships:* This correction reduces accumulated toxic substrate(s) through diet restriction. Examples for which this is used are phenylketonuria (PKU),[12] maple syrup urine disease (MSUD),[13] galactosemia,[14] and mitochondrial medium-chain, long-chain, and very-long-chain fatty acid oxidation[15] defects where phenylalanine; leucine, isoleucine, and valine; galactose; and long-chain fatty acids are limited, respectively.
- *Providing alternate metabolic pathways to decrease accumulated toxic precursors in blocked reaction sequences:* For example, innocuous isovalerylglycine is formed from accumulating isovaleric acid if supplemental glycine is provided to drive glycine-N-transacylase.[13] Isovalerylglycine is excreted in the urine.
- *Supplying products of blocked primary pathways:* Some examples are arginine in most disorders of the urea cycle,[3] cystine in homocystinuria,[5,16] tyrosine in PKU,[6,12] and BH_4[7] in biopterin synthesis defects.
- *Supplementing conditionally essential nutrients:* Examples are carnitine,[4] cystine,[5,16] and tyrosine[6] in secondary liver disease or with excess excretion of carnitine in organic acidemias.[17]
- *Stabilizing altered enzyme proteins:* The rate of biologic synthesis and degradation of holoenzymes is dependent on their structural conformation. In some holoenzymes, saturation by a coenzyme increases their biologic half-life and, thus, overall enzyme activity at the new equilibrium. This therapeutic mechanism is illustrated in homocystinuria and MSUD. Pharmacologic intake of pyridoxine in homocystinuria[16] and of thiamine in MSUD[2,13] increases intracellular pyridoxal phosphate and thiamine pyrophosphate, respectively, and increases the specific activity of any functional cystathionine β-synthase and branched-chain α-ketoacid dehydrogenase complex, respectively. BH_4 is available for use in patients with

non-PKU hyperphenylalaninemia (HPA or mild PKU) to enhance phenylalanine hydroxylase activity.[18]

- *Replacing deficient coenzymes:* Many vitamin-dependent disorders are due to blocks in coenzyme production and are "cured" by pharmacologic intake of a specific vitamin precursor. This mechanism presumably involves overcoming a partially impaired enzyme reaction by mass action. Impaired reactions required to produce methylcobalamin and adenosylcobalamin result in homocystinuria and methylmalonic aciduria/acidemia. Daily intakes of appropriate forms of milligram quantities of vitamin B_{12} may cure the disease.[19]
- *Inducing enzyme production:* If the structural gene or enzyme is intact but suppressor, enhancer, or promoter elements are not functional, abnormal amounts of enzyme may be produced. The structural gene may be "turned on" or "turned off" to enable normal enzymatic production to occur. In the acute porphyria of type I tyrosinemia, excessive δ-aminolevulinic acid (ALA) production may be reduced by suppressing transcription of the δ-ALA synthase gene with excess glucose.[2,20] Another suggested form of enzyme induction may be phenylalanine hydroxylase (PAH) where phenylalanine (PHE) loading with intact protein for 3 days induces a consistent decline in plasma PHE concentration in some patients.[21–25]
- *Supplementing nutrients that are inadequately absorbed or not released from their apoenzyme:* An example is biotin in biotinidase deficiency.[26]
- *Preventing absorption of a nutrient that may be toxic in excess:* Phenylalanine ammonia lyase, a plant enzyme that functions to catabolize PHE, is undergoing clinical studies for possible use in patients with mild PKU.[27] Norleucine, a structural analog of leucine, has been tried in mice with intermediate MSUD as a means of preventing leucine transport to the brain and brain injury.[28] Large neutral amino acids (LNAA) other than PHE are available for preventing absorption of PHE from the intestinal tract and passage across the blood–brain barrier (BBB).[29] Long-term side effects of these high intakes of amino acids have not been studied.

Practical Considerations in Nutrition Support

The primary approach to therapy of patients with an IEM is via nutrition management.

Nutrients

The problem of ensuring adequate nutrition for infants and children with IEMs may be decreased by the use of a protocol or plan for treatment. Each patient requires individualized medical and nutrition care. Diet restrictions required to correct imbalances in some metabolic relationships usually require the use of elemental medical foods. These medical foods are normally supplemented with small amounts of intact protein that supply the restricted nutrient(s). These foods may supply up to 90%, but sometimes less, of the protein requirement of patients with disorders of amino acid or nitrogen metabolism. Other nitrogen-free foods that provide energy are limited in their range of nutrients. Consequently, care must be taken to provide nutrients previously considered to be food contaminants because their essentiality has been demonstrated through long-term use of total parenteral nutrition.[30] Thus, in addition to nutrients for which recommended dietary allowances (RDAs)[1] are established, including fat, linoleic acid, and α-linolenic acid, other nutrients must be supplied in adequate amounts. These include minerals and vitamins. To ensure normal nutrition status indices, most mineral intakes must be greater than RDAs due to poor absorption by patients ingesting elemental diets; they also should be ingested in at least three meals per day for best absorption.[31]

Osmolality

Elemental medical foods used in amino acid disorders consist of small molecules that may result in an osmotic load greater than the physiologic tolerance of the patient. Abdominal cramping, diarrhea, distention, nausea, or vomiting may result from use of hyperosmolar feeds. More serious consequences can occur in infants, such as hypertonic dehydration, hypovolemia, hypernatremia, and death. A mathematical formula for estimating approximate osmolality of medical food mixtures is given in the chapter *Practical Aspects of Nutrition Management.*[32] The neonate should not be fed an elemental formula that contains greater than 450 mOsm/kg water.

Maillard Reaction

Medical foods for inborn errors of amino acid or nitrogen metabolism are formulated from free amino acids, carbohydrates, and often fat, minerals, and vitamins. The Maillard reaction is a complex group of chemical reactions in foods in which reacting amino acids, peptides, and protein condense with sugars, forming bonds for which no digestive enzymes are available. The Maillard reaction is accelerated by heat and is characterized in its initial stage by a light brown color, followed by buff yellow and dark brown in the intermediate and final stages. Caramel-like color and roasted aromas develop. Those who prepare medical foods must be able to recognize the Maillard reaction because it causes loss of some sugars and amino acids. For this reason, medical foods should not be heated beyond 100°F (37.8°C).[33,34]

Introduction of Puréed Foods

Puréed foods (beikost baby foods) should be introduced into the diet at about 4 months of age if the infant shows developmental readiness by a decrease in tongue thrust. Beikost is important in the diet to provide unidentified nutrients and fiber, to enhance the infant's acceptance of a variety of tastes and textures, and, when table foods are eaten, to develop jaw muscles important for speech.[34]

Changes in Nutrition Support Prescription

As soon as nutrition support is well established in an infant or child, the prescription should be fine-tuned frequently. The frequency depends on the age of the child; infants require at least weekly changes in prescription whereas older children who are growing more slowly may not require a diet change more than monthly or every 2 to 3 months. Small, frequent changes in prescription prevent "bouncing" of plasma amino acid, glucose, organic acid, or ammonia concentrations and allow the intake to grow with the child, thus precluding the child's "growing out of the prescription."[34] This fine tuning is especially important in the preteen and teenage years to prevent inadequate intake of nutrients that result in poor linear growth. Pregnant women also require frequent diet changes based on biochemical indices.[34]

Monitoring

Successful management of IEMs requires frequent monitoring, which provides the physician and dietitian data that verify the adequacy of the nutrition support prescription. This data also motivates patient/parents to be compliant with the prescription. Premature and full-term infants to at least 6 months of age require twice weekly monitoring. Thereafter, weekly monitoring may be adequate if the patient is compliant with the diet prescription.

Some centers may wish to draw blood when the patient is fasting to monitor plasma analyte concentrations. Prolonged fasting (over 8 hours) may cause spurious elevations of plasma amino acid concentrations that could lead to unwarranted diet changes,[35] and blood drawn 15 minutes to 1 hour after a meal may also yield spuriously high values[36] in patients with amino acid disorders.

Inborn Errors of Amino Acid Metabolism

Most of the organic acid disorders, both in the core and secondary targets for newborn screening, require restriction of a branched-chain amino acid as part of nutrition management, so all except biotinidase deficiency and malonic acidemia are included in **Tables 9-2 through 9-6** with branched-chain amino acids. Patients with cystic fibrosis are usually treated by a gastroenterologist, and their nutrition management is addressed in Chapter 11, Pulmonary Diseases.

Information in Table 9-2 describes various inborn errors, nutrients to modify, vitamin responsiveness, and medical foods available that contain minerals and vitamins. Data in Table 9-3 outline recommended nutrient intakes for beginning therapy. Table 9-4 describes information on nutrition support during acute illness, medication and nutrient interactions, and nutrition assessment parameters. Sources of medical foods, their ingredients, and their composition may be obtained from information in Table 9-5.

Data outside the parentheses in Table 9-3 describe amounts of amino acids with which to begin nutrition support. For some disorders in which the initial plasma concentration(s) of toxic amino acid is 14 to 20 times the upper limit of the normal reference range, after 2 to 3 days of no intake of the amino acid, it should be introduced with the lowest recommended amount for age in parentheses. Data within the parentheses indicate the possible range of amino acid requirements, depending on the gene mutation and extent of the enzyme deficit. Only frequent monitoring of plasma concentrations of amino acids and other analytes, nutrient intake, and growth can verify the adequacy of intake.[34]

When specific amino acids require restriction, total deletion for 1 to 3 days or until the plasma concentration reaches the upper limit of the reference range is the best approach to initiating therapy. Longer term deletion or overrestriction may precipitate deficiency of the amino acid(s). The most limiting nutrient determines growth rate in all disorders, and overrestriction of an amino acid, nitrogen (N), or energy will result in further intolerance of the toxic nutrient. Results of amino acid and N deficiencies are described in Table 9-6.

Restricted amino acid requirements are based on genotype, age, gender, health status, and amount of total protein fed (intact and protein equivalent = N, g × 6.25 = g protein equivalent from elemental medical food containing free amino acids). For example, patients with PKU may fall into one of the following three classifications depending on genotype:[37]

- *Classical PKU:* Blood/plasma PHE concentration greater than 1200 μmol/L if untreated
- *Mild PKU:* Blood/plasma PHE concentration 600–1199 μmol/L if untreated
- *Non-PKU hyperphenylalaninemia (HPA):* Blood/plasma PHE concentration 120–599 μmol/L if untreated

Patients with classical PKU and some with mild PKU excrete phenylpyruvic acid (PPA) in the urine if the blood/plasma PHE concentration is elevated. According to one group of investigators, PPA excretion occurred when blood PHE concentration was greater than 424 μmol/L.[38] Because of the urinary loss of PPA and mental retardation found in patients with PKU, the disease was initially called imbecillitis phenylpyruvica or phenylpyruvic oligophrenia (little brains because of phenylpyruvic acid).[39]

Other patients with IEMs have variable nutrient requirements based on the same factors as patients with HPA.

TABLE 9-2 Nutrition Support of Inborn Errors of Metabolism

Inborn Error and Defect	Nutrient(s) to Modify	Vitamin Responsive?	Medical Foods Available
Inborn Errors of Amino Acid Metabolism			
Aromatic Amino Acids[2,12]			
Phenylketonuria, classical (phenylalanine hydroxylase)	Restrict PHE, increase TYR, provide protein, mineral, and vitamin intakes greater than RDA.	No	See Table 9-5.
Phenylketonuria, mild (phenylalanine hydroxylase)	Same as for PKU, classical.	±, Yes, BH_4 10–20 mg/day	See Table 9-5.
Non-PKU hyperphenylalaninemia (phenylalanine hydroxylase)	Same as for PKU, if needed.	Yes, BH_4 10–20 mg/day	See Table 9-5.
Hyperphenylalaninemia (dihydropteridine reductase)	Same as for PKU, if needed.	Yes, 1–10 mg/kg/day	See Table 9-5.
GTP cyclohydrolase I, (6-pyruvoyltetrahydropterin synthase, sepiapterin reductase)	Seldom necessary to provide diet.	Yes, 1–10 mg/kg/day	See Table 9-5 if diet needed.
Tyrosinemia type I (fumarylacetoacetate hydrolyase)	Restrict PHE and TYR. Provide greater than RDA for protein, energy, mineral, and vitamin intakes.	No	See Table 9-5.
	Drug: 2-(2-nitro-4-trifluromethylbenzyl)-1-3-cyclohexanedione.	—	
Tyrosinemia type II (tyrosine aminotransferase)	Restrict PHE and TYR. Provide protein, mineral, and vitamin intakes greater than RDA.	No	See Table 9-5.
Tyrosinemia type III (phenylpyruvic acid dioxygenase)	Same as for tyrosinemia type II.	No	See Table 9-5.
Branched-Chain Amino Acids[2,13]			
Maple syrup urine disease (branched-chain ketoacid dehydrogenase complex)	Restrict ILE, LEU, and VAL. Provide protein energy, mineral, and vitamin intakes above RDA.	Yes, thiamine-responsive if any residual enzyme activity. Response to thiamine inadequate to alleviate need for restriction of BCAAs.	See Table 9-5.
Isovaleric acidemia (isovaleryl-CoA dehydrogenase); β-methylcrotonylglycinuria (β-methylcrotonyl-CoA carboxylase)	Restrict LEU; supplement with L-carnitine and GLY. Provide protein, energy, mineral, and vitamin intakes above RDA.	No	See Table 9-5.
β-methylglutaconic aciduria type I (β-methylglutaconyl-CoA hydratase)	Same as for isovaleric acidemia except no GLY supplement. Unknown if beneficial if started neonatally.	No	See Table 9-5.
β-ketothiolase deficiency (mitochondrial acetoacetyl-CoA thiolase deficiency)	Restrict ILE, supplement L-carnitine. Provide protein, energy, vitamin, and mineral intakes above RDA. Supplement L-LEU and L-VAL.	No	See Table 9-5.
HMG-CoA lyase deficiency (β-hydroxy-β-methylglutaryl-CoA lyase deficiency)	Restrict LEU and fat; avoid fasting, supplement L-carnitine, provide protein, energy, minerals, and vitamins greater than RDA.	No	See Table 9-5.
Isobutyryl-CoA dehydrogenase deficiency	As yet unknown whether VAL should be restricted, L-carnitine supplemented, or protein, energy, minerals, and vitamins should be increased. If yes, supplement L-LEU and L-ILE.	No	See Table 9-5.

Inborn Error and Defect	Nutrient(s) to Modify	Vitamin Responsive?	Medical Foods Available
Sulfur Amino Acids[2,16]			
Homocystinuria, pyridoxine-nonresponsive (cystathionine-β-synthase)	Restrict MET, increase CYS, supplement folate, and betaine. Provide protein, energy, mineral, and vitamin intakes above RDA.	No	See Table 9-5.
Homocystinuria, pyridoxine-responsive (cystathionine-β-synthase)	None unless plasma homocystine remains elevated. If so, treat as B_6 nonresponsive.	Yes, vitamin B_6	See Table 9-5.
Hypermethioninemia I/III (methionine-s-adenosyltransferase deficiency)	Not treated by diet but with oral adenosylmethionine.	No	None
Other Inborn Errors of Amino Acid Metabolism[2,17]			
Glutaric acidemia type I (glutaryl-CoA dehydrogenase)	Restrict LYS and TRP. Supplement L-carnitine. Provide protein, energy, mineral, and vitamin intakes above RDA.	Yes. Some patients have a partial response to oral riboflavin 100–300 mg daily. Administer 15–25 mg, with food, several times daily.	See Table 9-5.
Methylmalonic acidemia (methylmalonyl-CoA mutase^0 or mutase-)	Restrict ILE, MET, THR, VAL, odd chain fatty acids, and long-chain unsaturated fatty acids. Supplement L-carnitine. Provide greater than RDA for protein, energy, mineral, and vitamin intakes.	No	See Table 9-5.
Methylmalonic acidemia (cobalamin reductase; adenosyltransferase)	Minimum restriction of ILE, MET, THR, and VAL. Supplement L-carnitine.	Yes, 1–2 mg hydroxycobalamin daily	See Table 9-5 if any used.
Propionic acidemia (propionyl-CoA carboxylase)	Restrict ILE, MET, THR, VAL, and long-chain fatty acids. Provide greater than RDA for protein, energy, mineral, and vitamin intakes. Supplement with L-carnitine daily.	Questionable. Some clinicians supplement D-biotin daily	See Table 9-5.
Cobalamin A and B	Vitamin B_{12}.	Yes, 1–2 mg hydroxycobalamin IM	
Cobalamin C and D	Supplement vitamin B_{12}, folate, betaine, and L-carnitine IM. Restrict ILE, MET, THR, VAL, if necessary.	Yes, hydroxycobalamin up to 20 mg as needed, and folate daily	
Inborn Errors of Nitrogen Metabolism[2,63-66]			
Carbamylphosphate synthetase deficiency; Ornithine transcarbamylase deficiency	Restrict protein. Add EAAs, L-carnitine, L-ARG, and L-CIT. Provide greater than RDA for energy, mineral, and vitamin intakes.	No	See Table 9-5.
Citrullinemia (argininosuccinate synthetase deficiency)	Restrict protein. Add EAAs, L-carnitine, and L-ARG. Provide greater than RDA for energy, mineral, and vitamin intakes.	No	See Table 9-5.
Argininosuccinic aciduria (arginonosuccinate lyase)	Restrict protein. Add EAAs and L-ARG. Provide greater than RDA for energy, mineral, and vitamin intakes.	No	See Table 9-5.
Citrin deficiency (aspartate-glutamate carrier)	High protein, low carbohydrate, L-ARG; increase water-miscible lipid-soluble vitamins until liver enzymes normal. MCT.	No	See Table 9-5.

(continued)

TABLE 9-2 *(Continued)*

Inborn Error and Defect	Nutrient(s) to Modify	Vitamin Responsive?	Medical Foods Available
Inborn Errors of Carbohydrate Metabolism[2,14,71,72]			
Galactosemias			
Epimerase deficiency	Delete galactose. Add specific known amount of galactose. Provide RDA for protein, energy, minerals, and vitamins.	No	Isomil powder, ProSobee powder.
Galactokinase deficiency	Delete galactose. Provide RDA for protein, energy, mineral, and vitamin intakes.	No	Isomil powder, ProSobee powder.
Galactose-1-phosphate uridyl transferase deficiency	Delete galactose. Provide RDA for protein, energy, mineral, and vitamin intakes. Administer daily 750 mg calcium, 10 μg vitamin D, and 1 mg vitamin K_1 in addition to RDA. Unknown how strict diet should be in adults.	No	Isomil powder, ProSobee powder. *Do not use* formulas designed and marketed for lactase deficiency.
Inborn Errors of Fatty Acid Oxidation (Mitochondrial)[15,81]			
Carnitine acylcarnitine translocase defect; Carnitine palmitoyltransferase I defect	Avoid fasting; use low-fat, MCT-supplemented diet. Administer linoleic and α-linolenic acids. Uncooked cornstarch for hypoglycemia. Water-miscible, fat-soluble vitamins.	L-carnitine therapy if plasma carnitine low	See Table 9-5.
Very-long-chain acyl-CoA dehydrogenase deficiency; Long-chain acyl-CoA dehydrogenase deficiency; Long-chain hydroxyacyl-CoA dehydrogenase deficiency; Trifunctional protein deficiency	Restrict long-chain fats, administer MCT, linoleic and α-linolenic acids. Uncooked cornstarch for hypoglycemia. Avoid fasting. Water-miscible fat-soluble vitamins. High-protein, moderate carbohydrates. Administer DHA for TFP.	No	See Table 9-5.
Medium-chain acyl-CoA dehydrogenase deficiency	Restrict long-chain and avoid medium-chain fats; administer linoleic and α-linolenic acids. Uncooked cornstarch for hypoglycemia. Avoid fasting.	Yes?	See Table 9-5.
Short-chain acyl-CoA dehydrogenase deficiency; Short-chain 3Hydroxyacyl CoA dehydrogenase deficiency	Restrict fat; administer linoleic and α-linolenic acids. Uncooked cornstarch for hypoglycemia. Avoid fasting, moderate protein.	No	Skim milk after 2 years of age.

Abbreviations: ALA, alanine; BCAAs, branched-chain amino acids; CYS, cystine; EAAs, essential amino acids (includes conditionally essential cystine and tyrosine); GLY, glycine; ILE, isoleucine; IM, intramuscular; LEU, leucine; LYS, lysine; MCT, medium-chain triglycerides; MET, methionine; MSUD, maple syrup urine disease; PHE, phenylalanine; THR, threonine; TRP, tryptophan; TYR, tyrosine; VAL, valine.

Sources: Anderson HC, Marble M, Shapiro E. Long-term outcome in treated combined methylmalonic acidemia and homcystinuria. *Genet Med.* 1999;1:146–150; Carrillo-Carrasco J, Sloan J, Valle D, Hamosh A, Venditti CP. Hydroxocobalimin dose escalation improves metabolic control in cblC. *J Inherit Metab Dis*. 2009;52:728–731; Huemer M, Simma B, Fowler B, Suormala T, Bodamer OA, Sass JO. Prenatal and postnatal treatment in cobalamin C defect. *J Pediatr*. 2005;147:469–472; Urbon Artero A, Aldona Gomez J, Reig Del Moral C, Nieto Conde C, Merinero Cortes B. Neonatal onset methylmalonic aciduria and clinical improvement with betaine therapy. *An Esp Pediatr*. 2002;56:337–341; Singh RH. Nutrition management of patients with inherited disorders of urea cycle enzymes. In Acosta PB, ed. *Nutrition Management of Patients with Inherited Metabolic Disorders*. Sudbury, MA: Jones and Bartlett Publishers; 2010:405–429; and Smith DL, Bodamer OA. Practical management of combined methylmalonic aciduria and homocystinuria. *J Child Neurol*. 2002;17:353–356.

TABLE 9-3 Recommended Nutrient Intakes (with Ranges) for Beginning Therapy

	Age (years)					
Nutrients to Modify	**0.0 < 0.5**	**0.5 < 1.0**	**1 < 4**	**4 < 7**	**7 < 11**	**11 < 19**
Inborn Errors of Amino Acid Metabolism						
Aromatic Amino Acids						
Phenylketonuria and hyperphenylalaninemia[2,11,12,34]						
PHE (mg)	55 (70–20)/kg	30 (50–15)/kg	325 (200–450)/d	425 (225–625)/d	450 (250–650)/d	500 (300–750)/d
TYR (mg)	195 (210–180)/kg	185 (200–170)/kg	2800 (1400–4200)/d	3150 (1750–4550)/d	3500 (2100–4900)/d	3850 (2100–5600)/d
Protein (g)	3.5–3.0/kg	3.0–2.5/kg	≥ 30/d	≥ 35/d	≥ 40/d	≥ 50–65/d
Energy (kcal)	120/kg	110/kg	900–1800/d	1300–2300/d	1650–3300/d	1500–3300/d
Tyrosinemia type I[2,11,12,34]						
PHE (mg)	100 (125–65)/kg	80 (105–45)/kg	600 (500–700)/d	650 (550–750)/d	700 (600–800)/d	800 (700–900)/d
TYR (mg)	75 (95–45)/kg	55 (75–30)/kg	400 (300–500)/d	450 (350–550)/d	500 (400–600)/d	550 (450–650)/d
Protein (g)	3.5–3.0/kg	3.0–2.5/kg	≥ 30/d	≥ 35/d	≥ 40/d	≥ 50–65/d
Energy (kcal)	← 100–120% of RDA →					
Tyrosinemia type II, III[2,11,12,34]						
PHE (mg)	100 (125–65)/kg	80 (105–45)/kg	450 (400–500)/d	500 (450–550)/d	550 (500–600)/d	600 (550–700)/d
TYR (gm)	75 (100–40)/kg	55 (80–20)/kg	400 (350–450)/d	450 (400–500)/d	500 (450–550)/d	475 (400–550)/d
Protein (g)	3.5–3.0/kg	3.0–2.5/kg	≥ 30/d	≥ 35/d	≥ 40/d	≥ 50–65/d
Energy (kcal)	120/kg	110/kg	900–1800/d	1300–2300/d	1650–3300/d	1500–3300/d
Branched–Chain Amino Acids						
Maple syrup urine disease[2,13,34]						
ILE (mg)	60 (90–30)/kg	50(70–30)/kg	50 (70–20)/kg	25 (30–20)/kg	25 (30–20)/kg	25 (30–10)/kg
LEU (mg)	80 (100–40)/kg	55 (75–40)/kg	55 (70–40)/kg	50 (65–35)/kg	45 (60–30)/kg	40 (50–15)/kg
VAL (mg)	70 (95–40)/kg	55 (80–30)/kg	50 (70–30)/kg	40 (50–30)/kg	28 (30–25)/kg	22 (30–15)/kg
Protein (g)	3.5–3.0/kg	3.0–2.5/kg	≥ 30/d	≥ 35/d	≥ 40/d	≥ 50–65/d
Energy (kcal)	← 100–125% of RDA →					
Isovaleric acidemia, β-methylglutaconyl hydratase deficiency type I[2,11,13,34]						
LEU (mg)	95 (110–65)/kg	75 (90–50)/kg	975 (800–1150)/d	1275 (1050–1500)/d	1445 (1190–1700)/d	1955 (1610–2300)/d
L-carnitine (mg)	300–100/kg	300–100/kg	300–100/kg	300–100/kg	300–100/kg	300–100/kg
GLY (mg)	← 125 (150–100)/kg →					
Protein (g)	3.5–3.0/kg	3.0–2.5/kg	≥ 30/d	≥ 35/d	≥ 40/d	≥ 50–65/d
Energy (kcal)	← 100–125% of RDA →					

(continued)

TABLE 9-3 *(Continued)*

Nutrients to Modify	Age (years) 0.0 < 0.5	0.5 < 1.0	1 < 4	4 < 7	7 < 11	11 < 19
HMG-CoA lyase deficiency[2,11,12,34]						
LEU (mg)	120 (140–100)/kg	110 (130–90)/kg	90 (100–80)/kg	80 (90–70)/kg	60 (80–40)/kg	50 (60–40)/kg
L-carnitine (mg)	← 50–100/kg →					
Protein (g)	3.5–3.0/kg	3.0–2.5/kg	≥ 30/d	≥ 35/d	≥ 40/d	≥ 50–65/d
Fat (g)	← 25–30% of energy →					
Energy (kcal)	← 100–125% of RDA →					
Avoid fasting	← →					
β-ketothiolase deficiency[2,11,13,34]						
ILE (mg)	70 (80–60)/kg	65 (75–55)/kg	60 (70–50)/kg	55 (65–45)/kg	55 (65–45)/kg	45 (55–35)/kg
L-carnitine (mg)	← 100–200 mg/kg →					
Protein (g)	3.5–3.0/kg	3.0–2.5/kg	≥ 30/d	≥ 35/d	≥ 40/d	≥ 50–65/d
Fat (g)	← 25–30% of energy →					
Energy (kcal)	← 100–125% of RDA →					
Avoid fasting	← →					
Supplemental L-LEU and L-VAL	← To maintain normal plasma concentrations →					
Isobutyryl-CoA dehydrogenase deficiency[13]						
ILE (mg)	70 (80–60)/kg	60 (70–50)/kg	55 (65–45)/kg	55 (65–45)/kg	50 (60–40)/kg	45 (55–35)/kg
GLY (mg)	100 (150–100)/kg	← 125 (150–100)/kg →				
L-carnitine (mg)	← 100–300/kg →					
Protein (g)	3.5–3.0/kg	3.0–2.5/kg	≥ 30/d	≥ 35/d	≥ 40/d	≥ 50–65/d
Energy (kcal)	← 100–125% of RDA →					
Sulfur Amino Acids						
Homocystinuria, cystathionine-β-synthase deficiency (pyridoxine nonresponsive)[2,11,16,34]						
MET (mg)	35 (50–20)/kg	28 (40–15)/kg	20 (30–10)/kg	15 (20–10)/kg	15 (20–10)/kg	15 (20–10)/kg
CYS (mg)	300–250/kg	250–200/kg	150 (200–100)/kg	150 (200–100)/kg	150 (200–100)/kg	75 (60–50)/kg
Betaine (g)	← 1–3/d →		← 3–6/d →			
Folate (mg)	← 0.5–1.0/d →		← 1–3/d →			
Protein (g)	3.5–3.0/kg	3.0–2.5/kg	≥ 30/d	≥ 35/d	≥ 40/d	≥ 50–65/d
Energy (kcal)	120/kg	115/kg	900–1800/d	1300–2300/d	1650–3300/d	1500–3300/d

Other Amino Acids						
Glutaric acidemia type I [2,11,17,34]						
LYS (mg)	85 (100–70)/kg	65 (90–40)/kg	55 (80–30)/kg	50 (75–25)/kg	45 (65–25)/kg	40 (60–20)/kg
TRP (mg)	25 (40–10)/kg	15 (30–10)/kg	12 (16–8)/kg	12 (16–8)/kg	8 (10–5)/kg	6 (8–4)/kg
L-carnitine (mg)	← 300–100/kg →					
Riboflavin (mg)	← 300–100 d, administer in 25-mg doses orally with food →					
Protein (g)	3.5–3.0/kg	3.0–2.5/kg	≥ 30/d	≥ 35/d	≥ 40/d	≥ 50–65/d
Energy (kcal)	120/kg	115/kg	900–1800/d	1300–2300/d	1650–3300/d	1500–3300/d
Do not overrestrict TRP	← →					
Propionic acidemia; methylmalonic acidemia [2,11,17,34]						
ILE (mg)	95 (120–60)/kg	70 (90–40)/kg	610 (485–735)/d	795 (630–960)/d	900 (715–1090)/d	1215 (956–1470)/d
MET (mg)	35 (50–15)/kg	25 (40–10)/kg	330 (275–390)/d	435 (360–510)/d	495 (410–580)/d	665 (550–780)/d
THR (mg)	90 (135–50)/kg	55 (75–20)/kg	505 (415–600)/d	660 (540–780)/d	745 (610–885)/d	1010 (830–1195)/d
VAL (mg)	85 (105–60)/kg	66 (75–30)/kg	690 (550–830)/d	900 (720–1080)/d	1020 (815–1225)/d	1380 (1105–1655)/d
D-biotin (mg)	← 5–10/d for propionic acidemia →					
Hydroxy-cobalamin (mg)	← 1–2/d for cobalamin-responsive methylmalonic acidemia →					
L-carnitine (mg)	← 300–100/kg →					
Protein (g)	3.5–3.0/kg	3.0–2.5/kg	≥ 30/d	≥ 35/d	≥ 40/d	≥ 50–65/d
Energy (kcal)	← 100–125% of RDA →					
Multiple carboxylase deficiency; Biotinidase deficiency [17]						
Biotin (mg)	← 10–20/d →					
Inborn Errors of Nitrogen Metabolism						
Citrullinemia; Argininosuccinic aciduria [2,11,34,63,66]						
L-ARG (mg)	700–350/kg	700–350/kg	500–250/kg	500–250/kg	500–250/kg	400–200/kg
Protein (g)	2.5–1.10/kg	1.9–1.0/kg	1.8–0.7/kg	1.3–0.7/kg	1.7–0.9/kg	1.4–0.8/kg
Energy (kcal)	← 125–150% of RDA →					
Carbamylphosphate synthetase deficiency; Ornithine transcarbamylase deficiency [2,11,34,63,66]						
L-CIT (mg)	700–350/kg	700–350/kg	500–250/kg	500–250/kg	500–250/kg	400–200/kg
Protein (g)	2.5–1.7/kg	1.9–1.0/kg	1.8–0.7/kg	1.3–0.7/kg	1.7–0.9/kg	1.4–0.8/kg
Energy (kcal)	← 125–150% of RDA →					

(continued)

TABLE 9-3 *(Continued)*

Nutrients to Modify	Age (years)					
	0.0 < 0.5	0.5 < 1.0	1 < 4	4 < 7	7 < 11	11 < 19
Argininemia[2,11,34,63,66]						
Protein (g)	2.5–1.0/kg	1.9–1.0/kg	1.8–0.7/kg	1.3–0.7/kg	1.7–0.9/kg	1.4–0.8/kg
Energy (kcal)	← 125–150% of RDA →					
Citrin deficiency[65]						
Protein (g)	4.5–4.0/kg	4.0–3.5/kg	3.5–3.0/kg	3.0–2.5/kg	3.0–2.5/kg	2.5–2.0/kg
L-ARG (mg)	← 600–100/kg →					
Carbohydrate (g)	← Low →					
Energy (kcal)	← 100–125% RDA for age →					
Inborn Errors of Carbohydrate Metabolism						
Galactosemias[2,11,14,71,72]						
Epimerase deficiency						
Galactose (mg)	← 1000–1500/d →		← 500–1000/d →			
Protein (g)	>2.2/kg	>2.0/kg	>23/d	>30/d	>35/d	>45–65/d
Energy (kcal)	120/kg	115/kg	900–1800/d	1300–2300/d	1650–3300/d	1500–3300/d
Galactokinase deficiency						
Protein (g)	>2.2/kg	>2.0/kg	>23/d	>30/d	>35/d	>45–65/d
Energy (kcal)	120/kg	115/kg	900–1800/d	1300–2300/d	1650–3300/d	>1500–3300/d
Galactose-1-phosphate uridyltransferase deficiency						
Calcium (mg)[a]	360	540	800	800	800	1200
Vitamin D (μg)[b]	10	10	10	10	10	10
Vitamin K (μg)[c]	30	4	5	6	7	8
Protein (g)	>2.2/kg	>2.0/kg	>30/d	>35/d	>40/d	>45–65/d
Energy (kcal)	120/kg	115/kg	900–1800/d	1300–2300/d	1650–3300/d	1500–3300/d
Inborn Errors of Fatty Acid Oxidation[11,15,34,90]						
Carnitine acylcarnitine translocase defect; Carnitine palmitoyltransferase defect						
Avoid fasting	← →					
Uncooked cornstarch	← To avoid hypoglycemia, 1 g/kg at bedtime →					
Protein (g)	← 15–20% of energy →					
Fat, long chain	← 10% of energy →					
Linoleic acid	← 3–4% of energy →					

α-linolenic acid	0.6–1% of energy
MCT oil	20% of energy
Energy	RDA for age. Avoid obesity.
Glucose	As needed for hypoglycemia
Water-miscible fat-soluble vitamins	RDA for age
Very-long-chain acyl-CoA dehydrogenase deficiency; Long-chain acyl-CoA dehydrogenase deficiency; Long-chain hydroxy-acyl-CoA dehydrogenase deficiency; Trifunctional protein defect	
As above except protein	30% of energy
Add docosahexaenoic acid (DHA)	
Medium-chain acyl-CoA dehydrogenase deficiency; Short-chain acyl-CoA dehydrogenase deficiency; Short-chain β-hydroxyacyl-CoA dehydrogenase deficiency	
Avoid fasting	
Protein (g)	15–20% of energy
Fat	20–30% of energy
Linoleic acid	3–4% of energy
α-linolenic acid	0.6–1% of energy
Uncooked cornstarch	To prevent hypoglycemia, 1 g/kg at bedtime
Energy (kcal)	RDA, avoid obesity

a. In addition to 750 mg/day after 1 year of age, should be given in addition to recommendations for at least 2 years.

b. 10 μg vitamin D should be given for at least 2 years after 1 year of age in addition to recommendations.

c. 1 mg vitamin K should be given for 2 years after 1 year of age in addition to recommendations.

Abbreviations: ARG, arginine; CIT, citrulline; CYS, cystine; GLY, glycine; ILE, isoleucine; LEU, leucine; LYS, lysine; MET, methionine; PHE, phenylalanine; THR, threonine; TRP, tryptophan; TYR, tyrosine; VAL, valine.

TABLE 9-4 Nutrition Support During Acute Illness; Medications and Nutrient Interactions and Nutrition Assessment Parameters

Inborn Error and Nutrient Support During Acute Illness	Medication and Nutrient Interaction	Nutrition Assessment Parameters
Inborn Errors of Amino Acid Metabolism Aromatic Amino Acids		
Phenylketonuria; Hyperphenylalaninemia[2,12,34]		
Delete dietary PHE 1–3 days *only*. For infant offer Pedialyte with added Polycose to maintain electrolyte balance, if needed. Give sugar-sweetened, caffeine-free soft drinks with added Polycose or Moducal to maintain energy intake at 100%. If necessary, give IV glucose, electrolytes at 150 mL/kg/24 hours to supply a glucose infusion rate of 10 mg/kg/min, and amino acids free of PHE to maintain anabolism. Return to oral medical food and complete diet as rapidly as tolerated.	Usually no medication required with early and continuing therapy throughout life.	Plasma PHE, transthyretin, albumin, ferritin, and TYR; bone radiographs of lumbar vertebrae; dietary intakes of PHE, TYR, protein, energy, minerals, and vitamins. See Chapter 3 nutrition assessment in this book for other routine assessment parameters and standards. Growth; see Chapter 2.
Hyperphenylalaninemias		
Same as above.	Same as above.	Plasma PHE, TYR, transthyretin, albumin, and ferritin; dietary intake of PHE, TYR, protein, energy, minerals, vitamins. See also Chapters 2 and 3 in this book and reference 42 (from this chapter) for other routine assessment parameters and standards. Bone radiographs of lumbar vertebrae.
Tyrosinemia type I[2,12,34]		
Delete dietary PHE and TYR, 1–3 days *only*. For infant, offer Pedialyte with added Polycose to maintain electrolyte balance, if needed. Give sugar-sweetened, caffeine-free soft drinks with added Polycose or Moducal to maintain energy intake at 120–130% of RDA. If necessary, give IV glucose and electrolytes at 150 mL/kg/24 hours to supply a glucose infusion rate of 10 mg/kg/min, and amino acids free of PHE and TYR to maintain anabolism. Return to oral medical food and complete diet as rapidly as tolerated.		Plasma PHE, TYR, transthyretin, albumin, ferritin, bicarbonate, phosphate, potassium, alkaline phosphatase, electrolytes, and liver enzymes; urinary succinylacetone; dietary intake of PHE, TYR, protein, energy, minerals, and vitamins. Growth. Liver imaging studies. Bone radiographs of lumbar vertebrae. See also Chapters 2 and 3 in this book and reference 42 (from this chapter) for other routine assessment parameters and standards.
Tyrosinemia type II, III[2,12,34]		
Same as for tyrosinemia type I.		Plasma PHE, TYR, transthyretin, albumin, ferritin, urinary N-acetyl-tyrosine, p-tyramine, p-hydroxyphenyl organic acids; bone radiographs of lumbar vertebrae; dietary intake of PHE, TYR, protein, energy, minerals, and vitamins. See also Chapters 2 and 3 in this book and reference 42 (from this chapter) for Chapter 3 nutrition assessment in this book for other routine assessment parameters and standards. Growth.

Branched-Chain Amino Acids		
Maple syrup urine disease[2,13,34]		
Delete dietary BCAAs 1–3 days *only*. For infant, offer Pedialyte with added Polycose to maintain electrolyte balance if needed. Give sugar-sweetened, caffeine-free soft drinks with added Polycose or Moducal to maintain energy intake at 100–125% of RDA. If necessary, give IV glucose and electrolytes at 150 mL/kg/24 hours to supply a glucose infusion rate of 10 mg/kg/min and amino acids free of BCAAs. Return to oral medical food and complete diet as rapidly as tolerated.	Anticonvulsants if seizures occur. Phenobarbital and phenytoin lead to accelerated metabolism of vitamin D and vitamin D deficiency that respond to 1,25-dihydroxyvitamin D. Valproate depresses appetite, and causes an increase in plasma GLY concentration and loss of carnitine.	Plasma BCAAs, ALA, ALLO, albumin, transthyretin, and ferritin; urine ketoacids of BCAAs. Bone radiographs of lumbar vertebrae, cation/anion gap; dietary intake of BCAAs, protein, energy, minerals, and vitamins. See also Chapters 2 and 3 in this book and reference 42 (from this chapter) for other routine assessment parameters and standards. Growth.
Isovaleric acidemia; β-methylcrotonyl-glycinuria; β-methylglutaconic aciduria type I		
Delete dietary LEU 1–3 days *only*. Increase GLY and L-carnitine. For infant, offer Pedialyte with Polycose to maintain electrolyte balance if needed. Give sugar-sweetened, caffeine-free soft drinks with added Polycose or Moducal to maintain energy intake at 100–125% of RDA. If necessary, give IV glucose and electrolytes at 150 mL/kg/24 hours to supply a glucose infusion rate of 10 mg/kg/min, and amino acids free of LEU. Return to oral medical food and complete diet as rapidly as tolerated.	Benzoates and salicylates are contraindicated.	Plasma BCAAs. Carnitine, GLY, isovalerylglycine, transthyretin, albumin, ferritin; CBC/differential. Bone radiographs of lumbar vertebrae. Urinary isovalerylglycine, hydroxyisovaleric acid, cation/anion gap. Dietary intakes of LEU, protein, energy, minerals, and vitamins. See also Chapters 2 and 3 in this book and reference 42 (from this chapter) for other routine assessment parameters and standards. Growth.
HMG-CoA lyase deficiency [2,13,34]		
Same as above.		Same as above.
Isobutyryl-CoA dehydrogenase deficiency [2,13,34]		
Same as above except restrict VAL.		Same as isovaleric acidemia.
β-ketothiolase deficiency		
Delete dietary ILE 1–3 days only, administer L-carnitine. For infant, offer Pedialyte with Polycose to maintain electrolyte balance, if needed. Give sugar-sweetened, caffeine-free soft drinks with added Polycose or Moducal to maintain energy intake at 100–125% of RDA. IV glucose and electrolytes at 150 mL/kg/24 hrs to supply a glucose infusion of 10 mg/kg/min, if required. Return to oral medical food and complete diet as rapidly as possible.		Same as isovaleric acidemia.
Homocystinuria, pyridoxine nonresponsive[2,16,34]		
Delete dietary MET 1–3 days *only*. For infant offer Pedialyte with added Polycose to maintain electrolyte balance if needed. Give sugar-sweetened, caffeine-free soft drinks with added Polycose or Moducal to maintain energy intake at 100%. If necessary, give IV glucose, lipid, and amino acids free of MET. Return to oral medical food and complete diet as rapidly as tolerated.	Anticonvulsants if seizures occur. Phenobarbital and phenytoin lead to accelerated metabolism of vitamin D and cause vitamin D deficiency that responds to 1,25-dihydroxy- vitamin D. Valproate depresses appetite and causes an increase in plasma GLY.	Plasma MET, CYS, HOMOCYS; trans-thyretin; albumin, erythrocyte folate; bone radiographs of lumbar vertebrae; dietary intake of MET, CYS, protein, energy, minerals, and vitamins. See also Chapters 2 and 3 in this book and reference 42 (from this chapter) for other routine assessment parameters and standards. Growth.

(continued)

TABLE 9-4 *(Continued)*

Inborn Error and Nutrient Support During Acute Illness	Medication and Nutrient Interaction	Nutrition Assessment Parameters
Other Inborn Errors of Amino Acid Metabolism		
Glutaric acidemia type I[17, 34]		
Delete LYS and TRP 1–3 days *only*. For infant offer Pedialyte with added Polycose to maintain electrolyte balance, if needed. Give sugar-sweetened, caffeine-free soft drinks with added Polycose or Moducal to maintain energy intake at 100%. If necessary, give IV glucose and electrolytes at 150 mL/kg/24 hours to supply a glucose infusion of 10 mg/kg/min, and amino acids free of LYS and TRP. Return to oral medical food and complete diet as rapidly as tolerated.	Baclofen-made by Geneva Generics, Inc. Valproate depresses appetite, and causes an increase in plasma GLY concentration and loss of carnitine.	Plasma LYS, TRP transthyretin, albumin, ferritin; free carnitine; urinary glutaric acid; dietary intake of LYS, TRP, protein, energy, minerals, and vitamins. Bone radiographs of lumbar vertebrae. See also Chapters 2 and 3 in this book and reference 42 (from this chapter) for other routine assessment parameters and standards. Growth.
Propionic acidemia; Methylmalonic acidemia[2,17,34]		
Delete ILE, MET, THR, VAL 1–3 days *only*. Increase L-carnitine. For infant, offer Pedialyte with added Polycose to maintain electrolyte balance, if needed. Give sugar-sweetened, caffeine-free soft drinks with added Polycose or Moducal to maintain energy intake at 100–125% of RDA. If necessary, give IV glucose at 150 mL/kg, to supply 10 mg/kg/min, electrolytes and amino acids free of ILE, MET, THR, and VAL to maintain anabolism. Return to oral medical food and complete diet as rapidly as tolerated.	Carbaglu® during illness if accompanied by elevated blood ammonia. Supplement folate, pantothenate, pyridoxine, and vitamin B_{12} at 3 to 5 times RDA when phenylbutyrate is used. Valproate depresses appetite and causes an increase in plasma GLY concentration and loss of carnitine.	Plasma ILE, MET, THR, VAL, albumin, transthyretin, GLY, free carnitine, blood ammonia, and cation/anion gap. Urinary metabolites of propionate or methylmalonate, CBC/differential; plasma transthyretin, or RBP. Bone radiographs of lumbar vertebrae. Dietary intake of ILE, MET, THR, VAL, protein, energy, minerals, and vitamins. See also Chapters 2 and 3 in this book and reference 42 (from this chapter) for other routine assessment parameters and standards. Growth.
Cobalamin A and B		
Delete ILE, MET, THR, and VAL 1–3 days *only*. Return to usual diet as rapidly as possible.		Plasma ILE, MET, THR, VAL, albumin, transthyretin, GLY, free carnitine, blood ammonia, cation/anion gap. Urinary metabolites of propionate or methylmalonate, CBC/differential; plasma transthyretin or RBP. Bone radiographs of lumbar vertebrae. Dietary intake of ILE, MET, THR, VAL, protein, energy, minerals, and vitamins. See also Chapters 2 and 3 in this book and reference 42 (from this chapter) for other routine assessment parameters and standards. Growth.
Multiple carboxylase deficiency; Biotinidase deficiency[2, 17, 34]		
Biotin, 10–20 mg/day. For infant offer Pedialyte with added Polycose to maintain electrolyte balance, if needed. Give sugar-sweetened caffeine-free soft drinks with added Polycose or Moducal to maintain energy at 100–125% of RDA. If necessary give IV glucose and electrolytes at 150 mL/kg/24 hours to supply a glucose infusion rate of 10 mg/kg/min. Return to complete diet as rapidly as tolerated.	Anticonvulsants if seizures occur. Phenobarbitol and phenytoin tend to accelerate metabolism of vitamin D and cause deficiency that responds to 1,25-dihydroxy-vitamin D. Valproate decreases appetite and causes loss of L-carnitine and an increase in plasma GLY.	Ketolactic acidosis, organic aciduria, hyperammonia, tachypnea and hyper-ventilation, skin rash, and alopecia. Growth.

Inborn Errors of Nitrogen Metabolism		
Urea cycle disorders[2,24,63,64,65]		
Blood $NH_3 > 200$ µmol/L: Delete protein 1–3 days only. Increase L-ARG or L-CIT if not arginase deficient. Give Pedialyte and sugar-sweetened, caffeine-free soft drinks with added Polycose or Moducal to maintain energy intake at 125–150% of RDA. If necessary give IV glucose, and electrolytes at 150 mL/kg/24 hours to supply 10 mg/kg/min. Return to oral medical food and complete diet as rapidly as tolerated.	Phenylbutyrate: folate, niacin pantothenate, pyridoxine, vitamin B_{12} (administer at 3–5 times RDA). Anticonvulsants for seizures; phenobarbital and metabolism of vitamin D and vitamin D deficiency that responds to 1,25-dihydroxyvitamin D. Valproate depresses appetite and causes an increase in plasma GLY concentration and loss of carnitine.	Plasma amino acids, ammonia, albumin, transthyretin, and triglycerides; dietary intake of protein, energy, minerals, and vitamins. See also Chapters 2 and 3 in this book and reference 42 (from this chapter) for other routine assessment parameters and standards. Growth.
Citrin deficiency[63,65]		
	Anticonvulsants for seizures; phenobarbital and ammonia, albumin, and phenytoin lead to accelerated metabolism of vitamin D and vitamin D deficiency that responds to 1,25-dihydroxyvitamin D. Valproate depresses appetite and causes an increase in plasma GLY concentration and loss of carnitine.	Plasma amino acids, transthyretin, and triglycerides; dietary intake of protein, energy, minerals, and growth. See also Chapters 2 and 3 in this book and reference 42 (from this chapter) for other routine assessment parameters and standards. Growth.
Inborn Errors of Carbohydrate Metabolism		
Galactosemias[2,14,34]		
Epimerase deficiency		
Same as for normal infant. Avoid food and drugs containing galactose or lactose.		Albumin, transthyretin. Bone radiographs of lumbar vertebrae. Dietary intake of galactose, protein, energy, minerals, and vitamins. See also Chapters 2 and 3 in this book and reference 42 (from this chapter) for other routine assessment parameters and standards. Growth.
Galactokinase deficiency		
Same as for normal infant. Avoid food and drugs containing galactose or lactose.		Urinary galactose; routine eye examinations for cataracts. See also Chapters 2 and 3 in this book and reference 42 (from this chapter) for other routine assessment parameters and standards. Growth.
Galactose-1-phosphate uridyl transferase deficiency		

(continued)

TABLE 9-4 *(Continued)*

Inborn Error and Nutrient Support During Acute Illness	Medication and Nutrient Interaction	Nutrition Assessment Parameters
Same as for normal infant. Avoid drugs containing galactose or lactose.		Albumin, transthyretin. Erythrocyte galactose-1 phosphate; plasma or urine galactol; routine eye examinations for cataracts. Liver enzymes, bone radiographs. Dietary intake of galactose, protein, energy, minerals, and vitamins. See also Chapters 2 and 3 in this book and reference 42 (from this chapter) for other routine assessment parameters and standards. Growth.
Inborn Errors of Fatty Acid Oxidation (Mitochondrial)[15,34]		
Carnitine transporter deficiency; Carnitine translocase deficiency; Carnitine palmitoyl transferase I, II deficiency; Long-chain acyl-CoA dehydrogenase deficiency; Very-long-chain acyl-CoA dehydrogenase deficiency; Trifunctional protein deficiency; Medium-chain acyl-CoA dehydrogenase deficiency; Short-chain acyl-CoA dehydrogenase deficiency; Short-chain β-hydroxy acyl-CoA dehydrogenase deficiency		
Uncooked cornstarch as needed to help prevent hypoglycemia. If necessary, give IV glucose at 150 mL/kg to supply a glucose infusion rate of 10 mg/kg/min. At home, frequent feeds of fluids containing 2.5 g carbohydrate per fluid ounce. Return to usual diet as rapidly as possible.	Valproate depresses appetite and causes an increase in plasma GLY concentration and loss of carnitine.[11]	Plasma essential fatty acid and fat-soluble vitamins. Plasma glucose and blood gases during illness. Bone radiographs. Nutrient intake. Plasma acylcarnitines. See also Chapters 2 and 3 in this book and reference 42 (from this chapter) for other routine assessment parameters and standards. Growth.

Abbreviations: ARG, arginine; ALLO, alloisoleucine; BCAAs, branched-chain amino acids; CBC, complete blood count; CIT, citrulline; CYS, cystine; GLY, glycine; GTP, guanosine triphosphate; HOMOCYS, homocystine; ILE, isoleucine; IV, intravenous; LEU, leucine; LYS, lysine; MET, methionine; PHE, phenylalanine; RBP, retinol-binding protein; THR, threonine; TRP, tryptophan; TYR, tyrosine; UDP, uridine diphosphate; VAL, valine.

TABLE 9-5 Selected Nutrient Composition (per 100 g powder) and Sources of Medical Foods for Patients with Disorders of Amino Acid, Nitrogen, and Fatty Acid Metabolism

Disorder/Medical Foods	Modified Nutrient(s) (mg/100 g, source)	Protein Equivalent[a] (g/100 g, source)	Fat (g/100 g, source)	Carbohydrate (g/100 g, source)	Energy (kcal/100 g)	Linoleic acid/ α-linolenic acid (mg/100 g)	Minerals/ Vitamins Not Added
Inborn Errors of Aromatic Amino Acids							
Phenylketonuria							
Abbott Nutrition[b]							
Phenex-®1	PHE 0, TYR 1500, L-carnitine 20, Taurine 40	15.0 Amino acids[c]	21.7 High oleic safflower, coconut, soy oils	53 Corn syrup solids	480	3500/350	None/none
Phenex-2 Unflavored	PHE 0, TYR 3000, L-carnitine 40, Taurine 50	30.0 Amino acids[c]	14.0 High oleic safflower, coconut, soy oils	35 Corn syrup solids	410	2200/225	None/none
Phenex-2 Vanilla	PHE 0, TYR 3000, L-carnitine 40, Taurine 50	30.0 Amino acids[c]	13.5 High oleic safflower, coconut, soy oils	36 Corn syrup solids	410	2200/225	None/none
Applied Nutrition Corp[d]							
PhenylAde Amino Acid Bars	PHE 20, TYR 1960, L-carnitine 20, Taurine 60	20.0 Amino acids[c]	34	38	540	0/0	None/none
PhenylAde Drink Mix Essential	PHE 0, TYR 3000, L-carnitine 20, Taurine 80	25.0 Amino acids[c]	13 Safflower, canola, soybean, coconut, flaxseed oils	45 Sucrose, modified food starch, dextrin, corn syrup solids	390	2025/525	None/none
PhenylAde 40 Drink Mix	PHE 0, TYR 3744, L-carnitine 20, Taurine 80	40.0 Amino acids[c]	2 Partially hydrogenated coconut oil	40 Sucrose, modified food starch	336	0/0	None/none
PhenylAde 60 Drink Mix	PHE 0, TYR 6990, L-carnitine added, Taurine added	60.0 Amino acids[c]	0	20 Sucrose, corn syrup solids, modified food starch	327	0/0	None/none
PKU Drink (per 100 mL)	PHE 0, TYR 1190, L-carnitine 10, Taurine 45	10.7 Amino acids[c]	0	18.6 Sugar	106	0/0	?
Mead Johnson Nutritionals[f]							
Phenyl-Free-1	PHE 0, TYR 1600, L-carnitine 51, Taurine 30	16.2 Amino acids[c]	26 Palm olein, soy, coconut, high oleic sunflower oils	51 Corn syrup solids, sugar, modified cornstarch, maltodextrin	500	4500/380	None/none

(continued)

TABLE 9-5 *(Continued)*

Disorder/Medical Foods	Modified Nutrient(s) (mg/100 g, source)	Protein Equivalent[a] (g/100 g, source)	Fat (g/100 g, source)	Carbohydrate (g/100 g, source)	Energy (kcal/100 g)	Linoleic acid/ α-linolenic acid (mg/100 g)	Minerals/ Vitamins Not Added
Phenyl-Free-2	PHE 0, TYR 2200, L-carnitine 49, Taurine 49	22.0 Amino acids[c]	8.6 Soy oil	60 Sugar, corn syrup solids, modified cornstarch	410	4600/651	None/none
Phenyl-Free-2HP	PHE 0, TYR 4000, L-carnitine 36, Taurine 63	40.0 Amino acids[c]	6.3 Soy oil	44 Sugar, corn syrup solids, modified cornstarch	390	3200/453	None/none
Nutricia North America[g]							
LoPhlex	PHE 0, TYR 1120, L-carnitine 70, Taurine 140	69.9 Amino acids[c]	< 0.21	< 0.98	287	0/0	None/none
Periflex Infant	PHE 0, TYR 1440, L-carnitine 10, Taurine 20	13.0 Amino acids[c]	19.1 Soy, coconut, high oleic, safflower, M. alpine, C. cohena oils	49.3 Corn syrup solids	421	3368/2850	None/none
XPHE Maxamaid	PHE 0, TYR 2650, L-carnitine 20, Taurine 140	25.0 Amino acids[c]	< 1.0 None added	56 Corn syrup solids, sugar	324	None/none	None/none
XPHE Maxamum	PHE 0, TYR 4000, L-carnitine 39, Taurine 140	40.0 Amino acids[c]	< 1.0 None added	34 Sugar	305	None/none	None/none
PKU 3 Milupa	PHE 0, TYR 6000, L-carnitine 0, Taurine 0	68.0 Amino acids[c]	0 None added	1.7 Sugar	280	None/none	Chromium, selenium/ None
Vitaflo US LLC[h]							
PKU Cooler (per 100 mL)	PHE 0, TYR 1370, L-carnitine 12.5, Taurine 25.7	11.5 Amino acids[c]	Trace	5.9 Sugar, maltodextrin	71	0/0	None/inositol
PKU Express	PHE 0, TYR 6590, L-carnitine 65.1, Taurine 129.6	60.0 Amino acids[c]	<0.5	15 Sugar, dried glucose syrup	302	0/0	None/inositol
PKU Gel	PHE 0, TYR 4630, L-carnitine 45.8, Taurine 91.1	42.0 Amino acids[c]	< 0.5	43 Sugar, dried glucose syrup	342	0/0	None/inositol

Tyrosinemia Types I, II, III Abbott Nutrition[b]							
Tyrex-1	PHE 0, TYR 0, L-carnitine 20, Taurine 40	15.0 Amino acids[c]	21.7 High oleic safflower, coconut, soy oils	53 Corn syrup solids	480	3500/350	None/none
Tyrex-2	PHE 0, TYR 0, L-carnitine 40, Taurine 50	30.0 Amino acids[c]	14.0 High oleic safflower, coconut, soy oils	35 Corn syrup solids	410	2200/225	None/none
Mead Johnson Nutritionals[f]							
Tyros 1	PHE 0, TYR 0, L-carnitine 50, Taurine 30	16.7 Amino acids[c]	26 Palm olein, soy, coconut, high oleic safflower oils	51 Corn syrup, cornstarch, sugar, maltodextrin	500	4500/380	None/none
Tyros 2	PHE 0, TYR 0, L-carnitine 49, Taurine 49	22.0 Amino acids[c]	8.5 Soy oil	60 Corn syrup solids, sugar, modified cornstarch	410	4600/651	None/none
Nutricia North America[g]							
XPHE, TYR Analog	PHE 0, TYR 0, L-carnitine 10, Taurine 20	13.0 Amino acids[c]	20.9 High oleic safflower, soy, coconut oils	59 Corn syrup solids	475	3025/428	None/none
XPHE, TYR Maxamaid	PHE 0, TYR 0, L-carnitine 20, Taurine 140	25.0 Amino acids[c]	< 1.0 None added	56 Sugar, corn syrup solids	324	None/none	None/none
VitaFlo USA LLC[h]							
TYR cooler (per 100 mL)	PHE 0, TYR 0, L-carnitine 13, Taurine 25	11.5 Amino acids[c]	Trace	5.9 Sugar, maltodextrin	71	ND/ND	None/inositol
TYR express	PHE 0, TYR 0, L-carnitine 143, Taurine 256	60.0 Amino acids[c]	< 0.5	15 Sugar, modified cornstarch, dried glucose syrup	302	0/0	None/inositol
TYR gel	PHE 0, TYR 0, L-carnitine 46, Taurine 90	42.0 Amino acids[c]	<0.5	43 Sugar, modified cornstarch, dried glucose syrup	342	ND/ND	None/inositol
Inborn Errors of Branched-Chain Amino Acids *Branched-Chain Ketoaciduria (MSUD)* Abbott Nutrition[b]							
Ketonex-1	ILE 0, LEU 0, VAL 0, L-carnitine 100, Taurine 40	15.0 Amino acids[c]	21.7 High-oleic safflower, coconut, soy oils	53 Corn syrup solids	480	3500/350	None/none

(continued)

TABLE 9-5 *(Continued)*

Disorder/Medical Foods	Modified Nutrient(s) (mg/100 g, source)	Protein Equivalent[a] (g/100 g, source)	Fat (g/100 g, source)	Carbohydrate (g/100 g, source)	Energy (kcal/100 g)	Linoleic acid/ α-linolenic acid (mg/100 g)	Minerals/ Vitamins Not Added
Ketonex-2	ILE 0, LEU 0, VAL 0, L-carnitine 200, Taurine 50	30 Amino acids[c]	14 High-oleic safflower, coconut, soy oils	35 Corn syrup solids	410	2200/230	None/none
Applied Nutrition Corp[d]							
Complex MSUD Drink Mix	ILE 0, LEU 0, VAL 0, L-carnitine 30, Taurine 100	25.0 Amino acids[c]	12 Safflower, canola, soybean, coconut oils	45 Sucrose, modified food starch, dextrin, corn syrup solids	384	1871/494	None/none
Cambrooke Foods[e]							
Camino pro MSUD Drink	ILE 0, LEU 0, VAL 0, L-carnitine 30, Taurine NA	15.0 Amino acids[c]	0	26 Sugar	149	None/none	?
Camino pro MSUD Bar	ILE 8, LEU 14, VAL 10, L-carnitine 9.57, Taurine NA	10.0 Amino acids[c]	3.6 ?	39 Sugar	165	NA	NA
Camino pro MSUD Sorbet Stix	ILE 0, LEU 0, VAL 0, L-carnitine 20.1, Taurine NA	10.0 Amino acids[c]	0	10.9 Sugar	70	0/0	NA
Mead Johnson Nutritionals[f]							
BCAD 1	ILE 0, LEU 0, VAL 0, L-carnitine 50, Taurine added	16.2 Amino acids[c]	26 Palm olein, soy, coconut, high oleic sunflower oils	51 Corn syrup solids, sugar, modified cornstarch, maltodextrin	500	4500/380	None/none
BCAD 2	ILE 0, LEU 0, VAL 0, L-carnitine 49, Taurine added	24.0 Amino acids[c]	8.5 Soy oil	57 Corn syrup solids, sugar, modified cornstarch	410	4600/610	None/none
Nutricia North America[g]							
Acerflex	ILE 0, LEU 0, VAL 0, L-carnitine 20, Taurine 140	20.0 Amino acids[c]	17 Canola, high oleic safflower oils	40.5 Corn syrup solids	395	2689/NA	None/none
MSUD Analog	ILE 0, LEU 0, VAL 0, L-carnitine 10, Taurine 20	13.0 Amino acids[c]	20.9 High oleic, safflower, coconut, soy oils	59 Corn syrup solids	475	3025/NA	None/none
Milupa MSUD 2	ILE 0, LEU 0, VAL 0, L-carnitine 0, Taurine 0	54.0 Amino acids[c]	0	21 Sugar	300	0/0	Chromium, selenium/ none

MSUD Maxamaid	ILE 0, LEU 0, VAL 0, L-carnitine 20, Taurine 140	25.0 Amino acids[c]	< 0.1	56 Sugar, corn syrup solids	324	0/0	None/none
MSUD Maxamum	ILE 0, LEU 0, VAL 0, L-carnitine 39, Taurine 140	40.0 Amino acids[c]	< 1	34 Sugar, corn syrup solids	305	0/0	None/none
Vitaflo USLLC [h]							
MSUD Gel	ILE 0, LEU 0, VAL 0, L-carnitine 12, Taurine 91.1	42.0 Amino acids[c]	< 0.5	43 Sugar, starch, modified cornstarch	342	NA	None/inositol
MSUD Express	ILE 0, LEU 0, VAL 0, L-carnitine 165.6, Taurine 129.6	60.0 Amino acids[c]	< 0.5	15 Dried glucose syrup	302	NA	None/inositol
MSUD Express Cooler (per 100 mL)	ILE 0, LEU 0, VAL 0, L-carnitine 0, Taurine NA	15.0 Amino acids[c]	< 0.1	7.8 Sugar	92	NA	None/inositol
Isovaleric Acidemia Abbott Nutrition[b]							
I-Valex-1	LEU 0, GLY 1000, L-carnitine 900, Taurine 40	15.0 Amino acids[c]	21.7 High-oleic safflower, coconut, soy oils	53 Corn syrup solids	480	3500/350	None/none
I-Valex-2	LEU 0, GLY 2000, L-carnitine 1800, Taurine 50	30.0 Amino acids[c]	14.0 High-oleic safflower, coconut, soy oils	35 Corn syrup solids	410	2200/230	None/none
Mead Johnson Nutritionals[f]							
LMD	LEU 0, GLY 1100, L-carnitine 50, Taurine added	16.2 Amino acids[c]	26 Palm olein, soy, coconut, high-oleic sunflower oils	51 Corn syrup solids, sugar, maltodextrin, modified cornstarch	500	4500/380	None/none
Nutricia North America[g]							
XLeu Analog	LEU 0, GLY 2050, L-carnitine 10, Taurine 20	13.0 Amino acids[c]	20.9 High oleic safflower, coconut, soy oils	59 Corn syrup solids, galactose	475	3025/NA	None/none
XLeu Maxamaid	LEU 0, GLY 3990, L-carnitine 10, Taurine 140	25.0 Amino acids[c]	< 0.1	56 Sugar, corn syrup solids	324	0/0	None/none
XLeu Maxamum	LEU 0, GLY 6300, L-carnitine 39, Taurine 140	40.0 Amino acids[c]	< 1	34 Sugar, corn syrup solids	305	0/0	None/none

(continued)

TABLE 9-5 *(Continued)*

Disorder/Medical Foods	Modified Nutrient(s) (mg/100 g, source)	Protein Equivalent[a] (g/100 g, source)	Fat (g/100 g, source)	Carbohydrate (g/100 g, source)	Energy (kcal/100 g)	Linoleic acid/ α-linolenic acid (mg/100 g)	Minerals/ Vitamins Not Added
Homocystinuria							
Abbott Nutrition [b]							
Hominex-1	MET 0, CYS 450, L-carnitine 20, Taurine 40	15.0 Amino acids[c]	21.7 High oleic safflower, coconut, soy oils	53 Corn syrup solids	480	3500/350	None/none
Hominex-2	MET 0, CYS 900, L-carnitine 40, Taurine 50	30.0 Amino acids[c]	14.0 High oleic safflower, coconut, soy oils	35 Corn syrup solids	410	2200/225	None/none
Mead Johnson Nutritionals[f]							
HCY 1	MET 0, CYS 600, L-carnitine added, Taurine 30	16.2 Amino acids[c]	26 Palm olein, soy, coconut, high-oleic sunflower oils	51 Corn syrup solids	500	4500/380	None/none
HCY 2	MET 0, CYS 810, L-carnitine added, Taurine 57	22.0 Amino acids[c]	8.5 Soy oil	61 Sucrose, corn syrup solids	410	4600/610	None/none
Nutricia North America[g]							
Methionaid Milupa	MET 0, CYS 3700, L-carnitine NA, Taurine NA	60.0 Amino acids[c]	0	3 Hydrolyzed cornstarch	250	0/0	Chromium, molybdenum, selenium/ Vitamins A, C, D, E, K, choline, inositol
XMET Analog	MET 0, CYS 390, L-carnitine 10, Taurine 20	13.0 Amino acids[c]	20.9 High oleic safflower, coconut, soy oils	59 Corn syrup solids	475	3025/ND	None/none
XMET Maxamaid	MET 0, CYS 750, L-carnitine 20, Taurine 140	25.0 Amino acids[c]	< 0.1	57 Sugar, corn syrup solids	324	0/0	None/none
XMET Maxamum	MET 0, CYS 1200, L-carnitine 390, Taurine 140	40.0 Amino acids[c]	< 1.0	34 Sugar	305	0/0	None/none
Milupa HOM 2	MET 0, CYS 3400, L-carnitine 0, Taurine 0	69.0 Amino acids[c]	0.0	3.8 Sugar	290	0/0	Chromium, selenium/ none

Vitaflo US LLC[h]							
HCU Cooler (per 100 mL)	MET 0, CYS 410, L-carnitine 13, Taurine 25	11.5 Amino acids[c]	Trace	5.9 Sugar, maltodextrin	71	0/0	None/inositol
HCU Express	MET 0, CYS 1920, L-carnitine 158, Taurine 238	60.0 Amino acids[c]	< 0.5	15 Sugar, starch, dried glucose syrup	302	0/0	None/inositol
HCU Gel	MET 0, CYS 1370, L-carnitine 50, Taurine 90	42.0 Amino acids[c]	< 0.5	43 Sugar, starch, dried glucose syrup	342	0/0	None/inositol
Propionic/Methylmalonic Acidemia Abbott Nutrition[b]							
Propimex-1	MET 0, VAL 0, ILE 120, THR 100, L-carnitine 900, Taurine 40	15.0 Amino acids[c]	21.7 High oleic safflower, coconut, soy oils	53.0 Corn syrup solids	480	3500/350	None/none
Propimex-2	MET 0, VAL 0, ILE 240, THR 200, L-carnitine 1800, Taurine 50	30.0 Amino acids[c]	14.0 High oleic safflower, coconut, soy oils	35.0 Corn syrup solids	410	2200/225	None/none
Mead Johnson Nutritionals[f]							
OA1	MET 0, VAL 0, ILE 0, THR 0, L-carnitine ND, Taurine ND	15.7 Amino acids[c]	26.0 Palm olein, soy, coconut, high oleic safflower oils	51.0 Corn syrup solids, sugar, modified cornstarch, maltodextrin	500	4500/380	None/none
OA2	MET 0, VAL 0, ILE 0, THR 0, L-carnitine ND, Taurine ND	21.0 Amino acids[c]	9.0 Soy oil	59.0 Corn syrup solids, sugar, modified cornstarch, maltodextrin	410	4600/608	None/none
Nutricia North America[g]							
XMTVI Analog	MET 0, VAL 0, ILE trace, THR 0, L-carnitine 10, Taurine 20	13.0 Amino acids[c]	20.9 High oleic safflower, coconut, soy oils	59.0 Corn syrup solids	475	3025/ND	None/none
XMTVI Maxamaid	MET 0, VAL 0, ILE trace, THR 0, L-carnitine 20, Taurine 140	25.0 Amino acids[c]	< 0.1	56.0 Sugar, corn syrup solids	324	0/0	None/none
XMTVI Maxamum	MET 0, VAL 0, ILE trace, THR 0, L-carnitine 39, Taurine 140	40.0 Amino acids[c]	< 1.0	34.0 Sugar, corn syrup solids	305	0/0	None/none

(continued)

TABLE 9-5 *(Continued)*

Disorder/Medical Foods	Modified Nutrient(s) (mg/100 g, source)	Protein Equivalent[a] (g/100 g, source)	Fat (g/100 g, source)	Carbohydrate (g/100 g, source)	Energy (kcal/100 g)	Linoleic acid/ α-linolenic acid (mg/100 g)	Minerals/ Vitamins Not Added
Milupa OS2	MET 0, VAL 0, ILE trace, THR 0, L-carnitine 0, Taurine 0	56.0 Amino acids[c]	0.0	18.9 Sugar	300	0/0	Chromium, selenium/ none
Vitaflo US LLC[h]							
MMA/PA Express	MET 0, VAL 0, ILE 0.22, THR 0, L-carnitine 28.88, Taurine 216.6	60.0 Amino acids[c]	< 0.5	15 Sugar, starch, dried glucose syrup	302	0/0	None/inositol
MMA/PA Gel	MET 0, VAL 0, ILE 0.15, THR 0, L-carnitine 50, Taurine 90	42.0 Amino acids[c]	< 0.5	43 Sugar, starch, dried glucose syrup	342	0/0	None/inositol
Glutaric aciduria type I Abbott Nutrition[b]							
Glutarex-1	LYS 0, TRP 0, L-carnitine 900, Taurine 40	15.0 Amino acids[c]	21.7 High oleic safflower, coconut, soy oils	53.0 Corn syrup solids	480	3500/350	None/none
Glutarex-2	LYS 0, TRP 0, L-carnitine 1800, Taurine 50	30.0 Amino acids[c]	14.0 High oleic safflower, coconut, soy oils	35.0 Corn syrup solids	410	2200/225	None/none
Mead Johnson Nutritionals[f]							
GA	LYS 0, TRP 0, L-carnitine ND, Taurine ND	15.1 Amino acids[c]	26.0 Palm olein, soy, coconut, high oleic safflower oils	52.0 Corn syrup solids, sugar, modified cornstarch, maltodextrin	500	4500/380	None/none
Nutricia North America[g]							
XLYS, XTRP Analog	LYS 0, TRP 0, L-carnitine 10, Taurine 20	13.0 Amino acids[c]	20.9 High oleic safflower, coconut, soy oils	59.0 Corn syrup solids	475	3025/ND	None/none
XLYS, XTRP Maxamaid	LYS 0, TRP 0, L-carnitine 20, Taurine 140	25.0 Amino acids[c]	< 0.3	56.0 Sugar, corn syrup solids	324	0/0	None/none

XLYS, XTRP Maxamum	LYS 0, TRP 0, L-carnitine 39, Taurine 140	40.0 Amino acids[c]	< 1.0	34.0 Sugar, corn syrup solids	305	0/0	None/none
Vitaflo US LLC[h]							
GA Gel	LYS 0, TRP 0, L-carnitine 46, Taurine 90	42.0 Amino acids[c]	0.0	43.0 Sugar, starch, dried glucose syrup	342	0/0	None/inositol
Urea Cycle Enzyme Defects Abbott Nutrition[b]							
Cyclinex-1	Non-essential amino acid-free, L-carnitine 190, Taurine 40	7.5 Amino acids[c]	24.6 High oleic safflower, coconut, soy oils	57.0 Corn syrup solids	510	3900/375	None/none
Cyclinex-2	Non-essential amino acid-free, L-carnitine 370, Taurine 60	15.0 Amino acids[c]	17.0 High oleic safflower, coconut, soy oils	45.0 Corn syrup solids	440	2800/275	None/none
Mead Johnson Nutritionals[f]							
WND®1	Non-essential amino acid-free, L-carnitine added, Taurine added	6.5 Amino acids[c]	26.0 Palm olein, soy, coconut, high oleic sunflower oils	60.0 Corn syrup solids, sugar, modified cornstarch	500	4500/ND	None/none
WND®2	Non-essential amino acid-free, L-carnitine added, Taurine added	8.2 Amino acids[c]	10.2 Soy oil	71.0 Corn syrup solids, sugar, modified cornstarch	410	5500/ND	None/none
Nutricia North America[g]							
Milupa UCD2	Non-essential amino acid-free, L-carnitine 0, Taurine 0	67.0 Amino acids[d]	0	4.4 Sugar	290	0/0	Chromium, selenium/ none
Fatty Acid Oxidation Defects Mead Johnson Nutritionals[f]							
Pregestimil Lipil	Medium-chain fatty acids 75.3, L-carnitine added, Taurine added	14.0 Casein hydrolysate, L-amino acids[c]	28.0 MCT, soy, high oleic, vegetable, single cell oils (ARA, DHA)	51.0 Corn syrup solids, dextrose, modified cornstarch	500	5200/590	None/none

(continued)

TABLE 9-5 *(Continued)*

Disorder/Medical Foods	Modified Nutrient(s) (mg/100 g, source)	Protein Equivalent[a] (g/100 g, source)	Fat (g/100 g, source)	Carbohydrate (g/100 g, source)	Energy (kcal/100 g)	Linoleic acid/ α-linolenic acid (mg/100 g)	Minerals/Vitamins Not Added
Portagen	Medium-chain fatty acids 19.1, L-carnitine added, Taurine added	16.5 Casein hydrolysate	22.0 MCT, corn oil	54.0 Corn syrup solids, sugar	470	1620/ND	None/none
Nutricia North America[g]							
Monogen®	Medium-chain fatty acids 10.6, L-carnitine added, Taurine added	11.4 Whey protein concentrate, L-amino acids[c]	11.8 Fractionated coconut oil, walnut oil	68.0 Corn syrup solids	424	473/101	None/none
Vitaflo US LLC[h]							
Lipistart	Medium-chain fatty acids 17.0, L-carnitine added, Taurine added	14.1 Whey protein isolate, sodium caseinate	21.7 Fractionated coconut oil, soy oil	56.0 Dried glucose syrup	466	1767/246	None/inositol

a. g protein equivalent = g nitrogen × 6.25.

b. Abbott Nutrition, 625 Cleveland Avenue, Columbus, OH 43215; 800-551-5838.

c. All except glycine are in the L-form.

d. Applied Nutrition Corp., 10 Saddle Road, Cedar Knolls, NJ 07927; 800-605-0410.

e. Cambrooke Foods, Two Central Street, Framingham, MA 01701; 866-456-9776.

f. Mead Johnson Nutritionals, 2400 W Lloyd Expressway, Evansville, IN 47721; 800-457-3550.

g. Nutricia North America, PO Box 117, Gaithersburg, MD 20884; 800-365-7354.

h. Vitaflo US LLC, 123 East Neck Road, Huntington, NY 11743; 888-848-2356.

Values listed, although accurate at time of publication, are subject to change. The most current information may be obtained by referring to product labels.

Abbreviations: ND, no data; NA, not available.

Source: Data supplied by each company.

TABLE 9-6 Results of Amino Acid and Nitrogen Deficiencies

Amino Acid	Manifestations of Deficiency
Arginine	Elevated blood ammonia
	Elevated urinary orotic acid
	Generalized skin lesions
	Poor wound healing
	Retarded growth
Carnitine	Fatty myopathy
	Cardiomyopathy
	Depressed liver function
	Neurologic dysfunction
	Defective fatty acid oxidation
	Hypoglycemia
	Hypertriacylglycerolemia
Citrulline	Elevated blood ammonia
Cysteine	Impaired nitrogen balance
	Impaired sulfur balance
	Decreased tissue glutathione
	Hypotaurinemia
Isoleucine	Weight loss or no weight gain
	Redness of buccal mucosa
	Fissures at corners of mouth
	Tremors of extremities
	Decreased plasma cholesterol
	Decreased plasma isoleucine
	Elevations in plasma lysine, phenylalanine, serine, tyrosine, and valine
	Skin desquamation, if prolonged
Leucine	Loss of appetite
	Weight loss or poor weight gain
	Decreased plasma leucine
	Increased plasma isoleucine, methionine, serine, threonine, and valine
Lysine	Weight loss or poor weight gain
	Impaired nitrogen balance
Methionine	Decreased plasma methionine
	Increased plasma phenylalanine, proline, serine, threonine, and tyrosine
	Decreased plasma cholesterol
	Poor weight gain
	Loss of appetite
Phenylalanine	Weight loss or poor weight gain
	Impaired nitrogen balance
	Aminoaciduria
	Decreased serum globulins
	Decreased plasma phenylalanine
	Mental retardation
	Anemia
Taurine	Impaired visual function
	Impaired biliary secretion
Threonine	Arrested weight gain
	Glossitis and reddening of the buccal mucosa
	Decreased plasma globulin
	Decreased plasma threonine
Tryptophan	Weight loss or no weight gain
	Impaired nitrogen retention
	Decreased plasma cholesterol
Tyrosine	Impaired nitrogen retention
	Catecholamine deficiency
	Thyroxine deficiency
Valine	Poor appetite, drowsiness
	Excess irritability and crying
	Weight loss or decrease in weight gain
	Decreased plasma albumin
Nitrogen	No or decreased weight gain
	Impaired nitrogen retention

Consequently, each patient's nutrition prescription must be individualized to her or his specific needs.

Tetrahydrobiopterin (BH_4) has been found to lower blood PHE concentration when administered to many patients with non-PKU HPA and some with mild PKU, but very few with classical PKU have been tested.[40,41] Large neutral amino acids (LNAAs) free of PHE, carbohydrate, fat, minerals, and vitamins have been fed to noncompliant adults at 0.5 g/kg of body weight daily and mean plasma PHE concentration decreased by 39%. Other actual food intake of the patients was not reported.[29]

Following the establishment of a firm diagnosis of classical PKU, a prescription must be given for the nutrition management of the patient. For the neonate who weighs 3.4 kg and has an initial blood PHE concentration of 1600 μmol/L with a blood tyrosine (TYR) concentration of 50 μmol/L, the initial prescription may be as follows for the first 3 days:

PHE, mg	0×3.4 kg	= 0 mg/day
TYR, mg	348×3.4 kg	= 1183 mg/day
Protein, g	3.5×3.4 kg	= 11.9 g/day
Energy, kcal	120×3.4 kg	= 408 kcal/day

Plan the diet by first determining which medical food (exempt infant formula) will be used.

Food	Amount	PHE (mg)	TYR (mg)	Protein (g)	Energy (kcal)
Phenex-1 powder	79 g	0	1185	11.9	379
Polycose powder[a]	6 g	0	0	0	30
Total		0	1185	11.9	409
Per kg body weight		0	348	3.5	120

Add water to make 621 mL (21 fl oz).

[a] 380 kcal/100 g powder.

PHE must be added to the diet to prevent its deficiency as blood/plasma PHE concentration declines.

PHE, mg 35 × 3.4 kg = 119 mg/day

TYR, mg 304 × 3.4 kg = 1034 mg/day

Protein, g 3.5 × 3.4 kg = 11.9 g/day

Energy, kcal 120 × 3.4 kg = 408 kcal/day

First add proprietary infant formula to supply the required PHE. Similac Advance with Iron powder contains 465 mg PHE, 10.8 g protein, and 521 kcal per 100 g powder. To determine the amount of Similac powder to add, divide 119 g by the 465 mg PHE and multiply by 100; this yields 26 g. To determine the remaining protein to give as medical food, subtract the 2.8 g protein in 26 g Similac powder from 11.9 g to get 9.1 g. Phenex-1 contains 1500 mg TYR, 15 g protein, and 480 kcal per 100 g powder. Divide 9.1 g protein by 15.0 to get 60.6 g powder. Round to 61 g. Multiply 480 kcal per 100 g by 0.61 g to obtain 293 kcal. Remaining energy, if any is required, is determined by adding 135 kcal of Similac with 293 kcal of Phenex-1. This yields 428 kcal. No further energy is required.

Food	Amount	PHE (mg)	TYR (mg)	Protein (g)	Energy (kcal)
Similac Advance with Iron powder	26 g	121	117	2.8	135
Phenex-1 powder	61 g	0	915	9.1	293
Total		121	1032	11.9	422
Per kg body weight		36	304	3.5	124

Add water to yield 628 mL (21 fluid ounces).

Several clinical phenotypes of branched-chain ketoaciduria (maple syrup urine disease [MSUD]) exist, and the amount of each branched chain amino acid required will differ by genotype, age, gender, state of health, and protein intake.[13] These phenotypes include intermediate, intermittent, classic, thiamine-responsive, and dihydrolipoyl dehydrogenase (E3)-deficient MSUD.

Patients with intermediate or intermittent MSUD will require less strict diet management than patients with classical MSUD. However, introduction of BCAA-free medical food to these patients with consistent daily use, especially during febrile illness, will help prevent acidosis. Nutrition therapy of the patient with classical MSUD should be introduced with the first suspicion of disease to prevent severe illness. The 3.4 kg child should be offered a BCAA-free medical food for the first 3 days of therapy. A prescription that includes protein and at least 140 kcal/kg should be written:

Protein, g 3.5 × 3.4 kg = 11.9 g

Energy, kcal 140 × 3.4 kg = 476 kcal

Food	Amount	Protein (g)	Energy (kcal)
Ketonex-1 powder	79 g	11.9	379
Polycose powder[a]	26 g	—	99
Total		11.9	478
Per kg body weight		3.5	140

Add water to yield 710 mL (24 oz).

a. 380 kcal/100 g powder

The three BCAAs must be added to the diet to prevent deficiency, and ILE must be added on or before day four to prevent skin desquamation (see Yannicelli,[17] Figure 8.2). The amount of LEU added at this time may be less than when the plasma concentration has reached the treatment range. The amount of VAL added may be the full prescription depending on the plasma concentration.

ILE, mg 60 × 3.4 kg = 204 mg

LEU, mg 75 × 3.4 kg = 255 mg

VAL, mg 70 × 3.4 kg = 238 mg

Protein, g 3.5 × 3.4 kg = 11.9 g

Energy, kcal 140 × 3.4 kg = 476 kcal

Fill the LEU prescription with Similac Advance with Iron powder, which contains 575 mg ILE, 1080 mg LEU, and 640 mg VAL per 100 g powder.

All other patients with IEMs have nutrient requirements that may differ widely. Thus, the diet prescription must be individualized to support normal growth of each patient.

Protein requirements of infants and children with IEMs are normal if liver or renal function is not compromised. However, the form in which the protein is administered must be altered in order to restrict specific amino acids. Consequently, medical foods formulated from free amino acids must be used with small amounts of intact protein to provide amino acid and N requirements. Because N retention from free amino acid mixes differs from that of amino acids derived from intact protein (as reviewed by Acosta[42]), recommended protein intakes of infants and children with

Food	Amount	ILE (mg)	LEU (mg)	VAL (mg)	Protein (g)	Energy (kcal)
Similac Advance with Iron powder	24 g	138	259	154	2.6	125
Ketonex-1 powder	62 g	0	0	0	9.3	298
ILE solution[a]	6.6 mL	66	0	0	0	0
VAL solution[a]	8.4 mL	0	0	84	0	0
Polycose powder[b]	14 g	0	0	0	0	53
Total		204	259	238	11.9	476
Per kg body weight		60	76	70	3.5	140

[a] 10 mg/mL

[b] 380 kcal/100 g powder

Add water to make 650 mL (22 fl oz). As plasma LEU concentration decreases a greater amount of Similac may be added to help maintain plasma ILE, LEU, and VAL in the treatment range and to support normal growth.

inborn errors of amino acid metabolism are 125–150% greater than RDAs.[1] Other factors may also contribute to the need by patients with inherited amino acid disorders for greater protein intakes than recommended for normal persons, as reported by Loots et al.[43] Conjugation of PHE in the liver and later excretion in the urine of the compounds produced was reported by Moldave and Meister.[44] **Table 9-7** describes urinary loss of some of these conjugates, but plasma concentrations at which these losses occur are not provided, nor is their total daily loss given. Medical food and intact protein should be given four to six times daily to enhance nitrogen retention.[45–47] According to Arnold et al,[48] plasma transthyretin concentrations are positively correlated with linear growth, with concentrations of at least 200 mg/L resulting in the greatest height for age. Acosta and Yannicelli[49] found similar correlations in 2- to 13-year-old children with PKU. Yannicelli et al.[50] reported poor linear growth in children with methylmalonic or propionic acidemia who failed to ingest adequate protein and energy. In fact, protein intake as recommended by Acosta leads to excellent growth with greater restricted amino acid tolerance than when RDA for protein is provided.

Fat intakes and the essential fatty acids, linoleic and α-linolenic, should meet RDAs,[1] except in mitochondrial fatty acid oxidation defects. Acosta et al.[51] found no essential fatty acid deficiency in patients with PKU undergoing nutrition therapy, except in those ingesting fat-free medical foods.

TABLE 9-7 Urinary Loss of Some Conjugated Amino Acids by Patients with Various IEMs

Inborn Error	Amino Acid Conjugate
β-ketothiolase	β-methylglutaconic acid (ILE)
Branched-chain ketoaciduria (MSUD)	Acetylleucine (LEU), acetylisoleucine (ILE), acetylvaline (VAL), lactylleucine (LEU), lactylisoleucine (ILE), lactylvaline (VAL), α-hydroxyisovaleryl conjugates of GLY, ILE, LEU, VAL
Isovaleric acidemia	Isovalerylalanine (LEU, ALA), isovalerylasparagine, (LEU, $ASPNH_2$), isovaleric-β-D-glucuronide (LEU), isovalerylglycine, isovalerylglutamic acid (LEU, GLY, GLU), isovalerylhistidine (LEU, HIS), isovaleryllysine (LEU, LYS), isovaleryltryptophan (LEU, TRP), β-hydroxy isovaleric acid (LEU), acetyltryptophan (TRP)
Methylmalonic acidemia	β-methylglutaconic acid (ILE)
Phenylketonuria	Phenylalanine (PHE), phenylacetylglutamine (PHE, $GLUNH_2$), phenyllactic acid (PHE), phenylpyruvic acid (PHE), acetylphenylalanine (PHE).
Propionic acidemia	β-methylglutaconic acid (ILE)
Tyrosinemia	Acetylphenylalanine (PHE), acetyltyrosine (TYR)

Abbreviations: ASPNH2, asparagine; GLU, glutamate; GLUNH2, glutamine; GLY, glycine; HIS, histidine; ILE, isoleucine; LEU, leucine; LYS, lysine; PHE, phenylalanine; TRP, tryptophan; TYR, tyrosine.

Sources: Dorland L, Duran M, Wadman SK, Niederwieser A, Bruinvis L, Ketting D. Isovaleryl-glucuronide, a new urinary metabolite in isovaleric acidemia. Identification problems due to rearrangement reactions. *Clin Chim Acta.* 1983;134(1–2):77–83; Duran M, Bruinvis L, Ketting D, Karmerling JP, Wadman SK, Schutgens RB. The identification of (E)-2-methylglutaconic acid, a new isoleucine metabolite in the urine of patients with beta-ketothiolase deficiency, propionic acidaemia and methylmalonic acidaemia. *Biomed Mass Spectrom.* 1982;9:1–5; Hagenfeldt L, Naglo AS. New conjugated urinary metabolites in intermediate type maple syrup urine disease. *Clin Chim Acta.* 1987;169:77–83; Jellum E, Horn L, Thoresen O, Krittingen EA, Stokke O. Urinary excretion of N-acetyl amino acids in patients with some inborn errors of amino acid metabolism. *Scand J Clin Lab Invest Suppl.* 1986;184:21–26; Lehnert W. N-isovalerylalanine and N-isovalerylsarcosine: two new minor metabolites in isovaleric acidemia. *Clin Chim Acta.* 1983;134(1–2):207–212; Lehnert W, Werle E. Elevated excretion of N-acetylated branched-chain amino acids in maple syrup urine disease. *Clin Chim Acta.* 1986;172:123–126; Loots DT, Erasmus E, Mienie LJ. Identification of 19 new metabolites by abnormal amino acid conjugation in isovaleric acidemia. *Clin Chem.* 2005;5:1510–1512; Loots DT, Mienie LJ, Erasmus E. Amino-acid depletion induced by abnormal amino-acid conjugation and protein restriction in isovaleric acidemia. *Eur J Clin Nutr.* 2007;61:1323–1327; and Woolf LI. Excretion of conjugated phenylacetic acid in phenylketonuria. *Biochem J.* 1951;49:ix–x.

Energy intakes of infants and children with inborn errors of metabolism must be adequate to help support normal rates of growth. Provision of apparently adequate amino acids and N without sufficient energy will lead to growth failure. Pratt and associates[52] suggested that energy requirements are greater than normal when L-amino acids supply the protein equivalent. Maintenance of adequate energy intake is essential for normal growth and development and to prevent catabolism. If RDA[1] for energy cannot be achieved through oral feeds, nasogastric, gastrostomy, or parenteral feeds must be employed. Mathematical formulas for calculating protein and energy requirements for the child with a metabolic disorder ingesting an elemental food with failure to thrive can be found in other sources.[11] Amino acid solutions designed for specific metabolic defects may be obtained from Apria Healthcare (http://apria.com/home/) if parenteral alimentation is required. Care must be taken to prevent overweight or obesity because weight loss results in elevated plasma amino acid concentrations. Fluid intake should be 1.5 mL/kcal for infants and 1.0 mL/kcal for children. Most adults will ingest adequate fluid.

Major, trace, and ultratrace mineral and vitamin intakes should exceed RDA for age.[1,53–56] If the medical food mixture fails to supply ≥ 100% of requirements for infants and children, appropriate supplements should be given. In patients with PKU, plasma phenylalanine concentrations > 480 μmol/L may lead to loss of bone matrix[49,50,54–56] in spite of adequate calcium, phosphorous, and vitamin D intakes. All organic acidemias, unless well controlled, will result in bone mineral loss.[57] Alexander et al.[31] reported poor absorption of a number of minerals when free amino acids were the primary protein source. Acosta and Yannicelli[49] and Pasquali et al.[56] reported increased bone collagen loss with age in children with PKU as plasma PHE increased, as compared to normal children. Nutrient intakes of calcium, phosphorus, and vitamin D met or exceeded RDA for age, and concentrations of plasma calcium, phosphorus, and serum vitamin D were adequate (see **Figure 9-1**).[49,56] Iron status is a problem in children with PKU.[53,58,59] Niacin[60,61] synthesis from tryptophan also appears to be a problem in patients with PKU and elevated plasma PHE. Elevated PHE concentrations may inhibit biotinidase activity.[62]

Inborn Errors of Nitrogen Metabolism

Eight enzyme defects have been reported in the urea cycle resulting in elevated concentrations of blood ammonia.[63,64] Four of the defects are suspected by elevated concentrations of blood arginine (ARG) or citrulline (CIT) on newborn screening (see Table 9-1). Consequently, differential diagnosis is essential for appropriate therapy.

The urea cycle normally contributes large amounts of ARG to the body ARG pool. When the urea cycle is nonfunctional, ARG becomes an essential amino acid.[2,63] Consequently, L-ARG must be administered in all disorders of the urea cycle except arginase deficiency (see Tables 9-2 and 9-3). In carbamyl phosphate synthetase (CPS) or ornithine transcarbamylase (OTC) deficiency, L-CIT may be given in place of or with L-ARG. When administered in adequate

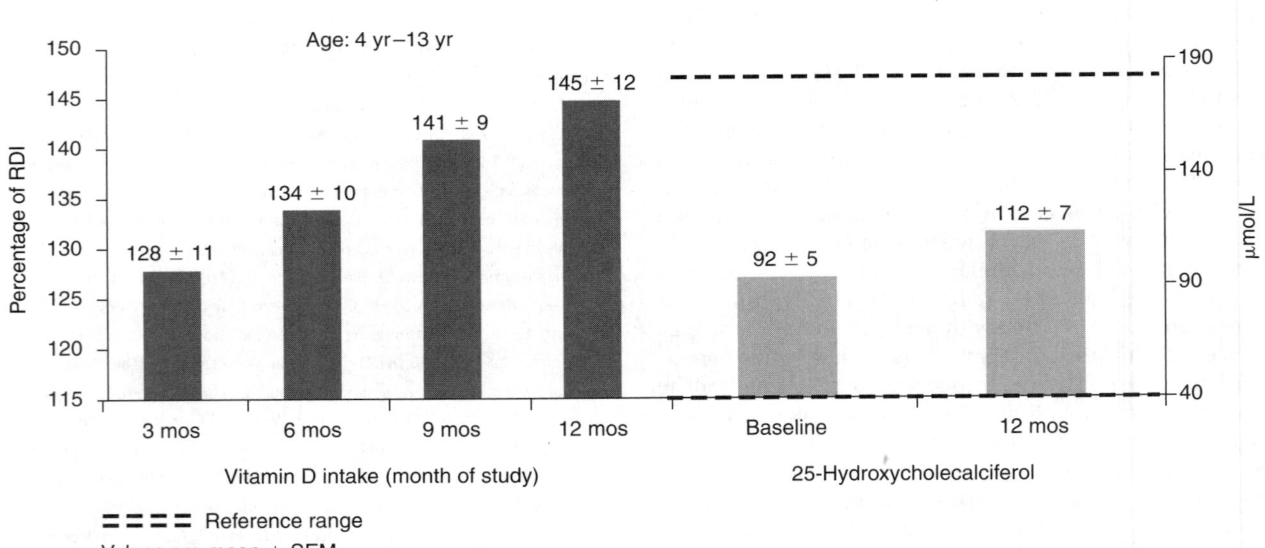

FIGURE 9-1 Vitamin D Intakes and Serum 25-Hydroxycholecalciferol Concentrations

amounts, these amino acids also enhance waste N excretion.[64] L-ARG, when given orally, should be in the base form because the hydrochloride form will cause acidosis.

Protein restriction resulting in N restriction is the primary approach to prevention of elevated blood ammonia (see Tables 9-2 and 9-3) in all except citrin deficiency (CIT II), which requires a high protein, low carbohydrate diet.[65] Citrin is an aspartate-glutamate carrier. Ornithine translocase transports ornithine into the mitochondria; a deficiency results in hyperornithinemia, hyperammonemia, and homocitrullinuria (HHH syndrome). Protein quality is determined by its essential amino acid content and completion of digestion. Protein synthesis and N utilization are more efficient when all amino acids are present in appropriate amounts at the same time. Severe restriction of intact protein leads to inadequate intake of several essential and conditionally essential amino acids, as well as minerals and vitamins. Because of this, medical foods consisting of essential and conditionally essential amino acids, minerals, and vitamins have been devised (see Table 9-5). Carnitine, cystine, taurine, and tyrosine may not be synthesized in adequate amounts when liver parenchymal cells are damaged. Thus, any medical food used for therapy of urea cycle disorders should contain carnitine, cystine, taurine, and tyrosine. Overrestriction of an essential amino acid or N leads to decreased protein synthesis or body protein catabolism and increased blood ammonia concentration. To provide adequate amounts of essential amino acids in the protein-restricted diet, from one-half to two-thirds of the protein prescription should be supplied by medical food,[34] as long as growth is proceeding. During the prepubertal growth spurt, greater amounts of protein may be required than previously needed. Maintenance of anabolism is essential to prevent hyperammonemia.

The protein quality of medical foods must be evaluated based on their amino acid, mineral, and vitamin content because intact protein sources (dairy products, meat, fish and other seafood, poultry) normally supply large amounts of minerals and vitamins. Intracellular minerals are important for protein synthesis. Medical foods devised for patients with urea cycle disorders must supply all minerals and vitamins not contributed by the small quantities of low-protein breads/cereals, fruits, fats, and vegetables the patient may ingest. Acosta et al.[66] reported that adequate intakes of protein and energy for 6 months in 17 patients resulted in a change in anthropometric Z scores of length from −1.2 to −0.8 ($p = 0.04$), a head circumference change from −1.0 to −0.68 ($p = 0.22$), and a weight change from −0.9 to −0.4 ($p = 0.01$). Plasma albumin concentration increased from 34 g/L at baseline to 38 g/L at 6 months. Mean protein intake in infants 0 < 6 months of age was 70% of Food and Agriculture Organization (FAO) recommendations and 62% in 6 < 12-month-old infants. Linear growth increased without an increase in plasma ammonia concentrations.

Because protein intake is severely restricted in urea cycle enzyme defects in all except CIT II, energy (kcal) intake should be increased to prevent use of muscle protein for energy purposes, thereby preventing catabolism of body protein (see Table 9-3). The best energy-to-protein ratio is unknown in these disorders; however, obesity should be avoided. Energy is the first requirement of the body, and inadequate energy intake for protein synthesis and other needs will lead to elevated blood ammonia concentration.[2]

Waste N excretion is enhanced through treatment with sodium benzoate, sodium phenylacetate, or sodium phenylbutyrate. Sodium benzoate is conjugated with glycine primarily in hepatic and renal cell mitochondria to form hippurate, which is cleared by the kidney.[44] Sodium phenylacetate conjugates with glutamine in kidney and liver cells to form phenylacetylglutamine, which is excreted by the kidney.[67,68] Phenylacetic acid conjugates with taurine in the kidney.[67] Glycine is readily made from serine. Tetrahydrofolate is required for this reaction to occur. Glycine also can be synthesized from glutamate. Pyridoxal phosphate (PLP) and an aldolase are required for this set of reactions. Because several coenzymes are required to maintain serine, nicotinamide-adenine dinucleotide (NAD), PLP, and glycine pools and the use of CoA in synthesis of hippurate, folate, pantothenate, pyridoxine, and niacin should be administered at greater than RDAs[1] for age when sodium benzoate is given therapeutically. Because dietary intake of potassium is often low and use of drugs to enhance waste N loss can lead to its urinary excretion, frequent monitoring of plasma potassium (K+) concentration is essential to maintain it within the normal range.[63] Daily supplements of KCl may be required because very low plasma K+ concentration can lead to death.

A protein-free prescription should be given for the 3.2 kg infant for 2 to 3 days to lower blood ammonia concentration to treatment range, and may be as follows:

L-ARG, mg	150 × 3.2 kg = 480 mg
Energy, kcal	140 × 3.2 kg = 448 kcal
Sodium phenylbutyrate, mg	450 × 3.2 kg = 1440 mg

Food	Amount	Energy
L-ARG base	480 mg	0
ProPhree powder	88 g	449
Total		449
Per kg body weight		140

Add water to make 650 mL (22 fl oz).

Protein must be added as soon as blood ammonia concentration reaches the upper limit of the treatment range, and may be as follows:

L-ARG base	150×3.2 kg = 480 mg
Protein, g	2.4×3.2 kg = 7.7 g
Energy, kcal	135×3.2 kg = 432 kcal
Sodium phenylbutyrate, mg	475×3.2 kg = 1520 mg

Two-thirds of prescribed protein may be given as medical food; 7.7 g × 0.67 yields 5.2 g protein as medical food. The remainder of protein may be given as Enfamil Lipil.

Food	Amount	ARG (mg)	Protein (g)	Energy (kcal)
Enfamil Lipil powder	22 g	60	2.2	103
Cyclinex-1 powder	73 g	—	5.5	372
L-ARG base	420 mg	420	—	—
Total		480	7.7	475
Per kg body weight		150	2.4	148

Add 1520 mg sodium phenylbutyrate. Add water to make 650 mL (22 fl oz).

Inborn Errors of Carbohydrate Metabolism: Galactosemias

Galactosemias have been screened for in the United States for almost as long as PKU. Three forms of galactosemia have been reported: galactokinase deficiency, galactose-4-epimerase deficiency, and galactose-1-phosphate uridyl transferase (GALT)[14] deficiency.

Deletion of galactose in all forms of galactosemia must be accompanied by adequate intakes of protein, energy, minerals, and vitamins (see Tables 9-2 and 9-3). Galactose binds with phosphate in patients with GALT deficiencies. This intracellular sequestering of phosphorus in combination with excess urinary phosphate loss (Fanconi syndrome) suggests the need for phosphorus intake greater than the RDA.[1] Inadequate calcium intake coupled with hypogonadism results in depressed bone mineral density in patients with galactosemia.[69,70] When GALT-deficient prepubertal patients were given 750 mg calcium, 1.0 mg vitamin K_1, and 10 μg vitamin D_3 daily for 2 years, in addition to their galactose-restricted diet, a significant increase in bone mineral content of the spine occurred.[71]

Therapy of galactosemia due to GALT deficiency, although lifesaving in the infant, has resulted in less than optimum outcomes. Poor outcomes may be the result of small but significant intakes of naturally occurring galactose in fruits, vegetables, grains, legumes (dried beans and peas), and other foods.[72] On the other hand, in vivo synthesis of galactose[73,74] may be responsible for long-term complications in patients with gene mutations resulting in no enzyme activity. Defective tissue galactosylation of proteins, carbohydrates, and lipids, which is depressed by elevated concentrations of erythrocyte galactose-1-phosphate in the patient, may contribute.[75,76]

Infant formula powders made from soy protein isolate without added lactose contain significantly less galactose than do liquid soy protein isolate formulas, formulas for lactase deficiency, or formulas made from hydrolyzed casein, due to the added carrageenan.[14] Milk products, including all soft cheeses and some hard cheeses, and organ meats must be eliminated. Careful label reading for the presence of lactose, casein, or whey and examination of all drug ingredients should be practiced before suggesting the use of any food or drug.[14] Lactobionic acid, found in Neo-calglucon, should not be used in patients with galactosemia due to the presence of galactose.[77]

Rates of decline in erythrocyte galactose-1-phosphate differ in infants with differing genotypes. Infants with a genotype of Q188R/Q188R, all receiving the same diet management, had an erythrocyte galactose-1-phosphate of 4.9 mg/dL at 5 to 8 months of age, and patients with a genotype of Q188R/other had a concentration of 3.3 mg/dL at the same age. Patients with a genotype of other/other had an erythrocyte galactose-1-phosphate of 2.5 mg/dL when in the same age range.[78] Use of the breath test to measure galactose oxidation also indicates differences in utilization of galactose in patients by genotype.[79] Whether to eliminate more than milk from the diet of adults with GALT deficiency is not known, but is now being discussed by some medical geneticists.

Inborn Errors of Fatty Acid Oxidation (Mitochondrial)

Fatty acids are a primary fuel for the body when fasting is prolonged, and are a direct source of fuel for heart and skeletal muscle. Ketones such as acetoacetate and β-hydroxybutyric acid, obtained during hepatic fat metabolism, are an important energy source for the brain and other tissues.[80] Consequently, all fat must not be removed from the diet and care must be taken to supply required energy, linoleic acid, and α-linolenic acid (see Table 9-3). Fat restriction in long-chain and very-long-chain fatty acid oxidation defects; replacement of most fat with MCT; addition of the docosahexaenoic acid precursor, α-linolenic acid, with the use of canola, soy, walnut, or flaxseed oils[15]; avoidance of fasting; glucose therapy as needed; and uncooked cornstarch have improved outcomes (see Table 9-3). Patients with a defect in medium- or short-chain fatty acid oxidation require avoidance of fasting and of MCT oil, addition of glucose for hypoglycemia, and uncooked cornstarch as needed. The recommendation for fat is 30–35% of energy for children and adults.

Patients with VLCAD, LCHAD, TFP, or CPT 2 deficiency require about 10% of energy as long-chain fats and about

20% of energy as MCT. With this restriction of long-chain fats, absorption of fat-soluble vitamins, especially vitamin E, may prove difficult. Thus, supplementation with a water-miscible form of vitamin E should be considered if plasma α-tocopherol concentrations are below reference range when frequently analyzed. Ingested vitamins A and D should remain in normal ranges.[42] MCT mixed with orange juice given prior to exercise to patients with LCHAD, LCAD, or TFP lowered muscle pain and the incidence of rhabdomyolysis more than in patients given only orange juice.[15]

Genetic Metabolic Dietitians International has developed resources for helping to manage patients with VLCAD or MCAD deficiency. These nutrition guidelines are available at http://www.gmdi.org/Resources/NutritionGuidelines/VLCADGuidelines/ and http://www.gmdi.org.

Protein intake at much greater than the RDA may be beneficial in helping to control hypoglycemia and in preventing the obesity that occurs in patients fed high-carbohydrate diets. Patients with LCHAD or TFP deficiency fed 30% of energy as protein[15] had higher resting energy expenditure and lower energy intake while on the high protein diet than on a diet containing only 11% of energy as protein. Patients with medium- and short-chain fatty acid oxidation defects may benefit with up to 20% of energy as protein to help control hypoglycemia. Some patients with SCAD deficiency have been found to respond to riboflavin supplementation. Because riboflavin is extremely insoluble, 15 to 25 mg should be given orally with meals up to three times daily.[1]

Malonyl-CoA decarboxylase is present in high amounts in human heart and skeletal muscle, and the liver, kidney, and pancreas.[81] Malonyl-CoA decarboxylase plays a key role in peroxysmal systolic and mitochondrial fatty acid oxidation, and appears to inhibit CPT I.[82] Malonyl-CoA decarboxylase deficiency results in variable clinical symptoms including hypoglycemia, hypotonia, cardiomyopathy, developmental delay, acidosis, seizures, and elevated urinary malonic acid.[83,84] Moderate long-chain fat restriction, MCT, and L-carnitine supplementation with frequent feedings appear to be beneficial (see Tables 9-2 and 9-3).[84,85]

Glutaric aciduria type II (multiple acyl-CoA dehydrogenase deficiency) is caused by defects in electron transport lipoprotein (ETF) or ETF-ubiquinone oxidoreductase (ETF-QO), and results in three main phenotypes: neonatal onset with congenital anomalies, neonatal onset without congenital anomalies, and mild or later onset.[86] Diets low in protein and fat with supplementation of L-carnitine and riboflavin have been tried with those who present neonatally with or without birth defects, but these infants usually die within the first months of life.[87] Patients with milder or later onset of symptoms treated with oral riboflavin, L-carnitine, and diets low in protein and fat (see Table 9-2) have had little better outcomes than infants who present neonatally.[86–89] The Europeans have developed an approach somewhat different than that used in the United States for managing patients with mitochondrial fatty acid oxidation defects.[90]

Areas Needing Further Research

In 1988, the National Institutes of Health recognized the need for research on nutrition therapy of inborn errors of metabolism by issuing a request for applications (RFA).[91] The goals listed in the RFA were (1) to improve the effectiveness of currently utilized nutrition therapies of inborn errors by making them safer, more palatable, and less likely to lead to secondary deleterious consequences; and (2) to develop new rational diet therapies based on knowledge of pathogenesis. Research approaches outlined in the following list were identified for support, and investigations utilizing these approaches were encouraged:

- Investigations of how vitamins may affect active coenzyme concentrations and activate specific deficient enzymes
- Studies of the pathogenesis of the clinical manifestations of inborn errors, designed to develop rationale for better diet therapy
- Longitudinal studies of the adequacy of nutrition therapies in maintaining normal growth and development while maximizing therapeutic response
- Studies of the development of secondary nutrient deficiencies in patients on therapeutic diets, due to interference with the availability of other nutrients, such as trace elements
- Investigation of possible injurious effects of specific components of therapeutic diets
- Attempts to improve nutrition therapies of inborn errors to eliminate metabolic problems not completely controlled, such as hyperlipidemia and hyperuricemia in glycogen storage disease or carnitine wasting in renal Fanconi syndrome or the organic acidemias
- Development of methods for improving the palatability or acceptability of nutrition therapy, such as by the substitution of specific amino acid–deficient peptides for amino acid mixtures
- Development of animal models for the study of nutrition therapies of inborn errors, either by a search for heterozygotes or through use of recombinant DNA methods

Other research needs include the following:

- Investigation of reasons for and methods to eliminate bone mineral loss in patients with PKU and other IEMs[54,56]
- Evaluation of reasons for and methods to prevent anemia in patients with PKU who are ingesting recommended iron for age[55,58]

- Examination of the effectiveness of different methods and approaches to educate the adolescent patient with an IEM to encourage diet compliance[92,93]
- Determination of whether the addition of prescribed cholesterol to the elemental diet of patients with PKU helps prevent osteopenia and abnormally low blood cholesterol concentrations and helps prevent spontaneous abortions in pregnant treated women with PKU[12,94,95]
- Investigation of how much niacin is required by the patient with PKU to maintain niacin status and whether elevated plasma PHE concentration is related to decreased metabolism of tryptophan to niacin[60,61]
- Evaluation of cause for seborrheic dermatitis in patients with elevated plasma PHE concentrations, low plasma tyrosine concentrations,[12] or low plasma biotin concentrations[62]

Functions of the Dietitian in Nutrition Support of Patients with an Inborn Error of Metabolism

The roles of the dietitian in nutrition support of patients with an inborn error of metabolism are outlined in **Table 9-8**. The dietitian, because of her or his central role in therapy, is often the case manager,[11] coordinating clinical care and acting as liaison with the public health nutritionist[96,97] or home health agency.[11] The crucial role of the dietitian in long-term management of the patient with an inborn error of metabolism mandates excellent interpersonal skills as well as a knowledge base far in excess of entry-level requirements. Without this knowledge and the capability to transmit this knowledge to patients, parents, and professionals, outcomes may be poor or death may occur.

TABLE 9-8 Functions of the Dietitian in Nutrition Support of Patients with Inborn Errors of Metabolism

During Diagnosis	Evaluate nutrient intake. Prepare nutrition support plan. Implement nutrition support plan. Evaluate nutrition support plan. Evaluate nutrition status. Record findings in medical records. Adjust amino acid prescription (e.g., glycine). Adjust selected medications (e.g., sodium benzoate, sodium phenylbutyrate).
During Critical Illness	Recommend composition of feedings. Develop tube feedings when needed. Monitor nutrition support. Record in medical record. Recommend amount to feed per hour. Recommend continuous or intermittent feedings. Recommend route of alimentation. Recommend necessary laboratory tests. Recommend peripheral or central line feeding. Recommend size of feeding tube.
During Long-Term Care	Formulate diet prescription/nutrition care plan. Record in medical record. Monitor for diet compliance. Revise nutrition care plan as needed. Evaluate effectiveness of nutrition care plan. Coordinate with other agencies. Prepare sample menus. Modify diet prescription during illness. Prescribe medical food. Prescribe very-low-protein foods. Recommend methods of feeding. Evaluate research findings and apply to clinical care. Fill diet prescription. Monitor for gastrointestinal complications. Refer to other specialists. Monitor potential nutrient–drug interactions. Help caretaker prepare patient-specific food lists, if needed. Help caretaker prepare shopping lists, if needed.

Source: Acosta PB. *Nutrition Management of Patients with Inherited Metabolic Disorders.* Sudbury, MA: Jones & Bartlett Learning, 2010.

Nutrigenomics

Some dietitians supply direct services to patients with a single gene defect and their families; these services have been provided for over 55 years in university hospital/clinic medical genetic services. Only in relatively recent years have some nutrients been considered capable of interacting with the genome to change gene expression, structure, and function.[98] Patients with multifactorial diseases usually not seen in medical genetics clinics are the usual persons for whom the dietitian provides diet counseling; these patients' diseases may include, among others, cancer, diabetes mellitus, heart disease, hypertension, osteomalacia, and ulcers. Diet alone is seldom the exclusive therapy, and if it must be followed long-term it is seldom adequately adhered to.

According to Bull and Fenech,[98] risk for developmental and degenerative diseases increases with increasing DNA damage, which is dependent on nutrition status and optimal concentration of micronutrients for prevention of genome damage. Overfeeding and failure to ingest foods with bioactive compounds, minerals, vitamins, and protein in adequate amounts may lead to DNA methylation and chronic disease,[99,100] whereas ingestion of a diet rich in minerals and vitamins may help prevent disease.[101,102]

REFERENCES

1. Otten JJ, Hellwig JP, Meyers LD. *Dietary Reference Intakes: The Essential Guide to Nutrient Requirements*. Washington, DC: National Academies Press; 2006.
2. Elsas LJ, Acosta PB. Inherited metabolic disease: amino acids, organic acids, and galactose. In: Shils ME, Shike M, Olson J, Ross AC, Caballero B, Cousins RJ, eds. *Modern Nutrition in Health and Disease,* 10th ed. Philadelphia: Lippincott Williams & Wilkins; 2005:909–959.
3. Goldblum OM, Brusilow SW, Maldonado YA, Farmer ER. Neonatal citrullinemia associated with cutaneous manifestations and arginine deficiency. *J Am Acad Dermatol.* 1986;14:321–326.
4. Borum PR, Bennett SG. Carnitine as an essential nutrient. *J Am Coll Nutr.* 1986;5:177–182.
5. Sansaricq C, Garg S, Norton PM, Phansalkar SV, Snyderman SE. Cystine deficiency during dietotherapy of homocystinemia. *Acta Paediatr Scand.* 1975;64:215–218.
6. Laidlaw SA, Kopple JD. Newer concepts of the indispensable amino acids. *Am J Clin Nutr.* 1987;46:593–605.
7. Blau N, Thony B, Cotton RGH, Hyland K. Disorders of tetrahydrobiopterin and related biogenic amines. In: Scriver CR, Beaudet AL, Sly WS, Valle D, eds. *The Metabolic and Molecular Bases of Inherited Disease,* 8th ed. New York: McGraw-Hill; 2001:1725–1776.
8. Acosta PB. Nutrition support for inborn errors. In: Samour PQ, King K, eds. *Handbook of Pediatric Nutrition,* 3rd ed. Boston: Jones & Bartlett Publishers; 2005:239–286.
9. Frazier DM. Newborn screening by mass spectrometry. In: Acosta PB, ed. *Nutrition Management of Patients with Inherited Metabolic Disorders.* Sudbury, MA: Jones & Bartlett Publishers; 2010:21–65.
10. American College of Medical Genetics. Newborn screening: toward a uniform screening panel and system. *Genet Med.* 2006;8(Suppl 1):1S–252S.
11. Acosta PB. *Nutrition Management of Patients with Inherited Metabolic Disorders*. Sudbury, MA: Jones & Bartlett Publishers; 2010.
12. Acosta PB, Matalon KM. Nutrition management of patients with inherited disorders of aromatic amino acids. In: Acosta PB, ed. *Nutrition Management of Patients with Inherited Metabolic Disorders.* Sudbury, MA: Jones & Bartlett Publishers; 2010:119–174.
13. Marriage B. Nutrition management of patients with inherited disorders of branched-chain amino acid metabolism. In: Acosta PB, ed. *Nutrition Management of Patients with Inherited Metabolic Disorders.* Sudbury, MA: Jones & Bartlett Publishers; 2010:175–236.
14. Acosta PB. Nutrition management of patients with inherited disorders of galactose metabolism. In: Acosta PB, ed. *Nutrition Management of Patients with Inherited Metabolic Disorders.* Sudbury, MA: Jones & Bartlett Publishers; 2010:343–367.
15. Gillingham MB. Nutrition management of patients with inherited disorders of mitochondrial fatty acid oxidation. In: Acosta PB, ed. *Nutrition Management of Patients with Inherited Metabolic Disorders.* Sudbury, MA: Jones & Bartlett Publishers; 2010:369–403.
16. van Calcar S. Nutrition management of patients with inherited disorders of sulfur amino acid metabolism. In: Acosta PB, ed. *Nutrition Management of Patients with Inherited Metabolic Disorders.* Sudbury, MA: Jones & Bartlett Publishers; 2010:237–281.
17. Yannicelli S. Nutrition management of patients with inherited disorders of organic acid metabolism. In: Acosta PB, ed. *Nutrition Management of Patients with Inherited Metabolic Disorders.* Sudbury, MA: Jones & Bartlett Publishers; 2010:283–341.
18. Blau N, Koch R, Matalon R, Stevens RC. Five years of synergistic scientific effort on phenylketonuria therapeutic development and molecular understanding. *Mol Genet Metab.* 2005;86:S1.
19. Rosenblatt DS, Fenton W. Inherited disorders of folate and cobalamin transport and metabolism. In: Scriver CR, Beaudet AL, Sly WS, Valle D, eds. *The Metabolic and Molecular Bases of Inherited Disease,* 8th ed. New York: McGraw-Hill; 2001:3897–3934.
20. Bonkowsky HL, Magnussen CR, Collins AR, Doherty JM, Hess RA, Tschudy DP. Comparative effects of glycerol and dextrose on porphyrin precursor excretion in acute intermittent porphyria. *Metabolism.* 1976;25:405–414.
21. Langenbeck U, Burgard P, Wendel U, Lindner M, Zschocke J. Metabolic phenotypes of phenylketonuria. Kinetic and molecular evaluation of the Blaskovics protein loading test. *J Inherit Metab Dis.* 2009;32:506–513.
22. Blaskovics ME, Schaeffler GE, Hack S. Phenylalaninaemia. Differential diagnosis. *Arch Dis Child.* 1974;49:835–843.
23. Blaskovics ME. Diagnostic considerations in phenylalaninemic subjects before and after dietary therapy. *Ir Med J.* 1976;69:410–414.
24. Bremer JH. Transitory hyperphenylalaninemia. In: Bickel H, Hudson FP, Woolf LI, eds. *Phenylketonuria and Some Other Inborn Errors of Amino Acid Metabolism.* Stuttgart: Georg Thieme Verlag; 1971:93–97.
25. Gjetting T, Petersen M, Guldberg P, Guttler F. Missense mutations in the N-terminal domain of human phenylalanine hydroxylase interfere with binding of regulatory phenylalanine. *Am J Hum Genet.* 2001;68:1353–1360.
26. Wolf B. Disorders of biotin metabolism. In: Scriver CR, Beaudet AL, Sly WS, Valle D, eds. *The Metabolic and Molecular Bases of Inherited Disease,* 8th ed. New York: McGraw-Hill; 2001:3935–3962.
27. Sarkissian CN, Gamez A, Wang L, et al. Preclinical evaluation of multiple species of PEGylated recombinant phenylalanine ammonia lyase for the treatment of phenylketonuria. *Proc Natl Acad Sci U S A.* 2008;105:20894–20899.
28. Zinnanti WJ, Lazovic J, Griffin K, et al. Dual mechanism of brain injury and novel treatment strategy in maple syrup urine disease. *Brain.* 2009;132:903–918.
29. Matalon R, Michals-Matalon K, Bhatia G, et al. Double blind placebo control trial of large neutral amino acids in treatment of PKU: effect on blood phenylalanine. *J Inherit Metab Dis.* 2007;30:153–158.
30. Rudman D, Feller A. Evidence for deficiencies of conditionally essential nutrients during total parenteral nutrition. *J Am Coll Nutr.* 1986;5:101–106.
31. Alexander JW, Clayton BE, Delves HT. Mineral and trace-metal balances in children receiving normal and synthetic diets. *Q J Med.* 1974;169:80–111.

32. Acosta PB. Rationales for and practical aspects of nutrition management. In: Acosta PB, ed. *Nutrition Management of Patients with Inherited Metabolic Disorders.* Sudbury, MA: Jones & Bartlett Publishers; 2010:99–118.
33. Erbersdobler HF, Somoza V. Forty years of furosine—forty years of using Maillard reaction products as indicators of the nutritional quality of foods. *Mol Nutr Food Res.* 2007;51:423–430.
34. Acosta PB, Yannicelli S. *Nutrition Support Protocols,* 4th ed. Columbus, OH: Ross Products Division, Abbott Laboratories; 2001.
35. Guttler F, Olesen ES, Wamberg E. Diurnal variations of serum phenylalanine in phenylketonuric children on low phenylalanine diet. *Am J Clin Nutr.* 1969;22:1568–1570.
36. Gropper SS, Acosta PB. Effect of simultaneous ingestion of L-amino acids and whole protein on plasma amino acid and urea nitrogen concentrations in humans. *J Parenter Enteral Nutr.* 1991; 15:48–53.
37. Scriver CR, Waters PJ, Sarkissian C, et al. PAHdb: a locus-specific knowledgebase. *Hum Mutat.* 2000;15:99–104.
38. Alvarez DL, Campistol PJ, Ribes RA, Riverola de Vecina AT [Phenylalanine metabolites in hyperphenylalaninemic children]. *An Esp Pediatr.* 1992;36:371–374.
39. Folling A. The original detection of phenylketonuria. In: Bickel H, Hudson FP, Woolf LI, eds. *Phenylketonuria and Some Other Inborn Errors of Amino Acid Metabolism.* Stuttgart: Georg Thieme Verlag; 1971:1–3.
40. Kure S, Hou DC, Ohura T, et al. Tetrahydrobiopterin-responsive phenylalanine hydroxylase deficiency. *J Pediatr.* 1999;135:375–378.
41. Hennermann JB, Buhrer C, Blau N, Vetter B, Monch E. Long-term treatment with tetrahydrobiopterin increases phenylalanine tolerance in children with severe phenotype of phenylketonuria. *Mol Genet Metab.* 2005;86(Suppl 1):S86–S90.
42. Acosta PB. Evaluation of nutrition status. In: Acosta PB, ed. *Nutrition Management of Patients with Inherited Metabolic Disorders.* Sudbury, MA: Jones & Bartlett Publishers; 2010:67–98.
43. Loots DT, Mienie LJ, Erasmus E. Amino-acid depletion induced by abnormal amino-acid conjugation and protein restriction in isovaleric acidemia. *Eur J Clin Nutr.* 2007;61:1323–1327.
44. Moldave K, Meister A. Synthesis of phenylacetylglutamine by human tissue. *J Biol Chem.* 1957;229:463–476.
45. Dangin M, Boirie Y, Garcia-Rodenas C, et al. The digestion rate of protein is an independent regulating factor of postprandial protein retention. *Am J Physiol Endocrinol Metab.* 2001;280:E340–E348.
46. Herrmann ME, Brosicke HG, Keller M, Monch E, Helge H. Dependence of the utilization of a phenylalanine-free amino acid mixture on different amounts of single dose ingested. A case report. *Eur J Pediatr.* 1994;153:501–503.
47. Schoeffer A, Herrmann ME, Brosicke HG, Moench E. Effect of dosage and timing of amino acid mixtures on nitrogen retention in patients with phenylketonuria. *J Nutr Med.* 1994;4:415–418.
48. Arnold GL, Vladutiu CJ, Kirby RS, Blakely EM, Deluca JM. Protein insufficiency and linear growth restriction in phenylketonuria. *J Pediatr.* 2002;141:243–246.
49. Acosta PB, Yannicelli S. Nutrient intake and biochemical status of children with phenylketonuria undergoing nutrition management. Unpublished data. Columbus, Ohio: Ross Products Division, Abbott Laboratories; 2003.
50. Yannicelli S, Acosta PB, Velazquez A, et al. Improved growth and nutrition status in children with methylmalonic or propionic acidemia fed an elemental medical food. *Mol Genet Metab.* 2003;80:181–188.
51. Acosta PB, Yannicelli S, Singh R, et al. Intake and blood levels of fatty acids in treated patients with phenylketonuria. *J Pediatr Gastroenterol Nutr.* 2001;33:253–259.
52. Pratt EL, Snyderman SE, Cheung MW, et al. The threonine requirement of the normal infant. *J Nutr.* 1955;56:231–251.
53. Acosta PB, Yannicelli S, Singh RH, Elsas LJ, Mofidi S, Steiner RD. Iron status of children with phenylketonuria undergoing nutrition therapy assessed by transferrin receptors. *Genet Med.* 2004;6:96–101.
54. Yannicelli S, Medeiros DM. Elevated plasma phenylalanine concentrations may adversely affect bone status of phenylketonuric mice. *J Inherit Metab Dis.* 2002;25:347–361.
55. Acosta PB, Yannicelli S. Plasma micronutrient concentrations in infants undergoing therapy for phenylketonuria. *Biol Trace Elem Res.* 1999;67:75–84.
56. Pasquali M, Singh R, Kennedy MJ, et al. Pyridinium cross-links: a parameter of bone matrix turnover in phenylketonuria. *Book of Abstracts,* 5th Meeting of the International Society for Neonatal Screening, June 26–29, 2002. Genoa, Italy.
57. Bushinsky DA. Acid-base imbalance and the skeleton. *Eur J Nutr.* 2001;40:238–244.
58. Bodley JL, Austin VJ, Hanley WB, Clarke JT, Zlotkin S. Low iron stores in infants and children with treated phenylketonuria: a population at risk for iron-deficiency anaemia and associated cognitive deficits. *Eur J Pediatr.* 1993;152:140–143.
59. Gropper SS, Yannicelli S, White BD, Medeiros DM. Plasma phenylalanine concentrations are associated with hepatic iron content in a murine model for phenylketonuria. *Mol Genet Metab.* 2004;82:76–82.
60. La Du BN, Zannoni VG. Basic biochemical disturbances in aromatic amino acid metabolism in phenylketonuria. In: Bickel H, Hudson FP, Woolf LI, eds. *Phenylketonuria and Some Other Inborn Errors of Amino Acid Metabolism.* Stuttgart: Georg Thieme Verlag; 1971:6–13.
61. Lewis JS, Loskill S, Bunker ML, Acosta PB, Kim R. N-methylnicotinamide excretion of phenylketonuric children and a child with Hartnup disease before and after phenylalanine and tryptophan load. *Fed Proc.* 1974;33:666A.
62. Schulpis KH, Nyalala JO, Papakonstantinou ED, et al. Biotin recycling impairment in phenylketonuric children with seborrheic dermatitis. *Int J Dermatol.* 1998;37:918–921.
63. Singh RH. Nutritional management of patients with urea cycle disorders. *J Inherit Metab Dis.* 2007;30:880–887.
64. Brusilow S, Horwich A. Urea cycle enzymes. In: Scriver CR, Beaudet AL, Sly WS, Valle D, eds. *The Metabolic and Molecular Bases of Inherited Disease,* 8th ed. New York: McGraw-Hill; 2001:1909–1963.
65. Dimmock D, Kobayashi K, Iijima M, et al. Citrin deficiency: a novel cause of failure to thrive that responds to a high-protein, low-carbohydrate diet. *Pediatrics.* 2007;119:e773–e777.
66. Acosta PB, Yannicelli S, Ryan AS, et al. Nutritional therapy improves growth and protein status of children with a urea cycle enzyme defect. *Mol Genet Metab.* 2005;86:448–455.
67. Ambrose AM, Powder FW, Sherwin CP. Further studies on the detoxification of phenylacetic acid. *J Biol Chem.* 1933;101:669–675.

68. James MO, Smith RL, Williams RT, Reidenberg M. The conjugation of phenylacetic acid in man, sub-human primates and some non-primate species. *Proc R Soc Lond B Biol Sci.* 1972;182:25–35.
69. Kaufman FR, Loro ML, Azen C, Wenz E, Gilsanz V. Effect of hypogonadism and deficient calcium intake on bone density in patients with galactosemia. *J Pediatr.* 1993;123:365–370.
70. Rubio-Gozalbo ME, Hamming S, van Kroonenburgh MJ, Bakker JA, Vermeer C, Forget PP. Bone mineral density in patients with classic galactosaemia. *Arch Dis Child.* 2002;87:57–60.
71. Panis B, Vermeer C, van Kroonenburgh MJ, et al. Effect of calcium, vitamins K_1 and D_3 on bone in galactosemia. *Bone.* 2006;39:1123–1129.
72. Acosta PB, Gross KC. Hidden sources of galactose in the environment. *Eur J Pediatr.* 1995;154:S87–S92.
73. Berry GT, Moate PJ, Reynolds RA, et al. The rate of de novo galactose synthesis in patients with galactose-1-phosphate uridyltransferase deficiency. *Mol Genet Metab.* 2004;81:22–30.
74. Schadewaldt P, Kamalanathan L, Hammen HW, Wendel U. Age dependence of endogenous galactose formation in Q188R homozygous galactosemic patients. *Mol Genet Metab.* 2004;81:31–44.
75. Charlwood J, Clayton P, Keir G, Mian N, Winchester B. Defective galactosylation of serum transferrin in galactosemia. *Glycobiology.* 1998;8:351–357.
76. Lai K, Langley SD, Khwaja FW, Schmitt EW, Elsas LJ. GALT deficiency causes UDP-hexose deficit in human galactosemic cells. *Glycobiology.* 2003;13:285–294.
77. Harju M. Lactobionic acid as a substrate of ß-galactosidases. *Milchwissenschaft.* 1990;45:411–415.
78. Singh RH, Kennedy MJ, Jonas CR, Dembure P, Elsas LJ. Whole body oxidation and galactosemia genotype: prognosis for galactose tolerance in the first year of life. *J Inherit Metab Dis.* 2003;26:123A.
79. Berry GT, Singh RH, Mazur AT, et al. Galactose breath testing distinguishes variant and severe galactose-1-phosphate uridyltransferase genotypes. *Pediatr Res.* 2000;48:323–328.
80. Roe CR, Ding J. Mitochondrial fatty acid oxidation disorders. In: Scriver CR, Beaudet AL, Sly WS, Valle D, eds. *The Metabolic and Molecular Bases of Inherited Disease,* 8th ed. New York: McGraw-Hill; 2001:2297–2326.
81. Sacksteder KA, Morrell JC, Wanders RJ, Matalon R, Gould SJ. MCD encodes peroxisomal and cytoplasmic forms of malonyl-CoA decarboxylase and is mutated in malonyl-CoA decarboxylase deficiency. *J Biol Chem.* 1999;274:24461–24468.
82. Saggerson D. Malonyl-CoA, a key signaling molecule in mammalian cells. *Annu Rev Nutr.* 2008;28:253–272.
83. Ficicioglu C, Chrisant MR, Payan I, Chace DH. Cardiomyopathy and hypotonia in a 5-month-old infant with malonyl-CoA decarboxylase deficiency: potential for preclinical diagnosis with expanded newborn screening. *Pediatr Cardiol.* 2005;26:881–883.
84. Salomons GS, Jakobs C, Pope LL, et al. Clinical, enzymatic and molecular characterization of nine new patients with malonyl-coenzyme A decarboxylase deficiency. *J Inherit Metab Dis.* 2007;30:23–28.
85. Yano S, Sweetman L, Thorburn DR, Mofidi S, Williams JC. A new case of malonyl coenzyme A decarboxylase deficiency presenting with cardiomyopathy. *Eur J Pediatr.* 1997;156:382–383.
86. Frerman FE. Defects of electron transfer lipoprotein and electron transfer lipoprotein oxidoreductase: glutaric acidemia type II. In: Scriver CR, Beaudet AL, Sly WS, Valle D, eds. *The Metabolic and Molecular Bases of Inherited Disease,* 8th ed. New York: McGraw-Hill; 2001:2357–2365.
87. Angle B, Burton BK. Risk of sudden death and acute life-threatening events in patients with glutaric acidemia type II. *Mol Genet Metab.* 2008;93:36–39.
88. Maillart E, Acquaviva-Bourdain C, Rigal O, et al. Multiple acyl-CoA dehydrogenase deficiency (MADD): a curable cause of genetic muscular lipidosis. *Rev Neurol (Paris).* 2010:166:289–294.
89. Vockley J. Glutaric aciduria type 2 and newborn screening: commentary. *Mol Genet Metab.* 2008;93:5–6.
90. Spiekerkoetter U, Lindner M, Santer R, et al. Treatment recommendations in long-chain fatty acid oxidation defects: consensus from a workshop. *J Inherit Metab Dis.* 2009;32:498–505.
91. Levin EY, de la Cruz F. *Nutritional Therapy of Inborn Errors of Metabolism.* Bethesda, MD: National Institutes of Child Health and Human Development; 1988.
92. Hummel SL, DeFranco AC, Skorcz S, Montoye CK, Koelling TM. Recommendation of low-salt diet and short-term outcomes in heart failure with preserved systolic function. *Am J Med.* 2009;122:1029–1036.
93. Coffen RD. The 600-step program for type 1 diabetes self-management in youth: the magnitude of the self-management task. *Postgrad Med.* 2009;121:119–139.
94. Colomé C, Artuch R, Lambruschini N, Cambra FJ, Campistol J, Vilaseca M. Is there a relationship between plasma phenylalanine and cholesterol in phenylketonuric patients under dietary treatment? *Clin Biochem.* 2001;34:373–376.
95. Acosta PB, Michals-Matalon K, Austin V, et al. Nutrition findings and requirements in pregnant women with phenylketonuria. In: Platt LD, Koch R, de la Cruz F, eds. *Genetic Disorders and Pregnancy Outcome.* New York: Parthenon Publishing Group; 1997:21–32.
96. Belsten LM, Rarback S, Wellman NS. The metabolic nutritionist as a team member and case manager. *Top Clin Nutr.* 1987;2:76–81.
97. Stephens-Hitchcock E, Walker EJ. The public health approach to the treatment and follow-up of children with metabolic disorders. *Top Clin Nutr.* 1987;2:82–86.
98. Bull C, Fenech M. Genome-health nutrigenomics and nutrigenetics: nutritional requirements or 'nutriomes' for chromosomal stability and telomere maintenance at the individual level. *Proc Nutr Soc.* 2008;67:146–156.
99. Ferguson LR. Nutrigenomics approaches to functional foods. *J Am Diet Assoc.* 2009;109:452–458.
100. Plagemann A, Harder T, Brunn M, et al. Hypothalamic proopiomelanocortin promoter methylation becomes altered by early overfeeding: an epigenetic model of obesity and the metabolic syndrome. *J Physiol.* 2009;587:4963–4976.
101. Jang SH, Lim JW, Kim H. Mechanism of beta-carotene-induced apoptosis of gastric cancer cells: involvement of ataxia-telangiectasia-mutated. *Ann N Y Acad Sci.* 2009;1171:156–162.
102. Kim KC, Friso S, Choi SW. DNA methylation, an epigenetic mechanism connecting folate to healthy embryonic development and aging. *J Nutr Biochem.* 2009; 20:917–926.

Developmental Disabilities

Harriet H. Cloud

The nutritional needs of children with developmental disabilities vary and primarily involve energy, growth, regulation of the biochemical processes, and repair of cells and body tissue. Nutritional risk factors often include growth deficiency, obesity, gastrointestinal disorders, metabolic problems, feeding problems, and drug–nutrient interaction problems. The Centers for Disease Control and Prevention have reported that 17% of children under age 18 have some type of developmental disability.[1]

Definition of Developmental Disabilities

A developmental disability was defined in Public Law 99-101-496 ed. (1990, revised in 2000 to PL 106-402), the Developmental Disabilities Assistance and Bill of Rights Act,[2] as a severe chronic disability of a person that is attributable to a mental or physical impairment or combination of mental and physical impairments with the following characteristics:

- Manifests before the person attains age 22
- Likely to continue indefinitely
- Results in substantial functional limitations in three or more areas of major life activity (self-care, receptive and expressive language, learning, mobility, self-direction, capacity for independent living, and economic self-sufficiency)
- Reflects the person's need for a combination of special interdisciplinary or generic care, treatments, or other services that are lifelong or of extended duration and are individually planned and coordinated

Children with special healthcare needs are those who have or are at increased risk for a chronic physical, developmental, behavioral, or emotional condition and who require health and related services of a type or amount beyond that required by children generally.[3]

The etiology of developmental disabilities has been traced to chromosomal aberrations such as Down syndrome (trisomy 21) and Prader-Willi syndrome, neurologic insults in the prenatal period, prematurity, infectious diseases, trauma, congenital defects such as cleft lip and palate, neural tube defects such as spina bifida, inborn errors of metabolism, and other syndromes of lesser incidence.[4]

Nutrition considerations that involve the child with developmental disabilities include assessment of growth and the problems surrounding energy balance. This can lead to failure to thrive, obesity, or slow growth rate in height. The second major consideration includes feeding from the standpoint of oral motor problems, developmental delays of feeding skills, inability to self-feed, behavioral problems, and tube feedings. Other areas for nutritional consideration include drug–nutrient interaction, constipation, dental caries, urinary tract infections, allergies, and food or nutrition information the parent has received related to hyperactivity, attention deficit disorders, and treatment of disorders such as Down syndrome and autism with alternative or complementary medicine. **Table 10-1** includes a list of developmental disorders and their nutrition considerations.[5]

Nutritional Needs of the Child with Developmental Disabilities

Energy needs for children with developmental disabilities vary as they do for normal children; very little specific information is available for either. A decreased energy need is most apparent in chromosomal aberrations such as Down syndrome, conditions accompanied by limited gross motor activity such as in spina bifida, and syndromes characterized by low muscle tone such as is found in Prader-Willi syndrome, Rubinstein-Tabyi syndrome, and Turner's syndrome.

Energy needs of infants and children with other developmental disabilities such as cerebral palsy and Rett syndrome are highly individualized and vary widely.[4]

The dietary reference intakes (DRIs) are a set of nutrient-based reference values that have replaced the recommended dietary allowances (RDAs) (see Appendix H). They

TABLE 10-1 Developmental Disorders and Corresponding Nutrition Considerations

Syndrome or Developmental Disability	Nutrition Diagnostic Terms	Indicators of this Nutrition Diagnosis
Autism spectrum disorders (ASD) Characterized by delayed speech and language development, ritualistic or repetitive behaviors, and impairments in social interactions.	Inadequate energy intake	Limited or restricted food choices
	Excessive energy intake	High intake of food (kcal) due to food obsessions or use of food by behavioral interventions
	Food-medication interactions	Potential interactions between food and a variety of medications used for individuals with ASD
	Underweight	Inadequate energy intake Body mass index (BMI) <5th percentile for children 2–19 y Refusal to eat Restricted or limited food choices that result in low energy intake
	Overweight	BMI >85th percentile for children 2–19 y Excessive energy intake Infrequent, low duration, and/or low intensity physical activity Large amounts of sedentary activities Limited food choices that result in excessive energy intake
	Harmful beliefs/attitudes about food	Eating behavior serves a purpose other than nourishment Pica Food fetish
	Undesirable food choices	Intake that reflects an imbalance of nutrients/food groups Avoidance of foods/food groups Complementary and alternative medicine treatments, often nutrition-based (vitamin B-6 supplements, gluten-free casein-free diet) may place child at risk for nutrient deficiencies Intake inconsistent with Dietary Reference Intakes, US Dietary Guidelines, MyPyramid, or other methods of measuring diet quality Inability, unwillingness, or disinterest in selecting food consistent with the guidelines Condition associated with diagnosis, ASD–food selectivity, rigid eating patterns
Cerebral palsy A disorder of muscle control or coordination resulting from an injury to the brain during early fetal, perinatal, and early childhood development. There may be associated problems with intellectual, visual or other system functions.	Increased energy expenditure	Unintentional weight loss Evidence of need for accelerated or catch-up growth or weight gain; absence of normal growth Condition associated with a diagnosis (eg. cerebral palsy)
	Inadequate energy intake	Failure to gain or maintain appropriate weight Insufficient energy intake from diet compared to needs Inability to independently consume foods/fluids
	Excessive energy intake	Increased body adiposity Weight gain greater than expected Enteral nutrition more than measured/estimated energy expenditure
	Swallowing difficulty	Abnormal swallow study Prolonged feeding time

		Coughing, choking, prolonged chewing, pouching of food, regurgitation, facial expression changes during eating Decreased food intake Avoidance of food Mealtime resistance
	Altered gastrointestinal (GI) function	Constipation Condition associated with diagnoses: internal muscle tone in cerebral palsy can be affected as well as more visible external muscle tone
	Food-medication interactions	Seizure medications: food and medication interactions
	Underweight	Inadequate energy intake BMI <5th percentile for children 2–19 years Decreased muscle mass, muscle wasting Inadequate intake of food compared to estimated or measured needs History of physical disability or malnutrition
	Overweight	BMI >85th percentile for children 2–19 years Excessive energy intake Infrequent, low duration and/or low-intensity physical activity Large amounts of sedentary activities
Cystic fibrosis An inherited disorder of the exocrine glands, primarily the pancreas, pulmonary system, and sweat glands, characterized by abnormally thick luminal secretions.	Increased energy expenditure	Unintentional weight loss Evidence of need for accelerated or catch-up growth or weight gain; absence of normal growth Condition associated with a diagnosis (eg. cystic fibrosis)
	Altered gastrointestinal function	Abnormal digestive enzyme and fecal fat studies Malabsorption Steatorrhea
	Impaired nutrient utilization	Abnormal digestive enzyme and fecal fat studies Growth stunting or failure Evidence of vitamin and/or mineral deficiency Steatorrhea Condition associated with diagnoses: cystic fibrosis
Down syndrome A genetic disorder that results from an extra no. 21 chromosome, causing developmental problems such as congenital heart disease, mental retardation, short stature, and decreased muscle tone	Excessive energy intake	Increased body adiposity Energy intake higher than estimated need Reduced energy needs related to short stature, low muscle tone
	Breastfeeding difficulty	Poor sucking ability as an infant (due to low tone) Poor weight gain
	Altered GI function	Constipation (related to low muscle tone, low activity, and/or low fiber intake) Celiac disease (higher incidence in Down syndrome)

(continued)

TABLE 10-1 *(Continued)*

Syndrome or Developmental Disability	Nutrition Diagnostic Terms	Indicators of this Nutrition Diagnosis
Prader-Willi syndrome (PWS) A genetic disorder marked by poor feeding skills in infancy, hypotonia, short stature hyperphagia, and cognitive impairment. When not carefully managed, hyperphagia leads to obesity. May be treated with growth hormone.	Excessive energy intake	Increased body adiposity Energy intake higher than estimated need Condition associated with diagnosis (eg. hyperphagia and PWS) Reduced energy needs related to short stature, low muscle tone
	Breastfeeding difficulty	Poor sucking ability as an infant (due to low tone) Poor weight gain
	Harmful beliefs/attitudes about food	Eating behavior serves a purpose other than nourishment Pica Food obsession
	Undesirable food choices	Intake inconsistent with diet quality guidelines Unable to select foods, independently, that are consistent with food quality, kcal controlled guidelines Condition associated with diagnosis, PWS-food hyperphagia, obsession with food
Spina bifida (myeolomeningocele) results from a midline defect of the skin, spinal column and spinal cord. It is characterized by hydrocephalus, lack of muscular control, and mental retardation	Excessive energy intake	Increased body adiposity Energy intake higher than estimated need Reduced energy needs related to altered body composition, short stature
	Swallowing difficulty	Abnormal swallow study Noisy wet upper airway sounds Condition associated with diagnosis of Arnold Chiari malformation of the brain
	Altered gastrointestinal function	Constipation Condition associated with diagnosis: neurogenic bowel

Source: Adapted from American Dietetic Association. Position of the America Dietetic Association: Providing Nutrition Services for Infants, Children and Adults with Developmental Disabilities.

were developed in response to a need for a more precise and customized approach to defining nutrient requirements. Criteria and dietary reference intake values for energy in the pediatric age group are shown in **Table 10-2**.[6] The adaptability of these reference sets to the special needs population requires further research.

Lowered Energy Needs

Children with Down syndrome, Prader-Willi syndrome, or spina bifida have been found to have a slower growth rate and lower basal energy needs and muscle tone, leading to diminished motor activity when compared to the child who is not developmentally disabled.[7] Not to be forgotten is a familial predisposition to obesity. As a result of these factors, children with developmental disabilities tend to become overweight and obese when fed according to normal standards. Recent studies have shown that children with disorders such as Down syndrome are frequently provided food intake greater than the DRI.[7,8] Monitoring the growth of these children is essential to prevent excessive weight gain or becoming overweight.

Higher Energy Needs

Children with cerebral palsy (CP) often tend to be seriously underweight for height.[9] One study found that poor growth was associated with increased occurrence of health problems.[10] Studies have been conducted to estimate the energy needs of the child with cerebral palsy and have utilized indirect calorimetry and the doubly labeled water method. Recent studies have found that adults with cerebral palsy have higher resting metabolic rates than their controls.[11] A previous study by Bandini and colleagues[12] found that the resting energy expenditure (REE) of adolescents with cerebral palsy was lower than in adolescent controls. Stallings and associates[13] completed a study of children ages 2 to 12 with spastic quadriplegia cerebral palsy compared with a normal control group. The conclusion was that growth failure and an abnormal pattern of REE are related to inadequate energy intake.[13,14]

Two other methods for determining the energy needs of this population include using a nomogram for calculating body surface area and standards based on kcal/m^2/hour (see Appendix F).[14] This method can be used for males and females who are 6 years of age and older. Indirect calorimetry is generally considered to be the most accurate method of determining energy requirements. However access to the equipment may be limited and its use impractical in this population.

The information in determining the basal energy need must be modified for growth and activity level. The DRIs are generally not appropriate to use in determining the energy levels of children with developmental disabilities. A more appropriate strategy would be to utilize basal energy needs with an individualized percentage added for growth rates and energy levels, which encompasses slower growth rates and lowered motor activity. The dearth of research in this area makes it difficult to develop standards and requires that the dietitian and physician evaluate the child's nutritional needs individually.

Protein, Carbohydrates, and Fats

Careful monitoring of protein intake is essential in the child with developmental disabilities. It is generally recommended that 15–20% of the total calories come from protein, which

TABLE 10-2 Criteria and Dietary Reference Intake Values for Energy by Active Individuals in the Pediatric Age Group[a]

Life Stage Group	Criterion	Active PAL[b] EER (kcal/d)	
		Male	Female
0 through 6 months	Energy expenditure plus energy deposition	570	520 (3 mo)
7 through 12 months	Energy expenditure plus energy deposition	743	676 (9 mo)
1 through 2 years	Energy expenditure plus energy deposition	1046	992 (24 mo)
3 through 8 years	Energy expenditure plus energy deposition	1742	1642 (6 years)
9 through 13 years	Energy expenditure plus energy deposition	2279	2071 (11 years)
14 through 18 years	Energy expenditure plus energy deposition	3152	2368 (16 years)
Over 18 years	Energy expenditure plus energy deposition	3067[c]	2403 (19 years)

[a]For healthy, moderately active Americans and Canadians.

[b]PAL = physical activity level, EER = estimated energy requirement, TEE = total energy expenditure.

[c]Subtract 10 kcal per day for males and 7 kcal per day for females for each year of age over 19 years.

Source: Institute of Medicine of the National Academies. *Dietary Reference Intakes for Energy, Carbohydrate, Fiber, Fat, Fatty Acids, Cholesterol, Protein and Amino Acids (Macronutrients).* Washington, DC: The National Academies Press; 2002.

may be difficult for a child with an oral motor feeding problem such as a child with cerebral palsy. These children often suffer from serious malnutrition manifested by little or no weight gain and limited growth in height. One study of 75 gastrostomy-fed children, ages 2 to 6 years, exhibited impressive growth in height and weight at 12 and 18 months after fundoplication surgery and initiation of the gastrostomy feeding.[15]

Carbohydrates are the primary source of energy for all individuals. According to the usual pediatric dietary recommendations, at least 50% of calories should come from carbohydrates with no more than 10% coming from sucrose. Children with developmental disabilities often have a high percentage of their carbohydrate calories coming from foods highly concentrated in sucrose, such as candy, carbonated beverages, cookies, and so forth. Dietary counseling related to better choices of carbohydrate foods is frequently required, just as it is for normal children.

Fats should provide 30–35% of the total caloric intake, increasing palatability and satiety, as well as providing a supply of the essential fatty acids. For the child who tends to be overweight or obese, fat intake should be carefully evaluated and controlled. For the underweight child, fat can provide an important source of supplemental calories. Infant formulas are now modified to include a higher percentage of the fatty acids arachidonic acid (ARA) and docosahexanoeic acid (DHA) based upon research indicating improvement in visual acuity and cognitive development.[16] These formulas should be used for the infant with special needs when the infant is not breastfed.

Vitamins, Minerals, and Botanicals

Research findings do not indicate that children with developmental disabilities have higher than normal vitamin and mineral needs. Studies have addressed the vitamin needs of children with Down syndrome, spina bifida, fragile X syndrome, and autism.[17–19] Children on anticonvulsant medications (such as phenobarbital, Dilantin, Depakote, Topamax, and others) may experience poor absorption of both vitamins and minerals.

Numerous studies[17] have searched for nutritional deficiencies as causative factors in Down syndrome. Traditionally, the studies have included numerous vitamins, minerals, fatty acids, digestive enzymes, lipotropic nutrients, and drugs. Media coverage has promoted the use of antioxidants (vitamins A, C, and E and minerals such as zinc, copper, manganese, and selenium) along with the amino acids glucosamine, tyrosine, and tryptophan. The expected outcomes are improved growth; increased cognition, alertness, and attention span; and changed facial features. The key concept in the nutritional intervention is metabolic correction of genetic overexpression. It is reported that presence of the third chromosome 21 causes overproduction of superoxide dismutase and cystathionine beta synthase, which disrupt active methylation pathways. Vitamin supplements of antioxidants are considered key to the treatment. At this point, nutritional supplements are considered an expensive, questionable approach.

In addition, parents of children with ADHD report that omitting sugar from the diet decreases hyperactivity. Historically this was reported, but is not found in the current literature.[20]

Blue green algae also has been promoted for children with Down syndrome and other developmental disabilities, purportedly to increase attention span and concentration. Of concern is that little monitoring is part of the initiation of these treatments. High-dose supplementation of vitamin B_6 and magnesium has been proposed for autism to diminish tantrums and self-stimulation activities, and improve attention and speech.[21] Other proposed treatments include dimethyl glycine (DMG), and gluten- and casein-free diets.[21] Limited research is available to substantiate anything other than subjective reports that the child is helped.[21,22]

Diminished bone density and a propensity to fracture with minimal trauma are common in children and adolescents with moderate to severe cerebral palsy. A recent study demonstrated that 77% of the children with CP had osteopenia correlated with medication, feeding problems, and lower triceps skinfold measures.[23]

Studies involving children with spina bifida have involved ascorbic acid saturation and the impact of supplementation of ascorbic acid for producing an acidic urinary pH. Concern was shown in recent studies related to the effect of supplemental ascorbic acid on serum vitamin B_{12} levels. No evident B_{12} deficiency developed in one study of 40 children receiving long-term vitamin C supplementation.[24]

Since 1980, the literature has reflected the growing interest in vitamin supplementation in the prevention of spina bifida.[24] Nutritional deficiencies identified as possible etiologic factors include folic acid, multivitamins, and zinc.[24] A British study[25] supplemented 234 mothers with a multivitamin/iron preparation 1 month prior to conception. Vitamins included were A, D, thiamine, riboflavin, pyridoxine, niacin, ascorbic acid, and folic acid. Supplemented mothers had a recurrence rate of 0.9% compared to 5.1% of the 219 mothers without supplementation. Homocysteine-methionine metabolism appears to be altered in women with pregnancies affected by neural tube defects; however, the specific mechanisms of causation are not yet known.

As a result of these studies, the U.S. Public Health Service recommends that all women between the ages of 14 and 45 get an extra 400 mcg of folate daily.[26] Recent data demonstrate that this public health action is associated with increased folate blood levels among U.S. women of childbearing age and that the national rate of spina bifida has decreased by 20%. The Food and Drug Administration approved fortification of all enriched cereal grain products with folic acid in 1998, although at a level that still requires folic acid supplementation.[26]

An additional concern related to children with spina bifida has been their allergic reaction to latex brought about by multiple surgeries.[27] For those children affected, it has been recommended that they avoid certain foods: bananas, water chestnuts, kiwi, and avocados. Mild reactions can occur from apples, carrots, celery, tomatoes, papaya, and melons.[27]

A special concern regarding adequacy of vitamin and mineral intake is the effect of certain medications commonly prescribed to developmentally disabled children on utilization of certain vitamins and minerals. Among these medications are antibiotics, anticonvulsants, antihypertensives, cathartics, corticosteroids, stimulants, sulfonamides, and tranquilizers (see **Table 10-3**). Their nutritional effects can include nausea and vomiting, gastric distress, constipation, and interference with the absorption of vitamins and minerals. In some cases, vitamin and mineral supplements are recommended.[28]

TABLE 10-3 Drug–Nutrient Interaction

Generic Name	Brand Name	Drug–Nutrient Interaction
Cardiovascular Disease		
Digoxin	Lanoxin	Anorexia Nausea
Furosemide	Lasix	Hyponatremia Hypokalemia Hypomagnesemia Calcium loss
Respiratory Disease		
Prednisone	Deltisone Orasone Liquid Prednisone	Weight gain due to drug-induced appetite increase or edema Stunting of growth in children Hyperglycemia
Trimethaprim	Bactrim	Can cause folate depletion Sulfa in the product can cause anemia
Amoxicillin	Amoxil	Absorption provided by increased fluids
Gastrointestinal Disease		
Ranitidine	Zantac	May cause nausea/diarrhea Constipation
Metoclopramide	Reglan	Nausea and diarrhea
Seizure Disorders		
Carbamazepine	Tegretol	Unpleasant taste Anorexia Sore mouth
Phenobarbital	Phenobarbital	Can induce folate deficiency vitamin D deficiency vitamin K deficiency High intake of folic acid (> 5 mg per day) can interfere with seizure control Folate depletion can lead to megaloblastic anemia
Phenytoin	Dilantin	Same as phenobarbital
Primidone	Mysoline	Folate depletion leading to megaloblastic anemia
Valproic Acid	Depakene and Depakote	Carnitine deficiency Coagulating defects may occur with risk of bleeding and anemia
Hyperactivity		
Methylphenidate	Ritalin	Anorexia when given before a meal

Source: Pronsky ZM, Redfern CM, Crowe J, Epstein J, Young V. *Food Medication Interactions*, 13th ed. Birchrunville, PA: Food-Medication Interactions; 2007.

Nutrition Assessment

Assessment of the child with developmental disabilities includes all components of nutrition assessment for normal children (as addressed in Chapter 3) plus the inclusion of an evaluation of feeding skills and development. Taking anthropometric measurements of children who are unable to stand and who have gross motor handicaps will require some ingenuity. Weights may be difficult to obtain on standing calibrated balance beam scales for the child with spina bifida or CP. Chair and bucket scales are available for use in both clinics and schools, and bed scales are indicated for the severely affected. Recumbent boards can be constructed or commercially obtained. Alternate measures for height measurements include arm span, knee-to-ankle height, or sitting height.[29]

Standards for comparison of weight, height, and head circumference are found on the 2000 Centers for Disease Control and Prevention (CDC) growth charts (see Appendix B).[30] Because these standards were developed using a normal population, the child with developmental disabilities may plot as short, especially when length or height for age is considered. This is particularly true for children with chromosomal aberrations such as Down syndrome[31] or those with a neural tube defect such as spina bifida. Growth charts have been developed for children with a number of disabilities (see **Table 10-4**), but for the most part the CDC charts are recommended. Copies of the Down syndrome growth curves are in Appendix C. Proper interpretation is needed.

Weight-for-age, interpreted for the developmentally disabled, is also an important indicator of nutritional status and requires comparison with height-for-age. Again, it is the child with Down syndrome, spina bifida, CP, Cornelia de Lange syndrome, Prader-Willi, or chromosomal aberrations in general whose height/weight relationship should be carefully monitored. Early identification of inappropriate relationships is critical so that nutrition counseling related to energy balance can be given. The CDC charts include the body mass index (BMI) as an indicator of overweight or risk for overweight. Using the BMI for age can be very helpful for the child with developmental disabilities; however, it may not always identify overweight in children who are overfat because of decreased muscle mass. Skinfold measures also should be used. Growth velocity is also an important anthropometric measurement as growth velocity information assists the dietitian in evaluating changes in rate of growth over a specified period of time. Incremental growth curves are available for plotting growth velocity.[32] Skinfold thickness is a useful measurement for estimating body fat and is recommended along with arm circumference.[33] (See Appendix D.)

Biochemical measures for the child with developmental disabilities should include at minimum hemoglobin and hematocrit levels, complete blood count, urinalysis, and semi-quantitative amino acid screening. The inclusion of this test in an assessment would depend upon biochemical testing the child received in the primary healthcare facility. Other tests may be indicated for children on an anticonvulsant medication who may have low serum levels of folic acid, carnitine, ascorbic acid, calcium, vitamin D, alkaline phosphatase, phosphorus, and pyridoxine. A glucose tolerance test is recommended for individuals with Prader-Willi syndrome.[34] Thyroid levels are part of the protocol for children with Down syndrome. After an initial screening, thyroid levels should be checked annually.

The methods used to obtain dietary information about a child with developmental disabilities are identical to those used with a normal child. The parent must be interviewed for the infant and young child. Often it is difficult to obtain the food intake for an older child who has a degree of mental retardation. It is highly recommended that written dietary records be analyzed with computer software.

In addition to dietary information, an assessment of feeding skills and identification of feeding problems that influence the child's food intake is indicated. This part of the evaluation may include such members of the healthcare team as the physical therapist, occupational therapist, dentist, and psychologist. Observation of an actual feeding session is critical and may utilize an evaluation tool such as the Developmental Feeding Tool (DFT) from the Boling Center for Developmental Disabilities, University of Tennessee (found in **Exhibit 10-1**).[35]

The feeding evaluation should include assessment of the oral mechanism, neuromuscular development, head and trunk control, eye–hand coordination, position for feeding, and social-behavioral components, which include the interaction between child and caregiver. Children with developmental disabilities frequently have oral motor feeding problems and positioning problems and tend to be very easily distracted.[36]

Management of Nutrition Concerns

Once the nutritional problems have been identified for the child with developmental disabilities, various types of intervention programs may be implemented. First, however, the motivation level and degree of understanding of the parents and the family must be taken into consideration. Indeed, the guidelines for intervention provided in the surgeon general's report[37] on case management for children with developmental disabilities specify that all approaches should be family-centered, community-based, comprehensive, and culturally competent. Intervention should include all aspects of a child's treatment program to avoid issuing an isolated set of instructions relevant only to the treatment goals of one discipline among the many involved in a child's care. This is an important consideration for

TABLE 10-4 List of Some Special Growth Charts

Condition	Reference(s)	Printed Copies Available
Achondroplasia	Horton WA, Rotter JI, Rimoin DL, Scott CI, Hall JG. Standard growth curves for achondroplasia. *J Pediatr*. 1978;93(3):435–438.	Cedars-Sinai Medical Center Birth Defects Center 444 S. San Vincente Blvd., Los Angeles, CA 90048 (213) 855-2211 Camera-ready copies
Brachmann-(Cornelia) de Lange syndrome	Kline AD, Stanley C, Belevich J, Brodsky K, Barr M, Jackson LG. Developmental data on individuals with the Brachmann-de Lange syndrome. *Am J Med Genet*. 1993;47(7):1053–1058.	
Cerebral palsy (quadriplegia)	Krick J, Murphy-Miller P, Zeger S, Wright E. Pattern of growth in children with cerebral palsy. *J Am Diet Assoc*. 1996:96:680–685.	Kennedy Krieger Institute 707 N. Broadway, Baltimore, MD 21205 www.kennedykrieger.org
Down syndrome	Cronk CE, Growth of children with Down's syndrome: birth to age 3 years. *Pediatrics*. 1978;61(4):564–568.	
Marfan syndrome	Pyeritz RE, Marfan Syndrome and Related Disorders In Emery AH, Rimoirn LD, eds; *Principles and Practice of Medical Genetics*. New York: Churchill Livingstone; 1983:3579–3624. Pyeritz RE, Murphy EA, Lin SJ, Rosell EM. Growth and anthropometrics in the Marfan syndrome. *Prog Clin Biol Res*. 1985;200:355–366.	Camera-ready copies in article
Myelomeningocele	Ekvall S, ed. *Ped Nutrition in Chronic Disease and Developmental Disorders: Prevention, Assessment and Treatment*. New York: Oxford Press; 1993: Appendix 2.	
Noonan syndrome	Witt DR, Keena BA, Hall JG, Allanson JE. Growth curves for height in Noonan syndrome. *Clin Genet*. 1986; 30(3):150–153.	Camera-ready copies in article
Prader-Willi syndrome	Greenswag L, Alexander R. *Management of Prader-Willi Syndrome*, 2nd ed. New York: Springer-Verlag; 1995: Appendix B growth chart.	
Sickle cell disease	Phebus CK, Gloninger MF, Maciak BJ. Growth patterns by age and sex in children with sickle cell disease. *J Pediatr.* 1984;105:28–33. Tanner JM, Davies PS. Clinical longitudinal standards for height and height velocity for North American children. *J Pediatr.* 1985;107:317–329.	

the dietitian working with this particular population.[38,39] A parent or other designated family member may be the individual's case manager, or another healthcare professional may be the case manager. Nutrition intervention would then become a part of the total intervention package rather than standing alone.

Another important consideration is whether the family gives a high priority to a particular intervention procedure. This applies to any discipline, but in this case particularly to nutrition. For example, consider an obese child with spina bifida who has frequent urinary tract infections and a major problem with constipation. The family of this child may give a lower priority to weight management until they take care of the other problems. If that is the case, then suggestions should be provided when the family is ready. When suggestions are given, the coping and educational level of the family should be considered. Often parents have difficulty accepting the fact that they have a child with a developmental disability and may not be able to deal with too many suggestions at once. Cultural competence requires sensitivity to

EXHIBIT 10-1 Developmental Feeding Tool

Parent/Guardian ____________________ Date ____________________

Address ____________________ Staff member ____________________

City __________ State ______ Zip ________ Child's name ____________________

County __________ Telephone __________ Birth date __________ Age ____ Sex ____ Race ______

Head circumference (cm) ________ (%ile CDC) __________ Hand dominance ____________

Height (cm) ________ (%ile CDC) __________ Weight (kg) __________ (%ile CDC) ____________

Weight for height (%ile CDC) ____________ Hematocrit __________ Urine screen ________

PHYSICAL

Yes	No	Size
____	____	1. Weight (Avg. %ile CDC)
____	____	2. Underweight
____	____	3. Overweight
____	____	4. Stature (Avg. %ile CDC)
____	____	5. Short (Below 5th %ile for ht. CDC)
____	____	6. Tall (Above 95th %ile for ht. CDC)
____	____	7. Abnormal body proportions*
____	____	8. Head circumference (Avg. %ile CDC)
____	____	9. Microcephalic
____	____	10. Macrocephalic
Laboratory		
____	____	11. Hematocrit (Normal)
____	____	12. Urine screen (Normal)*
Health Status		
____	____	13. Bowel problems*
____	____	14. Diabetes
____	____	15. Vomiting
____	____	16. Dental caries
____	____	17. Anemia
____	____	18. Food allergies/intolerance*
____	____	19. Medications*
____	____	20. Vitamin/mineral supplements*
____	____	21. Ingests nonfood items
____	____	22. Therapeutic diet*
____	____	23. General appearance (Normal)*
____	____	24. Head (Normal)*
____	____	25. Eyes (Normal)*
____	____	26. Ears (Normal)*
____	____	27. Nose (Normal)*
____	____	28. Teeth/gums (Normal)*
____	____	29. Palate (Normal)*
____	____	30. Skin (Normal)*
____	____	31. Muscles (Normal)*
____	____	32. Arms/hands (Normal)*
____	____	33. Legs/feet (Normal)*

NEUROMOTOR/MUSCULAR

Yes	No	Tonicity
____	____	34. Body tone (Normal)*
Head and Trunk Control		
____	____	35. Head control (Normal)*
____	____	36. Lifts head in prone
____	____	37. Head lags when pulled to sitting
____	____	38. Head drops forward
____	____	39. Head drops backward
____	____	40. Trunk control (Normal)*
Upper Extremity Control		
____	____	41. Range of motion (Normal)*
____	____	42. Approach to object (Normal)*
____	____	43. Grasp of object (Normal)*
____	____	44. Release of object (Normal)*
____	____	45. Brings hand to mouth
____	____	46. Dominance established
Reflexes		
____	____	47. Grossly normal
____	____	48. Asymmetrical tonic neck reflex*
____	____	49. Symmetrical tonic neck reflex*
____	____	50. Moro reflex*
____	____	51. Grasp reflex*
Body Alignment		
____	____	52. Scoliosis
____	____	53. Kyphosis

EXHIBIT 10-1 (*Continued*)

____ ____ 54. Lordosis
____ ____ 55. Hip subluxation or dislocation suspected

Position in Feeding

____ ____ 56. Mother's lap
____ ____ 57. Infant seat
____ ____ 58. High chair
____ ____ 59. Table and chair
____ ____ 60. Wheelchair
____ ____ 61. Other adaptive chair*

ORAL/MOTOR

Yes No Facial Expression

____ ____ 62. Symmetrical structure/function*
____ ____ 63. Muscle tone lips/cheeks (Normal)
____ ____ 64. Hypertonic muscle tone of lips
____ ____ 65. Hypotonic muscle tone of lips

Oral Reflexes

____ ____ 66. Gag (Normal)*
____ ____ 67. Bite (Normal)*
____ ____ 68. Rooting (Normal)*
____ ____ 69. Suck/swallow (Normal)*

Respiration

____ ____ 70. Mouth
____ ____ 71. Nose
____ ____ 72. Thoracic
____ ____ 73. Abdominal
____ ____ 74. Regular rhythm*

Oral Sensitivity

____ ____ 75. Inside mouth (Normal)*
____ ____ 76. Outside mouth (Normal)*
____ ____ 77. Hypersensitivity*
____ ____ 78. Hyposensitivity*
____ ____ 79. Intolerance to brushing teeth

FEEDING PATTERNS

Yes No Bottle-Feeding

____ ____ 80. Suckling tongue movements
____ ____ 81. Sucking tongue movements
____ ____ 82. Firm lip seal*
____ ____ 83. Coordinated suck-swallow-breathing
____ ____ 84. Difficulty swallowing*

Cup-Drinking

____ ____ 85. Adequate lip closure*
____ ____ 86. Loses less than ½ total amount*
____ ____ 87. Wide up-and-down jaw movements
____ ____ 88. Stabilizes jaw by biting edge of cup
____ ____ 89. Stabilizes jaw through muscle control
____ ____ 90. Drinks through a straw

Feeding Patterns—Spoon-Feeding

____ ____ 91. Suckles as food approaches
____ ____ 92. Cleans food off lower lip
____ ____ 93. Cleans food off spoon with upper lip
____ ____ 94. Munching pattern

Lateralizes Tongue

____ ____ 95. When food placed between molars
____ ____ 96. When food placed center of tongue
____ ____ 97. To move food from side to side
____ ____ 98. Vertical jaw movements
____ ____ 99. Rotary jaw movements

Feeding Patterns—Chewing

____ ____ 100. Lip closure during chewing*

Isolated, Voluntary Tongue Movements

____ ____ 101. Protrudes/retracts tongue
____ ____ 102. Elevates tongue outside mouth
____ ____ 103. Elevates tongue inside mouth
____ ____ 104. Depresses tongue outside mouth
____ ____ 105. Depresses tongue inside mouth
____ ____ 106. Lateralizes tongue outside mouth
____ ____ 107. Lateralizes tongue inside mouth

Special Oral Problems

____ ____ 108. Drools*
____ ____ 109. Thrusts tongue when utensil placed in mouth*
____ ____ 110. Thrusts tongue during chewing/swallowing*
____ ____ 111. Other oral-motor problem*

NUTRITION HISTORY

Yes No Past Status

____ ____ 112. Feeding problems birth–1 year*
____ ____ 113. Breast-fed
____ ____ 114. Bottle-fed
____ ____ 115. Weaned

(continued)

EXHIBIT 10-1 *(Continued)*

Yes	No	Current Status
____	____	116. Eats blended food
____	____	117. Eats limited texture
____	____	118. Eats chopped table foods
____	____	119. Eats table foods
____	____	120. Feeds unassisted
____	____	121. Feeds with partial guidance
____	____	122. Feeds with complete guidance
____	____	123. Drinks from a cup unassisted
____	____	124. Drinks from a cup assisted
____	____	125. Finger feeds
____	____	126. Uses a spoon
____	____	127. Uses a fork
____	____	128. Uses a knife
____	____	129. Average rate of eating
____	____	130. Fast rate of eating
____	____	131. Slow rate of eating
Diet Review		
____	____	132. Appetite normal
____	____	133. Eats 3 meals/day
____	____	134. Snacks daily
Dietary Intake, Current		
____	____	135. Milk/dairy products, 3–4/day
____	____	136. Vegetables, 2–3/day
____	____	137. Fruit, 2–3/day
____	____	138. Meat/meat substitute, 2–3/day
____	____	139. Bread/cereal, 3–4/day
____	____	140. Sweets/snacks, 1–2/day
____	____	141. Liquids, 2 cups/day

SOCIAL/BEHAVIORAL

Yes	No	Child–Caregiver Relationship
____	____	142. Child responds to caregiver
____	____	143. Caregiver affectionate to child
Social Skills		
____	____	144. Eye contact
____	____	145. Smiles
____	____	146. Gestures, i.e., waves bye-bye
____	____	147. Clings to caregiver
____	____	148. Interacts with examiner
____	____	149. Responds to simple directions
____	____	150. Seeks approval
____	____	151. Toilet trained
____	____	152. Knows own sex
Behavior Problems		
____	____	153. Self-abusive
____	____	154. Hyperactive
____	____	155. Aggressive
____	____	156. Withdrawn
____	____	157. Other*
Play		
____	____	158. Plays infant games, i.e., pat-a-cake
____	____	159. Solitary play
____	____	160. Parallel play
____	____	161. Cooperative play
____	____	162. Additional comments*

COMMENTS

Source: From Smith MAH, Connolly B, McFadden S, Nicrosi CR, Muckolls J, Russell FF, Wilson WM. *Feeding Management for a Child with a Handicap: A Guide for Professionals*. Memphis, TN: Memphis University of Tennessee Center for the Health Sciences Child Development Center; 1982. Used with permission.

expectations and perspectives related to childcare within a given culture. Increasing numbers of diverse populations are moving into this country and often are non-English-speaking. This requires an interpreter to ensure that the family understands and accepts the intervention suggested.[39]

It is better to give one or two specific nutrition activities for a parent to work on at first. More evaluation and suggestions can be given at frequent follow-up visits. Also, it is important to communicate with the parent or caregiver by telephone for reinterpretation of what was said during the visit. This is particularly true when parents are distraught and find it difficult to follow through on several suggestions given at once. As a result, they may not attempt anything. In addition, increasing numbers of parents have computer access to the Internet, a new avenue for communication; however, misinformation often is provided online.

An important consideration for this particular population is the cost of some of the nutrition intervention suggestions. The nutritionist should determine whether there is a community resource or insurance that can help pay. Variability in state coverage requires research on the part of the nutritionist.

The general principle in the management of nutritional concerns is the importance of the interdisciplinary team approach.[39] Again, it has been the author's experience that most children with developmental disabilities have problems that require input from the physician, physical therapist, occupational therapist, social worker, psychologist, and nurse, in addition to the nutritionist. Pulling that team together is important in order to have successful nutrition intervention. Some examples of the interdisciplinary approach include working with the occupational therapist or speech pathologist in control of oral motor problems and the positioning of the child with a feeding problem or working with a psychologist on behavioral problems. These problems influence how nutrition is addressed. Communication is a key element in the success of the interdisciplinary approach; group discussions, correspondence between groups, and good documentation are vital. The success of an interdisciplinary effort can be phenomenal and bring about positive changes in the nutritional problems, so it is worth the effort to ensure lines of communication are maintained.

Nutritional Problems

Many infants and children with developmental disabilities develop other problems such as obesity, failure to thrive, constipation, and dental diseases.

Obesity

Weight management of the child with developmental disabilities is indicated for any child who tends to plot higher than the 75th percentile for BMI. Conditions that predispose a child to obesity are low muscle tone, limited physical activity, isolation, lack of knowledge about food, and slow growth in height, all of which are found in children with Down syndrome, Prader-Willi syndrome, spina bifida, Turner's syndrome, Myelomeningocele, and Cerebral Palsy. The energy needs of such children are outlined in Table 10-4.

Prevention is the best way to avoid obesity. Counseling in appropriate feeding practices, increasing physical activity, and frequent monitoring of height and weight are essential in a prevention program. Important topics to cover in counseling the parent for preventive weight management include:

- Assessing growth curves and growth rates
- Identifying true hunger cues
- Increasing activity
- Selecting nutritious low-calorie foods
- Identifying food preparation practices
- Placing emphasis on food in the family
- Estimating serving sizes
- Having mealtime structure

Successful programs for the obese individual should be individually planned and include a written meal plan. For the school-age child, successful management will require contact with the child's school to determine which foods are available through the school food service.[4] Often the family is unaware that Section 504 of the 1973 Rehabilitation Act provides for modified school lunches when a prescription is submitted for a child with special needs. Dietary modification of the school meal can be ordered by the physician or a registered dietitian and may address calories, protein, carbohydrates, and allergy/food intolerances. The prescription is generally submitted on a form that can be provided by the school or state child nutrition program.

Childhood weight management must be carefully planned in order to avoid poor growth or nutritional deficiencies. In the school setting, it should become a part of the individualized education plan. Dietary records maintained by the parent and others caring for the child such as teachers, day care workers, family, and friends are useful for monitoring intake. The diet plan for the older developmentally disabled child who is also mentally retarded must be presented in a way the child can understand. The interdisciplinary approach of working with a special education teacher to present written or pictorial information in an understandable format is helpful for success in this area.

Lack of exercise is often common in the child or adolescent with developmental disabilities. The availability of exercise programs for such children varies from school system to school system, as does the availability of general community-based programs of exercise. Exploring and coordinating community exercise resources is an important part of the dietitian's role in providing good nutritional care. Special Olympics events exist in almost all states and are associated with school sports in which the child with developmental disabilities can participate and compete.

Behavioral considerations are also an important aspect of weight management programs for the child with developmental disabilities. Important behavioral assessments to make include:

- Speed of eating
- Meal frequency
- Length of time spent eating
- Where meals are eaten

Frequently used behavior strategies include establishing a reward system for compliance with diet, increasing exercise, and targeting eating behaviors to change.

Prader-Willi Syndrome

Intervention for obesity for the child with Prader-Willi syndrome requires special involvement of both the family and healthcare providers.[40] Total environmental control of food access plus a low-calorie diet combined with consistent behavior management techniques and physical exercise are necessary. Environmental control may include locking the refrigerator, cupboards, and kitchen. Individuals with Prader-Willi syndrome often hide and hoard food and exhibit emotional outbursts when food is withheld. Physical exercise is challenging due to the hypotonia that is characteristic of the syndrome, a poor sense of balance, and reluctance to exercise. The individual tires easily and often has limited gross motor skills.

It has been estimated that the caloric needs of the child with Prader-Willi syndrome are 37–77% of normal for weight maintenance, that weight loss occurs at 8 to 9 calories per centimeter of height, and that maintenance of appropriate weight can be accomplished at 10 to 11 calories per centimeter of height.[40]

Several hypocaloric regimens have been used in various centers with variable success. The use of a modified diabetic exchange list has been successful along with a balanced low-calorie diet, a ketogenic diet, and a protein-sparing modified fast.[34]

Increasing physical activity and exercise are important strategies, and daily exercise routines should be begun early to prevent problems secondary to hypotonia. Adaptive physical education programs in the school should be used with the school-age child with Prader-Willi. Recent treatment has included growth hormone therapy to increase stature.[41] Short-term studies have shown favorable results of growth hormone therapy. In one Japanese study, clients were assessed for 1 and 5 years and mean height velocity improved significantly.[42] Advances in the early diagnosis of infants with Prader-Willi syndrome is an important factor in beginning an early intervention program that includes working with failure to thrive followed by hyperphagia and weight management concerns.

Failure to Thrive

Failure to thrive, defined as inadequate weight gain for height, is frequently found in the child with developmental disabilities. It may result from the following:

- Impaired oral motor function and resultant feeding problems
- Excessive energy needs, such as occur in cerebral palsy, pulmonary problems, and heart disease
- Gastrointestinal problems such as reflux, diarrhea, and malabsorption
- Infections and frequent illnesses
- Medications that may affect appetite
- Pica consumption leading to lead intoxication or parasites such as giardia
- Parental/caretaker inadequacy related to feeding

Nutrition intervention must begin with a careful assessment, including a feeding evaluation with the opportunity for observation of parent/caregiver–child interaction and environmental concerns. Management strategies will be individualized, but will generally require increasing calories by providing concentrated formula for the infant, using supplemental formulas, or providing energy-dense foods through carbohydrate or fat supplements (see **Table 10-5**).

Some children with developmental disabilities and failure to thrive require medical evaluations to determine the existence of gastroesophageal reflux and aspiration leading to a need for tube feeding or total parenteral nutrition on a temporary basis following a surgical procedure for a gastrointestinal disorder. Usually this will be followed with a return to oral feeding (see Chapters 19 and 20).

Constipation

Constipation, defined as infrequent bowel movements of hard stools, often afflicts children with developmental disabilities due to lack of activity, generalized hypotonia, or limited bowel muscle function. It can also result from insufficient fluid intake, lack of fiber in the diet, frequent vomiting, and medications. Parents frequently report using laxatives, mineral oil, and enemas on a regular basis to correct the problem. As a rule, laxatives and enemas are not recommended because they can lead to dependency, and mineral oil decreases the absorption of the fat-soluble vitamins A, D, E, and K.

TABLE 10-5 Foods that Can Be Added to Pureed Foods to Increase Calories

Food	Calories
Infant cereal	9/tbsp
Nonfat dry milk	25/tbsp
Cheese (melted)	120/oz
Margarine	101/tbsp
Evaporated milk	40/oz
Vegetable oils	110/tbsp
Strained infant meats	100–150/jar
Glucose polymers, powdered or liquid	30/tbsp

Treatment includes adjusting the diet to increase fiber and fluid content. Usual recommendations are as follows:

- Maintain adequate fluid intake, exceeding the daily requirement for age, including water and diluted fruit juice.
- Increase fiber content of the diet by replacing white bread and canned fruits with whole-grain breads and cereals, raw vegetables, fresh fruits, dried fruits, commercial fiber-rich beverages, and cereals fortified with 1 to 2 tablespoons of unprocessed bran. Fiber can also be increased successfully by adding fiber supplements. One of the newer fiber products used successfully in children and occasionally in toddlers is Benefiber, a water-soluble powder of partially hydrolyzed guar gum, which can be added to beverages or soft food. Generally it is used from the age of 6 years on; however, exceptions have been made under medical supervision.
- Yogurt now manufactured with pre- and probiotics has been successful in improving the intestinal function of children.
- Increase daily exercise.

Feeding Problems

Feeding problems are defined as the inability or refusal to eat certain foods because of neuromotor dysfunction, obstructive lesions, or psychosocial factors. Most feeding problems are the result of oral motor difficulties (see **Table 10-6**) caused by neuromotor dysfunction, developmental delays, positioning problems, a poor mother–child relationship, or sensory defensiveness.[36] All of these problems may contribute to such behavioral problems as a refusal to eat, mealtime tantrums, resistance to texture changes, and the like.

Intervention for feeding problems lends itself best to the team approach, utilizing occupational therapy, physical therapy, speech, nursing, psychology, nutrition, and social work.[36] A single written care plan developed by the team, prioritized with the parent's assistance according to the child's needs, should be provided. Nutritional intervention may involve increasing calories, altering the texture of foods offered, and determining tube-feeding formulas. Additional nutrition education and counseling, oral motor therapy, and behavior management counseling are part of the feeding plan. Many children with feeding problems of an oral motor nature will benefit from a modified barium swallow in order to detect the possibility of aspiration. This will allow the team to determine the necessity of thickening liquids. A number of products have been developed for thickening and generally consist of a corn starch base, which has advantages over the use of cereal. New technology now exists allowing specially trained speech therapists to treat dysphagia with the VitalStim collar.

Dental Disease

Dental health care contributes to overall improved nutritional status, but is often an unmet need in children and adolescents who are developmentally disabled. Dental caries and gum disease are prevalent in this population and are caused by plaque formation, tooth susceptibility, sugar

TABLE 10-6 Oral Motor Problems and Affect on Food Intake

Problem	Description	
Tonic bite reflex	Strong jaw closure when teeth and gums are stimulated	Interferes with actual intake of food
Tongue thrust	Forceful and often repetitive protrusion of an often bunched or thick tongue in response to oral stimulation	Parent or care taker may misinterpret as child's dislike of food
Jaw thrust	Forceful opening of the jaw to the maximal extent during eating, drinking, attempts to speak, or general excitement	Interferes with acceptance of food and swallowing
Tongue retraction	Pulling back the tongue within the oral cavity at the presentation of food, spoon, or cup	Makes swallowing and chewing difficult along with cup drinking
Lip retraction	Pulling back the lips in a very tight, smile-like pattern at the approach of the spoon or cup toward the face	Makes food intake difficult and requires facilitation to relax the lips
Sensory defensiveness	A strong adverse reaction to sensory input (touch, sound, light)	Can lead to refusal to accept a variety of foods due to oral sensitivity

Source: Cloud, Harriet. *Feeding a Priority for the Dietetic Professional.* 2009. www.nutritionmatters.us

consumption, and medication. Prevention includes home care, professional treatment, and nutritional intervention.

Nutritional intervention involves decreasing the sucrose intake of the diet by eliminating candy, sugar-containing gum, sugar-containing carbonated beverages, cookies, cakes, and highly sweetened foods. Supplying adequate fluoride in the drinking water is helpful in the prevention of caries. In communities where the water supply is not fluoridated, toothpaste and topical application of fluoride can be used. Many families drink bottled water, which may not contain fluoride; however, some manufacturers are now adding fluoride and list it on the food label.

Gingival disease is often found where dental hygiene is poor. Children taking Dilantin for seizures may suffer gingival hyperplasia, a side effect of the drug. Nutrition counseling to increase intake of raw fruits and vegetables and improve snacking practices, coupled with good dental hygiene instruction from the dentist and regular dental care, are important components of dental intervention problems. One additional concern for the child with developmental disabilities is late weaning from the bottle and extended use of the "sippy" cup filled with juice, tea, or other sweetened beverages. Permitting a child to constantly drink from this cup can contribute to an increase in dental caries.

Seizures

The ketogenic diet has been developed and used in the treatment of epileptic seizures nonresponsive to anticonvulsants.[43] Traditionally, the diet is recommended for children under age 5 with myoclonic, absence, and atonic seizures that are medically nonresponsive. This diet is high in fat and very low in protein and carbohydrates, and is designed to increase the body's reliance on fatty acids rather than glucose for energy. The classic fat-to-carbohydrate ratio is 4:1. It is thought that the ketosis produced by the high fat to low carbohydrate ratio decreases the number and severity of the seizures. Typically, the diet provides 1 gram of protein per kilogram of body weight, although protein can be increased if linear growth slows unacceptably.[43] To achieve dehydration and reduce urinary loss of ketones, fluids were limited; however, this led to constipation and kidney stones and is no longer considered beneficial.[44] Historically, the diet is high in saturated fat content; however, in recent years, corn oil and MCT oil have been used, but protocols also contain whipping cream, bacon, butter, margarine, and mayonnaise.[43]

The child under 18 months of age, older than 12 years, or obese may be started on a 3:1 ratio. Other variants of the ketogenic diet include the MCT diet originated in 1970;[46] the modified Atkins diet; and the low glycemic index treatment, which stabilizes blood glucose and allows more carbohydrate than the classic ketogenic diet. Infants and children fed by either bottle or tube can be given the ketogenic diet as a liquid feeding. A powdered formula is available (Ketocal, Scientific Hospital Supplies; other products include KetoVolve and Ketonia).

Numerous studies have evaluated the effectiveness of the ketogenic diet. The largest study, completed by Johns Hopkins Hospital, enrolled 150 children.[47,48] Daily carbohydrate-free vitamin and mineral supplements are required because the diet is low in calcium, magnesium, iron, vitamin C, and other water-soluble vitamins and minerals. The expense of the diet, compliance problems, and lack of palatability have made its use controversial. Concerns also have been raised related to growth.

Like all children on metabolic diets, the child requires close monitoring and frequent follow-up visits. Routine laboratory studies are required at clinic visits following initiation on months 1, 2, 6, 9, and 12, including urinalysis, electrolytes, transaminates, bilirubin, glucose, serum calcium, lipid profile, and prealbumin. The diet may be discontinued for children who are seizure-free for 2 years. Although this diet is high in fat and low in protein and carbohydrates, it is different from the Atkins diet and parents should be so advised.

Autism, Attention Deficit Disorder, and Attention Deficit Hyperactivity Disorder

There is an increased incidence in the frequency of children with these disorders that affects their nutritional status.

Autism

Autism is one of five disorders under the category pervasive developmental disorders (PDD) and has grown in incidence since 1980. All types of PDD are neurologic disorders that are usually evident by age 3. In general, children who have one of the types of PDD have difficulty in talking, playing with other children, and relating to others including their family. The five types of PDD are autistic disorder, Rett's disorder, childhood disintegrative disorder, Asperger's syndrome, and pervasive developmental disorder not otherwise specified. PDDs are four times more common in boys, with the exception of Rett's disorder, which is more commonly found in girls.

Autistic disorders or autism spectrum disorders (ASD) affect 3.4 per 1000 children per year.[48] Children with autistic disorder also have mental retardation. The term *Asperger's syndrome* is most often used to describe children with the problems of ASD but who have normal to high cognitive levels.[48] Efforts to find the cause of ASD have led to many studies involving a toxic environment, toxic food, nutritional deficiencies, immune system problems, oxidative stress, gastrointestinal problems, allergies, and emotional stress. The definition of a toxic environment or toxic food when applied to ASD includes air pollution, lead in the soil, manipulation of food production with chemical spraying, hormones added to meat, and so on. The role of nutrition has involved neurotransmitters; essential fatty acids; nutrients with antioxidant qualities such as vitamins A, C, E, and selenium; mineral supplementation with zinc, calcium, and magnesium; a mercury-free diet; or an allergy elimination diet. So many possible causes have led to many proposed diets but little research on the various therapies and their outcomes.

Nutrition and eating problems may affect up to three-quarters of children with ASD. Some of these problems include routine intake and refusal to try new foods; short attention span; increased sensitivity to food textures, color, taste, or temperature; food obsessions or ritual; eating nonfood items; compulsive eating or drinking; packing the mouth with food; vomiting; and gag reflex. For some children, gastrointestinal problems similar to celiac disease have occurred. GI problems include constipation, diarrhea, reflux, vomiting, bloating, pain, and feeding problems. Intolerance to gluten and casein has been identified as a contributor to inflammation of the intestine and the occurrence of brain opioids, but there has been very little research. As a result, the gluten-free, casein-free diet is considered a complementary and alternative therapy and has gained increasing popularity with parents of children with ASD.[49]

Intervention Strategies

No one therapy works for all individuals with ASD. Medical nutrition therapy should be individualized and used along with behavior management, speech therapy, occupational therapy, and counseling. Various diets have been described on the Internet and include a gluten-free, casein-free diet; specific carbohydrate diets; and the body ecology diets.[49] Numerous Websites exist for ordering these products. When these diets are chosen the dietitian needs to work with the parents to ensure that their energy needs and other nutrient needs are being met. Additional help may be required in label reading, meal preparation, and shopping for food sources. Extensive research is needed in keeping up with all of the products appearing on the market, in order to effectively counsel the parent.

Attention Deficit Hyperactivity Disorder and Attention Deficit Disorder

Attention deficit hyperactivity disorder (ADHD) or ADD is a neurobehavioral problem being seen with increasing frequency in children. It has been associated with learning disorders, inappropriate degrees of impulsiveness, hyperactivity, and attention deficit. Causes of ADHD are unclear. There are three subtypes of ADHD developed by the American Psychiatric Association: (1) combined type of hyperactivity and attention deficit, (2) predominately inattentive type, and (3) predominately hyperactive-impulse behavior.[50]

Many of these children are on medications that may affect their weight and growth in height. Medications used to treat these disorders often cause anorexia, so the child's nutrition assessment and follow-up should include anthropometric measures. If the child is on medications, the time of administration is important, generally after eating.

Many dietary treatments have been proposed, starting in 1973 when Feingold proposed removing food coloring and naturally occurring salicylates from the diet. This was followed by eliminating sugar and caffeine and the addition of large doses of vitamins. Feingold's treatments have been discounted as lacking scientific validity and effectiveness. The need for additional research is indicated.

It has been suggested that a lack of essential fatty acids (EFAs) is a possible cause of hyperactivity in children. Some children given omega-3 fatty acids showed improvement in hyperactivity.[51] Various biochemical reasons for a deficiency of the fatty acids could be a lack of ability to metabolize linoleic acid normally, an inability to absorb EFAs effectively, or because EFA requirements for these children are higher than normal. The dosage for omega-3 supplementation ranges from 20 to 60 mg/kg.[51] Because the supplement is in capsule form it lends itself to research studies, which are anticipated in the future.

The most effective treatment for the child with ADHD or ADD is a diet based on the Dietary Guidelines or the Food Guide Pyramid with mealtime structure, small amounts of food followed by refills, a distraction-free environment, and no "grazing" on food or liquids throughout the day.

Community Resources and Cost

Several federal programs provide financial coverage for nutrition services for children with developmental disabilities and special healthcare needs. Title V of the Social Security Act provides funding for maternal and child health services including children with special healthcare needs. Title XIX of the Social Security Act funds Medicaid, which funds medical services for low income individuals and families. In addition, Medicaid has funded tube feeding formulas, dietary supplements, eating devices, and in some states formulas for inherited disorders of metabolism. Nutrition services are included in the legislation passed in 1985 for early intervention programs serving infants and toddlers from birth to age 5. Project Head Start was created in 1965 to promote school readiness among preschool children from low income families, and is mandated to include children with special needs.[52]

One of the programs that provides actual formulas and food for children from low income families is the Supplemental Program for Women, Infants and Children (WIC).

Infants and children from birth to 5 years of age with inherited disorders of metabolism can receive dietary supplements and special formulas. Children with special needs and developmental disabilities of school age are eligible for meal modification under Section 504 of the Rehabilitation Act of 1973 and the Americans with Disabilities Act of 1990.

Other legislation that provides funding for children with developmental disabilities and funding of nutrition services includes the Child Health Act of 2000 and State Children's Health Insurance Programs. All of these programs are possible sources of dietary needs; however, programs vary from state to state.

Conclusion

The nutritional needs of children with developmental disabilities are important considerations in treatment and program planning. The goal is to ensure a nutritional intake adequate for growth and to provide enough energy for participation in therapy. Research is needed to better define the nutritional requirements of this population and the use of the DRIs for this population.

Dietitians in programs serving this population are challenged to defend the cost effectiveness of nutritional care and to develop nutrition education materials and programs specifically adapted for these children and adolescents in collaboration with special education professionals.

Case Study

Nutrition Assessment

Patient history: A 14-year-old girl with Down syndrome was admitted to a mental health services facility for treatment of sleep apnea, prediabetes, and severe behavioral activities. The contributing factor to the medical problems was her severe obesity. Prior to her admission to the facility she had been in public school in their special education programs, but her behavior was so difficult to control that the school transferred her to the mental health facility. She is the only individual in her family with Down syndrome and was born when her mother was 40. There is a history of diabetes in the family, and food has always been used as a reward for this girl.

Food/nutrition-related history: This child's birth weight was 7 lb., 8 oz, birth length was 19″, and the pregnancy was full term. She was breastfed until 3 months of age, when she was transferred to Similac and reportedly had no feeding problems other than consuming over 36 oz. of milk daily and eating baby food in unusual amounts. Her weaning to a cup was late, at 18 months, and her motor skill development was late with an inability to walk until 28 months of age. She also had low muscle tone.

By the time she was 12 months of age her weight was 28 lbs., placing her above the 95th percentile, and each subsequent year she remained between the 75th and 95th percentile for her weight, but at the 10th percentile for her height.

During her preschool and school years the child's intake was reported as very limited in variety with a heavy concentration of foods from fast food restaurants, and little intake of fruits and vegetables. She drank milk but preferred soft drinks and sweetened tea. She also consumed many sweetened desserts, cookies, and bakery products. Although her mother reported trying to control this behavior, a grandparent was very indulgent. She also developed behavioral problems with a great deal of acting out behavior both at home and at school. It was this behavior that led to her referral to the mental health facility.

Anthropometric Measurements

Weight: 247 pounds > 97th percentile

Height: 56″ 50th–75th percentile

H/W relationship: > 97th percentile

BMI: > 97%

Estimated energy needs: 1716 kcal

Estimated energy intake at home: 3000 kcal (based on maternal report)

Estimated protein needs: 52 g

Biochemical Data

Hgb: 14 mg

Hct: 36 mg

Cholesterol: 210

Glucose: 120 mg

Medications: Topomax, Clonidine for seizures and behavioral problems

Diet order following physical examination: 1500 calories plus exercise

Nutrition-Focused Physical Findings

1. Excessive appetite
2. Dry skin
3. Inactivity with behavioral outbursts related to walking
4. Feeding problems—very rapid eating with possibility of choking
5. Low muscle tone
6. Constipation

Nutrition Diagnoses

1. Obesity.
2. Excessive intake of carbohydrates.
3. Inadequate fluid intake due to refusal to eat raw fruits, vegetables and whole grains.

Intervention Goals

1. Weight loss and acceptance of difference in food provided.
2. Increase consumption of high fiber foods.
3. Limit midmeal snacks to fruit and vegetables. Counsel parents related to meal management and poor behavior related to food.
4. Increase physical activity at school and home.

Nutrition Interventions

1. Modify the menus to provide 1500 calories including snacks.
2. Provide copies of menu to group home staff and parents.
3. Increase availability of fresh fruit and raw vegetables for snacks.
4. Increase water intake.

Monitoring and Evaluation

1. Weigh monthly and plot continuously with report to parents.
2. Counsel parents monthly or as necessary related to food intake and exercise at home.
3. Walking at school with teachers and other students.

Questions for the Reader

1. Teachers report that student eats only part of the meal provided and refuses the snacks offered. What would be your response?
2. The parents report in their monthly conference that the student is very rebellious and refuses to participate in the family activities unless provided with a trip to a fast food restaurant for hamburgers and French fries. What could you suggest?
3. Monthly weights show a loss of 2–3 pounds each month. Should there be a reward system followed by motivational interviewing?

REFERENCES

1. Centers for Disease Control and Prevention. Developmental disabilities. Available at: http://www.cdc.gov/ncbddd/dd/default.htm. Accessed December 14, 2009.
2. *Developmental Disabilities Assistance and Bill of Rights Act*, Public Law 106-402; 2000.
3. McPherson M, Arango P, Fox H, et al. A new definition of children with special health care needs. *Pediatrics*. 1998;102:137–140.
4. Cloud H. Update on nutrition for the children with special needs. *Top Clin Nutr*. 1997;13(1):21–32.
5. Van Riper, C, Wallace, L. Position of the American Dietetic Association: providing nutrition services for people with developmental disabilities and special health care needs. *J. Am. Diet. Assoc.* 110:296–307.
6. Institute of Medicine of the National Academies. *Dietary Reference Intakes for Energy, Carbohydrate, Fiber, Fat, Fatty Acids, Cholesterol, Protein and Amino Acids*. Washington, DC: National Academies Press; 2002.
7. Luke A, Roizen NJ, Sutton M, Schoeller DA. Energy expenditure in children with Down syndrome: correcting metabolic rate for movement. *J Pediatr*. 1994;125:829–838.
8. Luke A, Sutton M, Raizen NJ, Schoeller DA. Nutrient intake and obesity in prepubescent children with Down syndrome. *J Am Diet Assoc*. 1996;12:1262–1267.
9. Sullivan PB, Juszczak E, Lambert BR, Rose M, Ford-Adams ME, Johnson A. Impact of feeding problems on nutritional intake and growth: Oxford Feeding Study II. *Dev Med Child Neurol*. 2002;44(7):461–467.
10. Stevenson RD, Conway M, Chumlea WC, et al. Growth and health in children with moderate to severe cerebral palsy. *Pediatrics*. 2006;118(3):1010–1018.
11. Johnson RK, Goran MI, Ferrara MS, Poehlman ET. Athetosis raises resting metabolic rate in adults with cerebral palsy. *J Am Diet Assoc*. 1996;96:145–148.
12. Bandini LG, Schneller DA, Fukagana NK, Wykes L, Dietz WH. Body composition and energy expenditure in adolescents with cerebral palsy or myelodysplasia. *Pediatr Res*. 1991;29:70–77.
13. Stallings VA, Cronk CE, Zemme BS, Charney EB. Body composition in children with spastic quadriplegic cerebral palsy. *J Pediatr.* 1995;126(5):833–839.
14. Stallings VA, Zemel BS, Davies JC, Cronk CE, Charney EB. Energy expenditure of children and adolescents with severe disabilities: a cerebral palsy model. *Am J Clin Nutr.* 1996;64(4):627–634.
15. Corwin DS, Isaacs JS, Georgeson KE, Bartolucci A, et al. Weight and length increases in children after gastrostomy placement. *J Am Diet Assoc*. 1996;96(9):874–879.
16. Holland M, Murray P. Diet and nutrition. In: Lucas BL, ed. *Children with Special Health Care Needs: Nutrition Care Handbook*. Chicago, IL: American Dietetic Association; 2004:5–22.
17. Bennett FC, McClelland S, Kriegsmann E, Andrus L, Sells C. Vitamin and mineral supplementation in Down's syndrome. *Pediatrics*. 1983;72:707–713.
18. Bidder RT, Gray P, Newcombe RG, Evans BK, Hughes M. The effects of multivitamins and minerals on children with Down syndrome. *Dev Med Child Neurol*. 1989;31:532–537.

19. Pueschel SM. General health care and therapeutic approaches. In: Pueschel SM, Pueschel JK, eds. *Biomedical Concerns in Persons with Down Syndrome*. Baltimore, MD: Brookes Publishing; 1992:273–287.
20. Ekvall V, Ekvall SW, Mays SD. ADHD. In: Ekvall SW, ed. *Pediatric Nutrition in Chronic Diseases and Developmental Disorders*. New York: Oxford Press; 2005:145–150.
21. Cornish E. Gluten and casein free diets in autism: a study of the effects on food choice and nutrition. *J Hum Nutr Diet*. 2002;15(4):261–269.
22. Quinn HP. Nutrition concerns for children with pervasive developmental disorder/autism. *Nutr Focus*. 1995;10(5):1–7.
23. Henderson RC, Kairalla JA, Barrington JW, Abbas A, Stevenson RD. Longitudinal changes in bone density in children and adolescents with moderate to severe cerebral palsy. *J Pediatr.* 2005;146:769–775.
24. Bergman KE, Makoseh J, Tews KH. Abnormalities of hair zinc concentrations in mothers of newborn infants with spina bifida. *Am J Clin Nutr*. 1980;33:2145–2150.
25. Smithells RN, Nevin NC, Seller MJ, et al. Further experience of vitamin supplementation for prevention of neural tube defect recurrences. *Lancet*. 1983;1:1027.
26. Green NS. Folic acid supplementation and prevention of birth defects. *J Nutr.* 2002;132(8 Suppl):2356S–2360S.
27. Pittman T. Latex allergy in children with spina bifida. *Ped Neurosurg*. 1995;22(2):96–100.
28. Pronsky ZM, Redfern CM, Crowe J, Epstein J, Young V. *Food Medication Interactions*, 13th ed. Birchrunville, PA: Food-Medication Interactions; 2007.
29. Chumlea WC, Guo SS, Steinbaugh ML. Prediction of stature from knee height for black and white adults and children with application to mobility-impaired or handicapped persons. *J Am Diet Assoc.* 1994;94(12):1385–1388.
30. National Center for Health Statistics in collaboration with National Center for Chronic Disease Prevention and Health Promotion. CDC growth charts. 2000. Available at: http://www.cdc.gov/growthcharts. Accessed August 31, 2010.
31. Cronk C, Crocker AC, Pueschel SM, et al. Growth charts for children with Down syndrome: 1 month to 18 years of age. *Pediatrics.* 1988;81:102.
32. Roche AF, Hines JH. Incremental growth charts. *Am J Clin Nutr*. 1980;33:2041–2052.
33. Frisancho AR. New norms of upper limb fat and muscle areas for assessment of nutritional status. *Am J Clin Nutr.* 1981;34:2540–2545.
34. Cassidy SB. Prader-Willi syndrome. *J Med Genetics*. 1997;34(11):917–923.
35. Smith MAH, Connolly B, McFadden S, et al. Developmental feeding tool. In: Smith MAH. *Feeding Management for a Child with a Handicap*. Memphis, TN: Boling Child Development Center, University of Tennessee Center for Health Sciences; 1982:69.
36. Cloud H, Ekvall S, Hicks L. Feeding problems of the child with special health care needs. In: Ekvall SW, Ekvall VK, eds. *Pediatric Nutrition in Chronic Diseases and Developmental Disorders*, 2nd ed. New York: Oxford University Press; 2005.
37. U.S. Department of Health and Human Services, Public Health Service. *Surgeon General's Report: Children with Special Health Care Needs*. Chicago: DHHS publication no. (HRS) D/MC, 87-2.
38. American Dietetic Association. Providing nutrition services for infants, children and adults with developmental disabilities and special health care needs. *J Am Diet Assoc*. 2009;104(1):97–106.
39. Terry RD. Needed: a new appreciation of culture and food behavior. *J Am Diet Assoc.* 1994;95(5):501–503.
40. Hoffman CJ, Abeltman D, Pipes P. A nutrition survey of and recommendations for individuals with Prader-Willi who live in group homes. *J Am Diet Assoc*. 1992;92(7):823–830.
41. Hauffa BP. One-year results of growth hormone treatment of short stature in Prader-Willi syndrome. *Acta Paedia*. 1997;423(Suppl):63–65.
42. Obata K, Sakazume S, Yoshino A, Murakami N, Sakuta R. Effects of 5 years' growth hormone treatment in patients with Prader-Willi syndrome. *J Pediatr Endocrinol Metab.* 2003;16(2):155–162.
43. Kelly MT, Hays TL. Implementing the ketogenic diet. *Top Clin Nutr*. 1997;13(1):53–61.
44. Huttenlocher PR, Wilbourn AJ, Signore JM. Medium chain triglycerides as a therapy for intractable childhood epilepsy. *Neurol.* 1971;21:1097–1103.
45. Sampath A, Kossoff EH, Furth SL, Pyzik PL, Vining EP. Kidney stones and the ketogenic diet: risk factors and prevention. *J Child Neurol*. 2007;4:375–378.
46. Freeman JM, Vining EP, Pillas DJ, Pyzik PL, Casey JC, Kelly LM. The efficacy of the ketogenic diet—1998: a prospective evaluation of intervention of 150 children. *Pediatrics*. 1998;102:1358–1363.
47. Neal EG, Chaffe H, Schwartz RH, et al. The ketogenic diet for the treatment of childhood epilepsy: a randomized controlled trial. *Lancet Neurol*. 2008;7:500–506.
48. Yeargin-Allsopp M, Rice C, Karapurkar T, Doerberg N, Boyle C, Murphy C. Prevalence of autism in a U.S. metropolitan area. *JAMA*. 2003;289:49–55.
49. Cornish E. Gluten and casein free diets in autism: a study of the effects on food choice and nutrition. *J Hum Nutr Diet*. 2002;15(4):261–269.
50. American Psychiatric Association. *Diagnostic and Statistical Manual of Mental Disorders,* 4th ed. Washington, DC: American Psychiatric Association; 1994.
51. Burgess JR, Stevens L, Zhang W, Peck L. Long-chain polyunsaturated fatty acids in children with attention-deficit hyperactivity disorder. *Am J Clin Nutr*. 2000;71(1 Suppl):30.
52. Office of Head Start, Administration for Children and Families, U.S. Department of Health and Human Services. About Head Start. Available at: http://eclkc.ohs.acf.hhs.gov. Accessed August 31, 2010.

Pulmonary Diseases

Erin Redding and Shannon Despino

Promoting optimal growth and development is important for any child, but it is especially important for the child with chronic pulmonary disease. In this chapter, the nutritional management of cystic fibrosis (CF), bronchopulmonary dysplasia (BPD), and asthma is discussed. Adequate nutrition in the care of the child with CF or BPD plays an important prognostic role in the outcome of these diseases. A discussion on asthma is included because it is one of the most common chronic diseases of childhood, and nutrition may play an important role in its management.

Cystic Fibrosis

CF, a genetic disorder characterized by widespread dysfunction of the exocrine glands, is the most common lethal hereditary disease of the Caucasian race.[1] The disease is characterized by an abnormality in the CF transmembrane conductance regulator (CFTR) protein, causing an increased sodium reabsorption and a decreased chloride secretion. The result is the production of abnormally thick and viscous mucus, which affects various organs of the body. In the lungs, the thick mucus clogs the airways; causing obstruction, subsequent bacterial infections, and progressive lung disease. In the pancreas, the thick mucus prevents the release of pancreatic enzymes into the small intestine for the digestion of foods. Blockage of ducts eventually causes pancreatic fibrosis and cyst formation. About 90% of CF patients have pancreatic insufficiency (PI),[2] exhibited by such gastrointestinal symptoms as frequent, foul-smelling stools; increased flatus; and abdominal cramping. In a small percentage of patients, 8% according to the 2008 CF Foundation Patient Registry,[3] the ducts and tubules of the liver are obstructed by mucus, resulting in liver disease that may progress to cirrhosis. Common complications in the older CF population include CF-related diabetes (CFRD) and bone disease. A unique characteristic of CF is an increased loss of sodium and chloride in the sweat. Sterility in males and decreased fertility in females is also seen.

The life expectancy of CF patients has greatly improved since the disease was first described as a distinct clinical entity by Andersen in 1938.[4] During the 1930s to 1950s, CF patients usually died at an early age, secondary to malabsorption and malnutrition. Pancreatic enzyme therapy, antibiotic therapy, nutrition therapy, and earlier diagnosis have been major contributory factors to the improvement in the prognosis for patients with CF. The CF Foundation currently reports the median age of survival to be 37.4 years.[3]

Genetics/Incidence

CF is transmitted as an autosomal recessive trait. Both parents are carriers of the defective gene but exhibit no symptoms of the disease themselves. Each offspring of two carriers of the defective gene has a 25% chance of having the disease, a 50% chance of being a carrier of the defective gene, and a 25% chance of neither having the disease nor being a carrier.

The CF gene was discovered in 1989 on the long arm of chromosome 7.[5] The CF gene product is a protein called the CFTR, which is a cyclic adenosine monophosphate (cAMP)-regulated chloride channel and regulator of secondary chloride and sodium channels normally present in epithelial cells.[6–11] The most common mutation is called DF508, and it accounts for the majority of CF alleles among the Caucasian population worldwide.[12] However, over 1500 mutations of the CFTR gene have been identified,[13] which accounts for the variability of disease symptoms and severity that is seen among patients with CF. It is hoped that these genetic discoveries will lead to improved treatment, including gene therapy and ultimately a cure for the disease.

Approximately 26,000 children and adults in the United States have CF. The incidence of CF is 1 in 3500 births each year. CF is most common in Caucasians, which account for about 95% of the affected population; however, CF can be diagnosed in all racial and ethnic groups.[3]

Manifestations/Diagnosis

Manifestations of the disease are numerous and vary greatly from patient to patient, due in part to the large numbers of mutations of the defective gene. A summary of common pulmonary and gastrointestinal manifestations of CF is depicted in **Table 11-1**. Any child who repeatedly exhibits any of these symptoms should be tested for CF. In addition, CF should be considered when a child tastes salty when kissed or experiences heat prostration. Other manifestations of CF include the bilateral absence of the vas deferens in males and decreased fertility in females.

According to the consensus statement on the diagnosis of CF published by the CF Foundation,[13] the diagnosis of CF should be based on the presence of one or more characteristic features of the disease:

- Evidence of chronic sinopulmonary disease
- Evidence of gastrointestinal (GI) and nutritional abnormalities
- Evidence of salt-loss syndromes
- Evidence of obstructive azoospermia in males
- Family history of the disease
- A positive newborn screening test result plus an elevated sweat chloride test

Sweat chloride is measured by a quantitative pilocarpine iontophoresis sweat test. A sweat chloride concentration greater than 60 mmol/L is indicative of the diagnosis of CF. Patients with an intermediate sweat chloride concentration (30–59 mmol/L for infants under 6 months of age and 40–59 mmol/L for individuals over 6 months of age) should undergo CFTR mutation analysis to rule out CF. The diagnosis can also be made with the identification of CF mutations on both alleles of the CFTR gene, which is sometimes even seen in patients who have a negative sweat test (< 39 mmol/L).[13]

TABLE 11-1 Manifestations of Cystic Fibrosis

Pulmonary	Gastrointestinal
Chronic cough	Failure to thrive
Repeated bronchial infections	Steatorrhea
Increased work of breathing	Hypoalbuminemia
Digital clubbing	Rectal prolapse
Bronchospasm	Frequent, foul-smelling stools
Cyanosis	Abdominal cramping
Chronic pneumonia	Voracious appetite
Nasal polyps	Anemia
Chronic sinusitis	Intussusception of the small and large bowel
	Vitamin deficiencies

The CF Foundation recommends that all states routinely conduct newborn screening for CF. Research has revealed that earlier diagnosis of CF is linked with improved growth and lung function, reduced hospital stays, and increased life expectancy. This is largely in part to more prompt medical treatment and nutrition intervention. A positive CF newborn screen does not always mean that the patient has CF, so further medical testing such as a sweat test must be done to confirm the diagnosis. With all states conducting routine newborn screening for CF, it is expected that the median age of survival will continue to increase combined with an increased quality of life.[13]

Management

Rigorous daily management is required to control the symptoms of the disease. Daily chest percussion therapy and postural drainage, along with aerosolized medications, help to clear the airways of mucus, improve existing lung compromise, and retard future deterioration. Aerosolized, oral, or intravenous antibiotics are used to control pulmonary infections. Pancreatic enzyme replacement therapy is a crucial part of the management of the GI symptoms in patients who exhibit PI. These patients are required to take pancreatic enzymes prior to each meal and snack containing fat, protein, and/or complex carbohydrates. Dosage of pancreatic enzymes is individualized, depending on factors such as the extent of pancreatic involvement, dietary intake, and the weight and age of the patient. Vitamin, mineral, and salt supplementation are also recommended and are discussed in detail in the nutrition management section of this chapter. Providing adequate nutrition for normal growth and development is one of the primary goals of disease management in CF, and the CF Foundation recommends that every patient with CF be assessed by a registered dietitian at least once a year. The complex and multifaceted nature of the disease requires an interdisciplinary team approach with patient and family involvement in decision making to optimize disease management and improve health outcomes.

Effects of CF on Nutritional Status

CF is a disease with many nutrition implications. The following section will further explain the nutritional manifestations of this disease and how and why it is important to monitor the nutritional status of patients with CF.

Chronic Energy Deficit

Many aspects of CF stress the nutritional status of the patient directly or indirectly by affecting the patient's appetite and subsequent intake. Aspects of pulmonary and GI involvement affecting nutritional status are summarized in **Table 11-2**. CFRD and liver disease also impact nutritional status. Bile salts and bile acid losses contribute to fat malabsorption.

TABLE 11-2 Aspects of Cystic Fibrosis that Affect Nutritional Status

Pulmonary	Gastrointestinal
Increased work of breathing	Malabsorption of fat
Chronic cough	Loss of fat-soluble vitamins
Cough-emesis cycle	Loss of essential fatty acids
Chronic antibiotic therapy	Malabsorption of protein
Fatigue, anxiety	Anorexia
Decreased tolerance for exercise	Gastroesophageal reflux/ esophagitis
Repeated pulmonary infections	Bile salts and bile acid loss
	Distal intestinal obstructive syndrome (DIOS)
	Fibrosing colonopathy

Gastrointestinal losses occur in spite of pancreatic enzyme replacement therapy. Also, the catch-up growth that is often needed after diagnosis requires additional calories. The energy metabolism of CF patients has been studied and generally an increase in resting energy expenditure has been found, as compared with controls and/or predicted resting energy expenditure.[14–18] It is estimated that energy requirements for patients with CF range from 110–200% of the calories recommended for healthy individuals of the same age, gender, and size.[19,20] All of these factors can contribute to a chronic energy deficit which, if left untreated, can lead to a marasmic type of malnutrition. The primary goal of nutritional therapy is to overcome this energy deficit and to promote normal growth and development for CF patients in an effort to optimize lung function and increase longevity.

Appetite

Many references have been made to the voracious appetites of CF patients. This may be true of undiagnosed and untreated patients, particularly infants. In practice, however, dietetics professionals often deal with patients with CF who have very poor appetites and early satiety. As previously mentioned, Table 11-2 delineates some aspects of CF that can contribute to poor appetite and failure to thrive. Psychosocial issues that the patient may be dealing with may cause depression, anxiety, fatigue, and anorexia that will also impact appetite and nutritional status. Behavioral issues related to eating and ineffective parenting strategies may play a role in a child's poor appetite and intake as well. Studies of the use of medications for appetite stimulation, such as megestrol acetate, as part of therapy for CF have been conducted with positive short-term results.[21] However, more study is needed to determine the long-term effects of megestrol acetate on growth, pulmonary function, and clinical stability in CF.[21]

Growth

The expectation of the CF Foundation is that children with cystic fibrosis should grow and develop like their peers without CF. In addition, adults are expected to maintain a nutrition status similar to healthy individuals of the same age. In 2005, the CF Foundation established the following updated age-specific goals for patients with CF:[19]

- *Infants and toddlers 2 years or younger:* Achieve weight for length at the 50th percentile by 2 years
- *Children and adolescents 2 years old to 20 years old:* Achieve or exceed the 50th percentile for body mass index (BMI) for age and gender
- *Females 20 years or older:* Achieve or exceed a BMI of 22
- *Males 20 years or older:* Achieve or exceed a BMI of 23

Growth studies in the past have found CF patients to be smaller and lighter than their age- and sex-matched peers. For example, in 1964 Sproul and Huang[22] found the 50th percentile for CF patients from infancy to adolescence for height and weight to be between the 3rd and 10th percentiles on the growth charts for healthy children. These same investigators noted an absence of the adolescent growth spurt in the CF population. Growth deficiencies significantly correlated with the severity of respiratory disease but did not correlate with PI.[22]

More recent reports are revealing improved growth and weight gain in people with CF. According to the 2008 CF Foundation Patient Registry,[3] the median BMI percentile for patients 2–20 years old was 48%, and the median BMI for patients 21 years or older was 21%. These improvements are likely multifactorial, but largely can be attributed to increased nutrition intervention and a more widespread understanding of the correlation between nutrition status and lung function.

Nutrition as a Prognostic Indicator

More and more studies are indicating that nutritional status is an important prognostic indicator in the outcome of CF. For example, Konstan and associates[23] evaluated the 1990s data from the Epidemiologic Study of Cystic Fibrosis (ESCF) and found that better growth parameters at age 3 years were associated with better pulmonary function at age 6 years. Furthermore, patients whose growth parameters improved between the ages of 3 and 6 years had better pulmonary function at age 6 years.[23] Peterson and colleagues[24] found that children who weighed more and who steadily gained weight at an appropriate and uninterrupted rate had better pulmonary function as measured by forced expiratory volume at 1 second (FEV_1) than did those children with CF who experienced periodic weight losses. Data from the German CF quality assurance project found a positive association of weight-for-height with lung function.[25] Patients with

CF who had weight-for-height less than 90% of predicted had significantly lower values on pulmonary function tests than those patients with normal weight-for-height.[25] Beker and colleagues[26] found height to be an important prognostic indicator of survival for both male and female patients with CF. Refer to **Figure 11-1** for a graph demonstrating the relationship between FEV_1 and BMI percentiles. It is clear that there is an association between growth parameters and lung function. Due to the fact that progressive lung disease is usually what causes the morbidity and mortality of CF, the CF Foundation recognizes the importance of nutrition intervention to optimize growth and help improve lung function.

Nutritional Screening and Assessment

Because nutrition plays such an important role in the treatment of CF, routine nutritional screenings and thorough assessments are very important. The CF Foundation recommends that every patient with CF should be assessed by a registered dietitian annually. Some patients who are at increased nutrition risk may benefit from meeting with a registered dietitian more frequently. In this section, anthropometric, biochemical, clinical, dietary, and drug–nutrient interaction evaluations will be discussed. The CF Foundation has published a consensus report on pediatric nutrition for patients with CF as well as the *Clinical Practice Guidelines for Cystic Fibrosis*, which includes nutrition management information.[27–29] Refer to **Exhibit 11-1** for the CF Foundation's recommendations for nutritional status assessment.

Anthropometric

Monitoring growth parameters is an important component of the screening, assessment, and follow-up of CF patients. As with any child, CF patients should be weighed and measured routinely by trained individuals using appropriate techniques and equipment, such as those described by Fomon[30] and the CF Foundation.[27,28] For children less than 36 months of age, weight-for-age, recumbent length-for-age, weight-for-height, and head circumference-for-age should

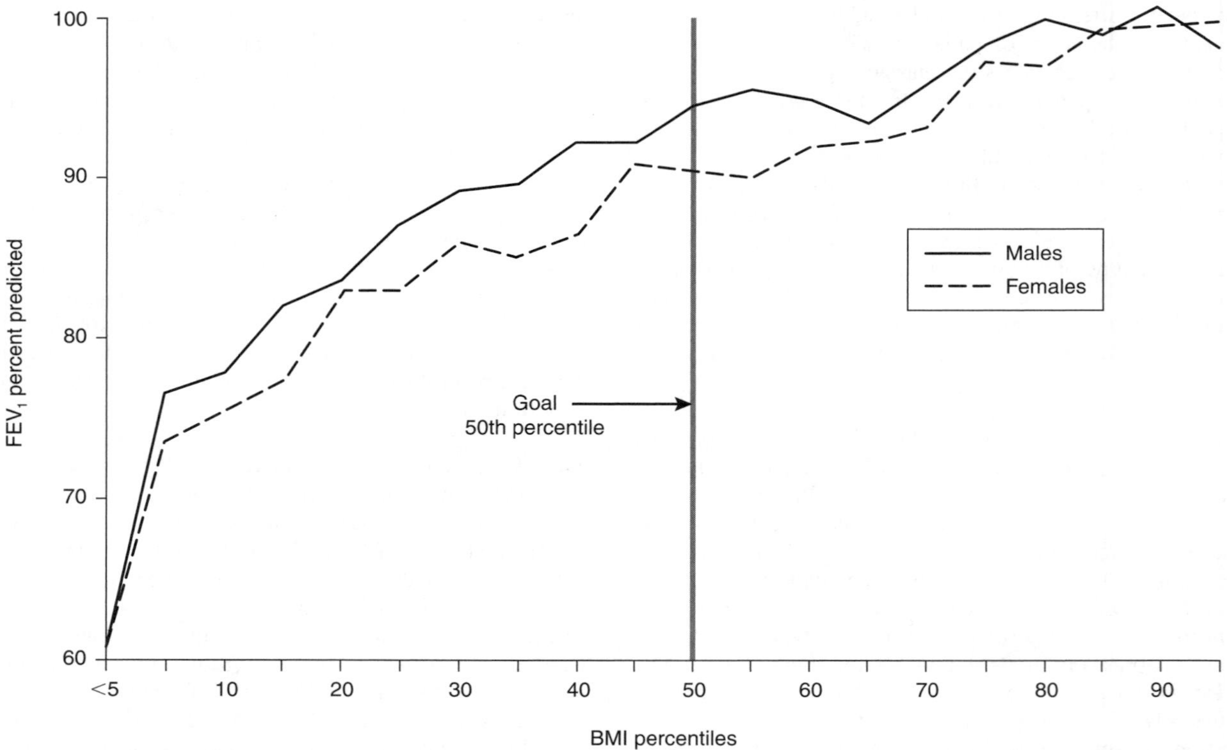

FIGURE 11-1 FEV_1 Percent Predicted vs. BMI Percentiles in Patients 6 to 20 Years

Source: Used with permission of the Cystic Fibrosis Foundation. Cystic Fibrosis Foundation Patient Registry, 2008 Annual Report. Bethesda, MD: Cystic Fibrosis Foundation, 2009.

EXHIBIT 11-1 Nutritional Assessment in Routine CF Center Care

	At Diagnosis	Every 3 Months Birth to 24 Months	Every 3 Months	Annually
Head circumference	x[a]	x		
Weight (to 0.1 kg)	x	x	x	
Length (to 0.1 kg)	x	x		
Height (to 0.1 cm)	x		x	
Mid-arm circumference (MAC) (to 0.1 cm)	x			x
Triceps skinfold (TSF) (to 1.0 mm)	x[b]			x
Mid-arm muscle area, mm^2 (calculated from MAC and TSF)	x[b]			x
Mid-arm fat area, mm^2 (calculated from MAC and TSF)	x[b]			x
Biological parents' heights[c]	x			
Pubertal status, female				x[d]
Pubertal status, male				x[e]
24-hour diet recall				x
Nutritional supplement intake[f]				x
Anticipatory dietary and feeding behavior guidance		x	x[g]	x

[a]If younger than 24 months of age at diagnosis.

[b]Only in patients older than 1 year of age.

[c]Record in cm and gender-specific height percentile; note patient's target height percentile on all growth charts.

[d]Starting at age 9 years, annual pubertal self-assessment form (patient or parent and patient) or physician examination for breast and pubic hair Tanner-stage determination; annual question as to menarchal status. Record month and year of menarche on all growth charts.

[e]Starting at age 12 years, annual pubertal self-assessment form (patient or parent and patient) or physician examination for genital development and pubic hair Tanner-stage determination.

[f]A review of enzymes, vitamins, minerals, oral and enteral formulas, herbal, botanical, and other CAM products.

[g]Routine surveillance may be done informally by other team members, but the annual assessment and every 3 month visits in the first 2 years of life and quarterly visits for patients at nutritional risk should be done by the center's registered dietitian.

Source: Borowitz D, Baker R, Stallings V. Consensus report on nutrition for pediatric patients with cystic fibrosis. *J. Pediatric Gastroenterology & Nutrition.* 2002;35(3):247.

be accurately measured and plotted on the National Center for Health Statistics (NCHS) growth curves at each clinic visit or hospitalization.[22] For children 2 years of age or older who are measured standing, weight-for-age, height-for-age, and BMI-for-age should be measured, plotted, and calculated. (See Appendix B for growth charts and Chapter 3 for additional information.)

Historically, % Ideal Body Weight (IBW) has been used as a method to classify nutrition risk status in children with CF. BMI percentile has been shown to be more sensitive to changes in percent predicted FEV_1 and has stronger association to percent predicted FEV_1 than %IBW. Therefore, the CF Foundation recommends that an age-appropriate BMI method be used to assess weight and height, instead of the %IBW method of assessment.[31]

According to the CF Foundation, anthropometric measurements, including mid-arm circumference and triceps skinfold thickness, should be obtained according to standard procedures by a registered dietitian at least once a year on all patients greater than 1 year of age.[27–29,32] From these measurements, mid-arm muscle circumference, mid-arm muscle area (mm^2) and mid-arm fat area (mm^2) should be calculated and compared with gender- and age-specific normative data.[33] (See Appendix D.) Measurements provide information about fat and somatic protein stores and are particularly beneficial when monitoring the effects of nutrition intervention over time. They are also useful in monitoring the nutrition status of CF patients with liver disease and ascites, in which case weight may not be a good indicator of nutrition status.

It is important to determine whether patients with CF are achieving their full genetic potential in terms of height growth. One method is to determine mid-parental height, plot this height on the growth chart at age 20, and use this percentile as the target for the individual patient. The CF Foundation suggests calculating target height as follows: Add 13 centimeters to the mother's height if the patient is a boy, or subtract 13 centimeters from the father's height if the patient is a girl. Obtain the average of the two parents' adjusted heights. To calculate the patient's target height range, adjust +/− 10 cm for a boy and +/− 9 cm for a girl.[27,28]

Biochemical

Laboratory monitoring of nutritional status as recommended by the CF Foundation at diagnosis and annually is outlined in **Exhibit 11-2**.

Protein Status

Undiagnosed infants, particularly those who are breastfed, often present with hypoalbuminemia and subsequent edema. The malabsorption that occurs in undiagnosed CF causes inadequate absorption of protein. The low protein content of breast milk as compared with modified cow's milk formulas further compromises the infant's protein status. Upon diagnosis of CF and the initiation of pancreatic enzyme therapy, hypoalbuminemia is usually corrected because the infant is no longer malabsorbing protein. It is wise to check a serum albumin level in newly diagnosed infants.

EXHIBIT 11-2 Laboratory Monitoring of Nutritional Status

	How Often to Monitor			
	At Diagnosis	Annually	Other	Tests
Beta Carotene			At physician's discretion	Serum levels
Vitamin A	x[1]	x		Vitamin A (retinol)
Vitamin D	x[1]	x		25-OH-D
Vitamin E	x[1]	x		α-tocopherol
Vitamin K	x[1]		If patient has hemoptysis or hematemesis; in patients with liver disease	PIVKA-II (preferably) or prothrombin time
Essential Fatty Acids			Consider checking in infants or those with FTT	Triene; tetraene
Calcium/Bone Status			> age 8 years if risk factors are present	Calcium, phosphorus, ionized PTH, DEXA scan
Iron	x	x	Consider in-depth evaluation for patients with poor appetite	Hemoglobin, hematocrit
Zinc			Consider 6-month supplementation trial and follow growth	No acceptable measurement
Sodium			Consider checking if exposed to heat stress and becomes dehydrated	Serum sodium; spot urine sodium if total body sodium depletion suspected
Protein Stores	x	x	Check in patients with nutritional failure or those at risk	Albumin

[1]Patients diagnosed by neonatal screening do not need these measured.

Abbreviations: FTT, failure to thrive; PTH, parathyroid hormone; DEXA, dual energy x-ray absorptiometry; PIVKA, protein induced by vitamin K antagonistism or absence.

Source: Borowitz D, Baker R, Stallings V. Consensus report on nutrition for pediatric patients with cystic fibrosis. *J. Pediatric Gastroenterology & Nutrition.* 2002;35(3):252.

Any time an inadequate protein intake is suspected, it may be beneficial to assess the albumin or prealbumin level. However, it is important to remember that other potential causes of an abnormal albumin value include infection and other physiologic stress, fluid overload, congestive heart failure, and severe hepatic insufficiency.[34] CF patients, who chronically have inadequate calorie intakes, usually have a marasmic type of malnutrition. Their visceral protein levels are usually in the normal range, whereas somatic protein stores are low.[34]

Iron Status

Hemoglobin and hematocrit are checked annually. If there is evidence of anemia, further iron studies should be obtained, including serum iron, iron-binding capacity, ferritin, transferrin, and reticulocyte count.[29] A trial of iron therapy will help determine if the anemia is caused by iron deficiency or anemia of chronic disease.

Fat-Soluble Vitamins

Even patients who are adequately treated with pancreatic enzymes may continue to malabsorb fat and consequently fat-soluble vitamins, so it is important that fat-soluble vitamin levels are checked annually. Vitamin A levels should not be drawn during an acute illness because vitamin A is a negative acute phase reactant and will be decreased with acute illness and inflammation.[27,28] Many CF patients, especially those in northern latitudes, among certain cultures, or with limited sun exposure, may not be exposed to enough sunlight to meet vitamin D needs. Measuring 25-hydroxyvitamin D and parathyroid hormone (PTH) annually in the late fall is recommended for monitoring bone disease (see the bone health section later in this chapter).[27,28] Reports of low vitamin E levels and symptomatic deficiency states have been reported.[27,28]

The long-term antibiotic therapy commonly used in the treatment of CF alters the gut flora. Because an important source of vitamin K is microbiologic synthesis in the gut, vitamin K status is often negatively affected. For this reason, it is important to monitor serum vitamin K levels. It is preferable to monitor proteins induced by vitamin K absence or antagonism (PIVKA-II), but this measurement is not always available. Prothrombin time (PT) is an indirect measurement of vitamin K status and is more widely utilized. PT may also be a useful measure of hepatic synthetic function in patients with nutritional failure or biliary cirrhosis.[27,28]

Essential Fatty Acids

Patients with CF are also at risk of essential fatty acid (EFA) deficiency. The etiology of EFA deficiency can be multifactorial, including fat malabsorption and abnormal fatty acid oxidation. It also has been associated with certain CF genotypes and pancreatic status. Some of the clinical manifestations of EFA deficiency include scaly rash, poor growth, and alopecia. EFA deficiency is also correlated with an increased inflammatory response in patients with CF. Checking a triene to tetraene ratio has often been the common way to assess for EFA deficiency in patients exhibiting poor growth; however, more recent studies have shown serum linoleic acid status to be associated with improved growth and pulmonary status.[35] The goal of nutrition care is to prevent EFA deficiency. A minimum of 3–5% of total calories should come from EFAs.[36] Some sources of EFAs include soybean oil, canola oil, walnuts, fatty fish, and flaxseed.

CF-Related Diabetes Screening

With the increased life expectancy of CF patients, the frequency of glucose intolerance in this population has increased.[37] One study estimated that up to 75% of adults with CF have some form of glucose intolerance and 15% have CFRD.[38] CFRD is a distinct clinical entity because it has features of both type 1 and type 2 diabetes.[37,38] Clinical symptoms of CFRD include polydipsia, polyuria, fatigue, unintentional weight loss, and decreased lung function. **Table 11-3** outlines how CFRD is diagnosed.

CFRD can be classified as CFRD with fasting hyperglycemia or CFRD without fasting hyperglycemia. CFRD with fasting hyperglycemia is characterized by a fasting blood glucose (FBG) equal to or greater than 126 mg/dL. CFRD without fasting hyperglycemia is characterized with a normal FBG but an oral glucose tolerance test (OGTT) equal to or greater than 200 mg/dL. The type of CFRD a patient is diagnosed with may affect their treatment plan.[37]

Pancreatic Function/Malabsorption

PI is often inferred based on a patient presenting with symptoms of malabsorption. Stool fecal elastase-I is considered a highly sensitive and specific way to measure pancreatic function and is generally tested at the time of diagnosis. Patients who are initially pancreatic sufficient can become pancreatic insufficient over time. This is especially true of those who have an identified mutation that is associated with PI. These patients should have their pancreatic function evaluated annually by checking a stool fecal elastase-I.[27,28]

When a patient is pancreatic insufficient and on pancreatic enzyme therapy, it is important to evaluate the appropriateness of their enzyme regimen at regular intervals. In some instances, a 72-hour fecal fat test is used to assess fat absorption. This test is conducted as follows:[36]

1. Patient's stool is collected for 72 hours and frozen.
2. An accurate food record must be kept for a minimum of the 3 days that stool is being collected. In addition,

TABLE 11-3 Diagnosis of Cystic Fibrosis Related Diabetes

Test	Time	Blood Glucose Level	Diagnosis	Action
Casual blood glucose	Done at any time regardless of eating	< 100 mg/dL (< 5.6 mmol/L)	CFRD is not likely	Do blood glucose levels every year or earlier if CFRD symptoms occur.
		100–199 mg/dL (5.6–1.0 mmol/L)	Gray zone	Do a fasting blood glucose test or an OGTT.
		≥ 200 mg/dL (≥ 11.1 mmol/L)	CFRD likely	Do a fasting blood glucose test or an OGTT.
Fasting blood glucose	Done in the morning before breakfast	< 100 mg/dL (< 5.6 mmol/L)	Normal	Do blood glucose levels every year or unless CFRD symptoms occur.
		100–125 mg/dL (5.6–6.9 mmol/L)	Impaired fasting glucose	Make sure the level was fasting. If so, an OGTT should be done.
		≥ 126 mg/dL (≥ 7.0 mmol/L)	CFRD with fasting hyperglycemia	Make sure the level was fasting. More testing may be done to confirm CFRD diagnosis unless patient has symptoms. Other tests may be another fasting glucose test or an OGTT. If the patient has CFRD, he or she will learn to manage it with insulin.
OGTT (with normal fasting glucose)	2 hours after glucose load	< 140 mg/dL (< 7.8 mmol/L)	Normal glucose tolerance	Do blood glucose levels every year or earlier if CFRD symptoms occur.
		140–199 mg/dL (7.8–11.0 mmol/L)	Impaired glucose tolerance	Do an OGTT every year or earlier if CFRD symptoms occur.
		≥ 200 mg/dL (≥ 11.1 mmol/L)	CFRD without fasting hyperglycemia	High risk of getting CFRD with fasting hyperglycemia. Patients will learn to use a blood sugar meter and how to count carbohydrates in the food they eat. The doctor may give insulin if the patient has symptoms, is ill, or is taking steroids.

Abbreviations: CFRD, cystic fibrosis related diabetes; OGTT, oral glucose tolerance test.

Source: Courtesy of Hardin D, Brunzell C, Schissel K, Schindler T, Moran A. *Managing Cystic Fibrosis Related Diabetes (CFRD): An Instruction Guide for Patients and Families*, 4th ed. Bethesda, MD: Cystic Fibrosis Foundation, 2008.

sometimes it may be useful to keep a food record 1–2 days prior to the stool collection to ensure the patient is consuming adequate fat for the test results to be accurate (goal: 2–3 g fat/kg/day). Using the food diary, the average fat intake per day is calculated in grams.

3. The coefficient of fat absorption (COA) is calculated:

$$\text{(grams of fat consumed} - \text{grams of fat excreted)/}$$
$$\text{grams of fat consumed} \times 100\% = \text{COA}$$

The normal COA for premature infants is 60–75%, for full-term newborns 80–85%, for age 10 months to 3 years 85–95%, and for age > 3 years 95%.[36] Any CF patient who demonstrates a percentage less than is deemed normal in correlation with their age may require an increased dosage of pancreatic enzymes or the initiation of pancreatic enzymes if not already prescribed. Although 72-hour fecal fat tests are an accurate way of assessing fat absorption, the steps that must be completed are cumbersome for patients and families. In addition, older patients are uncomfortable or embarrassed collecting their stools. For these reasons, it can be difficult to complete a 72-hour fecal fat test, and adjustments are often made to pancreatic enzyme dosages based on reported symptoms of malabsorption or poor weight gain in the setting of adequate caloric intake.

Clinical

An assessment of the patient's overall health status should be obtained. Questions about activity and energy levels should be asked. Any missed school or work days should be noted. A general review of systems should be performed by the physician and a description of the patient's Tanner stage should be noted.[27–29] (See Appendix E, Progression of Sexual Development.) Co-morbid medical conditions such as active pulmonary or sinus disease, gastroesophageal reflux disease (GERD), CFRD, hepatobiliary disease, or history of gut resection should be noted.[27–29] These conditions will also have a direct impact on the patient's nutritional status by affecting appetite, intake, and disease state. Questions about the patient's use of alternative/complementary medicine therapies should be asked in addition to questions about the use of routine medications.

Stool Pattern

Information about the patient's stool pattern should be monitored carefully at each clinic visit because this is a good indication of the adequacy of the enzyme therapy. Questions to be asked during a nutrition screening and assessment should include the following:

- Number of stools per day
- Consistency of stools
- Presence of oily discharge
- Rectal prolapse
- Foul-smelling, floating stools and/or flatus
- Abdominal cramping
- Protruding abdomen

Increased frequency or volume of stool output, notable oil in stools or in toilet water, extremely malodorous stools, increased gassiness and abdominal distention, and/or stools that float instead of sinking to the bottom of the toilet are all signs that a patient may be experiencing malabsorption. Some patients with persistent malabsorptive symptoms should also be evaluated for nonpancreatic causes of malabsorption such as lactose intolerance, bacterial overgrowth of the small intestine, giardia or other parasites, celiac disease, or inflammatory bowel disease.[27,28] It is also important to ask about constipation. Constipation can be a symptom of distal intestinal obstructive syndrome (DIOS), which is also a complication of PI.

Enzyme Therapy

Important aspects of enzyme replacement therapy that need to be checked during every clinic visit and hospitalization are:

- Type of enzymes
- Brand
- Amount taken
- When taken
- Method of administration
- Timing with meals
- Calculation of units of lipase/kilogram body weight/meal and total units of lipase/kilogram body weight/day
- Compliance
- Where enzymes are being stored

Enzymes should be stored at room temperature because they may be deactivated by extreme heat or cold. The expiration date should be monitored closely because enzymes become less potent when expired.

Other Medications

It is important to note other medications the patient may be taking at each clinic visit, including antibiotics, bronchodilators, H_2 blockers, antacids, prokinetic agents, steroids, diuretics, cardiac medications, appetite stimulants, probiotics, vitamins, and minerals.

Pulmonary Status

The pulmonary status of the patient will directly influence the patient's nutritional status. The dietetics professional should note the presence of an acute pulmonary exacerbation and chronic disease. CF patients older than about 6 years of age will be able to perform pulmonary function tests to assess the extent of their pulmonary involvement.

Bone Health Indices

Patients with CF are at risk for developing osteopenia and osteoporosis. The origin of bone disease in CF appears to be multifactorial (**Figure 11-2**). Important contributing factors include malabsorption of vitamins D and K, failure to thrive, delayed puberty, physical inactivity, and use of corticosteroid medications. The prevalence of bone disease appears to increase with severity of lung disease and malnutrition.[39] Several studies have demonstrated a positive correlation between bone mineral density (BMD) Z-scores, FEV_1, and BMI.[40–43] Patients with severe pulmonary disease ($FEV_1 < 30\%$) often have severe bone disease with a high rate of kyphosis and fractures of long bones, vertebrae, and ribs.[41,44]

According to the 2004 *Guide to Bone Health and Disease in CF: A Consensus Statement*, patients older than 8 years of age should have a dual energy x-ray absorptiometry (DXA) as a measure of bone mineral density if $< 90\%$ ideal body weight, $FEV_1 < 50\%$ predicted, glucocorticoids ≥ 5 mg/day for ≥ 90 days/yr, delayed puberty, or history of fractures.[39] In addition to the DXA, children at risk for poor bone health should have annual tests for serum calcium, phosphorus, intact parathyroid hormone, and 25-hydroxyvitamin D level.[45] Normative data are not available for children younger than 8 years of age. All patients should have DXA scans by age 18 years if the scans have not been previously obtained for other reasons.

Dietary

As part of the nutritional assessment, dietary analysis provides important information about what, where, and how

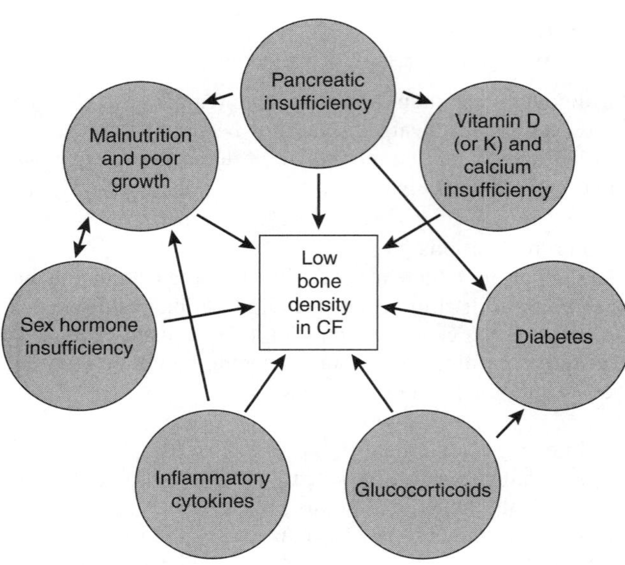

FIGURE 11-2 Pathogenesis of Bone Disease in CF

Source: Courtesy of Aris RM, Merkel PA, Bachrach LK, et al. Consensus statement: guide to bone health and disease in cystic fibrosis. *J Clin Endocrinol Metab.* 2005;90:1888–1896.

much the CF patient is eating. Several methods of gathering the data can be utilized, including a 24-hour dietary recall, a 3- to 5-day food record, and a food frequency questionnaire. The dietetics professional should analyze the diet's adequacy in terms of energy, protein, and other key nutrients such as calcium and iron by looking for a variety of foods in adequate amounts. During this interview, information about the patient's appetite, eating patterns, consumption of sweetened beverages, and behavioral issues related to feeding should be noted.[27–29] The Behavioral Pediatrics Feeding Assessment Scale, which is a self-report measure of meal-time problems, may be administered to identify and evaluate behavioral issues related to eating.[27,28,46]

Drug–Nutrient Interactions

It is important to consider drug–nutrient interactions when assessing any patient, and CF patients are often on a long list of medications. A dietitian or other healthcare provider should take into account how these medications may impact the patient's appetite, if there are dietary restrictions related to any of the patient's medications, and/or what biochemical data may need to be evaluated with the use of certain medications. For example, prolonged antibiotic therapy can alter the gut flora and subsequently influence vitamin K status. In addition, some of the intravenous antibiotics can cause nausea in a number of patients. CF patients with an asthma component of their disease may be on steroids periodically. As the CF patient's pulmonary disease progresses, issues with fluid status may develop. If diuretics are prescribed, fluid and electrolyte status need to be carefully monitored.

Nutritional Management

The overall goal of nutrition management is to promote normal growth and development for the patient with CF. The main components of nutrition management in CF are the provision of adequate energy, protein, and nutrients; pancreatic enzyme therapy; and vitamin and mineral supplementation.

Adequate Diet for Normal Growth and Development

In the past, the GI symptoms of the disease, such as increased number of bulky, foul-smelling stools; increased flatus; and abdominal cramping, were treated with a low-fat diet. Today, with the advent of better enzyme replacement therapy, fat restriction is no longer routinely imposed on all patients. Health professionals now appreciate the tremendous energy demands of the disease, and there is good evidence to support that higher energy intake results in improved weight gain.[31] Estimated energy recommendations to support age-appropriate growth in children with CF over the age of 2 years range from 110% to 200% of energy needs for the healthy population of similar age, gender, and size.[31] This can be accomplished by increasing both the amount and caloric density of foods consumed. To achieve this energy goal, patients with CF often require a greater amount of dietary fat, 35–40% of total energy.[28] It is appropriate to encourage the use of polyunsaturated fats that are good sources of the EFAs, linoleic acid and alpha-linolenic acid, rather than saturated fats. Vegetable oils such as flax, canola, and soy and cold-water marine fish are high in calories and a good source of these fats.[27,28] Limited information is available describing specific dietary protein recommendations for children with CF;[35] however, protein intake is correlated with overall calorie intake and, in general, patients with CF who consume adequate calories also consume adequate protein.[47,48] Defining energy needs in patients with CF can be a challenge due to many individual variables. It is suggested that formulas be used as a starting point, but gain in weight and height, velocity of weight and height gain, and fat stores may provide a more objective measure of energy balance.[35]

Age-specific considerations in the nutritional management of CF are summarized in **Exhibit 11-3**. Infants with CF may be successfully breastfed, as long as pancreatic enzymes are administered prior to each feeding. Standard iron-fortified infant formulas are alternatives to breast milk but also require the administration of pancreatic enzymes prior to each feeding. A study of newly diagnosed infants

EXHIBIT 11-3 Nutritional Management of CF Patients

1. Infant
   - Breast milk or standard iron-fortified infant formula should be recommended. Special formulas such as Alimentum (Abbott Laboratories) and Pregestimil (Mead Johnson Nutritionals), protein hydrolysate formulas containing medium-chain triglycerides, can be recommended for infants in special situations, such as gut resection or increased fat malabsorption.
   - Pancreatic enzymes should be given prior to feedings.
   - Vitamin supplements and a source of fluoride should be given.
   - Introduction of solid foods and advancement of diet should proceed as recommended by the American Academy of Pediatrics (AAP). The RD should guide parents toward foods that will enhance weight gain. Meat, a good source of iron and zinc, may be recommended as a first food for infants consuming human milk.
   - Salt should be added to breast milk or infant formula, particularly in hot weather. When solid foods are added to the infant's diet, salt should be added to these foods.
   - Referrals should be made to community programs such as the WIC program.
2. Toddler
   - Toddlers' diets should be based on a normal healthy diet for age with a variety of foods.
   - Parents should be forewarned of the normal decrease in growth and appetite during this age.
   - Regular meal and snack times should be encouraged.
   - Constant snacking or "grazing" should be discouraged.
   - Drinking of sweetened beverages should be discouraged.
   - Pancreatic enzymes and vitamins are continued.
   - Continue communication with community programs such as the WIC program.
3. Preschool and school age
   - A normal healthy diet with a variety of foods should continue to form the basis of the diet.
   - Limit sweetened beverages.
   - Parents lose control of what child eats away from home at preschool, child care, and school.
   - Arrangements need to be made for child to take enzymes during the school day.
   - Vitamin therapy is continued.
   - Diet prescriptions for a high-calorie, high-protein, high-salt diet can be sent to the school.
4. Adolescent
   - Patients are exercising more independence in food choices.
   - Parents can provide appropriate food environment at home.
   - Patients can be taught to include quick-to-prepare high-calorie foods in daily diet.
   - Snack and fast foods can add a significant amount of calories to the diet and should not be discouraged.
   - Limit sweetened beverages.
   - Health professionals should emphasize the importance of high-calorie intake and enzyme and vitamin therapy directly to the patient and not via the parents.
   - Nutrition needs increase prior to and during adolescent growth spurt.

with CF compared nutrition and growth parameters of those infants fed standard infant formula with those fed a protein hydrolysate formula.[49] There was no significant difference in growth parameters between the two groups of infants. Therefore, standard infant formulas should be used for the routine care of newly diagnosed infants with CF, rather than expensive hydrolyzed formulas.[49]

To close the gap between energy needs and the amount of calories the patient is able to consume, energy-dense foods can be added to the patient's diet. For example, butter, cheese, sour cream, and peanut butter can easily be added to the patient's favorite foods, as tolerated. **Exhibit 11-4** depicts one approach to increasing calories and protein.

A meta-analysis of the literature has been conducted on the various treatment approaches to the nutrition management of CF patients including oral supplementation, enteral nutrition, parenteral nutrition, and behavioral intervention, and their effectiveness on weight gain. Weight gain was produced in CF patients with all interventions. The behavioral

EXHIBIT 11-4 Instructional Handout on Increasing Calories

Calorie-Protein Boosters

—Some ways to hide extra calories and protein—

Powdered milk (33 cal/tbsp, 3 g pro/tbsp)
Add 2–4 tbsp to 1 cup milk. Mix into puddings, potatoes, soups, ground meats, vegetables, and cooked cereal.

Eggs (80 cal/egg, 7 g pro/tbsp)
Add to casseroles, meat loaf, mashed potatoes, cooked cereal, and macaroni & cheese. Add extra to pancake batter and french toast. (Do not use raw eggs in uncooked items.)

Butter or margarine (45 cal/tsp)
Add to puddings, casseroles, sandwiches, vegetables, and cooked cereal.

Cheeses (100 cal/oz, 7 g pro/oz)
Give as snacks or in sandwiches. Add melted to casseroles, potatoes, vegetables, and soup.

Wheat germ (25 cal/tbsp)
Add a tablespoon or two to cereal. Mix into meat dishes, cookie batter, casseroles, etc.

Mayonnaise or salad dressings (45 cal/tsp)
Use liberally on sandwiches, on salads, as a dip for raw vegetables, or as a sauce on cooked vegetables.

Evaporated milk (25 cal/tbsp, 1 g pro/tbsp)
Use in place of whole milk, in desserts, baked goods, meat dishes, and cooked cereals.

Sour cream (26 cal/tbsp)
Add to potatoes, casseroles, dips; use in sauces, baked goods, etc.

Sweetened condensed milk (60 cal/tbsp, 1 g pro/tbsp)
Add to pies, puddings, milkshakes. Mix 1–2 tbsp with peanut butter and spread on toast.

Peanut butter (95 cal/tbsp, 4 g pro/tbsp)
Serve on toast, crackers, bananas, apples, and celery.

Carnation Instant Breakfast (130 cal/pckt, 7 g pro/pckt)
Add to milk and milkshakes.

Gravies (40 cal/tbsp)
Use liberally on mashed potatoes and meats.

High Protein Foods

- MEATS—Beef, Chicken, Fish, Turkey, Lamb
- MILK & CHEESE—Yogurt, Cottage Cheese, Cream Cheese
- EGGS
- PEANUT BUTTER (with Bread or Crackers)
- DRIED BEANS & PEAS (with Bread, Cornbread, Rice)

Source: Courtesy of Pediatric Pulmonary Center, ©1990, University of Alabama at Birmingham, Birmingham, Alabama.

interventions were found to be as effective as more invasive medical procedures.[50] The best choice of intervention for a CF patient needs to be made on an individual basis.

Pregnancy

With the increased life expectancy of patients with CF, more women with the disease are becoming pregnant. In addition to the usual nutrient recommendations of CF, the increased energy needs of pregnancy must be taken into consideration. Emphasis needs to be put on proper weight gain. The woman's weight before and during pregnancy has a tremendous impact on the outcome for both mother and infant.[51] A pregnant woman with CF must add between 340 and 1000 kcal/day to her usual diet, depending on her weight at conception, degree of malabsorption, and level of pulmonary function and infection.[51] A diet sufficient in iron and calcium should be emphasized, and salt intake should not be restricted except for medical reasons.[45]

Intake of vitamins and minerals should be monitored and blood levels of fat-soluble vitamins should be obtained before and during pregnancy to determine the correct vitamin dose.[45] Mothers with CF have successfully breastfed their infants.[52] Breastfeeding further increases the energy demands on the patient with CF and needs to be considered on an individual basis.

CF-Related Diabetes

As with any patient with CF, the treatment goal for CFRD is to provide a diet that promotes optimal growth and development in children and adolescents, achievement and maintenance of normal weight in adults, and optimal nutritional status.[37,53] Other treatment goals include controlling hyperglycemia to reduce diabetes complications, avoiding severe hypoglycemia, and assisting the patient in adapting to another chronic illness from a psychological standpoint.[37] The patient with CFRD should be allowed as much flexibility as possible in the nutrition management of these two diseases.[37] The primary goal remains meeting the patient's energy needs.[37] Foods with carbohydrates have the greatest impact on blood sugar. Simple sugars can be included in the diet plan, but regular sodas and other sweetened beverages should be discouraged. The patient needs to learn how to recognize the carbohydrate content of foods, such as with the carbohydrate counting method, which is used when taking rapid acting insulin to cover meals.[37,53] For those on a fixed insulin regimen, blood sugars can be better managed by eating a consistent amount of carbohydrate at each of the three meals and three snacks in addition to eating at the same time each day.[38] Eating protein and fat-containing foods along with simple sugars slows the absorption of the simple sugars from the intestinal tract. Fat should continue to contribute about 40% of total calories, and protein intake should provide about 20% of total calories.[37]

Patient/Family Education

Patient and family education on nutrition management and its importance in the patient's overall health care is an integral component of the individual patient's care plan. A qualified, registered dietitian should be available to the patient and family to assist them in meeting the nutritional needs of the patient in the least invasive way possible. Information about the nutrient content of foods and suggestions for increasing the patient's caloric intake should be available.

Luder and Gilbride[54] studied the effects of nutrition counseling that was provided quarterly for a 4-year period, based on self-management skills in a group of patients with CF. These patients had significant increases in their energy intakes as well as in their body mass index values, without decline in pulmonary function over this time period.[54] Considerable emphasis should be placed on anticipatory guidance as an integral part of nutrition management.[27–29]

Feeding issues are prominent in this patient population, and the health professional needs to provide anticipatory guidance to the parents/caretakers of these patients to try and avoid battles over eating.[55,56] The importance of behavioral programs in the nutritional care of CF patients is receiving more and more recognition.[56]

For children with CF ages 1–12 years with or at risk of growth deficits, the CF Foundation recommends that intensive treatment with behavioral intervention in conjunction with nutrition counseling be used to promote weight gain.[19] Some strategies include complimenting children for appropriate feeding behaviors (e.g., trying a new food, taking consecutive bites), paying minimal attention to behaviors not compatible with eating (e.g., refusing food), and limiting mealtimes to 15 minutes specifically for toddlers.[57]

Supplemental Nutrition

Milkshakes and other high-calorie drinks can be used to supplement oral intake. Commercial oral beverages (such as Ensure or Boost) can also be used to boost calories, but they require additional expense.

Oftentimes, in spite of vigorous efforts by the patient, the patient's family, and dietetics professionals, it is very difficult to meet the patient's energy needs by the oral route alone. The CF Consensus Conference on pediatric nutrition for patients with CF suggests that the use of supplemental tube feedings be considered when optimization of feeding behaviors and addition of oral supplements have not achieved adequate weight gain or growth parameters. The patient and family need to be given the facts about available adjunct therapies in a positive way and be involved in the decision making.[27,28] CF centers have reported using various forms of tube feedings, including nasogastric, gastrostomy, and jejunostomy feedings. Tube feedings are often administered on a continuous basis while the patient is asleep. There are a variety of formulas available, some with fairly high concentrations of MCT oil, which can be helpful with fat absorption issues. Intact formulas of various caloric concentrations can be used. Hydrolyzed or elemental formulas can be used when appropriate and may reduce the amount of pancreatic enzyme replacement therapy needed; however, they are more costly than intact formulas. Both types of formulas have been associated with successful nutrition repletion.[45] Pancreatic enzyme administration with overnight tube feeds will be discussed briefly in the "Pancreatic Enzyme Replacement Therapy" section of this chapter.

Vitamin and Mineral Supplementation

Vitamins

Recommendations of the CF Consensus Conference for pediatric nutrition for patients with CF regarding vitamin supplementation can be found in **Exhibit 11-5**.[27,28] CF-specific multivitamin preparations are available on the market that contain high amounts of the fat-soluble vitamins A, D, E, and K in a water-miscible form to meet the needs of patients with CF. **Table 11-4** compares the amounts of fat-soluble vitamins in different CF-specific vitamins to a standard multivitamin. The use of the CF-specific multivitamins simplifies patients' vitamin regimen and helps to improve patient compliance.[30] Not all of the commercially available products contain the recommended level of vitamin K, so vitamin K status needs to be monitored carefully. Often additional vitamin K is given to patients as a prophylactic measure to prevent vitamin K deficiency, especially given the frequent usage of antibiotics.[24,25]

Vitamin D deficiency is common in CF and is found in infants diagnosed by newborn screening and in children and young adults.[35] The CF Foundation has specific recommendations in regard to treating a 25-OH vitamin D level that is less than 30 ng/mL.[53] The recommendation is to treat with Ergocalciferol for 8 weeks according to the following dosing schedule: 12,000 IU weekly for patients less than 5 years of age and 50,000 IU weekly for patients over 5 years of age. If 25-OH vitamin D levels remain less than 30 ng/mL 2–4 weeks after completion of treatment, then the vitamin D dose is increased to twice per week for 8 weeks. When repleting vitamin D levels it is always important to make sure the patient is also getting adequate calcium. If after this additional treatment, the levels are still less than 30 ng/mL, then phototherapy or increased sunlight exposure should be considered or a referral to endocrinology for consideration of use of more polar vitamin D supplements, which may be better absorbed.[53]

Vitamin D treatment recommendations as outlined by the CF Foundation Bone Consensus report may not correct low vitamin D levels.[58] A study by Green and colleagues at the Johns Hopkins Medical Institutions demonstrated the success of treatment with 50,000 IU of ergocalciferol once, twice, or three times weekly as 33%, 26%, and 43%,

EXHIBIT 11-5 Recommendations for Vitamin Supplementation

In addition to a standard, age-appropriate dose of nonfat-soluble multivitamins, the following should be given:

	Individual Vitamin Daily Supplementation			
	Vitamin A (IU)	Vitamin E (IU)	Vitamin D (IU)	Vitamin K (mg)
0–12 months	1500	40–50	400	
1–3 years	5000	80–150	400–800	
4–8 years	5000–10000	100–200	400–800	At least 0.3 mg*
> 8 years	10000	200–400	400–800	

*Currently, commercially available products do not have ideal doses for supplementation. In a recent review, no adverse effects have been reported at any dosage level of vitamin K. Clinicians should try to follow these recommendations as closely as possible until better dosage forms are available. Prothrombin time or, ideally, PIVKA-II levels should be checked in patients with liver disease, and vitamin K dose titrated as indicated.

Source: Borowitz D, Baker R, Stallings V. Consensus report on nutrition for pediatric patients with cystic fibrosis. *J. Pediatric Gastroenterology & Nutrition*. 2002;35(3):251.

respectively. This institution has since changed its practice to treating vitamin D deficiency with 50,000 IU daily for 4 weeks in both adult and pediatric patients, though there is no long-term data available yet to evaluate the success of this regimen.[58] Another study by Boas and colleagues evaluated the safety and efficacy of a 2-week trial of very high dose ergocalciferol (50,000 IU/day for 14 days) for children and adults with CF and PI, all of whom had 25-OH vitamin D levels < 30 ng/mL. When post-treatment vitamin D levels were measured, 94% of the participants demonstrated a significant increase in 25-OH vitamin D levels within the therapeutic (30–50 ng/mL) or high therapeutic (50–100 ng/mL) range, without any potentially toxic vitamin D levels noted.[59]

More institutions are now developing their own vitamin D treatment protocols in CF patients; further studies are needed to determine the appropriate treatment strategies.

Minerals

Minerals such as zinc, iron, and selenium have been studied in the CF population. Additional study is needed before specific supplementation recommendations can be made. A trial of zinc supplementation for 6 months may be initiated for patients with CF who have poor growth.[27,28] All patients with CF should be encouraged to consume at least the DRIs for calcium for their age group. For example, the DRI for calcium for children older than 9 years of age is 1300 mg.[60] CF patients who are on steroids, who have decreased dietary intake of calcium, and/or who are found to have decreased bone density may benefit from calcium supplementation. These minerals as well as other macro- and micronutrients are important to the overall nutritional status of the patient with CF. Therefore, eating a variety of foods should be encouraged.

Additional salt should be added to the diet during times of increased sweating, such as

- During hot weather
- With fevers
- During strenuous physical activity
- With profuse diarrhea

The additional salt compensates for the increased losses of sodium and chloride through perspiration. In most instances, liberal use of the salt shaker and the inclusion of high-salt foods in the diet will supply the needed sodium and chloride. Salt supplements may be used in instances of very heavy sweating. Both breastfed and formula-fed infants need supplementation with sodium chloride, particularly during hot weather.[27,28] Infants without CF require 2 to 4 mEq/kg/day of sodium; infants with CF are likely to require the upper end of this normal range, even when not exposed to heat stress.[27,28] In practice, ⅛ teaspoon per day of table salt is recommended for infants less than 6 months of age, and ¼ teaspoon per day is recommended for infants greater than 6 months of age. The table salt is typically added to the infant's formula throughout the day.[35]

Pancreatic Enzyme Replacement Therapy

Types of Available Enzymes

In an effort to confirm safety and efficacy of pancreatic enzymes, a new rule was issued in 2004 requiring makers of pancreatic enzyme products to obtain approval by the U.S.

TABLE 11-4 Comparison of Cystic Fibrosis–Specific Vitamin and Mineral Supplements in United States to Non–Cystic-Fibrosis–Specific Products[a]

Age	SourceCF[b,c] Drops, Chewables, and Softgels	ADEK Chewables[b,d]	AquADEKs[b,e] Drops and Softgels	Vitamax[b,f] Drops and Chewables	Poly-Vi-Sol Drops[g] and Centrum Chewables and Tablet
Vitamin A (IU): Retinol and Beta Carotene					
0–12 mo	4627 (1 mL) 75% BC[h]	—	5751 (1 mL) 87% BC	3170 (1 mL) 0% BC	1500 (1 mL) 0% BC
1–3 y	9254 (2 mL) 75% BC	—	11502 (2 mL) 87% BC	6340 (2 mL) 0% BC	3000 (2 mL) 0% BC
4–8 y	16,000/chewable 88% BC	9000/chewable 60% BC	Ages 4–10 y: 18,167/1 softgel 92% BC	5000/chewable 50% BC	3500/chewable 29% BC
> 9 y	32,000/2 softgels 88% BC	18,000/2 chewables 60% BC	Ages 10 and up: 36,334/2 softgels 92% BC	10,000/2 chewables 50% BC	7000/2 tablets 29% BC
Vitamin E (IU)[i]					
0–12 mo	50 (1 mL)	—	50 (1 mL)[i]	50 (1 mL)	5 (1 mL)
1–3 y	100 (2 mL)	—	100 (2 mL)[i]	100 (2 mL)	10 (2 mL)
4–8 y	200/chewable	150/chewable	Ages 4–10 y: 150/1 softgel[i]	200/chewable	30/chewable
> 9 y	400/2 softgels	300/2 chewables	Ages 10 and up: 300/2 softgels[j]	400/2 chewables	60/2 tablets
Vitamin D (IU)					
0–12 mo	500 (1 mL)	—	400 (1 mL)	400 (1 mL)	400 (1 mL)
1–3 y	1000 (2 mL)	—	800 (2 mL)	800 (2 mL)	800 (2 mL)
4–8 y	1000/chewable	400/chewable	Ages 4–10 y: 800/1 softgel	400/chewable	400/chewable
> 9 y	2000/2 softgels	800/2 chewables	Ages 10 and up: 1600/2 softgels	800/2 chewables	800/2 tablets
Vitamin K (μg)					
0–12 mo	400 (1 mL)	—	400 (1 mL)	300 (1 mL)	0
1–3 y	800 (2 mL)	—	800 (2 mL)	600 (2 mL)	0
4–8 y	800/chewable	150/chewable	Ages 4–10 y: 700/1 softgel	200/chewable	10/chewable
> 9 y	1600/2 softgels	300/2 chewables	Ages 10 and up: 1400/2 softgels	400/2 chewables	50/2 tablets
Zinc (mg)					
0–12 mo	5 (1 mL)	—	5 (1 mL)	7.5 (1 mL)	0
1–3 y	10 (2 mL)	—	10 (2 mL)	15 (2 mL)	0
4–8 y	15/chewable	7.5/chewable	Ages 4–10 y: 10/softgel	7.5/chewable	15/chewable
> 9 y	30/2 softgels	15/2 chewables	Ages 10 and up: 20/2 softgels	15/2 chewables	22/2 tablets

[a] The content of this table was confirmed December 2008. Products also contain a full range of water-soluble vitamins; see SourceCF.com for content.

[b] CF-specific products.

[c] SourceCF Liquid, Chewables, and Softgels are registered trademarks of SourceCF Inc., a subsidiary of Eurand Pharmaceuticals, Inc.

[d] ADEK Chewables is a registered trademark of Axcan Pharma, Inc.

[e] AquADEKs Liquid and Softgels are registered trademarks of Yasoo Health Inc.

[f] Vitamax Drops and Chewables are registered trademarks of Shear/Kershman Labs, Inc.

[g] Poly-Vi-Sol Drops is a registered trademark of Mead Johnson and Company. Centrum Chewables and Tablets are registered trademarks of Wyeth Consumer Care.

[h] Beta carotene.

[i] α-Tocopherol.

[j] Contains mixed tocopherols.

Abbreviation: BC, beta carotene.

Source: Reprinted from Pediatric Clinics of North America, Vol. 56, Michel S, Maqbool A, Hanna M, Mascarenhas M. Nutrition management of pediatric patients who have cystic fibrosis. *Pediatric Clin N Am.* 2009;56:1123–1141. Copyright 2009, with permission from Elsevier.

Food and Drug Administration (FDA) by April 28, 2010. There are 3 brands which received FDA approval (**Table 11-5**), and they contain varying amounts of lipase, which breaks down fat; protease, which breaks down protein; and amylase, which breaks down carbohydrate.

The nonproprietary name of these products is pancrelipase. The products are available in capsule form and feature an enteric coating that protects the enzymes from inactivation in the acid environment of the stomach. The enzymes become activated in the alkaline pH of the duodenum.

Dosage/Administration

There is a CF consensus statement on the use of pancreatic enzyme supplements.[61,62] Extremely high doses of pancreatic enzymes have been associated with fibrosing colonopathy or strictures in the colon in CF patients.[63,64] A recommended starting dose for infants is 2000 to 5000 units of lipase per 4 oz feeding, though this may be less in newborns who take less volume at each feeding.[57] Another proposed weight-based enzyme dosing schedule is starting with 1000 units of lipase/kg body weight/meal for children younger than 4 years of age and 500 units of lipase/kilogram body weight/meal for those over age 4.[61,62] The usual enzyme dose for snacks is one-half of the mealtime dose. It is recommended not to exceed 2500 units of lipase/kg body weight/meal, with a maximum daily dose of 10,000 units lipase/kg body weight. Calculating units of lipase/kilogram body weight/meal has become an integral component of routine care. For example, a 10-year-old child weighing 35.7 kg who takes a mealtime dose of three capsules of a pancreatic enzyme preparation containing 20,000 units of lipase per capsule will receive 1681 units of lipase/kg body weight/meal (60,000 units of lipase divided by 35.7 kg = 1681 units of lipase/kg body weight/meal). Careful monitoring of the patient's growth, stool pattern, and the absence or presence of gastrointestinal symptoms is necessary to determine the adequacy of therapy. Monitoring and adjusting the dosage as needed should be continued throughout the patient's treatment. If the patient with CF is still exhibiting symptoms of malabsorption after reaching a maximum enzyme dose, it may be because the stomach contents are too acidic when reaching the small intestine and are inactivating the enzymes. In these cases, the addition of bicarbonate or other drugs that inhibit gastric acidity may be helpful.[61,62] Nonpancreatic reasons for malabsorption should also be considered.

Enzymes should be taken immediately prior to meals and snacks that contain fat, protein, and complex carbohydrate. The enterically coated enzymes should not be chewed or crushed. For infants and small children who are unable to swallow a capsule, the capsule can be opened and the contents mixed with a soft, acidic food such as applesauce. Enzymes mixed with food should be used within 30 minutes of mixing. When the enterically coated enzymes are mixed with a higher pH food such as pudding or milk, the enzymes will become activated and begin breaking down the food. Older patients swallow their enzymes whole prior to eating a meal or snack.

There is currently no consensus on enzyme dosing for gastrostomy tube feedings, and often it can be difficult to dose enzymes appropriately. The CF Foundation recommends that

TABLE 11-5 Examples of Pancreatic Enzymes

Enzyme	Form*	Lipase USP Units	Protease USP Units	Amylase USP Units
Creon 6[1]	Delayed release capsules	6000	19,000	30,000
Creon 12[1]	Delayed release capsules	12,000	38,000	60,000
Creon 24[1]	Delayed release capsules	24,000	76,000	120,000
Pancreaze MT4[2]	Delayed release capsules	4200	10,000	17,500
Pancreaze MT10[2]	Delayed release capsules	10,500	25,000	43,750
Pancreaze MT16[2]	Delayed release capsules	16,800	40,000	70,000
Pancreaze MT20[2]	Delayed release capsules	21,000	37,000	61,000
ZENPEP 5[3]	Delayed release capsules	5000	17,000	27,000
ZENPEP 10[3]	Delayed release capsules	10,000	34,000	55,000
ZENPEP 15[3]	Delayed release capsules	15,000	51,000	82,000
ZENPEP 20[3]	Delayed release capsules	20,000	68,000	109,000

*Form as described by respective company

[1]Solvay Pharmaceuticals: http://www.creon-us.com/default.htm

[2]Ortho-McNeil-Janssen Pharmaceuticals: http://www.pancreaze.net

[3]Eurand: http://www.zenpep.com/pdfs/zenpep_PI_09.pdf

patients take their usual meal dose of pancreatic enzymes by mouth prior to the initiation of the feeding.[27,28] If receiving continuous overnight tube feeds, some patients may need to take additional enzymes during the middle of the night or at the end of their feeding.[27,28] Giving enterically coated microspheres or microtablets via the feeding tube as a med during a feed or prior to a feed is another option but may result in clogging of the feeding tube. Unfortunately, there is currently no optimal way to dose enzymes during continuous tube feeds. A patient's tolerance to their tube feeds, as well as if the patient will be able to comply with the enzyme regimen at home need to be assessed. It is important to tailor the enzyme regimen to the individual needs of each patient.

Patient Compliance

Administering enzymes to an extremely young infant can be a frustrating endeavor for the parent or caretaker, primarily because of the young infant's natural extrusion reflex. After a few months of age, taking enzymes becomes part of a patient's daily routine. Parents of toddlers should be warned against allowing the child to "graze" throughout the day because this makes enzyme dosing difficult. In the preadolescent and adolescent age groups, patient compliance with enzyme administration can become a big issue. Some schools require the child to come to the school office for medications, and this may be a source of embarrassment and alienation from peers for the child with CF. The lack of compliance needs to be discussed with the child and a solution must be found that is agreeable to the child, parents, and school authorities.

Pancreatic enzyme therapy is very expensive and contributes significantly to the overall cost of the disease management. Enzymes are often covered by third-party payers and some state programs for children with special healthcare needs.

Referral to Food/Nutrition and Other Resources

Referral to food and nutrition resources such as the USDA's Special Supplemental Nutrition Program for Women, Infants, and Children (WIC) program and the Food Stamp Program should be made based on the individual's needs. In some states, referrals can be made to the state program for children with special healthcare needs for aid in obtaining supplemental feedings, enzymes, and vitamins. Children who participate in the Child Nutrition Program at their school will need diet prescriptions for high-calorie, high-protein diets sent to their schools.

CF has a tremendous impact on patients and their families emotionally, physically, and financially. Most CF centers provide an interdisciplinary team approach to the care of these children and their families to better help them meet their many needs.

Alternative/Complementary Medicine

As with other chronic diseases, the use of alternative/complementary medicine in CF care has sparked the interest of patients with CF, their families, and health professionals. To date, little published science-based research exists in the area of alternative and complementary medicine in CF care. More and more CF centers are surveying their patients to ascertain the extent of alternative medicine practices. Currently, patients with CF are obtaining a lot of their information from the Internet, with many CF Internet sites having links to alternative medicine sites. CF centers need to study alternative medicine practices further so that CF caregivers can advise patients and their families as to the safety and efficacy of various therapies.

Patients at three CF centers participated in a survey regarding the use of nonmedical treatment.[65] Nonmedical treatment was used by 66% of the population; 57% of the population used at least one religious treatment; 27% used at least one nonreligious treatment.[65] Group prayer (48%) was the most common nonmedical therapy, and 92% of those participating in group prayer perceived benefit. Chiropractors were consulted by 14%, with 69% of these patients perceiving benefit. Nutrition modalities other than those prescribed by the CF caretakers were employed by 11% of the population; 78% of these patients used these treatments frequently (more than five times); 87% perceived benefit. Meditation was used by 5%, with 94% reporting perceived benefit.

It is important that CF caregivers ask questions about alternative/complementary medicine practices when interviewing patients with CF and their family members, especially in regard to ingested substances. This is especially important information to obtain from patients who may be participating in studies with experimental drugs because the possibility exists that substances such as unregulated botanical products may confound the study results.

Identification of Areas Needing Further Research

There are many unanswered questions about CF in general and, more specifically, in regard to nutrition. Additional research is needed to determine specific nutrient requirements of patients with CF in regard to energy, protein, vitamins, minerals, and EFAs. The most appropriate method for delivering these nutrients must be determined. Further study on the psychosocial and emotional benefits and drawbacks of invasive nutritional therapy and the effect of improved nutritional status on body composition and the progression of the pulmonary disease would be beneficial. More study is needed on the role of anabolic agents such as insulin and growth hormone and on appetite stimulants, such as megastrol acetate, to determine the cost/benefits of these adjunct therapies. With lung transplantation becoming more available to CF patients, appropriate nutrition management pre- and posttransplantation will need further study.

CF is a complicated disease, affecting many organs of the body, and the disease process is highly variable. Proper nutritional care is an integral part of its therapy. Therefore, every patient and family deserves individualized treatment and support from an interdisciplinary team of health professionals, including a qualified dietetics professional, trained in the care of patients with CF.

Bronchopulmonary Dysplasia

Bronchopulmonary dysplasia (BPD) was first described by Northway and colleagues[66] in 1967 as a form of chronic lung disease seen in infants with severe hyaline membrane disease who required mechanical ventilation and high concentrations of oxygen for prolonged periods of time. Since that time, improvements in neonatal intensive care and changing epidemiology or prematurity have resulted in changes in both the definitions of BPD and the pathology of the lung disease. Most recently, clinical practice has advanced, resulting in a decrease in lung injury in larger (greater than 1200 gram birth weight) and more mature infants. At the same time, more and more premature infants are surviving at earlier gestational ages and lower birth weights. The National Institute of Child Health and Human Development/National Heart, Lung and Blood Institute refined the definition of BPD to reflect differing criteria for infants born at less than or greater than 32 weeks gestation.[67] The expanded definition includes different diagnostic criteria for mild, moderate, and severe forms of the disease.[67] For example, the definition of severe BPD for an infant with a gestational age of less than 32 weeks is the need for 30% oxygen or more and/or positive pressure at 36 weeks postmenstrual age or discharge, whichever comes first.[67]

Today's definition of BPD includes infants who have had an acute lung injury with minimal clinical and radiographic findings, as well as those with major radiographic abnormalities. BPD represents a continuum of lung disease. The pathogenesis of BPD is multifactorial but includes primarily arrested lung development due to the necessary accelerated maturation of the lungs due to premature birth. Severe, diffuse, acute lung injury and an early inflammatory response exacerbate the abnormal lung development due to primary injury and inadequate immature repair mechanisms. The lungs may be damaged by the barotrauma from the use of intermittent positive pressure ventilation (IPPV) and by oxygen toxicity from the high concentrations of oxygen required by these infants early in life.[68,69] Infection may play a role in the pathogenesis of BPD.[68] Other factors that may contribute to the development of the disease include increased fluids contributing to pulmonary edema[70] and inadequate early nutrition impeding lung reparative processes.[71,72]

Today, younger and smaller preterm infants are surviving with the aid of mechanical ventilation. Consequently, BPD has become one of the most common sequelae of newborn intensive care unit stays. BPD has become rare in premature infants weighing 1500 grams or more with uncomplicated respiratory distress syndrome. This is due to the use of antenatal steroids, surfactant replacement therapy, gentler ventilation that reduces barotrauma, better nutrition, and careful use of supplemental oxygen.[73] However, the incidence of BPD is about 30% of infants with birth weight under 1000 grams and is higher in lower birth weight infants. As BPD patients are followed over time, chronic lung disease remains a major clinical problem for many of these patients into late childhood and early adolescence.[68,74]

Signs of respiratory distress, such as chest retractions, tachypnea, crackles, and wheezing, characterize BPD. Supplemental oxygen therapy may be required, and there may be changes on the patient's chest radiograph. Pulmonary complications of BPD may include recurrent atelectasis, pulmonary infections, and respiratory failure requiring mechanical ventilation. Other complications of BPD include pulmonary edema, cor pulmonale, poor growth, neurodevelopmental delays including delayed feeding skills, and cardiovascular problems.

The primary goal of BPD management is to provide the patient with the necessary pulmonary support during the acute and chronic phases of the disease to minimize lung damage and to maintain optimal oxygen saturation. This may include mechanical ventilation, supplemental oxygen, anti-inflammatory and β-adrenergic aerosols, and diuretic therapy. Of equal importance is the provision of adequate nutrition, not only for growth and development, but also to compensate for the demands of the disease. Growth of new lung tissue can occur in humans until about 8 years of age. Theoretically, a BPD patient can "outgrow" the disease if adequate pulmonary and nutritional support can be provided.

Increased Nutrient Requirements

Adequate nutrition is important for patients with BPD but can often be a challenge for parents and health providers. The following section will further explore the nutrition implications of BPD.

Effects of Prematurity

Most babies who develop BPD are premature infants, so it is easy to see that these infants have little fat, glycogen, or other nutrients in reserve, particularly iron, calcium, and phosphorus. Faced with the demands of prematurity and the stress of BPD, the infant can quickly develop a state of negative nutrient balance.

Effects of Bronchopulmonary Dysplasia

Several factors increase the energy and nutrient requirements of BPD patients, including the following:

- Increased basal metabolic rate
- Increased work of breathing
- Chronic hypoxia
- Chronic illness/infections
- Respiratory distress/metabolic complications
- Tissue repair/catch-up growth
- Drug–nutrient interactions

Weinstein and Oh[75] reported that resting oxygen consumption was approximately 25% higher in eight infants with BPD, when compared with controls. Kurzner and colleagues[76] found that infants with BPD and growth failure had increased resting oxygen consumption, as compared with control infants and infants with BPD and normal growth. Other investigators have also found an increase in resting energy expenditure in infants with BPD as compared to controls, ranging from 125–150%.[77–79]

Treatment of the BPD patient usually includes a wide array of medications, including diuretics, steroids, and bronchodilators. The impact of these drugs on the patient's nutritional status is further discussed in **Table 11-6**.

Decreased Nutrient Consumption

Infants with BPD are extremely fluid sensitive because of the acute lung disease and the possible complication of cor pulmonale, or right-sided heart failure. When fluid restrictions are imposed, this places a limitation on the provision of energy and nutrients. One study[78] showed that infants with BPD had significantly lower energy intakes, as compared to controls. Thus, infants with BPD often require a calorically enhanced formula in order to meet their energy needs for adequate growth.

TABLE 11-6 BPD Drug–Nutrient Interactions

Medication	Nutrients Affected (lowers all)	Other Effects
Diuretics (e.g., furosemide)	Na, K, Cl, Mg, Ca, Zn	Volume depletion Metabolic alkalosis Anorexia Diarrhea Hyperuricemia Gastrointestinal irritant
Bronchodilators (e.g., theophylline)		Gastrointestinal distress Nausea Vomiting Diarrhea
Steroids (e.g., dexamethasone)	Ca, P	Growth suppression

Frequent intubations and mechanical ventilation interfere with the normal feeding sequence and feeding-skill development. Therefore, these infants may be poor oral feeders and develop aversive oral behavior.[80] Also, these patients may experience fatigue or decreased oxygen saturation during feeding because of their underlying pulmonary disease.[81,82] Infants with BPD also may have associated gastroesophageal reflux, causing an impediment to feeding.[83]

Growth of Infants with BPD

It is unrealistic to expect true growth to occur when life-threatening events, such as respiratory failure, necrotizing enterocolitis, or other serious problems of prematurity, are taking place. The patient must be fairly stable in order for growth to occur. Growth failure is a complication of BPD. A poor pattern of growth in patients with BPD is often related to the severity of pulmonary disease.[84] One study found that resting metabolic rate is inversely correlated with body weight in infants with BPD.[76] These investigators also found that infants with BPD who had growth failure had significantly lower birth weights, younger gestational ages, increased duration of oxygen therapy, and increased duration of mechanical ventilation as compared to those infants with normal growth.[76] Yeh and colleagues[78] found a significantly smaller rate of weight gain (grams/day) in infants with BPD as compared to a control group of premature infants who had mild transient pulmonary problems and did not require mechanical ventilation.

DeRegnier and colleagues[85] studied 16 very-low-birth-weight infants who developed BPD and compared them to birth-weight-matched control infants without BPD during the first 6 postnatal weeks. At the end of the study period, the infants with BPD had lower Z-scores for weight and head circumference, lower arm muscle area, and lower arm fat area than the control group. However, length Z-scores were not significantly different between the two groups. When the BPD infants achieved full enteral feedings, they gained weight at the same rate as the controls but did not achieve catch-up growth. These investigators speculated that early reductions in muscle and fat accretion and growth velocity may contribute to the long-term growth failure of BPD patients, thus emphasizing the need for optimal nutrition intake early in the postnatal period.[85]

Forty infants with BPD were studied for 7 months after initial hospital discharge. During this period, 73% of the infants experienced a decrease in weight-for-age Z-score; 20% experienced a decrease in length-for-age Z-score; and 65% experienced a decrease in weight-for-length Z-score. Low socioeconomic status, days of postdischarge illness, and "suspect" development were associated with a significantly increased risk of growth failure.[86] Another study of preterm infants with BPD noted they had lower weights, lengths, total body fat, and fat-free mass than the control group at 6 weeks after term. Fat-free mass and total body fat of the patients with BPD remained lower than normal during the first year of life.[87]

In a longer follow-up study of patients with BPD, 12 school-age children with BPD were compared to a preterm control group matched for birth weight, gestational age, and gender, as well as with an age-matched control group. Both the BPD group and the preterm group were shorter than the healthy term control group. The BPD group also had lower lean body mass and lower bone mineral content when compared to the control.[74] Another study of school-age children with BPD compared children who had been born prematurely with and without the development of BPD. The children with BPD were significantly smaller in weight and head circumference but not height. However, when possible confounders that are known to be correlates of poor growth were applied, the differences were no longer significant. These investigators suggest that the poor growth reported in children with BPD may be related to other factors besides BPD.[88]

Adequate oxygenation must be maintained in the patient with BPD for growth to occur. Studies have shown that desaturation may occur during feeding and sleeping.[81,82,89] Positive growth can occur in infants with BPD who maintained an oxygen saturation of greater than 92% while sleeping. However, short-term pulse oxygen saturation studies were not always reliable predictors of oxygen saturation during prolonged periods of sleep. Another study found that patients with BPD who were maintained on home oxygen therapy maintained their original weight percentiles whereas those infants who discontinued oxygen therapy experienced significant decreases in weight gain.[90]

Nutritional Screening and Assessment

It is important to monitor the nutritional status of patients with BPD to ensure they are receiving adequate nutrition for growth and development and to compensate for the demands of the disease. The following section will explain markers of nutritional status in patients with BPD and how to perform a nutritional assessment.

Anthropometric

Obtaining daily weights in a BPD patient is essential during the early hospitalization(s) and critical stages of the disease. Weight data help to identify fluid overload in a patient, as well as growth.

Monitoring weight, length, and head circumference on a regular basis during the follow-up period is needed to assess whether the infant or child is achieving expected growth. Measurements should be made using appropriate techniques and equipment (see Chapter 3) and be plotted on appropriate growth charts, using either the NCHS growth charts and correcting for gestational age or growth charts that allow assessment of infants of varying gestational age, such as those by Babson and Benda.[22,91] When using NCHS growth charts, weight should be corrected for gestational age until 24 months, length until 36 months, and head circumference until 18 months.[45] Additional measurements such as mid-arm circumference and triceps skinfold can be useful in determining whether weight gain is secondary to growth or edema. See also Appendix B for growth charts and arm and triceps measurement tables.

Biochemical

Biochemical monitoring of the BPD patient is individualized based on the patient's clinical status, the type and amount of diuretic therapy, and the protocol of the individual institution. During diuretic therapy, electrolytes need to be monitored, especially sodium, chloride, and potassium. Mineral status should be monitored including calcium, phosphorus, and magnesium. Other helpful measurements include prealbumin or albumin as a measure of visceral protein stores; a complete blood count; alkaline phosphatase, parathyroid hormone, and 25-hydroxyvitamin D for monitoring for rickets of prematurity; and urine specific gravity, especially if the patient is fluid restricted and/or a concentrated formula is being given.

Clinical

The patient's pulmonary status will have an impact on nutritional needs and intake. If a patient with BPD is ventilator dependent, this is an indication of respiratory failure and severe lung disease. Ventilator-dependent BPD patients require close follow-up because it may be difficult initially to determine their nutritional needs. Many chronic ventilator-dependent patients with BPD have very low energy needs and yet their other nutrient needs are the same as other infants with BPD. For these patients, feedings must be adjusted to meet nutrient needs without providing too many calories, which often requires vitamin and mineral supplementation. A patient who has a low arterial partial pressure of oxygen is not properly oxygenating tissue, which may contribute to growth failure. These patients may require supplemental oxygen for tissue oxygenation and growth. Noting a patient's oximetry reading is important. An increase in pulmonary symptoms such as the presence of tachypnea, rales, rhonchi, and bronchiolitis/pneumonia is indicative of active pulmonary disease. The presence of chronic pulmonary disease and acute pulmonary exacerbations in BPD patients increases energy needs and at the same time may increase their sensitivity to fluids.

Other medical conditions, such as cor pulmonale, gastroesophageal reflux with or without aspiration, esophagitis, repeated emesis, and the patient's medication regimen, should also be noted. Table 11-6 lists drug–nutrient interactions of medications commonly prescribed for BPD patients. It is important to note a patient's input and output to complete the clinical assessment.

Dietary

The BPD patient's dietary intake needs to be evaluated for calories; protein; fluid; electrolytes; key minerals such as calcium, phosphorus, and iron; and caloric distribution of fat, protein, and carbohydrate. The type of feeding—enteral versus parenteral—should be noted, as well as the route of administration and vitamin and mineral supplementation. This can then be compared to the patient's estimated nutrient and fluid requirements.

Of particular importance in the nutrition assessment of BPD patients is careful monitoring of the patient's ability to suck and swallow and the patient's feeding skill development. The sucking reflex does not develop until about 34 weeks gestation. Alternate methods of feeding are required until this reflex develops. Neurologic impairment may prevent the patient from being able to coordinate sucking and swallowing. Noxious stimuli to the patient's mouth, such as frequent intubations and suctioning, may seriously affect normal feeding skill development. Maintaining adequate oxygenation during feedings is essential.[81,82] It is important to note whether the patient tires during feedings and whether he or she turns blue around the mouth or fingertips, indicating a drop in oxygen saturation. It is imperative that these problems be identified early and appropriate intervention instituted.

Nutrition Management

After the nutritional assessment of a patient with BPD is complete, it is important to provide appropriate nutrition interventions that will support the infant's nutritional requirements. There are many factors that need to be taken into consideration when establishing these interventions. The next section will explore in more detail the nutrition management of patients with BPD.

Nutrients of Concern

It is important to assess and monitor intake of macronutrients as well as several key micronutrients in the BPD patient.

Energy and Protein

The caloric requirement for infants with BPD is higher than normal and ranges from 120–150 kcal/kg/day; those with severe BPD may need more than 150 kcal/kg/day.[83] Meeting these high levels of intake can be a challenge, especially when other problems exist such as fluid restrictions, gastrointestinal immaturity, and renal immaturity. Dr. Oh[92] describes three phases of nutritional management of infants with BPD. The estimated energy requirements of each phase and the components of the energy expenditure are depicted in **Table 11-7**.

- *Acute phase:* The BPD patient during this phase is critically ill and at risk for clinical morbidities, such as patent ductus arteriosus and necrotizing enterocolitis. No calories are needed for specific dynamic action or for growth. Efforts should be made to keep thermal losses to a minimum. Possible feeding complications during this phase include fluid overload and hyperglycemia. The BPD patient has decreased fluid tolerance because of pulmonary edema and reduced cardiac output. Caloric provision is often relegated to secondary importance, behind these two problems and electrolyte imbalance.
- *Intermediate phase:* This phase is characterized by a period of clinical improvements and a gradual introduction of oral feeding. Again, thermal losses should be kept to a minimum. Fluid overload continues to be a possible complication, but generally the BPD patient is able to tolerate an increase in fluid during this phase.
- *Convalescent phase:* This is a period of recovery when the patient is usually feeding orally. Minimizing thermal losses continues to be important, as well as monitoring activity, growth, and adequate oxygenation of tissues. Continued monitoring of intake, growth, and development is important.

The immature kidney cannot handle high-protein loads, so protein should constitute about 8% to 12% of the total calories, with the remainder of the calories evenly divided between carbohydrate and fat.[93]

TABLE 11-7 Calorie Requirements (kcal/kg/d) of Infants with Bronchopulmonary Dysplasia at Various Stages of Nutritional Management

Component	Acute	Intermediate	Convalescent
Basal metabolic rate	45	60	60
Stool losses	0–10	10	60
Thermal stress	0–10	0–10	10
Activity	5	5	10
Specific dynamic action	0	0–5	10
Growth allowance	0	20–30	20–30
Total	50–70	95–120	120–130

Acute = clinical illness, oral feeding difficult; intermediate = clinical improvement, gradual introduction of oral feeding; convalescent = recovery, oral feeding exclusively.

Source: Used with permission of Ross Products Division, Abbott Laboratories, Inc., Columbus, OH 43216. From *Bronchopulmonary Dysplasia and Related Chronic Respiratory Disorders*, © 1986, Ross Products Division, Abbott Laboratories, Inc.

Vitamins A and E

Many studies have examined the role of vitamin A (retinol) in animals and premature infants who develop chronic lung disease.[94] Vitamin A is essential in the respiratory tract for maintenance of the integrity and differentiation of epithelial cells. Deficiency of vitamin A results in loss of cilia and other changes in the airways, which resemble the changes seen in BPD. Vitamin A adequacy may decrease the incidence of BPD in infants with very low birth weight, and thus, plasma serum vitamin A levels should be monitored.[95] Administering 5000 IU vitamin A intramuscularly three times a week to infants at risk for developing BPD may be advantageous.[96,97] Some newborn intensive care units administer vitamin A in an attempt to protect against BPD.[98]

Adequate vitamin E status is particularly important in premature infants with BPD who are on oxygen therapy because vitamin E is a major antioxidant. Vitamin E acts as an oxygen free radical scavenger and membrane stabilizer, protecting lipid-containing cell membranes from oxidation. Infants are most likely to receive adequate vitamin E when fed human milk or commercial formulas. Large doses of vitamin E appear to offer no additional protection against BPD.[99]

Trace Minerals

Particular attention should be given to the following trace minerals, which are components of an antioxidant enzyme system: copper, zinc, selenium, and manganese.[93] No specific recommendations for these minerals have been established for the infant with BPD. Zinc can be decreased with diuretic therapy and premature infants often are in negative zinc balance.[100] Infants with BPD may be at risk for toxic accumulation of certain trace elements, such as copper and manganese, especially if the patient has cholestasis or other liver disease.[93]

Iron

The recommended iron intake is 2 to 4 mg of elemental iron/kg/day,[101] and the supplementation should begin no later than 2 months of age. Iron can be provided through a supplement or through the use of iron-fortified formulas. Adequate iron status is especially important in patients with BPD in order to maximize tissue oxygenation and minimize oxygen consumption.[69]

Calcium and Phosphorus

Infants born prematurely are born without the benefit of the calcium and phosphorus accretion of the third trimester of gestation. In addition, the calcium and phosphorus status of premature infants with BPD can be further compromised by diuretic therapy, steroid therapy, long-term use of parenteral nutrition, and feeding delays. Consequently, infants with BPD are at risk for developing rickets of prematurity or osteopenia, which is diagnosed by decreased bone density on X-rays and an alkaline phosphatase level over 400 units/L. Therefore, the adequacy of calcium and phosphorus intake requires special attention. Preterm human milk can be fortified with a commercial human milk fortifier. Premature formulas and premature transitional formulas provide higher concentrations of these minerals. Adequate vitamin D (400 IU/d) intake is also important.[101]

Electrolytes

Electrolyte imbalance may result, especially when the infant is receiving diuretic therapy. The infant with BPD can usually tolerate a sodium intake of 1.5 to 3.5 mEq/kg/d.[69] Potassium (3 mEq/kg/d) and chloride may need to be supplemented depending on the diuretic therapy.[69,70] The infant should be closely monitored when sodium chloride and/or potassium chloride are being added to the infant's feedings.

Barriers to Meeting Increased Needs

Many barriers must be overcome in order to meet the increased nutrient needs of the infant with BPD. These barriers include:

- Fluid restriction for infants with cor pulmonale with or without right-sided heart failure and those who are fluid sensitive
- Gastrointestinal limitations such as an immature gut and gastroesophageal reflux
- Immature renal function, making renal solute load of feedings an issue
- Chronic hypoxia, especially during feedings and sleep
- Feeding difficulties, including lack of sucking reflex and feeding aversions
- Significant GERD resulting in vomiting or discomfort with feeding

Meeting Nutritional Needs

Translating these energy, protein, and other nutrient needs into a feeding order can be challenging.

Parenteral Nutrition (PN)

During the acute phase of BPD, parenteral nutrition is often employed. See also Chapter 4 for specific guidelines for PN in the early postnatal period for premature infants.

The deleterious effects of intravenous fat in pulmonary-compromised patients has been noted in some studies.[102,103] Other studies have shown that the possible adverse effect of lipid infusion is related to the maturity of the infant and the rate of the infusion.[104,105] The American Academy of Pediatrics recommends starting lipids in the low-birth-weight infant at 0.5 to 1.0 g/kg/day and slowly increasing to a maximum of 2.0 to 3.0 g/kg/day.[101] Serum triglyceride levels should be kept below 150 mg/dL.[101]

For preterm infants, the American Academy of Pediatrics recommends starting glucose infusions at a rate less than 6 mg/kg/minute and steadily increasing to an infusion rate of 11–12 mg/kg/minute.[101] High glucose loads in patients with BPD have been shown to increase resting energy expenditure, basal oxygen consumption, and carbon dioxide production.[77] Infants with borderline respiratory function may not be able to excrete this additional carbon dioxide, and respiratory acidosis can result.

Enteral Nutrition

Enteral feedings must be begun at a slow rate to allow the immature intestine of the premature infant to adapt to the feedings (refer to Chapter 4). During this transitional phase, PN is often continued in order to meet the increased energy needs of the patient. It is very important to maintain the delivery of adequate energy and protein while tolerance to enteral feedings is being established.

This transitional phase can become very complicated. An infant must be hungry before an oral feeding will be readily accepted. Continuous infusions of nutritional solutions may suppress natural hunger sensations. Hunger is particularly important when feeding skills are being developed. An appropriate schedule of parenteral feedings, enteral tube feedings, and oral feedings must be determined by members of the interdisciplinary healthcare team, including family members and caregivers, to best suit the individual patient's needs.

Fortified breast milk or premature infant formulas, which have higher concentrations of vitamins and minerals, may be used. Breast milk is preferred initially for the premature gastrointestinal tract because it is easily tolerated and associated with decreased incidence of necrotizing enterocolitis.[83] The infant should continue with breast milk fortified with a human milk fortifier or with premature formula until reaching a weight of 2000 to 2500 g. At this point, the infant can most likely be transitioned to a premature follow-up formula or a standard infant formula concentrated to 22 or 24 Kcal/oz. Both premature formulas and premature follow-up formulas have the fatty acids docosahexaenoic acid (DHA) and arachidonic acid (ARA) added. To meet some infants' very high energy needs, it may become necessary to further concentrate the formula to 26 to 30 kcal/oz. Currently, there is some controversy as to the best approach for further concentration of the formula. Some registered dietitians prefer to further concentrate the formula by adding less water. The proponents of this method argue that by concentrating formula in this manner, protein, vitamins, and mineral contents per volume are not diluted. Another approach is using a 24 kcal/oz formula as a base and adding carbohydrate in the form of glucose polymers or rice cereal, with or without added fat. When modulating formulas, it is important to maintain a proper balance of nutrients. Caloric distribution should continue to be approximately 8% to 12% protein, 40% to 50% carbohydrate, and 40% to 50% fat.[93] An example of a modulated formula is given in **Table 11-8**.

Care should be taken not to dilute the protein content to a level that is inadequate for growth.[106] Fat should not provide more than 60% of total calories because ketosis may be induced. Fat delays gastric emptying, and a high fat content may be contraindicated in patients who have gastroesophageal reflux.[106] Boehm and associates[107] showed decreased fat absorption in patients with BPD that may contribute to inadequate weight gain. Regardless of the approach taken, excessive osmolality and renal solute load should be avoided. It is important to maintain adequate vitamin and mineral intakes. Once an infant is on standard formula or breast milk, a supplement of a standard infant multivitamin preparation may be recommended until the infant is taking about 1 L of formula. The usual recommendation is 1 cc of a standard infant multivitamin with breast milk or formula intakes over 16 ounces per day and 0.5 cc for intakes between 16 and 30 ounces per day.[108]

Brunton and colleagues[109] studied preterm infants with BPD fed either a standard formula or an enriched formula. The enriched formula had the same caloric concentration as the standard formula (27 Kcal/oz), but had higher concentrations of protein, calcium, phosphorus, and zinc. The study was conducted from 37 weeks postmenstrual age to 3 months chronological age. The results included greater linear growth, greater radial bone mineral content, and greater lean mass in the infants who were fed the enriched formula. This study suggests that, in addition to calories,

TABLE 11-8 Examples of a Modulated Formula

	Carbohydrate (g)	Protein (g)	Fat (g)
30 mL NeoSure ADVANCE 24*	2.49	0.69	1.32
1 g Polycose* powder	0.94	—	—
1 mL Microlipid[1]	—	—	0.50
Total	3.43	0.69	1.82
Kilocalories per gram	× 4	× 4	× 9
Kilocalories	13.72	2.76	16.38
% Total kilocalories	42	8	50
Total kilocalories = 32.86/31 mL 1.06 Kcal/mL			

*Ross Laboratories, Columbus, Ohio

[1]Microlipid, Mead Johnson, Evansville, Indiana

greater concentrations of protein and selected minerals may be necessary for catch-up growth in patients with BPD.[109]

When infants are receiving high-calorie formulas, careful monitoring is warranted. Increasing the caloric density may increase the potential renal solute load if fluid intake is limited. When the infant is growing and nitrogen is being utilized to form new tissue, the infant usually handles the solute load. However, if growth ceases or if there is increased fluid loss, such as with a febrile illness, renal solute load may become a problem for these infants, and azotemia may result. Urine specific gravity should be monitored.[106]

The infant may be unable to consume an adequate amount of formula by mouth. It may be necessary to deliver the balance of the formula via tube feeding to achieve adequate intake. Oral gastric or nasogastric feedings are commonly used for short-term supplementary feedings, whereas gastrostomy feedings are used for long-term tube feeding.

Addressing Feeding Difficulties

The patient's ability to suck and swallow must be assessed. Abnormalities in the developmental patterns of suck-and-swallow rhythms during feeding in preterm infants with BPD have been reported.[110] Feeding behavior should be assessed for age appropriateness based on corrected age.

Patients with BPD are susceptible to developing feeding difficulties because of their usual prematurity and because of the nature of the life-sustaining respiratory therapy that they receive. Intubations and suctioning are noxious stimuli to the oral area and can interfere with normal feeding development. Supplemental oxygen is usually delivered by nasal cannula and does not interfere with oral feedings.

Occupational therapists and speech pathologists identify feeding problems and design treatment plans. Nonnutritive sucking can be instituted during a tube feeding so that the infant can begin to associate feelings of satiety with sucking. In some instances, feedings thickened with rice cereal may be easier for infants to handle. Overlooking problems in the development of feeding skills can result in serious aversions to eating or decreased and inadequate intake.

When critical steps in feeding skill development have been missed, it may be necessary to design a program that breaks eating down into small steps and to orient the child to each step. Instead of feeding according to chronological age, it is more important to feed the child according to the stage of feeding development. A behavioral program may be necessary to help the patient overcome fears related to eating or when food refusal is used manipulatively.

Singer and associates[111] found that mothers of infants with BPD spent more time prompting the infants to feed, but these infants took in less formula and spent less time sucking than the two control groups of premature infants without BPD and term infants. In another study, parents often expressed concern about getting their infant with BPD to take enough food and reported long feeding times.[86] Problematic feeding interactions between the caregiver and the infant may develop. It is important that the health-care professional be aware of this potential problem and provide the family with anticipatory guidance in this area. If the patient's oral intake is not adequate to meet nutritional needs, then tube feedings are necessary. A plan for balancing tube feedings with oral feedings must be designed to establish hunger and appetite for feedings by mouth but providing the balance of nutrition via the tube feeding. Tube feedings can be nasogastric, oral gastric, trans pyloric, or gastrostomy. Drip, bolus, or a combination tube feeding schedule can be developed based on the patient's individual needs.

Family/Caretaker Education

The home care of the patient with BPD can be quite complex and may include supplemental oxygen and multiple medications and therapies as well as nutrition management. Family and caretaker education by a registered dietitian is an important component of the nutrition care plan, and adequate time must be devoted to education during the discharge-planning process. Written instructions for mixing formulas in common household measures for volumes that will be used in 24 hours or less should be given to families. It is best to have the family member or caretaker demonstrate the proper mixing of formulas, especially formula that is being concentrated or contains additives. Reinforcement of these instructions needs to take place on an ongoing basis in outpatient follow-up. It is important to consistently ask the family how they are mixing the formula at home to ensure that they are following the correct recipe and the infant is getting the calories that he or she needs to demonstrate adequate growth.

Referral to Food/Nutrition Resources

Caring for a patient with BPD can be very draining for the patient's family from emotional, physical, and financial standpoints. It is important to assess the patient's and family's needs with regard to food and nutrition resources. Appropriate referrals must be made. Often, this can be done in cooperation with the nurse and/or social worker.

Medical and Nutrition Follow-up

After discharge from the hospital, the infant with BPD will require regular medical and nutrition follow-up. Feedings will need to be adjusted as the patient grows and develops. Many patients benefit from being enrolled in early intervention programs, which can provide nutrition, occupational therapy, physical therapy, and speech therapy as needed by the individual patient.

Identification of Areas Needing Further Research

Effects of early onset of respiratory failure and vigorous ventilator support on nutrient and energy requirements for patients with BPD should be assessed at various stages of the disease, particularly regarding energy, protein, vitamins A and E, and minerals such as calcium, phosphorus, and zinc. Assimilation and absorption of nutrients in patients with BPD and whether a deficiency of one of these nutrients plays a role in the etiology of the disease also must be determined. General growth studies, including studies that establish appropriate growth for patients with BPD at various stages of the disease, would provide guidance for healthcare practitioners. Nutritional requirements of BPD patients at various stages of the disease and appropriate methods and timing of nutrition intervention in BPD treatment require further study. The long-term sequelae of BPD and its current treatment modalities require ongoing investigation.

Asthma

Asthma is the most common chronic disease of childhood, affecting an estimated 7 million children from birth to 18 years of age.[112] The prevalence of childhood asthma has been increasing, as it has for adults, since 1980 and has become a major public health problem.[113] Asthma is the most common cause of school absenteeism in the United States with about 14 million lost school days per year.[113] In 2004, children up to 17 years old had 7 million ambulatory visits, 750,000 emergency department visits, and nearly 200,000 hospitalizations because of asthma.[113] Disparities exist among racial/ethnic populations, with a higher prevalence seen in non-Hispanic blacks and Puerto Ricans compared to non-Hispanic white children.[113] Non-Hispanic blacks have more emergency department visits, more hospitalizations, and an increase in asthma mortality, which are not explained entirely by higher asthma prevalence.[114] There is increased prevalence in childhood among males, children of lower socioeconomic groups, African Americans, and those with a family history of asthma or allergies.[115,116] Underdiagnosis and inappropriate treatment are major contributors to morbidity and mortality.[116]

Eight objectives of the Healthy People 2010[117] health objectives for the nation are related to asthma. These objectives are:

1. Reduce asthma deaths (objective 24-1).
2. Reduce hospitalizations for asthma (objective 24-2).
3. Reduce hospital emergency department visits for asthma (objective 24-3).
4. Reduce activity limitations among persons with asthma (objective 24-4).
5. Reduce number of school or work days missed (objective 24-5).
6. Increase the proportion of persons with asthma who received formal patient education (objective 24-6).
7. Increase the proportion of persons with asthma who receive appropriate care (objective 24-7).
8. Establish in at least 15 states a surveillance system for tracking asthma data (objective 24-8).

Asthma is defined by the National Heart, Lung and Blood Institute (NHLBI)[118] as a chronic inflammatory disorder of the airways. Symptoms of this inflammation include recurrent episodes of wheezing, breathlessness, chest tightness, and cough, particularly at night and early in the morning. These asthma episodes are associated with widespread but variable obstruction of airflow, which is often reversible either spontaneously or with treatment. Inflammation of the airways also causes an associated increase in airway responsiveness to a variety of stimuli.[118] Inflammation causes airway narrowing and increased airway secretions. Chronic inflammation can lead to airway remodeling, which can cause progressive loss of pulmonary function.[116] Airway obstruction is caused by bronchoconstriction, airway edema, chronic mucus plug formation, and airway remodeling.[116,118]

According to the NHLBI guidelines,[118] asthma management consists of four components:

1. Assessment and monitoring
2. Control of environmental factors and co-morbid conditions that affect asthma
3. Pharmacologic therapy
4. Education for a partnership in asthma care

The diagnosis of asthma can be made when the clinician determines that episodic symptoms of airflow obstruction are present, that airflow obstruction is at least partially reversible, and when alternative diagnoses have been excluded.[118] Diagnostic tools available to the clinician include obtaining a thorough history; spirometry, which measures pulmonary function but is not feasible to measure in young children up to 5 to 6 years of age; chest radiograph; and pulse oximetry, a measure of oxygen saturation, to evaluate hypoxemia during an acute episode. Other diagnostic tests available include allergy testing, nasal and sinus evaluation, and gastroesophageal reflux assessment.[118] Differential diagnoses include aspiration, cystic fibrosis, cardiac or anatomical defects, and upper and lower respiratory tract infections.[116] The NHLBI guidelines include a classification system of asthma severity: intermittent, mild persistent, moderate persistent, and severe persistent. These classifications reflect the clinical manifestations of asthma and are based on frequency of daytime and nighttime symptoms, spirometry if available, and severity of asthma flare-ups.[118]

According to the NHLBI guidelines, the goals of asthma therapy are to:[118]

- Reduce impairment
  - Prevent chronic and troublesome symptoms
  - Require infrequent use ($\leq$ 2 days a week) of inhaled short-acting beta$_2$-agonist (SABA) for quick relief of symptoms (not including prevention of exercise-induced bronchospasm [EIB])
  - Maintain (near) normal pulmonary function
  - Maintain normal activity levels (including exercise and other physical activity and attendance at work or school)
  - Meet patients' and families' expectations of and satisfaction with asthma care
- Reduce risk
  - Prevent recurrent exacerbations of asthma and minimize the need for emergency department (ED) visits or hospitalizations
  - Prevent progressive loss of lung function; for children, prevent reduced lung growth
  - Provide optimal pharmacotherapy with minimal or no adverse effects

A major goal of asthma treatment is to reduce inflammation. The first step toward this is for the patient to recognize and avoid the triggers of asthma. Triggers may include indoor allergens such as dust mites, cockroaches, mold, and animal dander, and outdoor allergens such as trees, grasses, weeds, and pollens.[116] Environmental tobacco smoke and air pollutants are major precipitants of asthma symptoms in children.[118] Viral respiratory infections are the primary cause of severe asthma flare-ups. Other factors contributing to asthma severity include rhinitis, sinusitis, gastroesophageal reflux, and sulfite sensitivity.[118] In some children, weather or humidity changes, or exercise—especially in cold and dry air—may produce inflammation of the airways.[121] Food allergies may also cause asthma symptoms.[119]

In addition to reducing factors that increase the patient's asthma symptoms, pharmacologic therapy is an important component of asthma management.[118,120] The choice of specific medicines is based on asthma severity and the classification of asthma. The goal is to optimize pharmacotherapy while minimizing side effects. Long-term control medicines are taken daily to achieve and maintain control of persistent asthma by reducing inflammation. Long-term control medicines include inhaled corticosteroids, long-acting beta$_2$ agonists, cromolyn sodium and nedocromil sodium (mast cell stabilizers), methylxanthine, leukotriene modifiers, oral corticosteroids, and inhaled corticosteroids and long-acting beta$_2$ agonists in combination. Quick-relief medications, inhaled short-acting beta$_2$ agonists, anticholinergics, and short-course systemic corticosteroids are used to treat acute symptoms and exacerbations. Additionally, short-acting beta$_2$ agonists are used to pretreat exercise-induced asthma.[116,118,120]

Patient and family education in asthma care is another integral part of treatment. As the NHLBI guidelines[118] recommend, the healthcare professional must build a partnership with the patient and family. The patient and family need to be involved in problem solving for appropriate solutions for asthma trigger control and medication options. They should be able to recognize asthma symptoms and to treat appropriately and early. The patient and family members should demonstrate the proper use of inhalers and exhibit understanding of the proper use of other medications. Written instructions should be provided.[118,120] Long-term follow-up is essential to adjust medication as needed and for education reinforcement. Tobacco smoke is a common irritant and asthma trigger; therefore, smoking cessation information and counseling should be made available to family members.[116,118]

Food Allergies and Asthma

The rates of food allergies and asthma are rising, and it appears there may be more of a correlation between the two than was once thought. Infants diagnosed with an allergy in early infancy have been shown to have an increased risk of asthma.[121,122] There appears to be an even stronger association between the diagnosis of food allergies and asthma in children who have multiple or more severe food allergies.[123]

The role of food allergies in the exacerbation of asthma symptoms is controversial.[116] In a study by Adler and associates,[124] 14.5% of children with asthma were reported by their parents to have food-provoked asthma symptoms. Several studies have been reported in the scientific literature investigating the true incidence of asthma symptoms caused by food allergies using double-blind, placebo-controlled food challenges.[125–127] The results of these investigations thus far include findings that IgE-mediated reactions to food can cause respiratory symptoms, including wheezing, but that this is uncommon, even in children with histories of other adverse reactions to food. According to Ozol and Mete, only 6–8% of children with asthma have respiratory symptoms triggered by foods.[121] Although rare, it should be noted that patients with asthma are more likely to have a life-threatening reaction if they are exposed to foods they are allergic to because of the potential for respiratory system involvement.[122] It is important that patients receive thorough education on how to safely avoid foods they have been diagnosed as allergic to while still maintaining a balanced diet. (Please refer to Chapter 7 for more information on food hypersensitivities.)

Milk and Mucus

It is a common misconception among lay people that drinking milk causes an increased production of mucus and may be a trigger for asthma. However, there is no scientific evidence to support this claim. This belief may persist because milk, particularly whole milk, coats the tongue and mouth and some people may have the sensation that they have an increase in mucus production or that their mucus is thicker after milk consumption. In an Australian study, believers and nonbelievers of the milk–mucus connection were studied.[128] Clearing their throats was the most common symptom described by both the believers and nonbelievers after drinking milk. Words commonly used to describe the sensation associated with drinking milk were "thick," "blocked," and "clogged."[128] These same researchers administered chocolate cow's milk or chocolate soy milk in a randomized trial.[129] They found that the same type of sensory perceptions of milk were described by believers and nonbelievers of the milk–mucus connection theory for both types of milk. These researchers concluded that these same perceptions extended to milk substitute beverages as well as milk. Further studies found the ingestion of a cow milk solution powder dissolved in a strawberry-flavored beverage to have no effect versus placebo on the pulmonary function in a group of adult mild asthmatics in a double-blind placebo-controlled study.[128,129] Individuals may have bona fide milk allergy, but these numbers are relatively low. Indiscriminate elimination of a whole food group such as dairy products from the diet of a child with asthma may be totally unnecessary and may deprive the child of an important source of nutrients such as calcium.

Role of Breastfeeding in the Prevention of Asthma

The relationship of breastfeeding to asthma prevention has been studied using data from the National Health and Nutrition Examination Survey (NHANES III) with conflicting interpretations. One group of investigators found that breastfed children as compared to never breastfed children "may" have a delay in the onset of asthma or recurrent wheeze or they "may" actually be actively protected against asthma.[130] However, Rust and colleagues[131] found that breastfeeding "did not appear" to have an impact on asthma prevention or a reduction in its severity. According to the NHANES III data, the relationship between breastfeeding and asthma prevention is not strong. Wright and associates[132] found that longer durations of exclusive breastfeeding increased the risk of reported asthma among children with asthmatic mothers.

Relationship Between Asthma and Obesity

Both asthma and obesity have been increasing at alarming rates in the United States. This epidemiological observation prompted studies conducted during the 1980s, which generated the hypothesis of an association between asthma and obesity.[133] This association has been studied in adults and children.

Studies in adults have found that obesity does affect pulmonary function. The prospective Nurses' Health Study II found that BMI was a strong, independent, positive risk factor for the onset of asthma.[134] Other investigators in Finland have shown improvements in lung function, symptoms, morbidity, and health status with weight reduction in obese patients with asthma.[135] Possible explanations for the association between asthma and obesity include the possibilities that gastroesophageal reflux as a result of obesity exacerbates asthma, that physical inactivity may promote both diseases, and that the high-fat diets of obese patients may promote airway inflammation and asthma.[133]

The relationship between asthma and obesity also has been studied in the pediatric population. Many of these studies have been conducted with inner city, minority populations because these populations have the highest prevalence of asthma and are at greatest risk of experiencing the morbidity and mortality of this chronic disease.

Luder and associates[136] compared a group of inner city children with asthma to a group of their peers. The prevalence of overweight was significantly higher in children with moderate to severe asthma than in their peers. In the asthma group, a higher BMI was associated with significantly more severe asthma symptoms, such as lower pulmonary function measurements, more school absenteeism, and a greater number of prescribed asthma medications.[136] These investigators recommend studying the effect of weight reduction in asthma patients with a high BMI on asthma symptoms. Gennuso and colleagues[137] studied urban minority children and adolescents who had asthma and nonasthma controls. These investigators found an increase in obesity among children with asthma for both sexes and across ages as compared to controls. The severity of asthma was not related to obesity. These investigators concluded that asthma is a risk factor for obesity in children. As part of the National Cooperative Inner City Asthma Study, Belamarich and colleagues[138] found that 19% of the asthma patients ages 4 to 9 years had BMIs over the 95th percentile, as compared to 11% of all children in the NHANES III survey. The investigators also found that obese children with asthma required more asthma medication, reported more days of wheezing, and visited the emergency department more than nonobese children with asthma.

The Tucson Children's Respiratory Study found that female subjects who were overweight or obese between 6 and 11 years of age were seven times more likely to develop new asthma symptoms at age 11 and 13 years.[139] These investigators hypothesized that being overweight may influence female sex hormones, which in turn increase asthma risk. Gilliland and associates[140] studied almost 4000 school-age children in the longitudinal Children's Health Study in southern California. These investigators found that overweight was associated with increased risk of new onset asthma in boys and in nonallergic children. Tantisira and colleagues[141] studied children with mild to moderate asthma who were enrolled in the Childhood Asthma Management Program (CAMP). They found that although an increasing BMI was associated with an increase in forced expiratory volume in 1 second (FEV_1) and forced vital capacity (FVC), the ratio of FEV_1 to FVC was reduced. There was a positive association between BMI and cough/wheeze with exercise. This study did not support the hypothesis that an increase in BMI increases asthma severity, but the increase in exercise-induced bronchospasm with increasing BMI suggests a relationship between increased airway responsiveness and BMI.

The conclusions that can be drawn regarding the association of overweight and asthma from these studies in pediatrics include:

- There is a higher prevalence of overweight in children with asthma.
- Overweight children with asthma have increased asthma symptoms.
- Overweight may influence asthma risk.

Effects of Nutrients on Asthma

Because asthma affects the lives of so many adults and children, much research has been done in the area of asthma treatment and the prevention of asthma exacerbations, including the impact of nutrition on asthma patients. Many studies have been performed investigating the role of various nutrients in protecting against asthma, as well as their effects on improving asthma symptoms. Nutrients that have been studied include vitamin C, fish oils, selenium, and electrolytes, including sodium and magnesium.[120]

Vitamin C

Antioxidants protect cell membranes from damage caused by free radicals and chemical oxidants. Of the antioxidant vitamins, vitamin C has received the most attention, with most of the studies involving adult subjects. According to NHANES I, lower dietary vitamin C intakes were associated with lower FEV_1. However, the difference in this pulmonary function test between the highest and lowest levels of dietary vitamin C was not great and the clinical significance of this finding was questioned.[142] Other studies of adult subjects showed that asthma patients had low blood levels of vitamin C and that low vitamin C intake was associated with weaker lung function.[120] In one pediatric study, children ages 8 to 11 years who never ate fresh fruit had 4.3% lower pulmonary function and had a 25.3% higher incidence of wheezing than did children who ate fruit more than once a day.[143] However, vitamin C intake was not specifically analyzed in this study. Other studies have suggested possible short-term protective effects of vitamin C on airway responsiveness.[120] No conclusive evidence links vitamin C levels to asthma or identifies the role that vitamin C may play in the treatment of asthma.[120] This area warrants further investigation before routine supplementation can be recommended for asthma patients. However, encouraging children with asthma to include a daily source of vitamin C in their diets is sound advice.

Fish Oils

The ingestion of fish oils, which contain omega-3 fatty acids, causes arachidonic acid (AA) to be replaced by eicosapentaenoic acid (EPA) and docosahexaenoic acid (DHA) in cell membranes. This replacement leads to a decrease in the production of the inflammatory metabolites of AA, including leukotrienes. It is thought that this change in metabolites could have potential effects on airway inflammation, which is why fish oil ingestion and its relationship to asthma has been studied.[120,144]

As with the antioxidants, most of the studies have been with adult asthma patients.[120] A positive relationship between dietary fish intake and higher pulmonary function was found when the data from NHANES I were examined.[145] Two studies of Australian schoolchildren found an association between oily fish intake (tuna, salmon, herring) and a reduction in prevalence of increased airway responsiveness and in the incidence of asthma.[146,147] This same group of investigators compared the clinical effects of fish oil supplementation and a diet that increases omega-3 polyunsaturated fatty acids with a diet enriched in omega-6 fatty acids in a double-blind, randomized trial of 39 children with asthma. No significant changes in clinical severity of asthma were found.[147] Another group of investigators found decreased asthma symptoms when fish oil capsules were given to 29 children with asthma who participated in a randomized controlled trial in a controlled environment in terms of inhalant allergens and diet.[148] The majority of the studies do not show significant clinical improvement in asthma patients with the use of fish oils, despite some changes seen in inflammatory cell functions.[149] Another question that remains is whether dietary fatty acids play a role in the development of asthma.[149] The data are inconclusive at this point and do not support the use of fish oil in the treatment of asthma.[120] Further investigation is warranted, but recommending the inclusion of fatty fish in the diets of children with asthma is simply consistent with current healthy diet recommendations.

Selenium

The relationship of selenium to asthma has been studied because of selenium's role as an antioxidant. No current data demonstrate a beneficial effect of selenium supplementation on pulmonary function tests in asthma patients. Although some studies have indicated a possible correlation between low serum levels of selenium and asthma symptoms, there is not sufficient evidence to advocate the use of selenium supplementation in the treatment of asthma.[120]

The role that specific nutrients may play in asthma has sparked much interest in the scientific community. More research in this area is needed before specific recommendations can be made. Interest in this area will probably continue to grow, especially as the practice of alternative/complementary medicine receives more attention. The data gathered to date reinforce the importance to asthma patients of a diet containing a variety of food sources.

Electrolytes

The relationship of increased sodium intake and asthma has been investigated by several groups of researchers.[120] These studies have been performed because it was hypothesized that diets high in salt may increase bronchial reactivity. Although the data have shown small adverse effects of increased sodium intake on bronchial reactivity, no significant effects on the clinical symptoms of asthma have been found.[120] Also, the data from many of the studies are confounded by other variables, such as other dietary constituents. Currently, there is little scientific data to support the use of low-salt diets in the treatment of asthma.[120]

Magnesium and its role in asthma has been studied in adult asthma patients. Clinical trials have been conducted on the effect of magnesium infusion during acute asthma exacerbations.[120] Small, transient improvements in pulmonary functions were observed with the magnesium infusions, but these changes were not as great as those seen with $beta_2$ agonist inhalation therapy.[120] One study in England[150] evaluated the relationship between magnesium intake, assessed from food frequency questionnaires, and pulmonary function FEV_1, airway reactivity to methacholine, and self-reported wheezing. A magnesium intake of 100 mg per day or higher was associated with a 27.7 mL higher FEV_1, a reduction in relative odds of airway hyperresponsiveness of 0.82, and a reduction in wheeze symptoms.[150] These studies indicate that although intravenous magnesium supplementation may have a minimal role in the treatment of acute asthma, further study is needed of the role of magnesium supplementation in the treatment of chronic asthma.[120]

Effects of Asthma Treatment on Nutritional Status

Most of the effects of asthma treatment on the nutritional status of patients are related to the use of oral steroids and high-dose inhaled steroids. According to the NHLBI guidelines, medium- to high-dose inhaled corticosteroids may be needed daily for long-term control in patients whose disease is classified as moderate persistent.[118] For patients whose disease is in the severe persistent classification, long-term control may require high-dose inhaled corticosteroids as well as a long-acting bronchodilator plus oral corticosteroids.[118] The primary goal is to treat the asthma with the smallest doses of medicines that will control the symptoms in order to minimize side effects.

Linear Growth

According to the NHLBI guidelines, poorly controlled asthma may delay growth in children.[118] In general, children with asthma tend to have longer periods of reduced growth rates prior to puberty.[118] However, this delay in puberty does not appear to affect final adult height.[151] This delay in puberty also is not associated with the use of inhaled corticosteroids.[152] The potential for adverse effects on linear growth from inhaled corticosteroids appears to be dose-dependent.[118,152–155] High doses of inhaled corticosteroids have greater potential for growth suppression than lower doses.[118] When inhaled corticosteroids are used as recommended, the majority of studies report no change in expected growth velocity.[153,154] In contrast, a few studies have demonstrated a small growth delay in children on inhaled corticosteroids, but the delay in growth velocity is not sustained, is not progressive, and may be reversible.[116,118] A meta-analysis of the effect of inhaled steroids found decreased growth velocity with inhaled steroids, but the effect on final adult height was unknown.[155] A study by Agertoft and Pedersen[156] in Denmark showed that expected adult height was attained for asthma patients on inhaled steroids. This is an area of asthma management that warrants further study, especially in young, preschool-age children.[157] Using high doses of inhaled corticosteroids with children having severe persistent asthma has less potential for decreasing linear growth than does using oral systemic corticosteroids.[118] The use of oral corticosteroids on a prolonged basis does stunt linear growth.[151]

Bone Density

Chronic corticosteroid use does induce osteoporosis.[158] Corticosteroids decrease calcium absorption from the gastrointestinal tract and decrease renal calcium reabsorption, which leads to a decrease in plasma calcium. At the same time, there is an increase in parathyroid hormone secretion and an increase in bone resorption, all of which lead to osteoporosis. That is why it is important that the smallest possible dose be used to control asthma symptoms. Many studies—again mainly in adults—have been performed on the effect of inhaled corticosteroids on bone density, with varying results reported. Short-term effects on markers of bone turnover, such as osteocalcin, have been reported, but the long-term risk of osteoporosis is not clear.[159,160] Collagen turnover was found to be reduced in children receiving long-term (over 12 months) inhaled steroid treatment.[161] Martinati and colleagues[162] found no adverse effect on bone mass in prepubertal children with mild to moderate asthma when treated with beclomethasone dipropionate, as compared to children treated with cromolyn sodium, a nonsteroidal anti-inflammatory drug. Most long-term studies indicate that inhaled corticosteroids have a negligible effect, if any, on bone mineral density.[157] However, more research is needed before there is agreement as to the effect of the dose and duration of inhaled corticosteroids on bone density in patients, especially children with asthma.

Investigators conclude that attention should be given to the maintenance of adequate calcium and vitamin D intake in patients on chronic steroid therapy.[158] Calcium supplementation may be necessary in some patients, especially if dietary intake of calcium is low.[160] Calcium supplementation alone may be insufficient to completely block the progression of corticosteroid-dependent osteoporosis.[163] Other factors that may benefit the patient are weight-bearing exercise and the avoidance of other inhibitors of osteoblast production, such as alcohol excess.[157] In a study of adult asthmatic patients, Gagnon and associates[164] did find a significant positive correlation between bone density and calcium intake in asthmatic patients. This is another compelling reason why indiscriminate elimination of dairy products from the diet of a child with asthma may be harmful.

Excessive Weight Gain

Common, well-known side effects of oral corticosteroid therapy include appetite stimulation, central distribution of fat, sodium and fluid retention, and steroid-induced glucose intolerance. For the asthma patient whose disease is in the persistent severe classification and who may require chronic oral steroid therapy to control asthma symptoms, anticipatory dietary guidance as to how to combat some of these side effects, such as limiting salt intake or limiting concentrated sweets, will be beneficial.

Nutritional Management

The growth of children with asthma should be monitored on a regular basis (see also Chapter 3). Any deviation in growth parameters should be investigated. BMI should be calculated and the BMI-for-age growth charts used to monitor overweight asthma patients and those at risk for overweight.[32] Nutrition counseling and lifestyle changes need to be emphasized by the healthcare practitioner at the first sign that an asthma patient may be at risk for overweight.

Based on the available data, a diet that provides a variety of foods, including fruits, vegetables, and dairy products, should be encouraged. Educational tools such as the USDA MyPyramid[165] or the USDA/HHS Dietary Guidelines for Americans[166] can be utilized. Patients and family members should be warned against eliminating whole food groups from the diet indiscriminately. Preadolescent and adolescent patients should receive information about healthy weight control practices, including regular exercise. Chronically ill adolescents, including asthma patients, were found to have increased body dissatisfaction and to be at increased risk of engaging in unhealthy weight-loss practices.[167]

Some patients with asthma who have a true food allergy will require an allergen elimination diet. (See Chapter 7, Food Hypersensitivities, for further details.)

Combating Steroid Side Effects

For those asthma patients who must take oral corticosteroids on a regular basis, additional factors should be closely monitored. An adequate calcium intake is essential. These patients should be receiving at least the DRIs[60] for calcium and in some instances may require calcium supplementation. Adequate vitamin D intake is also important.[158] The patient may need to modify kilocalorie intake to maintain weight control. The registered dietitian can assist the patient in identifying ways to accomplish a healthy diet, especially if the patient develops steroid-induced hyperglycemia. Moderate exercise should be encouraged because this will help maintain bone density and will assist with weight control.

Alternative/Complementary Medicine

Many asthma patients and their families have turned to alternative/complementary medicine therapies. Relaxation techniques, such as biofeedback training and yoga, are commonly practiced. Acupuncture has also been tried and although there is a very low risk associated with acupuncture in pediatrics, controlled studies of acupuncture for asthma in children are limited.[168] It is important to ask about the use of specific herbal products when obtaining a diet history. Several recent studies reported that traditional Chinese medicine (TCM) herbal formulas are safe and had a positive effect on symptoms and/or lung function in children when used as monotherapy or complementary therapy.[168] Investigation of TCM herbal therapy for children with asthma is an active area of research and may have potential as a complementary and alternative medicine therapy for asthma.[168]

Identification of Areas for Further Research

The areas needing further research have been indicated throughout this section. Additional scientific study of the role of specific nutrients in asthma must be done before precise recommendations for supplementation can be made. The effects of chronic steroid therapy and chronic inhaled steroid therapy on growth in children, especially in infants and young children, and on bone density require continued study. The relationship between being overweight and asthma requires further investigation. It is exciting to realize that nutrition may play a major role in the treatment of this significant public health problem.

Case Study

Nutrition Assessment

Client history: GB is an 11.5-year-old male with cystic fibrosis, mild lung disease, and PI. He presents to the outpatient nutrition clinic for annual nutrition evaluation.

Food/nutrition-related history: Patient reports that he generally has a good appetite. He always eats three meals per day and two to three snacks. Dietary intake from yesterday reported as:

- *Breakfast:* 1 slice of toast with peanut butter, 8 oz whole milk with chocolate syrup, ½ banana
- *Snack:* 1 cup pretzels, water
- *Lunch:* ½ hamburger, 1 cup French fries, ½ cup peaches, 8 oz apple juice
- *Dinner:* 1 cup spaghetti with beef marinara sauce, ½ cup cooked carrots, 8 oz whole milk
- *Snack:* apple with peanut butter

Patient and mom both agree that above intake is consistent with a typical day of eating for GB. Caloric intake is estimated approximately 1900 kcal/day. He appears to be eating a variety of foods and choosing some higher fat options for additional calories.

GB is currently swimming three to four times a week outdoors on his local swim team. He also plays basketball and baseball with his friends for fun. Mom reports that he is usually pretty active and likes to be outside with his friends.

Current nutrition-related medications include 1 AquADEK gel tab daily, ZENPEP 20 (3 with meals, 1 with snacks), and Prevacid. GB reports compliance with these meds as they are ordered every day. Mom confirms his compliance and states, "He always takes his enzymes before eating. I don't even have to remind him." He has been taking all of these medications at their current dosage for at least a year.

Nutrition-related physical findings: He complains of increased gassiness and abdominal pain after some of his meals over the past 3–4 months. He is stooling 2–3×/day. He reports that his stools float about half of the time and recently he's noticed that there is an oil ring in the toilet. He denies weight loss.

Biochemical data, medical tests, and procedures: Chem 10 WNL, CRP WNL, vitamin A slightly low, vitamin E slightly low, vitamin D (WNL), PT WNL

Anthropometric Measurements

35 kg, 144 cm

Comparative Standards

REE: (Schofield) 1289 kcal/day (37 kcal/kg) × 1.5–1.7 = 1950–2190 kcal/day
Estimated protein needs: (RDA) 1 g protein/kg/day

Nutrition Diagnosis

Nutrition Intervention

Nutrition prescription: High-calorie, high-protein diet, compliance with enzymes, and CF-specific vitamin

Monitoring and Evaluation

1. Growth pattern indices/percentile rankings
2. Biochemical data (vitamins A and E)
3. Total energy intake
4. Intestinal (signs and symptoms of malabsorption)

Questions for the Reader

1. How many units of lipase/kg/meal is GB's current enzyme regimen providing? What is the maximum recommended unit of lipase/kg/meal?
2. His serum vitamin A and E are slightly low. Is he on the recommended dose of his CF-specific MVI (AquADEK gel tab) for his age?
3. Calculate GB's BMI and plot on the correct NCHS growth chart to determine his BMI percentile for age. What is the CF Foundation's goal BMI percentile for his age? Is he currently meeting this goal?
4. Using this data and taking into account the information presented above, please develop at least one appropriate Nutrition Diagnosis.
5. Using NCP terminology, identify an appropriate nutrition intervention based on the etiology of your PES statement(s). Define an ideal goal of your intervention based on the signs and symptoms mentioned in your PES statement.

REFERENCES

1. Welsh MJ, Tsui L, Boat TF, Beaudet AL. Cystic fibrosis. In: Scriver CR, ed. *The Metabolic Basis of Inherited Disease*. New York: McGraw-Hill; 1989:3799–3876.
2. Borowitz D, Durie PR, Clarke LL, et al. Gastrointestinal outcomes and confounders in cystic fibrosis. *J Pediatr Gastroenterol Nutr*. 2005;41:273–285.
3. Cystic Fibrosis Foundation. *Cystic Fibrosis Foundation Patient Registry 2008 Annual Data Report*. Bethesda, MD: Cystic Fibrosis Foundation; September 2009.
4. Andersen DH. Cystic fibrosis of the pancreas and its relation to celiac disease: a clinical and pathologic study. *Am J Dis Child*. 1938;56:344–399.
5. Riordan JR, Rommens JM, Kerem B, et al. Identification of the cystic fibrosis gene: cloning and characterization of complementary DNA. *Science*. 1989;245:1066–1073.
6. Anderson MP, Gregory RJ, Thompson S, et al. Demonstration that CFTR is a chloride channel by alteration of its anion selectivity. *Science*. 1991;253:202–205.
7. Bear CE, Li CH, Kartner N, et al. Purification and functional reconstitution of the cystic fibrosis transmembrane conductance regulator (CFTR). *Cell*. 1992;68:809–818.
8. Cheng SH, Rich DP, Marshall J, et al. Phosphorylation of the R domain by cAMP-dependent protein kinase regulates the CFTR chloride channel. *Cell*. 1991;66:1027–1036.
9. Schwiebert EM, Egan ME, Hwang TH, et al. CFTR regulates outwardly rectifying chloride channels through an autocrine mechanism involving ATP. *Cell*. 1995;81:1063–1073.
10. Stutts MJ, Canessa CM, Olsen JC, et al. CFTR as a cAMP-dependent regulator of sodium channels. *Science*. 1995;269:847–850.
11. Welsh MJ, Smith AE. Molecular mechanisms of CFTR chloride channel dysfunction in cystic fibrosis. *Cell*. 1993;73:1251–1254.
12. Cystic Fibrosis Genetic Analysis Consortium. Population variation of common cystic fibrosis mutations. *Hum Mutat*. 1994;4:167–177.
13. Farrell PM, Rosenstein BJ, White TB, et al. Guidelines for diagnosis of cystic fibrosis in newborns through older adults: Cystic Fibrosis Foundation consensus report. *J Pediatr*. 2008;153(2):4–14.
14. Tomezsko JL, Stallings VA, Kawchak DA, et al. Energy expenditure and genotype of children with cystic fibrosis. *Pediatr Res*. 1994;35:451–460.
15. O'Rawe A, McIntosh I, Dodge JA, et al. Increased energy expenditure in cystic fibrosis is associated with specific mutations. *Clin Sci*. 1992;82:71–76.
16. Murphy M, Ireton-Jones CS, Hilman BC, et al. Resting energy expenditures measured by indirect calorimetry are higher in preadolescent children with cystic fibrosis than expenditures calculated from prediction equations. *J Am Diet Assoc*. 1995;95:30–33.
17. Shepherd RW, Vasques-Velasquez L, Prentice A, et al. Increased energy expenditure in young children with cystic fibrosis. *Lancet*. 1988;135:1300–1303.
18. Vaisman N, Pencharz PB, Corey M, et al. Energy expenditure of patients with cystic fibrosis. *J Pediatr*. 1987;111:137–141.
19. Stallings VA. New nutrition guidelines. Presented at North American Cystic Fibrosis Conference, Baltimore, MD; October 22, 2005.
20. Food and Nutrition Board. *Recommended Dietary Allowances*, 10th ed. Washington, DC: National Academies Press; 1989.
21. Eubanks V, Koppersmith N, Wooldridge N, et al. Effects of megestrol acetate on weight gain, body composition, and pulmonary function in patients with cystic fibrosis. *J Pediatr*. 2002;140:393–395.
22. Sproul A, Huang N. Growth patterns in children with cystic fibrosis. *J Pediatr*. 1964;65:664–676.
23. Konstan MW, Butler SM, Wohl MEB, et al. Growth and nutritional indexes in early life predict pulmonary function in cystic fibrosis. *J Pediatr*. 2003;142:624–630.
24. Peterson ML, Jacobs DR, Milla CE. Longitudinal changes in growth parameters are correlated with changes in pulmonary function in children with cystic fibrosis. *Pediatrics*. 2003;112:588–592.
25. Steinkamp G, Wiedemann B, on behalf of the German CFQA Group. Relationship between nutritional status and lung function in cystic fibrosis: cross sectional and longitudinal analyses from the German CF quality assurance (CFQA) project. *Thorax*. 2002;57:596–601.
26. Beker LT, Russek-Cohen E, Fink RJ. Stature as a prognostic factor in cystic fibrosis survival. *J Am Diet Assoc*. 2001;101:438–442.
27. Cystic Fibrosis Foundation. *Pediatric Nutrition for Patients with Cystic Fibrosis. Consensus Conferences: Concepts in CF Care*. Bethesda, MD: Cystic Fibrosis Foundation; 2001:1–39.
28. Borowitz D, Baker RD, Stallings V. Consensus report on nutrition for pediatric patients with cystic fibrosis. *J Pediatr Gastroenterol Nutr*. 2002;35:246–259.
29. Cystic Fibrosis Foundation. *Clinical Practice Guidelines for Cystic Fibrosis*. Bethesda, MD: Cystic Fibrosis Foundation; 1997.
30. Fomon SJ. *Nutrition of Normal Infants*. Philadelphia, PA: Mosby; 1993.
31. Stallings VA, Stark LJ, Robinson KA, et al. Evidence-based practice recommendations for nutrition-related management of children and adults with cystic fibrosis and pancreatic insufficiency: results of a systematic review. *J Am Diet Assoc*. 2008;108:832–839.
32. Centers for Disease Control and Prevention, National Center for Health Statistics. CDC growth charts: United States. Available at: http://www.cdc.gov/growthcharts/clinical_charts.htm Accessed August 16, 2010.
33. Frisancho AR. New norms of upper limb fat and muscle areas for assessment of nutritional status. *Am J Clin Nutr*. 1981;34:2540–2545.
34. Heimburger DC, Weinsier RL. *Handbook of Clinical Nutrition*, 3rd ed. St. Louis, MO: Mosby; 1997.
35. Michel SH, Maqbool A, Hanna MD, et al. Nutrition management of pediatric patients who have cystic fibrosis. *Pediatr Clin N Am*. 2009;56:1123–1141.
36. Hendricks K, Duggan C. *Manual of Pediatric Nutrition*, 4th ed. Hamilton, Ontario: BC Decker; 2005.
37. Hardin DS. The diagnosis and management of cystic fibrosis related diabetes. *The Endocrinologist*. 1998;8:265–272.
38. Brunzell C, Hardin D, Schissel K, Schindler T, Moran A. Managing cystic fibrosis related diabetes (CFRD). In: *An Instruction Guide for Patients and Families*, 4th ed. Bethesda, MD: Cystic Fibrosis Foundation; 2008.

39. Aris RM, Merkel PA, Bachrach LK, et al. Consensus statement: guide to bone health and disease in cystic fibrosis. *J Clin Endocrinol Metab.* 2005;90:1888–1896.
40. Elkin SL, Fairney A, et al. Vertebral deformities and low bone mineral density in adults with cystic fibrosis: a cross sectional study. *Osteoporos Int.* 2001:12;366–372.
41. Aris R, Renner JB, Winders AD, Buell HE, et al. Increased rate of fractures and severe kyphosis: sequelae of living to adulthood with cystic fibrosis. *Ann Intern Med. 1998*;128:186–193.
42. Henderson R, Madsen C. Bone mineral content and body composition in children and young adults with cystic fibrosis. *Pediatr Pulmonol.* 1999;27:80–84.
43. Haworth C, Selby PL, Webb AK, Dodd ME, Musson H, et al. Low bone mineral density in adults with cystic fibrosis. *Thorax.* 1999;54:961–967.
44. Shane E, Silverberg S, Silverberg SJ, Donovan D, Papadopoulos A, et al. Osteoporosis in lung transplantation candidates with end stage pulmonary disease. *Am J Med.* 1996;101:262–269.
45. American Dietetic Association, Pediatric Nutrition Practice Group. *Pediatric Manual of Clinical Dietetics,* 2nd ed. Washington, DC; 2008.
46. Crist W, McDonnell P, Beck M, et al. Behavior at mealtimes in the young child with cystic fibrosis. *J Devel Behav Pediatr.* 1994;15:157–161.
47. Kawchak D, Zhoa H, Scanlin TF, Tomezsko JL, et al. Longitudinal, prospective analysis of dietary intake in children with cystic fibrosis. *J Pediatr.* 1996;129:119–129.
48. White H, Morton A, Peckham DG, Conway SP, et al. Dietary intakes in adult patients with cystic fibrosis—do they achieve guidelines? *J Cystic Fibrosis.* 2003;3:1–7.
49. Ellis L, Kalnins D, Corey M, et al. Do infants with cystic fibrosis need a protein hydrolysate formula? A prospective, randomized, comparative study. *J Pediatr.* 1998;132:270–276.
50. Jelalian E, Stark LJ, Reynolds L, Seifer R. Nutrition intervention for weight gain in cystic fibrosis: a meta analysis. *J Pediatr.* 1998;132:486–492.
51. Winick M. *Nutrition and Pregnancy and Early Infancy.* Baltimore, MD: Williams and Wilkins; 1989.
52. Michel SH, Mueller DH. Impact of lactation on women with cystic fibrosis and their infants: a review of five cases. *J Am Diet Assoc.* 1994; 94:159–165.
53. Cystic Fibrosis Foundation. *Consensus Document: Diagnosis, Screening, and Management of Cystic Fibrosis Related Diabetes Mellitus. Consensus Conferences: Concepts in CF Care.* Bethesda, MD: Cystic Fibrosis Foundation; 1999;1–26.
54. Luder E, Gilbride JA. Teaching self-management skills to cystic fibrosis patients and its effect on their caloric intake. *J Am Diet Assoc.* 1989;89:359–364.
55. Stark LJ, Jelalian E, Mulvihill MM, et al. Eating in preschool children with cystic fibrosis and healthy peers: behavioral analysis. *Pediatrics.* 1995;95:210–215.
56. Stark LJ, Mulvihill MM, Jelalian E, et al. Descriptive analysis of eating behavior in school-age children with cystic fibrosis and healthy control children. *Pediatrics.* 1997;99:665–671.
57. Borowitz D, Robinson KA, Rosenfield M, et al. Cystic Fibrosis Foundation evidence-based guidelines for management of infants with cystic fibrosis. *J Pediatr.* 2009;155:S73–S93.
58. Green D, Carson K, Leonard A, et al. Current treatment recommendations for correcting vitamin D deficiency in pediatric patients with cystic fibrosis are inadequate. *J Pediatr.* 2008;153:554–559.
59. Boas SR, Hageman JR, Ho LT, et al. Very high-dose ergocalciferol is effective for correcting vitamin D deficiency in children and young adults with cystic fibrosis. *J Cystic Fibrosis.* 2009;8:270–272.
60. Institute of Medicine, Food and Nutrition Board. *Dietary Reference Intakes for Calcium, Phosphorus, Magnesium, Vitamin D, and Fluoride.* Washington, DC: National Academies Press; 1997.
61. Cystic Fibrosis Foundation. *Use of Pancreatic Enzyme Supplements for Patients with Cystic Fibrosis in the Context of Fibrosing Colonopathy. Consensus Conferences: Concepts in Care.* Bethesda, MD: Cystic Fibrosis Foundation; 1995:1–11.
62. Borowitz DS, Grand RJ, Durie PR, Consensus Committee. Use of pancreatic enzyme supplements for patients with cystic fibrosis in the context of fibrosing colonopathy. *J Pediatr.* 1995;127:681–684.
63. FitzSimmons SC, Burkhart GA, Borowitz D, et al. High-dose pancreatic enzyme supplements and fibrosing colonopathy in children with cystic fibrosis. *N Eng J Med.* 1997;336:1283–1289.
64. Schwarzenberg SJ, Wielinski CL, Shamieh I, et al. Cystic fibrosis-associated colitis and fibrosing colonopathy. *J Pediatr.* 1995;127:565–570.
65. Stern RC, Canda ER, Doershuk CF. Use of nonmedical treatment by cystic fibrosis patients. *J Adol Health.* 1992;3:612–615.
66. Northway WH, Rosan RCC, Porter DY. Pulmonary disease following respiratory therapy of hyaline membrane disease. *N Engl J Med.* 1967;276:357–368.
67. Jobe AH, Bancalari E. Bronchopulmonary dysplasia. *Am J Respir Crit Care Med.* 2001;163:1723–1729.
68. Abman SH, Groothius JR. Pathophysiology and treatment of bronchopulmonary dysplasia. Current issues. *Pediatr Clinics.* 1994;41:277–315.
69. Cox JH. Bronchopulmonary dysplasia. In: Groh-Wargo S, Thompson M, Cox J, eds. *Nutritional Care for High-Risk Newborns,* 3rd ed. Chicago: Precept Press; 2000:369–390.
70. Tammela OKT, Lanning FP, Koivisto ME. The relationship of fluid restriction during the 1st month of life to the occurrence and severity of bronchopulmonary dysplasia in low birth weight infants: a 1-year radiological follow up. *Eur J Pediatr.* 1992;151:367–371.
71. Wilson DC, McClure G, Halliday HL, et al. Nutrition and bronchopulmonary dysplasia. *Arch Dis Child.* 1991;66:37–38.
72. Frank L, Sosenko IR. Undernutrition as a major contributing factor in the pathogenesis of bronchopulmonary dysplasia. *Am Rev Respir Dis.* 1988;138:725–729.
73. Northway WH. Bronchopulmonary dysplasia: thirty-three years later. *Pediatr Pulmonol.* 2001; Suppl 23:5–7.
74. Giacoia GP, Venkataraman PS, West-Wilson KI, Faulkner MJ. Follow-up of school-age children with bronchopulmonary dysplasia. *J Pediatr.* 1997;130:400–408.
75. Weinstein MR, Oh W. Oxygen consumption in infants with bronchopulmonary dysplasia. *J Pediatr.* 1981;99:958–960.
76. Kurzner WI, Garg M, Bautista DB, et al. Growth failure in infants with bronchopulmonary dysplasia: nutrition and elevated resting metabolic expenditure. *Pediatrics.* 1988;81:379–384.
77. Yunis KA, Oh W. Effects of intravenous glucose loading on oxygen consumption, carbon dioxide production, and resting energy

expenditure in infants with bronchopulmonary dysplasia. *J Pediatr*. 1989;115:127–132.

78. Yeh TF, McClenan DA, Ajayi OA, Pildes RS. Metabolic rate and energy balance in infants with bronchopulmonary dysplasia. *J Pediatr*. 1989;114:448–451.
79. deGamarra E. Energy expenditure in premature newborns with bronchopulmonary dysplasia. *Biol Neonate*. 1992;61:337–344.
80. Farrell PA, Fiascone JM. Bronchopulmonary dysplasia in the 1990s: a review for the pediatrician. *Curr Probl Pediatr*. 1997;27:129–163.
81. Singer L, Martin RJ, Hawkins SW, et al. Oxygen desaturation complicates feeding in infants with bronchopulmonary dysplasia after discharge. *Pediatrics*. 1992;90:380–384.
82. Garg M, Kurzner SI, Bautista DB, Keens TG. Clinically unsuspected hypoxia during sleep and feeding in infants with bronchopulmonary dysplasia. *Pediatrics*. 1988;81:635–642.
83. Biniwale MA, Ehrenkranz RA. The role of nutrition in the prevention and management of bronchopulmonary dysplasia. *Semin Perinatol*. 2006;30:200–208.
84. Shankaran S, Szego E, Eizert D, Siegel P. Severe bronchopulmonary dysplasia: predictors of survival and outcome. *Chest*. 1984;86:607.
85. DeRegnier RA, Guilbert TW, Mills MM, Georgieff MK. Growth failure and altered body composition are established by one month of age in infants with bronchopulmonary dysplasia. *J Nutr*. 1996;126:168–175.
86. Johnson DB, Cheney C, Monsen ER. Nutrition and feeding in infants with bronchopulmonary dysplasia after initial hospital discharge: risk factors for growth failure. *J Am Diet Assoc*. 1998;98:649–656.
87. Huysman WA, deRidder M, deBruin NC, et al. Growth and body composition in preterm infants with bronchopulmonary dysplasia. *Arch Dis Child Fetal Neonatal Ed*. 2003;88:F46–F51.
88. Vrlenich LA, Bozynski ME, Shyr Y, et al. The effect of bronchopulmonary dysplasia on growth at school age. *Pediatrics*. 1995;95:855–859.
89. Moyer-Mileur LJ, Nielson DW, Pfeffer KD, et al. Eliminating sleep-associated hypoxemia improves growth in infants with bronchopulmonary dysplasia. *Pediatrics*. 1996;98:779–783.
90. Groothuis JF, Rosenberg AA. Home oxygen promotes weight gain in infants with bronchopulmonary dysplasia. *Am J Dis Child*. 1987;141:992–995.
91. Babson SG, Benda GI. Growth graphs for the clinical assessment of infants of varying gestational age. *J Pediatr*. 1976;89:814–820.
92. Oh W. Nutritional management of infants with bronchopulmonary dysplasia. In: Farrell PM, Taussig LM, eds. *Bronchopulmonary Dysplasia and Related Chronic Respiratory Disorders*. Columbus, OH: Ross Laboratories; 1986;96–101.
93. Niermeyer S. Nutritional and metabolic problems in infants with bronchopulmonary dysplasia. In: Bancalari E, Stocker JT, eds. *Bronchopulmonary Dysplasia*. Washington, DC: Hemisphere Publishing; 1988;313–336.
94. Zachman RD. Role of vitamin A in lung development. *J Nutr*. 1995;125:1634S–1638S.
95. Robbins ST, Fletcher AB. Early vs. delayed vitamin A supplementation in very-low-birth-weight infants. *J Parenter Enteral Nutr*. 1993;17:220–225.
96. Kennedy KA, Stoll BJ, Ehrenkranz RA, et al. Vitamin A to prevent bronchopulmonary dysplasia in very-low-birth-weight infants: has the dose been too low? *Early Human Dev*. 1997;49:19–31.
97. Tyson JE, Wright LL, Oh W, et al. Vitamin A supplementation for extremely-low-birth-weight infants. *New Eng J Med*. 1999;340:1962–1968.
98. Shenai JP. Vitamin A supplementation in very low birth weight neonates: rationale and evidence. *Pediatrics*. 1999;104:1369–1374.
99. Atkinson SA. Special nutritional needs of infants for prevention of and recovery from bronchopulmonary dysplasia. *J Nutr*. 2001;131:942S–946S.
100. Higashi A, Ikeda T, Iribe K, Matsuda I. Zinc balance in premature infants given the minimal dietary zinc requirement. *J Pediatr*. 1988;112:262–266.
101. American Academy of Pediatrics, Committee on Nutrition. Kleinman RE, ed., *Pediatric Nutrition Handbook*, 5th ed. Elk Grove Village, IL: American Academy of Pediatrics; 2004.
102. Green HL, Hazlett D, Demarec R. Relationship between intralipid-induced hyperlipemia and pulmonary function. *Am J Clin Nutr*. 1976;29:127–135.
103. Friedman Z, Marks KH, Maisels J, et al. Effect of parenteral fat emulsion on the pulmonary and reticuloendothelial systems in the newborn infant. *Pediatrics*. 1978;61:694.
104. Perira GR, Foxx WW, Stanely CA, et al. Decreased oxygenation and hyperlipemia during intravenous fat infusions in premature infants. *Pediatrics*. 1980;66:26–30.
105. Stahl GE, Spear MC, Egler JM, et al. The effect of lipid infusion rate on oxygenation in premature infants. *Pediatr Res*. 1984;18:406A.
106. Reimers KJ, Carlson SJ, Lombard KA. Nutritional management of infants with bronchopulmonary dysplasia. *Nutr Clin Prac*. 1992;7:127–132.
107. Boehm G, Bierbach U, Moro G, Minoli I. Limited fat digestion in infants with bronchopulmonary dysplasia. *J Pediatr Gastroenterol Nutr*. 1996;22:161–166.
108. Johnson D. Gaining and growing: assuring nutritional care of preterm infants. University of Washington. Available at: http://depts.washington.edu/growing. Accessed August 16, 2010.
109. Brunton JA, Saigal S, Atkinson SA. Growth and body composition in infants with bronchopulmonary dysplasia up to 3 months corrected age: a randomized trial of a high-energy nutrient-enriched formula fed after hospital discharge. *J Pediatr*. 1998;133:340–345.
110. Gewolb IH, Bosma JF, Taciak VL, Vice FL. Abnormal developmental patterns of suck and swallow rhythms during feeding in preterm infants with bronchopulmonary dysplasia. *Dev Med Child Neur*. 2001;43:454–459.
111. Singer LT, Davillier M, Preuss L, et al. Feeding interactions in infants with very low birth weight and bronchopulmonary dysplasia. *J Dev Behav Pediatr*. 1996;17:69–76.
112. Centers for Disease Control and Prevention, National Center for Health Statistics. Summary health statistics for U.S. children: National Health Interview Survey, 2008. Available at: http://www.cdc.gov/nchs/data/series/sr_10/sr10_244.pdf. Accessed January 14, 2010.
113. Centers for Disease Control and Prevention, National Center for Health Statistics. The state of childhood asthma, United States,

1980–2005. Available at: http://www.cdc.gov/nchs/data/ad/ad381.pdf. Accessed January 27, 2010.

114. Centers for Disease Control and Prevention. Asthma prevalence and control characteristics by race/ethnicity—United States, 2002. *MMWR.* 2004;53:145–148.

115. Rodriguez MA, Winkleby MA, Ahn D, et al. Identification of population subgroups of children and adolescents with high asthma prevalence. *Arch Pediatr Adolesc Med.* 2002;156:269–275.

116. Johnston J. Lower respiratory disorders. In: Millonig VL, Mobley C. eds. *Pediatric Nurse Practitioner Certification Review Guide*, 4th ed. Potomac, MD: Health Leadership Associates, Inc. 2004;135–151.

117. U.S. Department of Health and Human Services. *Healthy People 2010*, Conference ed. Washington, DC: USDHHS; January 2000.

118. National Heart, Lung and Blood Institute. Expert panel report 3: guidelines for the diagnosis and management of asthma. August 2007. Available at: http://www.nhlbi.nih.gov/guidelines/asthma/asthgdln.htm. Accessed January 27, 2010.

119. Sampson HA. IgE-mediated food intolerance. *J Allergy Clin Immunol.* 1988;81:495–504.

120. National Asthma Education and Prevention Program, National Heart, Lung and Blood Institute. *Expert Panel Report: Guidelines for the Diagnosis and Management of Asthma—Update of Selected Topics 2002.* Bethesda, MD: National Institutes of Health; 2002. Pub no. 02-5075.

121. Ozol D, Mete E. Asthma and food allergy. *Curr Opin Pulm Med.* 2008;14(1):9–12.

122. Beausoleil J, Fiedler J, Spergel J. Food intolerance and childhood asthma: what is the link? *Paediatr Drugs.* 2007;9(3):157–163.

123. Schroeder A, Kumar R. Food allergy is associated with an increased risk of asthma. *Clin Exp Allergy.* 2009;39(2):261–270.

124. Adler BR, Assadullahi T, Warner JA, Warner JO. Evaluation of a multiple food specific IgE antibody test compared to parental perception, allergy skin tests and RAST. *Clin Exp Allergy.* 1991;21:683–688.

125. Bock SA. Respiratory reactions induced by food challenges in children with pulmonary disease. *Pediatr Allergy Immunol.* 1992;3:188–194.

126. James JM, Berhisel-Broadbent J, Sampson HA. Respiratory reactions provoked by double-blind food challenges in children. *Am J Respir Crit Care Med.* 1994;149:59–64.

127. Onorato J, Merland N, Terral C, et al. Placebo-controlled double-blind food challenge in asthma. *J Allergy Clin Immunol.* 1986;78:1139–1146.

128. Pinnock CB, Arney WK. The milk-mucus belief: sensory analysis comparing cow's milk and a soy placebo. *Appetite.* 1993;20:61–70.

129. Nguyen MT. Effect of cow milk on pulmonary function in atopic asthmatic patients. *Ann Allergy Asthma Immunol.* 1997;79:62–64.

130. Chulada PC, Arbes SJ, Dunson D, Zeldin DC. Breast-feeding and the prevalence of asthma and wheeze in children: analyses from the Third National Health and Nutrition Examination Survey. *J Allergy Clin Immunol.* 2003;112:328–336.

131. Rust GS, Thompson CJ, Minor P, et al. Does breastfeeding protect children from asthma? Analysis of NHANES III survey data. *J Nat Med Assoc.* 2001;93:139–148.

132. Wright AL, Holberg CJ, Taussig LM, Martinez F. Maternal asthma status alters relation of infant feeding to asthma in childhood. *Advances Exp Med Biol.* 2000;478:131–137.

133. Chinn S. Obesity and asthma: evidence for and against a causal relation. *J Asthma.* 2003;40:1–16.

134. Camargo CA, Weiss ST, Zhang S, Willett WC, Speizer FE. Prospective study of body mass index, weight change, and risk of adult-onset asthma in women. *Arch Intern Med.* 1999;159:2582–2588.

135. Stenius-Aarniala B, Poussa T, Kvarnstrom J, et al. Immediate and long term effects of weight reduction in obese people with asthma: randomized controlled study. *BMJ.* 2000;320:827–832.

136. Luder E, Melnik TA, DiMaio M. Association of being overweight with greater asthma symptoms in inner city black and Hispanic children. *J Pediatr.* 1998;132:699–703.

137. Gennuso J, Epstein LH, Paluch RA, Cerny F. The relationship between asthma and obesity in urban minority children and adolescents. *Arch Pediatr Adolesc Med.* 1998;152:1197–1200.

138. Belamarich PF, Luder E, Kattan M, et al. Do obese inner-city children with asthma have more symptoms than nonobese children with asthma? *Pediatrics.* 2000;106:1436–1441.

139. Castro-Rodriguez JA, Holbert CJ, Morgan WJ, Wright AL, Martinez FD. Increased incidence of asthmalike symptoms in girls who become overweight or obese during the school years. *Am J Respir Crit Care Med.* 2001;163:1344–1349.

140. Gilliland FD, Berhane K, Islam T, et al. Obesity and the risk of newly diagnosed asthma in school-age children. *Am J Epi.* 2003;158:406–415.

141. Tantisira KG, Litonjua AA, Weiss ST, Fuhlbrigge AL, for the Childhood Asthma Management Program Research Group. Association of body mass with pulmonary function in the Childhood Asthma Management Program (CAMP). *Thorax.* 2003;58:1036–1041.

142. Schwartz J, Weiss ST. Relationship between dietary vitamin C intake and pulmonary function in the first National Health and Nutrition Examination Survey (NHANES I). *Amer J Clin Nutr.* 1994;59:110–114.

143. Cook DG, Carey IM, Whincup PH, et al. Effect of fresh fruit consumption on lung function and wheeze in children. *Thorax.* 1997;52:628–633.

144. Spector SL, Surette ME. Diet and asthma: has the role of dietary lipids been overlooked in the management of asthma? *Ann Allergy Asthma Immunol.* 2003;90:371–377.

145. Schwartz J, Weiss ST. The relationship of dietary fish intake to level of pulmonary function in the first National Health and Nutrition Examination Survey (NHANES I). *Eur Respir J.* 1994;7:1821–1824.

146. Peat JK, Salome CM, Woolcock AJ. Factors associated with bronchial hyperresponsiveness in Australian adults and children. *Eur Respir J.* 1992;5:921–929.

147. Hodge L, Salome CM, Hughes JM, et al. Effect of dietary intake of omega-3 and omega-6 fatty acids on severity of asthma in children. *Eur Respir J.* 1998;11:361–365.

148. Nagakura T, Matsuda S, Shichijyo K, et al. Dietary supplementation with fish oil rich in omega-3 polyunsaturated fatty acids in children with bronchial asthma. *Eur Respir J.* 2000;16:861–865.

149. Morris A, Noakes M, Clifton PM. The role of ω-6 polyunsaturated fat in stable asthmatics. *J Asthma.* 2001;38:311–319.

150. Britton J, Pavord I, Wisniewski A, et al. Dietary magnesium, lung function, wheezing, and airway hyperreactivity in a random adult population. *Lancet.* 1994;344:357–363.
151. Price JF. Asthma, growth and inhaled corticosteroids. *Resp Med.* 1993;87:23–26.
152. Merkus PJFM, van Essen-Zandvliet EEM, Duiverman EJ, et al. Long-term effect of inhaled corticosteroids on growth rate in adolescents with asthma. *Pediatrics.* 1993;91:1121–1126.
153. Agertoft L, Pedersen S. Effects of long-term treatment with an inhaled corticosteroid on growth and pulmonary function in asthmatic children. *Resp Med.* 1994;88:373–381.
154. Allen DB, Bronshky EA, LaForce CF, et al. Growth in asthmatic children treated with fluticasone propionate. *J Pediatr.* 1998;132:472–477.
155. Sharek PJ, Bergman DA. The effect of inhaled steroids on the linear growth of children with asthma: a meta-analysis. *Pediatr.* 2000;106. Available at: http://www.pediatrics.org/cgi/content/full/106/1/e8. Accessed February 1, 2002.
156. Agertoft L, Pedersen S. Effect of long-term treatment with inhaled budesonide on adult height in children with asthma. *N Eng J Med.* 2000;343:1064–1069.
157. Allen DB. Inhaled corticosteroid therapy for asthma in preschool children: growth issues. *Pediatrics.* 2002;109:373–380.
158. Hosking DJ. Effects of corticosteroids on bone turnover. *Resp Med.* 1993;87:15–21.
159. Barnes NC. Safety of high-dose inhaled corticosteroids. *Resp Med.* 1993;87:27–31.
160. Boner AL, Piacentini GL. Inhaled corticosteroids in children. Is there a "safe" dosage? *Drug Safety.* 1993;9:9–20.
161. Crowley S, Trivedi P, Risteli L, et al. Collagen metabolism and growth in prepubertal children with asthma treated with inhaled steroids. *J Pediatr.* 1998;132:409–413.
162. Martinati LC, Bertoldo F, Gasperi E, et al. Effect on cortical and trabecular bone mass of different anti-inflammatory treatments in preadolescent children with chronic asthma. *Am J Respir Crit Care Med.* 1996;153:232–236.
163. Picado C, Luengo M. Corticosteroid-induced bone loss. *Drug Safety.* 1996;15:347–359.
164. Gagnon L, Boulet LP, Brown J, Desrosiers T. Influence of inhaled corticosteroids and dietary intake on bone density and metabolism in patients with moderate to severe asthma. *J Amer Diet Assoc.* 1997;97:1401–1406.
165. U.S. Department of Agriculture. Mypyramid.gov: steps to a healthier you, 2005. Available at: http://www.mypyramid.gov. Accessed January 27, 2010.
166. U.S. Department of Agriculture, U.S. Department of Health and Human Services. Dietary guidelines for Americans, 2005. Available at: http://www.health.gov/dietaryguidelines/dga2005/document/default.htm. Accessed January 27, 2010.
167. Neumark-Sztainer D, Story M, Resnick MD, et al. Body dissatisfaction and unhealthy weight-control practices among adolescents with and without chronic illness: a population-based study. *Arch Pediatr Adolesc Med.* 1995;149:1330–1335.
168. Xiu-Min L. Complementary and alternative medicine in pediatric allergic disorders. *Curr Opin Allergy Clin Immunol.* 2009;9:161–167.

Gastrointestinal Disorders

Amanda Croll, Sarah Weston, Jennifer Autodore, and Jenni Beary

Introduction

The gastrointestinal tract may be thought of as a tube that processes and absorbs nutrients. The function of the gastrointestinal tract may be disrupted by disease, injury, drugs like chemotherapy or antibiotics, parasites, environmental toxins, or bacterial overgrowth, and result in alterations in nutritional requirements. Many nutrients are absorbed throughout the intestinal tract, whereas others are absorbed only at specific sites. Absorption of the latter class of nutrients is particularly vulnerable to disease or surgical resection. **Figure 12-1** graphically portrays the principal sites of absorption of macro- and micronutrients, vitamins, and minerals.

Symptoms of gastrointestinal disease can arise from disorders located in a specific region of the bowel, the entire bowel, or distant sites (for example, vomiting can occur due to pyloric stenosis, gastroenteritis, or a brain tumor). Common pediatric disorders are listed in **Table 12-1** and common diagnostic tests are given in **Table 12-2**. Many tests are available to evaluate gastrointestinal function as well as the presence or absence of disease.

Common gastrointestinal problems will be discussed in the first section of this chapter. These include acute diarrhea, chronic diarrhea, constipation, gastroesophageal reflux, and lactose intolerance. Discussions of celiac disease, inflammatory bowel disease, pancreatitis, cholestatic liver disease, liver transplant, short bowel syndrome, and intestinal transplant follow.

Acute Diarrhea

Diarrhea has been defined as passage of three or more loose, watery stools per day or as 10 mL/kg liquid stool per day.[1,2] A child having diarrhea for 3–7 days is among the most common reasons for seeking the assistance of a pediatrician and is estimated to cost at least $1.5 billion for evaluation and treatment.[3,4] The American Academy of Pediatrics (AAP) and the Centers for Disease Control and Prevention (CDC) have issued practice parameters and guidelines delineating treatment depending on the presence of dehydration.[3,5,6] "Gut rest," in which food is restricted, is an outdated concept and may result in malnutrition. General principles of diarrhea management are replacement of fluid and electrolyte losses and nutritional therapy with early age-appropriate feeding.[1] The composition of commonly used oral maintenance and rehydration solutions is presented in **Table 12-3**.

Nutrition Management

Nutrition management varies with the degree of dehydration. The AAP has distinguished stages of dehydration using the following physical signs:

- *Mild:* Slightly dry mucous membranes, increased thirst
- *Moderate:* Sunken eyes, sunken fontanelle, loss of skin turgor, dry mucous membranes
- *Severe:* Signs of moderate dehydration plus one or more of the following: rapid thready (scarcely perceptible) pulse, cyanosis, rapid breathing, delayed capillary refill time, lethargy, coma[3]

Mild Diarrhea with No Dehydration

The AAP encourages continuing a normal diet throughout the acute illness, including breastfeeding or full strength infant formula and a regular diet, excluding beverages high in sugar (resulting in high osmolality) such as juices and sodas. Increased fluid intake is necessary to compensate for losses. Infants and children who are not dehydrated can be kept hydrated using frequent breastfeeding, usual infant formula, and milk. The use of lactose-free formula is no longer recommended in management of acute diarrhea.[3,7] Using a regular diet as treatment for mild diarrhea does not change the volume of diarrhea and requires education of parents concerning treatment goals of maintaining a regular diet and hydration.[3] Most infants and children demonstrate hunger and thirst during mild, acute diarrheal illness, and parents

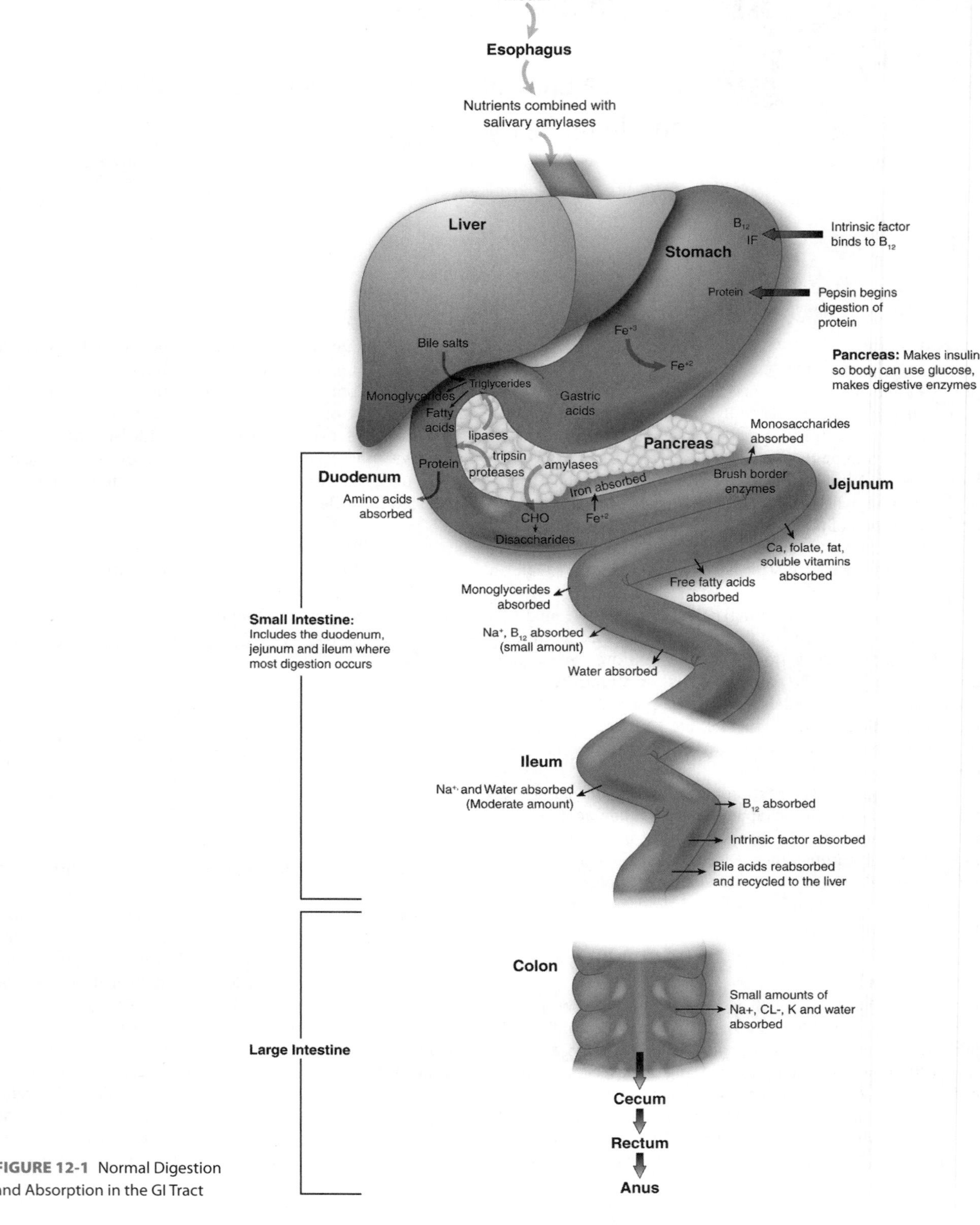

FIGURE 12-1 Normal Digestion and Absorption in the GI Tract

TABLE 12-1 Common Pediatric Gastrointestinal Disorders

Presenting Symptom	Differential Diagnosis	Treatment
Stomach and Esophagus		
Vomiting/regurgitation	Congenital anomaly of the gastrointestinal tract	Surgery
	Gastroesophageal reflux	Infants: positioning, medications such as antacids, H2 blockers, and proton pump inhibitors (PPI). If preceding fails, consider surgical treatment. All ages: medications, antacids, H2 blockers, PPI, avoid caffeine-containing foods and other personal triggers
	Eosinophilic esophagitis	Elimination diet, swallowed steroids
	Eosinophilic gastritis	Steroids, immunosuppressive medication
	Peptic disease	Medications such as antacids, H2 blockers, and PPI; avoid caffeine-containing foods and other personal triggers
	H. pylori	Antibiotics, PPI
	Gastroparesis	Prokinetics, diet changes such as multiple small low-fat meals per day, or postpyloric feeds
Dysphagia (choking after eating), odynophagia (pain with swallowing)	Congenital anomalies, strictures, webs	Surgery
	Eosinophilic esophagitis	Elimination diet, swallowed steroids
	Esophageal spasms/dysmotility	Calcium channel blockers and nitrates; avoid extreme temperatures in foods
	Peptic strictures	Medications such as antacids, H2 blockers, and PPI; dilation
Liver and Pancreas		
Jaundice	Extrahepatic biliary tract obstruction, such as biliary atresia	Surgical correction; diet/formula with medium chain triglycerides (MCT), fat-soluble vitamin supplementation, choleretic agents such as ursodeoxycholate
	Autoimmune hepatitis	Steroids, evaluation for fat malabsorption, fat-soluble vitamin supplementation, protein restriction only if encephalopathic
Jaundice with recurrent abdominal pain	Gallstones	Surgery
	Choledochal cyst	Surgery
Nausea, vomiting, abdominal pain	Pancreatitis	NPO; if severe or prolonged course expected then postplyoric tube feeds or parenteral nutrition; pain control, H2 blockers; when clinically able, resume low-fat oral diet
	Pancreatic pseudocyst	Monitor cyst size; if cyst increases with enteral nutrition, may require parenteral nutrition
Chronic diarrhea, failure to thrive	Pancreatic insufficiency, such as cystic fibrosis	Enzyme replacement therapy, fat-soluble vitamin supplementation, high calorie balanced diet
	Cholestatic disease	Diet/formula with MCT, fat-soluble vitamin supplementation
Small Bowel and Colon		
Anemia, gastrointestinal bleeding	Congenital malformations, such as Meckel's diverticulum, duplication cysts	Surgery
Vomiting	Food allergies	Hydrolysate formula, elimination diet
	Infectious enteropathies	Oral rehydration solutions, followed by lactose and/or sucrose restrictions
Diarrhea in neonatal period	Congenital disorders of carbohydrate absorption and transport	Restriction of the problematic carbohydrate, balanced nutrition, vitamin/mineral supplementation, enzyme replacement
Diarrhea, perioral and perianal rash	Zinc deficiency	Zinc supplementation

(continued)

TABLE 12-1 *(Continued)*

Presenting Symptom	Differential Diagnosis	Treatment
Diarrhea	Food allergies	Elemental formula and/or elimination diet
	Infectious enteropathies	Intravenous fluids, oral rehydration solutions, followed by lactose and/or sucrose restrictions if clinically indicated
	Crohn's disease	Enteral feeds for therapy and/or malnutrition, replete iron, fat-soluble vitamins, and zinc as necessary; monitor vitamin B_{12} if severe ileal disease or resection
	Ulcerative colitis	Enteral feeds for weight gain, replete iron as necessary, low-residue diet if strictures
	Celiac disease	Gluten-free diet
	Short bowel syndrome	Parenteral nutrition progressing to enteral nutrition to oral feeds; vitamin and mineral supplements specific to patient's condition
	Fructose intolerance	Dietary restrictions of fructose-containing foods
	Lactose intolerance	Dietary restrictions of lactose-containing foods
Diarrhea, normal growth pattern	Irritable bowel syndrome, chronic nonspecific diarrhea, toddler's diarrhea	Normal diet for age, increased soluble fiber intake, decreased intake of sorbitol-containing beverages (apple and pear juice) and other personal triggers
Abdominal distention/pain	Celiac disease	Gluten-free diet
	Short bowel syndrome	Total parenteral nutrition progressing to MCT-predominate hydrolysate formula; vitamin and mineral supplements
	Functional constipation	Complete bowel clean-out using saline enemas, mineral oil, Miralax; high-fiber diet and adequate fluids; bowel habit training
	Congenital disorders of carbohydrate absorption and transport	Restriction of the problematic carbohydrate, balanced nutrition, vitamin/mineral supplementation, enzyme replacement
	Fructose intolerance	Dietary restrictions of fructose-containing foods
	Lactose intolerance	Dietary restrictions of lactose-containing foods
Constipation	Hirschsprung's disease; post-NEC strictures	Surgery
	Functional constipation	Complete bowel clean-out using saline enemas, mineral oil, Miralax; high-fiber diet and adequate fluids; bowel habit training

TABLE 12-2 Common Diagnostic Tests for Pediatric Gastrointestinal Disorders

Test	Description	Useful to Help Diagnose
Barium enema	Barium sulfate administered by enema; colonic lumen and mucosa visualized by fluoroscopy.	• Colonic strictures and obstructions • Hirschsprung's disease • Polyps
Barium swallow	Barium sulfate administered orally; upper gastrointestinal tract is visualized by fluoroscopy.	• Aspiration • Dysmotility disorders • Hiatal hernias • Strictures • Varices
Breath hydrogen test	Oral administration of sugar and expiratory collection of hydrogen as an indirect measure of bacterial fermentation of unabsorbed carbohydrate.	• Fructose malabsorption • Lactose malabsorption • Bacterial overgrowth
DXA (dual energy X-ray absorptiometry)	Measures bone density in the spine, hip, or forearm.	• Osteomalacia • Osteopenia • Osteoporosis

TABLE 12-2 *(Continued)*

Test	Description	Useful to Help Diagnose
Colonoscopy	Insertion of flexible fiber optic tube via anus into large bowel; visual examination of colonic lining, biopsies obtained.	• Colitis • Polyps
CT (computed tomography scan) of abdomen	Multiple radiographs of abdomen with or without intraluminal and/or intravenous contrast; computer reconstructs multiple images to generate "slices" through the abdomen.	• Areas of inflammation (e.g., abscess) • Blood vessel anatomy and obstructions • Organ size and consistency • Tumors
EGD (esophagogastroduodenoscopy)	Fiber optic tube is inserted into upper gastrointestinal tract allowing mucosal lining of upper GI tract to be visualized and biopsies to be taken.	• Celiac disease • Duodenitis • Esophagitis, including esosinophilic esopahgitis (EE) • Gastritis • Peptic ulcer disease
Fecal fat test	Concurrent 3-day diet record of fat intake and stool collection; comparison as percentage of total fat in 24 hours excreted in stool. Malabsorption indicated in children if greater than 7% of fat is excreted; for infants less than 6 months of age if greater than 15% of fat is excreted.	• Fat malabsorption • Pancreatic insufficiency
pH probe	Tube with pH sensor is inserted into esophagus for 24 hours with feeding at regulated intervals.	• Gold standard for gastroesophageal reflux
Scintigraphy ("milk scan")	Barium ingested with X-rays capturing movement through upper GI tract	• Delayed gastric emptying • Pulmonary aspiration
Ultrasound	Can be of all abdominal organs or individual organs such as the stomach, intestines, gallbladder, liver, spleen, pancreas, kidney, and bladder	• Anatomical abnormalities • Cysts • Obstructions • Stones • Tumors
Upper GI/upper GI with small bowel follow-through:	Barium ingested with X-ray monitoring of path in GI tract to duodenum or to ileum if small bowel follow through.	• Anatomical abnormalities • Inflammation • Tumors
X-ray of abdomen		• Bowel dilatation or obstruction • Calcified gall bladder stones • Gas patterns and free air • Presence of stool in GI tract • Pnuematosis • Toxic megacolon

Sources: Corkins MR, Scolapino J. Diarrhea. In: Merritt R, ed. *The ASPEN Nutrition Support Practice Manual,* 2nd ed. Silver Spring, MD: ASPEN; 2005:207–210; Graham-Maar RC, French HM, Piccoli DA. Gastroenterology. In: Frank G, Shah SS, Catallozzi M, Zaoutis LB, eds. *The Philadelphia Guide: Inpatient Pediatrics.* Philadelphia, PA: Lippincott, Williams, and Wilkins; 2003:100–115; and Leonberg BL. *ADA Pocket Guide to Pediatric Nutrition Assessment.* Chicago: American Dietetic Association; 2008:106.

can respond to these cues. The BRAT(T) diet (bananas, rice, applesauce, tea, and toast) should be avoided because it is low in calories and is not a balanced source of nutrition. However, foods that are high in carbohydrates, such as rice, wheat, peas, and potatoes, may slow diarrheal output.

Diarrhea with Mild to Moderate Dehydration

Increased fluid intake is necessary to compensate for losses and may require the use of oral rehydration solutions (ORS) in addition to the regular diet.[3] The use of ORS helps to replace fluid and electrolyte losses from diarrhea. Dehydration

TABLE 12-3 Oral Rehydrating Solutions (ORS)

Solution	Glucose/ CHO (g/L)	Sodium (mEq/L)	Potassium (mEq/L)	Osmolality (mmol/L)	CHO/Sodium
Pedialyte (Abbott, Columbus, Ohio)	25	45	20	250	3.1
Pediatric Electrolyte (PendoPharm, Montreal, Quebec)	25	45	30	250	3.1
Kaolectrolyte (Pfizer, New York, New York)	20	48	20	240	2.4
Rehydralyte (Abbott, Columbus, Ohio)	25	75	20	310	1.9
WHO, ORS, 2002 (reduced osmolarity)	75	75	30	224	1
WHO, ORS, 1975 (original formulation)	111	90	20	311	1.2
Cola*	126	2	0.1	750	1944
Apple juice*	125	3	32	730	1278
Gatorade* (Gatorade, Chicago, Illinois)	45	20	3	330	62.5
Whole cow's milk	12 (lactose)	40	1226	285	Not available

*Cola, juice, and Gatorade are shown for comparison only; they are not recommended for use.

Abbreviations: CHO, carbohydrate; WHO, World Health Organization.

Sources: Adapted from Oral therapy for acute diarrhea. In: Kleinman RE, ed. *Pediatric Nutrition Handbook*, 6th ed. Elk Grove Village, IL: American Academy of Pediatrics; 2009:651–659; and Roberts J, Shilkofski N. *The Harriet Lane Handbook*, 17th ed. Elsevier Mosby; 2005:559,Table 20–14a.

can be treated at home by giving an ORS solution by syringe at the rate of 1 teaspoon (5 mL) per minute over 4 hours for a child less than 15 kg or 2 teaspoons (5-10 mL) for children 15–20 kg. This method of fluid administration is adequate to replace the fluid deficit within a 4-hour period. After 1–2 hours of this treatment, the infant or child may begin voluntarily accepting the rehydration liquid. If the child or infant is unable to cooperate, a nasogastric (NG) tube may be used at home or in the hospital. After correction of dehydration, age-appropriate feeding should be initiated as described above.[3]

Diarrhea with Severe Dehydration

Severe dehydration in infants and children is a medical emergency and requires immediate hospitalization. Once rehydration is complete, age-appropriate feeding can be initiated.

Lactose-Containing Products

Lactose-containing products, especially when given with complex carbohydrates, are no longer thought to increase diarrheal output or prolong the illness unless stool output clearly increases on a lactose-containing diet.[8]

Fiber

Infant formulas with added soy fiber have been reported to reduce liquid stools with no change in overall stool output in acute diarrhea and to reduce the length of antibiotic-associated diarrhea.[5,9,10] Use of soy formula with added fiber is not a standard of care because continuation of breast feeding or usual formula works to correct dehydration in most cases. Fiber has been used as part of a food-based regimen in several studies in underdeveloped countries for chronic diarrhea. The World Health Organization has developed an algorithm for the treatment of persistent diarrhea using locally available foods and simple clinical guidelines for use in underdeveloped countries.[11] Kolacek and colleagues compared a modular diet using food with a semi-elemental infant formula in the treatment of chronic diarrhea. The modular diet was found to decrease the duration of diarrhea and the time to nutritional recovery.[12,13] The modular diet included boiled minced chicken meat, sunflower oil emulsion, sucrose, corn flour, and a full range of vitamins and minerals. The success with this diet demonstrates the importance of returning to age-appropriate feeding as soon as rehydration is accomplished.

Prebiotics and Probiotics

Use of probiotics and prebiotics in infant and enteral formulas and in foods has been proposed as beneficial in the treatment of acute and chronic diarrhea of infancy and childhood. *Probiotics* are live microorganisms, historically available in fermented foods such as yogurt, that promote health by improving the balance of healthy organisms in the intestinal tract.[5] Additional proposed mechanisms are preventing adhesion of microbes to the gut mucosa, down regulation of inflammatory responses, and stimulation of immunoglobulin A production.[14,15] Technology has allowed beneficial bacteria to be freeze-dried, added to formula or foods, and be reactivated in the gut when consumed.[16]

Prebiotics are complex carbohydrates, not microorganisms, that promote the growth of healthy microorganisms in the intestinal tract.[5] Human milk contains oligosaccharides (a type of prebiotic) that promote the growth of *lactobacilli* and *bifidobacteria* in the colon of breastfed infants.[5,17] Higher intake of breast milk has been associated with a lowered incidence of acute diarrhea.[18]

Questions about consuming live probiotic bacteria and prebiotics include whether long-term consumption is safe and whether consumption has positive health effects. A randomized controlled trial has reported that healthy infants consuming a formula supplemented with prebiotic mixtures achieved normal growth and had stools more similar to breastfed infants when compared to infants fed an unsupplemented formula. The prebiotic mixtures included polydextrose and galactooligosaccharides in one group and polydextrose, galactooligosaccharides, and lactulose in the second group.[19] A double-blind randomized placebo-controlled trial evaluated the tolerance and safety of long-term consumption of different levels of cow's milk formula not supplemented and supplemented with different levels of *Bifidobacterium lactis* and *Streptococcus thermophilis* in infants 3–18 months of age. Healthy infants consuming the probiotic-supplemented formula reported a lower frequency of colic or irritability, and reduced severity of antibiotic-induced acute diarrhea.[20] Another study reported safe consumption by healthy infants of a formula containing *Bifidobacterium lactis* and *Streptococcus thermophilus.*[21] It has also been reported in a multicenter randomized double-blind trial that infants and children with mild diarrhea for longer than 3 days had a slightly decreased duration of acute diarrhea when treated with killed *lactobacillus.*[22] Another double-blind, placebo-controlled, randomized trial reported that infants in child care centers fed a standard cow's milk formula supplemented with *L. reuteri* or *B. lactis* had fewer and shorter episodes of diarrhea compared to infants fed the same formula without added probiotics.[23] There is still no consensus concerning the types and amounts of probiotics that are beneficial. More research is needed.

Infant formulas with prebiotics and probiotics include Nutramigen with Enflora LGG (probiotic, *Lactobacillus rhamnosus* GG) by Mead Johnson, Similac Advance Early-Shield (galactooligosaccharide) by Abbott, and Enfamil PREMIUM with Triple Health Guard (galactooligosaccharide) by Mead Johnson.

An example of an enteral formula for children over 1 year of age supplemented with probiotics is Boost Kids Essentials 1.0 and 1.5 (*L. reuteri* inserted in optional straw to use for drinking) by Nestlé. Examples of products using prebiotics include Pediasure enteral formula with fiber (NutraFlora and scFOS) by Abbott; Vital Jr (NutraFlora and scFOS), also from Abbott; and Peptamen Jr with fiber (contains insoluble fiber and Prebio, a blend of FOS and inulin) and Peptamen Jr with Prebio (no insoluble fiber) by Nestlé.

Chronic Diarrhea

Diarrheal illnesses in children follow a continuum from acute to chronic or persistent diarrhea. In 1982, the World Health Organization defined persistent or chronic diarrhea as "diarrhea episodes of presumed infectious etiology that begin acutely but last at least 14 days."[24] Persistent diarrhea has also been defined as "the passage of ≥ 3 watery stools per day for > 2 weeks in a child who either fails to gain or loses weight."[11] Persistent diarrhea has many triggers, including acute diarrhea caused by an enteric infection, and more recently HIV infection and AIDS.[11]

In a discussion of chronic diarrheal disease, the AAP distinguishes four kinds:

- Osmotic
- Secretory
- Dysmotility
- Inflammatory

Osmotic diarrhea may result from congenital or acquired disease and is often associated with failure to absorb a specific carbohydrate such as lactose or with excessive carbohydrate intake, such as excessive juice intake in toddlers or dietary fructose intolerance.[25] Diarrhea stops when the dietary cause is removed. *Secretory diarrhea* does not respond to cessation of oral intake. Disorders include congenital choridorrhea and neural crest tumors.[25] *Diarrhea from dysmotility* may be associated with rapid transit or irritable bowel syndrome.

Inflammatory diarrhea may result from enteric infection, inflammation secondary to celiac disease, or inflammatory bowel disease. Chronic or persistent diarrhea (also called intractable diarrhea of infancy) has been thought of as a nutritional disorder, and certainly requires nutritional treatment for recovery.[26–30]

Malnutrition is considered the most important epidemiologic risk factor for persistent diarrhea worldwide when no specific congenital, inherited, or acquired disorders are identified. Other associated risk factors are:

- Age less than 6 months
- Acute diarrheal episodes within the past 2 months
- Zinc deficiency
- Lack of breastfeeding
- Male sex
- Infection with enteropathogenic or enteroaggregative *Escherichia coli* or *Cryptosporidium*
- A history of intrauterine growth retardation[11]

If infection as a cause is excluded, other etiologies must be considered. These include food allergy, dietary protein intolerances, celiac disease, lactose or other disaccharide intolerances, cystic fibrosis and other causes of pancreatic insufficiency, and inflammatory bowel disease.[13] Lactose intolerance, celiac disease, and inflammatory bowel disease are discussed later in this chapter. Food allergy and dietary protein intolerances are discussed in Chapter 7, and cystic fibrosis is discussed in Chapter 11.

As with all diarrheal illnesses in infants, chronic diarrhea is dangerous if not treated promptly and appropriately, because it can result in dehydration and severe malnutrition.[28] Recent reports indicate that the incidence of chronic diarrhea has declined in the United States over the past two decades due to better treatment of acute diarrheal episodes.[25]

Nutrition Management

The first step is appropriate fluid resuscitation. Next, cautious refeeding through a combination of enteral feedings and/or parenteral nutrition is started slowly due to the possibility of metabolic alterations from refeeding syndrome.[31] Refeeding protocols may be required depending upon the degree of malnutrition, with monitoring of potassium, phosphorus, magnesium, calcium, and trace elements. Continued use of breast milk is recommended during infancy.[11] Continuously infused breast milk loses calories through adherence of protein and lipids on the tube walls; this factor should be considered when making calorie determinations.[32,33] Alterations in the continuous infusion-feeding method can be made to maximize nutrient delivery by using the shortest amount of tubing available and slanting the feeding syringe.[34] Another option is to use a formula for the continuous infusion for greater lipid delivery, saving the expressed breast milk for oral feedings.[35] In developed countries, specialized enteral formulas that are lactose-free and/or elemental may be preferred; however, research in developing countries has shown success using more readily available foods and formula.[11] Oral zinc supplementation is also recommended by WHO in developing countries.[36] Both a meta-analysis and Cochrane Review also recommend oral zinc supplementation, especially in those patients with malnutrition or history of multiple episodes of acute or persistent diarrhea.[37,38] Carbohydrate intolerance may or may not exist, and tolerance should be monitored. Adequate normal levels of protein, lipids, and vitamins can be given.[39]

Absorption of many nutrients may be improved by using continuous enteral feedings. A crossover study in infants with protracted diarrhea showed greater absorption of zinc, calcium, copper, fat, and nitrogen during continuous enteral feedings than with bolus enteral feedings.[40] Small bolus oral feedings may be retained for oral motor stimulation. The calories needed for catch-up growth may be in the range of 140–200 kcal/kg.[41] Nutritional support may start at 75 kcal/kg/day and increase over 5–7 days to 130–150 kcal/kg/day. Protein is started at 1–2 g/kg/day, increasing to 3–4 g/kg/day as caloric intake increases.[24] Mild zinc deficiency may play a role in both acute and chronic diarrhea. Zinc supplementation in developing countries has been associated with a decrease in number of stools per day and decreased number of days with watery diarrhea in acute diarrhea and reduction of the duration of persistent diarrhea.[42] Two pooled analyses of randomized controlled trials in developing countries found oral zinc supplementation benefited children with both acute and persistent diarrhea.[43,44] WHO/UNICEF have issued a statement recommending zinc supplementation: 10 mg/day for 10–14 days for infants $<$ 6 months of age and 20 mg/day for 10–14 days for infants and children $>$ 6 months of age.[36] A randomized double-blind placebo-controlled trial of zinc supplementation in breastfed infants in the United States showed no significant difference in diarrhea frequency in the supplemented and not supplemented groups.[45] Recommendations for use of zinc supplementation in developed countries need further research and evaluation.[45] Cereal and other infant foods should be continued as tolerated; however, juices and sodas should be avoided due to their high osmolality. For infants with malnutrition or who are severely dehydrated, use of a lactose-free formula may lead to quicker recovery.[8] Semi-elemental protein hydrolysate formulas such as Alimentum (Abbott) or Pregestimil (Mead Johnson) may also be used. Elemental formulas are commonly used in many hospitals, although short peptides are absorbed better than an equimolar amount of amino acids.[46,47] A semi-elemental formula may be superior to an elemental amino acid–based formula such as Neocate (SHNA), Elecare (Abbott), or Nutramigen AA (Mead Johnson).

As the infant improves, parenteral nutrition or IV hydration, if needed, is weaned, and enteral nutrition gradually increased in the form of continuous feedings. Gradually larger bolus oral feedings are added as tolerated. If this period of progressing from parenteral to enteral nutrition is prolonged, the transition from continuous feeding to oral bolus feedings can often be accomplished in the home setting.

Constipation

Constipation is common in childhood. The North American Society for Pediatric Gastroenterology, Hepatology and Nutrition (NASPGHAN) defines constipation as "a delay or difficulty in defecation, present for two or more weeks and sufficient to cause significant stress to the patient."[48]

Treatment in infants may include juices that contain natural sorbitol such as apple, pear, or prune (0.5 g/100 g, 2.1 g/100 g, and 12.7 g/100 g, respectively), increasing fluids, and verifying that infant formula is mixed correctly.[48] Rice cereal, a common first food for infants, may also cause constipation that resolves when infant oatmeal is used instead. Inadequate fluid intake also can be a cause of constipation.[49] High fiber diets with adequate fluids are recommended as the first line of therapy in children. Recommended fiber intake for children by age is listed in **Table 12-4**. Dwyer recommends "age plus 5" as an easy way to estimate fiber intake.[50] This estimation never exceeds, but may underestimate, fiber requirements as given in the DRIs' Adequate Intake (AI). For example, AI for an 8-year-old is 14 g/1000 kcal or 25 g/day. Dwyer's estimate of fiber needs is expressed as age 8 years + 5 grams = 13 g/day. Fiber supplements may be used when dietary intake is inadequate. When fiber alone fails, lubricants and laxatives may be required. The fiber content of common foods is presented in **Table 12-5**.

Medications such as phenytoin may slow peristalsis, and diuretics that alter fluid balance may cause constipation as well.[49] Mothers may believe the iron contained in formula causes constipation because of their experience with iron supplementation in pregnancy, but iron in formula has not been associated with adverse side effects including constipation.[49,51–54] Iron-fortified formula is recommended by the American Academy of Pediatrics for the first year of life to prevent anemia.[54] Standard infant low-iron formulas are no longer made in the United States.

When stooling is chronically difficult or painful, children may withhold stool, aggravating the existing problem. Encopresis may result due to the stretched rectal wall, allowing softer stool to leak out involuntarily.[49] A bowel program after a thorough clean-out often includes a high-fiber diet, adequate fluid, and increased physical activity.

Gastroesophageal Reflux

Gastroesophageal reflux (GER) is the passage of gastric contents into the esophagus and is a normal physiologic process that occurs throughout the day in healthy infants and children.[55] GER may include regurgitation and vomiting. Recurrent vomiting usually peaks at 4 months of age and resolves by 10–12 months when the infant achieves a more upright posture. When gastroesophageal reflux causes multiple vomiting episodes or interferes with growth, it is called gastroesophageal reflux disease (GERD).[55]

In 2009 a joint committee of NASPGHAN and the European Society for Pediatric Gastroenterology, Hepatology, and Nutrition (ESPGHAN) revised the 2001 clinical practice guidelines on pediatric GER and GERD.[56,57] The "happy spitter" is an infant who has frequent episodes of regurgitation but continues to grow well. Parental education concerning the expected improvement as the infant develops is all that is necessary. If the infant is not growing well or has increased irritability, changes in feeding are recommended. If GER is a symptom of an allergy to cow's milk protein, symptoms may resolve with a change to an extensively hydrolyzed or amino acid formula. If the infant is breastfed, elimination of cow's milk and egg from the mother's diet may also improve symptoms. Discontinuation of breastfeeding is rarely recommended. No data exist to support allergy to soy protein in infants causing regurgitation and vomiting. Decreasing volume of each feeding and offering more frequent feedings may also improve GER symptoms; however, total intake may decrease with this change.[57] Thickened formula may decrease the number of vomiting episodes but does not reduce the number of reflux episodes.[57,58] Use of infant rice or oatmeal cereal to thicken formula may result in too rapid weight gain and decrease the percentage of calories provided by protein and fat. Use of antiregurgitant formulas such as Enfamil AR (Mead Johnson) may similarly reduce the number of vomiting episodes but not decrease the number of reflux episodes. If the infant is diagnosed with failure to thrive, increasing the caloric density of formula is recommended, especially if extensively hydrolyzed or amino acid formulas have improved symptoms. Although GER symptoms do improve in the flat prone position, prone positioning is not recommended with infants because of its association with SIDS. The semi-supine position, such as in a car seat, worsens symptoms. Simple GER usually resolves around 18 months of age. GERD usually requires medical management.[57] In older children and adolescents there is no evidence that changes in diet improve symptoms, although in adults late night eating and obesity are associated with GER. Expert opinion suggests that children and adolescents eliminate caffeine, chocolate, and spicy foods. Alcohol use may also increase symptoms.[57] Left-sided sleeping in adolescents also may improve symptoms.

TABLE 12-4 Adequate Intake of Fiber for Children

Age (in years)	Total Fiber Intake (g/day)
1–3	19
4–8	25
Boys	
9–13	31
14–18	38
Girls	
9–13	26
14–18	26

Fiber recommendations are based on data for adults, 14 grams fiber/1000 kcal, using median energy intake from United States, Continuing Survey of Food Intakes by Individuals (CSFII), 1994–1996, 1998.

Source: Information compiled from http://www.nal.usda.gov/fnic/DRI//DRI_Energy/339-421.pdf.

Lactose Intolerance

Lactose intolerance is the inability to metabolize and digest lactose, which is the sugar most commonly found in

TABLE 12-5 Good Sources of Dietary Fiber

	Grams of Fiber	Serving Size		Grams of Fiber	Serving Size
Fruit			*Ready-to-Eat Cereal*		
Apple	2.2	1 med. w/skin	FiberOne (General Mills)	14	½ cup
Apple	2	1 med. w/o skin	All-Bran (Kellogg's)	10	½ cup
Apricot	7.8	dried, 3 oz	100% Bran (Post)	9	⅓ cup
Blueberries	4.4	1 cup raw	Shredded Wheat and Bran (Post)	8	1¼ cup
Dates, dried	4.2	10	Raisin Bran (Post)	8	1 cup
Kiwi	3.4	3 oz	Grape-Nuts (Post)	7	½ cup
Pear	4.1	1 med. raw	Multi Bran Chex (General Mills)	6	¾ cup
Prunes, dried	7.2	3 oz	Cracklin' Oat Bran (Kellogg's)	6	¾ cup
Prunes, stewed	6.6	3 oz	Mini Wheats (Kellogg's)	6	1 cup (30 biscuits)
Raisins	5.3	3 oz	Frosted Mini Wheats with raisins (Kellogg's)	6	¾ cup (24 biscuits)
Raspberries	5.8	1 cup	Shredded Wheat (Post)	6	1 cup
Strawberries, raw	2.8	1 cup	Mini Wheats with strawberries (Kellogg's)	5	¾ cup (24 biscuits)
Vegetables and Legumes			Wheat Chex (General Mills)	5	¾ cup
Avocado, California, raw	3	1 med.	Bran Flakes (Post)	5	¾ cup
Beans, black, boiled	7.2	1 cup	Banana Nut Crunch (Post)	4	1 cup
Beans, great northern, boiled	6	1 cup	Raisin Bran Pecan Date Crunch (Post)	4	½ cup
Beans, kidney, boiled	6.4	1 cup	Cranberry Almond Crunch	3	¾ cup
Beans, lima, boiled	6.2	1 cup	Low Fat Granola (Kellogg's)	3	½ cup
Beans, baby lima, boiled	7.8	1 cup	Grape-Nut Flakes (Post)	3	¾ cup
Beans, navy, boiled	6.6	1 cup			
Beans, green, canned	6.8	½ cup			
Broccoli, boiled	2.2	½ cup			
Chickpeas (garbanzo beans)	5.7	1 cup			
Cowpeas (black-eyed peas)	4.4	1 cup			
Lentils, boiled	7.9	1 cup			

Source: Data for sections on fruits and vegetables/legumes from Pennington JAT. *Bowes and Church's Food Values of Portions Commonly Used*, 15th ed. Philadelphia: JB Lippincott; 1989; and U.S. Department of Agriculture. *USDA Provisional Table on the Dietary Fiber Content of Selected Foods*; 1988. HNIS/PT-106; data for section on ready-to-eat cereals from a survey of manufacturer's Websites as of November 2009.

milk and milk products. It is caused by a shortage of the enzyme lactase, which is produced by the cells that line the small intestine.[59] People who lack this enzyme are unable to metabolize and completely digest lactose into its simpler forms—glucose and galactose—following the ingestion of a lactose-containing food or beverage. This results in digestive discomfort such as abdominal cramping, bloating, flatulence, and diarrhea. The Nutrition Committee of the American Academy of Pediatrics has published a thorough and complete review of lactose intolance.[59]

Lactose intolerance is commonly diagnosed noninvasively via a breath hydrogen test. Following the ingestion of a lactose-containing beverage, the patient blows into a balloon-like bag at intervals for a specified amount of time. Intermittent samples are taken and analyzed. Carbohydrate that is malabsorbed in the small intestine is fermented by colonic bacteria and releases hydrogen gas.[60] A raised hydrogen breath level signifies the inability to digest lactose. For details on a lactose-controlled diet, please refer to the *Pediatric Manual of Clinical Dietetics*.[61]

Primary Lactase Deficiency

Primary lactase deficiency is believed to be present in 70% of the world's population.[59,62,63] Prevalence and age of onset vary secondary to ethnicity and overall use of dairy products in the diet.[63] It is estimated that 20% of Hispanic, Asian, and black children under the age of 5 "have evidence of lactase deficiency and lactose malabsorption" as opposed to Caucasian children who traditionally do not develop symptoms of lactose intolerance until after the age of 4 or 5.[59,64] It is recommended that children who present with symptoms of lactose intolerance before the age of 2 to 3 receive more complete evaluation because secondary lactase deficiency may have developed from an unknown etiology.[59]

Secondary Lactase Deficiency

Secondary lactase deficiency may occur if the lining of the small intestine that houses lactase-containing epithelial cells is destroyed as a direct result of underlying disease (e.g., celiac disease), small intestinal resection, gastrectomy, chemotherapy treatments, parasitic infections (e.g., giardiasis), or acute diarrheal disease.[65] A study conducted by Nicols further confirmed that infants with severe malnutrition, especially those from developing countries, present with hypolactasia secondary to "suppression of lactase mRNA," which is regulated at the transcriptional level.[59,66,67]

According to the American Academy of Pediatrics Committee on Nutrition, elimination of lactose from the diet is generally not required for the treatment of secondary lactase deficiency and lactose malabsorption.[59] Treatment of the underlying condition is key. Once the primary issue is resolved, lactose-containing products can be reintroduced according to individual tolerance.[59]

Developmental (Neonatal) Lactase Deficiency

In the developing fetus/preterm infant, lactase is the last of the major intestinal disaccharidases to develop.[68] Lactase activity is low prior to gestational week 24.[69] It then begins to increase but remains deficient until 34 weeks gestation.[59,69] As a direct result, premature infants have lower levels of lactase activity and may be unable to digest and absorb lactose as well as their term counterparts.[68,70] Carlson demonstrated that the "addition of lactase to preterm formula reduces the amount of lactose by 70% after a two hour incubation period at room temperature."[68,71] Therefore, the use of lactase to hydrolyze lactose in preterm formulas and maternal breast milk may aid in decreasing "lactose malabsorption in preterm infants" and further lead to enhanced weight gain and improved feeding tolerance.[68]

Congenital Lactase Deficiency

Congenital lactase deficiency is an extremely rare autosomal recessive disorder that primarily affects those of Finnish decent.[72] It is caused by "mutations in the gene coding for the lactase enzyme (LC)."[73] Affected newborn infants present with severe diarrheal disease that occurs immediately following introduction of maternal breast milk or lactose-containing formula.[59,72] If left untreated, congenital lactase deficiency can be life threatening as a result of dehydration and loss of electrolytes.[59] Treatment includes complete removal of lactose from the diet and consumption of a lactose-free formula during infancy and lactose-free milk products after infancy.[59]

Celiac Disease

Celiac disease (CD) is a multisystem, T-cell-mediated chronic autoimmune intestinal disorder that occurs in genetically predisposed individuals.[74–76] At-risk populations include first-degree relatives of people with celiac disease, along with those previously diagnosed with type 1 diabetes mellitus, autoimmune thyroid disease, selective IgA deficiency, trisomy 21, Turner syndrome, or Williams syndrome.[74,75,77]

Emerging research shows that celiac disease is no longer considered an Irish or Celtic condition; nor is it considered to be a rare childhood disease.[78] Studies conducted in the United States and in Europe estimate prevalence in children between the ages of 2.5 and 15 years at 3 to 13 per 1000 children, or approximately 1:300 to 1:80.[74,77]

The clinical presentation of celiac disease is ever changing. Classic gastrointestinal-related symptoms include diarrhea, constipation, chronic abdominal pain, abdominal distention, and vomiting with associated failure to thrive.[74,77] Nongastrointestinal or extraintestinal symptoms include short stature, inadequate weight gain, weight loss, delayed puberty, dental enamel defects, dermatitis herpetaformis, and reduced bone mineral density. In addition, iron deficient anemia that is resistant to oral iron supplementation, fatigue, migraines, and joint pain may also present as symptoms.[74–77]

Those who present with symptoms suspicious of celiac disease must first receive serology testing, which includes immunoglobulin A (IgA) antibody and tissue transglutaminase (TTG), along with tissue transglutaminase immunoglobulin G (TTG IgG) if IgA deficiency is present. It is important that gluten remain in the diet to ensure reliable serology testing. Formal diagnosis must be further confirmed via intestinal biopsy. In some cases, diagnosis may be uncertain. If this is the case, human leukocyte antigen (HLA) typing and repeat biopsy can be performed. Trialing the gluten-free diet may also be considered. After trialing the gluten-free diet, repeat serology testing and intestinal biopsy are recommended. If once positive serology tests become negative following the trial of the gluten-free diet, this is tangible and supportive evidence for the diagnosis of celiac disease.[74,77]

Once formal diagnosis has been made, it is understood that individuals with celiac disease have a permanent intolerance to gluten and must adhere to a gluten-free diet. When nutritive sources of gluten (e.g., wheat, rye, barley, and its derivatives) and nonnutritive sources of gluten (e.g., toothpaste) are completely eliminated from the diet, gastrointestinal and often extraintestinal symptoms, serologic test results, histology, and growth and development should normalize as celiac symptoms improve and move into a state of remission.[74,75]

In both wealthy and developing countries, celiac disease remains underdiagnosed.[78] The only known treatment for celiac disease is the gluten-free diet. Strict dietary adherence proves beneficial. If left untreated, celiac disease can result in nutritional deficiencies, decreased bone mineral density, and neurological disorders. Scientific research further suggests that if left untreated, affected individuals are at increased risk for developing intestinal lymphoma, infertility, spontaneous abortion, and the delivery of low-birth-weight infants.[74,79,80] A gluten-free diet will allow for normal growth and development as well as relief from symptoms. Alternative therapeutic treatments are currently under development.[75,81]

Gluten is composed of two proteins, gliadin and glutenin. Gluten is the general name for storage proteins, referred to as prolamins, that are found in wheat, rye, and barley. Gliadin is the specific prolamin found in wheat, secalin in rye, and hordein in barley.[75,79,80] When ingested, it is these specific prolamins that cause villous atrophy, which may further result in nutrient malabsorption and/or deficiency.

Iron, calcium, and folate are key nutrients often affected in those with celiac disease, because these nutrients are absorbed in the proximal small bowel.[75,79,82] If the disease progresses further down the small intestinal tract, malabsorption of carbohydrates, fat, fat-soluble vitamins, and protein may also occur. The most common causes of anemia in those with celiac disease are iron, folate, or vitamin B_{12} deficiency. Calcium, phosphorus, and vitamin D deficiencies may also occur secondary to malabsorption or decreased intake of dairy products if lactose intolerance is present.[75] Secondary lactose intolerance is commonly observed as the enterocytes at the tips of damaged villi are absent, and therefore unable to produce the enzyme lactase.[75,79,83] Those diagnosed with celiac disease are considered at higher risk for developing bone disease and should receive dual energy x-ray absorpiometry (DXA scan), quantitative CT scan, or computerized bone age estimation at the time of diagnosis.[74,75,84] Strict adherence to the gluten-free diet during childhood will result in improved bone mineral density in adulthood.[74,84]

Whether or not an individual with celiac disease can safely consume oats remains controversial because oats may become contaminated by gluten during the harvesting and milling process.[74,75,79] Clinical research supports the safe consumption of 20–25 grams per day (¼ cup dry rolled gluten-free oats) in *most* children with celiac disease.[80] The patient should discuss the inclusion of gluten-free oats with his or her gastroenterologist and/or registered dietitian prior to ingestion because individual tolerance varies and monitoring of antibody levels is required.

Immediately following diagnosis, affected individuals should be referred to a registered dietitian with expertise in celiac disease to receive comprehensive nutrition education with emphasis on the importance of adhering to a gluten-free diet and the gluten-free lifestyle.[74,75,79,82] Attendance of all primary caregivers should be encouraged during the initial nutrition consultation. Nutrition counseling should focus on nutritive and non-nutritive sources of gluten, gluten-free alternatives, hidden sources of gluten, various aspects of cross-contamination, where one can purchase gluten-free products; credible resources and support groups, eating outside of the home, and identified age-related social situations.[74,75,79,82] Close attention should also be paid to anthropometric assessment, growth trends, nutritional intake, and need for multivitamin and mineral supplementation to aid in preventing and/or correcting nutrient deficiency.[74,75,79,82] Subsequent visits should encompass medical nutrition therapy components previously mentioned along with determining dietary compliance. One should also assess the comprehension level of the patient and family, along with addressing individual questions/concerns and providing continued support in an effort to achieve improved quality of life.[74,75,79,82]

Evidence-based nutrition practice guidelines have been published by the American Dietetic Association (ADA) for the dietary treatment of celiac disease. These formal guidelines can be viewed online at http://www.eatright.org within the Evidence Analysis Library (EAL).[82]

Inflammatory Bowel Disease

The two major types of inflammatory bowel disease (IBD) are Crohn's disease and ulcerative colitis (UC). Crohn's disease may occur in any portion of the gastrointestinal tract. Ulcerative colitis is by definition confined to the colon with minimal involvement of the terminal ileum.[85] Patients who develop nonspecific IBD-like symptoms are often temporarily termed as having indeterminate colitis. The two diseases have many features in common: diarrhea, gastrointestinal blood and protein loss, abdominal pain, weight loss, anemia, and growth failure. Children with IBD may experience growth failure due to inadequate intake, malabsorption, excessive nutrient losses, drug–nutrient interaction, and increased nutrient needs. Inadequate intake may be due to abdominal pain, gastritis, personal effort to decrease the incidence of diarrhea, and taste changes with zinc deficiency.

Nutrition Assessment

Nutrient deficits have been noted in 30–40% of adolescents and children with IBD.[86] At the time of diagnosis, about 85% of pediatric patients with Crohn's disease and 65% with ulcerative colitis present with weight loss.[87] A study by Burnham found pediatric/young adult Crohn's patients have a lower lean body mass than healthy controls, although they maintain a similar fat mass.[88]

Patients who present in a flare, or active disease state, often have multiple macro- and micronutrient losses. Inflammation of the mucosa and bowel resections can lead to general malabsorption. Depending on the location and length of the bowel resection, specific nutrients may no longer be absorbed and will need to be supplemented. Bacterial overgrowth due to altered motility or strictures can also lead to malabsorption.

Nutrition Therapy

There is lack of consensus for estimated caloric needs in pediatric patients with IBD. In a pediatric study, the REE (resting energy expenditure) of Crohn's patients was noted to be similar to that of the control group per kg of lean body mass. The REE per kg of body mass was not down regulated as it is in the starvation state.[89] In the adult population, it is documented that total energy expenditure is not significantly elevated in active disease compared to remission or inactive disease.[90]

Protein requirements are likely elevated due to protein losses as well as increased needs for healing, especially in post-op patients. In patients with IBD who present with protein-losing enteropathy, the body cannot synthesize new proteins as fast as they are lost through the gastrointestinal tract.[91] The resulting hypoalbuminemia cannot be corrected by the addition of protein to the diet.

Bile malabsorption leads to decreased absorption of long-chain fatty acids but not medium chain fatty acids, because bile is not required for the transport of medium-chain fatty acids through the mucosa. Fat malabsorption contributes to the malabsorption of fat-soluble vitamins.

All patients should be assessed for micronutrient deficiencies and repleted as necessary. Blood losses via the stool can lead to iron deficiency. Folate deficiency can result from drug–nutrient interactions as well as decreased intake of folate-rich food sources such as green leafy vegetables. The fat-soluble vitamins A, D, E, and K as well as zinc, magnesium, and calcium are lost when steatorrhea is present. Zinc deficiency may be related to diarrheal, high-output fistula losses and inadequate dietary intake. Magnesium and potassium also are lost via diarrhea. Patients with resections of the stomach or ileum, or severe disease of the terminal ileum may not be able to absorb sufficient vitamin B_{12}.[92,93] Patients should be on a daily multivitamin unless they are receiving enteral formula, which provides the equivalent of a multivitamin.[94] A study of 54 adults with Crohn's disease revealed that although those patients in clinical remission for longer than 3 months were able to meet macronutrient needs via food intake, micronutrient deficiencies remained. Low plasma levels of vitamin C, copper, niacin, and zinc were found in greater than 50% of patients.[95]

Although bone disease in IBD is multifactorial, vitamin D and calcium are important nutrients to monitor. Steroids are known to affect bone mineral density,[96] and new research shows that inflammatory cytokines lead to lower bone mineral density.[97] Even though calcium and vitamin D are not the sole answer in IBD-related low bone mineral density, blood levels should be kept within the normal range. Fat malabsorption can lead to low vitamin D levels, and vitamin D plays many roles beyond bone health in the body. A review article recommends 50,000 units of vitamin D_2 every week up to every day depending on the degree of fat malabsorption, or up to 10,000 units of vitamin D_3 every day for up to 5 months. This is followed by a maintenance dose of 50,000 units of vitamin D_2 every week. For children and adults without fat malabsorption, the recommendation ranges from 400–1000 units of vitamin D_3 every day.[98]

Drug–nutrient interaction from the pharmacotherapy used in the treatment of IBD may negatively affect nutrition. Sulfasalazine (azulfidine) interferes with folate absorption.[99] Methotrexate is a folic acid antagonist, and supplementation of folic acid helps to reduce methotrexate's hepatic side effects.[100,101] Corticosteroid therapy interferes with absorption of calcium, phosphate, and zinc.

Controlled studies have not supported the use of a low-residue, high-fiber, or low-refined-sugar diet to maintain remission of Crohn's disease.[102,103] Dairy products need not be restricted in patients with IBD; however, lactose malabsorption is more common in patients with small bowel Crohn's disease than in patients with disease involving the colon or UC. Lactose intolerance is often temporary during times of active disease. Advice concerning the intake of dairy products should be individualized to avoid unnecessary dietary restrictions.[104]

Nutrition support has both a primary and an adjunctive role in the treatment of IBD.[86] Primary nutrition therapy appears to be more effective in the treatment of Crohn's disease than of ulcerative colitis.[86,105] In a pediatric study, patients with active Crohn's disease were treated with exclusive enteral nutrition therapy (multiple formulas) versus corticosteroids. The duration of clinical remission, degree of mucosal healing, improvement in mucosal inflammation, and improvements to linear growth were greater with any of the enteral formulas than with steroids.[106] These results are similar to another pediatric study that showed exclusive enteral feeds with intact proteins were just as effective as corticosteroids in inducing remission, and had a lower rate of relapse.[107] Borelli also looked at a polymeric diet versus corticosteroid therapy, and found that the use of polymeric formulas led to increased mucosal healing at the end of the 10-week study.[108] A randomized controlled trial of a polymeric enteral formula and an elemental formula found similar results in inducing remission in children with Crohn's disease. Children given a polymeric diet, however, achieved better weight gain.[109]

Despite these positive studies in the pediatric population, a Cochrane Review, including both pediatric and adult studies, reported that corticosteroids were more effective in inducing remission. The protein composition of the formulas did not reveal any difference in the effectiveness of the enteral nutrition therapy.[110] However, for the maintenance of remission in Crohn's disease, enteral feeds were found to be beneficial in all age groups with no known side effects.[111]

Due to lifestyle changes that accompany exclusive enteral nutrition therapy, there is interest in the effectiveness of partial enteral nutrition therapy. A pediatric study using elemental formula provided as either 50% or 100% of calorie needs showed higher remission rates and improved hemoglobin, albumin, and erythrocyte sedimentation rate (ESR) in those receiving 100% of their calorie needs from formula.[112] However, in a study of patients with steroid-dependent Crohn's disease in a state of remission, the addition of enteral formula (either elemental or polymeric) taken orally along with a regular diet allowed 43% of patients to discontinue steroids and remain in remission at the 12-month follow-up.[113]

Bamba looked at elemental diets containing different amounts of long-chain triglycerides (LCT). The high LCT diet had a remission rate of 25% at 4 weeks, whereas the low LCT diet had a remission rate of 80%.[114] Other studies have found that formulas containing higher amounts of medium-chain triglycerides (MCT) have resulted in remission rates comparable to low-fat formulas or steroid therapy.[115,116] Per a Cochrane Review, there is inadequate evidence to support the use of omega-3 fatty acids for the induction or maintenance of remission of ulcerative colitis,[117,118] nor do they appear to be effective in the maintenance of remission in Crohn's disease.[119] Probiotics have not been shown to be effective for the induction or maintenance of remission of Crohn's disease,[120,121] but when added to standard therapy for ulcerative colitis, they may lead to a reduction of disease activity.[122]

Enteral feeding has been shown to reduce inflammation and improve well-being, nutrition, and growth, but the exact mechanism is unknown. A study on the use of enteral feeding showed that inflammatory markers were significantly improved over the first 7 days of treatment; significant improvement in growth-related proteins and nutritional markers was not seen until day 14 or later.[123]

In patients not treated with enteral nutrition therapy during periods of active disease and/or weight loss, oral nutritional beverages in addition to food can be useful. Because protein composition does not affect rates of remission or disease improvement, formula choice should be based on palatability and patient tolerance. If voluntary intake is insufficient, nasogastric enteral supplementation may be considered. Parenteral nutrition (PN) should be reserved for patients who have bowel obstructions or short bowel syndrome, or are unable to tolerate a sufficient quantity of enteral nutrition because of active disease. PN comes with a greater risk as well as a higher cost.

Pancreatitis

Pancreatitis can be divided into two groups: mild and severe. Approximately 70–80% of all cases are mild and will often resolve within 5–7 days.[124,125] The remaining cases are severe and require medical and nutritional therapy. Severe pancreatitis creates a state of hypermetabolism and catabolism with significant nitrogen losses, and results in an elevated systemic inflammatory response. It is often associated with infectious complications.[124,125]

Nutrition Therapy for Mild Pancreatitis

Traditionally in clinical practice, patients were often initially made NPO, and then advanced to a clear liquid diet as pain resolved. In a randomized controlled trial, patients with mild pancreatitis who resumed oral intake of liquids and solid foods prior to the resolution of pain were able to advance to a solid food diet sooner than those on bowel rest, thereby decreasing length of stay.[126] A study compared the initiation of a clear liquid diet versus soft solid food diet and found no significant difference between the two groups in cessation of feeds due to pain. Also, patients started on the soft solid diet took in significantly more calories and protein overall, with a decreased length of stay.[127] This research supports the initiation of oral feeds, both liquids and solids, during the first few days with the benefit of improved nutrient intake.

Nutrition Therapy for Severe Pancreatitis

Traditionally, severe pancreatitis has been treated with bowel rest and parenteral nutrition. Multiple studies now show that parenteral nutrition increases the pro-inflammatory response and contributes to gut atrophy, likely leading to bacterial translocation and increased infection rates.[128,129] A systematic review of 11 randomized controlled trials showed a statistically significant reduction in the risk of infectious complications and a statistically nonsignificant reduction in the risk of death with enteral feedings compared to parenteral nutrition.[130] The benefits of using enteral nutrition over parenteral nutrition include a decrease in systemic inflammation markers[131] and a decrease in expense.[132–134] If parenteral nutrition must be used, it should not be initiated within the first 5 days of admission due to the higher inflammatory response that is present in the beginning of the disease process.[135]

The timing of the start of nutrition support, either parenteral or enteral, varies widely in clinical practice. A systematic review that evaluated the timing of the initiation of enteral nutrition support found that initiation within the first 48 hours of admission showed significant benefits over the use of PN.[136] A review of several randomized controlled trials found a decreased risk of death in studies where enteral nutrition was started within 48 hours of admission.[129]

The feasibility of placing a nasogastric versus nasojejunal tube is important when considering the route of enteral feeding. In a study comparing nasoduodenal feeds in healthy volunteers versus patients with pancreatitis, those with pancreatitis had decreased pancreatic secretions.[137] This may in part contribute to the success seen in two trials with nasogastric feeds. There were no differences in clinical outcomes, pain medication requirements, or differences in C-reactive protein (CRP) in nasogastric- versus nasojejunal-fed patients with severe pancreatitis.[138,139] Another review of 20 randomized controlled trials reported that use of polymeric versus semi-elemental formula showed no statistically significant difference in feeding tolerance, infectious complications, and mortality. There is a lack of sound clinical evidence to support the recommendations for immunonutrition and probiotics.[140]

As the patient improves clinically, low-fat oral feeds are initiated, and slowly advanced, as enteral feeds are weaned to a normal diet.

Cholestatic Liver Disease

Biliary atresia is one of the more common chronic cholestatic liver diseases that presents in infants, and requires surgical intervention. Alagille syndrome, Byler syndrome, primary biliary cirrhosis, and primary sclerosing cholangitis are cholestatic liver diseases seen in childhood through adulthood. Long-term use of parenteral nutrition can lead to cholestasis; a complete discussion of parenteral nutrition–induced cholestasis is found in Chapter 20, Parenteral Nutrition. In cholestatic disease, a decrease in biliary bile acids results in fat and fat-soluble vitamin malabsorption. As the liver damage progresses leading to cirrhosis, there is decreased synthesis of albumin and transport proteins, causing laboratory protein markers to become low. Nutritional concerns progress from fat malabsorption to protein-energy malnutrition.[141]

Nutrition Assessment

Patients with chronic cholestasis/cirrhosis can present with ascites and/or organomegaly, which will falsely elevate the patient's weight. Use of this elevated weight would skew the results of a calculated BMI or the weight-for-length or weight/height assessment on a growth chart. These measurements can underestimate the degree of malnutrition.[142] The use of tricep skinfold thickness and mid-arm circumference to assess subcutaneous fat and skeletal muscle mass has been suggested, but these measurements can also be skewed by edema.[141] These anthropometric measurements require calipers that are regularly recalibrated and staff that are trained in proper technique.

Nutrition Therapy

Chronic cholestasis in infancy and early childhood leads to increased calorie needs. Calorie needs have been suggested to be 125–150% of the RDA for ideal body weight in children.[143] Infants with biliary atresia require calories in the range of 120–200 kcal/kg/day.[144] Protein requirements should focus on providing equal to or greater than the RDA for protein in the nonencephalopathic patient. Recommendations for protein in infants have been made at 2–3 g/kg/day.[143] With encephalopathy, protein should be temporarily restricted below the RDA until mental status returns to normal.[145]

Cholestatic liver disease leads to decreased biliary bile acids, resulting in malabsorption of LCT. Bile is not required for solubilization of MCT, which are absorbed unmodified into the portal circulation. Formulas containing a high percentage of MCT oil or supplementing foods with MCT oil is often recommended to provide fat and calories, while minimizing steatorrhea.[143] MCTs do not, however, provide essential fatty acids or aid in the absorption of fat-soluble vitamins;[146] thus, a source of linoleic acid is essential. In a study of infants on a formula containing 3% of calories from linoleic acid, they developed essential fatty acid deficiency. These results show that due to malabsorption with hepatobiliary disease, infants should receive well above 3% of calories from linoleic acid.[147] For infants with biliary atresia receiving formulas, those containing 40–60% of the fat from MCT are recommended.[148] For premature infants, the formula Similac Special Care (Abbott) provides half of its fat source as MCT. For term infants, the formula Pregestimil (Mead Johnson) contains 55% of its fat source as MCT. For children over 1 year of age and older, Peptamen Junior (Nestlé) contains 60% of its fat as MCT.

In liver disease, the prevalence of fat-soluble vitamin deficiencies correlates with increasing bilirubin levels.[145] There is a wide array of supplemental and deficiency treatment doses throughout the literature. It is important to remember that the degree of fat malabsorption is unique to each patient's disease state and can change as treatments or medications are changed.

Vitamin A is stored in the liver, and requires retinol-binding protein to circulate throughout the body. As liver disease progresses, there is impaired synthesis of retinol-binding protein, which leads to low vitamin A levels without a true deficiency. Clinical judgment needs to be used in the review of both serum retinol and retinol-binding protein laboratory results. Supplementation recommendations range from 5000–15,000 international units (IU)/day orally. For severe deficiency, intramuscular injections may be used.[141,143]

Vitamin E is stored in the liver and transported via lipoproteins. In patients with high triglycerides and cholesterol levels, the vitamin E level may be falsely elevated. It is best to check serum vitamin E levels in conjunction with total serum lipids to assess for deficiency. In children less than 12 years of age, a ratio of less than 0.6 mg/g and in children over 12 years of age, a ratio less than 0.8 mg/g are indicative of a deficiency. Supplementation recommendations in pediatrics range from 20–25 IU/kg/day of vitamin E or 10–200 IU/kg/day of alpha-tocopherol or intramuscular injections. Recommendations in adults range from 400–800 IU/day of alpha-tocopherol. The use of D-alpha-tocopheryl polyethylene glycol 1000 succinate TPGS vitamin E enhances the absorption of other fat-soluble vitamins.[141,143]

In cholestatic and noncholestatic liver disease, metabolic bone disease has a multifactorial etiology that includes a decrease in insulin-like growth factor 1, hypogonadism, malnutrition, low BMI, loss of muscle mass, low calcium, and vitamin D deficiency. Vitamin D is hydroxylated in the liver, as one of the steps to forming its active state. Increased vitamin D levels lead to increased calcium and phosphorus absorption in the intestine. In cholestatic patients with fat malabsorption, less vitamin D is absorbed, which decreases calcium and phosphorus absorption. The nonabsorbed fatty acids bind to calcium in the intestine, further decreasing calcium absorption. Absorption of calcium is also reduced by corticosteroid therapy.[149,150] A 25-OH vitamin D level shows the pool of both dietary and endogenous vitamin D. One study recommends checking vitamin D levels every 1 to 2 months until it is within an appropriate range.[143] DEXA scans are the gold standard for assessing bone density, and all patients at risk should be screened.

Recommendations for supplementation of vitamin D differ significantly in light of the emerging research on vitamin D. Ng and Balistreri have recommended a standard dose of 400 units/day of cholecalciferol in cholestatic infants and children.[143] In adults with primary biliary cirrhosis and primary sclerosing cholangitis, 400–800 IU/day of vitamin D in conjunction with TPGS vitamin E to enhance absorption has been recommended. In an adult-based review article by Holick, he recommends 50,000 units of vitamin D_2 every week up to every day depending on the degree of fat malabsorption, or up to 10,000 units of vitamin D_3 every day for up to 5 months, then a maintenance dose of 50,000 units of vitamin D_2 every week.[98] The vast differences in these recommendations point to the importance of trending laboratory values and making dosage adjustments based on each patient's clinical response to supplementation.

Vitamin K deficiency is due to fat malabsorption and decreased absorption from gut flora alterations. This deficiency, as well as impaired hepatic synthesis of clotting factors, leads to prolonged prothrombin time (PT). If the abnormal PT is thought to be related to a vitamin K deficiency, the medical team can prescribe oral or intravenous supplementation. In a study of cholestatic children taking vitamin K supplementation with normal or near-normal PT, 54% were found to be vitamin K deficient per measure of a PIVKA-II level (protein induced by vitamin K absence).[151] Although following a PIVKA-II level is not widely done in clinical practice, it should be considered to assess for subclinical signs of vitamin K deficiency.

Zinc, magnesium, and calcium are also lost in the presence of fat malabsorption. Supplementation should be given, and adjusted as necessary to maintain adequate levels.

Liver Transplant

The most common disease requiring liver transplantation in childhood is biliary atresia (over 50% of cases). Other less prominent causes are inherited metabolic disorders (e.g., alpha-1-antitrypsin deficiency, tyrosinemia, and urea cycle defects), intra-hepatic cholestasis syndromes (e.g., Alagille syndrome, Byler syndrome), chronic hepatitis with cirrhosis, and all forms of acute liver failure. Indications for transplantation include hepatic failure, complications of portal hypertension (e.g., variceal bleeding, ascities), specific metabolic disorders, and malignancy.

The patient with end-stage liver disease awaiting transplantation presents a formidable challenge to the medical and nutritional team. The particular liver disease involved, the magnitude of liver dysfunction, the presence of complications, and the transplantation procedure itself combine to present a complex treatment process including meeting nutritional needs for healing and growth.

Nutrition Assessment

Pretransplant nutritional care involves assessment of the current status and development of a therapeutic nutritional plan tailored to the liver disease and degree of debilitation.

Patients with chronic cholestasis/cirrhosis can present with ascites and/or organomegaly, which will falsely elevate the patient's weight as occurs in patients with cholestatic liver disease. (See also the discussion under "Cholestatic Liver Disease.")

Pretransplant Nutrition Therapy

End-stage liver disease creates a hypermetabolic state that elevates the REE.[152] In the hypermetabolic state, once the body's glucose stores are exhausted, lean body mass and proteins will be broken down for gluconeogenesis. Long periods of fasting are not recommended. Protein should not be restricted in infants and children with end-stage liver disease and is often provided at levels above the RDA, unless encephalopathy is present.[143,144] If the end-stage liver disease is related to a cholestatic liver disease, then the decreased pool of bile acids will result in malabsorption of long-chain triglycerides. Medium-chain triglycerides should be used to provide calories and minimize steatorrhea, but MCTs do not provide essential fatty acids or aid in the absorption of fat-soluble vitamins.[143] For more specific macro- and micronutrient information, please refer to the "Cholestatic Liver Disease" section of this chapter.

Multiple studies have shown that preoperative malnutrition negatively affects the outcome of liver transplant. Height Z-score is a good indicator of pretransplant malnutrition. Severe growth retardation is linked to increased length of stay and increased hospital costs after transplant.[153] In a study of infants with bilary atresia listed for liver transplant, researchers found the post-transplant mortality and graft failure risks include weight/height that is below two standard deviations at the time of listing.[154] Close nutrition monitoring in end-stage liver disease and optimizing nutritional intake will maximize growth potential and nutritional status going into transplant.

Post-Transplant Nutrition Therapy

In many cases, the underlying disease is corrected by transplant; therefore, calorie and protein needs should be individualized to the patient's specific postoperative needs and nutritional status.

Immediately after transplant, early nutritional support should be implemented due to preoperative malnutrition, surgical stress, and postoperative catabolism.[155] Nutrition support should be initiated and slowly advanced to meet calorie and protein needs. The enteral formula should be chosen based on each patient's protein and fat composition needs. In a study evaluating tube feedings, nasointestinal tube feedings that were started post-transplant versus maintenance intravenous fluids maintained until an oral diet could be initiated showed improved nitrogen balance by the fourth postoperative day and less overall infections.[156]

The nutritional goal is catch-up growth to achieve an age-appropriate weight and height. Post-transplant studies show growth-retarded children transplanted after 2 years of age continue to have some linear growth retardation.[157,158] If transplanted prior to 2 years of age, patients are able to achieve heights similar to their age-matched peer group.[157] A 4-year pediatric study reported catch-up growth and normal neurodevelopment in infants transplanted prior to 1 year of age.[159] Linear growth achievements can also be analyzed by the underlying disease that necessitated transplant. Patients with biliary atresia and alpha-1-antitrypsin achieve better linear growth post-transplant than patients with fulminant liver failure or chronic hepatitis.[159]

Drug–nutrient interactions are key considerations post-transplant. Steroids are known to affect linear growth and bone health, and to contribute to hyperglycemia and diabetes mellitus.[160] Immunosuppressive medications also contribute to electrolyte and magnesium losses.

Concern regarding metabolic bone disease continues after liver transplant. Risk factors include continued corticosteroid use, malnutrition, muscle wasting, preexisting osteopenia/osteoporosis, and immunosuppressive agents. Bone loss is greatest in the first year after transplant.[161] Patients with cholestatic liver disease who undergo liver transplant improve their bone mineral density.[162] In a prospective pediatric study an increase in bone mineral density was noted at 3 months post-transplant along with improvements in 25-OH vitamin D levels.[163]

Another possibility that the dietitian and medical transplant team must keep in mind is transplant-acquired food allergies (TAFA). The first reported allergy post-transplant was a passive transfer of a peanut allergy from donor to liver recipient. Two more case studies were reported in children with no food allergies prior to transplant who developed food allergies 12 months and 7 months after transplant. Both children were on tacrolimus and all allergy symptoms were resolved on an elimination diet.[164] A newer study suggests risk factors for developing food allergies post-transplant include patients who are under the age of 1 year, have hypereosinophilia, or have Epstein-Barre virus (EBV) viremia.[165]

Short Bowel Syndrome

Short bowel syndrome (SBS) is a condition in which the patient has an anatomic or functional loss of more than 50% of the small intestine.[166] Typically SBS results from necrotizing enterocolitis (NEC), volvulus, intestinal atresias, gastroschisis, ruptured omphalocele, or vascular infarct.[166–168] The result of the injury and/or resection is decreased small intestine surface area, which leads to malabsorption and large volume watery diarrhea.[169] Although most patients have had a significant bowel resection, some patients may have had a rather small amount of bowel removed, but have poor motility and absorption by the remaining intestine.[169,170] The degree of malabsorption is dependent upon the extent of missing or injured bowel; most affected individuals have difficulty sustaining appropriate growth and development without nutritional support. Growth is a major concern in this population, affected not only by adequate nutrient provision, but also by absorption.

Intestinal adaptation is the process by which the remaining intestine grows, dilates, and changes via cellular hyperplasia and villous hypertrophy in order to compensate for its loss of surface area or function. Adaptation is the ultimate goal of treatment and is the key to successful withdrawal of parenteral nutrition (PN). This period of adaptation begins soon after resection and continues for the first few years postresection.[2,168] The ability of the intestine to adapt is largely dependent on how much intestine remains, the health of the remaining intestine, the presence or absence of the ileocecal valve (ICV), and whether the colon is in continuity with the small bowel. In infants, it is possible to survive with 20 to 40 cm of small bowel if the colon is present. Without a colon, at least 40 cm of small bowel is needed to survive.[2]

Nutrient and Fluid Absorption

Absorption of fluids and nutrients occurs throughout the small intestine and colon. Half of the mucosal surface is contained within the proximal one-fourth of the small intestine.[169] Figure 12-1 illustrates sites of nutrient absorption in the small intestine and colon, as well as the possible implications of intestinal resections of these areas.

The duodenum and jejunum are the primary sites of digestion and absorption of proteins, carbohydrates, lipids, and most vitamins and minerals. Resections in these areas result in decreased surface area for absorption, causing increased osmotic diarrhea and loss of water-soluble vitamins.[171] Loss of calcium, iron, and magnesium can occur, as well as losses of trace minerals such as copper, chromium, and manganese. Decreased secretin, cholecystokinin, and pancreatic/biliary secretions result in decreased digestion and absorption of fats, proteins, and fat-soluble vitamins. Decreased disaccharidase secretion allows increased substrate for bacterial overgrowth because carbohydrates are not fully metabolized when these enzymes are decreased.

Decreased surface area from ileal resection results in decreased vitamin B_{12} absorption. Decreased bile salt reabsorption in the ileum increases bile acid in the stool and decreases enterohepatic circulation.[171] This causes decreased bile acid pools and decreased micelle formation. Decreased absorption of long chain fats results, as well as decreased absorption of fat-soluble vitamins. There is increased steatorrhea, and the potential for cholelithiasis and renal oxalate stones. Many gut hormones that affect GI motility are produced in the ileum, including enteroglucagon and peptide YY. Resection of the ileum can impair the nutrient-regulated gut motility.[172]

With jejunal resection, the ileum can assume the place of the jejunum in some ways to absorb less site-specific nutrients such as electrolytes and fluid, which the jejunum is responsible for when the bowel is intact.[173] However, due to some of the specific roles of the ileum, the jejunum cannot assume the role of the ileum. For example, loss of the terminal ileum requires B_{12} provision via intramuscular or nasal route for absorption because there are no other sites for B_{12} absorption in the proximal ileum, duodenum, or jejunum. With loss of the jejunum there are no absolute requirements for supplementation, because absorption will vary depending on the individual child.

The ileocecal valve (ICV) slows transit time and acts as a barrier to bacteria moving into the small bowel from the colon.[171] Resection of the ICV leads to vitamin B_{12} and possibly folate deficiency because sites for absorption are often lost with adjacent ileum resection. Combined ICV and ileum resections lead to decreased transit time and a large influx of nutrients into the large intestine, which can result in malabsorption. Bacterial overgrowth in the small bowel can be a major problem and lead to increased diarrhea and malabsorption.[166] Some centers routinely cycle patients on either a single antibiotic such as metronidazole for 1 to 2 weeks every month or a combination of two alternating antibiotics such as metronidazole and neomycin for overgrowth treatment. Length of treatment for overgrowth varies depending on the response to treatment; some children will continue treatment for only a few weeks whereas others can continue for several years.

The colon absorbs water, salvages malabsorbed carbohydrate, and absorbs sodium. Colonic resection decreases water and sodium reabsorption and increases risk for dehydration.[171]

Nutritional Adequacy

Growth is the ultimate measurement of nutritional adequacy. Caloric and protein needs are dependent on age and state of growth, as well as degree of overall malabsorption. Caloric needs vary from child to child, and can be as low as normal for age or quite increased. No good studies or data exist for recommendations on specific calorie levels, and clinical judgment along with known intake levels and growth outcomes for the specific child should be used. Adequate carbohydrate, fat, micronutrients, and fluid provision are also dependent on age and state of growth; however, they are more influenced by resection site. Micronutrients should be monitored routinely depending upon the specific anatomy of the individual and should be replaced as needed in available forms (enteral, intramuscular, or parenteral). The most common deficiencies are the fat-soluble vitamins, vitamin B_{12}, zinc, and iron.

Phases of Nutrition Therapy

Nutritional management of the pediatric patient with short bowel syndrome can be divided into four phases. The first phase involves fluid, electrolyte, and hemodynamic stability, and PN initiation. The second phase is the initiation of enteral nutrition (EN). The third phase is weaning of PN and advancing oral nutrition and EN. The fourth phase is long-term nutrient provision and growth monitoring.

Phase 1: Fluid, Electrolyte, and Hemodynamic Stability and PN Initiation

The first phase in the treatment of a new patient with SBS is PN while the GI tract is recovering postoperatively. PN should be started as soon as possible via central line.[170] Initial PN macronutrient needs vary depending on the infant and the clinical situation. Initiation of dextrose should be at 5–7 mg/kg/min and advancement by 1–3 mg/kg/min to an endpoint goal of 12–14 mg/kg/min.[170] Various institutions are reporting anecdotal success with pushing the endpoint goal to as much as 16 mg/kg/min to use as little lipid as possible while providing adequate calories. Initiation of lipid at 1 g/kg/day advancing 1 g/kg/day to an endpoint of no more than 3 g/kg/day is recommended.[170] Initiation of protein at 1–2 g/kg/day and advancement by 1–2 g/kg/day to an endpoint of 3–3.5 g/kg/day is recommended.[170]

Initial stool output, whether per rectum or ileostomy, typically increases needs for sodium, magnesium, and zinc to compensate for losses.[170,174] Serum zinc is not always reflective of zinc status, but monitoring trends can be helpful. An infant not responding to adequate caloric and protein provision, but with high output stool volume may benefit from additional zinc supplementation despite normal serum values. PN should be monitored carefully to minimize complications associated with PN therapy. Parenteral nutrition associated liver disease (PNALD) is a major cause of death in patients with SBS.[175] See Chapter 20 for PN management details for maximizing calcium and phosphorus and for preventing associated complications with use of PN.

Phase 2: Initiation of Enteral Nutrition

EN is the next phase of nutrition therapy, and should be started as soon as the patient is stable and gastrointestinal motility has returned as a necessary component to promote intestinal adaptation.[2,168] There is consensus that at least initially, EN infusion should be continuous via the gastric route.[2,168,176] A slow continuous infusion is thought to bathe the lumen and allow for better nutrient absorption.[2,168] In some conditions, if infants have a proximal high ostomy and a mucous fistula connected to a substantial portion of the bowel, refeeding the mucous fistula with the proximal bowel content can be done to prevent diffuse atrophy.[177]

If available from mom or via donor, breast milk should be used in infants with SBS to initiate EN. The abundance of growth factor and nucleotides available in breast milk versus formula makes it the ideal choice for these children.[168,170] If breast milk is unavailable, however, controversy exists as to the ideal formula for infants with SBS. Each infant is different, and a formula should be selected to start EN depending on his or her clinical situation.

Polymeric formulas have been shown to be better for mucosal adaptation in adults and in animal studies.[168,178,179] In pediatrics, hydrolyzed and even amino acid formulas are often preferred. In this population, mucosal breakdown, bowel dilation, and bacterial overgrowth all predispose the infants to higher rates of food allergies; thus, the provision of an amino acid formulation is a considerable advantage.[180] A 2001 prospective, randomized, cross-over trial involving 10 children with SBS and lasting 60 days found no difference in energy and nitrogen balance when using a hydrolyzed protein formula versus an intact protein formula. This study is often cited in pediatric SBS guides.[181] It should be noted, however, that the study did not measure adaptation, diarrhea, or perceived tolerance of formulas. Some advocate amino acid formulations for infants and more intact formulations for toddlers and older children, whereas others recommend use of a protein hydrolysate formula.[2,176]

If fat malabsorption exists from bile acid hypersecretion, PNALD, or pancreatic insufficiency, use of a formula with a higher percentage of fat from MCTs is preferred.[180] Even though MCTs increase the osmotic load slightly and offer fewer calories per gram than LCTs, the lack of a micelle needed for absorption makes them the ideal fats in this situation.[180] If bilirubin levels are elevated, use of a very high MCT formula such as Mead Johnson's Pregestimil (55% MCT oil) is recommended.[180,182]

In rat studies, the use of LCTs have facilitated better adaptation of the remaining bowel than the use of MCTs.[182,183] Many have extrapolated this to indicate that LCTs are better than MCTs for infants with SBS and facilitate better intestinal adaption.[168,176,179] Interesting work has been done recently in adults with SBS indicating that use of oleic acid (LCT) supplementation actually did not cause a delay in transit time (which is thought to stimulate adaption better) and actually decreased energy absorption by 14% versus placebo overall.[185]

The fact that this is an adult study with a small sample size ($n = 7$) poses limitations for its use in pediatrics. However, it does make an argument in the setting of a human model with LCTs. Several institutions advocate using a blend of both MCTs and LCTs.[180,182] Most typically in practice, amino acid formulations with higher MCT content such as Elecare (33% MCT, Abbott Labs) and Neocate Infant DHA/ARA (33% MCT, Nutricia) are preferred over lower MCT oil formulations such as standard Neocate Infant (5% MCT, Nutricia).

Phase 3: Advancement of EN and Oral Feeding While Weaning PN

The third stage of nutritional management should be started while the infant is still hospitalized, if possible. PN should be weaned as EN and oral tolerance increases, stool output decreases, and growth is achieved. The ultimate goal is elimination of PN because cholestasis occurs in 30% to 60% of children with SBS; liver failure develops in 3% to 19% of children who acquired SBS in the neonatal period.[186–188] Gradual advances in EN/oral intake are dependent upon gastric tolerance, stool output (frequency and consistency), and rate of growth.[2] This stage can be quite lengthy, depending on setbacks and rate of advancement. Stool should be monitored for frequency, acidosis, and reducing substances as EN and oral intake advances. PN should be cycled when 35–50% of EN goal has been achieved and if blood sugar levels are stable. Two to 6 hours off of PN each day allow for GI hormone release.[170,180] As PN is weaned, vitamin and mineral status should be closely monitored and supplemented as needed because the absorption route has changed and the potential for malabsorption has increased.

Oral feedings, even the smallest of volumes, should be started as soon as clinically stable and feasible, to prevent oral aversion.[2,168,176,180] Feeding aversions are common in this population for many reasons. First and foremost, prematurity and severe illness delay oral attempts and result in immature feeding skills.[170] Furthermore, frequent vomiting and diarrhea prevent pleasurable associations with food.[168] Oral feeds can be introduced as developmentally appropriate, and general precautions regarding monitoring for food allergies should be practiced. If the infant is unable to take any oral feedings, an oral motor stimulation program should be in place to help develop feeding skills. Feeding aversion in patients with SBS is notoriously difficult to treat, and the focus is on prevention of aversion as feasible.[2,179,189]

Phase 4: Maximizing Oral and Enteral Nutrition

The fourth phase of management is long-term advancement of EN and maximizing oral intake. Once EN is at goal, it may be beneficial to start fiber therapy if the colon (or most of it) is present. The conversion of complex carbohydrate to short-chain fatty acids (SCFAs; acetate, propionate, and butyrate) in the colon can cause significant caloric reuptake by colonic cells.[2,179,188] Additionally, SCFAs also stimulate sodium and water reabsorption, which aids in fluid management. Addition of a 1–3% pectin solution can decrease reducing substances and improve pH to allow for more fermentation of carbohydrates.[170] In orally fed patients, use of guar gum fiber such as Nestlé's Resource Benefiber (hospital grade) at 0.5 g/kg/day may be used as a more palatable replacement to pectin.

As the intestine adapts, the goal is to normalize the EN schedule while promoting oral intake and growth. If possible, EN should be cycled overnight to maximize oral intake in the daytime hours. It is necessary that children find palatable beverages providing complete nutrition to help lessen EN dependence and increase oral intake. Higher calorie formulas typically have higher osmolality and may interfere with desired gain. However, products such as Boost Kids Essentials 1.5 (Nestlé) provide a high percentage of calories from fat, with a lower osmolality.

Overly strict guidelines for oral intake should be discouraged. Each child needs to be carefully assessed because nutrient needs differ due to the amount and location of the resection. General guidelines include limiting simple sugars (juice, candy) in order to minimize osmotic diarrhea.[2,168,170,179,180,182,190] Fat and protein should be adequate to support growth. Soluble fiber of at least 5–10 g/day as pectin/guar gum is beneficial to slow the gut transit time.[168,176,182] Those with a colon have an additional bonus of caloric reuptake from provision of soluble fiber in the diet. Lactose should be avoided only if symptoms are reported with ingestion.[2,182] Liberal salt intake at meals helps make the meal bolus isotonic in the gut.[182]

Much has been reported on the guidelines for adults with SBS, and many of these have been adapted to the child.[182] In adults with a colon, 50–60% of kcal from CHO and 20–30% of kcal from fat is recommended as a balance of LCT and MCT. Those without a colon are encouraged to consume 40–50% kcal from carbohydrates and 30–40% of kcal from fat with more LCTs than MCTs. Isotonic fluids are always encouraged, regardless of the presence or absence of a colon. However, hypo-osmolar fluids and higher sodium-containing fluids are encouraged for those without a colon. Sometimes oral rehydration solutions (ORS) are recommended for those without a colon (see Table 12-3).

Increased renal oxalate stones occur with intestinal resections because of increased enteric absorption of oxalate (enteric hyperoxaluria).[191] Renal oxalate stones are well documented in the literature for adults with SBS, and up to 30% of this population develop stones.[2,182] However, the incidence is relatively rare in children.[191,192] A retrospective 5-year review at a tertiary pediatric medical center by Chang-Kit reported 72 cases of urolithiasis. Of note, seven patients had Crohn's disease, seven had cystic fibrosis, and four had SBS.[192] It is not routine to restrict oxalates in patients with Crohn's disease or cystic fibrosis. Thus, empiric restrictions, especially in the setting of a history of food aversions, are not necessary. A low oxalate diet or provision of extra calcium is recommended if 24-hour urinary oxalate levels are elevated.[182] Urinary oxalate levels should be monitored annually in this population.

Other Treatments

Although growth hormone and glutamine have been used in some adult studies,[193–195] more research is needed and there are no current recommendations for their use in pediatrics.[182,193–196] Alternative surgical procedures such as bowel lengthening, tapering enteroplasty, or intestinal transplant may be considered for those patients who are not making progress.[172,197–199]

Intestinal Transplantation

Small bowel transplantation may be indicated for patients who have attempted and failed standard medical, nutritional, and surgical management, especially in the setting of life-threatening liver dysfunction.[167,178] Surgical transplant can involve the isolated intestine, liver and intestine, or multivisceral transplantation that includes stomach, pancreas, and the entire small bowel, which can include or preclude the liver as well.[167] Small bowel with a concurrent liver transplant is more frequent in children because of the association of PNALD in children.[178] A handful of centers in the United States specialize in small bowel transplants. Care for the post-transplant patient varies from center to center. Management involves immunosuppression and nutritional rehabilitation with PN, EN, and oral feeding post-operatively.[167,178] Evaluation and monitoring similar to any transplant should occur in each child by an RD after transplant. Chronic rejection remains an issue, with centers of excellence reporting a 1-year survival rate of 95% compared to the 5-year survival rate of 77%.[167]

Case Study

Nutrition Assessment

Client history: PL is a 14-year-old male who presents with diarrhea for 3 weeks that has recently become bloody. He now has more than five bowel movements per day. PL complains of fatigue and per mother has experienced an 8-pound weight loss since pediatrician's appointment 2 months prior.

Food/nutrition-related history: PL reports not feeling as hungry as usual. His mother states he is only eating about 50–75% of what he used to. PL does not take any vitamin, mineral, or herbal supplements. He also does not drink any oral nutritional supplements.

Biochemical data, medical tests, and procedures:
(↓= below normal)
Na: 142 Cl: 102 BUN: 7 Glucose: 82 Ca: 8.9 ↓
H/H: 10.2 ↓ / 34.3 ↓ MCV: 74.1 ↓
K: 3.6 ↓ CO_2: 27 ↑ Cr: 0.6
Albumin: 3.1 CRP: 5.9 ↑

Medical Workup

EGD and colonoscopy: visual inflammation throughout small bowel and colon; biopsies pending. Findings consistent with Crohn's disease per attending. Plan to start Pentasa and enteral nutrition therapy to treat suspected disease and malnutrition.

Anthropometric Measurements

Weight: 36.3 kg

BMI: 15.3 (< 5%)

Height: 154 cm

Std Ht for age: 164 cm

% of Std Ht for age: 94%

Estimated Nutrition Needs

Calories: REE (1286) × 1.7–1.9 = 2185–2445 per day

Protein: 1–1.8 g/kg/day

Fluid: 1825 mL/day

Assessment

Percentage of ideal body weight and percentage of standard height for age indicate mild wasting and mild stunting of growth. Significant weight loss of 9% of his usual body weight has been observed over the past 2 months. Per patient and family, his diet prior to admission was likely hypocaloric, with possible dehydration due to diarrhea. Labs reflect low potassium and albumin levels, elevated CO_2 and CRP levels, as well as microcytic anemia. Per hospital protocol, PL may benefit from receiving 80% of estimated total caloric goal via enteral nutrition because this is believed to induce remission of disease and to aid in the treatment of malnutrition.

Nutrition Diagnoses

Based on the above information, a nutritional problem or diagnosis can be made.

Nutrition Interventions

Initiate EN: Recommend Peptamen 1.5 starting at 25 mL/hr, advancing by 25 mL every 5 hours, to a goal of 125 mL/hr × 10 hours per night, via nasogastric tube.

Initial/Brief Nutrition Education

Help patient to identify foods and nutritional supplement to meet 20% of estimated calorie needs orally. Outcome: patient will consume 20% of estimated calorie needs orally.

Coordination of Other Care During Nutrition Care

Discuss need for vitamin D and zinc levels on nutrition support rounds and signout to outpatient RD via email after patient's discharge. Outcome: labs ordered and evaluated, supplementation started if indicated. Outpatient appointment and email confirmed.

Questions for the Reader

1. What is the patient's IBW and percentage of IBW?
2. What is his estimated energy needs per kg?
3. Write at least one PES statement.
4. How many calories, how much protein, and how much free water are provided in this amount of tube feeding?
5. What would you want to monitor and evaluate during his hospitalization, and what are your plans for discharge?

Websites

Websites that provide additional information on the various GI conditions are listed below.

General Gastrointestinal

http://www.healthsystem.virginia.edu/internet/digestive-health/nutrition/resources.cfm
http://www.naspghan.org

Celiac

National Foundation for Celiac Awareness (NFCA)
http://www.celiaccentral.org
Celiac.com
http://www.celiac.com
Clan Thompson's Celiac Site
http://www.celiacsite.com
Online sources for gluten-free food/recipes
http://www.glutenfree.com
http://www.glutenfreemall.com
http://www.glutenfreeda.com

Magazines for People with Food Allergies and Sensitivities

http://www.glutenfreeliving.com
http://www.livingwithout.com

Crohn's and Colitis Foundation of America

http://www.ccfa.org

REFERENCES

1. World Health Organization, Department of Child and Adolescent Health and Development. *The Treatment of Diarrhoea—A Manual for Physicians and Other Senior Health Care Workers*, 4th ed. rev. Geneva: World Health Organization; 2005.
2. Corkins MR, Scolapino J. Diarrhea. In: Merritt R, ed. *The ASPEN Nutrition Support Practice Manual*, 2nd ed. Silver Spring, MD: ASPEN; 2005:207–210.
3. American Academy of Pediatrics. Oral therapy for acute diarrhea. In: Kleinman RE, ed. *Pediatric Nutrition Handbook*, 6th ed. Elk Grove Village, IL: American Academy of Pediatrics; 2009:651–659.
4. Glass RI, Lew JF, Gangarosa RE, LeBaron CW, Ho MS. Estimates of morbidity and mortality rates for diarrhea diseases in American children. *J Pediatr*. 1991;118:S27–S33.
5. King CK, Glass R, Breese JS, Duggan C. Management of acute gastroenteritis among children: oral rehydration, maintenance and nutritional therapy. *MMWR* 2003;52:1–16.
6. American Academy of Pediatrics, Provisional Committee on Quality Improvement, Subcommittee on Acute Gastroenteritis. Practice parameter: the management of acute gastroenteritis in young children. *Pediatrics*. 1996;97:424–435
7. Brown KH. Appropriate diets for the rehabilitation of malnourished children in the community setting. *Acta Paediatr Scand*. 1991;374(Suppl):151.
8. Brown KH, Peerson JM, Fontaine O. Use of non-human milks in the dietary management of young children with acute diarrhea: a meta-analysis of clinical trials. *Pediatrics*. 1994;93: 17–27.
9. Brown KH, Perez F, Peerson J, et al. Effect of dietary fiber (soy polysaccharide) on the severity, duration, and nutritional outcome of acute, watery diarrhea in children. *Pediatrics*. 1993;92:241–247.
10. Burks AW, Vanderhoof JA, Mehra S, Ostrom KM, Baggs G. Randomized clinical trial of soy formula with and without added fiber in antibiotic-induced diarrhea. *J Pediatr*. 2001;139:578–582.
11. Bhutta ZA, Ghishan F, Lindley K, Memon IA, Mittal S, Rhoads JM. Persistent and chronic diarrhea and malabsorption: working group report of the Second World Congress of Pediatric Gastroenterology, Hepatology, and Nutrition. *J Pediatr Gastroenterol Nutr*. 2004;39:S711–S716.
12. Kolacek S, Grguric J, Perci M, et al. Home-made modular diet versus semi-elemental formula in the treatment of chronic diarrhoea of infancy: a prospective randomized trial. *Eur J Pediatr*. 1996;155:997–1001.
13. Burpee T. Diarrheal diseases. In: Duggan C, Watkins, JB, Walker W, eds. *Nutrition in Pediatrics*, 4th ed. Hamilton, Ontario: BC Decker; 2008:631–640.
14. Uauy R. Novel oligosaccharides in human milk: understanding mechanisms may lead to better prevention of enteric and other infections. *J Pediatr*. 2004:145(3):283–285.
15. Van Niel CW. Probiotics: not just for treatment anymore. *Pediatrics*. 2004;115(1):174–177.
16. Hattner JA. Digestive health: probiotics and prebiotics for children. *Nutr Focus*. 2009;24(3):1–2.
17. Dai D, Walker WA. Protective nutrients and bacterial colonization in the immature human gut. *Adv Pediatr*. 1999;46:353–382.
18. Morrow AL, Ruiz-Palacios GM, Altaye M, et al. Human milk oligosaccharides are associated with protection against diarrhea in breast-fed infants. *J Pediat*. 2004;145:297–303.
19. Ziegler E, Vanderhoof JA, Petschow B, Mitmesser SH et al. *J Pediatr Gastroenterol Nutr*. 2007;44;359–364.
20. Thibault H, Aubert-Jacquin C, Goulet O. Effects of long-term consumption of a fermented infant formula with (Bifidobacterium breve c50 and Streptococcus thermophilus 065) on acute diarrhea in healthy infants. *J Pediatr Gastroenterol Nutr*. 2004;39(2):147–152.
21. Saavedra JM, Abi-Hanna A, Moore N, Yolken RH. Long-term consumption of infant formulas containing live probiotics bacteria: tolerance and safety. *Am J Clin Nutr*. 2004;79:261–279.
22. Salazar-Lindo E, Figueroa-Quintanilla D, Caciano MI, Reto-Valiente V, Chauviere G, Colin P. Effectiveness and safety of Lactobacillus LB in the treatment of mild acute diarrhea in children. *J Pediatr Gastroenterol Nutr*. 2007;44:571–576.
23. Weizman A, Asli G, Alsheikh A. Effect of a probiotics infant formula on infections in child care center: comparison of two probiotics agents. *Pediatrics*. 2004;115(1):5–9.

24. Snyder JD, Merson MH. The magnitude of the global problem of acute diarrhea disease: a review of active surveillance data. *Bull World Health Organ*. 1982;60:605–613.
25. American Academy of Pediatrics. Chronic diarrhea disease. In: Kleinman RE, ed. *Pediatric Nutrition Handbook*, 6th ed. Elk Grove Village, IL: American Academy of Pediatrics; 2009:637–649.
26. Klish WJ. Chronic diarrhea. In: Walker WA, Watkins JB, eds. *Nutrition in Pediatrics: Basic Science and Clinical Applications*. Hamilton, ON: Decker; 1997:603.
27. Chronic diarrhea in children: a nutritional disorder [editorial]. *Lancet*. 1987;1:143.
28. Lo CW, Walker WA. Chronic protracted diarrhea of infancy: a nutritional disorder. *Pediatrics*. 1983;72:786.
29. Evaluation of an algorithm for the treatment of persistent diarrhea: a multicentre study. *Bull World Health Organ*. 1996;74(5):479–489.
30. Baker SS, Davis AM. Hypocaloric oral therapy during an episode of diarrhea and vomiting can lead to severe malnutrition. *J Pediatr Gastroenterol Nutr*. 1998;27:1–5.
31. Solomon SM, Kirby KF. The refeeding syndrome: a review. *J Parenter Enteral Nutr*. 1985;85:28–36.
32. Stocks RJ, Davies DP, Allen F. Loss of breast milk nutrients during tube feeding. *Arch Dis Child*. 1985;60:164.
33. Greer FR, McCormick A, Loker J. Changes in fat concentration of human milk during the delivery by intermittent bolus and continuous mechanical pump infusion. *J Pediatr*. 1984;105:745.
34. Narayan I, Singh B, Harvey D. Fat loss during feeding of human milk. *Arch Dis*. 1984;59:475.
35. Lavin M, Clark RM. The effect of short-term refrigeration of milk and the addition of breast milk fortifier on the delivery of lipids during tube feeding. *J Pediatr Gastroenterol Nutr*. 1989;8:496.
36. WHO/UNICEF joint statement. Clinical management of acute diarrhea. 2005. Available at: http://www.WHO/FCH/CAH/04.7 or http://www.unicef.org/publications/index_21433. Accessed August 10, 2010.
37. Lukacik M, Thomas L, Aranda JV. A meta-analysis of the effects of oral zinc in the treatment of acute and persistent diarrhea. *Pediatrics*. 2008;121(2):326–336. unicef.org/publications/index_21433.html
38. Lazzerini M, Ronfani L. Oral zinc for treating diarrhea in children [review]. *Cochrane Library*. 2009;4:1–67.
39. Lee PC, Werlin SL. Carbohydrates. In: Baker RD Jr, Baker SS, Davis AM, eds. *Pediatric Parenteral Nutrition*. New York: Chapman and Hall; 1997:103.
40. Parker P, Stroop S, Greene H. A controlled comparison of continuous versus intermittent feeding in the treatment of infants with intestinal disease. *J Pediatr*. 1987;99:360.
41. Thobani S, Molla AM, Snyder JD. Nutritional therapy for persistent diarrhea. In: Baker SS, Baker RD Jr., Davis AM, eds. *Pediatric Enteral Nutrition*. New York: Chapman and Hall; 1994:291.
42. Sazawal S, Black RE, Bhan MK, Bhandari N, Sinha A, Jalla S. Zinc supplementation in young children with acute diarrhea in India. *N Engl J Med*. 1995;333:839–844.
43. Bhutta ZA, Black RE, Brown KH, et al. Prevention of diarrhea and pneumonia by zinc supplementation in children in developing countries: pooled analysis of randomized controlled trials. Zinc Investigators' Collaborative Group. *J Pediatr*. 1999;135:689–697.
44. Bhutta ZA, Bird SM, Black RE, et al. Therapeutic effects of oral zinc in acute and persistent diarrhea in children in developing countries: pooled analysis of randomized controlled trials. *Am J Clin Nutr*. 2000;72:1516–1522.
45. Heinig MJ, Brown KH, Lonnerdal B, Dewey KG. Zinc supplementation does not affect growth, morbidity or motor development of US term breastfed infants at 4–10 mo of age. *Am J Clin Nutr*. 2006;84:594–601
46. Keohane PP, Grimble CK, Brown B, et al. Influence of protein composition and hydrolysis method on intestinal absorption of protein in man. *Gut*. 1985;26:907.
47. Hegarty JE, Fairclough PD, Moriarity KJ, et al. Comparison of plasma and intraluminal amino acid profiles in man after meals containing a protein hydrolysate and equivalent amino acid mixture. *Gut*. 1982;23:670.
48. Baker SS, Liptak GS, Colletti RB, et al. Constipation in infants and children: evaluation and treatment. A medical position statement of the North American Society for Pediatric Gastroenterology and Nutrition, *J Pediatr Gastroenterol Nutr*.1999;29(5):612–626. Erratum in: *J Pediatr Gastroenterol Nutr*. 2000;30(1):109.
49. Goldberg D. Clinical assessment. In: Cox JH, ed. *Nutrition Manual for At-Risk Toddlers and Infants*. Chicago: Precept Press; 1997:59.
50. Dwyer JT. Dietary fiber for children: how much? *Pediatrics*. 1995;96(5):1019–1022.
51. Oski FA. Iron fortified formulas and gastrointestinal symptoms in infants: a controlled study. *Pediatrics*. 1980;66:168–170.
52. Reeves JD, Yip R. Lack of adverse side effects of oral ferrous sulfate therapy in 1 year old infants. *Pediatrics*. 1985;75:352–355.
53. Nelson SE, Ziegler EE, Copeland AM, et al. Lack of adverse reactions to iron fortified formula. *Pediatrics*. 1988;81:360–364.
54. American Academy of Pediatrics, Committee on Nutrition American Academy of Pediatrics. Iron fortified formulas. *Pediatrics*. 1999;104:119–123 (reaffirmed November 2002).
55. Sherman PM, Hassall E, Fagundes-Neto U, et al. A global, evidence-based consensus on the definition of gastroesophageal reflux disease in the pediatric patient. *Am J Gastroenterol*. 2009;104(5):1278–1295.
56. Rudolph CD, Mazur LJ, Liptak GS, et al. Guidelines for evaluation and treatment of gastroesophageal reflux in infants and children: recommendations of the North American Society for Pediatric Gastroenterology and Nutrition. *J Pediatr Gastroenterol Nutr*. 2001;32(Suppl 2):S1–S31.
57. Vandenplas Y, Rudolph CD, Di Lorenzo C, et al. Pediatric gastroesophageal reflux clinical practice guidelines: joint recommendations of the North American Society for Pediatric Gastroenterology, Hepatology, and Nutrition and the European Society for Pediatric Gastroenterology, Hepatology, and Nutrition. *J Pediatr Gastroenterol Nutr*. 2009;49(4):498–547.
58. Horvath A, Dziechciarz P, Szajewska H. The effect of thickened-feed interventions on gastroesophageal reflux in infants: systematic review and meta-analysis of randomized, controlled trials [review]. *Pediatrics*. 2008;122(6):e1268–e1277. Erratum in: *Pediatrics*. 2009;123(4):1254.
59. Heyman, MB, Committee on Nutrition. Lactose intolerance in infants, children, and adolescents. *Pediatrics*. 2006;118:1279–1286.
60. Lifshitz CH. Breath hydrogen testing in infants with diarrhea. In: Lifshitz F, ed., *Carbohydrate Intolerance in Infancy*. New York: Marcel Dekker; 1982:31–42.

61. Nevin-Folino N. Pediatric Nutrition Practice Group. Lactose controlled diet. *Pediatric Manual of Clinical Dietetics,* 2nd ed. Chicago: American Dietetic Association, 2008:635–640.
62. Kretchmer N. Lactose and lactase: a historical perspective. *Gastroenterology*. 1971;61:805–813.
63. Sahi T. Genetics and epidemiology of adult-type hypolactasia. *Scand J Gastroenterol Suppl*. 1994;202:7–20.
64. Paige DM, Bayless TM, Mellitis ED, Davis L. Lactose malabsorption in preschool black children. *Am J Clin Nutr*. 1977;30:1018–1022.
65. Lloyd ML, Olsen WA. Disaccharide malabsorption. In: Haubrick WS, Schaffner F, Berk JE, eds. *Bockus Gastroenterology*, 5th ed. Philadelphia, PA: Saunders; 1995:1087–1100.
66. Nichols BL, Dudley MA, Nichols VN, et al. Effects of malnutrition on expression and activity of lactase in children. *Gastroenterology*. 1997;112:742–751.
67. World Health Organization, International Working Group on Persistent Diarrhoea. Evaluation of an algorithm for the treatment of persistent diarrhoea: a multicenter study. *Bull World Health Organ*. 1996;74:479–489.
68. Erasmus H, Ludwig-Auser H, Paterson P, Sun Dongmei, Sankaran K. Enhanced weight gain in preterm infants receiving lactase-treated feeds: a randomized, double-blind, controlled trial. *J Pediatr.* 2002;141:532–537.
69. Mobassaleh M, Montgomery R, Biller J, Grand R. Development of carbohydrate absorption in the fetus and neonate. *Pediatrics*. 1985;75(1 Pt 2):160–166.
70. MacLean WC, Fink BB. Lactose malabsorption by premature infants: magnitude and clinical significance. *J Pediatr*. 1980;97:383.
71. Carlson SJ, Rogers RR, Lombard KA. Effect of a lactase preparation on lactose content and osmolality of preterm and term infant formulas. *J Parenteral Enteral Nutr*. 1991;15:564–566.
72. Savilahti E, Launiala K, Kuitunen P. Congenital lactase deficiency: a clinical study on 16 patients. *Arch Dis Child*. 1983;58:246–252.
73. Torniainen S, Savilahti E, Jarvela I. Congenital lactase deficiency—a more common disease than previously thought. *Duodecim*. 2009;125(7):766–770.
74. Hill ID, Dirks MH, Liptak GS. Guidelines for the diagnosis and treatment of celiac disease in children: recommendations of the North American Society for Pediatric Gastroenterology, Hepatology and Nutrition. *J Ped Gastroenterol Nutr*. 2005;40(1):1–19.
75. Niewinski M. Advances in celiac disease and gluten free diet. *J Am Diet Assoc.* 2008;108(4):661–672.
76. Alehan F, Canan O, Cemil T, Erol I, Ozcay F. Increased risk for coeliac disease in paediatric patients with migraine. *Cephalalgia*. 2008;28:945–949.
77. Lurz E, Scheidegger U, Schibli S, Schoni, Spalinger J. Clinical presentation of celiac disease and the diagnostic accuracy of serologic markers in children. *Eur J Pediatr*. 2009;168:839–845.
78. Anderson R. Coeliac disease: current approach and future prospects. *Intern Med J*. 2008;38:790–799.
79. Murray J, See J. Gluten-free diet: the medical and nutrition management of celiac disease. *Nutr Clin Prac*. 2006;21:1–15.
80. Case S. *The Gluten Free Diet: Comprehensive Resource Guide*. Regina, Saskatchewan, Canada: Case Nutrition Consulting; 2006.
81. Sollid LM, Khosla C. Future therapeutic options for celiac disease. *Nat Clin Pract Gastroenterol Hepatol*. 2005;2(3):140–147.
82. American Dietetic Association. Celiac disease. ADA Evidence Analysis Library. Available at: http://www.adaevidencelibrary.com. Accessed September 9, 2009.
83. Cammarota G, Danese S, De Lorenzo A, et al. High prevalence of celiac disease in patients with lactose intolerance. *Digestion*. 2005;71:106–110.
84. Pellerin G, Turner J. Prevalence of metabolic bone disease in children with celiac disease is independent of symptoms at diagnosis. *J Ped Gastroenterol Nutr*. 2009;49:1–5.
85. Motil KJ, Grand RJ. Inflammatory bowel disease. In: Walker WA, Watkins JB, eds. *Nutrition in Pediatrics: Basic Science and Clinical Applications*. Hamilton, ON: Decker; 1997:516.
86. Motil KJ, Grand RJ. Nutritional management of inflammatory bowel disease. *Pediatr Clin North Am*. 1985;32:447.
87. Motil KJ, Grand RJ, Davis-Kraft L, Ferlic LL, Smith EO. Growth failure in children with inflammatory bowel disease: a prospective study. *United States Department of Agriculture/Agricultural Research Service Children's Nutrition Research Center, Houston, Texas Gastroenterology.* 1993;105(3):681–691.
88. Burnham JM, Shults J, Semeao E, et al. Body-composition alterations consistent with cachexia in children and young adults with Crohn disease. *Am J Clin Nutr.* 2005;82(2):413–420.
89. Azcue M, Rashid M, Friffiths A, Pencharz PB. Energy expenditure and body composition in children with Crohn's disease: effect of enteral nutrition and treatment with prednisolone. *Gut*. 1997;41:203–208.
90. Stokes MA, Hill GL. Total energy expenditure in patients with Crohn's disease: measurement by the combined body scan technique. *J Parenter Enteral Nutr.* 1993;17:3–7.
91. Takeda H, Ishihama K, Fukui T, et al. Significance of rapid turnover proteins in protein-losing gastroenteropathy. *Hepatogastroenterology*. 2003;50(54):1963–1965.
92. Hartman C, Eliakim R, Shamir R. Nutritional status and nutritional therapy in inflammatory bowel diseases. *World J Gastroenterol*. 2009;15(21):2570–2578.
93. Parrish CR, Krenitsky J, Willcutts K, Radigan AE. Gastrointestinal disease. In: Gottschlich MM, ed. *The ASPEN Nutrition Support Core Curriculum*. Silver Spring, MD: ASPEN; 2007:508–539.
94. Vagianos K, Bector S, McConnell J, Bernstein CN. Nutrition assessment of patients with inflammatory bowel disease. *J Parenter Enter Nutr*. 2007;31(4):311–319.
95. Filippi J, Al-Jaouni R, Wiroth JB, Hebuterne X, Schneider SM. Nutritional deficiencies in patients with Crohn's disease in remission. *Inflamm Bowel Dis*. 2006;12(3):185–191.
96. Semeao EJ, Jawad AF, Stouffer NO, Zemel BS, Piccoli DA, Stallings VA. Risk factors for low bone mineral density in children and young adults with Crohn's disease. *J Pediatr*. 1999;135(5):593–600.
97. Paganelli M, Albanese C, Borrelli O, et al. Inflammation is the main determinant of low bone mineral density in pediatric inflammatory bowel disease. *Inflamm Bowel Dis*. 2007;13(4):416–423.
98. Holick MF. Vitamin D deficiency. *N Engl J Med*. 2007;357(3):266–280.
99. Davis AM, Baker SS, Baker RD Jr, et al. Pediatric gastrointestinal disorders. In: Meritt RM, ed. *The ASPEN Nutrition Support Practice Manual*. Silver Spring, MD: ASPEN; 1998:27–30.

100. Prey S, Paul C. Effect of folic or folinic acid supplementation on methotrexate-associated safety and efficacy in inflammatory disease: a systematic review. *Br J Dermatol*. 2008;160(3):622–628.
101. Hyams JS. Crohn's disease. In: Hyams WS, Hyams JS, eds. *Pediatric Gastrointestinal Disease: Pathophysiology, Diagnosis, Management*. Philadelphia, PA: WB Saunders; 1993:750–764.
102. Levenstein S, Prantera C, Luzi C, et al. A low residue or normal diet in Crohn's disease: a prospective controlled trial of Italian patients. *Gut*. 1985;26:989.
103. Levi AJ. Diet in the management of Crohn's disease. *Gut*. 1985;26:985.
104. Mishkin S. Dairy sensitivity, lactose malabsorption, and elimination diets in inflammatory bowel disease. *Am J Clin Nutr*. 1997;65:564–567.
105. Siedman EG, Leliedo N, Ament M, et al. Nutritional issues in pediatric inflammatory bowel disease. *J Pediatr Gastroenterol Nutr*. 1991;12:424.
106. Berni Canani R, Terrin G, Borrelli O, et al. Short- and long-term therapeutic efficacy of nutritional therapy and corticosteroids in paediatric Crohn's disease. *Dig Liver Dis*. 2006;38(6):381–387.
107. Ruuska T, Savilahti E, Maki M, et al. Exclusive whole protein enteral diet versus prednisolone in the treatment of acute Crohn's disease in children. *J Pediatr Gastroenterol Nutr*. 1994;19(2):175–180.
108. Borrelli O, Cordischi L, Cirulli M, et al. Polymeric diet alone versus corticosteroids in the treatment of active pediatric Crohn's disease: a randomized controlled open-label trial. *Clin Gastroenterol Hepatol*. 2006;4(6):744–753.
109. Ludvigsson JF, Krantz M, Bodin L, et al. Elemental versus polymeric enteral nutrition in pediatric Crohn's disease: a multicentre randomized controlled trial. *Acta Paediatr*. 2004;93:327–335.
110. Zachos M, Tondeur M, Griffiths AM. Enteral nutritional therapy for induction of remission in Crohn's disease. *Cochrane Database of Systematic Reviews*. 2007;1:CD000542.
111. Akobeng AK, Thomas AG. Enteral nutrition for maintenance of remission of Crohn's disease. *Cochrane Database of Systematic Reviews*. 2007;3:CD005984.
112. Johnson T, Macdonald S, Hill SM, Thomas A, Murphy MS. Treatment of active Crohn's disease in children using partial enteral nutrition with liquid formula: a randomized controlled trial. *Gut*. 2006;55:356–361.
113. Verma S, Holdsworth CD, Giaffer GH. Does adjuvant nutritional support diminish steroid dependency in Crohn's disease? *Scand J Gastroenterol*. 2001;36:383–388.
114. Bamba T, Shimoyama T, Sadaki M, et al. Dietary fat attenuates the benefits of an elemental diet in active Crohn's disease: a randomized controlled trial. *Eur J Gastroenterol Hepatol*. 2003;15:151–157.
115. Gassull MA, Fernandez-Banares F, Cabre E, et al. Fat composition may be a clue to explain the primary therapeutic effect of enteral nutrition in Crohn's disease: results of a double blind randomized multicentre European trial. *Gut*. 2002;51(2):164–168.
116. Sakurai T, Matsui T, Yao T, et al. Short-term efficacy of enteral nutrition in the treatment of active Crohn's disease: a randomized, controlled trial comparing nutrient formulas. *J Parenter Enteral Nutr*. 2002;26(2):98–103.
117. DeLey M, de Vos R, Hommes DW, Stokkers P. Fish oil for induction of remission of ulcerative colitis. *Cochrane Database of Systemic Reviews*. 2007;4:CD005573.
118. Turner D, Steinhart AH, Griffiths AM. Omega 3 fatty acids for maintenance of remission of ulcerative colitis. *Cochrane Database of Systemic Reviews*. 2007;3:CD006443.
119. Turner D, Zlotkin SH, Shah PS, Griffiths AM. Omega 3 fatty acids for maintenance of remission of Crohn's disease. *Cochrane Database of Systemic Reviews*. 2009;1:CD006320.
120. Butterworth AD, Thomas AG, Akobeng AK. Probiotics for induction of remission in Crohn's disease. *Cochrane Database of Systemic Reviews*. 2008;3:CD006634.
121. Rolfe VE, Fortun PJ, Hawkey CJ, Bath-Hextall F. Probiotics for maintenance of remission in Crohn's disease. *Cochrane Database of Systematic Reviews*. 2006;4:CD004826.
122. Mallon P, McKay D, Kirk S, Gardiner K. Probiotics for induction of remission in ulcerative colitis. *Cochrane Database of Systematic Reviews*. 2007;4:CD005573.
123. Bannerjee K, Camacho-Hubner C, Babinska K, et al. Anti-inflammatory and growth-stimulating effects precede nutritional restitution during enteral feeding in Crohn disease. *J Parenter Enteral Nutr*. 2004;38:270–275.
124. Abou-Assi S, O'Keefe SJ. Nutrition support during acute pancreatitis. *Nutrition*. 2002;18(11–12):938–943.
125. Frossard JL, Steer ML, Pastor CM. Acute pancreatitis. *Lancet*. 2008;371(9607):143–152.
126. Eckerwall GE, Tingstedt BB, Bergenzaun PE, Andersson RG. Immediate oral feeding in patients with mild acute pancreatitis is safe and may accelerate recovery—a randomized clinical study. *Clin Nutr*. 2007;26(6):758–763.
127. Sathiaraj E, Murthy S, Mansard MJ, Rao GV, Mahukar S, Reddy DN. Clinical trial: oral feeding with a soft diet compared with clear liquid diet as initial meal in mild acute pancreatitis. *Aliment Pharmacol Ther*. 2008;28(6):777–781.
128. Marik PE, Zaloga GP. Meta-analysis of parenteral nutrition versus enteral nutrition in patients with acute pancreatitis. *BMJ*. 2004;328(7453):1407.
129. Marik PE. What is the best way to feed patients with pancreatitis? *Curr Opin Crit Care*. 2009;15(2):131–138.
130. Petrov MS, Pylypchuk RD, Emelyanov NV. Systematic review: nutritional support in acute pancreatitis. *Aliment Pharmacol Ther*. 2008;28(6):704–712.
131. Windsor AC, Kanwar S, Li AG, et al. Compared with parenteral nutrition, enteral feeding attenuates the acute phase response and improves disease severity in acute pancreatitis. *Gut*. 1998;42(3):431–435.
132. McClave SA, Greene LM, Snider HL, et al. Comparison of the safety of early enteral vs. parenteral nutrition in mild acute pancreatitis. *J Parenter Enteral Nutr*. 1997;21(1):14–20.
133. Hernandez-Aranda JC, Gallo-Chico B, Ramirez-Barba EJ. Nutrition support in severe acute pancreatitis. Controlled clinical trial. *Nutr Hosp*. 1996;11(3):160–166.
134. Kalfarentzos F, Kehagias J, Mead N, Kokkinis K, Gogos CA. Enteral nutrition is superior to parenteral nutrition in severe acute pancreatitis: results of a randomized prospective trial. *Br J Surg*. 1997;84(12):1665–1669.

135. McClave SA, Chang WK, Dhaliwal R, Heyland DK. Nutrition support in acute pancreatitis: a systematic review of the literature. *J Parenter Enteral Nutr.* 2006;30(2):143–156.
136. Petrov MS, Pylypchuk RD, Uchugina AF. A systematic review on the timing of artificial nutrition in acute pancreatitis. *Br J Nutr.* 2009;101(6):787–793.
137. O'Keefe S, Abou-Assi S, Lee R, Siebel N. Impairment of nutrient-stimulated pancreatic trypsin and lipase secretion in patients with acute pancreatitis. *Gastroenterology.* 2000;118:4.
138. Eatock FC, Chong P, Menezes N, et al. A randomized study of early nasogastric versus nasojejunal feeding in severe acute pancreatitis. *Am J Gastroenterol.* 2005;100(2):432–439.
139. Kumar A, Singh N, Prakash S, Saraya A, Joshi YK. Early enteral nutrition in severe acute pancreatitis: a prospective randomized controlled trial comparing nasojejunal and nasogastric routes. *J Clin Gastroenterol.* 2006;40(5):431–434.
140. Petrov MS, Loveday BP, Pylypchuk RD, McIlroy K, Phillips AR, Windsor JA. Systematic review and meta-analysis of enteral nutrition formulations in acute pancreatitis. *Br J Surg.* 2009;96(11):1243–1252.
141. Alnounou M, Munoz SJ. Nutrition concerns of the patient with primary biliary cirrhosis or primary sclerosing cholangitis. *Pract Gastroenterol.* 2006;37:92–100.
142. Sokol RJ, Stall C. Anthropometric evaluation of children with chronic liver disease. *Am J Clin Nutr.* 1990;52:203–208.
143. Ng VL, Balistreri WF. Treatment options for chronic cholestasis in infancy and childhood. *Curr Treat Options Gastroenterol.* 2005;8(5):419–430.
144. Baker A, Amoroso P, Wilson S, et al. Increased resting energy expenditure: a cause of undernutrition in pediatric liver disease. *J Pediatr Gastroenterol Nutr.* 1991;13:318.
145. Delich PC, Siepler JK, Parker P. Liver disease. In: Gottschlich MM, ed. *The ASPEN Nutrition Support Core Curriculum.* Silver Spring, MD: ASPEN; 2007:540–557.
146. Kleiman R, Warman KY. Nutrition in liver disease. In: Baker SS, Baker RD Jr, Davis AM, eds. *Pediatric Enteral Nutrition.* New York: Chapman and Hall; 1994:261.
147. Pettei MJ, Daftary S, Levine JJ. Essential fatty acid deficiency associated with the use of a medium-chain-triglyceride infant formula in pediatric hepatobiliary disease. *Am J Clin Nutr.* 1991;53:1217–1221.
148. Kelly DA, Davenport M. Current management of biliary atresia. *Arch Dis Child.* 2007;92:1132–1135.
149. Sanchez AJ, Aranda-Michel J. Liver disease and osteoporosis. *Nutr Clin Pract.* 2006;21(3):273–278.
150. O'Brien A, Williams R. Nutrition in end-stage liver disease: principles and practice. *Gastroenterology.* 2008;134(6):1729–1740.
151. Mager DR, McGee PL, Furuya KN, Roberts EA. Prevalence of vitamin K deficiency in children with mild to moderate chronic liver disease. *J Pediatr Gastroenterol Nutr.* 2006;42(1):71–76.
152. Greer R, Lehnert M, Lewindon P, Cleghorm GJ, Shepard RW. Body composition and components of energy expenditure in children with end-stage liver disease. *J Pediatr Gastroenterol Nutr.* 2003;36(3):358–363.
153. Barshes NR, Chang IF, Karpen SJ, Carter BA, Goss JA. Impact of pretransplant growth retardation in pediatric liver transplantation. *J Pediatr Gastroenterol Nutr.* 2006;43(1):89–94.
154. Utterson EC. Shepherd RW, Sokol RJ, et al. Biliary atresia: clinical profiles, risk factors, and outcomes of 755 patients listed for liver transplantation. *J Pediatr.* 2005;147(2):180–185.
155. Stickel F, Inderbitzin D, Candinas D. Role of nutrition in liver transplantation for end-stage chronic liver disease. *Nutr Rev.* 2008;66(1):47–54.
156. Hasse JM, Blue LS, Liepa GU, et al. Early enteral nutrition support in patients undergoing liver transplantation. *J Parenter Enteral Nutr.* 1995;19(6):437–443.
157. Renz JF, de Roos M, Rosenthal P, et al. Posttransplantation growth in pediatric liver recipients. *Liver Transpl.* 2001;7(12):1040–1055.
158. McDiarmid SV, Gornbein JA, DeSilva PJ, et al. Factors affecting growth after pediatric liver transplantation. *Transplantation.* 1999;67(3):404–411.
159. Van Mourik ID, Beath SV, Brook GA, et al. Long-term nutritional and neurodevelopmental outcome of liver transplantation in infants aged less than 12 months. *J Pediatr Gastroenterol Nutr.* 2000;30(3):269–275.
160. Viner RM, Forton JT, Cole TJ, Clark IH, Noble-Jamieson G, Barnes ND. Growth of long-term survivors of liver transplantation. *Arch Dis Child.* 1999;80(3):235–240.
161. Sanchez AJ, Aranda-Michel J. Liver disease and osteoporosis. *Nutr Clin Pract.* 2006;21(3):273–278.
162. Gasser RW. Cholestasis and metabolic bone disease—a clinical review. *Wein Med Wochenschr.* 2008;158(19–20):553–557.
163. Okajima H, Shigeno C, Inomata Y, et al. Long-term effects of liver transplantation on bone mineral density in children with end-stage liver disease: a 2-year prospective study. *Liver Transpl.* 2003;9(4):360–364.
164. Ozdemir O, Arrey-Mensah A, Sorensen RU. Development of multiple food allergies in children taking tacrolimus after heart and liver transplantation. *Pediatr Transplant.* 2006;10(3):380–383.
165. Ozbek OY, Ozcay F, Avci Z, Haberal A, Haberal M. Food allergy after liver transplantation in children: a prospective study. *Pediatr Allergy Immunol.* 2009;20(8):741–747.
166. Ziegler MM. Short bowel syndrome in infancy: Etiology and management. *Clin Perinatol.* 1986;13:167.
167. Mazariegos GV, Squires RH, Sindhi RK. *Curr Gastroenterol Rep.* 2009;11(3):226–233.
168. King KL, Phillips SM. The ins and outs of pediatric short bowel. *Support Line.* 2009;31(3):18–26.
169. Taylor SF, Sokol RJ. Infants with short bowel syndrome. In: Hay WW, ed. *Neonatal Nutrition and Metabolism.* St. Louis, MO: Mosby Year Book; 1991;437.
170. Abad-Sinden A, Sutphen J. Nutritional management of pediatric short bowel syndrome. *Pract Gastro.* 2003;12:28–48.
171. Wessel JJ. Short bowel syndrome. In: Groh-Wargos S, Thompson M, Cox JH, eds. *Nutritional Care for High Risk Newborns,* 3rd ed. Chicago, IL: Precept Press; 2000:469–488.
172. Vanderhoof JA. Short bowel syndrome. In: Walker WA, Watkins JB, eds. *Nutrition in Pediatrics: Basic Science and Clinical Applications.* Hamilton, ON: Decker; 1997:610.
173. Klish WJ. The short gut. In: Walker WA, Watkins JB, eds. *Nutrition in Pediatrics.* Boston: Little, Brown; 1985:561.
174. Fleming CR, George L, Stoner GL, et al. The importance of urinary magnesium values in patients with gut failure. *Mao Clin Proc.* 1996;71:21–24.

175. Farrell MK. Physiologic effects of parenteral nutrition. In: Baker RD Jr, Baker SS, Davis AM, eds. *Pediatric Parenteral Nutrition.* New York: Chapman and Hall; 1997:36.
176. Abad-Jorge A, Roman B. Enteral nutrition management in pediatric patients with severe gastrointestinal impairment. *Support Line.* 2007;29(2):3–11.
177. Wong KY, Lan LC, Lin SC, et al. Mucous fistula refeeding in premature neonates with enterostomies. *J Pediatr Gastroenterol Nutr.* 2004;39:43–45.
178. Matarese LE, Costa G, Bond G, et al. Therapeutic efficacy of intestinal and multivisceral transplantation: survival and nutrition outcome. *Nutr Clin Pract.* 2007;22:474–481.
179. Parekh NR, Seidner DL. Advances in enteral feeding of the intestinal failure patient. *Support Line.* 2006;28(3):18–24.
180. Ching YA, Gura K, Modi B, Jaksic T. Pediatric intestinal failure: nutritional and pharmacological approaches. *Nutr Clin Pract.* 2007;22:653–663.
181. Ksiazyk J, Piena M, Kierkus J, Lyszkowska M. Hydrolyzed versus nonhydrolyzed protein diet in short bowel syndrome in children. *J Pediatr Gastroenterol Nutr.* 2002;35(5):615–618.
182. Matarese LE, O'Keefe SJ, Kandil HM, Bond G, Costa G, Abu-Elmagd K. Short bowel syndrome: clinical guidelines for nutrition management. *Nutr Clin Pract.* 2005;20:493–502.
183. Vanderhoof JA, Grandjean CJ, Kaufman SS, Burkley KT, Antonson DL. Effect of high percentage medium-chain triglyceride diet on mucosal adaptation following massive bowel resection in rats. *J Parenter Enteral Nutr.* 1984;(8):685–689.
184. Vanderhoof JA, Blackwood DJ, Mohammadpour H, Park JH. Effect of dietary menhaden oil on normal growth and development and on ameliorating mucosal injury in rats. *Am J Clin Nutr.* 1991;54:346–350.
185. Compher CW, Kinosian BP, Rubesin SE, Ratcliffe SJ, Metz DC. Energy absorption is reduced with oleic acid supplements in human short bowel syndrome. *J Parenter Enteral Nutr.* 2009;33:102–108.
186. Galea MH, Holliday H, Carachi R, et al. Short bowel syndrome: a collective review. *J Pediatr Surg.* 1992;27:592–596.
187. Cooper A, Floyd TF, Ross AJ. Morbidity and mortality of short bowel syndrome acquired in infancy: an update. *J Pediatr Surg.* 1984;19:711–717.
188. Linsheid TR, Tarnowski KJ, Rasnake LK, et al. Behavioral treatment of food refusal in a child with short gut syndrome. *J Pediatr Psych.* 1987;12:451.
189. Nordgaard I, Hansen BS, Mortensen PB. Importance of colonic support for energy absorption as small-bowel failure proceeds. *Am J Clin Nutr.* 1996;64:222–231.
190. Byrne, TA, Veglia L, Camelio M, et al. Clinical observations: beyond the prescription: optimizing the diet of patients with short bowel syndrome. *Nutr Clin Pract.* 2000;15:306–311.
191. Rahman N, Hitchcock R. Case report of paediatric oxalate urolithiasis and a review of enteric hyperoxaluria. *J Pediatr Urol.* 2010:6(2):112–116.
192. Chang-Kit L, Filler G, Pike J, Leonard MP. Pediatric urolithiasis: experience at a tertiary care pediatric hospital. *Can Urol Assoc J.* 2008;2(4):381–386.
193. Bryne TA, Morrissey TB, Nattakom TV, et al. Growth hormone, glutamine, and a modified diet enhance nutrient absorption in patients with severe short bowel syndrome. *J Parenter Enteral Nutr.* 1995;19:296–302.
194. Szkudlarek J, Jeppesen PB, Mortensen PB. Effect of high dose growth hormone with glutamins and no change in diet on intestinal absorption in short bowel patients: a randomized, double blind, crossover, placebo controlled study. *Gut.* 2000;47:199–205.
195. Scolapio JS. Effect of growth hormone, glutamine, and diet on body composition in short bowel syndrome: a randomized, controlled study. *J Parenter Enteral Nutr.* 1999;23:309–312.
196. Jeppesen PB, Hartmann B, Thulesen J, et al. Glucagon-like peptide 2 improves nutrient absorption and nutritional status in short-bowel patients with no colon. *Gastroenterology.* 2001;120:806–815.
197. Chaet MS, Warner BW, Farrell MF. Intensive nutritional support and remedial surgical intervention for extreme short bowel syndrome. *J Pediatr Gastroenterol Nutr.* 1994;19:295–298.
198. Thompson JS. Surgical management of short bowel syndrome. *Surgery.* 1993;113:4–7.
199. Warner BW, Chaet MS. Nontransplant surgical options for management of the short bowel syndrome. *J Pediatr Gastroenterol Nutr.* 1997;17:1–12.

Chronic Kidney Disease

Linda A. Phelan

Infants and children with chronic kidney disease (CKD) face multiple and frequent dietary manipulations throughout their course of treatment. This occurs at a time when growth and development are at their most dynamic stages and behavioral adaptations to eating and making food choices are greatly influenced. Dietary modifications, along with the physical and emotional effects of chronic illness, can result in outcomes counterproductive to these activities. However, with better understanding of the particular disease and its medical and nutritional management (including the timely initiation of recombinant human growth hormone, rhGH), it is possible to overcome what not too long ago were negative, though tolerated, outcomes: growth retardation and metabolic bone disease.

Stages, Etiology, and Consequences of Chronic Kidney Disease

The National Kidney Foundation has defined stages of CKD to help identify the progression of the disease toward end stage kidney failure. These stages progress from mild CKD (stages 1 and 2), to moderate (stage 3), severe (stage 4), and end stage (stage 5). At stage 5 the treatment options are dialysis (stage 5D) and transplant (stage 5T).[1] Diagnostic criteria used for placement in one of the CKD stages is based on presence of kidney damage (e.g., proteinuria) and functional impairment defined by the estimate of glomerular filtration rate (GFR).[2] Designation of a CKD stage is useful in estimating the degree of medical nutrition therapy necessary for controlling uremia, managing electrolyte balance, and setting goals for calorie, protein, and other nutrients. Achievement of normal growth and bone health are the desired outcomes in infants and children with CKD.

CKD in infants and children is almost equally represented by acquired and congenital etiologies.[3] Acquired diseases, such as chronic glomerulonephritis, fortunately have less impact on growth, due to their more insidious onset. Congenital diseases, however, can result in early and severe growth retardation.

Indeed, in the 2005 North American Pediatric Renal Transplant Cooperative Study annual report, of the 5927 children enrolled, more than one-third had significant growth failure.[4] Therefore, infants and toddlers (ages birth to 4 years) presenting with CKD must be aggressively nourished in order to promote at least a normal growth rate, preferably greater than the fifth percentile of length for age.[5,6] The earlier the age of onset of renal failure (GFR less than 30% of normal), the more potentially severe its impact on growth will be.[7–10]

The consequences of chronic kidney disease and its treatments for infants and children all potentially influence growth (see **Table 13-1**). If any of these conditions are left inadequately managed, linear growth of the child will be delayed.[11,12] Medical nutrition therapy that includes adequate calories and protein for growth, interventions to control renal osteodystrophy, management of electrolyte balance via addition and/or restriction of minerals and fluid, and finally control of uremia and anemia play a vital role in the control and progression of CKD and the ability of the child to grow normally. If properly treated, growth retardation can be arrested; however, catch-up growth is difficult to achieve.

The characteristic symptoms of CKD in children signaling increasing uremia are noted in **Table 13-2**. Several of those listed, including nausea, growth retardation, swelling, and shortness of breath, may respond favorably to some dietary modification(s). When, despite aggressive attempts at optimizing nutritional intake and preventing renal osteodystrophy, normal growth velocity is unattainable, the initiation of rhGH becomes necessary.[13,14] Of note is that adequate nutrition and control of renal bone disease continue to be significant therapies in the management of children with CKD.

In 1997, the National Kidney Foundation published the *Dialysis Outcomes Quality Initiative (K/DOQI) Clinical Practice Guidelines*, which were updated in 2001. The guidelines include the areas of chronic kidney disease, hemodialysis,

TABLE 13-1 Consequences of Chronic Kidney Disease

- Water/electrolyte imbalance
- Accumulation of endogenous/exogenous toxins
- Hypertension
- Acidosis
- Anemia
- Renal osteodystrophy
- Anorexia/undernutrition
- Need for steroid therapy

TABLE 13-2 Symptoms of Uremia in Children

- Nausea
- Weakness
- Fatigue
- Decreased school performance
- Loss of attention span
- Growth retardation
- Changes in urine output
- Shortness of breath
- Swelling of face/extremities/abdomen
- Amenorrhea in adolescent girls

peritoneal dialysis, vascular access, nutrition, bone metabolism and disease, and dyslipidemias. Within the nutrition guidelines is a section devoted to the pediatric patient.[15] The nutrition guidelines for children with CKD were updated in 2008.[16] The guidelines are based on a comprehensive review of available evidence and on the opinion of experienced practitioners. As such, the quantity of available evidence in pediatric CKD continues to be lacking or sparse due to small sample sizes and lack of randomized controlled trials. Often management decisions are made by the available evidence in adults with CKD and what we know about normal growth and development in non-CKD children. These guidelines are meant to be used as a starting point for assessment and intervention steps of medical nutrition therapy. They are meant to complement and not replace clinical judgment. Adjustments in the recommendations set forth by these guidelines may be necessary, based on clinical judgment, to achieve the ultimate goals of normal growth and development and bone health. It is strongly recommended that the reader refer to these guidelines for a comprehensive review of available evidence and opinion to date on nutrition as it applies to pediatric CKD.[16]

To summarize, the impact of CKD on growth in children depends upon the severity and duration of the renal insufficiency, the diagnosis, and the age of onset. The treatments for CKD, namely dialysis and transplantation, will affect growth as well.

Conservative Management

Treating children with CKD without dialysis requires judicious and frequent monitoring of diet intake, biochemical parameters, and growth.[16–18] Any chronic disease in children requires the historical, accurate recording of growth measurements. In CKD, weight and weight-for-height are particularly difficult to assess given the often insidious accumulation of extracellular fluid not always apparent in children. Also, the normal ranges for a number of laboratory values are different for children of different ages and should be considered whenever assessing a child's metabolic status and whether the restriction and/or addition of minerals is warranted.

Breast milk, if available, is the preferred feeding for infants with CKD. Formula selection in the past favored the use of PM 60/40 by Abbott Nutrition, given its preferred calcium to phosphorus ratio of 2:1 and low mineral content. However, now that normal growth can be obtained in infants with CKD and waste products significantly reduced, formula choice does not need to be limited unless the infant has other intolerances or conditions such as lactose intolerance or GI disorders. Although PM 60/40 may still be considered initially, the infant should be transitioned to a standard infant formula once growth is evident and electrolytes are within normal ranges, in order to provide adequate intake of nutrients. This is particularly important to consider in fluid-restricted infants whose volume of formula may need to be reduced.[5]

Calcium and Phosphorus

It has long been recognized that renal osteodystrophy contributes significantly to growth retardation in children with renal insufficiency.[19] Early in the course of renal disease, synthesis of 1,25-dihydroxycholecalciferol ($1{,}25(OH)_2D_3$) and the excretion of excessive dietary phosphate decrease, leading to the development of renal osteodystrophy and secondary hyperparathyroidism if left untreated. This often occurs before derangements in calcium, phosphorous, and parathyroid hormone levels are detected.[20–22] Hyperphosphatemia is considered a late indicator of bone deformities. Recently, vitamin D deficiency and insufficiency have been found to be increasingly prevalent in healthy children.[23–26] This is also true in children with CKD.[20,23] Insufficient vitamin D can exacerbate the suppression of calcitriol in CKD patients; therefore, recent K/DOQI recommendations advocate the assessment of vitamin D levels early in the course of CKD and supplementation of vitamin D if insufficiency or deficiency is confirmed.[16,27] Along with supplementation of vitamin D, current therapy may include any or all of the following: dietary restriction of high-phosphorus foods and fluids (primarily dairy products, chocolate, nuts, and colas), supplementation of vitamin D (1,25 $(OH)_2D_3$) and calcium, and the prescription of nonaluminum-, nonmagnesium-containing phosphate binders (calcium carbonate, acetate, glubionate, and/or sevelamer hydrochloride) to be taken with meals.[28–32]

In infants, PM 60/40 by Abbott Products may be the initial formula of choice; however, it contains less phosphorus than the more common infant formulas and it may be inadequate in providing sufficient phosphorus for the growing infant.[5] Changing formula to one containing more phosphorous or starting a phosphorous supplement may be necessary in infants with CKD who exhibit lower than normal phosphorous levels.

Sodium, Potassium, and Fluid

Sodium and fluid restriction might be necessary to prevent or control the incidence of hypertension and edema commonly associated with CKD. Usually, a no-added-salt diet is sufficient. Limitation of fluid should be based on the child's urine output and insensible losses. Hyperkalemia is rarely a problem as long as kidney function is greater than 5% of normal. However, some children may be prescribed medications such as ACE (angiotensin-converting enzyme) inhibitors (used to reduce proteinuria), which cause a reduction in GFR and concomitant reduction in the excretion of potassium (K). Should potassium restriction become necessary, limiting high-potassium foods in the diet is generally adequate. It is necessary to assess and monitor the potassium content of infant formula and nutritional supplements in addition to that of solid foods as blood levels are monitored.

For infants requiring sodium and/or potassium restriction, formulas such as PM 60/40 or Carnation Good Start are appropriate. Furthermore, if the volume of formula must be restricted, it is unlikely that any significant contribution of sodium or potassium will come from formula. It should be noted that infants with increased urine losses of sodium and/or potassium will need supplementation to their usual diet. Attention to the causes of CKD is particularly important in infants and young children. Obstructive uropathy and renal dysplasia are often accompanied with defects in the kidney tubule's ability to concentrate the urine. Increased excretion of water and sodium chloride are the result. Careful attention to providing increased fluid and salt supplementation becomes necessary. Infants and young children with excessive losses of fluid and salt experience growth retardation and vomiting due to dehydration.[33]

Protein/Energy

There is no evidence to suggest that the energy needs of children with CKD are elevated above the DRI for age. Energy needs are at least 80% of the recommended dietary allowance for height age and may be greater than 100% depending on activity level.[34] It is generally accepted that protein restriction much below the DRI for age is contraindicated in growing children. Current K/DOQI recommendations are to provide 100% of the DRI for chronological age.[16,18] Monitoring of energy intake over the course of CKD should be ongoing with the goal of providing DRI for chronological age, sex, and physical activity. Formulas to calculate DRI are found in Appendix H. Equations to adjust calorie needs for obese children are available. These equations should be implemented in calorie prescriptions for CKD children with BMI's above the 95th percentile. As with healthy children, the prevalence of obesity is increasing in children with CKD, and attention should be paid to better estimating calorie needs (see **Figure 13-1**).

Because of the prevalence of cardiovascular lesions in children with CKD, caloric distribution recommendations have been published recently for children at high risk for cardiovascular disease (CVD).[35] Indeed, children with CKD are at highest risk for pediatric CVD due to the frequency of dyslipidemia[34] and extra skeletal calcification, including vascular calcification.[20]

Children with CKD need caloric guidelines that primarily allow for proper growth and control the uremia and/or electrolyte abnormalities, but the guidelines also reduce or limit the risk of CVD, which is the leading cause of mortality in children with CKD.

$$\text{Boys: TEE} = 114 - [50.9 \times \text{age (y)} + \text{PA} \times [19.5 \times \text{weight (kg)} + 1161.4 \times \text{height (m)}]]$$

$$\text{Girls: TEE} = 389 - [41.2 \times \text{age (y)} + \text{PA} \times [15.0 \times \text{weight (kg)} + 701.6 \times \text{height (m)}]]$$

FIGURE 13-1 Equations to Estimate Energy Requirements for Children Between 3 and 18 Years of Age Who Are Overweight

Abbreviation: TEE, total energy expenditure.

Source: Food and Nutrition Board. *Dietary Reference Intakes for Energy, Carbohydrate, Fiber, Fat, Fatty Acids, Cholesterol, Protein, and Amino Acids (Macronutrients).* Washington, DC: National Academies Press; 2002.

Anytime protein, phosphorous, or potassium is restricted in the diet it reduces sources of calories. If these restrictions must be in place and extra simple sugars and fat must be increased to provide adequate calories, then guidelines that advise on using heart-healthy fats may be the only dyslipidemic choice available to use.[16] However, if the child with CKD is growing well and is stable, further dyslipidemia guidelines may be appropriate to use.

It is generally accepted that protein restriction much below the DRI for chronological age is contraindicated in growing children with CKD. With dietary phosphate restriction alone, a considerable limitation of protein intake could occur without restriction of protein per se. The recent K/DOQI nutrition guidelines for children with CKD have made recommendations regarding the levels of protein intake for pediatric CKD patients.[16] Protein is generally unrestricted at CKD stages 1 and 2, 100–140% of the DRI at CKD stages 3 and 4 and 100–120% of the DRI at CKD stages 4 and 5.[16] There is no evidence to suggest that restricting protein below the DRI will slow down the progression of CKD in children; however, restricting protein below the DRI can have adverse consequences by causing growth failure. Routine nutritional assessment including anthropometric measurements and dietary intake will indicate whether the prescribed protein and calorie levels are adequate.[36]

Providing optimal nutrition within the limitations of fluid restriction (voluntary or involuntary) is possible only by caloric supplementation of the formula to as much as 60 kcal/oz. Increasing caloric density by three times normal dilution requires a methodical approach.[5] Attempts should be made to maintain caloric distribution as follows, with the lower intakes of fat calories recommended for children over the age of 2 years:

Carbohydrate	35–65%
Protein	5–16%
Fat	30–55%

Carbohydrate sources such as Polycose (Abbott Laboratories) and Moducal (Mead Johnson) are coupled with an oil (canola oil, corn oil, or medium-chain triglyceride [MCT] oil for premature infants), as illustrated in **Figure 13-2**. Concentration of the formula with or without the addition of a protein supplement such as Beneprotein (Nestle Nutrition) increases protein content. Caloric density can be advanced 2 to 4 calories/day as tolerated.[5] A number of manipulations may be considered in addition to these, such as using Duocal, a powdered calorie supplement containing both carbohydrate and fat (Nutricia North America). Diluting adult renal formulas such as Suplena Carb Steady or Nepro Carb Steady (Abbott Laboratories) also has been

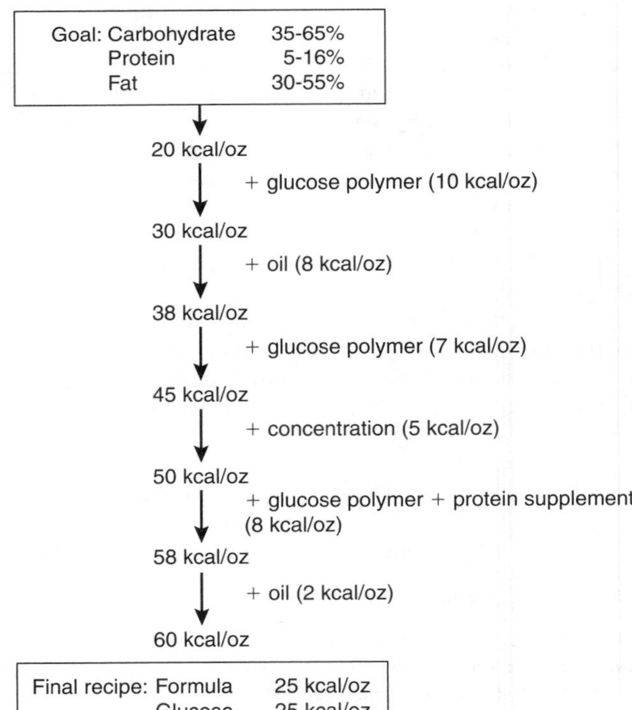

FIGURE 13-2 Increasing Caloric Density of Formula: An Example

(*Note:* Very low fat intake in children less than 2 years of age may compromise the development of the brain and the central nervous system.)

done for CKD infants as young as 6.9 months.[37] Ensuring the consistent daily intake of a sufficient volume of formula to meet an infant's nutritional goals for growth most often can be achieved only after the initiation of enteral tube feedings.[36–40] The presence of gastroesophageal reflux in infants with CKD is considered a major factor contributing to feeding problems in this age group.[41] However, continuous nighttime infusions of formula via feeding pump allow maximum tolerance of formula.

Once nutritional goals are realized and a feeding regimen established, additional oral stimulation through non-nutritive sucking can begin.[42] In the author's experience, once children are successfully transplanted they eventually return to normal feeding practices.

Vitamins and Minerals

Because few children with CKD have consistently adequate diets, it is suggested that a multivitamin be routinely recommended. Additionally, 0.5–1 mg folic acid per day should be included. Iron supplementation may be indicated as well, especially if the child is receiving erythropoietin, and ferritin and/or transferrin saturation levels are depressed.[43,44]

Dialysis

Dialysis is indicated once a child experiences symptoms that significantly interfere with activities of daily living. Peritoneal dialysis (continuous cycling or continuous ambulatory) is the preferred choice of dialytic care for infants and small children. Both hemodialysis and peritoneal dialysis are options for bigger children. Nutritional management is dictated by the type of dialytic therapy chosen; however, the principles are similar to those described for conservative management. Nutrient losses via dialysate (in particular, protein, phosphorus, sodium, and potassium) must be considered when assessing nutritional adequacy of the diet.[45]

Calcium and Phosphorus

Management of calcium and phosphorus balance continues to be necessary even while on dialysis, and is the same as stated previously.

Sodium, Potassium, and Fluid

A child's recommended intake for sodium and potassium is directly related to his or her residual renal function and the type and effectiveness of dialysis. Likewise, the degree of ultrafiltration possible and the child's urine output will dictate an advisable fluid intake. If restriction of sodium and potassium is necessary, which usually happens with hemodialysis, the elimination or limitation of foods containing especially large amounts of sodium and potassium is generally sufficient. Severely restricted diets often encourage noncompliance and dull a child's interest in food. Individualization of diet, taking into consideration the child's food preferences, is essential to successful control of sodium, potassium, and fluid intake.[46] With peritoneal dialysis, restriction of potassium often is not necessary except with anuric children. Infants on peritoneal dialysis often require continued sodium supplementation and/or phosphorous supplementation. Indeed, an infant with CKD stages 1 to 5 on a low mineral formula, such as PM 60/40, may be able to switch to a standard infant formula once started on peritoneal dialysis due to increased losses of sodium and phosphorous in the dialysate.

Protein/Energy

The nutritional requirements for protein and energy for patients undergoing peritoneal dialysis are not clear, and the historical reliance on serum albumin levels in the pediatric patient may be in question when assessing adequacy. It is known that some protein is lost to the dialysate, while glucose is absorbed from the dialysate. The degree to which these changes occur can be determined only through measurement of individual patients. Periodic calculations of urinary and dialysate urea nitrogen, dialysate protein and amino acids, and miscellaneous nitrogen losses are necessary.[47] The most current recommendation on protein needs for infants and children on dialysis is lower than previous recommendations. For hemodialysis, the addition of 0.1 g protein/kg/day to the DRI for chronological age is recommended. For peritoneal dialysis, the addition of 0.15–0.35 g protein/kg/day to the DRI for chronological age is suggested. For a detailed review of protein recommendations see the updated K/DOQI guidelines on nutrition for children with CKD.[16] The opinion of the K/DOQI workgroup is to start with the protein levels recommended and make adjustments as needed for factors such as adequate growth, infection, and peritonitis. Diets can then be developed and altered when measurements indicate the need, promoting growth while preventing obesity.[48] During periods of peritonitis, there is an increased loss of protein to the dialysate, and the child usually feels ill. Careful attention to dietary intake is important to prevent a potentially significant loss of lean body weight during this time of infection.

Protein and energy requirements for children on hemodialysis have been studied using urea kinetic modeling, as well as actual nitrogen balance techniques.[49,50] It was concluded that a protein intake of 0.3 g/cm/day and an energy intake of 10 kcal/cm/day produced positive nitrogen balance. The protein catabolic and urea generation rates of the children in positive balance were uniformly lower; therefore, no increase in dialysis requirements was necessary with these levels of intake.

The routine use of urea kinetic modeling is especially helpful in determining dialysis and nutritional adequacy in children.[51–53] Monthly monitoring of protein catabolic rates and urea generation provides insight into subtle changes in dialysis treatment and/or diet intake that otherwise might go unnoticed. Kinetic modeling, usually conducted by the dietitian, allows the dietitian access to the fundamental parameters and concepts of dialysis prescription, ensuring maximum confidence in the nutrition counseling of patients.

Lipids

Hyperlipidemia remains a problem in children on dialysis, particularly peritoneal dialysis.[54] Treatment in growing children remains controversial.[46]

Vitamins

It is advisable that children on both hemodialysis and peritoneal dialysis be provided water-soluble vitamins and folate, which are lost to dialysate.[55] Although studies have not been conducted in children, it is common practice to supplement dialysed children with water-soluble vitamins to account for vitamin losses in the dialysate. Care should be taken not to exceed the tolerable upper intake levels of vitamins when dietary and supplement sources of vitamins are provided.[16] There are specially formulated dialysis vitamin preparations on the market such as Nephro-Vite Rx (R&D Laboratories) and Nephrocaps (Fleming & Co.) that fulfill most patients' needs. Infants can be given less frequent dosing or partial dosing of the adult renal vitamin supplements on the market. If the dialysed child is receiving 100% of his or her nutritional needs via baby formulas or adult renal formulas, vitamin supplementation may not be necessary if the formula composition is meeting or exceeding the DRI for chronological age.

Carnitine

Secondary carnitine deficiency has been noted in patients receiving dialysis.[56] Treatment remains somewhat controversial, especially in pediatric programs. It is the opinion of the K/DOQI workgroup that there is insufficient evidence to recommend carnitine supplementation for children on dialysis.[16] This opinion is echoed by the European Pediatric Peritoneal Dialysis Working Group.[57]

Transplantation

The ultimate goal of all pediatric end-stage renal disease programs is transplantation. This is the only treatment option thus far that provides children with the opportunity for normal growth and development and potentially for catch-up growth.[58] Clinicians must be constantly vigilant for signs of rejection and infection, especially in the first postoperative year. Immunosuppression and antibiotic therapy result in side effects related to inefficient digestion and metabolism of nutrients, as well as to growth retardation.[59] The advent of new immunosuppressants, while providing increased protection from rejection, also increases the risk of the patient developing hyperglycemia (due to insulin resistance), hyperlipidemia, and hypercholesterolemia. Alternate-day steroid therapy has been shown to promote normal and, at times, catch-up growth. The medical course of the patient and the individual transplant program's protocol for immunosuppression will dictate just how quickly a patient can begin tapering to alternate-day dosing.

For small children receiving adult kidneys, parenteral nutrition may be considered immediately postoperatively. Surgically implanting an adult-size kidney into a very small child usually requires significant bowel manipulation to make enough room for the organ and an ileus may result.

Once oral feedings are resumed, the dietary recommendations are once again individualized. If kidney function is not normal, attention to sodium, potassium, phosphorus, and fluid will be necessary. A rise in blood urea nitrogen (BUN) level and a slow recovery to normal is usual even with normal kidney function due to the catabolic stress of surgery. If it is possible, aggressive nutritional support of the patient should resume soon after transplant.[60]

With the attainment of normal kidney function, a no-added-salt diet is still advisable. Hypertension, now a potential result of high-dose steroid therapy, is frequently seen after transplantation, and sodium restriction, at least during the acute phase (first 6 to 8 months after transplant), is helpful. Also, tubular loss of phosphate and magnesium is often present, requiring phosphorus and magnesium supplementation. Dietary phosphorus intake usually is not adequate to maintain blood levels above 3.0 mg/dL.

Perhaps the most important aspect of the diet at this time is instruction in appropriate portion sizes and a heart-healthy diet. Most children with CKD have never learned to eat nutritionally balanced meals. Additionally, the increased appetite accompanying steroid therapy should be manipulated in a positive, healthy fashion, before a taste develops for high-carbohydrate, high-fat foods. It is common to hear parents describe the mealtimes of their newly transplanted children as lasting all day with one meal overlapping another.

Once steroids are tapered to levels where hypertension and hyperglycemia are no longer problematic, a diet appropriate for chronological age is indicated. Because of the hyperlipidemic side effects of immunosuppressive drugs and the already deranged lipid levels of children with CKD, a heart-healthy diet with attention to low saturated and trans fats, low simple sugar, and low cholesterol should be advised. Please refer to the American Heart Association (AHA) guidelines for cardiovascular risk reduction in high risk pediatric patients for a comprehensive review of lipid-lowering diets for children.[34] The use of omega-3 fatty acids has been promoted in adult populations with hypertriglyceridemia. To date there is insufficient evidence to recommend omega-3 fatty acids to treat children with CKD.[16,61] Continued assessment of nutritional adequacy of the diet is necessary even with normal kidney function.

TABLE 13-3 Major Nutritional Considerations

Nutrient	Indication for Treatment	Modification
Phosphorus	CKD, elevated parathyroid hormone level, with or without hyperphosphatemia	Phosphate binders; low-phosphate diet; calcium and vitamin D supplement
	Posttransplant tubular loss; hypophosphatemia	Add supplement
Sodium	Hypertension; fluid retention	No added salt
	Daily steroid therapy	No added salt
	Increased urine losses	Add supplement
	Increased peritoneal dialysate losses	Add supplement
Potassium	$<$ 5% GFR; hyperkalemia	Restrict diet
	Diuretic therapy; hypokalemia; diarrhea	Add supplement
Protein	Infants with CKD (no dialysis)	DRI
	Children with CKD (no dialysis)	Limit to DRI
	Children on hemodialysis	DRI
	Infants/children on peritoneal dialysis	$>$ DRI
	Posttransplant	
Energy	Undernutrition/anorexia	$\geq$ DRI
	Infants with CKD (no dialysis)	$\geq$ DRI
	Children on hemodialysis	$\geq$ DRI
	Dextrose absorption from peritoneal dialysate	$\leq$ DRI
	Posttransplant steroid therapy	Varies
	Steroid-induced hyperglycemia	No concentrated sweets

Abbreviation: GFR, glomerular filtration rate.

Conclusion

The nutritional intake of the child is especially important in order to ensure optimal growth and development during all stages of renal disease. The diet must be adequate and consistent. This is no easy task in light of the symptomatology accompanying the disease. Anorexia and taste changes commonly associated with CKD[62,63] constantly challenge attempts to promote optimal nutritional care. Additionally, dietary modification (see **Table 13-3**) and implementation must be individualized for all age groups, taking into account developmental levels, growth potentials, and renal functional limitations. Input from the entire renal team at all times is critical to ensuring successful nutritional management of this population. Frequent evaluation of food intake, growth, kidney function, and developmental stages is essential to adequate care.

Case Study

JA is an 8-year-old girl who was referred to pediatric nephrology because of lack of weight gain for the previous 6 months, a poor appetite with some nausea and fatigue, and elevated blood pressures on two previous visits to her pediatrician. Labs were drawn at her initial visit, which included BUN 30, Cr 2.0, Ca 7.8, Phos 8.2, Na 139, K 4.9, albumin 2.3, and hematocrit 25. Anthropometric measurements included height of 120 cm, weight of 17 kg, and BMI of 11.8. Her blood pressure was checked and again found to be elevated at 130/92. Urinalysis showed proteinuria of 200 mg/dL. When asked if anyone in the family had high blood pressure or a kidney disease, the parents spoke of JA's grandfather, who was on dialysis before he died.

The dietitian was asked to meet with the family to assess JA's dietary intake. The RD reported that JA was described as a "picky" eater. She eats very small portions and often felt "full" before she finished a meal. Her typical calorie intake was estimated to be 1000 kcal/day. Her parents reported that over the past few months, JA tires easily and generally is not the active child they were used to when she was younger.

The nephrologist estimated JA to be in CKD stage 3 with an estimated GFR of 50. An ACE inhibitor was prescribed for hypertension and to control her proteinuria. The nephrologist also ordered a low phosphorous diet; the RD instructed patient and family.

Plans were made to admit JA to the hospital in 2 weeks for a kidney biopsy and to recheck her labs including % iron saturation, ferritin, vitamin D_{25}, and PTH.

Labs upon admit to the hospital showed a BUN of 29, creatinine 1.8, Ca 8.0, phos 7.5, hct 25, and alb 2.5. Her vitamin D_{25} level was low at 20, PTH high at 250, and iron studies showed 18% iron saturation and a ferritin of 82.

The biopsy showed membroproliferative glomerulonephritis type 2. The nephrologist advised JA's parents to return to the clinic in 2 weeks to begin training for EPO injections, another lab check for a phosphorous level, and follow-up with the dietitian. A 3-day food record was to be brought to the visit. Upon evaluation of the food record, the RD learned that JA's calorie intake remained at an average of 1000 kcal/day. Looking at the K/DOQI guidelines, the protein needs for stage 3 CKD were estimated to be 1–1.2 g protein/kg/day. Her food records showed adequate protein intake but inadequate calorie intake. JA's phosphorous level that day was 7.6.

Questions for the Reader

1. What are JA's height, weight, and BMI percentiles on the growth chart?
2. What is her desirable weight-for-height?
3. What is her estimated energy requirement (EER) based on desirable body weight?
4. Give an example of a PES statement for this initial assessment of JA.
5. What other nutrition intervention(s) should the RD address at this time? Mark all that apply.
   a. Potassium-restricted diet
   b. Sodium-restricted diet
   c. Increased calorie intake
   d. Decreased protein intake
6. What specific vitamin and mineral supplements should the RD recommend upon hospital admission?
7. What recommendations should the RD make at the final clinic visit? Mark all that apply.
   a. Start an oral nutritional supplement to increase calorie intake.
   b. Start a potassium-restricted diet.
   c. Initiate phosphorous binders.
   d. Restrict protein.

REFERENCES

1. Hogg RJ, Furth S, Lemley KV, et al. National Kidney Foundation's kidney disease outcomes initiative clinic practice guidelines for chronic kidney disease in children and adolescents: evaluation, classification and stratification. *Pediatrics*. 2003;111:1416–1421.
2. Mahan JD, Warady BA. Assessment and treatment of short stature in pediatric patients with chronic kidney disease: a consensus statement. *Pediatr Nephrol*. 2006;21;917–930.
3. Fine RN. Growth in children with renal insufficiency. In: Nissenson A, Fine RN, Gentile D, eds. *Clinical Dialysis*. New York: Appleton-Century Crofts; 1984:661.
4. North American Pediatric Renal Transplant Cooperative Study. Annual report. Renal transplantation, dialysis, chronic renal insufficiency. 2005. Available at: http://spitfire.emmes.com/study/ped/resources/annlrept2005.pdf. Accessed September 2, 2005.
5. Spinozzi NS, Nelson P. Nutrition support in the newborn intensive care unit. *J Renal Nutr*. 1996;6:188–197.
6. Ellis EN, Yiu V, Harley F, et al. The impact of supplemental feeding in young children on dialysis: a report of the North American Pediatric Renal Transplant Cooperative Study. *Pediatr Nephrol*. 2000;16:404–408.
7. Betts PR, White RHR. Growth potential and skeletal maturity in children with chronic renal insufficiency. *Nephron*. 1976;16:325–332.
8. Broyer M. Growth in children with renal insufficiency. *Pediatr Clin North Am*. 1982;29:991–1003.
9. Rizzoni G, Broyer M, Guest G. Growth retardation in children with chronic renal disease: scope of the problem. *Am J Kidney Dis*. 1986;7:256–261.
10. Seikaly MG, Salhab N, Gipson D, Yiu V, Stablein D. Stature in children with chronic kidney disease: analysis of NAPRTCS database. *Pediatr Nephrol*. 2006;21:793–399.
11. Rizzoni G, Basso T, Setari M. Growth in children with chronic renal failure on conservative treatment. *Kidney Int*. 1984;26:52–58.
12. Kleinknecht C, Broyer M, Hout D, et al. Growth and development of nondialyzed children with chronic renal failure. *Kidney Int*. 1983;24(S15):40–47.
13. Fine RN, Kohout EC, Brown D, Perlman AJ. Growth after recombinant human growth hormone treatment in children with chronic renal failure: report of a multicenter randomized double-blind placebo-controlled study. *J Pediatr*. 1994;124:374–382.
14. Berard E, Crosnier H, Six-Beneton A, et al. Recombinant human growth hormone treatment of children on hemodialysis. *Pediatr Nephrol*. 1998;12:304–310.
15. National Kidney Foundation. K/DOQI clinical practice guidelines for nutrition in chronic renal failure. *Am J Kidney Dis*. 2000;35(6):S105–S136.
16. National Kidney Foundation. K/DOQI clinical practice guideline for nutrition in children with CKD: 2008 update. *Am J Kidney Dis*. 2009;53(3, Suppl 2):S1-S124.
17. Hellerstein S, Holliday MA, Grupe WE, et al. Nutritional management of children with chronic renal failure. *Pediatr Nephrol*. 1987;1:195–211.

18. Rock J, Secker D. Nutrition management of chronic kidney disease in the pediatric patient. In: Ham-Gray L, Wiesenk K, eds. *A Clinical Guide to Nutrition Care in Kidney Disease*, 3rd ed. Chicago: American Dietetic Association; 2004:127–149.
19. Salusky IB, Goodman WG. The management of renal osteodystrophy. *Pediatr Nephrol.* 1996;10:651–653.
20. Wesseling K, Bakkaloglu S, Saluskey I. Chronic kidney disease mineral and bone disorder in children. *Pediatr Nephrol.* 2008;23:195–207.
21. Martinez I, Saracho R, Montenegro J, Llach F. A deficit of calcitriol synthesis may not be the initial factor in the pathogenesis of secondary hyperparathyroidism. *Nephrol Dial Transplant.* 1996;11(Suppl 3):22–28.
22. Levin A, Bakris GL, Molitch M, et al. Prevalence of abnormal serum vitamin D, PTH, calcium and phosphorus in patients with chronic kidney disease: results of the study to evaluate early kidney disease. *Kidney Int.* 2007;71:31–38.
23. Seeherunvong W, Abitbol CL, Chandar J, Zilleruelo G, Freundlich M. Vitamin D insufficiency and deficiency in children with early chronic kidney disease. *J Pediatr.* 2009;154:906–911.
24. Holick MF. Resurrection of vitamin D deficiency and rickets. *J Clin Invest.* 2006;116:2062–2072.
25. Looker AC, Dawson-Hughes B, Calvo MS, Gunter EW, Sahyoun NR. Serum 25-hydroxyvitamin D status of adolescents and adults in two seasonal subpopulations from NHANES III. *Bone.* 2002;30:771–777.
26. Gordon CM, Feldman HA, Sinclair L, et al. Prevalence of vitamin D deficiency among healthy infants and toddlers. *Arch Pediatr Adolesc Med.* 2008;162:505–512.
27. National Kidney Foundation. K/DOQI clinical practice guidelines for bone metabolism and disease in children with chronic kidney disease. *Am J Kidney Dis.* 2005;46:S1–S122.
28. Brookhyser J, Pahre SN. Dietary and pharmacotherapeutic considerations in the management of renal osteodystrophy. *Adv Renal Replace Ther.* 1995;2:5–13.
29. Tamanah K, Mak RH, Rigden SP, et al. Long-term suppression of hyperparathyroidism by phosphate binders in uremic children. *Pediatr Nephrol.* 1987;1:145–149.
30. Schiller LR, Santa Ana CA, Sheikh MS, Emmett M, Fordtran, JS. Effect of the time of administration of calcium acetate on phosphorus binding. *New Engl J Med.* 1989;320:1110–1113.
31. Schmitt J. Selecting an appropriate phosphate binder. *J Renal Nutr.* 1990;1:38–40.
32. Bleyer AJ, Burke SK, Dillon M, et al. A comparison of the calcium-free phosphate binder sevelamer hydrochloride with calcium acetate in the treatment of hyperphosphatemia in hemodialysis patients. *Am J Kidney Dis.* 1999;33:694–701.
33. Parekh RS, Flynn JT, Smoyer WE, et al. Improved growth in young children with severe chronic renal insufficiency who use specified nutritional therapy. *J Am Soc Nephrol.* 2001;12:2418–2426.
34. Betts PR, Macgrath G. Growth pattern and dietary intake of children with chronic renal insufficiency. *Br Med J.* 1974;2:189.
35. Kavey R-EW, Kavey RE, Allada V, Daniels SR, et al. Cardiovascular risk reduction in high risk pediatric patients. *Circulation.* 2006;114:2710–2738.
36. Nelson P, Stover J. Nutritional recommendations for infants, children and adolescents with ESRD. In: Stover, J, ed. *A Clinical Guide to Nutrition Care in End-Stage Renal Disease*, 2nd ed. Chicago: American Dietetic Association; 1994:79–97.
37. Hobbs DJ, Gast TR, Furguson KB, Bunchman TE, Barletta GM. Nutritional management of hyperkalemic infants with chronic kidney disease using adult renal formulas. *J Renal Nutr.* 2010;20(2):121–126.
38. Yiu VWY, Harmon WE, Spinozzi NS, et al. High-calorie nutrition for infants with chronic renal disease. *J Renal Nutr.* 1996;6:203–206.
39. Ledermann SE, Spitz L, Malony J, et al. Gastrostomy feeding in infants and children on peritoneal dialysis. *Pediatr Nephrol.* 2002;17:246–250.
40. Reed EE, Roy LP, Gaskin KJ, Knight JF. Nutritional intervention and growth in children with chronic renal failure. *J Renal Nutr.* 1998;8:122–126.
41. Ruley EJ, Boch GH, Kerzner B, Abbott AW. Feeding disorders and gastroesophageal reflux in infants with chronic renal failure. *Pediatr Nephrol.* 1989;3:424–429.
42. Bebaum JC, Pererra GR, Watkins JB, et al. Non-nutritive sucking during gavage feeding enhances growth and maturation in premature infants. *Pediatrics.* 1983;71:41–45.
43. Eschbach MD, Egrie JC, Downing MR, et al. Correction of the anemia of end-stage renal disease with recombinant human erythropoietin. *N Engl J Med.* 1987;310:73–78.
44. Van Wyck DB, Stivelman JC, Ruiz J. Iron status in patients receiving erythropoietin for dialysis-associated anemia. *Kidney Int.* 1989;35:712–716.
45. Wolfson M. Nutritional management of the continuous ambulatory peritoneal patient. *Am J Kidney Dis.* 1996;27: 744–749.
46. Secker D, Pencharz MB: Nutritional therapy for children on CAPD/CCPD: theory and practice. In: Fine RN, Alexander SR, Warady BA, eds. *CAPD/CCPD in Children*. Boston, MA: Kluwer Academic; 1998:567–603.
47. Schleifer CR, Teehan BP, Brown JM, Raimondo J. The application of urea kinetic modeling to peritoneal dialysis: a review of methodology and outcome. *J Renal Nutr.* 1993;3:2–9.
48. Harvey E, Secker D, Braj B, Picone G, Balfe JW. The team approach to the management of children on chronic peritoneal dialysis. *Adv Renal Replace Ther.* 1996;3:3–13.
49. Spinozzi NS, Grupe WE. Nutritional implications of renal disease. *J Am Diet Assoc.* 1977;70:493–497.
50. Grupe WE, Harmon WE, Spinozzi NS. Protein and energy requirements in children receiving chronic hemodialysis. *Kidney Int.* 1983;24:S6–S10.
51. Harmon WE, Spinozzi NS, Meyer A, Grupe WE. The use of protein catabolic rate to monitor pediatric hemodialysis. *Dial Transplant.* 1981;10:324.
52. Goldstein SL, Sorof JM, Brewer ED. Natural logarithmic estimates of Kt/V in the pediatric hemodialysis population. *Am J Kidney Dis.* 1999;33:518–522.
53. Juarez-Congelosi M, Orellana P, Goldstein SL. Normalized protein catabolic rate versus serum albumin as a nutrition status marker in pediatric patients receiving hemodialysis. *J Renal Nutr.* 2007;17:269–274.
54. Querfeld U, Salusky IB, Nelson P, et al. Hyperlipidemia in pediatric patients undergoing peritoneal dialysis. *Pediatr Nephrol.* 1988;2:447–452.

55. Warady BA, Kriley M, Alon U, Hellerstein S. Vitamin status of infants receiving long-term peritoneal dialysis. *Pediatr Nephrol.* 1994;8:354–356.
56. Matera M, Bellinghieri G, Costantino G, et al. History of L-carnitine: implications for renal disease. *J Renal Nutr.* 2003;13:2–14.
57. Schruder CH. The management of anemia in pediatric peritoneal dialysis patients. *Pediatr Nephrol.* 2003;18:805–809.
58. Fine RN. Renal transplantation for children—the only realistic choice. *Kidney Int Suppl.* 1985;17:515–517.
59. Neu AM, Warady BA. Dialysis and renal transplantation in infants with irreversible renal failure. *Adv Renal Replace Ther.* 1996;3:48–59.
60. Seagraves A, Moore EE, Moore FA, et al. Net protein catabolic rate after kidney transplantation: impact of corticosteroid immunosuppression. *J Parenter Enteral Nutr.* 1986;10:453–455.
61. Chronic Kidney Disease (CKD) evidence based nutrition practice guideline. Available at: http://www.adaevidencelibrary.com/topic.cfm?cat=3927. Accessed August 11, 2010.
62. Spinozzi NS, Murray CL, Grupe WE. Altered taste acuity in children with ESRD. *Pediatr Res.* 1978;12:442.
63. Shapera MR, Moel DI, Kamath SK, et al. Taste perception of children with chronic renal failure. *J Am Diet Assoc.* 1986;86:1359–1365.

Cardiology

Melanie Savoca, Monica Nagle, and Susan Konek

Congenital Heart Disease

Congenital heart disease (CHD) is one of the most common congenital defects in the United States with an incidence of approximately 8 per 1000 live births.[1] Malnutrition and growth disturbances are especially prevalent in this population and have been well documented in the literature. Research has demonstrated that failure to thrive in cardiac patients is attributed to a variety of factors and is often multifactorial. Some of these factors include inadequate energy intake, poor feeding skills, increased metabolic demands, and disturbances in gastrointestinal (GI) function, as well as type and clinical impact of the cardiac lesion.[2] The combination of chronic disease and malnutrition in the pediatric population can have a detrimental effect on growth, development, and disease-related morbidity and mortality.[3]

Nutrition support for infants and children with CHD covers a wide range of topics from acute care in infancy to chronic care in childhood. The magnitude of the effect of the cardiac defect on growth, development, and nutritional status depends on the particular lesion and its severity.[4] Malnutrition and growth retardation are common worldwide in infants and children with CHD.[5–16] Although some types of CHD are not found until older infancy, adolescence, and even adulthood, the majority of defects are diagnosed during routine prenatal care or soon after birth.[17]

Corrective surgeries for CHD have become increasingly common at an earlier age and can improve the nutritional status of infants with CHD by eliminating cardiac factors that contribute to failure to thrive.[18] If early cardiac surgery is not an option for an infant, then aggressive nutrition intervention and special nutrition considerations are required to prevent unsuccessful outcomes associated with malnutrition. Despite improvements in surgical palliation, nutritional problems contributing to malnutrition often emerge shortly after surgery and persist throughout the first year or years of life. Failure to thrive in pediatric patients with CHD results in more frequent hospital admissions with longer lengths of stay, ultimately increasing the cost of their care.[19] More alarming is the finding by Eskedal and colleagues[20] that a strong association exists between a decrease in weight-for-age following surgical correction of CHD and late mortality during the first year of life.

Factors Associated with Malnutrition

Inadequate energy intake has been frequently cited as a component of the growth failure in infants and children with CHD.[18,21–28] In one study by Barton and colleagues,[25] energy intake of children with CHD was 76% of the intake of unaffected children of the same age; eight infants with CHD had an intake of 82% of the estimated average requirements.

A study by Mitchell and associates[16] evaluated the nutritional status of 48 children admitted for surgical repair of CHD. All of the children were markedly malnourished; 83% had at least five biochemical or hematologic indices of malnutrition, and 52% had weights below the third percentile. Controversy exists concerning the etiology of growth failure and the role of inadequate energy intake, hypermetabolism, malabsorption, and cardiac anomaly.

Hypermetabolism has been described in CHD.[25] Total daily energy expenditure (TDEE) was measured in infants with CHD by the doubly labeled water method. TDEE includes basal metabolism as well as the energy of activity, sweating, and the mechanical labor of the heart and lungs.[29] A significantly higher TDEE was found for infants with CHD (101 ± 3 kcal/kg/day), as compared with the TDEE for healthy infants (67 ± 14 kcal/kg/day).[25] The calculated increase in TDEE was 36% above that of healthy infants, except for one infant who had a very high TDEE.[29] Another study did not find significantly higher resting energy expenditure (REE), measured by respiratory gas exchange method, in infants with CHD, except in a subgroup of infants with pulmonary hypertension and cardiac failure.[30] Leitch and associates found increased TDEE but not increased REE as a primary factor in reduced growth of infants with CHD as compared to age-matched controls.[31] Energy expenditure before and after cardiac surgery was measured in a doubly labeled water technique in 18 children with CHD, ages 4 to 33 months. Preoperative energy expenditures were clearly elevated in one-third of the children. This suggests that in a proportion of infants and children with CHD, increased basal metabolic rate is a contributing factor in the failure to thrive that is observed.

De Wit and colleagues[32] determined pre- and postoperative predictors of energy expenditure in children with CHD requiring open-heart surgery and compared measured REE with current predictive equations. Prospective REE data were collected using indirect calorimetry for 21 mechanically ventilated children (17 boys, 4 girls) admitted consecutively to the pediatric intensive care unit after surgery for CHD. Results indicated that most children had inadequate delivery of nutrients compared with actual requirements. Furthermore, cardiopulmonary bypass had a significant influence on energy expenditure after surgery; in patients who underwent cardiopulmonary bypass during surgery, mean REE was 26% higher than in patients undergoing non-bypass surgery. Children who were malnourished preoperatively had greater REE postoperatively. None of the current predictive equations predicted energy requirements within acceptable clinical accuracy.[32]

The type of cardiac lesion also significantly impacts the pattern of growth failure. Cardiac lesions are designated as cyanotic or acyanotic (**Table 14-1**), depending on the hemodynamic effect. Cyanotic heart diseases are characterized by insufficient pulmonary blood flow. Acyanotic heart diseases consist of lesions with left-to-right shunting, resulting in pulmonary overcirculation and signs of congestive heart failure. Other acyanotic lesions are those associated with compromised systemic output and include aortic stenosis, coarctation of the aorta, and interrupted aortic arch. Patients with cyanotic heart lesions usually exhibit reduced height and weight.[5–7,15,33,34] Modi and associates[35] found the basal metabolic state of the heart in infants and children to be significantly greater in the presence of cyanosis compared to acyanosis. Acyanotic lesions with a large degree of left-to-right shunting typically affect only weight while sparing height in the early stages.[5,33,36] One study found suboptimal recovery of somatic growth following corrective surgery for ventricular septal defects in infants with severe preoperative malnutrition. For both boys and girls, weight on follow-up was significantly lower when compared with healthy children from the same geographical area.[37]

Congestive heart failure (CHF) also may cause growth failure. Heart failure is thought to increase metabolic rate, therefore increasing the energy required for growth. Some cardiac diseases that may cause CHF include atrioventricular canal defects, cardiomyopathy, or CHD causing chronic hypoxemia. Additionally, patients with pulmonary hypertension in combination with CHD, particularly left-to-right shunts, have a higher risk for growth failure.[38] These children tend to weigh less than do children with cyanotic heart lesions.[26,28] One study found that growth retardation was proportional to the size of the shunt.[12] Another study using Waterlow's criteria for failure to thrive found the prevalence of malnutrition in children with left-to-right intracardial shunting to be 83%; children with pulmonary hypertension had even greater nutritional problems.[9] Obstructive malformations, such as pulmonary stenosis and coarctation of the aorta, typically result in impaired linear growth, with linear growth more affected than weight.[5,38,39] Strategies to nourish these infants and children in the acute and chronic aspects of care will be discussed in the following sections.

Acute Care

Nutrition support is essential during infancy due to the rapid increase in growth velocity. Nutrition is an integral component of care during all stages of treatment, including the acute phase when metabolic responses to stress are more profound.[40–42] Some infants with cardiac problems are

TABLE 14-1 Congenital Heart Defects

Cyanotic	Acyanotic
Ebstein's Anomaly of the Tricuspid Valve	Atrial Septal Defect (ASD)
Hypoplastic Left Heart Syndrome (HLHS)	Atrioventricular Septal Defect
Pulmonary Atresia with Intact Ventricular Septum (PA/IVS)	Patent Ductus Arteriosus (PDA)
Pulmonary Stenosis (PS)	Truncus Arteriosus
Tetralogy of Fallot (TOF)	Ventricular Septal Defect (VSD)
Total Anomalous Pulmonary Venous Return (TAPVR)	Aortic Stenosis (AS)
Transportation of the Great Arteries (TGA)	Coarctation of the Aorta (CoA)
Tricuspid Atresia	Interrupted Aortic Arch (IAA)

Source: George Ofori-Amanfo, MD, and Melanie Savoca, MS, RD, CNSC, LDN, Children's Hospital of Philadelphia.

admitted to the newborn or cardiac intensive care unit in an acutely ill state within the first days of life. Some can be stabilized and surgery may be deferred for weeks; others may need immediate surgery. Many infants with CHD require surgery before 1 year of age.[43] Depending on the type of cardiac defect, multiple surgeries may be planned for a staged palliation throughout childhood. As in any surgery, the best outcome is achieved in the patient who has a good nutritional status and positive nitrogen balance. Research has shown that preoperative malnutrition is associated with a longer intensive care unit length of stay.[44] The immediate goal for nutrition support in infants is to achieve the best nutritional status possible in preparation for surgery as well as during postoperative recovery.[45] Other less immediate nutrition support goals are to encourage normal growth velocity and support normal feeding skill development. Optimal nutrition support may be unattainable at times due to the many complicating factors in these patients in the acute care setting.[45] Nutrition goals should include adequate provision of nutrients for maintenance of lean body mass and wound healing.

For neonates diagnosed with CHD, the primary nutrition goal after birth is to minimize neonatal weight loss during the preoperative period. Controversy exists regarding route of nutrition for these patients. Nutritional practice varies among institutions, but many cardiac intensive care units initiate enteral feeds after cardiac surgery. This practice is the result of concerns of increased risk of necrotizing enterocolitis (NEC) from cyanosis, prostaglandin (PGE) administration, or the presence of umbilical arterial catheters (UAC) prior to surgery. However, feeding of infants with cyanosis has not been shown to be associated with elevated incidence of NEC, and in hemodynamically stable infants, PGE administration has not been shown to be a risk factor for adverse events associated with enteral feeding.[46] Although the presence of UAC has been a theoretical risk factor for gut hypoperfusion, in one large series there was no significant increase in NEC in infants fed with UAC in place,[47] irrespective of placement: high versus low lying.[48] Furthermore, early initiation of minimal enteral nutrition in newborns appears to enhance functional maturation of the GI tract.[46] In some infants, this period of enteral nutrition deprivation is inevitable. However, literature has shown that a cautious introduction of early postnatal enteral nutrition may be largely beneficial.

During the immediate postoperative period, nutrition support should be initiated to promote wound healing, minimize loss of lean body mass, and support vital organ function. Barriers may preclude the delivery of adequate calories for growth at this time. These barriers include hemodynamic instability, hypotension, hyperglycemia, electrolyte derangements, fluid restrictions, impaired renal function, and mechanical ventilation.[45] Although infants have a fundamental need to grow, growth is not a critical priority during the immediate postoperative period. Growth cannot occur until the infant begins to recover from the postoperative stress response and positive nitrogen balance is achieved.[40] Additionally, overfeeding is associated with increased carbon dioxide (CO_2) production, difficulties weaning from ventilatory support, and impaired immune and organ function.[45] Nutrition support in the acutely ill infant typically involves the use of parenteral nutrition (PN) and intravenous (IV) fluids and requires careful attention. The infant may be fluid restricted; there may be multiple lines requiring 0.5–1 mL/hr each for patency. Medications and infusions may use a significant amount of fluid. It is not uncommon to have only 60–80 mL/kg of fluid allotted for nutrition support.

Laboratory values may be abnormal. The use of diuretics may deplete total body sodium and potassium; calcium, phosphorus, and magnesium levels may also be abnormal.[49] Due to the need for fluid restriction, the renal lab values may reflect some degree of dehydration, with elevated sodium and blood urea nitrogen. Acid–base status may also be altered, complicating electrolyte management.

Furthermore, other end organ dysfunction is often common. Renal problems, such as acute tubular necrosis or renal insufficiency, may develop. Some infants may temporarily need dialysis, further complicating nutrition support (see Chapter 13, Chronic Kidney Disease). For infants and children needing support prior to surgery or those unable to be weaned from the bypass pump after surgery, extracorporeal life support may be used.[50,5152]

As determined appropriate by a multidisciplinary medical team, enteral nutrition (EN) should be introduced as tolerated. PN and EN should be used simultaneously in the gradual transition to full enteral feedings. Once full EN is achieved, nutrition support should provide adequate calories and protein for optimal growth. Anthropometric measurements and growth trends should be regularly monitored. Development of feeding skills may also be an integral component of care at this point. A speech-language pathologist should be consulted if difficulties or concerns are noted in oral feeds.

Extracorporeal Life Support

Extracorporeal life support (ECLS), also called extracorporeal membrane oxygenation (ECMO) is an advanced form of cardiopulmonary support for acute reversible cardiac or respiratory failure that is unresponsive to conventional medical management. ECLS is a supportive intervention, not a therapeutic intervention. It allows for cardiopulmonary rest to support the resolution of a reversible lung and/or heart pathology. If function does not recover, ECLS may be used as a bridge to transplant. Indications for ECLS in the cardiac population include acute cardiac arrest or being unable to separate from cardiopulmonary bypass. The physiologic goal of ECLS is to improve systemic oxygen delivery and allow normal aerobic metabolism to continue while allowing the lungs and/or heart to "rest." ECLS is achieved by draining venous blood, removing CO_2, adding oxygen through an artificial lung, and returning the blood to the circulation via a vein (veno-venous [VV]) or an artery (veno-arterial [VA]).[52] There is no difference in nutrition support for VV or VA ECLS.[53]

Nutrition goals for patients on ECLS are to provide adequate calories and protein to minimize catabolism and promote wound healing. Although critically ill patients on ECLS are severely stressed, catabolic, and have an increased metabolic burden of wound healing,[54] caloric requirements are decreased as neonates redirect energy, normally used for growth, to fuel the stress response.[53] ECLS replaces native pulmonary function and approximately 80% of cardiac function. The majority of thermoregulation is also provided by the ECLS circuit.[54] Research has estimated calorie needs for infants on ECLS to range between 70 and 80 kcal/kg. For older children, estimated energy needs may be 70–90% the REE.[53,55,56] Shew and colleagues[57] evaluated the effect of caloric intake on protein catabolism in 12 parenterally fed neonates on ECMO to determine whether higher calories would worsen or improve protein catabolism in critically ill neonates. They concluded that patients on ECMO are in negative nitrogen balance (mean -2.3 ± 0.6 g/kg/day), and higher caloric intake was positively correlated with negative protein balance, increased amino acid oxidation, increased protein breakdown and turnover, and increased CO_2 production.[57]

Nevertheless, provision of adequate caloric intake is paramount in this patient population. Fluid restriction, problems with glucose control, end organ dysfunction, and concerns of effects of IV lipids on the ECLS membrane pose challenges of meeting the calorie and protein needs. The key to nutritional management of the patient on ECLS is to provide optimal nutrition within the limits of restricted fluid intake. Total PN is initiated as early as possible with maximized caloric density. IV fat emulsion may be used to enhance caloric supply; however, fat emulsion should be administered through separate IV access during ECMO. Infusion directly through the ECMO circuit can cause agglutination and clot formation, which may result in disruption of normal ECMO blood flow and impaired delivery of calories.[58] Due to fluid restrictions, glucose infusion rate (GIR) should be calculated with each fluid change. A low-volume amount of 25% dextrose may yield a modest GIR; care should be taken if fluids are liberalized to adjust dextrose percentage. GIR should be limited to approximately 7 mg/kg/min (~10 g/kg/day) because excess carbohydrate intake may increase CO_2 production and respiratory quotient. Due to renal dysfunction, fluid resuscitation, and endocrine problems, electrolyte derangements are frequent occurrences among patients on ECMO. Careful attention to electrolyte needs and appropriate supplementation is of prime importance to avoid dysrhythmias. The electrolyte composition of PN should be determined by the patient's current serum electrolytes, prior need, and current clinical condition, particularly renal function. Problems have been noted with potassium, calcium, and magnesium. There may be an increased need for potassium in most infants and children undergoing ECLS, but vigilant monitoring of serum levels and urine output is needed. Sodium levels may initially be elevated secondary to sodium-containing resuscitation medications. Therefore, PN is often written with lower sodium and higher potassium.

Multiple complications can arise after initiation of ECMO support. Capillary leak syndrome is caused by increased vascular permeability due to prolonged hypoxia and hypotension, and can cause severe edema, particularly in neonates, with as much as a 50–75% weight increase. A systemic inflammatory response syndrome most often occurs related to blood exposure to foreign material, but is self-limited to 24–72 hours after initiation of ECLS or after a circuit change. Hemorrhagic or bleeding complications can also occur and are related to systemic heparization, which makes the blood twice as thin as normal. Cholestasis may be seen, but often resolves without long-term hepatic complications.[59] Gastroesophageal reflux (GER), delayed gastric emptying, and reduced gut motility are also seen in critically ill patients.[60]

In the past, EN has been restricted in patients on ECMO. This practice has been based on concerns of compromised splanchnic perfusion secondary to periods of hypoxia and vasopressor therapy in patients on ECMO. These factors may result in increased risk of NEC, bacterial translocation, and sepsis.[61] However, recent data show that EN in ECMO patients is not only safe,[62] but also maintains gut mucosal integrity, improves GI immunologic function, and minimizes the risk of sepsis.[63]

The practice of EN in patients on ECMO varies widely among centers. Initiation of EN is highly recommended because research has indicated that early initiation of enteral feeds is associated with the following findings: gut mucosal integrity and GI blood flow, secretion of GI hormones that enhances cell growth and development, improved glucose tolerance, stimulation of motor activity, improved GI mucosal immune function, and reduced morbidity in critically ill patients.[64–66] Research has determined that pediatric patients on ECMO have adequate gut hormone profiles, and enteral nutrition may be safely administered in this population.[67,68] EN may be instituted via the nasogastric route, initially as minimal or trophic feeds (10–15 mL/kg/day), and advanced slowly as tolerated.[69] Postpyloric feeding is suggested only if patients fail to tolerate gastric feeds. While on enteral nutrition, the patients should be monitored very closely for early signs of feeding intolerance.

Parenteral Nutrition Support

To plan the nutrition support for an acutely ill infant, the multidisciplinary team should review all fluids objectively. PN is driven by the total fluid limit of each patient. Laboratory tests, including basic metabolic and renal panels, glucose, and ionized calcium, should be monitored daily. Phosphorus and magnesium should be monitored daily until stable, and liver function should be checked weekly or as indicated. A bed scale can be helpful for the nursing staff to obtain daily weights used to evaluate fluid status. The pharmacist can determine whether the medications are concentrated appropriately to maximize fluid allotted for PN. Any dextrose used in fluid administration should be counted toward the overall GIR and carbohydrate and calorie intake. Sodium used in these fluids should be calculated because it can represent a significant and unexpected amount. Line patency fluids should be counted toward electrolyte, carbohydrate, calorie (if dextrose is a component), and fluid intake. PN fluids should be written last, accounting for the content of the other fluids. Because fluid is such an issue and may require altering in the course of the day, it may be helpful if total PN admixtures are not used and lipids run separately. PN is usually very concentrated in the cardiac infant, due to fluid restrictions. Central lines are generally used because peripheral PN lines should not contain more than 12.5% dextrose. With increasing dextrose concentrations, the osmolarity of solutions increases dramatically. Typically, the maximum dextrose concentration used in central lines is 25%. Higher dextrose percentages increase the risk of thrombosis. The tip of venous lines should be verified by radiology film prior to initiation of PN to determine the maximum dextrose concentration that can be safely infused. The risks and benefits of providing higher calories through a higher percentage of glucose should be considered carefully. GIR should be calculated daily or with every dextrose-containing fluid change. Postoperative infants may tolerate a GIR of only 10–12 mg glucose/kg/minute.

IV lipids are a concentrated source of calories and a source of essential fatty acids. Typically, 20% lipids are used (see Chapter 20). A 30% lipid solution is available for three-in-one mixtures, but pediatric applications for this product have not been seen in the literature. Lipids should be used over the greatest amount of time possible (24-hour infusion, if not contraindicated by a lipid-incompatible medication). Triglyceride levels should be monitored to assess tolerance to this therapy.

Protein needs are important to consider in this stressed population. Chaloupecky and colleagues[70] found that the provision of a small amount of IV protein, 0.8 g/kg/day, blunted the muscle proteolysis hypercatabolic response in infants after cardiac surgery, in contrast to an isocaloric maintenance dextrose solution. Starting PN with protein immediately postoperatively would seem to be warranted, even if only half of maintenance fluids can be used for this endeavor, due to electrolyte fluctuations. Careful attention to limited dextrose, protein, and electrolytes should be made because renal output may be temporarily reduced after cardiopulmonary bypass. Hyperglycemia is also common early after infant cardiac surgery. Insulin is not often used because glucose levels usually improve within 24–48 hours. Ballweg and associates[71] also found that hyperglycemia early after infant cardiac surgery was not associated with worse neurodevelopmental outcome at 1 year of age, but delayed sternal closure was associated with a statistically significant relationship among initial, minimum, and maximum glucose values.

In addition, it may not be possible for mineral needs for bone development to be met in the short term, due to the use of PN and fluid limitations. Diuretic use may alter calcium status. Premature and term infant calcium and phosphorus requirements for bone mineralization often cannot be realized until later. The use of premature infant or premature follow-up formulas may be considered as a component of the nutrition support for a fluid-restricted infant with higher mineral needs. Signs of cholestasis and bone demineralization should be monitored closely for patients requiring long-term PN.[72]

Gastrointestinal Function

As has been noted, major and frequently seen complications of hospitalized infants with CHD are inadequate enteral intake, GI morbidity, and feeding problems.[8] These affect growth and recovery and can influence short- and long-term outcomes.[38] The challenges of supporting nutrition in children with CHD are discussed in the sections highlighting specific conditions and points in the course of treatment. A number of GI concerns are common in many of these infants. Malabsorption, including fat and/or protein malabsorption, is a common feature.[18,73] Protein-losing enteropathy is a condition reported in patients with increased right-sided heart pressures, especially young children who have undergone the Fontan operation. Decreased cardiac output, in addition to causing early satiety and vomiting, may also cause decreased nutrient absorption.[28] Furthermore, some children with CHD have GI malformations that will affect their ability to be nourished. These may include pyloric stenosis, duodenal atresia, malrotation, and severe defects such as gastroschisis, all requiring surgical repair. Reduced gut perfusion is another factor recognized as a complication often present in infants with cardiac insufficiency. The risk of NEC is increased and care must be taken to avoid this serious condition.

Inadequate energy intake is felt to be the predominant cause of growth failure in infants with CHD. Achieving adequate calories through oral feedings is difficult. Oral feeding, even if the patient's condition allows, requires a great deal of energy expenditure and may result in tachypnea and fatigue. It is difficult to achieve adequate intake to support nutritional needs. Other factors contributing to inadequate intake include early satiety, decreased gastric capacity related to hepatomegaly, and delayed gastric emptying as a result of low cardiac output or medication side effect.

A study by Jadcherla, Vijayapal, and Leuthner[74] compared the impact of acyanotic and cyanotic CHD in neonates on enteral feeding milestones. Those children with cyanotic CHD had significant delays in time to initiate and achieve maximal gavage feeds and maximal nipple feeds, and prolonged lengths of hospital stay. Even so, a high percentage of infants in both groups eventually were able to achieve adequate nipple feedings upon discharge. This study also found that prolonged respiratory support had a negative effect in groups, affecting maximal nippling skills, but also delaying achievement of maximal tube feeds. It was noted in another study of infants with cyanotic and acyanotic heart lesions that feeding practices, rather than type of heart defects, predicted weight gain postoperatively.[75] Use of the needed feeding modalities will support weight gain and growth.

In planning for transition to enteral feeding, it is important to remember the impact of the cardiorespiratory system on the achievement of enteral nutrition support.[74] Infants with a history of cardiopulmonary bypass and prolonged respiratory support showed abnormalities in oromotor feeding skills. For pediatric patients intubated for more than 7 days, the risk of dysphagia increases, as does the inability to feed orally by hospital discharge.[76,77] The Jadcherla study noted other covariates including narcotic use, vasopressor support, and cardiopulmonary bypass. Tachypnea may also cause an uncoordinated suck, swallow, and breathe pattern necessary for successful oral feeding. Fatigue is common in these infants. They often cannot feed long enough to support their nutritional needs.

Sluggish reflexes, decreased sensory input, hypoxemia, neurological insults, or bowel ischemia may impair the GI system. In the event of gut hypoperfusion, waiting for bowel recovery may cause delayed initiation of EN. GER, which is common in up to 65% of healthy infants,[78,79] may play a role in CHD. The use of a nasogastric tube may result in increased reflux symptoms.

Neurologic maturation is another key factor that should be considered in the ability of an infant to reach optimal intake.[80] Infants with CHD have higher risk for neurologic sequelae, including bleeds or strokes. Children with CHD are often found to have neurologic disabilities.[81] Although neurologic deficits result from a variety of causes, infants with these complications are most often supported by long-term tube feedings. An acquired neurologic complication in patients with hypoplastic left heart syndrome (HLHS) may have a profound effect on the ability to feed. During surgery, the recurrent laryngeal nerve is at risk for injury. Although injury to this nerve can be caused by a variety of operative events, such as arch augmentation, the result is vocal cord paresis or paralysis and often GER.[82] It has been reported that laryngopharyngeal dysfunction presents after the Norwood procedure in about 48% of patients, with resultant dysphagia, aspiration, and left recurrent laryngeal nerve injury.[83] For these reasons, vocal cord dysfunction will often result in the need for gavage feedings to support nutrition.

Other complicating factors to achievement of EN goals were reported by Kogon and colleagues[84] in a review of 83 patients who underwent surgery for congenital heart defects within 15 days of life and survived to hospital discharge. Feeding difficulties included: 10.8% had prolonged time to reach full feeds, 44.6% had prolonged time to transition to oral feeds, and 9.6% required subsequent procedures to facilitate feeding. Significant risk factors for these individual endpoints included increased risk-adjusted congenital heart surgery (RACHS) score[85] and prolonged intubation. It was noted that the premature infant has greater challenges in the achievement of postoperative feeding. Premature infants with chronic hypoxia and poor pulmonary function had higher energy expenditure and greater caloric requirement.

These factors that affect GI function require consideration in plans to support the CHD infant with enteral feedings.

Enteral Nutrition Support

As previously noted, GI function may not be optimal in some infants with cardiac anomalies. Therefore, a slow, cautious approach to enteral feeding, such as a protocol used for feeding premature infants, is reasonable.[50] PN can be the supplemental nutrition source until full volume enteral feeding has been established. In the transition from PN to EN, caution should be used with the addition of hyperosmolar medications.[86,87] NEC also has been associated with hyperosmolar formulas, and the addition of medications can make an isotonic feeding hypertonic.[88,89] Hyperosmolar medications have also been known to cause osmotic diarrhea.

Many infants with CHD will need additional calories, so it may be necessary to increase the caloric density of infant formulas from 20 kcal/oz to 30 kcal/oz. Once full volume of enteral feeds is achieved, caloric density can be increased gradually. The multidisciplinary team should determine the volume of enteral fluid tolerated by each patient; however, the amount of fluid used is often related to the amount of diuretic therapy. Diuretics may be used to lessen the effects of high-volume feedings, although side effects of potassium wasting, acid–base problems,[90] and potential for altered calcium and magnesium excretion exist. The literature indicates infants tolerate feeds if the calorie increase is done slowly, increasing by approximately 2 kcal/oz at a time.[87] The enteral formulas used for infants and children with CHD are the same as for other children. To increase the caloric density of formulas, they can be made using less water with formula powder or liquid concentrate, which keeps the original proportion of carbohydrate, protein, and fat the same. However, when the caloric density of formulas is increased, the amount of electrolytes and minerals is also increased, and should be taken into consideration. Although this change does increase the osmolality of the formula, in practice, the medications added to formulas alter the osmolality to a much greater extent than the formula alone.[54] Osmolality of products commonly used in intensive care nurseries is discussed elsewhere.[87,89,91,92] In practice, some clinicians use an IV preparation of a medicine, such as IV potassium chloride instead of the oral form, which has a greater osmolality due to the syrup suspension of the medication.[87]

Calorie needs of infants and children with CHD are most often greater than those without cardiac problems. Studies using nutrition intervention in either the inpatient or outpatient setting have shown that normal growth can be achieved using higher calorie intakes. Continuous intragastric infusion of an average of 137 kcal/kg/day in 146 mL/kg/day of formula was used with a small group of 2- to 24-week-old infants with normal growth in weight and length.[93] Partial (12-hour) and total (24-hour) continuous nasogastric tube feedings of 31.8 kcal/oz formulas were compared with oral feedings in a group of young infants over a 5-month period. The formulas were made using a cow's milk- or soy protein–based formula with added rice cereal and glucose polysaccharides. Approximately 147 kcal/kg and 167 mL/kg were given in the 24-hour infusion group and 70 kcal/kg from tube feeding plus oral intake, for a total of 122 kcal/kg in the 12-hour infusion group; the oral feeding control group averaged 95 kcal/kg. Comparing Z-scores, only the 24-hour infusion group had improvement in length and weight.[94] Another study using 24-hour continuous infusion showed a growth improvement of 198% with infants age 1 week to 9 months who had previously displayed poor growth. The calorie range used was 120–150 kcal/kg with a 24–30 kcal/oz range in caloric densities of the formulas.[95] Infants with mild CHD were given higher calorie formula recipes to increase calorie intake by 20% in oral feedings. Favorable growth was seen in 60% of the group with the higher calorie intake.[96] Higher calorie formulas were used in a study with oral feedings and infants with CHD. Calories were increased by 32%, and weight gain improved significantly. The authors' recommendation is to begin supplementation from the time of diagnosis to optimize growth.[97] A study using nutritional counseling in underweight infants and children with CHD showed increased oral calorie intake and improved anthropometric studies over a 6-month period of counseling.[98] Interestingly, a small study reviewing feeding and growth of breastfed versus bottle-fed infants with CHD showed better growth in the breastfed infants.[99] A naturalistic study reviewing the behavioral and physiologic response of infants during feeding did not show a pattern in infants with CHD, as compared with healthy controls, but there was a wide range of individual differences among the 20 infants studied.[100]

The precise energy needs of infants with CHD are difficult to estimate, but many infants will need 120–150 kcal/kg or greater in EN. Toddlers and children may need 20–33% more than normal estimated needs. Post-cardiac repair, the calorie needs will usually decrease[16] but may stay 10–15 kcal/kg above the average for some infants or children. Calorie needs may also remain increased for catch-up growth for patients malnourished prior to surgery. Calorie needs may be estimated using indirect calorimetry while in the hospital; however, many nurseries do not have the equipment to accurately assess infants under 5 kg or infants who are mechanically ventilated. The best method is to set an estimated goal, assess growth parameters, and make adjustments as needed until appropriate growth velocity is achieved.

Pediatric Cardiomyopathy

Pediatric cardiomyopathy is a serious disorder of the heart muscle that is responsible for significant morbidity and mortality among affected children. The estimated incidence is between 1.13 and 1.24 cases per 100,000 children 18 years of age and younger, with the highest incidence among children less than 1 year of age.[101–103] Despite the low incidence, children with cardiomyopathy have some of the worst clinical outcomes compared to other heart diseases in children. Nearly one-third of all children diagnosed with pediatric cardiomyopathy prior to 1 year of age will die within 1 year of diagnosis, and approximately one-third will receive pediatric heart transplants.[104] Cardiomyopathy predominates at 64% as the most common indication for heart transplantation in older children.[104] Heart transplantation remains the standard of care for children who fail medical therapy.

The World Health Organization classifies cardiomyopathy into four distinct categories:[105]

1. Dilated cardiomyopathy is characterized by pathologic stretching of the myocardial fibers, causing dilatation of the ventricles and decreased contractility.
2. Hypertrophic cardiomyopathy is an abnormal growth or arrangement of myocardial fibers that leads to a thickening of the ventricular walls and reduction in size of the

pumping chamber; it is often associated with obstruction of the left ventricular outflow tract.

3. Restrictive cardiomyopathy is stiffening of the walls of the ventricles and loss of ventricular compliance, resulting in decreased cardiac filling and hence decreased cardiac output.
4. Arrythmogenic right ventricular cardiomyopathy is characterized by the replacement of myocytes in the right ventricle with fatty, fibrous tissue.

Malnutrition is one of the most significant clinical problems in children with cardiomyopathy due to an imbalance between nutritional intake and requirement. The disease is associated with increased caloric demands of the failing heart, increased work of breathing, and a general catabolic state of chronic illness. The patients have decreased oral intake from decreased appetite, feeding intolerance, and poor gastrointestinal absorption. Nearly one-third of children with this disorder will manifest some degree of growth failure during the course of their illness.[105] The fundamental cause is primarily persistent CHF, which can result in increased metabolic demands, GI issues, malabsorption, and decreased food intake. Although it is apparent that cardiomyopathy may lead to malnutrition, it is important to consider that malnutrition may further lead to complications that may directly or indirectly impact heart function and overall clinical status.[105] Infants, children, and adolescents with cardiomyopathy may also have need for a ventricular assist device (VAD) as a bridge to transplantation. Little is known about VAD-related gastroenterologic complications; however, because of its intra-abdominal placement, the potential exists for major abdominal complications, including intra-abdominal infections, delayed gastric emptying, gastritis, and pancreatitis.[106,107]

One study evaluating cardiac outcomes in chronically ill children revealed nutritional status was a strong and independent predictor of mortality and cardiac function.[108] Adequate nutrition forms an integral part of the management of heart failure associated with cardiomyopathy. Nutritional rehabilitation should be instituted early and aggressively to prevent a vicious downward cycle of growth failure and worsened clinical outcome. Optimal nutrition is critical in providing affected children the means to withstand the detrimental metabolic effects of the disease, participate in rehabilitation, and recover from their illness. The goal of therapy is adequate EN; however, the hospitalized acutely ill patient with decompensated heart failure may not tolerate enteral feeds. In such cases, PN should be instituted with transition to enteral feeds as soon as possible.

Chylothorax

Chylothorax is the presence of lymphatic fluid in the pleural space caused by a leak in the thoracic duct or because of lymphatic abnormalities. It is usually a result of iatrogenic complications of cardiac or thoracic surgery, commonly trauma to the thoracic duct or other surrounding vessels.[109,110] It also has been described in children with syndromes associated with CHD, including trisomy 21, Noonan's and Turner's syndromes, and cardio-facio-cutaneous syndrome.[111–117] Sometimes chylothorax can result from high pressure within the superior vena cava (SVC), thereby affecting the pressure in the lymphatic system.[109,118] This is seen mainly in operations that cause increased SVC pressure, such as the hemi-Fontan, bidirectional Glenn, Fontan, and Senning procedures, and can also be seen in patients with thrombus occluding the SVC or subclavian vessels.[118]

Chyle is a white, milky-appearing substance composed of chylomicrons and lymph, which is transported to the systemic circulation via the thoracic duct. The primary purpose of chyle is the absorption and transportation of long-chain triglycerides (LCT) in the intestines. Chyle is formed in the lacteals of the intestines during digestion in response to the presence of intraluminal fat. The chyle binds with LCT to form chylomicrons, which are then absorbed and transported by the intestinal lymphatics to the bloodstream. Chyle also contains protein and is responsible for absorption of fat-soluble vitamins; therefore, high losses are of great nutritional concern.[110] When a person is not being fed, the fluid can appear less white, and more yellowish or clear. Diagnosis of chylothorax can be made if there are elevated lymphocytes, triglycerides, and high total protein content in a sample of the pleural fluid.[110,118–120]

Treatment of chylothorax can be multifactorial. Pleural drainage, a very low-fat diet and/or a diet containing the majority of fats as medium-chain triglycerides (MCT), gut rest, or PN are the main modalities used in treating chylous effusions.[121] MCTs are absorbed directly into the portal system, as are carbohydrates and amino acids, and thus do not stimulate an increase in lymphatic flow. Nutritional management usually starts with trialing a low-fat or MCT-enriched formula, observing for a reduction in chylous output, and if ineffective, providing gut rest with PN.[110,122] Formulas containing high amounts of MCT may not meet patients' essential fatty acid (EFA) needs, because MCT does not contain EFAs. Therefore, supplementation with small amounts of LCT to meet 2–4% of total calories may be necessary to prevent EFA deficiency[110,122] in patients that are fed long term with these specialty formulas. An elevated triene-to-tetraene ratio is one clinical indicator of an EFA deficiency.[123] Good sources of EFA that include both linoleic and linolenic acids are walnut oil and flaxseed oil.[124] Formulas commonly used for the management of chylothorax are listed in **Table 14-2** for comparison purposes. Some patients are successfully fed using skimmed breast milk, which has been supplemented in calories using MCT, protein powder, and a source of EFA.[124,125]

TABLE 14-2 Selected Formulas with High MCT Content for Chylothorax

Formula	Type	Calories per 100 g Powder	MCT:LCT Ratio	Fat % of Calories	Protein g per 100 g Powder	n6:n3 Ratio
Monogen (Nutricia)	Powder	470	87:13	40	16.5	40.5:1
Portagen* (Mead Johnson)	Powder	424	90:10	25	11.4	4.6:1
Vivonex Pediatric** (Néstle)	Powder	412	68:32	25	12.4	7.7:1

*Not intended as a sole source of nutrition. For chronic (long-term) use: supplementation of essential fatty acids and other nutrients should be considered [manufacturer's notation]. Only contains vitamins and minerals, no trace elements.

**1 packet of Vivonex Pediatric contains 48.5 g powder.

Abbreviations: MCT, medium chain triglycerides; LCT, long chain triglycerides; n6, omega-6; n3, omega-3; g, grams.

Source: Data from manufacturers' product labels.

Medical management of chylous effusions may include use of somatostatin and its analogue octreotide. It is known to reduce intestinal secretions and inhibit lymph excretion.[126] Caution must be used when enterally feeding patients receiving somatostatin or octreotide because splanchnic circulation may be diminished; GI side effects should be closely monitored.[126]

High losses of chylous pleural fluid can result in deficiencies in fat-soluble vitamins.[110,120,122] Large volume output from chylothorax can cause high protein losses, resulting in low albumin levels and losses of electrolytes and immunoglobulins. Sodium and calcium levels may be decreased, and metabolic acidosis may be seen in patients with high outputs. Hypovolemia can also occur, which can lead to hemodynamic instability.[110]

Genetic Syndromes and Chromosome Anomalies

Many genetic syndromes and chromosome anomalies are associated with congenital heart defects, including Down syndrome (trisomy 21), trisomy 13 and 18, Turner's syndrome, William's syndrome, DiGeorge and/or velo-cardio-facial syndrome, Marfan syndrome, Ellis-van Crevald syndrome, Noonan's syndrome, VACTERL syndrome (tracheal and esophageal malformations associated with vertebral, anorectal, cardiac, renal, radial, and limb abnormalities), and CHARGE syndrome (coloboma, heart defect, atresia choanae, retarded growth and development, genital hypoplasia, ear anomalies/deafness).

Within the spectrum of genetic syndromes, many of these infants and children are likely to have feeding difficulties and may be genetically prone to growth delays. For infants with Down syndrome, low muscle tone may contribute to poor oromotor skills, as well as constipation and other digestive problems.[127,128] DiGeorge syndrome is a genetic disorder with varying conditions present in each infant with the syndrome. An estimated 90% of patients with DiGeorge syndrome have a chromosomal 22q11 deletion, which is associated with a wide range of CHD.[129,130] Other conditions common to this syndrome include hypocalcemia, immunodeficiency, dysmorphic facial appearance, palate anomalies, speech and feeding disorders, lack of or underdeveloped thymus and parathyroid glands, and neurocognitive and behavioral disorders.[131,132]

Infants and children with CHARGE syndrome should also be monitored closely for growth and adequacy of nutrition intake.[133] At birth, children with CHARGE syndrome usually have normal weights and lengths; however, growth and development retardation may become more apparent as the child matures.[134] These children have a higher incidence of aspiration and GER. Influence of feeding problems on growth in infancy should not be underestimated. Approximately 90% of children with CHARGE syndrome have received tube feedings at some point in time.[134]

Feeding in children with genetic and chromosomal anomalies can be a significant challenge for families and medical professionals. These children may require aggressive medical nutrition management, often requiring long-term enteral access via gastrostomy and jejunostomy feeding tubes. Gastroesophageal fundoplication may be indicated for GER that does not respond to conventional medical therapy.

Chronic Care

Feeding methodology often becomes a concern in the follow-up care of infants and children with cardiac anomalies. In infancy, when caloric needs are very high, an infant may eat eagerly for a short time and then quit. Parents and caregivers may assume the infant is full, but it may be that the infant lacks the energy needed to adequately feed. Other infants and children may refuse to eat or feed very poorly. Thommessen and associates[135] found 65% of parents of infants and children with CHD document feeding problems. The reported feeding problems were a good predictor of low voluntary food intake and suboptimal growth outcome.

As previously noted, higher calorie formulas or supplements may be used to decrease the volume needed for optimal caloric intake. For infants who may orally feed, oral feedings should typically not exceed 30 minutes in length. If an infant is unable to take a desired volume within that time, an indwelling nasogastric tube may be used to give the remainder of the feed. If an infant is close to goal, he or she may be able to feed by mouth during the day and receive overnight tube feedings to make up the daytime deficit. Frequent follow-up care with an outpatient dietitian should be recommended to ensure projected goal volumes and rate of growth are still appropriate for age. For some infants, 24-hour infusions may be needed. Attempts can be made to compress feedings into a shorter infusion time, giving a few hours off for social and developmental purposes. For infants and children not able to take oral feeds, an oral stimulation program should be initiated, and oral motor therapies can be instituted by an experienced occupational therapist or speech-language pathologist.

For infants and children who are thought to need tube feeding assistance for more than 3 months, a gastric tube (G-tube) is a positive step toward simplifying the care. G-tubes can be inserted surgically or endoscopically (percutaneous endoscopic gastrostomy). G-tubes and tube feedings should be viewed as tools to improve the quality of life. Without the pressure of forced or unpleasant mealtimes or around-the-clock marathons, feeding can be pleasurable, with the best possible behavioral and developmental outcome. Oral feedings should be a pleasant time for both the caregiver and the infant or child.

Monitoring growth has long been mandatory in infants and children with CHD. In the heterogeneous population of children with CHD, it is important to screen those at risk for malnutrition during follow-up care. Preventive measures and early nutritional intervention is the best approach to correcting growth problems in childhood. Multidisciplinary teamwork is again important; growth or appetite problems can be caused by a change in clinical course or by a change in medication. It is necessary to consider all possibilities for failure to thrive when cardiac status is stable and calorie intake appears sufficient for good growth. Reevaluation of all parameters on an ongoing basis provides the best outcome.

Pediatric Hyperlipidemia

Hyperlipidemia is an elevation of lipids in the bloodstream. These lipids include cholesterol, cholesterol esters, phospholipids, and triglycerides. They are transported in the blood as part of lipoproteins. The aim of nutrition support in pediatric hyperlipidemia is to provide nutrition for normal growth and development, as well as to normalize lipid levels as much as possible to decrease the risk of cardiovascular disease.[136] The Centers for Disease Control and Prevention analyzed results from the National Health and Nutrition Examination Survey (NHANES) for 1999–2006. The results of that analysis found the prevalence of abnormal lipid levels among youth ages 12–19 years was 20.3%.[137] The National Cholesterol Education Program (NCEP) and the American Heart Association (AHA) advocate dietary changes for all healthy children over 2 years of age and for adolescents.[138,139] The Therapeutic Lifestyle Changes (TLC) diet macronutrients recommendations are 50–60% of total calories from carbohydrates, 15% of total calories from protein, and limiting total fat to 25–35% of total calories.[138] Saturated fat and dietary cholesterol, which are LDL-raising nutrients, should be limited to less than 7% of total calories and 200 mg/day, respectively. Therapeutic options for lowering LDL cholesterol include consuming 2 g/day of plant stanols/sterols and increased viscous (soluble) fiber.[138] The dietary changes suggested for all individuals are similar to the TLC diet guidelines and can be incorporated into the use of the food pyramid.[138] Before the age of 2 years, restriction of fat intake may result in altered growth.[140] The American Academy of Pediatrics recommends that total fat intake should not fall below 20% of total calories for children and adolescents.[140]

The AHA heart-healthy dietary guidelines were revised in 2000 and emphasize the importance of a diet low in saturated and trans fat, and rich in fruits, vegetables, whole grains, fat-free and low-fat dairy products, and lean meat, fish, and poultry.[139] For children at higher risk, the new NCEP TLC guidelines offer dietary therapy for subgroups of people with specific medical conditions and risk factors, which include high LDL cholesterol, dyslipidemia, coronary heart disease or other cardiovascular disease, diabetes mellitus, insulin resistance, or metabolic syndrome. Refer to the NCEP guidelines for medical and dietary management of lipid serum levels.[138] If serum levels are not improved with dietary intervention alone, medication may be considered for children over 10 years of age.[140]

Increasing fiber intake is advocated for all children over 2 years of age. The American Dietetic Association recommends children consume a number of grams of fiber each day that equals their age plus 5 additional grams.[141] This rule should be applied throughout adolescence until the age of 20, at which time adult guidelines should be followed. Fiber may be helpful in reducing serum cholesterol. Studies on the lipid-lowering effect of fiber in children have been inconclusive.[142] However, one study found water-soluble fibers such as psyllium enhanced the hypocholesterolemia effect of NCEP dietary changes by lowering LDL cholesterol an additional 5–10%.[143] A dietary intervention program designed for preschoolers, Healthy Start has been shown to reduce serum cholesterol when measured over the course of the school year. This program in a largely minority Head Start preschool population reduced the total and saturated fat content of snacks and meals.[144]

A few studies indicate that nutrition education and dietary intervention can improve weight loss in obese children, reduce obesity-related health risks, and improve dyslipidemias.[144–148] In a study by Reinehr and Andler,[149] weight loss and a reduction in body mass index was shown to improve the atherogenic profile and insulin resistance in children 4–15 years of age. Activity is important in reducing the likelihood of childhood obesity, and it is also an important facet of promoting cardiovascular health.[150] Playing outdoors and high-activity playing have been shown to have positive effects on risk factors for CHD in children ages 4–7.[151] The activity level of the family influences the activity of the children. A family commitment to a healthy lifestyle, including diet and physical activity, is essential.

Case Study

Nutrition Assessment

Client history: JT is a 1-day-old male delivered at an outside hospital by vaginal delivery at 38 weeks gestation and birth weight of 3200 grams (25th percentile). He had a prenatal diagnosis of congenital heart disease. He was transported to a pediatric tertiary care facility on the day of birth in anticipation of corrective cardiac surgery. He arrived intubated and mechanically ventilated. His echocardiogram upon arrival confirmed a diagnosis of hypoplastic left heart syndrome (HLHS). He underwent Norwood procedure on day of life (DOL) #2. JT initially came off cardiopulmonary bypass but had open sternum due to profound hypoxemia associated with chest closure. He underwent delayed sternal closure on post-operative day (POD) #4 after aggressive dieresis had been accomplished.

Food/nutrition-related history: No enteral feeds were started in the preoperative period because surgery was planned for the following day. Parenteral nutrition was started on POD#1. JT was to receive 45 kcal/kg/day, 2 g protein/kg/day, and 2 g fat/kg/day from TPN. This was advanced to 60 kcal/kg/day on POD#2 and #3. Once his chest was closed and urine output improved, fluids were liberalized and TPN was advanced to 75 kcal/kg/day, 3 g/kg/day of protein, and 3 g/kg/day of lipid on POD#4.

On POD#5, the patient was started on trophic nasogastric (NG) feedings of maternal breast milk at 2 mL/hr. On POD#6, his umbilical arterial catheter was removed and a peripheral arterial line was placed. Feeds were then advanced by 30 mL/kg/day over the next few days to a goal of 100 mL/kg. The parenteral nutrition was weaned as the enteral feeding was advanced. Lipids were maintained at 3 g/kg/day to support calorie needs as the team was made aware that the child would not meet calorie needs if he was only at 100 mL/kg of enteral feedings of breast milk (20 kcal/oz). JT was slowly weaned off the ventilator and extubated onto nasal continuous positive airway pressure (NCPAP). Patient was made NPO peri-extubation. Once respiratory status was stable, enteral nutrition was resumed and enteral feeds were increased to 150 mL/kg/day. At this point, maternal breast milk was fortified with a standard infant formula liquid concentrate to 24 kcal/oz and lipids were discontinued. As of POD#12, JT was receiving 120 kcal/kg/day of current body weight, which had increased to 3.25 kg, up 100 grams from birth weight. By POD#18, JT had weaned off NCPAP, and continuous enteral feedings were condensed to bolus feeds every 3 hours. Oral feedings were attempted by the speech therapist, but found to be inappropriate at this time secondary to his increased work of breathing and uncoordinated suck and swallow patterns.

Anthropometric Measurements

Birth	Weight: 3.20 kg	Length: 49 cm	Wt/length: 50th–75th percentile
DOL#14	Weight: 3.25 kg	Length: 50 cm	Wt/length: 25th–50th percentile
DOL#28	Weight: 3.45 kg	Length: 51 cm	Wt/length: 25th–50th percentile
	Std Ht for age: 54.5 cm	% of Std Ht for age: 94%	

Estimated Nutrition Needs

Calories: WHO × 1.2–1.3 = 130–140 kcal/kg/day
Protein: 2–3 g/kg/day
Fluid: < 150 mL/kg/day for enteral nutrition

Biochemical Data, Medical Tests, and Procedures

Labs on DOL#28: (↓ = below normal; ↑ = above normal)

Na: 134	Cl: 91 ↓	BUN: 17	Gluc: 98	Mg: 1.9	H/H: 14.5/42.2 ↓
K: 3.7 ↓	CO_2: 36 ↑	Creat: 0.4	Ca: 9.3	Phos: 5.7	Alb: 2.8 ↓

Gastroesophageal Reflux Study/ Gastric Emptying Study

Studies showed multiple episodes of gastroesophageal reflux to the level of lower to mid esophagus, no evidence of pulmonary aspiration, and the rate of gastric emptying was within normal limits.

Current Medications

Captopril, furosemide, pantoprazole, aspirin, cholecalciferol 400 units/day

Assessment on DOL 28

Patient is currently receiving breast milk fortified to 24 kcal/oz at 60 mL every 3 hours. Current weight is 3.45 kg. Work of breathing has improved. Speech therapist continues to work with JT on oral feeding skills.

Percentage of IBW indicates weight is within normal limits, but percentage of standard height for age indicates mild stunting of growth. JT may benefit from increasing total caloric intake to achieve optimal growth. JT is on a proton pump inhibitor for reflux precautions. Labs reflect low potassium, chloride, and albumin, and elevated CO_2 levels.

Nutrition Diagnosis

Based on the information detailed above, a nutritional problem or diagnosis is made.

Nutrition Interventions

Because JT's weight gain has been suboptimal, recommend breast milk fortified to 27 kcal/oz and adjust volume to provide 150 mL/kg (65 mL every 3 hr) at JT's current body weight of 3.45 kg. Recommend limiting oral intake to ≤ 30 minutes, with the remainder of bolus feeds through the NG tube.

Questions for the Reader

1. What is JT's ideal body weight (IBW) and % of IBW on DOL#28?
2. How many calories and how much fluid per kilogram did JT's original regimen provide?
3. On average, how many grams per day of weight has JT gained over the past 14 days (between DOL#14 and #28)?
4. Write one PES statement.
5. How many calories per kg are provided in his current feeding regimen?
6. What would you want to monitor?
7. What rate of weight gain would be ideal for an infant of this age?
8. What are your goals for nutrition before discharge?

REFERENCES

1. Kay JD, Colan SD, Graham TP. Congestive heart failure in pediatric patients. *Am Heart J.* 2001;142(5):923–928.
2. Nydegger A, Bines JE. Energy metabolism in infants with congenital heart disease. *Nutrition.* 2006;22:697–704.
3. Steltzer M, Rudd N, Pick B. Nutrition care for newborns with congenital heart disease. *Clin Perinatol.* 2005;32:1017–1030.
4. Carlson SJ, Ryan JM. Congenital heart disease. In: Groh-Wargo S, Thompson M, Cox J, eds. *Nutritional Care for High Risk Newborns*, rev ed. Chicago: Precept Press, Inc.; 2000:397–408.
5. Mehrizi A, Drash A. Growth disturbance in congenital heart disease. *J Pediatr.* 1962;61:418–429.
6. Glassman MS, Woolf PK, Schwarz SM. Nutritional considerations in children with congenital heart disease. In: Baker SB, Baker RD Jr, Davis A, eds. *Pediatric Enteral Nutrition.* New York: Chapman & Hall; 1994:340.
7. Venogopalan P, Akinbami FO, Al-Minai KM, et al. Malnutrition in children with congenital heart disease. *J Saudi Med J.* 2001;22:1964–1967.
8. Cameron JW, Rosenthal A, Olson AD. Malnutrition in hospitalized children with congenital heart disease. *Arch Pediatr Adolesc Med.* 1995;149:1098–1102.
9. Villasis-Keever MA, Aquiles Pineda-Cruz R, Halley-Castillo E, et al. Frequency and risk factors associated with malnutrition in children with congenital cardiopathy. *Saluda Publica Mex.* 2001;43:313–323.
10. Thompson Chagoyan OC, Reyes Tsubaki N, Rubiela Barrios OL, et al. The nutritional status of the child with congenital cardiopathy. *Arch Inst Cardiol Mex.* 1998;68:119–123.
11. Dimiti AI, Anabwani GM. Anthropometric measurements in children with congenital heart disease at Kenyatta National Hospital (1985–1986). *East Afr Med J.* 1991;68:757–764.
12. Leite HP, de Camargo Carvalho AC, Fisberg M. Nutritional status of children with congenital heart disease and left-to-right shunt. The importance of the presence of pulmonary hypertension. *Arq Bras Cardiol.* 1995;65:403–407.
13. Miyague NI, Cardoso SM, Meyer F, et al. Epidemiological study of congenital heart defects in children and adolescents. Analysis of 4,538 cases. *Arq Bras Cardiol.* 2003;80:269–278.
14. Jacobs EG, Leung ML, Karlberg JP. Postnatal growth in southern Chinese children with symptomatic congenital heart disease. *J Pediatr Endocrinol Metab.* 2000;3:387–401.
15. Tambic-Bukovac L, Malcic I. Growth and development in children with congenital heart disease. *Lijec Vjesh.* 1993;115:79–84.
16. Mitchell IM, Logan RW, Pollock JCS, et al. Nutritional status of children with congenital heart disease. *Br Heart J.* 1995;73(3):277–283.

17. Levey A, Glickstein JS, Kleinman CS, et al. The impact of prenatal diagnosis of complex congenital heart disease on neonatal outcomes. *Pediatr Cardiol.* 2010;31(5):587–597.
18. Leitch CA. Growth, nutrition and energy expenditure in pediatric heart failure. *Prog Pediatr Cardiol.* 2000;11:195–202.
19. Silberback M, Shumaker D, Menshe V, Cobanoglu A, Morris C. Predicting hospital discharge and length of stay for congenital heart surgery. *Am J Cardiol.* 1993;72:958–963.
20. Eskedal LT, Hagemo PS, Seem E, et al. Impaired weight gain predicts risk of late death after surgery for congenital heart defects. *Arch Dis Child.* 2008;93(6):495–501.
21. Krieger I. Growth failure and congenital heart disease. Energy and nitrogen balance in infants. *Am J Dis Child.* 1970;120:497–502.
22. Huse DM, Feldt RH, Nelson RA, et al. Infants with congenital heart disease. *Am J Dis Child.* 1975;129:65–69.
23. Yahav J, Avigad S, Frand M, et al. Assessment of intestinal and cardiorespiratory function in children with congenital heart disease on high calorie formulas. *J Pediatr Gastroenterol Nutr.* 1985;4:778–785.
24. Hansen SR, Dorup I. Energy and nutrient intakes in congenital heart disease. *Acta Paediatr.* 1993;82:166–172.
25. Barton JS, Hindmarsh PC, Scrimgeour CM, et al. Energy expenditure in congenital heart disease. *Arch Dis Child.* 1994;70:59.
26. Van Der Kuip M, Hoos MB, Forget PP, Westerterp KR, Gemke RJ, De Meer K. Energy expenditure in infants with congenital heart disease, including a meta-analysis. *Acta Paediatr.* 2003;92:921–927.
27. Davis D, Davis S, Cotman K, et al. Feeding difficulties and growth delay in children with hypoplastic left heart syndrome versus d-transposition of the great arteries. *Pediatr Cardiol.* 2008;29(2):328–333.
28. Kelleher D, Lauseen P, Teixeira-Pinto M, Duggan C. Growth and correlates of nutrition status among infants with hypoplastic left heart syndrome (HLHS) after stage 1 Norwood procedure. *Nutrition.* 2006;22:237–244.
29. Broekhoff C, Houwen RHJ, de Meer K. Energy expenditure in congenital heart disease [commentary]. *J Pediatr Gastroenterol Nutr.* 1995;21:322–323.
30. Menon G, Poskitt EME. Why does congenital heart disease cause failure to thrive? *Arch Dis Child.* 1985;60:1134–1139.
31. Leitch CA, Karn CA, Peppard RJ, et al. Increased energy expenditure in infants with cyanotic congenital heart disease. *J Pediatr.* 1998;133:755–760.
32. De Wit B, Meyer R, Desai A, Macrae D, Pathan N. Challenge of predicting resting energy expenditure in children undergoing surgery for congenital heart disease. *Pediatr Crit Care Med.* 2010;11(4):496–501.
33. Forchielli ML, McColl R, Walker WA, et al. Children with congenital heart disease: a nutrition challenge. *Nutr Rev.* 1994;52:348–353.
34. Cheung MMH, Davis AM, Wilkinson JL, Weintraub RG. Long term somatic growth after repair of tetralogy of Fallot: evidence for restoration of genetic growth potential. *Heart.* 2003;89:1340–1343.
35. Modi P, Suleiman MS, Reeves BC, et al. Basal metabolic state of hearts of patients with congenital heart disease: the effects of cyanosis, age, and pathology. *Ann Thorac Surg.* 2004;78(5):1710–1716.
36. Umansky R, Hauck AJ. Factors in the growth of children with patent ductus arteriosis. *Pediatrics.* 1992;146:1078–1084.
37. Vaidyanathan B, Nair SB, Sundaram KR, et al. Malnutrition in children with congenital heart disease (CHD) determinants and short term impact of corrective intervention. *Indian Pediatr.* 2008;45(7):541–546.
38. Varan B, Tokel K, Yilmaz G. Malnutrition and growth failure in cyanotic and acyanotic congenital heart disease with and without pulmonary hypertension. *Arch Dis Child.* 1999;81(1):49–52.
39. Stranway A, Fowler R, Cunningkam K, et al. Diet and growth in congenital heart disease. *Pediatrics.* 1976;57:75–86.
40. Agus MS, Jaksic T. Nutritional support of the critically ill child. *Curr Opin Pediatr.* 2002;14:470–481.
41. Wang KS, Ford HR, Upperman JS. Metabolic response to stress in the neonate who has surgery. *Neoreviews.* 2006;7:410–418.
42. Madhok AB, Ojamaa K, Haridas V, Parnell VA, Pahwa S, Chowdhury D. Cytokine response to children undergoing surgery for congenital heart disease. *Pediatr Cardiol.* 2006;27:408–413.
43. Roth SJ, Adatia I, Pearson GD, Members of the Cardiology Group. Summary proceedings from the cardiology group on postoperative cardiac dysfunction. *Pediatrics.* 2006;117:S40–S46.
44. Gillespie M, Kuijpers M, Van Rossem M, et al. Determinants of intensive care unit length of stay for infants undergoing cardiac surgery. *Congenit Heart Dis.* 2006;1:152–160.
45. Owens JL, Musa N. Nutrition support after neonatal cardiac surgery. *Nutr Clin Pract.* 2009;24:242–249.
46. Bellander M, Ley D, Polberger S, Hellström-Westas L. Tolerance to early human milk feeding is not compromised by indomethacin in preterm infants with persistent ductus arteriosus. *Acta Paediatrica.* 2003;92(9):1074–1078.
47. Davey AM, Wagner CL, Cox C, Kendig JW. Feeding premature infants while low umbilical artery catheters are in place: a prospective, randomized trial. *J Pediatr.* 1994;124:795–799.
48. Barrington KJ. Umbilical artery catheters in the newborn: effects of position of the catheter tip. *Cochrane Database Syst Rev.* 1999;1:CD000505. DOI: 10.1002/14651858.CD000505.
49. Pronsky ZM. *Food-Medication Interactions*, rev ed. Birchrunville, PA: Food-Medication Interactions; 2004.
50. Walters HL III, Hakimi M, Rice MD, et al. Pediatric cardiac surgical ECMO: multivariate analysis of risk factors for hospital death. *Am Thorac Surg.* 1995;60:329–336.
51. Ishino K, Wong Y, Alexi-Meskishvili V, et al. Extracorporeal membrane oxygenation as a bridge to cardiac transplantation. *Artif Organs.* 1996;30:728–732.
52. Keckler SJ, Laituri CA, Ostlie DJ, Peter SD. A review of venovenus and venoarterial extracorporeal membrane oxygenation in neonates and children. *Eur J Pediatr Surg.* 2010;20(1):1–4.
53. Jaksic T, Shew SB, Keshen TH, Dzakovic A, Jahoor F. Do critically ill surgical neonates have increased energy expenditure? *J Pediatr Surg.* 2001;36(1):63–67.
54. Gravlee GP, Davis RF, Stammers AH, Ungerleider RM. *Cardiopulmonary Bypass: Principles and Practice.* Philadelphia, PA: Lippincott, Williams & Wilkins; 2008:155–171.
55. Brown RL, Wessel J, Warner BW. Nutrition considerations in the neonatal extracorporeal life support patient. *Nutr Clin Pract.* 1994;9(1):22–27.
56. Keshen TH, Miller RG, Jahoor F, Jaksic T. Stable isotopic quantitation of protein metabolism and energy expenditure in

neonates on- and post-extracorporeal life support. *J Pediatr Surg.* 1997;32(7):958–962.
57. Shew SB, Keshen TH, Jahoor F, Jaksic T. The determinants of protein catabolism in neonates on extracorporeal membrane oxygenation. *J Pediatr Surg.* 1999;34(7):1086–1090.
58. Buck ML, Wooldridge P, Ksenich RA. Comparison of methods for intravenous infusion of fat emulsion during extracorporeal membrane oxygenation. *Pharmacotherapy.* 2005;25(11):1536–1540.
59. Abbasi S, Stewart DL, Radmacher P, Adamkin D. Natural course of cholestasis in neonates on extracorporeal membrane oxygenation (ECMO): 10-year experience at a single institution. *Am Soc Artif Org J.* 2008;54(4):436–438.
60. Ukleja A. Altered GI motility in critically ill patients: current understanding of pathophysiology, clinical impact, and diagnostic approach. *Nutr Clin Pract.* 2010;25:16–25.
61. Crissinger KD. Regulation of hemodynamics and oxygenation in developing intestine: insight into the pathogenesis of necrotizing enterocolitis. *Acta Paediatr Suppl.* 1994;396:8–10.
62. Pettignano R, Heard M, Davis R, Labuz M, Hart M. Total enteral nutrition versus total parenteral nutrition during pediatric extracorporeal membrane oxygenation. *Crit Care Med.* 1998;26(2):358–363.
63. Hanekamp MN, Spoel M, Sharman-Koendjbiharie I, Peters JW, Albers MJ, Tibboel D. Routine enteral nutrition in neonates on extracorporeal membrane oxygenation. *Pediatr Crit Care Med.* 2005;6(3):275–279.
64. Tyson JE, Kennedy KA. Trophic feedings for parenterally fed infants. *Cochrane Database Syst Rev.* 2005;3:CD000504.
65. Okada Y, Klein N, van Saene HK, et al. Small volumes of enteral feedings normalise immune function in infants receiving parenteral nutrition. *J Pediatr Surg.* 1998;33:16–19.
66. Hadfield RJ, Sinclair DG, Houldsworth PE, Evans TW. Effects of enteral and parenteral nutrition on gut mucosal permeability in the critically ill. *Am J Respir Crit Care Med.* 1995;152:1545–1548.
67. Hanekamp MN, Spoel M, Sharman-Koendjbiharie M, et al. Gut hormone profiles in critically ill neonates on extracorporeal membrane oxygenation. *Pediatr Gastroenterol Nutr.* 2005; 40(2):175–179.
68. Piena M, Albers MJ, Van Haard PM, et al. Introduction of enteral feeding in neonates on extracorporeal membrane oxygenation after evaluation of intestinal permeability changes. *J Pediatr Surg.* 1998;3:30–34.
69. Mishra S, Agarwal R, Jeevasankar M, Deorari AK, Paul VK. Minimal enteral nutrition. *Indian J Pediatr.* 2008;75(3):267–269.
70. Chaloupecky V, Hucin B, Tlaskal T, et al. Nitrogen balance, 3-methylhistidine excretion, and plasma amino acid profile in infants after cardiac operations for congenital heart defects: the effect of early nutritional support. *J Thorac Cardiovasc Surg.* 1997;14:1053.
71. Ballweg JA, Ittenbach RF, Bernbaum J, et al. Hyperglycaemia after stage I palliation does not adversely affect neurodevelopmental outcome at 1 year of age in patients with single-ventricle physiology. *Eur J Cardiothorac Surg.* 2009;36(4):688–693.
72. Hartl WH, Jauch KW, Parhofer K, Rittler P. Working group for developing the guidelines for parenteral nutrition of the German Association for Nutritional Medicine. Complications and Monitoring—Guidelines on Parenteral Nutrition, Chapter 11. *GMS Ger Med Sci.* 2009;7.
73. Vaisman N, Leigh T, Voet H, et al. Malabsorption in infants with congenital heart disease with diuretic treatment. *Pediatr Res.* 1994;36:545–549.
74. Jadcherla SR, Vijayapal AS, Leuthner S. Feeding abilities in neonates with congenital heart disease: a retrospective study. *J Perinatol.* 2009;29:112–118.
75. Boctor DL, Pillo-Blocka F, McCrindle BW. Nutrition after cardiac surgery for infants with congenital heart disease. *Nutr Clin Pract.* 1999;14(3):111–115.
76. Einerson KD, Arthur HM. Predictors of oral feeding difficulty in cardiac surgical infants. *Pediatr Nurs.* 2003;29:315–319.
77. Kohr L, Dargan M, Hauge A, et al. The incidence of dysphagia in pediatric patients after open heart procedures with transesophageal echocardiography. *Ann Thorac Surg.* 2003;76:1450–1456.
78. Krebs N. Gastrointestinal problems and disorders. In: Kessler D, Dawson P, eds. *Failure to Thrive and Pediatric Undernutrition: A Transdisciplinary Approach.* Baltimore, MD: Paul H. Brookes; 1999:215–226.
79. Jung AD. Gastroesophageal reflux in infants and children. *Am Fam Physician.* 2001;64(11):1853–1860.
80. Medoff-Cooper B, Irving SY. Innovative strategies for feeding and nutrition in infants with congenitally malformed hearts. *Cardiol Young.* 2009;19(Suppl 2):90–99.
81. Maher KO, Giddings SS, Baffa JM, Pizzaro C, Norwood WI Jr. New developments in the treatment of hypoplastic left heart syndrome. *Minerva Pediatr.* 2004;56(1):41-49.
82. Daya H, Hosni A, Bejar-Solar J, Evans M. Pediatric vocal fold paralysis: a long-term retrospective study. *Arch Otolaryngol Head Neck Surg.* 2000;126:21–25.
83. Skinner ML, Halstead LA, Rubinstein CS, Atz AM, Andrews D, Bradley SM. Laryngopharyngeal dysfunction after Norwood procedure. *J Thoracic Cardiovasc Surg.* 2005;130:1293–1301.
84. Kogon BE, Ramaswamy V, Todd K, et al. Feeding difficulty in newborns following congenital heart surgery. *Congenit Heart Dis.* 2007;2(5):332–337.
85. Jenkins KJ, Gauvreau K, Newburger JW, Spray TL, Moller JH, Iezzoni LI. Consensus-based method for risk adjustment for surgery for congenital heart disease. *J Thorac Cardiovasc Surg.* 2002;123(1):110–118.
86. Pereira-da-Silva L, Henriques G, Videira-Amaral JM, Rodrigues R, Ribeiro L, Virella D. Osmolality of solutions, emulsions and drugs that may have a high osmolality: aspects of their use in neonatal care. *J Matern Fetal Neonatal Med.* 2002;11(5):333–338.
87. Sapsford A. Enteral nutrition products. In: Groh-Wargo S, Thompson M, Cox J, eds. *Nutritional Care for High Risk Newborns,* rev ed. Chicago: Precept Press; 1994:176.
88. White KC, Harkavy KL. Hypertonic formula resulting from added oral medications. *Am J Dis Child.* 1982;136:931.
89. Zenk L, Hutzable R. Osmolality of infant formulas, tube feedings, and total parenteral solutions. *Hosp Form.* 1978;577:8.
90. Cavell B. Gastric emptying in infants with congenital heart disease. *Acta Paediatr Scand.* 1981;70:517–520.
91. Ernst JA, Williams JM, Glick MR, et al. Osmolality of substances used in the intensive care nursery. *Pediatrics.* 1983;72:347.
92. Jew R. Osmolality of medications and formulas used in the newborn intensive care nursery. *Nutr Clin Pract.* 1997;12:158–163.
93. Bougle D, Iselin M, Kahyat A, et al. Nutritional treatment of congenital heart disease. *Arch Dis Child.* 1986;61:799–801.

94. Schwarz SM, Gewitz MH, See CC, et al. Enteral nutrition in infants with congenital heart disease and growth failure. *Pediatrics*. 1990;86:368–373.
95. Vanderhoof JA, Hofshire PJ, Baluff MA, et al. Continuous enteral feedings: an important adjunct in the management of complex congenital heart disease. *Am J Dis Child*. 1982;136:825–827.
96. Khajuria R, Grover A, Bidwai PS. Effect of nutritional supplementation on growth of infants with congenital heart diseases. *Indian Pediatr*. 1989;26:76–79.
97. Jackson M, Poskitt EM. The effects of high energy feeding on energy balance and growth in infants with congenital heart disease and failure to thrive. *Br J Nutr*. 1991;65:131–143.
98. Unger R, DeKleermaeker M, Gidding SS, Christoffel KK. Calories count. Improved weight gain with dietary intervention after cardiac surgery in children. *Am J Dis Child*. 1992;146:1078–1084.
99. Combs VL and Marino BL. A comparison of growth patterns in breast and bottle-fed infants with congenital heart disease. *Pediatr Nurs*. 1993;19:175–179.
100. Lobo ML and Michel Y. Behavioral and physiological response during feeding in infants with congenital heart disease: a naturalistic study. *Prog Cardiovasc Nurs*. 1995;10:26–34.
101. Nugent AW, Daubeney PE, Chondros P, et al. The epidemiology of childhood cardiomyopathy in Australia. *N Engl J Med*. 2003;348(17):1639–1646.
102. Lipchultz SE, Sleeper LA, Towbin JA, et al. The incidence of pediatric cardiomyopathy in two regions of the United States. *N Engl J Med*. 2003;348(17):1647–1655.
103. Grenier MA, Osganian SK, Cox GF, et al. Design and implementation of the North American Pediatric Cardiomyopathy Registry. *Am Heart J*. 2000;129:S86–S95.
104. Kirk R, Edwards LB, Aurora P, et al. Registry of the International Society for Heart and Lung Transplantation: twelfth official pediatric heart transplantation report—2009. *J Heart Lung Transplant*. 2009;28(10):993–1006.
105. Miller TL, Neri D, Extein J, Somarriba G, Strickman-Stein N. Nutrition in pediatric cardiomyopathy. *Prog Pediatr Cardiol*. 2007;24(1):59–71.
106. Costantini TW, Taylor JH, Beilman GJ. Abdominal complications of ventricular assist device placement. *Surg Infect (Larchmt)*. 2005;6(4):409–418.
107. Arabía FA, Tsau PH, Smith RG, et al. Pediatric bridge to heart transplantation: application of the Berlin Heart, Medos and Thoratec ventricular assist devices. *J Heart Lung Transplant*. 2006;25(1):16–21.
108. Al-Attar I, Orav EJ, Exil V, Vlach SA, Lipshultz SE. Predictors of cardiac morbidity and related mortality in children with acquired immunodeficiency syndrome. *J Am Coll Cardiol*. 2003;41(9):1598–1605.
109. Beghetti M, La Scala G, Belli D, et al. Etiology and management of pediatric chylothorax. *J Pediatr*. 2000;136:653–658.
110. Spain DA, McClave SA. Chylothorax and chylous ascites. In: Gottschlich MM, ed. *The ASPEN Nutrition Support Core Curriculum: A Case Based Approach—The Adult Patient*. Silver Spring, MD: ASPEN; 2007:477–486.
111. Prasad R, Singh K, Singh R. Bilateral congenital chylothorax with Nona syndrome. *Indian Pediatr*. 2002;39:975–976.
112. Lanning P, Simia S, Saramo I, et al. Lymphatic abnormalities in Noonan's syndrome. *Pediatr Radiol*. 1978;7:106–109.
113. Munoz Conde J, Gomez de Terroros I, Sanchez Ruiz F. Chylothorax associated with Turner's syndrome in a child. *An Esp Pediatr*. 1975;8:449–454.
114. Goens MB, Campbell D, Willins JW. Spontaneous chylothorax in Noonan syndrome. *Am J Dis Child*. 1992;146:1453–1456.
115. Hamada H, Fujita K, Kubo T, et al. Congenital chylothorax in a trisomy 21 newborn. *Arch Gynecol Obstet*. 1992;252:55–58.
116. Chan PC, Chiu HC, Hwu WL. Spontaneous chylothorax in a case of cardio-facio-cutaneous syndrome. *Clin Dysmorph*. 2002;11:297–298.
117. Bellini C, Mazzella M, Arioni C, et al. Hennekam syndrome presenting as non immune hydrops fetalis, congenital chylothorax, and congenital lymphangiectasis. *Am J Med Genetics*. 2003;120A:92–96.
118. Suddaby E and Schiller S. Management of chylothorax in children. *Pediatr Nurs*. 2004;30(4):290–295.
119. Büttiker V, Fanconi S, Burger R. Chylothorax in children: guidelines for diagnosis and management. *Chest*. 1999;116:662–687.
120. Winkler MF. Nutrition management of the patient with chylous fistula. *Support Line*. 2003;25:8–13.
121. Chan EH, Russell JL, Williams WG, Van Arsdell GS, Coles JG, McCrindle BW. Postoperative chylothorax after cardiothoracic surgery in children. *Ann Thorac Surg*. 2005;80:1864–1871.
122. Parrish C, McCray SR. When chyle leaks: nutrition management options. *Pract Gastroenterol*. 2004;26(5):60–76.
123. Sardesai VM. The essential fatty acids. *Nutr Clin Pract*. 1992;7(4):179–186.
124. Lessen R. Use of skim breast milk for an infant with chylothorax. *Infant Child Adolesc Nutr*. 2009;1(6):303–310.
125. Chan GM, Lechtenberg E. The use of fat-free human milk in infants with chylous pleural effusion. *J Perinatol*. 2007;27:434–436.
126. Roehr CC, Jung A, Proquitté H, et al. Somatostatin or octreotide as treatment options for chylothorax in young children: a systematic review. *Intensive Care Med*. 2006;32:650–657.
127. Hawli Y, Nasrallah M, El-Hajj Fuleihan G. Endocrine and musculoskeletal abnormalities in patients with Down syndrome. *Nat Rev Endocrinol*. 2009;5(6):327–334.
128. Mizuno K, Ueda A. Development of sucking behavior in infants with Down's syndrome. *Acta Paediatr*. 2001;90(12):1384–1388.
129. Thomas JA, Graham JM Jr. Chromosomes 22q11 deletion syndrome: an update and review for the primary. *Clin Pediatr (Phila)*. 1997;36(5):253–266.
130. Khositseth A, Tocharoentanaphol C, Khowsathit P, Ruangdaraganon N. Chromosome 22q11 deletions in patients with conotruncal heart defects. *Pediatr Cardiol*. 2005;26(5):570–573.
131. Goldmuntz E. DiGeorge syndrome: new insights. *Clin Perinatol*. 2005;32(4):963–978, ix–x.
132. Eicher PS, McDonald-McGinn DM, Fox CA, Driscoll DA, Emanuel BS, Zackai EH. Dysphagia in children with a 22q11.2 deletion: unusual pattern found on modified barium swallow. *J Pediatr*. 2000;137(2):158–164.
133. Blake KD, Prasad C. CHARGE syndrome. *Orphanet J Rare Dis*. 2006;1:34.
134. Dobbelsteyn C, Peacocke SD, Blake K, Crist W, Rashid M. Feeding difficulties in children with CHARGE syndrome: prevalence, risk factors, and prognosis. *Dysphagia*. 2008;23(2):127–135.

135. Thommessen M, Heiberg A, Kase BF. Feeding problems with children with congenital heart disease: the impact on energy intake and growth outcomes. *Eur J Clin Nutr*. 1992;46:457–464.
136. American Academy of Pediatrics Committee on Nutrition. Statement on cholesterol. *Pediatrics*. 1992;90:469–473.
137. Centers for Disease Control and Prevention. Prevalence of abnormal lipid levels among youths—United States, 1999–2006. *MMWR*. 2010;59(2):29–33.
138. National Cholesterol Education Program Expert Panel Detection, Evaluation, and Treatment of High Blood Cholesterol in Adults (Adult Treatment Panel III). Third report of the National Cholesterol Education Program (NCEP) Expert Panel on Detection, Evaluation, and Treatment of High Blood Cholesterol in Adults (Adult Treatment Panel III): final report. *Circulation*. 2002;106:3143–3421.
139. Krauss RM, Eckel RH, Howard B, et al. AHA dietary guidelines: revision 2000: a statement for healthcare professionals from the Nutrition Committee of the American Heart Association. *Circulation*. 2000;102(18):2284–2299.
140. NCEP Expert Panel on Blood Cholesterol Levels in Children and Adolescents. National cholesterol education program (NCEP). Highlights of the report of the Expert Panel on Blood Cholesterol Levels in Children and Adolescents. *Pediatrics*. 1992;89:525–527.
141. Marcason W. What is the "age+5" rule for fiber? *J Am Diet Assoc*. 2005;105(2):301–302.
142. Kwiterovitch PO. The role of fiber in the treatment of hypercholesterolemia in children and adolescents. *J Pediatr*. 1995;96:1005–1009.
143. Kwiterovich PO Jr. Recognition and management of dyslipidemia in children and adolescents. *J Clin Endocrinol Metab*. 2008;93(11):4200–4209.
144. Williams CL, Stobino BA, Bollella M, et al. Cardiovascular risk reduction in preschool children: the "Healthy Start" project. *J Am Coll Nutr*. 2004;23:117–123.
145. Wabitsch M, Hauner H, Heinze E, et al. Body fat distribution and changes in atherogenic risk factor profile in obese adolescent girls during weight loss. *Am J Clin Nutr*. 1994;60:54–60.
146. Sothern MS. Obesity prevention in children: physical activity and nutrition. *Nutrition*. 2004;20(7–8):704–708.
147. Cotts TB, Goldberg CS, Palma Davis LM, et al. A school-based health education program can improve cholesterol values for middle school students. *Pediatr Cardiol*. 2008;29(5):940–945.
148. Bond M, Wyatt K, Lloyd J, Taylor R. Systematic review of the effectiveness of weight management schemes for the under fives. *Obes Rev*. 2010 Feb 8. [Epub ahead of print]
149. Reinehr T, Andler W. Changes in the atherogenic risk factor profile according to degree of weight loss. *Arch Dis Child*. 2004;89:419–422.
150. Nutrition management of hyperlipidemia. In: William CP, ed. *Pediatric Manual of Clinical Dietetics*. Chicago: American Dietetic Association; 1998:265–283.
151. Saakslahti A, Numminen P, Varstala V, et al. Physical activity as a preventive measure for coronary heart disease risk factors in early childhood. *Scand J Med Sci Sports*. 2004;14:143–149.

Diabetes

Laurie Anne Higgins

Introduction

Through considerable research and new technologies during the last 20 years, the knowledge base regarding childhood diabetes has been extended, giving healthcare professionals new tools to help this population balance and improve their diabetes management. These tools include intensive insulin therapy, new medications, blood glucose self-monitoring devices, continuous blood glucose monitoring, psychological intervention, inclusion and education for family and support persons, insulin/food adjustment for exercise, and state-of-the-art medical nutrition therapy. The challenge to the dietitian on the diabetes team is to support the family's efforts and to help promote healthy eating habits by using information gained from current research coupled with insight into family dynamics.

Empowering parents to care for their child with type 1 diabetes (T1D) is the ultimate challenge for many healthcare professionals dealing with pediatric patients. Families already faced with altering their lifestyle to include insulin injections, blood glucose monitoring, and scheduled meals must face these challenges in combination with feelings of anger, fear, denial, and guilt.

Meal planning is one of the most important tools of diabetes self-management. However, studies have shown that diet is overwhelmingly the number one problem in diabetes care.[1] Many factors associated with poor adherence to diabetes-related meal planning are psychosocial in nature (e.g., anger, denial, frustration, poor understanding, social pressures, and restriction of favorite foods).[1] The American Diabetes Association's Nutrition Principles and Recommendations in Diabetes[2] provides a positive approach to this potentially overwhelming topic. Educators on the diabetes team must not lose sight of the fact that food provides more than nutrients, especially for children. Changes in eating should not be viewed as restrictions and losses, but rather as a healthful way for the whole family to eat. To be successful, the meal plan must not only meet nutritional requirements, but also be realistic and workable, without requiring major routine changes from those involved. Every attempt should be made to establish a meal plan that reflects the youth's food preferences and the family's social and cultural attitudes. Flexibility and graduated goal setting are important keys to success, increasing the chances of the youth's achieving optimal management and decreasing the development of complications. The goals for medical nutrition therapy are listed in **Table 15-1**.

The Diabetes Team

Management of diabetes requires teamwork. This was clearly demonstrated in the 1993 published results of the landmark Diabetes Control and Complications Trial (DCCT).[3] The DCCT supported the importance of a coordinated team approach to achieve nutrition goals. The ultimate therapeutic diabetes team utilized in the DCCT consisted of the patient and family as the primary players, along with the diabetes nurse educator, dietitian, behaviorist, and diabetologist.[4] The DCCT also provided important information specific to successful nutrition intervention strategies firmly based on scientific evidence. In 1994, shortly after the DCCT clinical findings were published, the American Diabetes Association (ADA) published a revised set of nutrition guidelines refocusing on an "individualized approach to nutrition self-management that is appropriate for the personal lifestyle and diabetes management goals of the individual with diabetes."[5]

Pediatric diabetes centers have built on the model of the DCCT to also include pediatric phlebotomists, child-life specialists, and care ambassadors (see **Figure 15-1**). Often the last part of an office visit is having the blood drawn, and that leaves the child very upset. The pediatric phlebotomist and child-life specialist can work with the family to reduce a child's anxiety, which can make this part of the visit much less traumatic. A child-life specialist can be instrumental in providing the family with therapeutic play and techniques

TABLE 15-1 Goals of Medical Nutrition Therapy for Children and Adolescents

- To provide adequate nutrition to maintain normal growth and development based on child's appetite, food preferences, and family lifestyle
- To maintain near-normal blood glucose levels and reduce/prevent the risks of short- and long-term diabetes
- To achieve optimal serum lipid levels
- To preserve social and psychological well-being
- To improve overall health through optimal nutrition
- To provide a level of information that meets the interest and ability of the family
- To provide information on current research to help the family make appropriate nutrition decisions

to help them with the often-difficult task of blood glucose checks and insulin injections. The care ambassador is usually a college graduate or a child-life specialist who is assigned to a family to help them navigate the healthcare system. The care ambassador will make sure the family has regular scheduled appointments and contacts the family between visits to assist them with whatever they need for their child's care,[6] such as changing or making their appointments with members of the diabetes team and renewing a prescription. Research has shown that patients with a care ambassador attend more clinic visits and have fewer severe hypoglycemic episodes and visits to the emergency room.[7]

Nutrition Principles for the Management of Diabetes and Related Complications

A positive approach to meal planning is to encourage family members and other support persons to follow the same lifestyle recommendations as the child with diabetes. In our attempt to maintain the "pleasures of the table," it is essential that the nutrition recommendations promote "normal" healthy eating and prevent isolating and dividing the child and family in their food choices. Research suggests that the nutrition needs of children with diabetes are no different than those of children without diabetes. They should follow the same Dietary Guidelines for Americans.[8] The current nutrition recommendations can only be defined as a nutrition prescription based on assessment, individual treatment goals, and outcomes (see **Table 15-2**).[9-10]

Calories

The meal plan should include enough calories (kcal) to maintain a consistent growth and to achieve and/or maintain a desirable body weight. In growing children, caloric

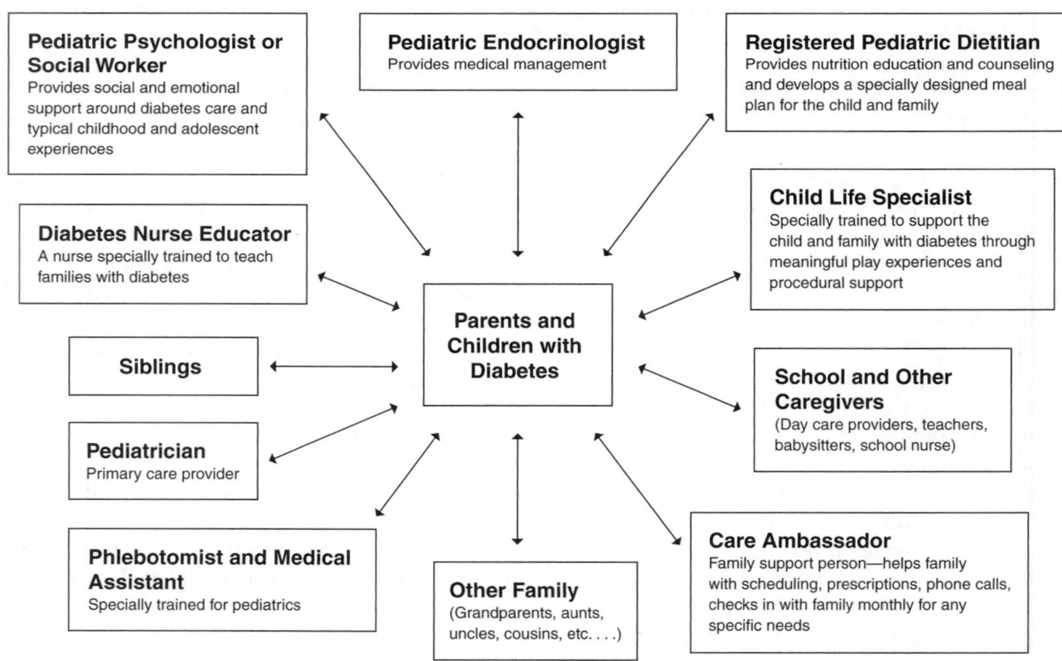

FIGURE 15-1 The Pediatric Diabetes Team

Source: Copyright © 2010 by Joslin Diabetes Center. All rights reserved. Reprinted with permission.

TABLE 15-2 Nutrition Recommendations Redistributed the Calories from Macronutrients

Acceptable Macronutrient Distribution Range (% of energy)			
	Children 1–3 Years	Children 4–18 Years	Adults
Protein	5–20	10–30	10–35
Carbohydrate	45–65	45–65	45–65
Fat	30–40	25–35	20–35
Fiber[11]	1–3 years of age		19 g/day
	4–8 years of age		25 g/day
	9–13 years of age Males Females		 31 g/day 26 g/day
	14–50 years of age Males Female		 38 g/day 26 g/day
Calories	Requirements for growth, based on nutrition assessment		

Fiber dietary reference intake = 14 g fiber/1000 kcal after 12 months of age
Source: Institute of Medicine of the National Academies. *Dietary Reference Intakes: The Essential Guide to Nutrient Requirements*. Washington, DC: National Academies Press; 2006.

intake should not be restricted and should be the same as for children without diabetes. Energy needs vary during periods of growth, so calorie needs should be compared and validated based on age, height, ideal body weight (IBW), activity, and average energy allowance per day. See **Table 15-3** for a variety of methods of estimating energy needs for an individual child. See also Appendix H for recommended dietary allowance (RDA) estimated energy requirement (EER) tables.

Nutrition management for children with diabetes continues to require carbohydrate counting and healthy eating. Mayer-Davis et al. demonstrated that in general, the dietary intake of youth with diabetes does not meet the current nutrition recommendations. Less than 50% of the participants met recommendations for total fat, vitamin E, fiber, fruits, or vegetables, and none of the participants met the whole grain recommendation of three servings a day.[11,12]

Carbohydrate and Sweeteners

The percentage of calories ingested from carbohydrate will vary and is individualized based on nutritional assessment and treatment goals. Many factors influence the glycemic response to foods, including the total amount of carbohydrate, type of carbohydrate (glucose, sucrose, fructose, lactose, or starch), degree of processing, glycemic index, glycemic load, and combination with other foods and ingredients. One of the most common misconceptions about carbohydrate is the belief that sugars are more rapidly digested and absorbed than are starches and therefore sugar contributes significantly to hyperglycemia. However, published research found little or no scientific evidence that supports this theory. Studies show a strong relationship between the total carbohydrate intake and the premeal insulin dose;[13] therefore, adjustment of the premeal insulin dose can allow a person with diabetes to incorporate most carbohydrates into the meal plan and still maintain appropriate blood glucose control. It is becoming common practice to encourage the family whenever possible to provide rapid insulin 20–30 minutes before the meal, especially when the meal is composed of mostly carbohydrates.

Glycemic Index and Glycemic Load

The glycemic index (GI) is the ranking of the glucose response after ingesting a 50-gram portion of carbohydrate of a food and comparing it to the glucose response of an index food.[14] The glycemic index is not a precise tool because the exact effect of foods on blood glucose differs significantly among individuals and is affected by many factors such as processing, preparation, and digestion.[5] On the other hand, the glycemic index can be used as an indicator of the general glucose response of an individual food. It can be a helpful tool when encouraging a child or adolescent to increase the amount of whole-grain products and fresh fruits and vegetables in their meal plan because these foods tend to demonstrate a slower glucose response and are healthier choices.

The glycemic load (GL) takes the GI into account but also uses the quantity of the carbohydrate eaten. This again can be used as a teaching tool to educate the youth and their family that when choosing a food with a high GI, having a smaller portion might be more manageable to cover with insulin.

Sucrose

Flexibility in allowing some sucrose into the meal plan may lead to better adherence. Sucrose can be incorporated into children's meal plans on a regular basis, assuming their intake is adequate and consists of foods from all of the essential food groups. To moderate the impact of these food choices on the blood glucose levels, it is advisable to substitute sucrose and sucrose-containing foods for other carbohydrates in the diet, and not simply to add these foods to the meal plan.[15] Because most sources of sugar for children under 10 years are from milk and milk products, fruit drinks, and carbonated soft drinks, it is important to promote overall healthy eating and optimal dental health by limiting empty calorie foods. Added sucrose-containing foods should be related to extra activity and special occasions. These foods should be promoted as a special "treat" or "once in a while" foods.

TABLE 15-3 Estimating Caloric Requirements

Based on nutrition assessment and typical day recall.
Validate caloric estimation.

Method 1: Dietary Reference Intakes: Estimated Energy Requirements (EER)[10]

Infants and Young Children

0–3 months	EER = (89 × weight [kg] − 100) + 175
4–6 months	EER = (89 × weight [kg] − 100) + 56
7–12 months	EER = (89 × weight [kg] − 100) + 22
13–35 months	EER = (89 × weight [kg] − 100) + 20

Children and Adolescents 3–18 Years

Boys

3–8 yrs	EER = 88.5 − (61.9 × age [y]) + PA × [(26.7 × weight [kg]) + (903 × height [m])] + 20
9–18 yrs	EER = 88.5 − (61.9 × age [y]) + PA × [(26.7 × weight [kg]) + (903 × height [m])] + 25

Girls

3–8 yrs	EER = 135.3 − (30.8 × age [yr] + PA × [(10.0 × weight [kg]) + (934 × height [m])] + 20
9–18 yrs	EER = 135.3 − (30.8 × age [yr] + PA × [(10.0 × weight [kg]) + (934 × height [m])] + 25

Adults 19 Years and Older

Men	EER = 662 − (9.53 × age [yr]) + PA × [(15.91 × weight [kg]) + (539.6 × height [m])
Women	EER = 354 − (6.91 × age [yr]) + PA × [(9.36 × weight [kg]) + (726 × height [m])

Method 2: Schofield Equation for Calculating Basal Metabolic Rate in Children[16]

Males

0–3 years	REE = 0.167W + 15.174H − 617.6
3–10 years	REE = 19.59W + 1.303H + 414.9
10–18 years	REE = 16.25W + 1.372H + 515.5
> 18 years	REE = 15.057W + 1.004H + 705.8

Females

0–3 years	REE = 16.252W + 10.232H − 413.5
3–10 years	REE = 16.969W + 1.618H + 371.2
10–18 years	REE = 8.365W + 4.65H + 200
> 18 years	REE = 13.623W + 23.8H + 98.2

REE × activity

Abbreviation: PA, physical activity coefficient (see **Table 15-4**).

TABLE 15-4 Physical Activity Coefficients (PA Values) for Use in EER Equations

	Sedentary (PAL 1.0–1.39)	Low Active (PAL 1.4–1.59)	Active (PAL 1.6–1.89)	Very Active (PAL 1.9–2.5)
	Typical daily living activities (e.g., household tasks, walking to the bus)	Typical daily living activities *plus* 30–60 minutes of daily moderate activity (e.g., walking 5–7 km/h)	Typical daily living activities *plus* At least 60 minutes of moderate activity	Typical daily living activities *plus* At least 60 minutes of moderate activity *plus* An additional 60 minutes of vigorous activity or 120 minutes of moderate activity
Boys 3–18 yrs	1.00	1.13	1.26	1.42
Girls 3–18 yrs	1.00	1.16	1.31	1.56
Men 19+ yrs	1.00	1.11	1.25	1.48
Women 19+ yrs	1.00	1.12	1.27	1.45

Abbreviation: PAL, physical activity level.
Source: Institute of Medicine of the National Academies. *Dietary Reference Intakes: The Essential Guide to Nutrient Requirements*. Washington, DC: National Academies Press; 2006.

Nutritive Sweeteners

Sweeteners other than sucrose also contain large amounts of carbohydrate and calories and can impact glycemic control. Common sweeteners such as fructose, corn syrup, honey, molasses, carob, dextrose, lactose, and maltose do not decrease calories or carbohydrate and offer no significant advantage over foods sweetened with sucrose.[9] Although fructose has been shown to produce a somewhat smaller rise in blood glucose compared to the other sweeteners listed, research evidence suggests potential negative effects of large amounts of fructose on plasma lipids, and it should not be added as a sweetening agent to foods.[17]

Commonly used sugar alcohols such as sorbitol, mannitol, xylitol, erthritol, lactitil, isomalt, maltitol, and hydrogenated starch hydrolysate may produce less of a glycemic response and average about 2.4 to 3.0 kcal/g, compared with 4 kcal/g from other carbohydrates.[18] However, gastrointestinal side effects such as stomach distress or diarrhea are noted when sugar alcohols are ingested in large amounts (50 g/day for sorbitol, 20 g/day for mannitol). Children may be more sensitive and have been shown to have diarrhea with intake as low as 0.5 or less g/kg body weight.[19]

Nonnutritive Sweeteners

Aspartame, acesulfame K, neotame saccharin, sucralose, and steviol glycosides are the most common noncaloric sweeteners used in the United States and have been approved by the Food and Drug Administration (FDA). The FDA determines an acceptable daily intake (ADI) for these sweeteners. ADI is defined as the amount of a food additive that can be safely consumed on a daily basis over a person's lifetime without any adverse effects, and includes a 100-fold safety factor (**Table 15-5**).

Aspartame contains 4 kcal/g but is 160 to 220 times sweeter than sucrose; therefore, aspartame provides negligible calories. Aspartame is rapidly metabolized in the gastrointestinal tract and does not accumulate in the system at recommended intakes. Aspartame is not heat stable and may decompose on long exposure to high temperatures. Aspartame safety data have been evaluated by regulatory agencies and expert committees, including the FDA, the EU Scientific Committee for Food (SCF), and the Joint FAO/WHO Expert Committee on Food Additives (JECFA), which have deemed it safe for its intended use. Aspartame was first approved by the FDA in 1981 for dry products and was expanded in 1983 to include carbonated beverages. Aspartame is presently approved in many countries and has been widely used by hundreds of millions of people over the last 20 years with no adverse effects.[20,21] However, because aspartame is composed of phenylalanine and aspartic acid, it should be restricted in those with phenylketonuria (PKU), a homozygous recessive inborn error of metabolism in which persons are unable to metabolize the amino acid phenylalanine. The FDA requires all products containing aspartame to display the words "Phenylketonurics: Contains Phenylalanine."

Acesulfame K has no caloric value and is 200 times sweeter than sucrose. Also, it is not metabolized by the body and is eliminated unchanged in the urine. Acesulfame K is heat stable and blends well with other sweeteners. The amount of potassium (K) in this sweetener is

TABLE 15-5 FDA ADI Guidelines for Non-Nutritive Sweeteners

	ADI (mg/kg body wt)	Average Amount (mg) in 12-oz. Can of Soda*	Cans of Soda to Reach ADI for 45-kg (100-lb.) Child	Amount (mg) in a Packet of Sweetener	Packets to Reach ADI for a 45-kg (100-lb.) Child
Acesulfame K	15	40⁺	17	50	13
Aspartame	50	200	11	35	63
Neotame	18	6[a]	135	N/A	N/A
Saccharin	5	140*	1.6	36	6.25
Sucralose	5	70	3.2	5	45
Stevioside (steviol glycosides)	4[b]	56	10	28	20

These recommendations are set by the Food and Drug Administration (FDA) for Acceptable Daily Intake (ADI) and include a 100-fold safety factor. The World Health Organization's Joint Expert Committee of Food Additives has set the ADI for saccharin. Use these as guidelines.[18]

*This number represents an average; different brand names and fountain drinks may have varied amounts of sweeteners.

⁺Based on the most common blend with 90 mg aspartame.

[a]http://www.neotame.com/pdf/neotame_science_brochure_US.pdf

[b]ADI is translated to 12 mg/kg/day for Rubiana (Truvia) and RebA (PureVia)

Source: Copyright © 1999 American Diabetes Association, Inc. *American Diabetes Association Guide to Medical Nutrition Therapy for Diabetes*, 1999. Reprinted and modified with permission from the American Diabetes Association.

minimal, with only 10 mg of potassium in one packet. No safety concerns have been raised about acesulfame K and it has been reported safe for all individuals.[5,18]

Saccharin is 200 to 700 times sweeter than sucrose and has no caloric value. Saccharin is heat stable, is not metabolized by the body, and is excreted unchanged in the urine. Parents often question whether it's safe for their child to ingest it, based on highly publicized research results in the 1970s suggesting a possible causal relationship between saccharin and bladder tumors in laboratory rats. It has been documented that the saccharin samples used in the studies were impure and the results were incorrectly interpreted.[18,22]

Sucralose is 600 times sweeter than sugar, is the only low-calorie sweetener made from sugar, and is excreted in the urine essentially unchanged.[18] Sucralose is not recognized by the body as either sugar or carbohydrate because it is not broken down or metabolized by the body. Furthermore, it does not affect blood glucose levels. Sucralose is marketed as Splenda, which contains a small amount of maltodextrin or dextrose and does provide some carbohydrate and calories. Individual packages contain less than 1 gram of carbohydrate, but 1 cup of Splenda granular contains 96 calories and 24 grams of carbohydrate. Sucralose is heat stable and may be used during cooking and baking. The FDA states that no adverse or carcinogenic effects are associated with sucralose consumption.

Neotame is 7000 to 13,000 times sweeter than sugar, partially digested in the small intestine, and excreted in the urine and the feces. Neotame does have a small amount of phenylalanine, but even when consumed at 90% of the estimated daily intake it was clinically not significant for individuals with PKU.[18] It is marketed as having a clean, sweet taste without the aftertaste associated with other noncaloric sweeteners, and is used in beverages and a variety of other foods. It is heat stable and can be used in a variety of products such as beverages, dairy products, and baked goods.

Stevioside is 250–300 times sweeter than sucrose and comes from the stevia plant. It is extracted from the leaf of the plant and is used as a noncaloric sweetener. It recently was given an ADI by the FDA and is being used in a variety of foods.[23] Steviosides are marketed as Rubiana (Truvia) and RebA (PureVia), both of which have zero calories per serving.

Fiber

Total dietary fiber consists of structural and storage polysaccharides and lignin in plants that are not well digested in humans.[24] Soluble fiber is made up of pectins, gums, mucilages, and some hemicelluloses. Insoluble fiber is made up of noncarbohydrate components, which include cellulose, lignin, and many hemicelluloses.

Increased intake of soluble fiber has been positively linked to improved glycemic control; however, interpretation of recent data collected in carefully controlled studies indicates that the effect of soluble fiber on blood glucose absorption, in the amounts consumed from foods, is probably clinically insignificant. Therefore, fiber recommendations for children with diabetes are the same as for children without diabetes: increase both types of fiber from a wide variety of food sources and base this increase upon the child's usual eating habits, glucose, and lipid goals.

Dietary fiber may be useful in the treatment or prevention of constipation, gastrointestinal disorders, and colon cancer. However, a high-fiber diet for some very young children may result in an insufficient caloric intake necessary for growth due to the satiety value provided by fiber, as well as possible impairment of mineral absorption. Therefore, the amount of dietary fiber recommended for children should be based upon individual eating habits and lipid goals. See also Chapter 12, Gastrointestinal Disorders, for further details about fiber.

Protein

Current nutrition recommendations for children with diabetes include protein from both animal and vegetable sources comprising 5–30% of calories per day. Protein intake in children and adolescents should be sufficient to ensure adequate growth and development, and maintenance of body protein stores. At this time, there are no data to support children with diabetes requiring a higher or lower protein intake than the RDA (see Appendix H). It is estimated that the average protein intake in the United States for all ages is about 15–20% of total daily calories, with the majority of protein intake coming from animal products. Diabetic nephropathy occurs in 20–40% of individuals with diabetes and is the leading cause of end-stage renal disease (ESRD).[25] Therefore, protein intake should be carefully assessed with a focus on overall healthy protein intake. Children engaging in consistent competitive exercise may need some additional protein due to increased energy needs, which can be met by increasing consumption of low-fat protein-rich foods rather than intake of liquid or powdered protein supplements.

Because most protein sources are low in carbohydrate, families sometimes consider these foods as a free option because they do not require insulin. Foods such as cheese, lean meats, and eggs do contain calories as well as saturated fat and cholesterol, and should not be considered a free food.

Total Fat

The primary dietary fat goal in children with diabetes is a healthy fat intake, sufficient to optimize growth and development. In 1991 the National Cholesterol Education Program

(NCEP) developed guidelines for fat intake for children over 2 years of age to decrease risk of cardiovascular disease.[26] Type 1 diabetes has been associated with an increased risk of cardiovascular disease, but evidence suggests that blood glucose control may directly influence the levels of several plasma lipids.[5]

Studies have shown intake levels for cholesterol, fat, and saturated fat in children with T1D are close to the recommendations for children without diabetes.[27] This is likely supported by the fact that the national trend has been leaning toward decreasing overall fat intake, but saturated fat intake is still high.[28] Unfortunately, some children and adolescents with diabetes consume fat levels well above what is recommended, and these individuals may be at an even greater risk for heart disease than children without diabetes. In 2004, the American Diabetes Association published guidelines for the management of dyslipidemia in children with diabetes (see **Table 15-6**).[29] Careful consideration should be given to providing enough fat in the diet for children less than 2 years of age, because the development of the brain and central nervous system are dependent on an adequate intake of fats.

TABLE 15-6 Management of Dyslipidemia in Children and Adolescents with Diabetes

Screening
After glycemic control is achieved:
Type 1
Obtain lipid profile at diagnosis and then, if normal, every 5 years
Begin at age 12 years (or onset of puberty, if earlier)
Begin prior to 12 years (if prepubertal) only if positive family history
Type 2
Obtain lipids profile at diagnosis and then every 2 years
Goals
Total cholesterol < 170 mg/dL
LDL < 100 mg/dL
HDL > 35 mg/dL
Triglycerides < 150 mg/dL
Treatment Strategies
Maximize glycemic control
Weight reduction, if necessary
Diet
< 7% of calories from saturated fat
< 200 mg cholesterol per day
Consider LDL-lowering dietary options
Increase soluble fiber
Limit intake of trans fatty acids
Emphasize weight management and physical activity
Medication in collaboration with a physician
Manage other cardiac disease risk factors
Blood pressure
Smoking
Obesity
Inactivity

Source: Adapted with permission from the American Diabetes Association. Management of dyslipidemia in children and adolescents with diabetes. *Diabetes Care.* 2003;26(7):2194–2197.

Vitamins and Minerals

Vitamins and minerals are necessary for normal growth and development. The majority of people with diabetes do not need additional vitamin and mineral supplements as long as their food intake is adequate and well balanced. However, a child's normal eating habits throughout the growth cycle may exclude or severely limit foods or food groups, and thus nutrient supplementation may be needed. The response to vitamin and mineral supplements will be favorable only when deficiencies are present; therefore, micronutrient adequacy should be evaluated periodically as a youth's food preferences change. Supplementation with certain vitamins and minerals, such as chromium, magnesium, zinc, and antioxidants, has been suggested as a treatment for diabetes and other health issues when a deficiency is present, but routine supplementation is not recommended by the American Diabetes Association because of lack of evidence and concern related to long-term safety.[25]

Vitamin D

Vitamin D and calcium are both very important for bone health and should be evaluated by the dietitian. Recent studies suggest that the general pediatric population is vitamin D deficient,[30] and youth with diabetes might be even more so.[30–33] The main sources of vitamin D are fortified milk (100 IU/8 oz.) and exposure to the sunlight (~20–30 minutes a day). The adequate intake for vitamin D is currently 5 mg (200 IU) from birth to 50 years. The American Academy of Pediatrics (AAP) has increased its recommendation to 400 IU per day for all infants, children, and adolescents.[34] If a child is not consuming adequate fortified milk or milk substitute, supplementation might be necessary to meet the new recommendations, especially during the winter months in northern areas.

Calcium

Calcium is a mineral that many children do not consume in adequate amounts, especially if they do not drink milk or consume any dairy products. Calcium intake for most ages still falls below estimated need, even with the increased number of calcium-fortified foods available.[35] Calcium intake is mainly determined by the consumption of milk and milk products, and if not consumed in adequate amounts, supplementation should be considered. See Chapter 6 (Table 6-1) for a listing of calcium sources.

Chromium

Chromium deficiency in both animal and human studies is associated with elevated blood glucose, cholesterol, and triglyceride levels, and with reduction in body growth and longevity. Populations at risk for chromium deficiency include the elderly and those on long-term total parenteral nutrition. Fortunately, most people with diabetes are not chromium deficient, and the ADA does not recommend chromium supplementation unless a deficiency is clearly documented.[9]

Magnesium

Magnesium deficiency has been associated with insulin resistance, carbohydrate intolerance, and hypertension, among other disorders. Only those patients at high risk should routinely be evaluated, such as those in poor glycemic control (diabetic ketoacidosis and prolonged glycosuria), those on diuretics, or those with intestinal malabsorption.

Sodium

Sodium recommendations for children and adolescents with diabetes are the same as for the general population. Current recommendations for children between 4 and 8 years of age is 1.2 g/day and for older children is 1.5 g/day, though intakes of the general population are much higher. The effect of sodium on blood pressure varies greatly depending on a person's level of sodium sensitivity. Research has not shown that those with diabetes are at a greater risk of developing hypertension if consuming a high-sodium diet. Routine monitoring of blood pressure is important and will help identify children and adolescents who may benefit from a reduction in sodium intake. Because sodium intake recommendations are the same as for the general population, guidelines should be directed toward the entire family.[36]

Zinc

Although insulin is stored as inactive zinc crystals in the beta cells and zinc is involved in insulin action, supplementation is only suggested to benefit those children with a zinc deficiency. When the dietary intake of children with type 1 diabetes was investigated, low intakes of zinc were noted in many 4- to 6-year-old children; however, a nationwide sample of all children also indicated inadequate zinc intake.[37] Low zinc intake may be attributed to limited consumption of animal products, particularly meat, in this age group. Poor growth also has been attributed to zinc deficiency in children with type 1 diabetes. Zinc supplementation in children with low zinc levels increased their rate of linear growth.[38] Zinc is found in red meats, some seafood, whole grains, and fortified breakfast cereals. Mayer-Davis et al. looked at youth with diabetes, and fewer than 20% met the recommended servings of fruits (≥ 2 servings/day), vegetables (≥ 3 servings/day), and grains (≥ 6 servings/day) and none met the recommended intake of whole grains (≥ 3 servings/day).[12] Youth with T1D and their families often avoid whole grain products in favor of more processed versions because they feel the lower carbohydrate levels are more healthful for diabetes.[39]

Antioxidants

The SEARCH for diabetes in youth study data suggest that many children with diabetes might not be meeting their recommendations for both vitamins E and C and might benefit from an age-appropriate multivitamin. The data also suggest working with the family to improve the variety of fruits and vegetables in the youth's meal plan, but it did not recommend additional supplementation at this time.[12,25]

Vitamin and Mineral Recommendations

Vitamin and mineral supplements should not be used in place of a varied, balanced meal plan to ensure that children and adolescents receive adequate nutrients. Inadequate nutrient intake is rare in children with diabetes as long as the child is eating a well-balanced diet, growing, gaining weight, and staying active. However, similar to children without diabetes, youth with diabetes are not meeting the present dietary recommendations, though in some areas their diets are even less healthful.[40] It is important that children with diabetes meet annually with a registered dietitian to ensure that their diet is nutritionally sound and no further recommendation is necessary. Those children at risk for nutrient deficiencies and who may benefit from a multivitamin supplement with antioxidants include those who are not consuming a variety of foods, are eliminating certain food groups, are strict vegetarians (vegans), are taking medications known to alter certain micronutrients, or who have consistently poor glycemic control, which can result in excess excretion of water-soluble vitamins.

Alcohol

Alcohol use and abuse should be discussed with the adolescent in an objective manner. Although the consumption of alcohol is illegal and is always discouraged for teens, facts about how alcohol affects blood glucose levels should be available to teens who express an interest in drinking. It should be made clear that alcohol lowers the blood glucose level and blocks gluconeogenesis, possibly leading to erratic behavior, loss of consciousness, or seizures, particularly if food is not consumed with the alcohol.[41] In addition, the teen should understand that glucagon is not effective in the treatment of alcohol-induced hypoglycemia because alcohol depletes glycogen stores.

Pointing out that alcohol alters the ability to think clearly may help the teen be more cautious about drinking alcohol or avoiding it altogether. It is important that those who choose to drink make sure that they wear diabetes identification because intoxication and symptoms of hypoglycemia can often be confused for one another. Drinking alone should always be discouraged.

If alcohol is consumed, it should be consumed in moderate amounts (no more than one drink per day for most females and no more than two drinks a day for most males) and only if diabetes is well managed. One drink or alcohol portion is defined as 12 oz. of beer, 5 oz. of wine, or 1.5 oz. of 80-proof distilled spirits. Each of these portions provides about 0.5 oz. of alcohol. As a general rule, it takes about 2 hours for the average 150-pound male to metabolize 1 oz. of alcohol.[2]

Designing the Meal Plan

The ultimate goals when designing a meal plan for a child who has been recently diagnosed with T1D are to:

- Provide healthy eating guidelines for the youth and family
- Promote positive behavioral changes
- Provide healthy meals and snacks
- Focus on healthy eating habits of the entire family

The amount of time required by the family to learn meal planning depends on multiple factors such as family dynamics, emotional status, extended support system, preconceived ideas about the "diabetic diet," and the family's social and cultural attitudes. The child should participate in the initial visit and be reassured that he or she will not be put on a "diet" or have many favorite foods taken away. Rather, healthy guidelines (a meal plan) will be provided based on the child's usual eating pattern to help promote healthy food choices. To avoid isolating the child and dividing the family, it should be emphasized that meal planning is simply a heart-healthy eating plan for both the child and the entire family. Eating the same foods provides a sense of unity within the family.

Nutrition Counseling

At the time of diagnosis, the parent and/or child may be asked to keep a record of what is eaten at each meal and snack. This helps establish the amount of food that is currently needed to satisfy the child's appetite. An accurate measurement of weight and height (or length), information on recent weight loss, and a calculation of IBW are needed to estimate the child's current nutrient and caloric needs. Determining the percentile of the height (length), weight, body mass index (BMI), and the range for IBW will identify the child's initial nutrition status and help guide the development of the meal plan. A newly diagnosed child is more likely to experience increased hunger due to glycosuria. It is important to respond to this stimulated appetite by providing sufficient food so that hunger and restriction are not associated with having diabetes. The appetite of most children will stabilize within the first few weeks after diagnosis, though it could take longer. If the youth has lost weight or not grown to their potential, their appetite may be higher than estimated needs. Within reason, the meal plan should reflect the amount of food the child desires and be readjusted once the appetite decreases. The family should be told that the meal plan might need to be adjusted 2 or 3 weeks after diagnosis once the child has returned to his or her growth potential.

Nutrition intervention at diagnosis should be based on the family's ability, interest, and readiness to learn. Attempts to present all concepts upon initial diagnosis may result in confusion and the family members' loss of confidence in their ability as caretakers. Provide only general guidelines such as consistency with timing, amount and types of foods, and the relationship among food, insulin, and exercise, and their effect on blood glucose (BG). The initial education might be in a hospital or an outpatient setting; routine follow-up visits or contact by phone may be beneficial. Many questions will arise when the child returns home and normal activity resumes. Above all, it should be stressed that:

- Parents should not limit food to maintain blood glucose control.
- Any changes associated with food choices should be made slowly.
- Ranges for food choices should be used with young children (i.e., 1–2 oz. protein, ½–1 fruit), offering smaller amounts first and using the larger end of the range if more food is requested.
- During initial education the length of time required to achieve nutrition management survival skills varies considerably between families and may require 2 to 4 hours of education in addition to time for menu writing and food selection using the meal plan.
- After the initial education, additional outpatient nutrition visits will be necessary to achieve ultimate nutrition education goals.

The initial visit in the outpatient setting should lay the groundwork in nutrition basics and serve to develop a sound and trusting relationship with the child and family. The Children's Checklist (**Exhibit 15-1**) offers a detailed analysis of the child's and family's eating habits and behaviors, food preferences, and family lifestyle, and will assist the registered dietitian in producing a realistic and workable meal plan for this very important population.

EXHIBIT 15-1 Children's Checklist: Assessing the Child Newly Diagnosed with Diabetes

Growth (Anthropometrics):

- Height
- Weight
- BMI or weight-for-height
- History of growth pattern
- Recent weight changes

Biochemical Indices:

- Blood glucose
- Glycosylated hemoglobin (A1C) and estimated average glucose (eAG)
- Lipid profile
- Microalbumin
- Ketones

Psychosocial Information:

- Identify the family unit at home (two parents, separated parents, single parent, divorced, siblings, other family, friends, or caretakers).
- Evaluate emotional state of parents, child, siblings (anger, fear, guilt, denial, anxiety).
- Assess child's interactions with parents and siblings.
- Identify person(s) responsible for shopping/cooking.
- Evaluate knowledge/comprehension levels and literacy.
- Identify cultural/religious systems that influence attitudes.
- Identify family members or friends with diabetes.
- Assess parents and family beliefs about the "diabetic diet."

Child's Usual Food Intake Prior to Symptoms of Diabetes

Home:

- Eats scheduled meals/snacks
- Includes staple foods, such as milk, cheese, yogurt, bread
- Eats meats, fruit, and vegetables on a regular basis
- Consumes beverages at meals/snacks other than milk
- Drinks soda/juice/water for thirst
- Follows special diet

School:

- Brings lunch from home or has school lunch.
- Beverage at lunch/snacks.
- Scheduled snacks are part of regular class activities.
- Obtains snack at school or snack sent from home.
- Frequency, length, and time of day of gym class.
- Participates in school sports or activities after school.

Weekends:

- Evaluate meals prepared or eaten with others on weekends.
- Identify meal schedule if different from weekdays.
- Determine restaurant eating habits on weekends.
- Assess sports/activities scheduled on weekends.

Eating Behaviors

Child:

- Overeats or undereats
- Relies on convenience and fast foods
- Experiences food jags often
- Refuses many of the family foods offered
- Finishes meals in reasonable amount of time
- Respects limits set for acceptable eating behavior at the table
- Location where meals and snacks are consumed
- Food allergies or intolerances

Family:

- Evaluate parents as role models.
- Healthy eaters, structured meals, planned meals, limit junk food in home.
- Unhealthy eaters, overweight, chronic dieters.
- Identify supervision at meals/snacks.
- Evaluate limit-setting around food choices.
- Assess cultural/religious eating behaviors.
- Identify whether food is used as a reward.

General guidelines to help develop a positive working relationship with the youth and their caretakers include:

- Include the youth in the interview to allow him or her to be part of the decision-making process. The youth will dictate the amount of food based on hunger and the parent will dictate the food choices.
- Do not refer to or label a youth as a diabetic but as a child or adolescent with diabetes.
- Interview the prepubertal child separately and then together with family to stimulate self-management.
- Provide reassurance that many of the youth's usual foods can be included in his or her meal plan.
- Describe the meal plan as a guideline for healthy eating rather than a diet.
- Stress healthy eating practices for the entire family rather than just focusing on the youth with diabetes.
- Avoid negative words when explaining meal planning such as *cannot, do not, never, should not, bad, restrict,* and especially the word *diet*. In a child's mind, *diet* connotes deprivation or a short-term process, rather than an ongoing process.

- Avoid using the terms *good* or *bad* for foods. Instead, use *healthy* and *not as healthy* to describe individual foods.
- Ask about favorite foods and avoid eliminating these foods. Instead, stress balance, moderation, and variety.
- Review the reality of special treats for birthday parties, holidays, and special occasions and relate "treat" foods with extra exercise and active days.
- Encourage the caregiver to include the youth in shopping and meal preparation.
- Revise or draft a realistic and workable meal plan with input from the parent and/or youth.
- Encourage the parents to always keep the lines of communication open so the youth can request special foods that he or she wants to eat and that can be worked into the meal plan. Avoid being the "food police." If the youth is always told "no," he or she may start to sneak food, which will cause unexplained high blood glucose levels.
- Advise the caregivers that it is not advisable to omit foods from the meal plan because of a single high blood glucose reading. An elevated BG level caused by stress may decrease rapidly when the stress is reduced, and hypoglycemia may occur if food is omitted.
- Continued nutrition follow-up and education are required every 6 months to 1 year as the child grows and develops and as the family works to gain expertise in the nutrition management of diabetes.

Meal-Planning Approaches

One of the primary reasons patients with diabetes have such a difficult time understanding food issues is due to a lack of nutrition education and counseling by a registered dietitian. Instead, patients may simply be told to restrict sugary foods or may be given a basic sample menu to follow without an adequate educational foundation. The DCCT provided important insight into the role of nutrition intervention in intensive diabetes management and stated that registered dietitians are best qualified to match appropriate meal-planning approaches to the needs of the patient. Today, there are several effective methods for teaching patients about food. Any method can be equally effective when "geared to the patient's intellectual level, repeated frequently, and evaluated."[42]

The two most common approaches used with children are advanced carbohydrate counting and basic carbohydrate counting. On occasion the family might request a food choice list (exchange list) for meal planning. These methods give structure to meal planning and provide the right balance among food, insulin, and exercise.

Carbohydrate Counting

The standard of care for children with T1D is to manage their diabetes on multiple daily injections (MDI) or continuous subcutaneous insulin infusion (CSII) using pump therapy. Advanced carbohydrate (carb) counting allows users greater flexibility in the timing of meals, the amount of food eaten at the meal, and the selection of specific foods. The meal-planning objective is to coordinate food intake (carbohydrate) by matching the peak activity of insulin with the peak levels of glucose resulting from the digestion and absorption of food. Only the carbohydrate value of the food is counted, which allows more accurate adjustment of premeal, rapid-acting insulin using an insulin-to-carb ratio. The insulin-to-carb ratio is based on the assumption that carbohydrate intake is the main consideration in determining meal-related insulin requirements together with self-monitored blood glucose (SMBG) values. Targeted blood glucose values are set by the diabetes team, the child, and his or her family. A general rule is that approximately 1 unit of rapid-acting insulin will be needed for every 10 to 15 grams of carbohydrate.[43] The child's insulin-to-carb ratio should be individually determined by the diabetes team based on the child's present insulin needs and meal plan. A youth's ratio can range from 1 unit of insulin for every 5 to 40 grams of carbohydrate depending on age, activity, and insulin needs.

In addition to covering the carbs at a meal, the youths are given a sensitivity factor (SF) and a target BG. This allows them to adjust the dose based on their BG prior to the meal or snack. If their BG is higher than target they will add some additional insulin, and if BG is lower than target subtract some insulin using the SF.

Special care must be given to prevent overeating because increased availability of insulin and food may promote unwanted weight gain. A good understanding of how carbohydrate affects blood glucose, what food groups contain carbohydrates, and the importance of portion control is necessary for carbohydrate counting to be effective. Reference books providing the carbohydrate content of specific foods are also helpful. Continuous reinforcement of healthy eating habits is advisable, because many young people tend to omit food groups as well as meals to accommodate busy schedules or to manage weight.

The Exchange/Choice or Food List

The lists of food choices (exchange lists) are based on the following food groups:

- *The carbohydrate group:* Starches (breads, cereals, grains, starchy vegetables, etc.), fruit, milk, nonstarchy vegetables, sweets, desserts, and other carbohydrates
- *The meat and meat substitute group:* Protein (meat, poultry, fish, dried peas, and beans)
- *The fat group:* Vegetable oils, avocado, and regular salad dressings.

Examples of the specific amount of carbohydrate, protein, fat, or combination of these nutrients in each food group are found in **Table 15-7**.[44] Foods with similar nutrient values are listed together and may be exchanged or traded for any other food on the same list. Exchange lists are used to achieve a consistent timing and intake of carbohydrate, protein, and fat and provide needed variety when planning meals. Exchange lists and a meal plan can be a starting point for those patients on intensive insulin management and can help them to understand and learn the carbohydrate content of foods.

Insulin Therapy

The standard of care for managing diabetes in children is called intensive management and uses a basal/bolus insulin plan. Intensive insulin therapy can include multiple daily injections (MDI) using rapid-acting insulin with either an intermediate or long-acting insulin or CSII pump therapy. A basal/bolus regimen allows more flexibility in the scheduling of meals and may eliminate the need for some snacks; however, intensive insulin therapy does increase the risk of hypoglycemia. The insulin action (onset, peak, and duration) of the insulin available is listed in **Table 15-8**. It is important to consider that insulin action will differ from person to person and can be affected by the injection site, activity level before and after the injection is given, and time of day.

Conventional insulin therapy is no longer the standard of care but is still used in practice. This therapy may include two daily injections of intermediate-acting insulin (NPH) or one injection of NPH with a long-acting/basal insulin (glargine [Lantus] or detemir [Levemir]), possibly combined with a small amount of rapid-acting insulin (lispro [Humalog], aspart [Novolog], or glulisine [Apidra]).

Many circumstances require permanent or temporary insulin adjustments to be made. As a child grows and food intake increases, the insulin dose also increases. During brief periods of illness, times of stress, or decreased activity, insulin needs may also increase. A change in the child's level of activity, which may be especially dramatic at the beginning and end of the school year, usually requires an adjustment in the insulin dosage. When these events resolve or change, the child's insulin dose will need to be readjusted. Otherwise, an increase of food in response to the higher insulin levels may result in inappropriate weight gain or hypoglycemia, whereas too little insulin may result in hyperglycemia.

Snacks

Snacks should be part of a healthy eating plan, and depending on the age of the child might be necessary. Snacks can help with maintaining the blood glucose and providing ad-

TABLE 15-7 Choose Your Foods: Exchange List for Diabetes

Foods List	Carbohydrates (grams)	Protein (grams)	Fat (grams)	Calories
Carbohydrate				
Starch: breads, cereals and grains, starchy vegetables, crackers, snacks, beans, peas, and lentils	15	0–3	0–1	80
Fruits	15	—	—	60
Milk				
Fat-free, low-fat, 1%	12	8	0–3	100
Reduced-fat, 2%	12	8	5	120
Whole	12	8	8	150
Sweets, Desserts, and Other Carbohydrates	15	Varies	Varies	Varies
Nonstarchy Vegetables	5	2	—	25
Meat and Meat Substitutes				
Lean	—	7	0–3	45
Medium-fat	—	7	4–7	75
High-fat	—	7	8+	100
Plant-based proteins	Varies	7	Varies	Varies
Fats	—	—	5	45
Alcohol	Varies	—	—	100

Source: © 2008 American Dietetic Association, American Diabetes Association. Reprinted with permission.

TABLE 15-8 Insulin Actions

Insulin	When to Take	Onset	Peak	Effective Duration
Rapid Acting Lispro (Humalog), Aspart (Novolog), Glulisine (Apidra)	0–15 minutes before the meal	10–30 minutes	30 minutes–3 hours	3–5 hours
Short Acting Regular (R)	30 minutes before the meal	30–60 minutes	2–5 hours	Up to 12 hours
Intermediate Acting NPH	Does not need to be given with food	90 minutes–4 hours	4–12 hours	Up to 24 hours
Long Acting Glargine (Lantus), Detemir (Levemir)	Does not need to be given with food	45 minutes–4 hours	Minimal	Up to 24 hours

equate calories during the day for growth and development. Snacking during the day is more desirable and will hopefully eliminate hunger in the evening hours. If the child is on a basal/bolus regimen then snacks before bedtime are not necessary unless the blood glucose is lower than desired or the child is hungry.

If the child is on conventional insulin therapy with NPH insulin it has a peaking action. To prevent hypoglycemia, the youth is encouraged to eat snacks between meals and at bedtime. Typically, a snack of 15 to 20 g of carbohydrate is recommended for young children and a snack of 20 to 30 g of carbohydrate or higher is recommended for adolescents. Snacking could also be necessary depending on activity such as length of time at recess and in physical education (PE) classes and the type and length of after-school activities. For example, if PE is offered only on Monday and Wednesday at 10:00 am, the child may need a larger snack on those days, preferably a snack with 20 to 30 g of carbohydrate and 1 to 2 oz. of protein. For very active days and extended appetite control, a long-lasting snack (2 to 3 hours) containing carbohydrate, protein, and fat can be given. For inactive children, whose main activity is not likely to increase beyond watching television and studying, snacks may contain only 10 to 20 g of carbohydrate.

CSII/Pump Therapy

Since the introduction of CSII in the 1970s, pump therapy has become very popular in patients with T1D. Diabetes centers around the country started using the pump on pediatric patients in the 1980s. Pump therapy demonstrated benefits such as improved glycemic control,[45,46] reduced episodes of hypoglycemia, improved linear growth, and decreased episodes of recurrent diabetic ketoacidosis (DKA).[47] Pumps are becoming more widely used even in children as young as 1 to 2 years of age. The advantage of the pump for the young child is that it offers the parents the ability to dose a very small amount of insulin and provide multiple doses throughout the day without having to give the child injections by syringe or pen.

Pump therapy provides only a rapid-acting insulin (Humalog, Novolog, or Apidra), which eliminates the unpredictable action of the longer-acting insulins. The pump delivers a small amount of insulin continuously (basal) and can be programmed to deliver boluses when eating a meal or snack, or for correcting high blood glucoses. There are pros and cons of pump therapy, which should be considered very carefully prior to putting any youth on an insulin pump.

Long-Acting Insulins

Long-acting insulins (basal) are becoming more popular in school-age children, adolescents, and young adults in place of the intermediate insulin NPH. They allow the child the flexibility of the pump without the additional equipment that comes with the pump. Long-acting insulin is given in one or two injections daily to meet the child's background or basal insulin needs. Additional injections of rapid insulin are given at meals and snacks to cover the carbohydrate and to correct the blood glucose. The long-acting insulin can last up to 24 hours and is usually started with one injection a day, usually given at dinner or bedtime for consistency. Some children have benefited from splitting the dose, due to the insulin possibly not lasting a full 24 hours or having some peaking action.

This insulin regimen can translate to at least four to five injections in an older child and as many as five to six in a younger child. To avoid additional insulin injections at school, NPH insulin can be added at breakfast with the rapid insulin to cover the morning snack and lunch. Long-acting insulin can be used at bedtime in place of NPH if there is concern of hypoglycemia in the middle of the night, and it will also give a little coverage in the late afternoon.

Before a family or child starts CSII or MDI, the child and the family must master advanced skills, including having a good understanding of advanced carbohydrate counting, which includes using insulin-to-carbohydrate ratios; understanding the sensitivity or correction factor to determine each insulin dose; and having the necessary math skills needed to calculate dosage.

Age-Specific Developmental Considerations

The most important psychosocial issues facing families with children with diabetes are:

- Defining responsibilities and support for diabetes management within the family
- Sharing treatment responsibilities among family members
- How and when these responsibilities are transferred from parent to child as the child develops[48]

As the child with diabetes progresses through the different stages of development, it is important to address how these changes affect the parents and/or the child and focus on the normal developmental issues of each stage. Encouraging parental involvement throughout childhood and early adulthood can be beneficial in the youth's diabetes management. See **Table 15-9**[49] for some of the development stages and how they relate to T1D.

Birth to 12 Months of Age

Initially, most infants consume 100% of their calories as breast milk or formula, eating every 3 to 4 hours. The AAP recommends that all babies be breastfed for the first 6 to 12 months of life; iron-fortified infant formula is the only acceptable substitute. Solids are typically introduced at 4 to 6 months and progress from cereal to fruits, meat, vegetables, and/or vegetable-meat dinners. Infants with diabetes do well following the same schedule. Eventually when the infant begins eating 2 to 3 tablespoons of baby foods and/or table food (other than low-calorie vegetables), basic carbohydrate counting can be introduced as a guideline. It is recommended to establish a feeding schedule despite somewhat erratic eating behaviors in the infant.

One to 4 Years of Age

A 1992 report in the *New England Journal of Medicine* proposed a possible link between drinking cow's milk as an infant and the development of type 1 diabetes. Upon further inspection the association of exposure to cow's milk and type 1 diabetes is unlikely.[50,51] Although whole cow's milk should not be given during the child's first year, after the first year, cow's milk should not be removed from the diets of infants who have a family history of type 1 diabetes.

Between 12 and 15 months of age, breastmilk (or formula) intake may begin to decrease and the intake of solid food increases. A total revision of the meal plan is needed at this time. During this time, a child may begin to be more accepting of meat and cheese, which can be added to the meal plan. Although fruits are included in the meal plan, fruit juice should be limited or avoided due to its effect on appetite, weight, and blood glucose.

As the toddler develops more mobility, interest in the environment also increases, and interest in food may wane. In some instances, getting the toddler to eat anything at a meal is an accomplishment. Erratic eating behaviors in toddlers require careful monitoring. In some cases, insulin is given after the meal, when the toddler has consumed the food and the dose of insulin can be titrated based on the amount of food consumed. This is also a very popular time for parents to transition their child to CSII, which will give them flexibility to split the insulin dose. For instance, they can give the amount of insulin to correct the BG if higher than desired and some of the insulin to cover the food as much as they feel comfortable giving and then make up the difference at the end of the meal.

Food-behavior guidelines for this young group, with or without diabetes, should be firmly established by caregivers at the time the child begins solid foods. Young children with T1D learn quickly how important it is for them to eat and it is very easy for parents to fall into behaviors of short order cooking or letting the child choose the foods.

School-Age Children

Adjusting diabetes around the school schedule rather than changing physical education classes or lunch periods to accommodate an insulin regimen communicates to the child that the child is more important than the diabetes. It is possible to arrange snacks and injections around most school schedules. Parents should be encouraged to address food and diabetes treatment issues with school personnel; however, some parents may require assistance from their diabetes care team. School-age children will ordinarily need three meals and two to three snacks a day, scheduled according to their insulin regimen. However, some children can omit the morning snack without creating a problem as long as lunch is not delayed. Children should be instructed to carry a fast-acting carbohydrate with them at all times in case of emergency. The use of chocolate candy bars or other high-fat items is discouraged as a treatment for hypoglycemia because fat ingestion slows the absorption of the carbohydrate needed to raise the blood glucose to a safe level. Most schools will offer lunch items appropriate to the needs of children following a meal plan, such as low-fat milk and fresh fruit. If school personnel are unwilling to cooperate, reference can be made to Section 504 of the Rehabilitation Act of 1973 and the Individuals with Disabilities Education Act of 1991 (originally the Education for All Handicapped Children Act of 1975), Public Law No. 94-142, which mandates that handicapped students, including children with diabetes, have access to all services necessary to assist in full participation in school.[52]

Adolescents

The advent of adolescence may bring a great deal of conflict into the lives of family members. Adolescents strive for independence and expect parents to trust them to manage

TABLE 15-9 Major Development Issues and Their Effect on Diabetes in Children and Adolescents

Developmental Stage (Approximate Ages)	Normal Developmental Tasks	T1D Management Priorities	Family Issues in T1D Management
Infancy (0–12 months)	Developing a trusting relationship/"bonding" with primary caretakers	• Preventing and treating hypoglycemia • Avoiding extreme fluctuations in the BG levels	• Coping with stress • Sharing the "burden of care" to avoid parent burnout
Toddler (13–36 months)	Developing a sense of mastery and autonomy	• Preventing and treating hypoglycemia • Avoiding extreme fluctuations in the BG levels due to irregular food intake	• Establishing a schedule • Managing the picky eater • Setting limits and coping with toddlers' lack of cooperation with regimen • Sharing the burden of care
Preschooler and early elementary age (3–7 years)	Developing initiative in activities and confidence in self	• Preventing and treating hypoglycemia • Unpredictable appetite and activity • Positive reinforcement for cooperation with regimen • Trusting other caretakers with diabetes management	• Reassuring the child that diabetes is no one's fault • Educating other caretakers about diabetes management
Older elementary school age (8–11 years)	• Developing skills in athletic, cognitive, artistic, and social areas • Consolidating self-esteem with respect to the peer group	• Making diabetes regimen flexible to allow for participation in school/peer activities • Child learning short- and long-term benefits of optimal control	• Maintaining parental involvement in insulin and BG monitoring tasks while allowing for independent self-care for "special occasions" • Continuing to educate school and other caretakers
Early adolescence (12–15 years)	Managing body changes Developing a strong sense of self-identity	• Managing increased insulin requirements during puberty • Diabetes management and blood glucose control become more difficult • Weight and body image concerns	• Renegotiating parents' and teen's role in diabetes management to be accepted by both • Learning coping skills to enhance ability to self-manage • Preventing and intervening with diabetes-related family conflict • Monitoring for signs of depression, eating disorders, and risky behaviors
Later adolescence (16–19 years)	Establishing a sense of identity after high school (decision about location, social issues, work, education)	• Begin discussion of transition to new diabetes team • Integrating diabetes into new lifestyle	• Supporting the transition to independence • Learning coping skills to enhance ability to self-manage • Preventing and intervening with diabetes-related family conflict • Monitoring for signs of depression, eating disorders, or risky behavior

Source: Reproduced with permission from the American Diabetes Association. Silverstein J, Klingensmith G, Copeland K, et al. Care of children and adolescents with type 1 diabetes: a statement of the American Diabetes Association. *Diabetes Care.* 2005;28(1):186–212.

their own diabetes. During the adolescent period they may vent their anger for the first time about having diabetes. The key to working successfully with adolescents is for the parents and the diabetes team to make every effort to provide positive reinforcement and negotiated support. Parents should continue their involvement and supervision of monitoring blood glucose and insulin administration at home. It is often more effective for team members to see adolescents and their parents individually, while at the same time respecting their confidentiality. More flexibility in food choices and an increase in calories during this period of growth is usually necessary. Food choices may improve in a nonjudgmental atmosphere and with assistance for the teen to work favorite foods into the meal plan. In clinic visits, teens should be routinely asked if they have any questions about their food choices. Focusing on the positive choices the adolescents are making and what they are doing right can lead to open discussion and follow-up visits.

Growth Maintenance

Routine charting of a child's height, weight, and BMI is an excellent way to monitor their growth pattern. Deviation from the child's normal growth curve (except for increased height or decreasing weight in a child who has reached full height potential) needs close monitoring. In a child whose diabetes is poorly controlled, weight percentile will often remain stationary or decrease. After about 6 months of little or no weight gain, height velocity may also begin to slow. Achieving optimal height potential can be used to motivate boys and girls to strive for better blood glucose control. Adolescents are more likely to be interested in improved self-care when they understand the relationship between good control, appropriate weight gain, consistent height increase, and/or normal menses.

Weight Control and Disordered Eating

Weight control can become an important issue to children prior to and when entering adolescence. Parents and the diabetes team must take concerns about body image seriously. Some weight gain is usually seen prior to growth spurts. If a youth's weight is disproportionate to height, the weight should be kept stable until the height fits the weight. Calorie reduction and food restriction are not recommended for children at any time during growth and development. Rather, the child should be encouraged to become involved in active play and physical exercise and to incorporate more fresh fruits and vegetables into his or her daily intake.

Youth who are overly concerned about weight gain but who find it hard to reduce their intake may choose to skip insulin injections to promote quick weight loss. Eating disorders in youth with diabetes can include anorexia nervosa, bulimia nervosa, and eating disorder not otherwise specified (ED-NOS).[53] Early identification of eating disorders by the diabetes team can help the individual to get the treatment necessary. Some of the signs are as follows:[54]

- Deterioration of psychosocial functions (school, work, interpersonal)
- Weight fluctuations of 10 pounds or more
- High glycosylated hemoglobin (A1C)
- Controlled diabetes only when hospitalized
- Unexplained diabetic ketoacidosis
- Reluctance or refusal to take more insulin or other medications
- Not checking BG
- Blaming insulin for weight problems
- Preoccupation with body image
- Engaging in excessive exercise
- Bingeing
- Restricting food
- Depression with low self-esteem

Referral to a registered dietitian or certified diabetes educator is the first line of defense when a child or adolescent exhibits weight dissatisfaction but does not exhibit clinical eating pathology. Strict guidelines regarding food and blood glucose should not be implemented because this may actually promote binge eating or weight gain. Adolescents should be advised that glucose fluctuations could create increased hunger and result in weight gain. Education should also be provided about serious short- and long-term consequences of destructive food behaviors. Referral to a mental health professional who is knowledgeable about diabetes and disordered eating, or hospitalization, is often necessary to break the disordered eating cycle.

Type 2 Diabetes

Type 2 diabetes (T2D) is increasing in our population, especially in high-risk ethnic groups.[55] The increased incidence of type 2 diabetes in children is proportional with the increased incidence of childhood obesity. Many of the cases occur in children of ethnic minorities including African American, Mexican American, Native American, and Asian American.[56] T2D in children, as in adults, is due to the combination of insulin resistance and beta-cell failure. Few studies have been done to determine the most effective way to manage these children. Incorporating physical activity and nutrition counseling to help the child or adolescent maintain or lose weight is often prescribed, coupled with either Metformin or insulin. Metformin is presently the only oral diabetes medication approved by the FDA for pediatric use.

Youth diagnosed with T2D have a greater incidence of co-morbidities at diagnosis. The ADA recommends that these children have blood pressure measurements, a fasting lipid profile, a microalbuminuria assessment, and a dilated eye examination at diagnosis.[25] Other issues that should be considered are co-morbidities associated with polycystic disease and obesity.

The increased rate of children being diagnosed with T2D is a public health problem. In a position statement of the American Diabetes Association and the National Institute of Diabetes, Digestive, and Kidney Diseases,[57] the following recommendations were made:

- Children of families at risk should be aware of the benefits of weight maintenance or moderate weight loss, and the health benefits of regular physical activity.
- Intervention strategies should involve counseling on weight loss and physical activity, with follow-up, which appears to be important for success.
- Drug therapy should not be routinely used to prevent diabetes until more information is known.

In 2002, the Diabetes Prevention Program published the results of a study comparing lifestyle intervention to administering Metformin in the prevention or delay of developing T2D in adults. There was a 58% reduction of diabetes progression in the lifestyle group as compared to a 31% reduction in the Metformin group.[58] These results are particularly important to those who are interested in preventing T2D in our youth. Providing education for a healthy and active lifestyle might be the best defense against this ever-growing public health epidemic.

Pregnancy

To help ensure a healthy pregnancy and a positive outcome for the woman with diabetes, optimal medical care must begin before conception. However, many unplanned pregnancies occur shortly after puberty among adolescents and young women with and without diabetes, putting those with pregestational diabetes mellitus (PGDM) at a higher risk for early pregnancy loss or congenital malformations. The deterioration of metabolic control in combination with other obstetric and medical complications during an unplanned pregnancy can lead to serious complications of diabetes such as retinopathy, nephropathy, hypertension, and neuropathy. It is the responsibility of the diabetes team to provide prepregnancy counseling, including information on the risk of congenital malformations, to those of childbearing age who have diabetes.

Unplanned pregnancies should be addressed immediately by a multidisciplinary team approach including a diabetologist, obstetrician, and diabetes educators, including a nurse, a registered dietitian, a social worker, and possibly an exercise physiologist. The team approach can guide the mother toward a goal of a healthy pregnancy and offspring.[59] Members of the adolescent or young adult's immediate family are encouraged to attend and participate in all learning sessions.

A preconception interactive care plan outlined by the ADA to facilitate reimbursement for all elements of the program by health insurance organizations includes the following:

- Patient education related to interaction of diabetes, pregnancy, and family planning
- Education in diabetes self-management skills
- Physician-directed medical care and laboratory testing
- Counseling by a mental health professional to reduce stress and improve adherence to the diabetes treatment plan

Nutrition management during pregnancy should begin at the earliest possible time. Caloric intake should be evaluated as soon as possible in the first trimester and at the start of each trimester thereafter to ensure adequate intake. Guidelines for medical nutrition therapy for pregnancy for preexisting diabetes are listed in **Exhibit 15-2**.

Breastfeeding

Breastfeeding is encouraged for mothers with diabetes and provides to the mother and infant the same benefits as it does for any woman and infant. Not only does breast milk contain immunoglobulins and antibodies, which protect the infant from diseases, intestinal distress, and allergic reactions, but the process of breastfeeding also encourages mother–infant bonding. Breastfeeding, however, increases the need for fluids, and mothers should be encouraged to drink 2 to 3 liters (8 to 12 cups) of caffeine-free liquids per day to cover the fluid needs of the mother and replace what is used in breast milk. Meal planning during breastfeeding requires assistance from a dietitian and physician. Insulin requirements are usually reduced during breastfeeding; however, caloric intake requires an additional 500 calories per day above what was consumed before the pregnancy. Extra calories may be added in the form of protein- and calcium-rich foods such as milk, yogurt, tofu, and cheese. The calcium requirement for lactating women is 1000 mg per day, unless the mother is under 18 years of age, in which case she would need 1300 mg/day.[10] Calcium intake should be routinely assessed by a dietitian to prevent calcium loss from the mother during breastfeeding. If the mother is not able to consume adequate sources of calcium-rich foods, a calcium supplement may be required. It is important to keep a carbohydrate food source (15 to 20 g) available while nursing because hypoglycemia may occur while breastfeeding. To prevent possible nocturnal hypoglycemia, an extra snack including 20 to 30 g of carbohydrate and a source of

EXHIBIT 15-2 Medical Nutrition Therapy Guidelines for Management of Diabetes in Pregnancy

Recommendations are the same for pre-existing diabetes and GDM except where noted.

Counseling and Education	• All pregnant women should receive MNT counseling by a registered dietitian (RD), Certified Diabetes Educator (CDE) preferred.
	• All pregnant women should receive SMBG training by a diabetes educator (DE), CDE preferred.
	• Daily food records and recorded SMBG are required to assess the effectiveness of MNT.
	• Carbohydrate counting skills are taught for either consistent carbohydrate intake or a personalized insulin-to-carbohydrate ratio so the patient can adjust insulin based on carbohydrate intake.
	• At least three encounters with a CDE are recommended:
	  • Visit 1 (60- to 90-minute individual or group visit with RD) for assessment and meal planning. This could be SMBG instruction if RD has received appropriate training.
	  • Visit 2 (30–45 min) with RD or RN in 1 week to assess and modify plan.
	  • Visit 3 (15–45 min) with RD or RN in 1–3 weeks to assess and modify plan as needed.
	• Additional visits every 2–3 weeks with RD or RN p.r.n. until delivery and one visit 6–8 weeks after delivery.

Calories	BMI Range	WHO BMI Range (kg/m²)	Prepregnancy Weight (kcal/kg)*	Recommended Weight Gain (lbs)
	Underweight (< 19.8)	(< 18.5)	36–40	28–40
	Normal weight (19.8–26.0)	(18.5–24.9)	30	25–35
	Overweight (26.1–29.0)	(25.0–29.9)	24	15–25
	Obese (> 29.0)	(≥ 30.0)	not < 1800 kcal	≥ 15
	Twins**			35–45
	Triplets**			45–55

Recommendations of kcal/kg and recommended weight gain apply only to the Institute of Medicine BMI criteria; the WHO BMI classification is included for comparison purposes only.

*An additional 150–300 kcal/day in the second and third trimesters.

**150 kcal/day above singleton pregnancy, or an amount consistent with target weight gain.

Distribution of Calories	• Individualize based on usual intake, preferences, and medical regimen. • Six to eight small meals/snacks. More frequent meals decrease postprandial hyperglycemia.

	GDM	Preexisting Diabetes
Carbohydrate Breakfast	40–45% total calories[†] 15–30 grams[‡]	45–55% total calories Individualize as per usual intake and BG levels
HS (before bed) Snack	15–30 grams carbs	15–30 grams carbs
Fiber	20–35 grams	20–35 grams
Protein	• 0.8 g protein/DBW plus an additional 25 g/day. • 20–25% of total calories is usual.	
Fat	• *Preexisting diabetes:* 30–35% total calories, with < 10% total calories from saturated fat. • *GDM:* < 40% total calories, with 10% total calories from saturated fat. • Encourage use of polyunsaturated and monounsaturated fats instead of saturated fats.	

EXHIBIT 15-2 *(Continued)*

Artificial sweeteners	• Sugar alcohols (sorbitol, mannitol, xylitol, maltitol) are safe for use in pregnancy, but may have a laxative effect if too much is consumed. Foods containing sweeteners still contain carbohydrate and must be counted in the meal plan. • Non-nutritive sweeteners considered safe during pregnancy: aspartame, acesulfame potassium (ace-K), and sucralose. • Because saccharin crosses the placenta and is cleared slowly by the fetus, it is not recommended during pregnancy.
Vitamin/mineral supplements	Prenatal multivitamin and mineral supplement including: • Iron (27 mg/day). • Folic acid (400 μg) to supplement average daily dietary intake of 400 μg for a total daily intake of 600 μg to 1 mg daily to decrease risk of neural tube defects. (Begin 400 μg prior to conception.) • Additional calcium supplementation may be needed to meet daily requirements of 1000 mg per day (1300 mg per day if under age 19). Begin prior to conception.
Physical activity	• Regular physical activity is recommended after clearance by provider. • Benefits include reducing insulin resistance, postprandial hyperglycemia, and excessive weight gain. • Hypoglycemia is more likely with prolonged exercise (> 60 minutes). • Encourage activity after meals to reduce postprandial hyperglycemia.

†Pregnant women should consume a minimum of 175 g carbohydrate per day.

‡May be increased if insulin is added.

Source: Reprinted with permission from Joslin Diabetes Center and Joslin Clinic Guideline for Detection and Management of Diabetes and Pregnancy (Rev. 09/14/2005). Joslin's Clinical Guidelines are reviewed periodically and modified as needed to reflect changes in clinical practice and available pharmacological information. Check Joslin's Website for the latest version (http://www.joslin.org).

protein may be added to the meal plan in the middle of the night.

Monitoring Blood Glucose

Glycosylated hemoglobin (A1C) measures the weighted average amount of glucose in the blood over a 2- to 3-month period. Used in conjunction with regularly monitored blood glucose, the A1C levels can help evaluate the level of control. However, the A1C level reflects an average amount of glucose in the blood and can be the result of very high and low blood glucose levels, which is not indicative of good control. Although "excellent control" for an adult with diabetes is 6% or less, the activity levels and eating habits of children and adolescents vary, so even a level under 7% can be unsafe and difficult to achieve in children. A1C goals should be set by the child's diabetes team and tailored to each individual case. Age-appropriate A1C goals are shown in **Table 15-10**.[60]

Home blood glucose monitoring meters provide the child and family with immediate feedback on the effects of food, exercise, insulin, and stress on blood glucose levels, allowing for more flexibility in lifestyle and food intake.

A youth with diabetes has many self-care responsibilities. Checking and recording the blood glucose levels may be one of the most bothersome responsibilities for a youth because it must be done so often and because others may inappropriately evaluate and judge the results. Blood glucose results are not totally reliable as a monitor of adherence to carbohydrate counting. If, by reporting a high blood glucose reading, a youth risks accusations of sneaking food or overeating, the youth may choose to record a more acceptable but false level. This practice may result in poor diabetes management. Establishing a nonjudgmental and honest atmosphere for the exchange of information is imperative for the parent, the dietitian, and other healthcare providers. When monitoring blood glucose, use the word "check" rather than "test" and use positive words to describe the results, such as "high" or "low" rather than "good" or "bad." Any information received from monitoring provides information with positive feedback, regardless of the number.[61]

TABLE 15-10 Age-Based A1C and eAG Goals

			Plasma BG Goal Range (mg/dL)*	
Age (years)	A1C	eAG (mg/dL)	Before Meals	Bedtime/Overnight
Toddlers and preschool (0–6)	< 8.5%	< 197	100–180	110–200
School age (6–12)	< 6–8%	< 126–183	90–180	100–180
Adolescents and young adults (13–19)	< 7.5%	< 169	90–130	90–150

*ADA goals

Estimated average glucose (eAG) is a new way to present the A1C. It is a number similar to the glucose meter readings. To determine average glucose the calculation is eAG = (28.7 × A1C) − 46.7. The American Diabetes Association has an eAG calculator available on its Website: http://www.diabetes.org/eag.jsp.

Source: Laffel LMB, Butler DA, Higgins LA, Lawlor MT, Pasquarello CA, eds. *Joslin's Guide to Managing Childhood Diabetes: A Family Teamwork Approach*. Boston, MA: Joslin Diabetes Center; 2009.

High or low blood glucose levels will still occur in most children even when insulin, exercise schedules, and carbohydrate counting are followed closely. When a high or low level occurs, it is useful to review the day's activities to see if there is an obvious explanation. The extent to which children should monitor blood glucose levels is variable, depending on many factors such as the type of insulin therapy, increased activity or exercise, sickness or infection, new food choices, change in lifestyle, increased stress, change in insulin type or dose, episodes of hypoglycemia, or overall control. A general guideline for blood glucose checking for most youth should be four BG checks daily, before each meal and before bedtime. Additional checks should be done before physical activity, if there is suspicion of hypoglycemia or hyperglycemia, or if the youth is ill.

Continuous Glucose Monitoring

Continuous glucose monitoring (CGM) is now widely available for the consumer, and some insurance companies are covering the system. The first generation of CGM was a masked system that provided retrospective data. The new real-time CGM allows the person with diabetes to have a complete picture of their blood glucose activity in real time. The system is made of three components: the sensor, transmitter, and receiver. The sensor is a small flexible electrode that sits under the skin in the interstitial fluid, which is the liquid that surrounds our cells. It is introduced by a needle, and then the needle is removed and the sensor can be worn 3–7 days depending on the CGM. The transmitter is a tiny computer attached to the sensor that sends the information from the sensor to a wireless receiver. The receiver is the size of a beeper or cell phone, and it will collect the information and display it on a screen. It will display the BG reading every 1–5 minutes and provide a directional trend of where the glucose is going. There is a slight delay in the reading, however, and the finger stick is still the gold standard when treating hypoglycemia. The devices also have arrows and alarms that can be set to warn the individual if their BG is rising or falling quickly so they can respond. This technology is very exciting and will allow educators to help youth cover meals (such as pizza, fast food, and Chinese food) that have been challenging in the past. Once the effect of the meal on the BG is viewed, the diabetes educator can help the youth determine the best way to cover the particular meal.

Exercise/Activity

Regular exercise or activity is an important element in controlling blood glucose, lowering lipid levels, and maintaining appropriate body weight. Aerobic exercise is necessary to maintain a healthy cardiovascular system as well as to improve glucose control. To prevent obesity in children, emphasis should be placed on the importance of routinely scheduled activity. A minimum of 30 minutes to 1 hour of daily activity is a reasonable goal. However, exercising when ketones are present, which may occur when the blood glucose level is above 240 mg/dL, or if the blood glucose is 400 mg/dL or higher without ketones, is not recommended.

To prevent hypoglycemia during activity, food intake may need to be increased or the dose of insulin decreased. Generally, children choose to increase food intake unless the activity occurs routinely, then the insulin can be adjusted accordingly. If the youth's overall activity increases and he or she is experiencing an increased number of hypoglycemic events, the diabetes team should be consulted for insulin adjustment. Older children may be instructed on how to reduce their own insulin dose when participating in sports. It is wise to avoid exercise when insulin is peaking, but it is not always preventable. If an unplanned activity occurs right after taking insulin, a larger snack, which includes carbohydrate as well as protein, may be needed. Some children may find it difficult to eat a large volume of food prior to prolonged activity and plan ahead to reduce their insulin dose.

The amount of insulin reduction depends on the results of blood glucose checks done before and after the activity.

Food adjustments will depend on the duration and intensity of the exercise and on the blood glucose level prior to the activity. A general rule is to add 10 to 15 g of carbohydrate for every 30 minutes of activity. Prolonged activity may utilize a majority of the glucose stores in the muscle. The body replaces these stores when blood glucose becomes available. It is important for the youth to realize that an adequate snack, probably containing protein as well as carbohydrate, may need to be eaten after prolonged exercise to avoid drops in blood glucose level, which may occur after the activity has stopped.

Hypoglycemia

The most common emergency in T1D is hypoglycemia. Hypoglycemia is defined for a child treated with insulin to be below 60 mg/dL, though some youth have symptoms at a higher number. Symptoms may occur when blood glucose levels are dropping rapidly even when the level is still in the normal range. Youth with diabetes should be instructed to wear medical alert identification at all times to ensure proper treatment of hypoglycemic reactions, which may render the child unable to communicate.

Treatment of mild hypoglycemia involves the 15-15 rule: Treat the low BG with 15 grams of fast-acting carbohydrate, wait 15 minutes, and then recheck the blood glucose. One gram of carbohydrate will bring the average adult's BG up ~3 mg/dL; younger children tend to be more sensitive, so 1 gram could bring their BG up 3–5 mg/dL. Because younger children are more sensitive to the fast-acting carbohydrates it is very easy to overtreat. Families are encouraged whenever possible to check the child's BG before treating so they can determine how much to treat. See **Table 15-11** for some hypoglycemia treatment options.

Illness

Illness in the child with diabetes always presents a challenge. Insulin must always be given and may need to be increased during these periods. The blood glucose should be monitored every 3 to 4 hours during illness. Parents need to know when to call the doctor for assistance in managing illness because certain symptoms, such as prolonged vomiting and fever, can lead to rapid dehydration and diabetic ketoacidosis. During a brief illness, the child's normal eating pattern should be maintained as much as possible, using foods that can be tolerated. Liquids also help to prevent dehydration, so the youth should have 6–8 oz. of fluids every 1–2 hours. If the child cannot tolerate food, it is important to replace some of the carbohydrate normally consumed with sugar-containing liquids that the body can easily use for energy. Some examples of easily tolerated liquids that contain 15 g of carbohydrate include 8 ounces of a regular carbonated beverage (with sugar), 4 ounces of fruit juice, a frozen fruit bar, or ½ cup of regular flavored gelatin. It is recommended to sip on room temperature liquids at a rate of about 15 g of carbohydrate per hour.

TABLE 15-11 Hypoglycemia Treatment for Youth with Diabetes

Item	5 Years of Age or Younger	6–10 Years of Age	Over 10 Years of Age
Amount recommended	5–10 g carbohydrate	10–15 g carbohydrate	15–20 g carbohydrate
Glucose tablets 4–5 g carb/each	1–2 tablets	2–3 tablets	3–4 tablets
Insta-glucose 24 g carb/tube	⅓–½ tube	½–⅔ tube	⅔–1 tube
Glutose 45 45 g/tube	⅙–¼ tube	¼–⅓ tube	⅓–½ tube
Regular soda or tonic water 1 fl oz = 3–4 g carb	2–3 fl oz	4–5 fl oz	5–6 fl oz
Table sugar 1 tsp = 4 g	2 tsp	3 tsp	4–5 tsp
Cake icing 1 tsp = 4 g	2 tsp	3 tsp	4–5 tsp
Orange juice ½ cup = 13–15 g carb	¼–½ cup	½–¾ cup	¾–1 cup
Apple juice ½ cup = 15 g carb	⅙–⅓ cup	⅓–½ cup	½–⅔ cup
Honey, maple, or Karo syrup 1 tsp = 4–5 g carb	2 tsp	3 tsp	4–5 tsp
LifeSavers 1 candy = 3 g	2–3 candies	4–5 candies	5–6 candies
Marshmallows, Mini (2 = 5 g) Large (1 = 5 g)	2–4 1–2	4–6 2–3	6–8 3–4
Raisins 1 Tbsp. = 7.5 g	1 Tbsp	1½–2 Tbsp	2½ Tbsp

Source: Reprinted with permission from Joslin Diabetes Center and Joslin Clinic. *Joslin's Guide to Managing Childhood Diabetes: A Family Teamwork Approach.* Boston, MA: Joslin Diabetes Center; 2009. Copyright © 2009 by Joslin Diabetes Center.

Conclusion

Nutrition management of the child with diabetes is one of the most important factors in attaining and maintaining metabolic control. Devising meal plans that provide flexibility while conforming to guidelines based on current research can be challenging for the dietitian. A thorough understanding of all the components of diabetes management will help the family adapt diabetes into their lifestyle instead of fitting their lifestyle into the diabetes. It is the role of the diabetes team members to empower the family and child with the knowledge to make healthy decisions in the management of diabetes.

Case Study

Nutrition Assessment

Patient history: JH is an 11-year-old male who's in the pediatrician's office this morning for a sick visit. Family just returned from Disneyworld on a 5-day vacation and the parents noticed while on vacation that JH was going to the bathroom often and had nocturnal enuresis the last two nights in Florida. They also reported that he had not been eating very well, had been drinking a lot of water, and had no energy. In the pediatrician's office it was noted that he had lost 5 lbs since his last well visit 4 months ago. His urine analysis was positive for glucose and negative for ketones. Pediatrician checked his BG, which was > 500 mg/dL, and referred the family to the local diabetes outpatient clinic on Friday afternoon before a 3-day holiday weekend for education. Additional lab work was done and it was determined JH was not in diabetic ketoacidosis (DKA) and it was not necessary to admit him to a hospital.

Family history: No family history for diabetes, auto-immune diseases, hyperlipidemia, hypertension, cardiac disease, or renal disease. Mom's family has history of breast cancer.

Nutrition history: JH has no food allergies or intolerances. He typically eats breakfast at home, brings his lunch to school, and eats his afternoon snack and dinner at home. JH and his parents provided a typical day dietary recall and daily schedule.

> **Breakfast:** 7–7:30 am on weekdays: 1½ cups cold cereal (Fruit Loops, Multigrain Cheerios), ½ cup 1% milk, and lately 6–8 oz. orange juice
>
> Weekends, 8–8:30 am: bagel (large), scrambled egg, and milk (6–8 oz.)
>
> **Morning snack at school:** 11 am: Kellogg's blueberry bar
>
> **Lunch:** 12 pm: usually brings—raisin bagel, grape juice pouch, raisins or a piece of fresh fruit (does not like school milk)
>
> School lunch: usually once a week: Domino's pizza (1 slice), juice box
>
> **Afternoon snack:** 3 pm: apple or grilled cheese sandwich or frozen pizza, water or milk to drink
>
> **Dinner:** 5:30–6:30 pm: ~3 oz chicken, ¼–½ cup green beans, ~¾–1 cup rice, pasta, or mashed potato. Mom tries to have 1–2 nights a week vegetarian, which is usually pasta ~1¼ cup with cheese, milk, or water, ½–¾ cup of chopped fruit or ice cream

Evening snack: usually none

Anthropometric Measurements

Weight:	30.2 kg
Height:	143.4 cm
BMI:	14.66
BMI Goal:	17.01
Other Labs:	A1C 10.8, Cholesterol 133, HDL 34, LDL 39, Trig 501

Insulin Plan

Basal insulin: 7 units at 9 am

Insulin-to-carbohydrate ratio (I:Carb): 1:30

Sensitivity factor (SF): 100

Target BG: 150 mg/dL

Nutrition Diagnosis/Problem

1. Weight loss
2. Food and nutrition-related knowledge deficit related to new diagnosis of type 1 diabetes

Nutrition Interventions

1. Comprehensive nutrition education
   a. Review advance carbohydrate counting.
   b. Review label reading.
      i. Weighing and measuring food
   c. Introduce calculating insulin doses using insulin-to-carbohydrate ratio.
2. Provide basic meal plan for weekend for family to use as a guide until they return at their next nutrition visit.
3. Reinforce education at following visit and build on the survival skills.
4. Goals of nutrition therapy:
   a. Advanced carb count
   b. Gain back lost weight and continue to grow along growth parameters
   c. Maintain blood glucose between 80 and 180 mg/dL
   d. Reinforce healthy eating

Questions for the Reader

1. What percentile on a growth chart are his weight, height, and BMI?
2. What are his estimated energy needs per day?
3. Write one PES statement.
4. What survival skills does the family have to learn to get them through the first weekend of diabetes?
5. Does the child need any further vitamin or mineral supplementation?

REFERENCES

1. Lockwood D, Frey ML, Gladish NA, Hiss RG. The biggest problem in diabetes. *Diabetes Educ.* 1986;12(1):30–33.
2. American Diabetes Association. Nutrition principles and recommendations in diabetes. *Diabetes Care.* 2004;27(Suppl 1):S36–S46.
3. Diabetes Control and Complications Trial Research Group. The effect of intensive treatment of diabetes on the development and progression of long-term complications in insulin-dependent diabetes mellitus. *N Engl J Med.* 1993;329(14):977–986.
4. Drash AL. The child, the adolescent, and the Diabetes Control and Complications Trial. *Diabetes Care.* 1993;16(11):1515–1516.
5. Franz MJ, Horton ES, Sr., Bantle JP, et al. Nutrition principles for the management of diabetes and related complications. *Diabetes Care.* 1994;17(5):490–518.
6. Butler DA, Lawlor MT. It takes a village: helping families live with diabetes. *Diabetes Spectrum.* 2004;17(1):26–31.
7. Laffel LM, Brackett J, Ho J, Anderson BJ. Changing the process of diabetes care improves metabolic outcomes and reduces hospitalizations. *Qual Manag Health Care.* 1998;6(4):53–62.
8. Dietary Guidelines Advisory Committee. Dietary guidelines for Americans 2005. 2005. http://www.health.gov/dietaryguidelines/dga2005/document/default.htm. Accessed August 12, 2010.
9. Bantle JP, Wylie-Rosett J, Albright AL, et al. Nutrition recommendations and interventions for diabetes: a position statement of the American Diabetes Association. *Diabetes Care.* 2008;31(Suppl 1):S61–S78.
10. Institute of Medicine of the National Academies. *Dietary Reference Intakes: The Essential Guide to Nutrient Requirements.* Washington, DC: National Academies Press; 2006.
11. Slavin JL. Position of the American Dietetic Association: health implications of dietary fiber. *J Am Diet Assoc.* 2008; 108(10):1716–1731.
12. Mayer-Davis EJ, Nichols M, Liese AD, et al. Dietary intake among youth with diabetes: the SEARCH for Diabetes in Youth Study. *J Am Diet Assoc.* 2006;106(5):689–697.
13. Sheard NF, Clark NG, Brand-Miller JC, et al. Dietary carbohydrate (amount and type) in the prevention and management of diabetes: a statement by the American Diabetes Association. *Diabetes Care.* 2004;27(9):2266–2271.
14. Jenkins DJ, Wolever TM, Taylor RH, et al. Glycemic index of foods: a physiological basis for carbohydrate exchange. *Am J Clin Nutr.* 1981;34(3):362–366.
15. Gillespie S. Implementing liberalized carbohydrate guidelines: nutrition free-for-all or a more rational approach to carbohydrate consumption? *Diabetes Spectrum.* 1996;9:165–167.
16. Schofield WN. Predicting basal metabolic rate, new standards and review of previous work. *Hum Nutr Clin Nutr.* 1985;39(Suppl 1):5–41.
17. Bantle JP, Swanson JE, Thomas W, Laine DC. Metabolic effects of dietary fructose in diabetic subjects. *Diabetes Care.* 1992; 15(11):1468–1476.
18. Position of the American Dietetic Association: use of nutritive and nonnutritive sweeteners. *J Am Diet Assoc.* 2004;104(2):255–275.
19. Payne ML, Craig WJ, Williams AC. Sorbitol is a possible risk factor for diarrhea in young children. *J Am Diet Assoc.* 1997; 97(5):532–534.
20. Butchko HH, Stargel WW, Comer CP, et al. Aspartame: review of safety. *Regul Toxicol Pharmacol.* 2002;35(2 Pt 2):S1–S93.
21. Wolf-Novak LC, Stegink LD, Brummel MC, et al. Aspartame ingestion with and without carbohydrate in phenylketonuric and normal subjects: effect on plasma concentrations of amino acids, glucose, and insulin. *Metabolism.* 1990;39(4):391–396.
22. Morrison AS, Buring JE. Artificial sweeteners and cancer of the lower urinary tract. *N Engl J Med.* 1980;302(10):537–541.
23. Chatsudthipong V, Muanprasat C. Stevioside and related compounds: therapeutic benefits beyond sweetness. *Pharmacol Ther.* 2009;121(1):41–54.
24. Marlett JA, McBurney MI, Slavin JL. Position of the American Dietetic Association: health implications of dietary fiber. *J Am Diet Assoc.* 2002;102(7):993–1000.
25. American Diabetes Association. Standards of medical care in diabetes—2010. *Diabetes Care.* 2010;33(Suppl 1):S11–S61.
26. National Cholesterol Education Program. *Report of the Expert Panel on Blood Cholesterol Levels in Children and Adolescents.* Bethesda, MD: U.S. Department of Health and Human Services; 1991. National Heart, Lung, and Blood Institute pub. no. 91-2732.
27. Virtanen SM, Ylonen K, Rasanen L, Ala-Venna E, Maenpaa J, Akerblom HK. Two year prospective dietary survey of newly diagnosed children with diabetes aged less than 6 years. *Arch Dis Child.* 2000;82(1):21–26.
28. U.S. Department of Agriculture, U.S. Department of Health and Human Services. Report of the Dietary Guidelines Advisory Committee on the Dietary Guidelines for Americans, 2000. Available at: http://www.health.gov/dietaryguidelines/dga2005/report/default.htm. Accessed August 12, 2010.
29. American Diabetes Association. Management of dyslipidemia in children and adolescents with diabetes. *Diabetes Care.* 2003;26(7):2194–2197.

30. Weng FL, Shults J, Leonard MB, Stallings VA, Zemel BS. Risk factors for low serum 25-hydroxyvitamin D concentrations in otherwise healthy children and adolescents. *Am J Clin Nutr* 2007; 86(1):150–158
31. Pozzilli P, Manfrini S, Crino A, et al. Low levels of 25-hydroxyvitamin D_3 and 1,25-dihydroxyvitamin D_3 in patients with newly diagnosed type 1 diabetes. *Horm Metab Res.* 2005;37(11):680–683.
32. Littorin B, Blom P, Scholin A, et al. Lower levels of plasma 25-hydroxyvitamin D among young adults at diagnosis of autoimmune type 1 diabetes compared with control subjects: results from the nationwide Diabetes Incidence Study in Sweden (DISS). *Diabetologia.* 2006;49(12):2847–2852.
33. Svoren BM, Volkening LK, Wood JR, Laffel LM. Significant vitamin D deficiency in youth with type 1 diabetes mellitus. *J Pediatr.* 2009;154(1):132–134.
34. Wagner CL, Greer FR. Prevention of rickets and vitamin D deficiency in infants, children, and adolescents. *Pediatrics* 2008; 122(5):1142–1152.
35. Forshee RA, Anderson PA, Storey ML. Changes in calcium intake and association with beverage consumption and demographics: comparing data from CSFII 1994–1996, 1998 and NHANES 1999–2002. *J Am Coll Nutr.* 2006;25(2):108–116.
36. National High Blood Pressure Education Program Working Group on High Blood Pressure in Children and Adolescents. The fourth report on the diagnosis, evaluation, and treatment of high blood pressure in children and adolescents. *Pediatrics.* 2004;114(Suppl 2):555–576.
37. Alaimo K, McDowell MA, Briefel RR, et al. Dietary intake of vitamins, minerals, and fiber of persons ages 2 months and over in the United States: Third National Health and Nutrition Examination Survey, phase 1, 1988–91. *Adv Data.* 1994;258:1–28.
38. Nakamura T, Higashi A, Nishiyama S, Fujimoto S, Matsuda I. Kinetics of zinc status in children with IDDM. *Diabetes Care.* 1991;14(7):553–557.
39. Mehta SN, Haynie DL, Higgins LA, et al. Emphasis on carbohydrates may negatively influence dietary patterns in youth with type 1 diabetes. *Diabetes Care.* 2009;32(12):2174–2176.
40. Rovner AJ, Nansel TR. Are children with type 1 diabetes consuming a healthful diet?: a review of the current evidence and strategies for dietary change. *Diabetes Educ.* 2009;35(1):97–107.
41. Madison LL, Lochner A, Wulff J. Ethanol-induced hypoglycemia. II. Mechanism of suppression of hepatic gluconeogenesis. *Diabetes.* 1967;16(4):252–258.
42. Arky RA. Current principles of dietary therapy of diabetes mellitus. *Med Clin North Am.* 1978;62(4):655–662.
43. Grinvalsky M, Nathan DM. Diets for insulin pump and multiple daily injection therapy. *Diabetes Care.* 1983;6(3):241–244.
44. Wheeler ML, Daly A, Evert A, et al. *Choose Your Foods: Exchange Lists for Diabetes*, sixth edition, 2008: description and guidelines for use. *J Am Diet Assoc.* 2008;5(108):883–888.
45. Tamborlane WV, Sherwin RS, Genel M, Felig P. Outpatient treatment of juvenile-onset diabetes with a preprogrammed portable subcutaneous insulin infusion system. *Am J Med.* 1980;68(2):190–196.
46. Tamborlane WV, Sherwin RS, Koivisto V, Hendler R, Genel M, Felig P. Normalization of the growth hormone and catecholamine response to exercise in juvenile-onset diabetic subjects treated with a portable insulin infusion pump. *Diabetes.* 1979;28(8):785–788.
47. Steindel BS, Roe TR, Costin G, Carlson M, Kaufman FR. Continuous subcutaneous insulin infusion (CSII) in children and adolescents with chronic poorly controlled type 1 diabetes mellitus. *Diabetes Res Clin Pract.* 1995;27(3):199–204.
48. Anderson BJ. Diabetes and adaptations in family systems. In: Holmes C, ed. *Neuropsychology and Behavioral Aspects of Diabetes.* New York: Springer-Verlag; 1990:85–101.
49. Silverstein J, Klingensmith G, Copeland K, et al. Care of children and adolescents with type 1 diabetes: a statement of the American Diabetes Association. *Diabetes Care.* 2005;28(1):186–212.
50. Couper JJ, Steele C, Beresford S, et al. Lack of association between duration of breast-feeding or introduction of cow's milk and development of islet autoimmunity. *Diabetes.* 1999;48(11):2145–2149.
51. Kimpimaki T, Erkkola M, Korhonen S, et al. Short-term exclusive breastfeeding predisposes young children with increased genetic risk of type I diabetes to progressive beta-cell autoimmunity. *Diabetologia.* 2001;44(1):63–69.
52. American Diabetes Association. Diabetes care in the school and day care setting. *Diabetes Care.* 2010;33(Suppl 1):S70-S74.
53. Colton P, Rodin G, Berenstal R, Parkin C. Eating disorders and diabetes: introduction and overview. *Diabetes Spectrum.* 2009;22(3):138–142.
54. Criego A, Crow S, Goebel-Fabbri AE, Kendall D, Parkin C. Eating disorders and diabetes: screening and detection. *Diabetes Spectrum.* 2009;22(3):143–146.
55. Dabelea D, Bell RA, D'Agostino RB, Jr., et al. Incidence of diabetes in youth in the United States. *JAMA.* 2007;297(24):2716–2724.
56. Fagot-Campagna A, Pettitt DJ, Engelgau MM, et al. Type 2 diabetes among North American children and adolescents: an epidemiologic review and a public health perspective. *J Pediatr.* 2000;136(5):664–672.
57. American Diabetes Association. The prevention or delay of type 2 diabetes. *Diabetes Care.* 2002;25(4):742–749.
58. Knowler WC, Barrett-Connor E, Fowler SE, et al. Reduction in the incidence of type 2 diabetes with lifestyle intervention or metformin. *N Engl J Med.* 2002;346(6):393–403.
59. American Diabetes Association. Gestational diabetes mellitus. *Diabetes Care.* 2004;27(Suppl 1):S88–S90.
60. Laffel LMB, Butler DA, Higgins LA, Lawlor MT, Pasquarello CA, eds. *Joslin's Guide to Managing Childhood Diabetes: A Family Teamwork Approach.* Boston, MA: Joslin Diabetes Center; 2009.
61. Lawlor MT, Anderson B, Laffel L. *Blood Sugar Monitoring Owner's Manual Booklet.* Boston, MA: Joslin Diabetes Center; 2007.

HIV and AIDS

Jill Rockwell

Overview

The first cases of acquired immune deficiency syndrome (AIDS) were reported in a small cohort of gay men in 1981.[1] Since that time, it is estimated that 65 million people worldwide have been infected with the human immunodeficiency virus (HIV, the virus that causes AIDS) and nearly 25 million people have died from AIDS.[2] According to the World Health Organization, approximately 33.4 million people worldwide were living with HIV in 2008, with 2.7 million of those people newly diagnosed with HIV.[3] AIDS has become a leading cause of death, and in some African countries it is actually lowering the life expectancy by as much as 15 years.[2,4,5]

HIV is a sexually transmitted and blood-borne disease. Modes of transmission include exposure to blood and body fluids such as sexual contact, breastfeeding, sharing of contaminated needles, and transmission from mother to child during the perinatal period or during labor and delivery. The greatest impact of the AIDS epidemic is among men who have sex with men (MSM); racial and ethnic minorities, with a growing number of infected minority women; and cases attributed to heterosexual transmission.[4] Nearly all transfusion-associated cases occurred prior to screening of the blood supply in 1985.[4]

The first pediatric cases of HIV were described in 1982.[6] The majority of pediatric cases were associated with perinatal transmission, which peaked in 1992 (901 cases) and sharply declined after 1994 with the advent of zidovudine therapy protocols to prevent/reduce perinatal transmission. From 1985 to 1999, AIDS cases among children declined 81%.[4] In 2004, children less than 19 years accounted for approximately 1820 cases or 1.2% of the cases of AIDS in the United States, which is a decrease of about 2000 cases from 2000.[7]

The prognosis of children with HIV and AIDS has improved tremendously in much of the developed world. Once a fatal disease, HIV can now be described as a chronic, manageable disease. Where treatment is available and affordable, most children are maintaining healthy states and thriving. Many children are reaching adulthood in a state of health, allowing them to attend college and gain employment.

The medical, nutritional, and social implications of pediatric HIV and AIDS are numerous and complex. Effective management of the disease requires a coordinated and comprehensive approach that involves early diagnosis and aggressive medical, nutritional, and psychosocial intervention. This chapter gives a brief overview of pediatric HIV infection and AIDS and an in-depth description of the goals and strategies of nutritional management of the pediatric patient with HIV infection and AIDS.

Immune Function and HIV/AIDS

HIV is a retrovirus that primarily infects cells of the immune system, a system composed of lymphocytes and other white blood cells. The lymphocytes are divided into two types, known as T-cells and B-cells. T-cells are responsible for cellular immunity or fighting off invading antigens; B-cells are responsible for humoral immunity or antibody (immunoglobulin) production. T-cells express different antigens; HIV targets T-cells expressing the CD4 antigen (referred to as CD4 cells). HIV integrates itself into the host CD4 cell's DNA and then replicates itself, creating additional virus that ultimately causes the immune cell's destruction and death, which leads to a weakened immune system without enough immune cells to fight infections.[8]

AIDS is an advanced disease caused by acquisition of the human immunodeficiency virus (HIV-1 or HIV-2) and subsequent destruction of the immune system. This decrease in cellular immunity impairs the host's ability to fight off infection and results in the host acquiring opportunistic infections and malignancies. Untreated HIV infection allows for the continued destruction of CD4 cells, resulting in a progression of HIV disease. When the immune system deteriorates to specified and measurable levels (described later in this chapter), the disease is termed acquired immune deficiency syndrome or AIDS.

Definitions of AIDS Surveillance of Children

Individuals with HIV disease range from healthy to seriously ill. The term *AIDS* is employed by the Centers for Disease Control and Prevention (CDC) to refer to those individuals who typically display specific "indicator" diseases as a result of HIV infection.[9]

As shown in **Table 16-1**, the current CDC definition criteria for children less than 13 years of age are based on clinical disease conditions/diagnoses and laboratory criteria. Only those children who meet the strict diagnostic criteria are classified as having AIDS. The classification categories include a letter designation (i.e., N, A, B, C) indicative of the presence of clinical conditions, and a number designation indicative of immune status, which is based on CD4 T-cell counts and the CD4 percentage of total lymphocytes. The immune categories (see **Table 16-2**) are further delineated by age groups, because CD4 T-cell norms differ according to age, usually being higher in younger children at baseline.[9]

As the immune system declines, the likelihood of symptomatic HIV infection increases. The AIDS diagnosis is reserved for those patients in category C: severely symptomatic. Today, the child carrying a diagnosis of AIDS may

TABLE 16-1 Clinical Manifestations/Categories for Children with HIV Infection and AIDS

Category N: Not Symptomatic Children who have no signs or symptoms considered to be the result of HIV infection or who have only one of the conditions listed in Category A.
Category A: Mildly Symptomatic Children with two or more of the conditions listed below but none of the conditions listed in Categories B and C. • Lymphadenopathy ($\geq$ 0.5 cm at more than two sites; bilateral = one site) • Hepatomegaly • Splenomegaly • Dermatitis • Parotitis • Recurrent or persistent upper respiratory infection, sinusitis, or otitis media
Category B: Moderately Symptomatic Children who have symptomatic conditions other than those listed for Category A or C that are attributed to HIV infection. Examples of conditions in clinical Category B include but are not limited to: • Anemia ($<$ 8 g/dL), neutropenia ($<$ 1000/mm^3), or thrombocytopenia ($<$ 100,000/mm^3) persisting $\geq$ 30 days • Bacterial meningitis, pneumonia, or sepsis (single episode) • Candidiasis, oropharyngeal (thrush), persisting $>$ 2 months in children over 6 months of age • Cardiomyopathy • Cytomegalovirus infection, with onset before 1 month of age • Diarrhea, recurrent or chronic • Hepatitis • Herpes simplex virus (HSV) stomatitis, recurrent (more than two episodes within 1 year) • HSV bronchitis, pneumonitis, or esophagitis with onset before 1 month of age • Herpes zoster (shingles) involving at least two distinct episodes or more than one dermatome • Leiomyosarcoma • Lymphoid interstitial pneumonia (LIP) or pulmonary lymphoid hyperplasia complex • Nephropathy • Nocardiosis • Persistent fever (lasting $>$ 1 month) • Toxoplasmosis, onset before 1 month of age • Varicella, disseminated (complicated chickenpox)
Category C: Severely Symptomatic Children who have any condition listed in the 1987 surveillance case definition for acquired immune deficiency syndrome, with the exception of LIP.

Source: Data from Centers for Disease Control and Prevention. Revised classification system for human immunodeficiency virus infection in children less than 13 years of age. *MMWR.* 1994;43(RR-12):1–10.

TABLE 16-2 Immunologic Categories Based on Age-Specific CD4+ T-Cell Counts and Percentage of Total Lymphocytes

Immunologic Category	< 12 Months μL (%)	1–5 Years μL (%)	6–12 Years μL(%)
1: No evidence of suppression	≥ 1500 (≥ 25)	≥ 1000 (≥ 25)	≥ 500 (≥ 25)
2: Evidence of moderate suppression	750–1499 (15–24)	500–999 (15–24)	200–499 (15–24)
3: Severe suppression	< 750 (<15)	< 500 (< 15)	< 200 (< 15)

Source: Data from Centers for Disease Control and Prevention. Revised classification system for human immunodeficiency virus infection in children less than 13 years of age. *MMWR*. 1994;43(RR-12):1–10.

be in significantly better health than in the days when treatment was unavailable. An undiagnosed infant may present to the medical system with *Pneumocystis carinii* pneumonia (PCP), an AIDS-defining illness. With the advent of medical therapies, that same child may have immune reconstitution (recovery of the CD4 T-cell number and percentage), which places the child in category 1 (no immune suppression), and remain quite healthy. The clinical category provides a snapshot for categorizing the historical "sickest" that the child has been. The immune category is a reflection of the child's current immune status.

Diagnosis

Ideally, pregnant women are screened for HIV infection as part of routine prenatal care. This screening provides for antenatal, peripartal, and neonatal HIV treatment that significantly decreases the rate of perinatal transmission to infants (approximately 1–4% versus 15–30% transmission without treatment).[10]

Infants are screened and diagnosed with laboratory testing that can usually confirm or exclude infection by 6 months of age. The DNA and RNA polymerase chain reaction (PCR) tests are used to determine an infant's HIV infection status. Children older than 18 months can be tested using the enzyme-linked immunosorbent assay (ELISA) and Western Immunoblotting (Western Blot) methods that screen for the presence of antibodies to HIV. This is the same test utilized for adult HIV testing. The ELISA and Western Blot cannot be used on children younger than 18 months because they give false positive readings by detecting maternal antibody that is passed to the infant in utero.[11] There should be a high index of suspicion when the mother's HIV status is unknown. Infants born to high-risk mothers or with symptoms as described in the clinical categories for children with HIV should be tested for HIV infection.

Clinical Manifestations of HIV Infection and AIDS

Children with HIV infection display a wide array of clinical features. Some untreated children have rapid disease progression whereas other children appear quite healthy and present after many years of immune decline. Presenting symptoms include lymphadenopathy, hepatosplenomegaly, failure to thrive, diarrhea, and multiple bacterial infections. As the clinical course progresses, the child may have severe cases of common childhood infections such as varicella (chicken pox), herpes simplex, and cytomegalovirus. With profound immunosuppression, severe infections such as disseminated mycobacterium avium complex (MAC/MAI), cryptococcal meningitis, and esophageal candidiasis may occur. Many of these infections and/or conditions are found in the description of the clinical categories as previously described in Table 16-1.[9,11]

In untreated children or children with advanced HIV disease or AIDS, conditions such as oral or esophageal candidiasis, diarrhea, severe bacterial infections, MAI, tuberculosis (both pulmonary and extrapulmonary), and encephalopathy can severely affect enteral intake and/or absorption of nutrients. Failure to thrive is a common issue in the untreated child, compounding the disease effects on the immune system.[9,11]

HIV treatment can also negatively impact the child's nutritional intake. Frequent doctor visits, blood draws, tests, and hospitalizations may result in emotional upset and decreased appetite. Medication regimens used to treat HIV infection and prophylactic medications used to prevent opportunistic infections may consist of several pills taken two to three times per day and may have gastrointestinal side effects such as nausea, vomiting, indigestion, and diarrhea. Some of the more severe medication side effects that can severely compromise intake include anemia, pancreatitis, and liver steatosis.[11]

Medications

Highly active antiretroviral therapy (HAART) is the hallmark of current treatment for HIV infection. HAART consists minimally of a three-drug regimen utilizing drugs from two different HIV drug classes. As of February 2009, there were 25 drugs available for treatment of HIV infection, although only 17 had approved pediatric indications.[11]

TABLE 16-3 Antiretrovirals and Common Side Effects (Nutritional Implications)

Class	Drug/Formulation	Side Effects
NRTI/NtRTI	Zidovudine (ZVD/AZT) capsule/liquid/tablets	Anemia, granulocytopenia, malaise, headache, nausea, vomiting, anorexia, myopathy, myositis, fat redistribution, lactic acidosis, liver toxicity
	Didanosine (ddl) capsule/liquid	Diarrhea, abdominal pain, nausea, vomiting, peripheral neuropathy, electrolyte abnormalities, hyperuricemia
	Lamivudine (3TC) tablet/liquid	Headache, fatigue, nausea, decreased appetite, diarrhea, skin rash, abdominal pain, pancreatitis, peripheral neuropathy, anemia, fat redistribution, lactic acidosis, hepatic steatosis
	Stavudine (d4T) capsule/liquid	Headache, GI disturbances, skin rashes, pancreatitis, peripheral neuropathy, lipodystrophy/lipoatrophy, lactic acidosis, hepatic steatosis
	Abacavir (ABC) tablet/liquid	Potentially lethal hypersensitivity reaction, nausea, vomiting, diarrhea, fever, rash, anorexia, headache
	Emtricitabine (FTC) capsule	Headache, insomnia, diarrhea, nausea, rash, skin discoloration, neutropenia, lactic acidosis, hepatic steatosis
	Tenofovir (TDF) tablet	Nausea, diarrhea, vomiting, flatulence, lactic acidosis, hepatic steatosis
NNRTI	Nevirapine (NVP) tablet/liquid	Skin rash, fever, nausea, headache, abnormal transaminase levels, hepatotoxicity
	Efavirenz (EFV) capsule/tablet	Skin rash, increased transaminase levels, central nervous system effects
	Etravirine (ETR) tablets	Nausea, rash, hypersensitivity reaction
PI	Nelfinavir (NFV) tablet/liquid	Diarrhea, asthenia, abdominal pain, rash, lipid abnormalities, fat redistribution
	Ritonavir (RTV) capsule/liquid	Nausea, vomiting, diarrhea, headache, abdominal pain, anorexia, circumoral paresthesias, lipid abnormalities, fat redistribution
	Lopinavir/ritonavir (LPV/RTV) tablet/liquid	Diarrhea, headache, asthenia, nausea, vomiting, rash, fat redistribution, lipid abnormalities
	Indinavir (IDV) capsule	Nausea, abdominal pain, headache, metallic taste, dizziness, hyperbilirubinemia, pruritis, rash, nephrolithiasis, fat redistribution
	Saquinavir (SQV) capsule/tablet	Diarrhea, abdominal discomfort, headache, nausea, paresthesias, skin rash, fat redistribution, lipid abnormalities
	Atazanavir (ATV) capsule	Elevation of indirect bili, jaundice, headache, fever, arthralgia, depression, insomnia, dizziness, nausea, vomiting, diarrhea, paresthesias, prolongation of PR interval (EKG changes)
	Fosamprenavir (f-APV) tablet/liquid	Vomiting, nausea, diarrhea, headache, perioral parasthesias, rash, lipid abnormalities, fat redistribution, neutropenia
	Darunavir (DRV) tablets	Diarrhea, nausea, vomiting, abdominal pain, headache, fatigue, skin rash, lipid abnormalities
	Tipranavir (TPV) capsule, liquid	Diarrhea, nausea, fatigue, headache, rash, vomiting, lipid abnormalities, fat redistribution
Entry inhibitor	Maraviroc (MVC) tablet	Cough, fever, upper respiratory tract infections, rash, musculoskeletal symptoms, abdominal pain, dizziness
Fusion inhibitor	Enfuvirtide (T-20) injection	Local injection site reactions
Integrase inhibitor	Raltegravir (RGV) tablet	Nausea, headache, dizziness, diarrhea, fatigue, itching, abdominal pain, vomiting

Source: Adapted from Working Group on Antiretroviral Therapy and Medical Management of HIV-Infected Children. Guidelines for the use of antiretroviral agents in pediatric HIV infection. February 23, 2009; 1–139. Available at: http://aidsinfo.nih.gov/ContentFiles/PediatricGuidelines.pdf. Accessed February 21, 2010.

Antiretroviral drug classes include six major categories, with the following five used in pediatrics:[11]

- Nucleoside/nucleotide analogue reverse transcriptase inhibitors (NRTIs/NtRTIs)
- Non-nucleoside analogue reverse transcriptase inhibitors (NNRTIs)
- Protease inhibitors (PIs)
- Entry inhibitors
- Integrase inhibitors

These drugs work on specific areas of the cell targeted by HIV and must be taken consistently and in combination to be effective. Efficacy of drug therapies is measured by clinical assessment, rebound, and/or maintenance of the CD4+ lymphocyte counts, and on the amount of HIV virus in the blood, commonly referred to as viral load. Effective medication therapy decreases the patient's viral load, allowing the CD4 cell counts to increase and be maintained. Common drug combinations include a protease inhibitor and two drugs from the NRTI class, NNRTI and two drugs from the NRTI class, or three NRTI drugs.[11] All of the drugs have significant side effects (see **Table 16-3**). Many are available in liquid and tablet/capsule formulation. The fusion inhibitors are injectable only. Rarely, patients may be on suboptimal therapy such as one or two drugs from the same class. This can be seen with patients with medication-related side effects or with poor adherence while medical, behavioral, psychiatric, and/or psychosocial interventions can be instituted. Monotherapy (the use of one drug) is utilized with neonates. Zidovudine (AZT/ZDV) is administered to the mother during labor and delivery and then to the neonate for 6 weeks to decrease the risk of perinatal transmission.

In addition to HAART, the pediatric patient may be taking medications regularly for prophylaxis or prevention of opportunistic infections. Many of the drugs used to treat HIV and prevent opportunistic infection have significant side effects and interactions. Foods, herbal treatments, and home remedies can significantly affect drug levels, leading to suboptimal drug levels or severe side effects. Although little research exists regarding pediatric HIV and the use of herbal treatments, thorough assessment of nutritional adjuncts is essential to optimize medical therapy.

Nutritional Implications

The growth and cellular immune function of HIV-infected children is impacted by their nutritional status. The majority of children infected with HIV will experience nutritional deficits during the course of their illness.[12] Pre-HAART nutritional issues affecting growth deficits and malnutrition include impaired absorption,[13] decreased dietary intake,[14] increased nutrient requirements, and the disease itself (see **Table 16-4**). Malnutrition has a deleterious effect on immune function, compromising the ability to produce effective antibodies; thus, it increases risks of life-threatening infections.[15]

In the current era of HIV and HAART, children in developed countries are living longer with fewer opportunistic infections. When seen, malnutrition is more likely associated with drug-resistant virus, noncompliance with therapy, and/or end-stage viral disease. Nutritional issues have become further complicated by potent drug therapies and possibly by the consequences of living longer with the disease itself. Some of the clinical and metabolic complications seen in adult HIV populations are now being seen in children. These include body fat redistribution, altered serum lipid levels, insulin resistance, and decreased bone mineral density.

Growth and Body Composition

Research results have demonstrated a variety of growth patterns in HIV-infected children, reflecting a broad spectrum of clinical course and disease activity. A large study in the United States reported that both HIV-positive and -negative children born to HIV-infected mothers are small at birth.[15] No significant differences in birth weights and lengths between HIV-infected and uninfected children born to these infected mothers were identified.[16] However, in this and a similar European study, infancy[16] and childhood[17] weights and heights were significantly lower in the HIV-infected group, and these differences persisted and increased with age. Several other studies of HIV-positive children reflect disturbed growth patterns including acute wasting, slow weight gain, and chronic slow linear growth.[14,18]

Growth can be an important prognostic indicator for children with HIV.[19–21] In particular, height velocity is an independent predictor of survival when controlling for age, viral load, and CD4+ count.[21] The presence of wasting syndrome classifies a child in clinical category C of the CDC criteria discussed earlier, which indicates a child is severely symptomatic.[11] With this in mind, maintenance of normal growth is taking on increased importance. Because

TABLE 16-4 Causes of Malnutrition

Causes	Etiology
Decreased intake	Nausea, anorexia, oral ulceration, esophagitis, chewing difficulties, pain, dementia, depression
Increased losses	Lactose intolerance, pancreatic insufficiency, malabsorption
Increased requirements	Fever, opportunistic infections, metabolic abnormalities
Psychosocial barriers	Inadequate access to food, unsafe food practices, caretaker substance abuse

children with HIV are living longer, studies have looked at antiretroviral therapy and its effects on growth. These data require careful consideration. Each study examines different patient populations with different drug treatment experience and various stages of the disease. For example, children receiving protease inhibitor–containing regimens experienced a wide spectrum of effects on growth ranging from weight gain,[22] improved height,[23] significantly improved height,[24] and small improvement in weight and height[25,26] to decline in weight and height.[27] Despite this wide range of findings, collectively these studies show a trend toward improved growth on PI-containing regimens. Virologic response to HAART may be a key factor to positive effect on weight and height.[28]

Growth failure can occur early in life and continues over time. A study comparing children infected with HIV to those exposed but not infected found HIV-infected children weighed 0.7 kg less and measured 2.2 cm shorter at 18 months than those exposed to the virus but not infected.[29] A study done in Europe compared growth in HIV-infected children to uninfected children over the first 10 years of life. At 10 years of age, children infected with HIV were found to weigh 7 kg less and be 7.5 cm shorter than the uninfected children. Children who received effective antiretroviral therapy were found to have better growth than those who received monotherapy.[30]

Insulin-like growth factor-1 (IGF-1) levels have been found to be low in children with HIV who have impaired growth. Effective antiretroviral therapy, leading to an increase in the percentage of lymphocytes that are CD4 cells (CD4%), appears to have an association with an improvement in IGF-1. One study found IGF-1 levels improved with initiation or change in antiretroviral medication regimens. An increase in lean body mass was associated with normalization of IGF-1 levels. Further research needs to be conducted to examine IGF-1 as a potential therapy to improve lean body mass in children with HIV.[31]

Lipodystrophy syndrome in HIV-positive adults is characterized by several changes in body composition. Classifications of lipodystrophy include lipoatrophy or arm, leg, buttock, and/or facial wasting; lipohypertrophy or truncal obesity; or mixed lipodystrophy including a combination of peripheral wasting and truncal obesity. In addition, affected individuals may exhibit metabolic complications including hypercholesterolemia, hyperlipidemia, and/or insulin resistance. Many, but not all, of these features have recently been described in children[32–37] using various methods of diagnosis including DXA (dual energy x-ray absorptiometry), magnetic resonance imaging (MRI),[33] and clinical assessment.[32] Although the causes of these abnormalities are not entirely clear, they seem to be at least in part due to drug therapies, particularly those containing protease inhibitors. Development of symptoms may be related to duration of HAART therapy[33] and increasing doses of medications.[32] Chemical abnormalities including high cholesterol and triglycerides have been described in children with or without clinical features of lipodystrophy,[36] and thus serial anthropometry, clinical assessment, and laboratory values can provide valuable information about a child trending toward lipodystrophy.

Bone Density

HIV-infected adults have increased rates of osteoporosis and osteopenia that may also be a side effect of HAART therapy. Lower bone mineral densities have also been found in HIV-positive children compared to healthy age-matched controls;[38–40] however, the relationship to drug therapy is still unclear. One study showed significantly lower bone mineral density among children on HAART with lipodystrophy compared to untreated HIV-positive children. A third group of HAART-treated children without lipodystrophy fell somewhere in between these two groups.[38] In contrast, others found that length of time on antiretroviral therapy and PI use were not significant factors in differences in bone mineral density between HIV-positive children and healthy controls.[39] Bone mineral density is best measured by DXA; however, it is too expensive and not widely available for routine use. Given the existing data just highlighted and the crucial time during childhood of laying down the majority of bone mass, thoughtful consideration should be given to dietary prevention of osteopenia and osteoporosis.

Caloric Requirements

Caloric requirements of HIV-infected children are not completely known. Although children with HIV were once thought to have an increased resting metabolic rate caused by viral infection, subsequent research suggests that clinically stable children have normal caloric needs.[41] Despite this fact, the benefit of caloric intake beyond the recommended dietary allowance (RDA) has been demonstrated. In a group of HIV-positive children consuming at least the RDA for calories,[14] children with normal growth patterns were shown to take in significantly more calories than those with poor growth. The resting energy expenditure (REE) and total energy expenditure (TEE) of both of these groups was similar.[17] It has been suggested to increase caloric intake by 50–100% over requirements for healthy children in HIV-positive children with weight loss.[42] Supplemental gastrostomy tube feeding restores weight gain but not subsequent height and lean body mass gains.[43,44] Therefore, lower caloric intake among growth failure/HIV-positive children is suggested as only one piece of the puzzle.[14] Weight loss in HIV-positive children can be linked to inadequate intake, increased requirements imposed by opportunistic infections, or malabsorptive losses.[45] Caloric requirements should be calculated according to additional needs subsequent to stress, fever, increased respiratory needs, and careful monitoring of serial growth measures.

Nutritional Intervention

The most appropriate nutrition plan for HIV-infected children is tailored to their clinical manifestations, growth, dietary history, gastrointestinal function, and social situation (**Table 16-5**). The child's caretakers should receive ongoing education to optimize growth, ensure access to food, promote safe food handling, and accommodate any necessary dietary modifications. Because of the risk of micronutrient deficiency in the HIV-infected child, it is prudent to consider a complete multivitamin/mineral supplement that provides one to two times the dietary reference intakes (DRIs).[46,47] Emerging data on risk of low bone mineral density suggest that attention should be given to ensure adequacy of calcium and vitamin D in the diet.

If an HIV-infected child is exhibiting slow growth, prescribing a high-calorie, high-protein, nutrient-dense diet early on is indicated. If enhancement of the typical diet is not sufficient to promote desired growth, oral nutritional supplementation, including shakes and commercial formulas, should be considered. When oral measures alone cannot achieve the nutritional goals, enteral tube supplementation should be administered. Gastrostomy (g) tubes are beneficial in providing both complete and supplemental feedings, as well as medication administration. Children with anorexia, neurological impairment, swallowing difficulty, or those taking a significant number of pills may benefit from a g-tube.

Nocturnal tube feedings are often preferred to daytime feedings because they can allow the child to eat normally during the day without interrupting daily activities. Formula selection should be determined based on the child's need for any modification from a polymeric formula. This may include fiber-containing, lactose-free, or more elemental formulas for those patients with enteropathy. Studies show improvements in weight gain (primarily as increased fat mass) in response to the increased caloric provisions, and suggest improvements in morbidity and mortality as a result of such nutritional rehabilitation.[44]

Parenteral nutrition (PN), despite its associated infection risks, may be warranted if hydration, electrolyte balance, or weight gain cannot be achieved through enteral means. Candidates for PN include children with intractable diarrhea with accompanying weight loss or severe recurrent or chronic pancreatic or biliary tract dysfunction.[10,44] For children experiencing oroesophageal ulcers, soreness, or inflammation, care should be given to selecting foods that are soft and nutrient dense, and not highly spiced or acidic. Drug side effects (see Table 16-3) may lead to anorexia, nausea/vomiting, epigastric distress, diarrhea, and/or glossitis and could result in a child's refusal to eat. Appetite stimulants such as megestrol acetate (Megace) increase oral intake in some anorectic children. Although Megace was associated with improvements in weight gain and increased fat mass, concurrent improvements in linear growth were not appreciated. In addition, weight-gain effects may not be sustained once the medication is discontinued.[48,49]

Dysphagia, developmental delay, and poor gross motor control secondary to neurologic complications associated with HIV may also contribute to poor intake. Neurologically impaired children should be closely monitored to ensure adequate intake and to prevent aspiration.

TABLE 16-5 Nutritional Evaluation and Management of the HIV-Infected Child

Nutritional Assessment

Dietary intake and nutrient analysis
- 24-hour diet recall or 3-day food diary
- Access to food
- Stability of home environment/caretakers

Anthropometry and body composition measurements
- Four-site skinfolds (if possible)
- Serial height (length), weight, and head circumference (until 36 months)
  - Z-scores (particularly with measurements $<$ 3rd percentile)
  - BMI and BMI percentage

Biochemical evaluation
- Albumin, lipid profile (fasting, if possible), fasting glucose/insulin, iron, other vitamin/mineral levels as indicated by degree of malnutrition and malabsorption

Drug–nutrient interactions
- Amprenavir: Avoid excess vitamin E supplementation because it contains ~100 IU/pill.

Nutritional Intervention

Diet modifications and education (based on growth, gastrointestinal function, and lipid abnormalities)
- Nutrient-dense with supplements as needed to optimize growth
- Lactose-free (if evidence of diarrhea/malabsorption)
- High fiber or low fiber
- Heart healthy, balanced with adequate calories for growth

Food safety assessment and counseling

Vitamin and mineral supplementation
- Multivitamin: 1 to 2 times RDA/DRI depending on diet
- Calcium and vitamin D supplement to achieve at least DRI

Tube feedings/total parenteral nutrition (when enteral diet alone fails)

Conclusion

Optimal nutritional status has been associated with improvements in immune function and morbidity in the HIV-infected child. Close nutrition surveillance and intervention results in improved clinical outcome and quality of life. Malnutrition in HIV-infected children is a serious complication. Early and aggressive nutritional support is indicated in all children infected with HIV and should include nutrient-dense oral feedings and enteral and parenteral supplementation when necessary. Anthropometric and body composition changes should be serially monitored, and biochemical parameters should be assessed so that necessary nutrition intervention can occur. These measures can provide crucial information regarding tendency towards some of the complications seen with HIV and HAART therapy such as fat redistribution, hyperlipidemias, and poor bone health. Ongoing research continues to augment the understanding of interrelationships between nutrition and HIV and will elucidate more definitive nutrition intervention strategies.

Case Study

Nutrition Assessment

Patient history: 15-year-old female recently diagnosed with HIV and started on HAART therapy. She has no past medical history.

Food/nutrition-related history: She had a good appetite and intake until HAART therapy was started. She has been experiencing nausea and anorexia since starting on HAART therapy and estimates she has lost 10 pounds over the past 3 weeks. Her usual weight is 105 pounds. She consumed three meals and one or two snacks per day prior to starting HAART therapy. She reports she has been unable to eat breakfast in the morning due to nausea and often does not eat lunch at school. Her symptoms usually improve in the afternoon and she is able to eat dinner with her family. She is not currently taking any vitamin, mineral, or herbal supplements.

Anthropometric Measurements

Weight: 43 kg (10th percentile)
Height: 162 cm (50th percentile)
BMI: 16.4 kg/m^2 (5th percentile)

Medications: Efavirenz, lamivudine, zidovudine

Labs: CD4 250 cells/mm^3

Diet order: High calorie, high protein

Nutrition Diagnoses

Based on the information provided above, a nutritional problem or diagnosis is made. Inadequate oral food/beverage intake.

Intervention Goals

Weight gain back to usual body weight of 105 pounds and improved oral intake to minimum three meals and two snacks per day.

Nutrition Interventions

Initial/brief nutrition education:
- Counsel to consume three meals and two snacks daily.
- Review sources of nutrient-dense foods.
- Review nutrition interventions for nausea.

Vitamin/mineral supplement:
- Start multivitamin to meet one to two times RDA/DRI for age.

Medical food supplements:
- Start one to two cans adult oral supplement to promote weight gain.

Monitoring and Evaluation

- **Weight change:** Monitor for improvement back to usual weight of 105 pounds.
- **Meal/snack pattern:** Goal of minimum three meals and two snacks per day.

Questions for the Reader

1. What are her estimated energy needs?
2. What are her estimated protein needs?
3. Write at least one PES statement.
4. What will you do during the follow-up visit 2 months later:
   a. If the teenager has not gained weight since her last visit?
   b. If the teenager develops diarrhea?

REFERENCES

1. Centers for Disease Control and Prevention. Pneumocystis pneumonia—Los Angeles. *MMWR*. 1981;30:250–252.
2. Centers for Disease Control and Prevention. The global HIV/AIDS pandemic. *MMWR*. 2006;55:841–844.
3. UNAIDS, World Health Organization. 09 AIDS Epidemic Update.2009. 1–100. Available at: http://data.unaids.org/pub/Report/2009/JC1700_Epi_Update_2009_en.pdf. Accessed August 12, 2010.
4. Centers for Disease Control and Prevention. HIV/AIDS—United States, 1981–2000. *MMWR*. 2001;50: 430–433.
5. Piot P, Bartos M, Ghys PD, Walker N, Schwartlander B. The global impact of HIV/AIDS. *Nature*. 2001;410:968–973.
6. Centers for Disease Control and Prevention. Unexplained immunodeficiency and opportunistic infections in infants—New York, New Jersey, California. *MMWR*. 1982;31(49):665–667.
7. Centers for Disease Control and Prevention. Epidemiology of HIV/AIDS—United States, 1981–2005. *MMWR*. 2006;55:589–592.
8. Weiss RA. Gulliver's travels in HIV land. *Nature*. 2001;410:963–967.
9. Centers for Disease Control and Prevention. Revised classification system for human immunodeficiency virus infection in children less than 13 years of age. *MMWR*. 1994;43(RR-12): 1–10.
10. Centers for Disease Control and Prevention. U.S. Public Health Service task force recommendations for use of antiretroviral drugs in pregnant HIV-1 infected women for maternal health and interventions to reduce perinatal HIV-1 transmission in the United States. *MMWR*. 2002;51:1–38.
11. Working Group on Antiretroviral Therapy and Medical Management of HIV-Infected Children. Guidelines for the use of antiretroviral agents in pediatric HIV infection. February 23, 2009; 1–139. Available at: http://aidsinfo.nih.gov/ContentFiles/PediatricGuidelines.pdf. Accessed February 21, 2010.
12. Miller TL. Nutritional aspects of pediatric HIV infection. In: Walker WA, Watkins JB, eds. *Nutrition in Pediatrics*, 2nd ed. Hamilton, Ontario, Canada: B. Dekker; 1996:534–550.
13. Miller TL, Orav EJ, Martin SR, Cooper ER, McIntosh K, Winter HS. Malnutrition and carbohydrate malabsorption in children with vertically transmitted human immunodeficiency virus 1 infection. *Gastroenterology*. 1991;100:1296–1302.
14. Arpadi SM. Growth failure in children with HIV infection. *J Acquir Immune Defic Syndr*. 2000;25(Suppl 1):S37–S42.
15. Chandra RK. Mucosal immune responses in malnutrition. *Ann NY Acad Sci*. 1983;409:345–352.
16. Miller TL, Easley KA, Zhang W, et al. Maternal and infant factors associated with failure to thrive in children with vertically transmitted human immunodeficiency virus-1 infection: the prospective, P2C2 human immunodeficiency virus multicenter study. *Pediatrics*. 2001;108:1287–1296.
17. Newell ML, Borja MC, Peckham C. Height, weight, and growth in children born to mothers with HIV-1 infection in Europe. *Pediatrics*. 2003;111:E52–E60.
18. Hilgartner MW, Donfield SM, Lynn HS, et al. The effect of plasma human immunodeficiency virus RNA and CD4(1) T lymphocytes on growth measurements of hemophilic boys and adolescents. *Pediatrics*. 2001;107:E56.
19. Benjamin DK Jr, Miller WC, Benjamin DK, et al. A comparison of height and weight velocity as a part of the composite endpoint in pediatric HIV. *AIDS*. 2003;17:2331–2336.
20. Carey VJ, Yong FH, Frenkel LM, McKinney RE Jr. Pediatric AIDS prognosis using somatic growth velocity. *AIDS*. 1998;12:1361–1369.
21. Chantry CJ, Byrd RS, Englund JA, Baker CJ, McKinney RE Jr. Growth, survival and viral load in symptomatic childhood human immunodeficiency virus infection. *Pediatr Infect Dis J*. 2003;22:1033–1039.
22. Wintergerst U, Hoffmann F, Solder B, et al. Comparison of two antiretroviral triple combinations including the protease inhibitor indinavir in children infected with human immunodeficiency virus. *Pediatr Infect Dis J*. 1998;17:495–499.
23. Fiore P, Donelli E, Boni S, Pontali E, Tramalloni R, Bassetti D. Nutritional status changes in HIV-infected children receiving combined antiretroviral therapy including protease inhibitors. *Int J Antimicrob Agents*. 2000;16:365–369.
24. Dreimane D, Nielsen K, Deveikis A, Bryson YJ, Geffner ME. Effect of protease inhibitors combined with standard antiretroviral therapy on linear growth and weight gain in human immunodeficiency virus type 1-infected children. *Pediatr Infect Dis J*. 2001;20:315–316.
25. Buchacz K, Cervia JS, Lindsey JC, et al. Impact of protease inhibitor-containing combination antiretroviral therapies on height and weight growth in HIV-infected children. *Pediatrics*. 2001;108:E72.
26. Miller TL, Mawn BE, Orav EJ, et al. The effect of protease inhibitor therapy on growth and body composition in human immunodeficiency virus type 1-infected children. *Pediatrics*. 2001;107:E77.
27. Nachman SA, Lindsey JC, Pelton S, et al. Growth in human immunodeficiency virus-infected children receiving ritonavir-containing antiretroviral therapy. *Arch Pediatr Adolesc Med*. 2002;156:497–503.
28. Verweel G, van Rossum AM, Hartwig NG, Wolfs TF, Scherpbier HJ, de Groot R. Treatment with highly active antiretroviral therapy in human immunodeficiency virus type 1-infected children is associated with a sustained effect on growth. *Pediatrics*. 2002;109:E25.
29. Moye J, Rich K, Kalish L, et al. Natural history of somatic growth in infants born to women infected by human immunodeficiency virus. *J Pediatr*. 1996;128:58–69.
30. European Collaborative Study. Height, weight, and growth in children born to mothers with HIV-1 infection in Europe. *Pediatrics*. 2003;111:e52–e60.
31. Chantry CJ, Hughes MD, Alvero C, et al. Insulin-like growth factor-1 and lean body mass in HIV-infected children. *J Acquir Immune Defic Syndr*. 2008;48:437–443.
32. Amaya RA, Kozinetz CA, McMeans A, Schwarzwald H, Kline MW. Lipodystrophy syndrome in human immunodeficiency virus-infected children. *Pediatr Infect Dis J*. 2002;21:405–410.
33. Vigano A, Mora S, Testolin C, et al. Increased lipodystrophy is associated with increased exposure to highly active antiretroviral therapy in HIV-infected children. *J Acquir Immune Defic Syndr*. 2003;32:482–489.

34. Arpadi SM, Cuff PA, Horlick M, Wang J, Kotler DP. Lipodystrophy in HIV-infected children is associated with high viral load and low CD41-lymphocyte count and CD41-lymphocyte percentage at baseline and use of protease inhibitors and stavudine. *J Acquir Immune Defic Syndr.* 2001;27:30–34.
35. Lainka E, Oezbek S, Falck M, Ndagijimana J, Niehues T. Marked dyslipidemia in human immunodeficiency virus-infected children on protease inhibitor-containing antiretroviral therapy. *Pediatrics*. 2002;110:E56.
36. Jaquet D, Levine M, Ortega-Rodriguez E, et al. Clinical and metabolic presentation of the lipodystrophic syndrome in HIV-infected children. *AIDS*. 2000;14:2123–2128.
37. Beregszaszi M, Jaquet D, Levine M, et al. Severe insulin resistance contrasting with mild anthropometric changes in the adipose tissue of HIV-infected children with lipohypertrophy. *Int J Obes Relat Metab Disord*. 2003;27:25–30.
38. Mora S, Sala N, Bricalli D, Zuin G, Chiumello G, Vigano A. Bone mineral loss through increased bone turnover in HIV-infected children treated with highly active antiretroviral therapy. *AIDS*. 2001;15:1823–1829.
39. Arpadi SM, Horlick M, Thornton J, Cuff PA, Wang J, Kotler DP. Bone mineral content is lower in prepubertal HIV-infected children. *J Acquir Immune Defic Syndr*. 2002;29:450–454.
40. O'Brien KO, Razavi M, Henderson RA, Caballero B, Ellis KJ. Bone mineral content in girls perinatally infected with HIV. *Am J Clin Nutr*. 2001;73:821–826.
41. Alfaro MP, Siegel RM, Baker RC, Heubi JE. Resting energy expenditure and body composition in pediatric HIV infection. *Pediatr AIDS HIV Infect*. 1995;6:276–280.
42. World Health Organization. Nutrient requirements for people living with HIV/AIDS: a report of technical consultation. 2003. Available at: http://www.who.int/nutrition/publications/Content_nutrient_requirements.pdf. Accessed August 12, 2010.
43. Henderson RA. Effect of enteral tube feeding on growth of children with symptomatic human immunodeficiency virus infection. *J Pediatr Gastroenterol Nutr*. 1994;18:429–434.
44. Miller TL, Awnetwant EL, Evans S, Morris VM, Vazquez IM, McIntosh K. Gastrostomy tube supplementation for HIV-infected children. *Pediatrics*. 1995;96:696–702.
45. Coodley GO, Loveless MO, Merrill TM. The HIV wasting syndrome: a review. *J Acquir Immune Defic Syndr*. 1994;7:681–694.
46. Heller LS, Shattuck D. Nutrition support for children with HIV/AIDS. *J Am Diet Assoc*. 1997;97:473–474.
47. Galvin T. Micronutrients: implications in human immunodeficiency virus disease. *Top Clin Nutr*. 1992;7:63–73.
48. Clarick RH, Hanekom WA, Yogev R, Chadwick EG. Megestrol acetate treatment of growth failure in children infected with human immunodeficiency virus. *Pediatrics*. 1997;99:354–357.
49. Antiretroviral therapy and medical management of pediatric HIV infection and 1997 USPHS/IDSA report on the prevention of opportunistic infections in persons infected with human immunodeficiency virus. *Pediatrics*. 1998;99:354–357.

Hematology and Oncology*

Paula Charuhas Macris and Kathryn Hunt

Introduction

Each year in the United States, more children die from cancer than from any other disease. In fact, cancer is the fourth overall leading cause of death in children under age 20, ranking behind only unintentional injury, homicide, and suicide.[1,2] Cancer accounts for 11% of the deaths by disease of all children 1 to 14 years old and 5% of adolescents 15 to 19 years old.[1,2] From 2001 to 2005, the annual incidence of cancer was 167 cases per million children from birth to age 19 years.[1,2] During the same period, the annual mortality rate due to cancer was 27 cases per million children from birth to age 19 years.[1,2] Leukemia constitutes the highest percentage of pediatric cancers, followed by children with central nervous system malignancies and lymphoma. The overall incidence rates of childhood cancers are shown in **Figure 17-1**.[1]

Despite these statistics, over the past three decades, the medical community has made tremendous improvements in both short-term and long-term survival rates of children with cancer. Thirty years ago, only 50% of children under age 15 could expect to survive cancer for 5 years or more. Today, the 5-year survival rate for these children is approaching 80%. The primary reason for the increase in childhood cancer survival is improved treatment protocols for acute lymphocytic leukemia (ALL), which comprises approximately one-third of all malignancies. A secondary reason for increased survival rates is high participation in randomized, cooperative group clinical trials, such as those of the Children's Oncology Group (COG). The COG is a consortium of pediatric institutions that provide care to children and adolescents with cancer. Multiple, sequential clinical trials have led to incremental improvements in the treatment of children with cancer. More recently, biologic and immunologic targeted therapies have been developed for neuroblastoma and relapsed leukemias. A final factor in improved survival rates has been the interdisciplinary nature of supportive care available to patients and families undergoing intense oncologic treatment. With the numerous nutritional implications of chemotherapy, surgery, radiation therapy, and hematopoietic cell transplantation (HCT), which can lead to malnutrition and other complications, families benefit from supportive care delivered by experienced pediatric oncology dietitians, social workers, advanced practice nurses, pharmacists, and other care team members, working with the physicians.

Childhood Cancer and Malnutrition

The incidence of malnutrition in children with newly diagnosed cancer is highly variable and dependent upon factors such as advanced or metastatic disease, the degree of tumor burden, histology, and treatment protocols. Certain types of treatment procedures promote the development of malnutrition: major abdominal surgery; radiation to the head, neck, esophagus, abdomen, or pelvis; or frequent (compressed) courses of chemotherapy (3-week intervals or less).[3]

Approximately 40% to 80% of children become malnourished during intensive cancer treatment, due to the aggressive nature of treatment protocols and the negative implications of therapy.[4] Characteristics of childhood malnutrition may include tissue wasting, anorexia, weakness, anemia, hypoalbuminemia, and skeletal muscle atrophy.[4] Medical researchers are divided over the extent to which malnutrition at diagnosis or during therapy impacts survival rates. However, the research has established that malnutrition is clearly associated with increased infection rates, decreased tolerance of chemotherapy, delays in treatment, and diminished quality of life.[5] Childhood cancers associated with high nutrition risk are presented in **Table 17-1**.[1,2,4–7]

*Parts of this chapter have been reprinted with permission from *Nutrition Focus*. 2009;24(1):1–8.

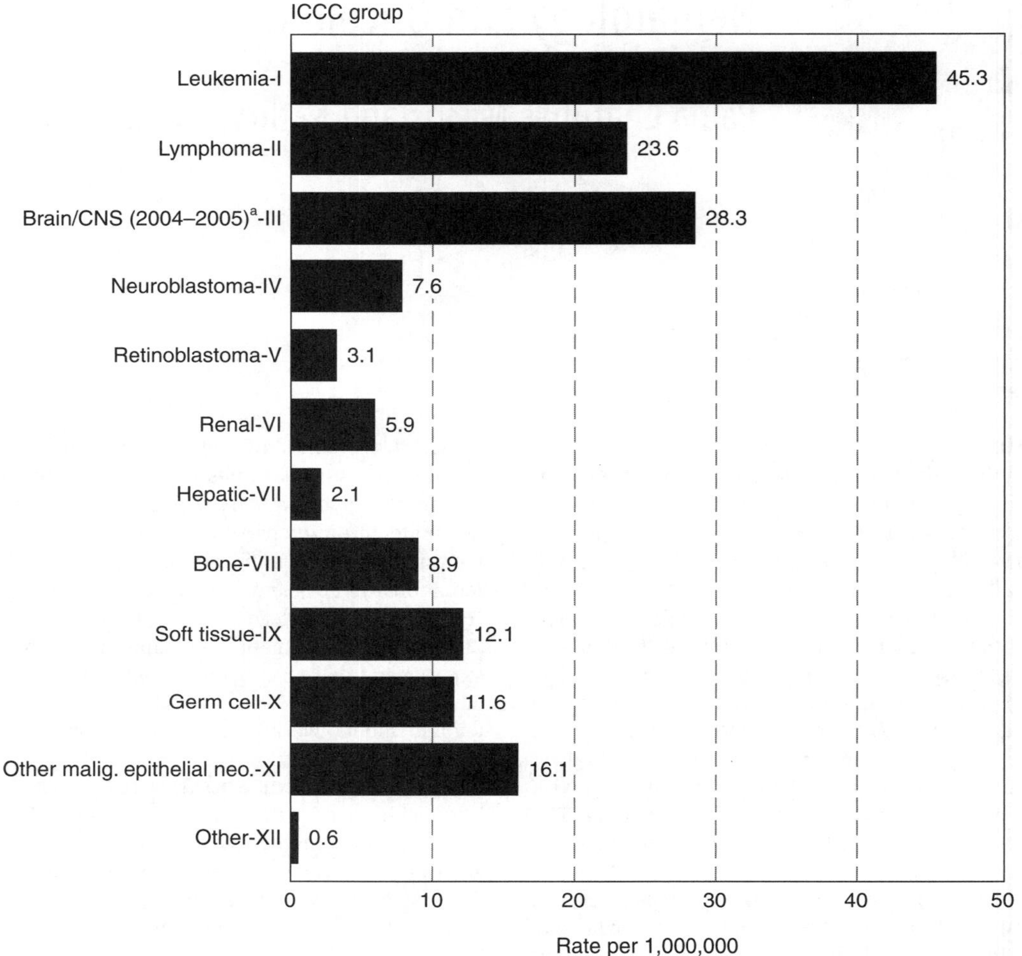

FIGURE 17-1 Childhood Cancer: SEER Incidence Rates 2002–2006 by ICCC Group (Includes Group III Benign Brain (2004–2006) and Myelodysplastic Syndromes) Under 20 Years of Age, Both Sexes, All Races

[a]Rate for Group III (Brain/CNS) includes benign brain tumors and is based only on cases diagnosed in 2004–2006.

Source: Reprinted with permission from Ries LAG, Smith MA, Gurney JG, et al., eds. *Cancer Incidence and Survival among Children and Adolescents: United States SEER Program 1975–1995*. Bethesda, MD: National Cancer Institute; 1999:1–15. NIH Pub. No. 99-4649.

Infants (birth to 12 months) with leukemia, hepatoblastoma, or brain tumors are highly vulnerable to malnutrition and chemotherapy-related toxicities, as are young toddlers, whose development of self-feeding skills is often interrupted. Children often suffer from pain, mucositis, and vomiting, and are therefore unable to accept breastmilk, infant formula, or solid foods at sufficient energy and protein levels needed to sustain growth and weight gain.

Adolescent cancer patients are equally vulnerable to therapy-induced malnutrition because adolescence is the

TABLE 17-1 Common Childhood Cancers, Standard Treatment Plans, and Factors Affecting Nutritional Status

Childhood Cancer	Factors Affecting Nutritional Status	5-Year Relative Survival Rates (1999–2005)
Acute lymphocytic leukemia High-risk categories: • White blood cell count ≥ 50,000 mm^3 and/or age ≥ 10 years • Infants < 12 months of age • Chromosomal abnormalities (Philadelphia+) • T-cell phenotype • Relapsed Lymphoblastic lymphoma	• Need for cranial radiation • Treatment with highly emetogenic and mucosal toxic chemotherapy • Asparaginase-induced pancreatitis • Steroid-induced hyperglycemia requiring insulin • Frequent NPO status for procedures and intrathecal chemotherapy • HCT often necessary for cure	83.8% Infant < 1 year: 51.7% 65–85%
Acute myelogenous leukemia • Newly diagnosed • Relapsed disease	• Prolonged immunosuppression • At risk for fungal infections • Prolonged hospitalizations ("same old food" burn-out); HCT may be necessary	56.7%
Brain tumors • Medulloblastoma • Ependymoma/choroid plexus (PNET) • Astrocytoma • Other gliomas	• Treatment consists of 6 weeks of radiation therapy • Younger children require sedation for radiation (prolonged NPO status) • Hypogeusia • Nausea, vomiting, fatigue • Increased risk for dysphagia	85% Metastatic: < 60%; localized, nonmetastatic: 69.6% 82.6% 52.8%
Hepatic tumors Hepatoblastoma • High risk: unresectable, metastatic, and prematurity	• Prematurity • Young age (< 2 years) • Liver transplant	69.2%
Neuroblastoma • High risk: stage III and IV • MYCN* amplification • Relapsed disease	• Young age (average age at diagnosis: 3.1 years) • Interruption in baseline feeding pattern • Significant nausea and vomiting • High need for enteral tube feeding • Postsurgery complication: high-output diarrhea • HCT • Prolonged transition to baseline oral intake after treatment	73.2% (also includes low risk)
Non-Hodgkin's lymphoma • Burkitts • Anaplastic large cell • Diffuse large B-cell	• Mucosal toxic chemotherapy (mouth and GI tract) • Frequent NPO status for intrathecal chemotherapy • Lack of interest in eating due to GI mucosal damage • Major nausea • At risk for infection	Burkitts: 80–90% Anaplastic large cell: 60–75% Diffuse large B-cell: 80–90%
Sarcomas • High risk: stage III and IV • Rhabdomyosarcoma (RMS) (especially parameningeal RMS) • Ewing's • Osteosarcoma • Metastatic disease	• Compressed chemotherapy cycles • Treatment with highly emetogenic and mucosal toxic chemotherapy • Lack of recovery time between chemotherapy cycles to regain lost weight • High energy and protein requirements	Osteosarcoma: 67.1% Ewing's: 63.1% Soft tissue and extraosseous sarcomas: 9.9% Rhabdomyosarcoma: 61.4%

(continued)

TABLE 17-1 *(Continued)*

Childhood Cancer	Factors Affecting Nutritional Status	5-Year Relative Survival Rates (1999–2005)
Wilms' tumor • High risk: stage III and IV • Unfavorable resection • Relapsed/metastatic disease	• Surgical resection of tumor and kidney • Postoperative ileus requiring PN support • Radiation therapy: younger patients often NPO several hours prior to treatment	87.1% (also includes low risk)
Other, rare childhood malignancies • Chronic myelogenous leukemia (CML) • Juvenile chronic myelogenous leukemia (JCML)	• Treatment for both CML and JCML is HCT	CML:70–75% JCML: 50%

*MYCN: An oncogene present on chromosome 2. The MYCN gene is amplified (has more than 10 copies instead of 2 copies) in a subset of neuroblastoma tumors; this amplification is associated with poor outcome.

Abbreviations: GI, gastrointestinal; HCT, hematopoietic cell transplantation; NPO, non per os (nothing by mouth); PN, parenteral nutrition.

Sources: Ries LAG, Smith MA, Gurney JG, et al., eds. *Cancer Incidence and Survival among Children and Adolescents: United States SEER Program 1975-1995.* Bethesda, MD: Gurney JG, Bondy ML. Epidemiology of childhood cancer. General principles of chemotherapy. In Pizzo PA, Poplac D, eds. *Principles and Practice of Pediatric Oncology,* 5th ed. Philadelphia, PA: Lippincott Williams & Wilkins; 2006:1–13; Mauer AM, Burgess JB, Donaldson SS, et al. Special nutritional needs of children with malignancies: a review. *J Parenter Enteral Nutr.* 1990;14:315–324; Ladas EJ, Sacks N, Meacham L, et al. A multidisciplinary review of nutrition considerations in the pediatric oncology population: a perspective from Children's Oncology Group. *Nutr Clin Pract.* 2005;20:377–393; Williams DM, Hobson R, Imeson J, Gerrard M, McCarthy K, Pinkerton CR. Anaplastic large cell lymphoma in childhood: analysis of 72 patients treated on the United Kingdom Children's Cancer Study Group chemotherapy regimens. *Br J Haematol.* 2002;117:812–820; and Cairo MS, Raetz E, Lim MS, Davenport V, Perkins SL. Childhood and adolescent non-Hodgkin lymphoma: new insights in biology and critical challenges for the future. *Pediatr Blood Cancer.* 2005;45:753–769.

second period in the human life cycle where significant gains in growth and development occur. Cancers that develop during the second decade of life (10 to 20 years), such as Ewing's sarcoma and osteosarcoma, pose special challenges for the adolescent patient and the care team. Adolescents have high growth demands, and therefore require nutrient-dense diets, which are especially important because the aggressive chemotherapy regimens used for this age group often cause rapid weight loss from nausea, vomiting, and mucositis.

Malnutrition, manifested by underweight status, is not the only risk factor for morbidity during cancer treatment. Childhood obesity presents its own set of risks during treatment, as obesity trends in North America are escalating to epidemic highs. Obese children with cancer, especially those with acute leukemias, may suffer increased toxicities from chemotherapy. The cause of increased morbidity is likely multifactorial including altered drug clearance due to increased body fat and co-morbidities associated with obesity such as obstructive sleep apnea and glucose intolerance.[5]

Nutritional Effects of Cancer Therapy

Children with cancer are often treated with multimodal therapies, depending on the type and stage of the malignancy. Cancer therapies may produce only mild, transient nutrition issues or may lead to severe, permanent problems, which impact nutritional status. The four main treatments are chemotherapy, surgery, radiation therapy, and HCT.

Chemotherapy

Chemotherapeutic agents work by inhibiting DNA synthesis of both normal tissues and malignant cells. Most of the adverse effects associated with chemotherapy stem from damage to rapidly proliferating cells including the epithelial cells of the gastrointestinal (GI) tract. The degree of the GI alterations depends upon the specific medication, dosage, duration, rate of metabolism, and the child's susceptibility.[8]

Nutritional and medical complications associated with chemotherapy are outlined in **Table 17-2**.[9–11] Nausea and vomiting, which are associated with chemotherapy, are the most common problems interfering with adequate oral intake. These symptoms occur as a result of a direct central nervous system effect as drugs are administered. Complications of chemotherapy-induced emesis include weight loss, dehydration, fluid and electrolyte imbalances, and metabolic alkalosis.[11] Management of chemotherapy-induced nausea and vomiting includes the judicious use of antiemetics. Single agent or combination antiemetics are frequently used and can decrease the child's discomfort. Nonpharmacologic interventions such as music therapy, hypnosis, and muscle relaxation have been described as effective techniques for treating nausea and vomiting.[12]

TABLE 17-2 Nutritional Implications of Chemotherapeutic Agents

Drug	Antitumor Spectrum	Nutritional Implications
Alkylating Agents		
Busulfan	Leukemias (HCT)	Nausea and vomiting, mucositis, hepatic (high dose)
Carboplatin	Brain tumors, germ cell tumors, neuroblastoma	Nausea and vomiting, hepatic (mild)
Cisplatin	Testicular and other germ cell tumors, brain tumors, osteosarcoma, neuroblastoma	Nausea and vomiting, renal
Cyclophosphamide	Lymphomas, leukemias, sarcomas, neuroblastoma	Nausea and vomiting, fluid retention
Ifosfamide	Sarcomas, germ cell tumors	Nausea and vomiting, renal
Lomustine	Brain tumors, lymphomas, Hodgkin's disease	Nausea and vomiting, renal
Melphalan	HCT	Nausea and vomiting, mucositis, diarrhea (high dose)
Procarbazine	Hodgkin's disease, brain tumors	Nausea and vomiting, mucositis
Temozolomide	Brain tumors	Nausea and vomiting
Antimetabolites		
Cladaribine	AML, CLL, indolent lymphomas	Mild nausea and vomiting
Cytarabine	Leukemia, lymphomas	Nausea and vomiting, mucositis, flu-like syndrome
Fludarabine phosphate	AML, CLL, indolent lymphomas	Mild nausea and vomiting
Fluorouracil	Carcinomas, hepatic tumors	Nausea and vomiting, mucositis, diarrhea
Mercaptopurine	ALL, CML	Hepatic, mucositis
Methotrexate	Leukemia, lymphomas, osteosarcoma	Mild mucositis, hepatic, renal
Thioguanine	ALL, AML	Nausea and vomiting, mucositis, hepatic (VOD)
Antitumor Antibiotics		
Bleomycin	Lymphoma, testicular and other germ cell tumors	Nausea and vomiting, mucositis
Dactinomycin	Wilms', sarcomas	Nausea and vomiting, mucositis, hepatic (VOD)
Daunomycin	ALL, AML, lymphomas	Nausea and vomiting, mucositis, diarrhea
Doxorubicin	ALL, AML, lymphomas, most solid tumors	Nausea and vomiting, mucositis, diarrhea
Idarubicin	ALL, AML, lymphomas	Nausea and vomiting, mucositis, diarrhea
Mitoxantrone	ALL, AML, lymphomas	Nausea and vomiting, mucositis
Plant Product		
Etoposide	ALL, AML, lymphomas, neuroblastoma, sarcoma, brain tumors	Nausea and vomiting, mucositis, diarrhea
Irinotecan	Rhabdomyosarcomas	Nausea and vomiting, diarrhea, hepatic, dehydration, ileus
Topotecan	Neuroblastoma, rhabdomyosarcoma	Nausea and vomiting, mucositis, diarrhea
Vincristine	ALL, lymphoma, most solid tumors	SIADH, constipation
Vinblastine	Histiocytosis, Hodgkin's disease, testicular	Mucositis, constipation
Miscellaneous		
All-trans retinoic acid	Acute promyelocytic leukemia	Hypertriglyceridemia
Dexamethasone	Leukemia, lymphomas, brain tumors	Highly variable*
Imatinib mesylate	Ph+ CML	Nausea and vomiting, fatigue, hepatic
Native asparaginase	ALL, lymphoma	Pancreatitis, hepatic
PEG-asparaginase	ALL, lymphoma	Pancreatitis, hepatic
Prednisone	Leukemia, lymphomas	Highly variable*
13-cis-retinoic acid	Minimal residual disease neuroblastoma	Xerostomia, hypertriglyceridemia, hypercalcemia

*Refer to Table 17-5, section on corticosteroids.

Abbreviations: ALL, acute lymphoblastic leukemia; AML, acute myelogenous leukemia; CLL, chronic lymphoblastic leukemia; CML, chronic myelogenous leukemia; HCT, hematopoietic cell transplantation; SIADH, syndrome of inappropriate antidiuretic hormone; VOD, veno-occlusive disease.

Sources: Adamson PC, Balis FM, Berg S, Blaney SM. General principles of chemotherapy. In Pizzo PA, Poplac D, eds. *Principles and Practice of Pediatric Oncology,* 5th ed. Philadelphia, PA: Lippincott Williams & Wilkins; 2006:290–365; Chu E, DeVita VT. *Physicians' Cancer Chemotherapy Drug Manual.* Sudbury, MA: Jones and Bartlett Publishers; 2006; and Charuhas PM, Aker SN. Nutritional implications of antineoplastic chemotherapeutic agents. *Clin Appl Nutr.* 1992;2:20–33.

Acupuncture, acupressure, and aromatherapy have also been reported to prevent and treat chemotherapy-induced nausea and vomiting.[13]

Alterations in taste and smell as a result of chemotherapy may persist well beyond periods of nausea and vomiting and result in prolonged anorexia.[14] In addition, children may develop food aversions that can limit oral intake.

Mucositis is a major GI complication and is usually intensified by concurrent radiation therapy.[15] Mucositis may affect any part of the GI tract and lead to ulceration, bleeding, and malabsorption. Chemotherapy-induced neutropenia accentuates these complications. Diligent mouth care may help to prevent additional oral breakdown. Fortunately, the renewal rate of the GI tract mucosa is rapid so that mucositis from chemotherapy is usually short-lived.

Certain chemotherapy and antibiotic agents may cause malabsorption and alterations in the gut flora, with subsequent weight loss and diarrhea.[11] Children who experience diarrhea either due to chemotherapy or from an infectious cause may benefit from probiotic replacement therapy in the setting of multiple antibiotic coverage.[16] Constipation related to the use of vincristine or narcotics or due to inactivity may result in significant abdominal discomfort and loss of appetite.

Surgery

Surgery is often the preferred method of therapy for solid tumors and tumors in the GI tract. Surgical removal of a tumor may lead to insufficient oral intake over several days during a time of increased requirements of energy and protein. Depending on the surgical site, nutrient intake and absorption may be significant. Surgery involving the head or neck area or the GI tract may result in profound nutritional implications including chewing and swallowing issues, diarrhea, malabsorption of vitamins and minerals, and fluid and electrolyte imbalances.

Radiation Therapy

Radiation therapy is a primary treatment modality for many brain tumors, and is used in combination with surgery and chemotherapy to treat other cancers, including unresectable tumors. The nutritional implications of radiation depend upon many factors, including:

- The region of the body radiated
- Dose, fractionation, length of time, and field size of the radiation administered
- Concurrent use of other antitumor therapy such as surgery or chemotherapy
- The child's initial nutritional status

As with chemotherapy, radiation destroys malignant cells as well as rapidly replicating normal tissues, including the GI tract. Nutritional sequelae associated with radiation therapy are detailed in **Table 17-3**.[8]

Hematopoietic Cell Transplantation

Treatment with HCT is an established therapeutic modality for certain pediatric hematologic and malignant disorders (see **Table 17-4**).[17] Children receiving a traditional myeloablative regimen are prepared with high doses of chemotherapy and possibly total body and local irradiation. In recent years, nonmyeloablative conditioning regimens, which deliver lower dose chemotherapy and radiation, have also been developed. Children with relapsed malignancy following myeloablative HCT or those with nonmalignant disorders may be candidates for the nonmyeloablative regimens. The intense conditioning regimen is designed to eliminate active and residual malignant cells or a defective hematopoietic system to restore normal hematopoiesis and immunologic function.[18] An intravenous infusion of autologous (child's own), syngeneic (identical twin), or allogeneic (from a histocompatible related or unrelated donor) stem cells follows conditioning. The source of the stem cells may be bone marrow, peripheral blood, or umbilical cord blood.

Posttransplant Course

Severe pancytopenia (low blood counts) lasts from 2 to 6 weeks posttransplant. Children are at the greatest risk for bacterial and fungal infections until the stem cells engraft.

TABLE 17-3 Nutritional Implications of Radiation Therapy

Radiation to the central nervous system
- Anorexia
- Nausea and vomiting

Radiation to the head and neck
- Nausea
- Mucositis, esophagitis
- Altered taste and smell
- Tooth decay
- Altered salivation (saliva becomes thick and viscous)
- Dysphagia

Radiation to the gastrointestinal system
- Nausea and vomiting
- Diarrhea
- Steatorrhea and malabsorption
- Fluid and electrolyte imbalances

Total body radiation
- Nausea, vomiting, diarrhea
- Mucositis, esophagitis
- Altered taste acuity and salivation
- Anorexia
- Delayed growth and development

Source: Barale KV, Charuhas PM. Oncology and hematopoietic cell transplantation. In: Queen PS, King K, eds. *Handbook of Pediatric Nutrition*, 3rd ed. Sudbury, MA: Jones and Bartlett Publishers; 2005:459–481.

TABLE 17-4 Conditions for Application of Pediatric Hematopoietic Cell Transplantation

Hematologic malignancies
• Acute leukemia
• Chronic leukemia
• Myelodysplastic syndrome
Malignant solid tumors
• Advanced-stage neuroblastoma
• Refractory Ewing's sarcoma
• Recurrent lymphomas
Immunodeficiency disorders
• Severe combined immunodeficiency disease
• Wiskott-Aldrich syndrome
• Hyper IgM syndrome
• Other cellular immunodeficiencies
Nonneoplastic disorders
• Severe aplastic anemia
• Thalassemia major
• Fanconi anemia
• Diamond-Blackfan syndrome
• Sickle cell disease
• Paroxysmal nocturnal hemoglobinuria
• Shwachman Diamond syndrome
• Lysosomal storage diseases (e.g., Gaucher's disease, metachromatic leukodystrophy, Niemann-Pick disease)
• Mucopolysaccharidoses (e.g., Hunter's disease, Hurler's disease)
• Infantile osteopetrosis
• Hemophagocytic lymphohistiocytosis
• Refractory autoimmune disorders

Source: Locatelli F, Giorgiani, Di Cesare-Merlone A, Merli PM, Sparta V, Moretta F. The changing role of stem cell transplantation in childhood. *Bone Marrow Transplant.* 2008;41:S3–S7.

During this period, supportive care including frequent red blood cell and platelet transfusions, systemic antibiotic therapy, and parenteral nutrition (PN) support are instituted.

Nutrition effects of HCT are due to the conditioning therapy, infections, graft-versus-host disease (GVHD), and medications, including anti-infectious and immunosuppressive agents.[18] Complications interfering with nutrient intake include mucositis; esophagitis; dysgeusia (impaired taste); xerostomia (oral dryness); thick, viscous saliva; nausea; vomiting; anorexia; diarrhea; steatorrhea; and multiple-organ dysfunction.[18] The duration and intensity of symptoms, as well as the stress of treatment, preclude oral intake for a minimum of 3 to 4 weeks posttransplant and necessitate the use of PN support. Oral intake is encouraged as soon as tolerated. Calorie, protein, and fluid goals should be defined for each child.

At hospital discharge, some children are still unable to eat an adequate amount of nutrients, and partial PN and/or enteral tube feeding may be prescribed, especially for children with chronic food aversions and long-term anorexia. Supplemental intravenous hydration may also be necessary. Follow-up nutrition counseling and assessment are imperative throughout the child's posttransplant course to ensure provision of adequate nutrition support.

Graft-Versus-Host Disease

Children who receive allogeneic transplants are at risk for the development of GVHD, an immunologic reaction in which the newly engrafted stem cells react against the host's tissue antigens following engraftment. The ensuing immunologic response can cause multiple-organ damage.[19] The GVHD may occur as an acute reaction early posttransplant or progress to a chronic condition. Because of its potentially devastating effects, efforts are directed at prevention of GVHD. Medications and therapy used for prophylaxis and treatment of GVHD are presented in **Table 17-5**.[20]

Acute GVHD can affect the skin, liver, or GI tract. Clinical symptoms include a maculopapular rash, cholestatic liver dysfunction, or nausea, vomiting, and diarrhea. Intestinal GVHD can involve either the upper or lower GI tract.[19] Upper intestinal GVHD symptoms include early satiety, anorexia, nausea, and vomiting. In lower intestinal GVHD, diarrhea may be severe and, at its worst, associated with crampy abdominal pain and bleeding. Children with severe disease often require a period of bowel rest with PN support. Refeeding guidelines include slow diet progression and feeding one new food at a time, as illustrated in **Table 17-6**.[21]

Nutrition Assessment

Nutritional status at diagnosis has been associated with treatment outcome in children with cancer.[22,23] Nutrition assessment should begin at diagnosis and continue throughout treatment.[8] Techniques for the newly diagnosed child do not differ from normal nutrition assessment recommendations as presented in Chapter 3. However, a clear understanding of the specific type and stage of cancer, treatment protocol, and effects of therapy are necessary to better formulate an appropriate nutrition care plan.

Anthropometry

Initial measurements should include age, height (recumbent length in children less than 2 years of age), weight, and in children younger than 2 years of age, occipital frontal head circumference (see growth charts, Appendix B). Any measurement below the 10th percentile should be investigated as a sign of growth impairment due to inadequate nutrition. Weight-for-height percentile is believed to be the most reliable anthropometric indicator of nutrition

TABLE 17-5 Therapies Used for Prophylaxis and Treatment of GVHD

Therapy	Nutritional Effects
Antithymocyte globulin	Nausea and vomiting, diarrhea, stomatitis
Azathioprine	Nausea and vomiting, anorexia, diarrhea, mucosal ulceration, esophagitis, steatorrhea
Beclomethasone dipropionate	Xerostomia, dysgeusia, nausea
Budesonide	None known
Corticosteroids	Sodium and fluid retention resulting in weight gain or hypertension, hyperphagia, weight gain, hypokalemia, skeletal muscle catabolism and atrophy, gastric irritation and peptic ulceration, osteoporosis, growth retardation in children, decreased insulin sensitivity and impaired glucose tolerance, hyperglycemia or steroid-induced diabetes, hypertriglyceridemia
Cyclosporine	Nausea and vomiting, renal insufficiency, magnesium wasting, potassium wasting
Extracorporeal photopheresis	Intravenous fluid may be necessary to maintain adequate hydration status; monitor calcium status if citrate anticoagulant is used because it may bind calcium and induce hypocalcemia
Methotrexate	Nausea and vomiting (mild to moderate); anorexia; mucositis and esophagitis; diarrhea; renal and hepatic changes; decreased absorption of vitamin B_{12}, fat, and D-xylose; hepatic fibrosis; change in taste acuity
Methoxsalen (in conjunction with Psoralen 1 ultraviolet A light)	Nausea, hepatotoxicity
Monoclonal antibodies	Nausea and vomiting
Mycophenolate mofetil	Nausea and vomiting, diarrhea
Sirolimus	Hypertriglyceridemia
Tacrolimus	Nephrotoxicity, hyperglycemia, hyperkalemia, hypomagnesemia
Thalidomide	Constipation, nausea, xerostomia
Ursodeoxycholic acid	Nausea and vomiting, diarrhea, dyspepsia

Source: Hematopoietic Stem Cell Transplantation, *Nutrition Care Criteria*. Seattle, WA: Seattle Cancer Care Alliance, 2002.

status in the child with cancer.[4] It can be used to reliably predict nutrition status because of its high direct correlation with triceps skinfold and mid-arm muscle circumference measurements. In the pediatric cancer patient, current or previous chemoradiotherapy may depress growth. Catch-up growth has been observed in these children;[24] however, children who receive cranial irradiation may develop long-term growth disturbances.[25] Children receiving long-term therapy or post-HCT should have their growth velocity plotted yearly to detect deviations from normal growth patterns.[18] From the baseline anthropometry information, the child's body surface area and ideal weight, which are often used to calculate medication dosages, can be determined.

For prepubertal children (females less than 12 years old; males less than 14 years old), ideal weight is determined by matching the weight at the 50th percentile for height on the age- and gender-specific Centers for Disease Control and Prevention (CDC) growth charts for the United States. For postpubertal children, an estimation of the ideal weight is determined using the body mass index (BMI) CDC growth charts for age. If the child's BMI is between the 25th and 75th percentiles, this may be considered an ideal weight. An adjusted weight is calculated for children greater than 120% ideal weight using the following equation:[26]

$$\text{Adjusted weight} = [\text{actual weight (kg)} - \text{ideal weight (kg)}] \times 0.25 + \text{ideal weight (kg)}$$

It is important to assess both growth history and the current height for age, weight for age, and weight for length or BMI. Arm anthropometry, to determine somatic muscle protein and adipose reserves, may also be assessed during the initial evaluation.

Biochemistry

Finding reliable measures to detect malnutrition in the pediatric cancer patient can be challenging. Both the disease itself and the treatment can affect laboratory data used for nutrition assessment. Hematologic parameters, such as hemoglobin and hematocrit, often reflect the disease state and treatment with blood transfusions, rather than nutritional status. Many chemotherapy agents will suppress bone marrow production and lower lymphocyte counts; therefore,

TABLE 17-6 Gastrointestinal GVHD Diet Progression

Phase	Clinical Symptoms	Diet	Nutrition Support
1. Bowel rest	GI cramping Large volume watery diarrhea or active GI bleeding Depressed serum albumin Severely reduced transit time Small-bowel obstruction or diminished bowel sounds Nausea and vomiting	Oral: NPO	PN with supplemental zinc and possibly copper
2. Introduction of oral feeding	Minimal GI cramping Diarrhea less than 500 mL/day Guaiac-negative stools Improved transit time (minimum 1.5 hours) Infrequent nausea and vomiting	Oral: Isosmotic, low-residue, low-lactose beverages, initially 60 mL every 2 to 3 hours, for several days	PN Trophic enteral feeds of semi-elemental formula if patient unable to eat
3. Introduction of solids	Minimal or no GI cramping Formed stool	Oral: Allow introduction of solid food, once every 3 to 4 hours: minimal lactose, low fiber, low fat (20–40 g/day), low total acidity, no gastric irritants	Begin to cycle and decrease PN Advance feeds slowly (small boluses or continuous infusion) if patient unable to eat
4. Expansion of diet	Minimal or no GI cramping Formed stool	Oral: Minimal lactose, low fiber, low total acidity, no gastric irritants; if stools indicate fat malabsorption, low fat	Nighttime supplemental PN if oral intake less than needs or patient unable to maintain weight owing to malabsorption Enteral feed schedule and formula dependent on any residual GI symptoms
5. Resumption of regular diet	No GI cramping Normal stool Normal transit time Normal albumin	Oral: Progress to regular diet by introducing one restricted food per day; acid foods with meals, fiber-containing foods, lactose-containing foods; order of addition will vary depending on individual tolerances and preferences Patients no longer exhibiting steatorrhea should have the fat restriction liberalized slowly	Discontinue PN Supplemental enteral feeds if patient unable to consume adequate nutrients

Abbreviations: GI, gastrointestinal; GVHD, graft-versus-host disease; NPO, nil per os (nothing by mouth).

Source: Gauvreau JM, Lenssen P, Cheney CL, Aker SN, Hutchinson ML, Barale KV. Nutritional management of patients with intestinal graft-versus-host disease. *J Am Diet Assoc.* 981;79:673–677.

the complete blood count must be interpreted cautiously once therapy begins. Biochemical indices on renal and hepatic function as well as serum lipids, glucose, and electrolytes should always be reviewed for detection of nutrient deficiencies.

Serum albumin is used to evaluate internal protein status. A concentration of less than 3.2 g/dL may reflect early malnutrition; however, the measurement does not necessarily establish malnutrition, because infection, excessive GI or renal losses, impaired liver function, certain chemotherapy agents, and overhydration each depress serum albumin levels.[27] Furthermore, because the half-life is 20 days or longer, serum albumin levels may not be as clinically useful as prealbumin, which has a much shorter biologic half-life of approximately 2 days. Prealbumin is less influenced by changes in body fluids than serum albumin is, making it a more reliable test with which to evaluate nutritional status. With a shorter half-life, prealbumin provides for more frequent measurements, which makes it more sensitive in identifying malnutrition that is otherwise undetectable by anthropometric data such as weight loss, BMI, or hypoalbuminemia. Therefore, the shorter half-life of prealbumin shows whether there is a correlation between the cancer treatment and improvements in calorie and protein intake as well as weight gain in pediatric cancer patients.[27] Like albumin, however, prealbumin measurements may also be influenced by infection and fever. Nevertheless, given its preferred biochemical attributes, prealbumin is the best available marker of nutritional status.

Nutrition History

The nutrition history includes a comprehensive assessment of current oral and GI symptoms including chewing or swallowing difficulties, mucositis and esophagitis, taste alterations, xerostomia, heartburn, nausea and vomiting, early satiety, changes in appetite, and altered bowel habits. Current dietary modifications including use of special diets, presence of food allergies, food aversions or intolerances, and use of vitamin, mineral, and herbal supplements should also be included in the initial evaluation. Stage of eating development (e.g., self-feeding skills, puree versus table food, bottle versus cup) and use of infant formulas or breastfeeding should also be assessed.

Physical Assessment

Careful clinical observation is valuable to detect the presence of obesity, emaciation, dehydration, or edema.

Other Assessment Tools

The child's medical history, physical strength, activity level, organ function, and level of pain and pain control, which may interfere with oral intake, should be evaluated.

Nutrient Requirements

Nutrient requirements during childhood cancer are described in **Table 17-7**. The goals are to:

- Provide adequate nutrition to preserve lean tissue and promote growth and development
- Identify and prevent or correct protein-energy malnutrition
- Prevent or correct metabolic abnormalities
- Maximize quality of life

Energy and Protein Requirements

Energy requirements should be based on age, weight, gender, therapy, and growth needs.[18] Although the dietary reference intakes (DRI) for energy and protein are categorized by age and gender, they may not be appropriate in this population. Factors affecting nutrient needs include inactivity, bacterial sepsis, fever secondary to neutropenia, or secondary complications such as neutropenic enterocolitis. Basal metabolic rate[28] with additions for growth, infection, and stress can be used to determine energy needs. Multiplying the basal metabolic rate by a factor of 1.6 to 1.8 for very young or malnourished children will allow for growth, stress, and light activity.[18] The Harris-Benedict formula and other equations have been used to estimate calorie needs in adults and may be appropriate for children who have completed their growth.[29]

Vitamins, Minerals, and Other Requirements

Vitamin and mineral requirements have not been determined for children with cancer. Recommendations are based on the DRI (Appendix H). Extensive radiation or surgical damage to the GI tract and treatment with long-term antibiotic therapy for chronic infections may also increase the child's need for vitamins and minerals. Specific nutrient deficiencies may occur from therapy-related treatments; however, they are difficult to identify without laboratory assay. Most children receiving cancer treatment benefit from taking an age-specific multivitamin/mineral supplement without iron, to prevent iron overload, which may develop due to red cell transfusions during therapy.

Children diagnosed with ALL, non-Hodgkin's lymphoma, or those who develop GVHD following HCT are especially at risk for developing osteopenia and fractures due to the use of corticosteroids during treatment.[9,30] Corticosteroids disrupt calcium absorption,[31] and the natural intake of calcium and vitamin D from the child's own diet is often insufficient to meet increased needs. Therefore, calcium and vitamin D supplementation, in addition to the multivitamin/mineral supplement, is often necessary to maintain bone health.

Children undergoing HCT require additional vitamin C to promote tissue recovery via collagen biosynthesis after cytoreductive therapy (see Table 17-7).[18] Some chemotherapies, as well as medications used to treat fungal and viral infections (e.g., ambisone, foscarnet) are nephrotoxic and may cause increased losses of certain minerals. For example, cisplatin commonly causes magnesium, phosphorus, potassium, and zinc wasting.[11] Children undergoing cancer treatment with nephrotoxic chemotherapy agents may require long-term supplementation of these nutrients.

Vitamin D

Vitamin D deficiency is pandemic across all age groups in industrialized nations and is now currently at the forefront of the medical and nutrition literature.[32] Historically, the majority of research has centered on the link between vitamin D deficiency and rickets in children and exacerbation of osteoporosis in adults. Currently, there are prospective

TABLE 17-7 Nutrient Requirements During Childhood Cancer

Nutrient Requirements	Recommendations

Calories	• Infants: Birth to 12 months: Use RDA for age for appropriate weight infants. Use catch-up growth calculation if underweight: (Kcal/kg/day = Kcal/kg/day for weight age × ideal weight age (kg) ÷ actual weight in kg)
	• Older children (> than 1 year): Use BMR table multiplied by additional factors:
	  • Appropriate weight for height: BMR × 1.6
	  • Obese: BMR × 1.3
	  • Sedentary with 5% weight loss: BMR × 1.4–1.6
	  • 10% weight loss from usual weight or weight is 90% or less of usual or ideal weight: BMR × 1.8–2.0
	• Use adjusted weight calculation for obese children; BMI weight at the 75th percentile may also be used to calculate energy needs in obese children
	• HCT: BMR × 1.6 during immediate posttransplant course; BMR × 1.4 following engraftment and medically stable

Protein	• Infants birth to 6 months: 3 g/kg/day • Infants 6 to 12 months: 2.5–3 g/kg/day • Children: 2–2.5 g/kg/day (in most cases) • Adolescents with increased lean body mass: 1.5–1.8 g/kg/day
Fat	• 10–30% total calories
Fluid	• 1–10 kg: 100 mL/kg/day • 11–20 kg: 1000 mL plus 50 ml for every kg > 10 per day • 21–40 kg: 1500 mL plus 20 mL for every kg > 20 per day • > 40 kg: 1500 mL/m^2 body surface area
Vitamins	• Use ASPEN[47] parenteral vitamin guidelines for age • After PN discontinued, oral multiple vitamin/mineral without iron, during antineoplastic therapy • Provide additional vitamin C during HCT: < 31 kg, additional 250 mg vitamin C per day > 31 kg, additional 500 mg vitamin C per day
Minerals and electrolytes	• Iron supplementation contraindicated during oncologic therapy and HCT • Eliminate copper and manganese from PN in presence of hepatic dysfunction (i.e., serum bilirubin > 10.0 mg/dL) • Closely monitor serum electrolytes during therapy

Abbreviations: ASPEN, American Society for Parenteral and Enteral Nutrition; BEE, basal energy expenditure; BMI, body mass index; BMR, basal metabolic rate; CDC, Centers for Disease Control and Prevention; PN, parenteral nutrition; RDA, recommended dietary allowance.

studies evaluating the relationship between vitamin D deficiency and risk for development of cancer and other chronic diseases.[33] Although determining a clear relationship between vitamin D deficiency and the development of certain diseases is in the early stages of research,[34] practitioners who care for children with cancer should routinely measure the serum 25-OH vitamin D level to evaluate for deficiency.

Omega-3 Fatty Acids

Certain medications, including tacrolimus, corticosteroids, and all-trans retinoic acid, are known to cause a fluctuation and possible increase in serum triglyceride levels.[35] Because clinical trials have shown that fish oil (omega-3 fatty acids including docosahexaenoic and eicosapentaenoic acid) supplementation can improve hypertriglyceridemia (≥ 500 mg/dL) in adults,[36] it is an accepted practice among pediatric practitioners to use this Food and Drug Administration approved therapy for children with cancer. It is provided when the child is tolerating oral medications.

Nutrition Support

There is a wide range of practices regarding the timing, duration, and method of nutrition intervention in children with cancer.[5] A paper published by the COG Nutrition Committee presented results from a survey involving 233 participating cancer institutions.[37] The results showed there is no uniform approach to nutrition assessment or intervention among various cancer centers. The primary goal of nutrition therapy for the pediatric oncology population is to sustain and promote normal growth and development while undergoing necessary anticancer therapy.

Oral Diet

Suboptimal oral intake of short duration during treatment is of less concern if the child is initially well-nourished and can compensate or eat more when feeling well. These children may benefit from high-density foods that increase energy and other nutrient levels of the diet. Suggestions for boosting the nutrient density of foods consumed are shown in **Table 17-8**. Dietary guidelines for managing common nutrition problems seen during and following therapy are addressed in **Table 17-9**.

Refeeding a child following intensive cancer therapy may be a slow process because the child's appetite and tolerance for food fluctuate widely. Young children with preexisting delays in feeding development should have intervention from a feeding team. Determination of feeding skills in the young child will facilitate choices for self-feeding because many young children's feeding skills will regress during intense oncologic therapy.

Individualizing the child's diet by including frequent servings of foods enjoyed (in the absence of oral and GI symptoms) may enhance oral intake. Although many commercial liquid medical nutritional supplements designed for pediatric patients are currently available, taste acceptance

TABLE 17-8 Guidelines for Increasing Nutrient Density

Butter, margarine, and oils • Add to soup, mashed and baked potatoes, hot cereal, grits, rice, noodles, and cooked vegetables.	• Stir into sauces and gravies.
Cream • Use on desserts, gelatin, pudding, fruit, pancakes, waffles, and mashed potatoes. • Use in soups, sauces, egg dishes, batters, puddings, and custards; put on cereals.	• Mix with pasta, mashed potatoes, and rice. • Substitute for milk in recipes. • Make cocoa with cream and add marshmallows.
Sour cream • Add to soups, baked potatoes, vegetables, sauces, salad dressings, gelatin desserts, bread, and muffin batter.	• Use as dip for raw fruits and vegetables.
Mayonnaise • Add to salad dressing. • Spread on sandwiches and crackers.	• Use in sauces and gelatin desserts.
Honey (use in children over 1 year of age) • Add to cereal, milk drinks, fruit desserts, smoothies, or yogurt.	• Use as a glaze for meats such as chicken.
Granola • Use in cookie, muffin, and bread batters. • Sprinkle on vegetables, yogurt, ice cream, pudding, custard, and fruit.	• Mix with dried fruits and nuts for a snack. • Substitute for bread or rice in pudding recipes.
Dried fruits and nuts • Cook and serve dried fruits for breakfast or as dessert. • Add to muffins, cookies, breads, cakes, rice and grain dishes, cereals, puddings, and stuffing.	• Bake in pies and turnovers. • Combine with cooked vegetables such as carrots, sweet potatoes, or acorn and butternut squash.
Milk and cheese • Mix one cup dry milk powder in four cups of liquid milk; use this milk for cooking and baking. • Add milk powder directly to hot or cold cereals, scrambled eggs, soups, gravies, casserole dishes, and desserts.	• Add grated cheese or chunks of cheese to sauces, vegetables, soups, salads, and casseroles. • Spread cream cheese on hot buttered bread.
Eggs • Add eggs to soups and casseroles.	• Slice boiled eggs in sauces and serve over rice, cooked noodles, buttered toast, or hot biscuits.
Peanut butter • Add peanut butter to sauces; use on crackers, waffles, or celery sticks.	• Spread peanut butter on hot buttered bread.

Source: Medical Nutrition Therapy Services, Seattle Cancer Care Alliance, Seattle, Washington.

TABLE 17-9 Dietary Guidelines for Managing Common Nutrition Problems of Children with Cancer

Oral and esophageal mucositis (inflammation of the oral and esophageal mucosa) • Try soft or pureed foods or a blenderized liquid diet. • Offer soft, nonirritating, cold foods (popsicles, ice cream, frozen yogurt, slushes) and smooth, bland, moist foods (custard, cream soups, mashed potatoes).	• Encourage frequent mouth rinsing to remove food and bacteria and promote healing.
Xerostomia (oral dryness) • Offer moist foods (stews, casseroles, canned fruit) and liquids. • Add sauce, gravy, margarine, butter, or broth to dry foods.	• Drink liquids with meals. • Offer sugar-free lemon-flavored candy to help stimulate saliva. • Encourage good oral hygiene.
Thick, viscous saliva and mucous • Try club soda, hot tea with lemon, or a beverage with citric acid. • Encourage adequate fluid intake.	• Encourage good oral hygiene.
Dysgeusia (impaired taste) • Enhance food taste with herbs, spices, flavor extracts, and marinades. • Offer cold foods. • Offer fruit-flavored beverages.	• Try tart foods like oranges or lemonade, which may have more taste. • Encourage good oral hygiene. • Offer fluids with meals to help take away a bad taste in the mouth.
Nausea and vomiting • Try high carbohydrate foods and fluids (crackers, toast, gelatin) and nonacidic juices. • Try small, frequent feedings. • Offer cold, clear liquids and solids. • Avoid overly sweet or high fat foods. • Avoid feeding in a stuffy, too-warm room or one filled with cooking odors or other odors that might be disagreeable.	• Encourage drinking or sipping liquids frequently throughout the day; using a straw may help. • Encourage rest periods after meals. • Avoid offering favorite foods when nauseated; it may cause a permanent dislike of the food.
Diarrhea • Try a low-fat, low-fiber, low-lactose diet. • Avoid caffeine.	• Eat warm or room temperature foods because hot foods may increase bowel motility • Encourage adequate fluids to prevent dehydration.
Constipation • Encourage fluids. • Drink hot liquids to increase bowel activity.	• Offer high-fiber foods.
Other helpful hints • Take the child's sports bottle filled with a favorite beverage when going shopping or to a clinic appointment. • If lack of appetite is a problem at mealtimes, limit snacks and fluids for 1 to 2 hours before the meal. • Serve food "family style" to allow the child to dish out his or her own food portions.	• Serve very small servings on a large dinner plate so that portions will not look as overwhelming. • Arrange foods creatively on plates. • Serve brightly colored foods and different food shapes together. • Offer new foods along with favorite foods. • Allow the child to help prepare the food.

Source: Medical Nutrition Therapy Services, Seattle Cancer Care Alliance, Seattle, Washington.

may be a limiting factor. Shakes made with familiar products and supplemented by glucose polymers or other nondetectable modular components (e.g., protein or fat) are usually best tolerated. Supplements are often acceptable if offered in an unobtrusive manner as part of the regular meal or snack pattern. For the lactose-intolerant child, lactose-free or soy-based products (e.g., soy milk, soy-based or milk-based lactose-free commercial medical nutritional supplements) can be useful. Oral and esophageal lesions may limit tolerance for oral supplements. Hyperosmolar or lactose-containing products may aggravate diarrhea. Encouragement from staff, parental involvement, patient education, and nutrition classes can help improve acceptance of supplements.

For a thorough evaluation of the child's intake, daily food intake records provide a basis for decisions regarding supplemental or nonvolitional feeding. Parenteral or enteral nutrient solutions, other intravenous fluids, and oral intake must all be included when evaluating intake. Older children and family members may assist with record keeping and provide valuable intake information.

Enteral Nutrition

Over the past 20 years, enteral tube feeding has become the primary nutrition intervention strategy for children and adolescents undergoing cancer treatment. Such children already require placement of a central line for chemotherapy, intravenous fluids, medications, and the administration of blood products. Therefore, because the central line was in place, medical oncologists and pediatric oncology dietitians formerly used the central line to also administer PN to those children who could not maintain their weight by eating. However, now that nutrition is an accepted supportive-care modality in the treatment of childhood cancer, enteral tube feeding has become the preferred method of providing the child with safe, beneficial, and physiologic nutrition support. Because tube feeding maintains the function and integrity of the GI tract, its other benefits include reduced risk for infection and that it is a more cost-effective therapy than PN. For children who have difficulty taking oral medications, enteral tube feeding provides a safe route for administration. Finally, feeding tubes can help reduce anxiety in children, parents, and providers from failing to meet nutrient and fluid goals via oral feeding.

Overcoming barriers to successful nasogastric (NG) tube placement requires skilled pediatric oncology dietitians, dedicated oncology nurses, nurse practitioners, and an educated medical staff. A team approach for NG tube placement can be highly effective. Child life specialists are invaluable in helping children better understand and cope with the fear and discomfort of the NG tube placement. Thus, the necessity for NG tube placement must be presented to the child and family in a positive manner to restore the malnourished child back to normal weight and health, or to prevent further nutrition deficits in at-risk children.

The following criteria may be useful when considering enteral tube feeding candidates:

- Interval or total weight loss of $>$ 5% of pre-illness body weight (usual weight).
- Weight for height reaches $\leq$ 90% of ideal weight for height, adjusted for height and age.
- BMI falls to or below the 10th percentile.
- Repeated attempts to meet nutrient needs orally have failed.
- Child or adolescent has functioning GI tract.
- Lowest weight threshold: an agreed upon weight, determined by healthcare providers and parents that if reached, is unsafe for the child or adolescent to proceed with therapy without enteral nutrition support intervention. This can be based on the above criteria.

Current practice at Seattle Children's Hospital is for NG tube placement in children, from birth to young adulthood, whose weight decreases to or below 90% of ideal weight for height for age. At our institution, we conducted a retrospective review of 57 children with nonmetastatic sarcoma (mean age 12 years; range 1 to 21 years) who received intensive chemotherapy during the period from 2002 to 2005.[38] Severe malnutrition (less than 80% of ideal weight for height for age) occurred in 2% at diagnosis, 9% at nadir (lowest recorded weight during treatment), and 4% at time of local radiation or surgery. Enteral tube feedings were used in 44% of patients for a mean of 138 days (range 1 to 310 days). Gastrostomy tubes were used in two children, both with parameningeal (tumor next to brain) primary sites. Additionally, PN was used in 21% of children for a mean of 11 days (range 3 to 38 days). We concluded that malnutrition during intensive chemotherapy for pediatric sarcomas can usually be prevented with aggressive enteral nutrition support, which proved to be feasible and well-tolerated for extended durations.[38]

Interest in the use of enteral nutrition support for children undergoing HCT has increased in the past decade due to the need to decrease cost and the desire to mitigate the risks associated with PN, especially infection.[16] Enteral feedings may also help to maintain mucosal integrity and further decrease infections and the inflammatory response.[39]

Despite this interest, case series and pilot studies have suggested major challenges when using enteral nutrition in the pediatric HCT population. Complications such as dislodgement of nasoenteral tubes;[40,41] delayed gastric emptying;[42] inadequate electrolyte and mineral intake, specifically calcium, magnesium, phosphorus, and zinc;[43] and inadequate energy intake[40,44,45] have been reported. The combined use of enteral feedings with PN during HCT is an acceptable and cost-effective alternative.[46] Candidates for enteral nutrition during HCT include children who:

- Receive nonmyeloablative or reduced-intensity conditioning regimen
- Fail to recover appetite and resume eating after engraftment and resolution of conditioning-related mucositis and esophagitis
- Have chronic GVHD (i.e., oral, esophageal, liver, pulmonary, weight loss, quiescent phases of GI)

- Have neurological complications that preclude safe swallowing
- Are ventilated[47,48]

Parenteral Nutrition

During cancer therapy, the child's GI tract may not be usable for oral diet or enteral feedings due to complications associated with surgery, nausea and vomiting, diarrhea, colitis, pancreatitis, intestinal GVHD, ileus, or radiation enteritis. In these situations, PN is indicated. The decision to use PN is often based upon the child's nutritional status, type of therapy, expected oral and GI complications associated with the chosen treatment, and availability of peripheral veins. Multiple lumen central venous catheters are often placed at the start of treatment for delivery of medications and blood products, so access is available for PN and hydration fluids. Cyclic or home PN can be used to provide nutrition support while allowing the child time out of the hospital. A home health agency can work with caregivers to provide PN solutions, education, and monitoring.

Children maintained on PN support must be closely monitored to ensure that nutrient and fluid requirements are met and that any serum electrolyte alterations, especially as a result of medications and/or GI losses, are corrected promptly. Early studies showed that nutrition support provided to children undergoing intense oncologic therapy resulted in improved treatment tolerance with fewer treatment delays and accelerated recovery of bone marrow function.[49,50]

Due to intensive treatment regimens, PN has been the standard nutrition support therapy for children undergoing HCT.[48] Improved visceral protein status,[51] maintenance of body weight,[52] and earlier engraftment following cytoreductive therapy[53] have been observed in pediatric transplant patients. Improved disease-free survival has been reported in allogeneic transplant patients who received prophylactic PN.[54]

Special Considerations

In addition to ongoing monitoring and assessment throughout the child's treatment course, the pediatric oncology dietitian must also be aware of special considerations that may impact the child's nutritional status.

Long-Term Nutritional Sequelae

Chronic complications associated with cancer therapy may impact a child's nutritional status and require intervention for several years. Endocrine and growth disorders (e.g., thyroid disease, obesity, alterations in pubertal development), osteonecrosis, cardiopulmonary disease, and neurologic or neurosensory disorders have been described.[25]

Growth hormone deficiency with decreased growth velocity and delayed onset of puberty have been observed in children following HCT.[55] Children who have received cranial irradiation prior to HCT show growth hormone deficiency with deceleration of normal growth rates.[55] Regular evaluations to determine occurrence of endocrine gland dysfunction are recommended.

Medical complications of long-term survivors of HCT are well-recognized,[56,57] and include chronic GVHD,[58] osteoporosis,[30] hyperlipidemia,[59] hyperglycemia,[59,60] and infection.[61]

Integrative Medicine

The use of complementary or integrative therapies by the pediatric oncology population is becoming increasingly more prevalent. Parents seek out these therapies for their children undergoing conventional cancer treatments for many reasons, including a desire to relieve the burden of side effects caused by chemotherapy, motivation to find a cure, pursuit of greater control over their child's disease, improved quality of life, and hope.[62] For these reasons, parents often choose nonconventional therapies such as herbs, high-dose antioxidants, homeopathy, and botanicals that they feel may help their child, but are unaware of potential harmful effects or if the therapy may interfere with conventional treatments. Parents of children with relapsed cancer will more frequently turn to use of alternative therapies than those with an initial diagnosis.[62] The integrative therapies that are frequently used and are reported to help alleviate treatment side effects, including nausea, vomiting, pain, and anxiety, are acupuncture and massage.[13]

The use of herbals and megavitamin therapy in the treatment of childhood cancer raises several concerns, including:

- Unexpected or undesirable interactions between preparations and prescribed medications may affect the action of drugs routinely used during the course of chemotherapy and HCT.
- Potential contamination of preparations derived from plants poses the risk of bacterial, fungal, or parasitic infections. A few specific preparations have been associated with serious toxic side effects or infections.[20]
- Alternative nutrition therapy may be chosen as the sole source of treatment.

There is ongoing debate regarding the concurrent use of dietary antioxidants and their potential interaction with chemotherapeutic agents,[62,63] Those who support the use of antioxidants believe there is evidence that they protect healthy cells from the toxic effects of chemotherapy drugs while at the same time leaving the cancer cells exposed to the drugs. A classic example is the use of the dietary antioxidant coenzyme Q10, which, when combined with doxorubicin, was touted to protect cardiac tissue.[64] Those who argue against the use of antioxidants during chemotherapy are concerned that these nutrients will interfere with or reduce the efficacy of chemotherapeutic agents that use reactive oxygen species as a mechanism for cytotoxicity.[63]

Herbal and botanical preparations are derived directly from plants and may be sold as tablets, capsules, liquids, extracts, teas, powders, or topical preparations; however, the dose is dependent on the potency of the preparation. The potential for herbs and other supplements to interact with chemotherapy has been reported only in adults. The sole clinical trial that has measured the interaction between a natural health product and chemotherapy examined the effect of St John's wort on plasma concentrations of SN38, the active metabolite of irinotecan.[62] The study concluded there was a reduction in systemic exposure to SN38 by 42%, when given concurrently with St. John's wort, which resulted in drug failure of irinotecan.[62]

Some herbals are contraindicated in children with cancer because of their association with serious side effects. Garlic and gingko biloba may reduce blood-clotting factors.[65,66] Other botanicals containing pyrrolizidine alkaloids, such as comfrey and maté tea, may induce hepatotoxicity.[67] Herbal preparations should be discontinued during HCT. The pediatric oncology dietitian must be sensitive to the family's views and biases and educate the healthcare team appropriately.

Diet for the Immunosuppressed Child

The goal of the diet for the immunosuppressed child is to maximize healthy food options while minimizing GI exposure to pathogenic organisms resulting in increased morbidity and mortality.[68] Although no empirical research exists on the relative benefits of restricting specific food groups, most facilities place restrictions ranging from no raw fresh fruits or vegetables to a specific low microbial diet.[68–70]

Table 17-10 shows an example of diet restrictions for immunosuppressed children. High-risk foods, identified as potential sources of organisms known to cause infection during immunosuppression, are restricted. In recent years, many transplant centers have liberalized their diets to allow well-washed raw fruits and vegetables. Recommendations on the duration of the diet are based on treatment and type of HCT.

Food Safety

Providing education on food safety may be more important in reducing food-borne illness than extensive diet restrictions.[71] A food-handling observational study showed that healthy people repeatedly made food-handling errors in their home, thus increasing risk.[71] Improper holding temperatures and/or personal hygiene of food handlers

TABLE 17-10 Diet Guidelines for Immunosuppressed Patients

These guidelines are intended to minimize the introduction of pathogenic organisms into the GI tract by food while maximizing healthy food options for immunosuppressed children. These guidelines should be coupled with food safety education to assume proper food preparation and storage in the home and hospital kitchen. High-risk foods, identified as potential sources of organisms known to cause infection in immunosuppressed children, are restricted.

In general, these guidelines should be followed by children who have an absolute neutrophil count of below 1×103 μl. Children receiving an autologous transplant should follow the diet for the first 3 months after HCT; children receiving an allogeneic transplant should follow the diet until off all immunosuppressive therapy (i.e., cyclosporine, tacrolimus, prednisone).

Food Restrictions

Contraindicated:

- Raw and undercooked meat (including game), fish, shellfish, poultry, eggs, sausage, and bacon
- Raw tofu, unless pasteurized or aseptically packaged
- Luncheon meats (including salami, bologna, hot dogs, ham, and others) unless heated until steaming
- Refrigerated smoked seafood typically labeled as lox, kippered, nova-style, or smoked or fish jerky (unless contained in a cooked dish); pickled fish
- Nonpasteurized milk and raw milk products, nonpasteurized cheese, and nonpasteurized yogurt
- Blue-veined cheeses, including blue, Gorgonzola, Roquefort, and Stilton
- Uncooked soft cheeses including brie, camembert, feta, and farmer's
- Mexican-style soft cheese, including queso blanco and queso fresco
- Cheese containing chili peppers or other uncooked vegetables
- Fresh salad dressings (stored in the grocer's refrigerated case) containing raw eggs or contraindicated cheeses
- Unwashed raw and frozen fruits and vegetables and those with visible mold; all raw vegetable sprouts (alfalfa, mung bean, all others)
- Raw or unpasteurized honey
- Unpasteurized commercial fruit and vegetable juices

Source: Medical Nutrition Therapy Services, Seattle Cancer Care Alliance, Seattle, Washington.

contribute most to disease incidence.[72] Education should emphasize hand washing; high-risk foods; proper temperatures for storage, defrosting, and cooking; cross-contamination issues; correct cooling and reheating procedures; and sanitation.

Several infections are of particular concern with the pediatric oncology population, including Salmonella enteritis, *Campylobacter jejuni, E. coli* 0157:H7, and *Listeria monocytogenes*. The CDC publishes food-borne illness diagnosis and management recommendations for healthcare professionals.[73]

Special Food Service Needs

The food service for pediatric oncology patients should be designed to provide a variety of foods served at frequent intervals to meet the child's tolerance. Traditional hospital food services with set menus, trayline service, rigid meal hours, and 24-hour advance menu selection often do not meet the needs of many pediatric oncology and transplant patients. A more flexible food service, such as unit nourishment centers or satellite kitchens, will provide opportunities for oral intake.[74]

Some facilities have implemented hotel-style room service with extended hours (up to 24 hours/day), telephone ordering systems, short delivery times, and elimination of wasted trays.[75] At one facility, children's caloric intake improved significantly and protein intake increased by 18% after the introduction of room service. Satisfaction with hospital food also improved, with excellent ratings increasing by 35%.[75]

Feeding Relationship and Family-Centered Care

An often overlooked and unintended consequence of pediatric cancer therapy is the disruption to the relationship between parents and their children in the area of food and nutrition. Because anticancer therapy often causes nausea, vomiting, loss of appetite, and taste alterations, children lose the pleasure of eating. By nature, children look to their parents for their daily food intake and parents instinctively assume and guard their nurturing role as the primary food provider. Frequently, neither children nor parents are prepared for the intervening influence and directives of the pediatric oncology dietitian, whose responsibilities include counseling parents and age-appropriate children in new eating habits, patterns, and food choices critical to cancer treatment. Parents can quickly sense a loss of control in their role as providers, and children can suffer from the loss of their comfort foods and mealtime rituals and routines. The potential disruption to eating patterns and habits can be a source of stress and anxiety for the child and can lead to a family that becomes overly focused on food. Therefore, it is essential that the pediatric oncology dietitian understand and appreciate the parent–child–food relationship and support both the parent's role and the child's need for his or her parent to continue as the food provider. While educating the parents and age-appropriate children on their essential diet and nutritional needs and the side effects of therapy, the pediatric oncology dietitian must reinforce and support both the parents' needs to make appropriate dietary decisions for their children and the child's needs for security, familiarity, and routine. Such family-centered care, including respect for the feeding dynamics between parents and children, is an essential component of pediatric cancer treatment.

Promoting Oral Intake During Hospitalization

Encouraging oral intake in a young child with cancer is challenging. Anxious, scared, or depressed children do not feel like eating. Chronic pain may also decrease the child's interest in eating. Providing a calm, relaxed hospital atmosphere for eating, with uninterrupted time for feeding (e.g., door closed, sign posted) may improve intake. Small children require a secure feeding position (e.g., high chair, toddler feeding table), a bib, towel, and covered floor area to limit anxiety over spills.

Children should not be forced to eat. A maximum mealtime of 20 to 30 minutes should be adequate, and the child should be provided with food textures and portion sizes that are age appropriate. Older children may benefit from group eating situations, such as a playroom area, or participatory food preparation times, as well as by knowing their oral intake goals for hospital discharge. Many facilities implement an outside food policy, allowing the child's family or caregivers to bring food that conforms to the medical diet order into the hospital. These items are usually not stored on the unit; perishable foods must be consumed immediately. Family education in food safety is vital.

For children refusing to eat, behavior modification techniques may be necessary.[76] Children transitioning from tube feeding may exhibit oral, motor, sensory, and developmental feeding problems that make weaning difficult. A weaning process based on developmental stages is recommended.[77]

Sickle Cell Disease

Sickle cell disease (SCD) is a genetic disorder characterized by the production of abnormal hemoglobin, which causes red blood cells to become sickle shaped. Sickle-shaped red blood cells trigger inflammation, coagulation, and platelet aggregation resulting in inadequate tissue blood flow and chronic anemia. Clinical manifestations of SCD include severe painful crises, acute chest syndrome, splenic sequestration, stroke, chronic pulmonary and renal dysfunction, delayed growth, neuropsychological deficits, and premature death.[78] According to the National Institutes of Health,[79] SCD affects approximately 70,000 individuals in the United States, primarily African Americans.

Paramount in supportive care for SCD is the prevention of pain crises. Chronic blood transfusions, pain management, antibiotics to prevent infections, and immunizations are also necessary. The only curative treatment for SCD is HCT.[80] Children receiving a matched sibling HCT have a > 80% overall disease-free survival rate.[80]

Nutrition assessment, nutrient requirements, and nutrition support practices for children with SCD do not differ from children with other oncologic or hematologic disorders; however, children with SCD may be at risk for specific nutrient deficiencies. Altered vitamin A,[81] vitamin B_6,[82] red blood cell folate,[83] and vitamin D[84] status have been described and emphasize the need for regular monitoring and supplementation as indicated. Most children with SCD do require folic acid supplementation. Delayed skeletal maturation with altered bone development has also been reported.[85] Hepatic iron overload is another serious complication of SCD due to chronic transfusion therapy.[86] Treatment for iron overload includes chelation therapy, which may cause depletion of divalent cations such as calcium and magnesium. Although delayed growth may be observed in children with SCD, one multi-center trial showed improved linear growth following HCT.[87]

Nutrition Education for Children with SCD

Oral intake may be compromised during acute pain crises, so a diet emphasizing nutrient-dense foods with provision of adequate calories and protein should be emphasized for children with SCD. Long-term suboptimal nutrition support may impact growth and development. Maintaining an adequate hydration status is also necessary because dehydration may cause sickling of red blood cells. An iron-free multivitamin/mineral supplement is recommended for all children with SCD.

Conclusion

The nutrition needs of the child with cancer are an important consideration in the overall treatment plan. Optimum nutrition management of this highly complex population is vital because children with cancer experience multiple adverse oral and GI nutritional complications as a result of both the disease and treatment. Dietary modifications, due to therapy-induced adverse nutritional effects, are frequently necessary to promote an appropriate intake while encouraging a well-balanced diet. Specialized nutrition support may be required to ensure that nutrient needs are met to promote adequate growth and development. Ongoing education provides an opportunity to teach age-appropriate nutrition and food safety concepts to support cancer therapies.

Case Study

Nutrition Assessment

A previously healthy 7-year-old female presented to her primary care physician for a well-child visit. During the appointment, it was observed that the child was pale. Parents gave a history of easy bruising, which had persisted for the past 2 months. A complete blood count with differential showed anemia, thrombocytopenia, and a white blood cell count of 65,000 thou/μL (normal: 4500–13,500 thou/μL).

Family history: negative for cancers.

Patient was referred to Seattle Children's Hospital for further evaluation.

A diagnosis of acute myelogenous leukemia (AML)-M4 (select marker) was confirmed by bone marrow biopsy. Other markers notable for central nervous system–negative disease with FLT 3 marker (poor prognostic indicator).

Anthropometric Measurements

Height: 128.1 cm

Weight: 24.2 kg

Ideal weight for height: 26 kg (50th percentile CDC height)

Nutrition History

No known allergies.

Typical day's intake: three meals with snacks throughout the day

Breakfast: pancakes or cereal with 2% milk or yogurt and cheese

Lunch: sandwich (ham or turkey with cheese and butter) or caesar salad with ranch dressing or macaroni and cheese

Dinner: chicken or pasta with butter (no sauce) or steak or pizza, vegetables

Snacks: carrots, broccoli, bananas, apples, melon, grapes, strawberries

Taking a pediatric multivitamin supplement

During the first round of induction chemotherapy, the patient's weight decreased to a nadir of 22.2 kg, 6 days into treatment (85% of ideal weight for height). Patient had symptoms of nausea, vomiting, and increased stooling.

A nasogastric (NG) enteral tube was placed for initiation of a 1 kcal/mL pediatric elemental formula; however, due to mucositis and bloody stools, she did not tolerate NG feeds well.

Computed tomography (CT) scan confirmed typhilitis and pancolitis. Patient placed NPO and maintained on full total parenteral nutrition (TPN) support.

Nutrition Diagnosis/Problem

The above items can now be used to determine a nutrition diagnosis or problem. Inadequate energy intake related to altered gastrointestinal function and increased energy needs as evidenced by bloody diarrhea and weight loss of > 8% of usual body weight in one week.

Nutrition Intervention

Goal: Patient will be able to regain weight lost and maintain an acceptable weight throughout therapy.

Food/nutrient delivery: Patient to be placed NPO and TPN instituted.

Nutrition education: Educate patient/caregivers on need to remain NPO, to allow gut rest for healing of current gastrointestinal symptoms.

Nutrition counseling: Patient to remain NPO with TPN support until resolution of typhilitis and pancolitis. When symptoms have resolved, reinstitute NG feeds as tolerated and educate patient/caregivers on appropriate food/fluid choices.

Coordination of nutrition care: Work regularly with medical team (e.g., primary provider, team nurse) following patient.

Monitoring and Evaluation

After placing patient NPO for 12 days, a low-lactose, low-fiber, low-acid diet, with three to four foods per tray, was instituted. NG feeds were reinitiated, with a 1 kcal/mL pediatric elemental formula, at an infusion rate of 10 mL/hour. Feeds were slowly advanced over 1 week until a goal of 65 mL/hour × 24 hrs was achieved, at which point TPN was discontinued.

Questions for the Reader

1. What are this patient's energy and protein needs per kg?
2. What are this patient's BMI, height, and weight percentiles on the CDC growth chart?
3. Write one PES statement for this patient.
4. What was the total number of calories once the full tube feeding goal was achieved?

REFERENCES

1. Ries LAG, Smith MA, Gurney JG, et al., eds. *Cancer Incidence and Survival among Children and Adolescents: United States SEER Program 1975–1995*. Bethesda, MD: National Cancer Institute; 1999:1–15. NIH Pub. No. 99-4649.
2. Gurney JG, Bondy ML. Epidemiology of childhood cancer. General principles of chemotherapy. In Pizzo PA, Poplac D, eds. *Principles and Practice of Pediatric Oncology*, 5th ed. Philadelphia, PA: Lippincott Williams & Wilkins; 2006:1–13.
3. Sala A, Pencharz P, Barr RD. Children, cancer, and nutrition—a dynamic triangle. *Cancer.* 2004;100:677–687.
4. Mauer AM, Burgess JB, Donaldson SS, et al. Special nutritional needs of children with malignancies: a review. *J Parenter Enteral Nutr.* 1990;14:315–324.
5. Ladas EJ, Sacks N, Meacham L, et al. A multidisciplinary review of nutrition considerations in the pediatric oncology population: a perspective from Children's Oncology Group. *Nutr Clin Pract.* 2005;20:377–393.
6. Williams DM, Hobson R, Imeson J, Gerrard M, McCarthy K, Pinkerton CR. Anaplastic large cell lymphoma in childhood: analysis of 72 patients treated on the United Kingdom Children's Cancer Study Group chemotherapy regimens. *Br J Haematol.* 2002;117:812–820.
7. Cairo MS, Raetz E, Lim MS, Davenport V, Perkins SL. Childhood and adolescent non-Hodgkin lymphoma: new insights in biology and critical challenges for the future. *Pediatr Blood Cancer.* 2005;45:753–769.
8. Barale KV, Charuhas PM. Oncology and hematopoietic cell transplantation. In: Queen PS, King K, eds. *Handbook of Pediatric Nutrition*, 3rd ed. Sudbury, MA: Jones and Bartlett Publishers; 2005:459–481.
9. Adamson PC, Balis FM, Berg S, Blaney SM. General principles of chemotherapy. In Pizzo PA, Poplac D, eds. *Principles and Practice of Pediatric Oncology*, 5th ed. Philadelphia, PA: Lippincott Williams & Wilkins; 2006:290–365.
10. Chu E, DeVita VT. *Physicians' Cancer Chemotherapy Drug Manual.* Sudbury, MA: Jones and Bartlett Publishers; 2006.
11. Charuhas PM, Aker SN. Nutritional implications of antineoplastic chemotherapeutic agents. *Clin Appl Nutr.* 1992;2:20–33.
12. Keller VE. Management of nausea and vomiting in children. *J Pediatr Nurs.* 1995;10:280–286.
13. Ladas EJ, Post-White J, Hawks R, Taromina K. Evidence for symptom management in the child with cancer. *J Pediatr Hematol Oncol.* 2006;28:601–615.
14. Sherry VW. Taste alterations among patients with cancer. *Clin J Oncol Nurs.* 2002;6:73–76.

15. Kennedy L, Diamond J. Assessment and management of chemotherapy-induced mucositis in children. *J Pediatr Oncol Nurs.* 1997;4:164–174.
16. Lipkin AC, Lenssen P, Dickson BJ. Nutrition issues in hematopoietic stem cell transplantation: state of the art. *Nutr Clin Pract.* 2005;20:423–439.
17. Locatelli F, Giorgiani, Di Cesare-Merlone A, Merli PM, Sparta V, Moretta F. The changing role of stem cell transplantation in childhood. *Bone Marrow Transplant.* 2008;41:S3–S7.
18. Charuhas PM. Pediatric hematopoietic stem cell transplantation. In Hasse JM, Blue LS, eds. *Comprehensive Guide to Transplant Nutrition.* Chicago, IL: American Dietetic Association; 2002:226–247.
19. Vogelsang GB, Lee L, Bensen-Kennedy DM. Pathogenesis and treatment of graft-versus-host disease after bone marrow transplant. *Annu Rev Med.* 2003;54:29–52.
20. Charuhas PM, ed. *Nutrition Care Criteria.* Seattle, WA: Seattle Cancer Care Alliance; 2002.
21. Gauvreau JM, Lenssen P, Cheney CL, Aker SN, Hutchinson ML, Barale KV. Nutritional management of patients with intestinal graft-versus-host disease. *J Am Diet Assoc.* 981;79:673–677.
22. Deeg HJ, Sediel K, Bruemmer B, Pepe MS, Appelbaum F. Impact of patient weight on non-relapse mortality after marrow transplantation. *Bone Marrow Transplant.* 1995;15:461–468.
23. Murry DJ, Riva L, Poplack DG. Impact of nutrition on pharmacokinetics of anti-neoplastic agents. *Int J Cancer Supp.* 1998;11:48–51.
24. Katz JA, Chambers B, Everhart C, Marks JR, Buchanan GR. Linear growth in children with acute lymphoblastic leukemia treated without cranial irradiation. *J Pediatr.* 1991;118:575–578.
25. Diller L, Chow EJ, Gurney JG, et al. Chronic disease in the childhood cancer survivor study cohort: a review of published findings. *J Clin Oncol.* 2009;14:2339–2355.
26. Wiggins KL, ed. *Guidelines for Nutrition of Renal Patients,* 3rd ed. Chicago, IL: American Dietetic Association; 2001:13.
27. Elhasid R, Laor A, Lischinsky S, Postovsky S, Weyl Ben Arush M. Nutritional status of children with solid tumors. *Cancer.* 1999;86:119–125.
28. Altman PL, Dittmer DS. *Metabolism.* Bethesda, MD: Federation of American Societies for Experimental Biology; 1968:344.
29. Bechard LJ, Adiv OE, Jaksic T, Duggan C. Nutritional supportive care. In: Pizzo PA, Poplac D, eds. *Principles and Practice of Pediatric Oncology,* 5th ed. Philadelphia, PA: Lippincott Williams & Wilkins; 2006:1330–1335.
30. Sanders JE, Hoffmeister PA, Storer BA. Treatment of osteopenia/osteoporosis in pediatric hematopoietic cell transplantation [abstract]. *Blood.* 2004;104:57.
31. Zeitler PS, Travers S, Kappy MS. Advances in the recognition and treatment of endocrine complications in children with chronic illness. *Adv Pediatr.* 1999;46:101–149.
32. Cannell JJ, Hollis BW. Use of vitamin D in clinical practice. *Altern Med Rev.* 2008;13:6–20.
33. Holick MF, Chen TC. Vitamin D deficiency: a worldwide problem with health consequences. *Am J Clin Nutr.* 2008;87(Suppl):1080S–1086S.
34. Lappe JM, Travers-Gustafson D, Davies KM, Recker RR, Heaney RP. Vitamin D and calcium supplementation reduces cancer risk: results of a randomized trial. *Am J Clin Nutr.* 2007;85:1586–1591.
35. Sadovsky R, Kris-Etherton P. Prescription omega-3-acid ethyl esters for the treatment of very high triglycerides. *Postgrad Med.* 2009;121:145–153.
36. Bays H. Clinical overview of omacor: a concentrated formulation of omega-3 polyunsaturated fatty acids. *Am J Cardiol.* 2006;98:71i–76i.
37. Rogers PC, Melnick SJ, Ladas EJ, Halton J, Baillargeon J, Sacks N. Children's Oncology Group (COG) Nutrition Committee. *Pediatr Blood Cancer.* 2008;50:447–450.
38. Hawkins DS, Ehling S, Gard K, Hunt K, Conrad C. Nasogastric nutritional support is feasible in pediatric sarcoma patients receiving intensive chemotherapy. Poster presentation at Connective Tissue Oncology Society. 12th Annual Meeting, November 2–4, 2006. Venice, Italy.
39. Johansson JE, Ekman T. Gastrointestinal toxicity related to bone marrow transplantation: disruption of the intestinal barrier precedes clinical finds. *Bone Marrow Transplant.* 1997;19:921–926.
40. Sefcick A, Anderton D, Byrne JL, Teahon K, Russell NH. Nasojejunal feeding in allogeneic bone marrow transplant recipients: results of a pilot study. *Bone Marrow Transplant.* 2001;28:1135–1139.
41. Lenssen P, Bruemmer B, McDonald GB, Aker SN. Nutrient support in hematopoietic cell transplantation. *J Parenter Enteral Nutr.* 2001;25:219–228.
42. Eagle DA, Gian V, Lauwers GY, et al. Gastroparesis following bone marrow transplantation. *Bone Marrow Transplant.* 2001;28:59–62.
43. Papadopoulou A, MacDonald A, Williams MD, Darbyshire PJ, Booth IW. Enteral nutrition after bone marrow transplantation. *Arch Dis Child.* 1997;77:131–136.
44. Langdana A, Tully N, Molloy E, Bourke B, O'Meara A. Intensive enteral nutrition support in paediatric bone marrow transplantation. *Bone Marrow Transplant.* 2001;27:741–746.
45. Szeluga DJ, Stuart RK, Brookmeyer R, Utermohlen V, Santos GW. Nutritional support of bone marrow transplant recipients: a prospective randomized clinical trial comparing total parenteral nutrition to an enteral feeding program. *Cancer Res.* 1987;47:3309–3316.
46. Hopman GD, Pena EG, Le Cessie S, Van Weel MH, Vossen JM, Mearin ML. Tube feeding and bone marrow transplantation. *Med Pediatr Oncol.* 2003;40:375–379.
47. Charuhas PM, Lipkin A, Lenssen P, McMillen K. Hematopoietic stem cell transplantation. In: Merritt R, ed. *The American Society for Parenteral and Enteral Nutrition Support Practice Manual,* 2nd ed. Silver Spring, MD: ASPEN; 2006:187–199.
48. American Society for Parenteral and Enteral Nutrition. Guidelines for the use of parenteral and enteral nutrition in adult and pediatric patients. *J Parenter Enteral Nutr.* 2002; (1Suppl):1SA–138SA.
49. Rickard KA, Detamore CM, Coates TD, et al. Effect of nutrition staging on treatment delays and outcome in stage IV neuroblastoma. *Cancer.* 1983;52(4):587–598.
50. Hays DM, Merritt RJ, White L, Ashley J, Siegel SE. Effect of total parenteral nutrition on marrow recovery during induction therapy for acute nonlymphocytic leukemia in childhood. *Med Pediatr Oncol.* 1983;11:134–140.
51. Uderzo C, Rovelli A, Bonomi M, Fomia L, Pirovano L, Masera G. Total parenteral nutrition and nutritional assessment in leu-

kaemia children undergoing bone marrow transplantation. *Eur J Cancer*. 1991;27:758–762.
52. Yokoyama S, Fujimoto T, Mitomi T, Yabe M, Yabe H, Kato S. Use of total parenteral nutrition in pediatric bone marrow transplantation. *Nutrition*. 1989;5:27–30.
53. Weisdorf S, Hofland C, Sharp HL, et al. Total parenteral nutrition in bone marrow transplantation: a clinical evaluation. *J Pediatr Gastroenterol Nutr*. 1984;3:95–100.
54. Weisdorf SA, Lysne J, Haake RJ, et al. Positive effect of prophylactic total parenteral nutrition on long-term outcome of bone marrow transplantation. *Transplantation*. 1987;43:833–838.
55. Sanders JE. Growth and development after hematopoietic cell transplant in children. *Bone Marrow Transplant*. 2008;41:223–337.
56. Charuhas PM. Chronic nutrition-related complications associated with pediatric hematopoietic stem cell transplantation. *Building Block*. 2005;28:1–6.
57. Faraci M, Bekassy AN, Defazio V, Tichelli A, Dini G. Non-endocrine late complications in children after allogeneic haematopoietic SCT. *Bone Marrow Transplant*. 2008;41:S49–S57.
58. Flowers MED, Storer B, Carpenter P, et al. Treatment change as a predictor of outcome among patients with classic chronic graft-versus-host disease. *Biol Blood Marrow Transplant*. 2008;14:1380–1384.
59. Taskinen M, Saarinen-Pihkala UM, Hovi L, Lipsanen-Nyman M. Impaired glucose tolerance and dyslipidaemia as late effects after bone-marrow transplantation in childhood. *Lancet*. 2000;356:993–997.
60. Hoffmeister PA, Storer BE, Sanders JE. Diabetes mellitus in long-term survivors of pediatric hematopoietic cell transplantation. *J Pediatr Hematol Oncol*. 2004;26:81–90.
61. Nichols WG. Combating infections in hematopoietic stem cell transplant recipients. *Expert Rev Anti Infect Ther*. 2003;1:57–73.
62. Seely D, Stempak D, Baruchel S. A strategy for controlling potential interactions between natural health products and chemotherapy. A review in pediatric oncology. *J Pediatr Hematol Oncol*. 2007;29:32–47.
63. Labriola D, Livingston R. Possible interactions between dietary antioxidants and chemotherapy. *Oncology*. 1999;13:1003–1011.
64. Lamson DW, Brignall MS. Antioxidants in cancer therapy: their actions and interactions with oncologic therapies. *Altern Med Rev*. 1999;4:304–329.
65. American Cancer Society. *American Cancer Society's Guide to Complementary and Alternative Cancer Methods*. Atlanta, GA: American Cancer Society; 2000:204–205.
66. Gardiner P, Kemper KJ. Herbs in pediatric and adolescent medicine. *Pediatr Rev*. 2002;21:44–57.
67. McGee J, Patrick RS, Wood CB, Blumgart LH. A case of veno-occlusive disease of the liver in Britain associated with herbal tea consumption. *J Clin Pathol*. 1976;29:788–794.
68. Moody K, Finlay J, Mancuso C, Charlson M. Feasibility and safety of a pilot randomized trial of infection rate: neutropenic diet versus standard food safety guidelines. *J Pediatr Hematol Oncol*. 2006;28:126–133.
69. French MR, Levy-Milne R, Zibrik D. A survey of the use of low microbial diets in pediatric bone marrow transplant programs. *J Am Diet Assoc*. 2001;101:1194–1198.
70. Restau J, Clark AP. The neutropenic diet. Does the evidence support this intervention? *Clin Nurse Spec*. 2008;22:208–211.
71. Anderson JB, Shuster TA, Hanson KE, Levy AS, Volk A. A camera's view of consumer food-handling behaviors. *J Am Diet Assoc*. 2004;104:186–191.
72. Collins JE. Impact of changing consumer lifestyles on the emergence/reemergence of foodborne pathogens. *Emerging Infect Dis*. 1997;3:471–479.
73. Diagnosis and management of foodborne illnesses: a primer for physicians and other health care professionals. *MMWR*. 2004;53:1–33.
74. Lowe M, Mortensen S. "Room service"—feeding on demand succeeds for cancer patients. *J Am Diet Assoc*. 1995;95(Suppl):A82.
75. Williams R, Virtue K, Adkins A. Room service improves patient food intake and satisfaction with hospital food. *J Pediatr Oncol Nurs*. 1998;15:183–189.
76. Handen BL, Mandell F, Russo DC. Feeding induction in children who refuse to eat. *Am J Dis Child*. 1986;140:52–54.
77. Schauster H, Dwyer J. Transition from tube feedings to feeding by mouth in children: preventing eating dysfunction. *J Am Diet Assoc*. 1996;96:277–281.
78. Bhatia M, Walters MC. Hematopoietic cell transplantation for thalassemia and sickle cell disease: past, present, and future. *Bone Marrow Transplant*. 2008;41:109–117.
79. National Heart, Lung and Blood Institute. Who is at risk for sickle cell anemia? Available at: http://www.nhlbi.nih.gov/health/dci/Diseases/Sca/SCA_WhoIsAtRisk.html. Accessed November 13, 2009.
80. Bolanos-Meade J, Brodsky RA. Blood and marrow transplantation for sickle cell disease: overcoming barriers to success. *Curr Opin Oncol*. 2009;21:158–161.
81. Schall JI, Zemel BS, Kawchak DA, Ohene-Frempong K, Stallings VA. Vitamin A status, hospitalizations, and other outcomes in young children with sickle cell disease. *J Pediatr*. 2004;145:99–106.
82. Nelson MC, Zemel BS, Kawchak DA, et al. Vitamin B_6 status of children with sickle cell disease. *J Pediatr Hematol Oncol*. 2002;24:463–469.
83. Kennedy TS, Fung EB, Kawchak DA, Zemel BS, Ohene-Frempong K, Stallings VA. Red blood cell folate and serum vitamin B_{12} status in children with sickle cell disease. *J Pediatr Hematol Oncol*. 2001;23:165–169.
84. Buison AM, Kawchak DA, Schall J, Ohene-Frempong K, Stallings VA, Zemel BS. Low vitamin D status in children with sickle cell disease. *J Pediatr*. 2004;145:622–627.
85. Buison AM, Kawchak DA, Schall JI, et al. Bone area and bone mineral content deficits in children with sickle cell disease. *Pediatrics*. 2005;116:943–949.
86. Brown K, Subramony C, May W, et al. Hepatic iron overload in children with sickle cell anemia on chronic transfusion therapy. *J Pediatr Hematol Oncol*. 2009;31:309–312.
87. Eggleston B, Patience M, Edwards S, et al. Effect of myeloablative bone marrow transplantation on the growth in children with sickle cell anaemia: results of the multicenter study of haematopoietic cell transplantation for sickle cell anaemia. *Br J Haematol*. 2007;136:673–676.

Nutrition for Burned Pediatric Patients

Michele Morath Gottschlich and Theresa Mayes

Trauma is a major cause of mortality in children, and a significant number of these deaths are from burns. Burn injury poses a complex metabolic challenge that is directly related to subsequent morbidity and mortality. As such, an important determinant of outcome is adequacy of energy and nutrient provision. If nutriture becomes impaired, wound healing and organ function will suffer. In addition, malnutrition will induce deterioration of immune defenses and profound catabolism of lean body mass and bone tissue.

The purpose of this chapter is to point out metabolic changes, physiologic deficiencies, and nutritional requirements of burned infants and children. Because the common denominator to which all nutrients are related is adequacy of energy intake, methods for evaluating caloric requirements will be emphasized. The basis for selecting the safest and most efficacious route of support and ratio of nutrients will be addressed. This chapter will also review enteral and parenteral feeding techniques, as well as present options available for assessing and monitoring the nutrition rehabilitation program.

Anatomic and Physiologic Considerations

Pediatric burn injury has a high mortality rate, compared with that of adults with equivalent burns,[1,2] although outcome has clearly improved with advancements in burn care.[3] The higher incidence of complications in pediatric burn patients is partially attributable to the fact that the unique physical and metabolic features of infants and children are frequently overlooked. It is important to recognize that the burned youngster in need of medical and nutritional therapy presents a separate and often much more complex therapeutic problem than does his or her adult counterpart.

Although the older child rapidly approaches the physical and metabolic makeup of the adult and responds to injury and treatment in a corresponding fashion, specialized nutritional care is required by younger age groups due to their anatomic and physiologic immaturity (**Table 18-1**). All burned children, however, pose a special challenge to meet obligatory growth needs. Burn injuries represent a particular threat to growth through imposition of a catabolic state. Bone growth is slowed during the acute phase postburn.[4] Furthermore, height and weight gain velocities have been documented during the first 3 years following the burn injury and showed no significant catch-up growth.[5]

A burned child, with more limited endogenous reserves and greater caloric and protein requirements than an adult, quickly reaches negative nitrogen balance with a smaller area of burn. Furthermore, the functional immaturity of the infant's gastrointestinal tract and renal system[6–8] poses a unique challenge to his or her ability to tolerate nonvolitional feeding regimens and nutrient-dense products. They are extremely susceptible to diarrhea, dehydration, and malnutrition, which only worsen the degree of catabolism.

Metabolic Manifestations of Thermal Injury

Extensive burn injury initiates the most marked alterations in body metabolism that can be associated with any illness. The pattern of physiologic events following thermal injury falls into two phases: the ebb response and the flow response.[9,10] The initial, or ebb, response of the burn syndrome is short, lasting 3 to 5 days postinjury. This phase is characterized by general hypometabolism and is manifested by reductions in oxygen consumption, cardiac output, blood pressure, and body temperature (**Table 18-2**). Fluid resuscitation is conducted during this time in response to the tremendous fluid losses that occur during the early postburn period.

With the resuscitative restoration of circulatory blood volume, the body advances to a prolonged state of hypermetabolism and increased nutrient turnover, termed the flow phase. This second phase is influenced by elevations in circulating levels of catecholamines,[11,12] glucocorticoids,[13–15] and glucagon.[16–20] Insulin levels are usually in the normal

TABLE 18-1 Anatomic and Physiologic Immaturities of Children of Various Ages

System	Deficit	Clinical Implications	Age of Maturation
Temperature regulation	Labile system Surface area/body weight ratio greatly increased	Increased radiant and evaporative heat loss Increased metabolic rate in an attempt to maintain core temperature	10–12 years
Integument	Thin skin	Heat penetrates more rapidly, with resultant deeper burn	16–18 years
Gastrointestinal	Immature tract Limited surface area of the small intestinal mucosa Decreased gastric volume capacity	Limited capacity to digest or assimilate some nutrients Prone to antigen absorption High incidence of diarrhea	1–2 years
Renal	Glomerular immaturity Young kidneys inefficient in excretion of sodium chloride and other ions, as well as in water resorption	Renal concentrating ability low; therefore, more water required to excrete the renal solute load produced by the metabolism of protein and electrolytes	1–2 years

TABLE 18-2 Metabolic Alterations Following Burns

		Flow Response	
	Ebb Response	Acute Phase	Adaptive Phase
Dominant factors	Loss of plasma volume Shock Low plasma insulin	Elevated catecholamines Elevated glucagon Elevated glucocorticoids Normal or elevated insulin High glucagon-to-insulin ratio	Stress hormones subsiding
Symptoms	Hyperglycemia Decreased oxygen consumption Depressed resting energy expenditure Decreased blood pressure Reduced cardiac output Decreased body temperature	Catabolism Hyperglycemia Increased respiratory rate Increased oxygen consumption Hypermetabolism Increased body temperature Increased cardiac output Redistribution of polyvalent cations, such as zinc and iron Mobilization of metabolic reserves Increased urinary excretion of nitrogen, sulphur, magnesium, phosphorus, and potassium Accelerated gluconeogenesis	Anabolism Normoglycemia Energy turnover diminished Convalescence

Source: Adapted from Gottschlich MM, Alexander JW, Bower RH. Enteral nutrition in patients with burns or trauma. In: Rombeau JL, Caldwell MD, eds. *Enteral and Tube Feeding.* With permission of WB Saunders Co., 1990.

range or even elevated. However, the rise in the glucagon/insulin ratio,[20] in combination with other hormonal derangements, initiates gluconeogenesis, lipolysis, and protein degradation. Hypermetabolism and hypercatabolism also vary with the time postburn. The classic studies of Wilmore and colleagues[12,21] show that, following the ebb phase, catabolic hormone production and oxygen consumption increase dramatically, peaking between the 6th and 10th day following burns.[12,21] Thereafter, metabolic rate slowly begins to decrease, and a gradual recession of catabolism occurs. These metabolic and hormonal sequelae have important implications from a nutritional perspective.

Fluid Requirements

Altered capillary permeability results in the escape of fluid, electrolytes, and protein from the vascular compartment to the interstitial area surrounding the burn wound. The injured area also loses its ability to act as a barrier to water evaporation. In children, with their relatively larger surface area per weight, the insensible water loss is of critical magnitude. Infants and young children are particularly susceptible to a lack of sufficient water intake because of their considerably higher obligatory urinary and insensible water losses, compared with those of adults. Hemodynamic dysfunction as a consequence of fluid shifts necessitates prompt provision of intravenous fluid resuscitation to restore tissue blood flow and to prevent shock following burns. Children require more fluid per square meter of body surface area than do adults with burns.[22]

The most popular pediatric fluid replacement formula is the Parkland formula,[23] modified for children (**Table 18-3**).

TABLE 18-3 Pediatric Fluid Calculations for Resuscitation and Maintenance

I. Resuscitation

A. Calculated resuscitation + basal requirement (less than 2 yrs: 2000 cc/m² BSA)

1. (4 cc × ____ kg × ____ % burn) + (1500 cc × _____ m² BSA)

(_______) + (_______) = _____cc/24 hours

B. Resuscitation fluid per 8 hours

1. 1st 8 hours: give ½ of total calculated cc/24 hours
2. 2nd 8 hours: give ¼ of total calculated cc/24 hours
3. 3rd 8 hours: give ¼ of total calculated cc/24 hours

II. Maintenance Fluids

A. Basal fluid requirement: 1500 cc/m² BSA (less than 2 yrs: 2000 cc/m² BSA)

1. Total body surface area ________ m² BSA
2. 24 hours _________cc

B. Evaporative water loss

1. Adults: (25 + % burn) m² BSA = cc/hr
   Children: (35 + % burn) m² BSA = cc/hr
2. Calculated evaporative water loss
   a. (_____ + _____ % burn) _____ m² BSA = _______cc/hr; ________ cc/24 hours

C. Total maintenance fluids = basal requirement + evaporate water loss

1. 24 hours _________ cc
2. Hourly _________ cc

Example calculation for a 7-year-old patient weighing 25 kg, with a 45% TBSA burn, 0.95 m² BSA

I. Resuscitation

A. Calculated resuscitation + basal requirement

1. (4 cc × 25 kg × 45% burn) + (1500 cc × 0.95 m² BSA)

(4500 cc) + (1425 cc) = 5925 cc/24 hours

B. Resuscitation fluid per 8 hours

1. 1st 8 hours: give ½ of total calculated cc/24 hours = 2962 cc, 370 cc/hr
2. 2nd 8 hours: give ¼ of total calculated cc/24 hours = 1481 cc, 185 cc/hr
3. 3rd 8 hours: give ¼ of total calculated cc/24 hours = 1481 cc, 185 cc/hr

II. Maintenance Fluids

A. Basal fluid requirement: 1500 cc/m² BSA

1. Total body surface area 0.95 m² BSA
2. 24 hours 1425 cc

B. Evaporative water loss

1. Adults: (25 + % burn) × m² BSA = cc/hr
   Children: (35 + % burn) × m² BSA = cc/hr
2. Calculated evaporative water loss
   a. (35 + 45% burn) × 0.95 m² BSA = 76 cc/hr; 1824 cc/24 hours

C. Total maintenance fluids = basal requirement + evaporate water loss

1. 24 hours: 1425 cc + 1824 cc = 3249 cc/24 hours
2. Hourly: 3249 cc/24 hours = 135 cc/hr

Abbreviations: BSA, body surface area; TBSA, total body surface area.

Source: Courtesy of the Shriners Hospitals for Children, Cincinnati, Ohio.

The modified Parkland formula includes a factor for basal fluid needs, in addition to compensation for losses from the burn wound. The application of this formula should not replace assessment of the patient's vital signs, blood pressure, and urinary output, because these are the ultimate determinants of the adequacy of replacement.

Caloric Needs

Increases in energy expenditure accompany burn injury. The degree of hypermetabolism is generally related to the size of the burn,[21] with burns of approximately 50% body surface area encountering a peak in energy expenditure. The root cause of hypermetabolism continues to be an active area of investigation. A number of studies support the role of cytokines in postburn metabolism.[24–28] Following injury, cytokines appear to produce neuromediators that activate endocrine organs to produce higher concentrations of catecholamines, glucagon, and cortisol. Sleep pattern disturbance has also been suggested as a factor contributing to increased metabolism following burn injury.[29] Elevations in catabolic hormones have been reported following sleep deprivation.[30,31] Furthermore, specific to burns, Gottschlich et al. report an inverse correlation between epinephrine and norepinephrine levels and rapid eye movement stage of sleep, suggesting a neuroendocrine response to lack of sleep as a contributor to postburn hypermetabolism and hypercatabolism.[32] Prevention of infection and reducing wound size are the primary means of decreasing metabolic rate. However, sufficient pain and anxiety control are crucial means of reducing metabolism in the pediatric population as well. Application of a reliable pain scale index is vital, so that severity of pain is understood and therefore treated appropriately. Age-appropriate explanations of procedures prior to performance may appear trivial, but offer huge rewards toward the reduction of anxiety. Finally, as a metabolic correlation with sleep is increasingly established, nightly promotion of uninterrupted sleep, with attention to duration and quality, should be viewed as an intricate component of the care plan.

The provision of sufficient calories to meet the increased metabolic expenditure is a critical factor in the management of the burned child. Energy needs may be estimated or measured. A number of pediatric energy equations have been applied successfully in burns (**Table 18-4**). Studies support reduced energy demands in this population.[38,39] It has been suggested that during stress, there is a shift in energy expenditure necessary for growth to that needed for acute illness. Energy needs for activity are also greatly reduced in the acute postburn phase.

The wide range of formulas for calculating energy needs is an indication of the uncertainties of this approach. Most mathematic derivations utilize body weight, age, and burn size as the only determinants of caloric requirements. Although these three factors represent significant effectors of metabolic rate, energy expenditure is also influenced by surgery, pain, anxiety, sepsis, body composition, gender, thermal effect of food, sleep deprivation, and physical activity. Therefore, mathematic formulas could derive fairly inaccurate caloric goals, considering the variability among individuals. If caloric needs are underestimated, some tissues, as well as exogenous substrates, will be consumed for energy. Although it is important to provide pediatric burn patients with the energy needed to compensate for hypermetabolism, as well as for growth and development, reports also caution against the delivery of an overabundance of calories. Administering a surfeit of calories has been associated with increased metabolic rate, hyperglycemia, and liver abnormalities and can cause an increase in carbon dioxide production.[40,41]

Indirect calorimetry remains a viable option in the assessment of energy expenditure in pediatric burn patients. The use of indirect calorimetry in burn care has been extensively reviewed elsewhere.[42,43] In general, the patient's caloric goal should be calculated at 120–130% of the measured resting energy expenditure (REE).[44–46] Although some degree of error is possible with this extrapolation, it is more accurate than estimates based solely on weight, age,

TABLE 18-4 Formulas for Calculating Energy Requirements of Burned Children

Reference	Age	%TBSA Burned	Calories/Day
Curreri[33]	0–1 yr	< 50	Basal + (15 × % BSAB)
	1–3 yr	< 50	Basal + (25 × % BSAB)
	4–15 yr	< 50	Basal + (40 × % BSAB)
Davies and Liljedal[34]	Child	Any	60W + (35 × % BSAB)
Hildreth[35–37]	< 15 yr	> 30	(1800/m² BSA) + (2200/m² burn)
Hildreth[38]	< 12 yr		(1800/m² BSA) + (1300/m² burn)
Mayes[39]	0–3 yr	10–50	108 + 68W + (3.9 × % BSAB)
			818 + 37.4W + (9.3 × % BSAB)

Abbreviations: W, weight in kg; BSA, body surface area burn; TBSA, total body surface area.

and burn size. To ensure the clinical validity of this goal, tests must be repeated regularly. Because hypermetabolism undergoes transient variation during the recovery phase, it is recommended that indirect calorimetry be conducted twice weekly, at minimum, for proper adjustment of the nutritional support regimen.

Carbohydrate Needs

Metabolic changes that occur following thermal injury include deranged carbohydrate metabolism. Early in the response to burns, glycosuria and hyperglycemia frequently occur. A similar response is observed in patients with supervening sepsis. Predisposition to glucose intolerance is correlated with the severity of the burn injury. Elevated blood glucose is also modulated by the phase of injury. During the shock phase, hyperglycemia is primarily caused by decreased peripheral tissue utilization in lieu of impaired tissue perfusion and low insulin levels.[47,48] Glucose intolerance typically persists during the flow phase, but it appears to be the result of enhanced hepatic glucose production and gluconeogenesis.[47]

Carbohydrate plays an important role in the nutritional support of the burned child. It appears to be the most important nonprotein calorie source in terms of nitrogen retention in burned patients,[49] although a limit exists to its effectiveness as an energy source.[40,41] Excessive glucose loads, which can increase carbon dioxide production, heighten glucose intolerance, and induce hepatic fat deposition, should be avoided.[50–52] Therefore, all burn patients should be monitored for hypercapnia and hyperglycemia. Exogenous insulin administration is often necessary to improve blood glucose levels and to achieve maximal glucose utilization. Intensive insulin therapy that maintains blood glucose levels significantly below previous thresholds has correlated with reduced morbidity and mortality in critical care.[53–56] As a result, insulin protocols are increasingly supported in the burn intensive care unit and have been associated with improved outcomes.[57–61]

Protein Requirements

The protein requirements of the burned infant and child are elevated because of accelerated tissue breakdown and exudative losses during a period of rapid repair and growth. Failure to meet heightened protein needs can be expected to yield suboptimal clinical results in terms of wound healing and resistance to infection. The infant and child further adapt to inadequate protein intake by curtailing growth of cells, conceivably sacrificing genetic potential.

Studies have shown that enteral fortification using large quantities of protein can accelerate the synthesis of visceral proteins and promote positive nitrogen balance and host defense factors.[44,62–67] For example, Alexander and colleagues[62] demonstrated that severely burned children on enteral diets containing approximately 22% of calories as protein had higher levels of total serum protein, retinol-binding protein, prealbumin, transferrin, C3, and immunoglobulin G (IgG), and better nitrogen balance than patients receiving 15% of calories as protein. In addition, the high-protein group had improved survival and fewer episodes of bacteremia. Therefore, in planning a nutritional intervention strategy for a burned youngster, an important goal is the provision of a sufficient quantity of protein. Patients greater than 6 months of age with burns in excess of 30% TBSA should receive 20–23% of calories as protein.[9,62,68] This translates to 2.5–4.0 g/kg, for a nonprotein calorie/nitrogen ratio of 80:1. The safe provision of this level of protein in those less than 3 years of age has been documented with evidence correlating decreased length of stay with higher protein provision.[69] Other factors that influence protein repletion, assuming an adequate intake of energy, include the quality of dietary protein; intact, whey protein is encouraged.

Close monitoring of protein intake is necessary because excessive protein loads or amino acid imbalances may result in azotemia, hyperammonemia, or acidosis. Particular care must be taken when administering high-protein feedings to children younger than 12 months of age because excessive amounts can have adverse effects on immature or compromised kidneys. Ongoing assessment of fluid status, blood urea nitrogen (BUN), plasma proteins, and nitrogen balance is recommended for individual evaluation of tolerance and adequacy. However, when fluid intake is adequate, renal or hepatic dysfunction does not exist, and pathways of intermediary metabolism are relatively mature, a high-protein diet is usually tolerated well.

Fat Needs

During the flow phase, burn-mediated increases in catecholamine and glucagon levels stimulate an accelerated rate of fat mobilization and oxidation. It is recognized, however, that lipid is important to the diet of the burned child because of its high caloric density, its role in myelination of nerve cells and brain development, the palatability it imparts to food, and its role as a carrier for the fat-soluble vitamins. In addition, fat in the form of the essential fatty acid linoleate provides vital components for cellular membranes and is a precursor for dienoic prostaglandin synthesis.

The minimum requirement for linoleic acid needed to prevent omega-6 fatty acid deficiency is considered to be approximately 2–3% of the calories consumed. This requirement is usually not difficult to accomplish because most enteral feeding supplements and intravenous fat emulsions contain high levels of fat and linoleic acid.[44,68,70] An overabundance of dietary lipid, however, can be detrimental to recovery from burns.[71] Complications ascribed to excessive fat intake have been reported. These include lipemia, fatty liver, diarrhea, and decreased resistance to infection.[70–72]

Furthermore, lipid appears to represent an inefficient source of calories for the maintenance of nitrogen equilibrium and lean body mass following major injury.[73–75]

Therefore, conservative administration of fat, particularly linoleic acid, given its immunosuppressive metabolites, is recommended to burned children greater than 6 months of age.[5,44] Given its competitive effects on the down-regulation of linoleic acid, provision of omega-3 fatty acid, a proven anti-inflammatory and immune-enhancing agent, is recommended.[44,72]

Micronutrient Needs

The functions of vitamins and trace elements pertinent to burn injury have been summarized elsewhere.[68,76–79] Optimal vitamin and mineral intake for the burned child remains to be determined, because few satisfactory data are available in this area of nutrition. Nevertheless, several facts are indisputable and bring to mind the importance of micronutrient supplementation. First, vitamin and mineral requirements increase with severity of thermal injury, related to heightened protein synthesis, enhanced caloric expenditure, and increased micronutrient losses. Second, individual vitamin and mineral needs are also dependent on preburn status.

Undoubtedly, a deficiency of vitamins and minerals would compromise reparative processes. However, oral, tube feeding, and intravenous hyperalimentation regimens frequently do not meet the heightened needs for certain micronutrients. Thus, it is recommended that additional supplementation be provided,[68,70,76–83] especially of those vitamins and trace elements associated with energy expenditure, wound healing, immune function, bone mineral density, coagulation, and those likely to have enhanced urinary and wound losses. Thiamine, riboflavin, niacin, folate, biotin, vitamin K, magnesium, phosphorus, chromium, and manganese are all cofactors for energy-dependent processes. The requirement for pyridoxine is closely related to dietary protein intake and protein metabolism. Vitamin B_{12}, folate, and zinc are cofactors necessary for collagen synthesis. Furthermore, inadequacy of many micronutrients, particularly vitamins A, C, E, and pyridoxine, as well as zinc, copper, and iron inadequacies, can adversely affect immune function. Iron supplementation, however, remains controversial,[44] because excessive iron also appears to enhance susceptibility to infection.[84]

Recently, a high incidence of hypovitaminosis D has been demonstrated in pediatric burn patients.[79,85] Evidence also suggests a high rate of bone demineralization and increased risk of fractures in the acute postburn phase.[86–88] Burn patients are at risk for bone disease from a variety of sources including extended bedrest, institutionalization, increased glucocorticoids, decreased growth hormone, and reduced serum cholesterol, a precursor of vitamin D. Vitamin D depletion is an additional causative factor.[79,85] The most effective means to treat this acute deficiency appears to be supplemental vitamin D_3; however, the effects of such treatment on outcomes is unknown.[89] In addition, vitamin D depletion has been reported well into convalescence, potentially impacting long-term bone growth and development in pediatric burns.[90,91]

Daily intakes of a multivitamin and supplemental vitamins A, C, D, and zinc (**Table 18-5**) are usually suggested. Many centers administer folate as well, although there is much less information on which to base levels of intake at this time. Extensive bleeding following burns and burn surgeries is common. The provision of therapeutic levels of intravenous vitamin K may be a helpful adjunct, specifically in the postoperative period or while on antibiotic therapy. Although select vitamin and mineral replacement in excess of RDAs appears to be justified in burned children, some micronutrients, particularly fat-soluble vitamins, are toxic in large amounts. Thus, all micronutrients should be administered judiciously.

Nutritional Intervention Strategies

The goal of nutritional support for the pediatric burn patient is to provide adequate calories and nutrients to facilitate wound healing, maximize immunocompetence, maintain or improve organ function, and prevent loss of lean body mass. Specific objectives vary, however, according to the underlying metabolic and nutritional status of each patient. Special consideration is indicated whenever fluid restriction,

TABLE 18-5 Vitamin and Trace Mineral Recommendations

Children and adolescents (3 years or older)

1. Major burn
   - One multivitamin daily
   - 500 mg ascorbic acid twice daily*
   - 10,000 IU vitamin A daily
   - 220 mg zinc sulfate daily*
   - 800 IU vitamin D_3 daily
2. Minor burn (< 20%) or reconstructive patient
   - One multivitamin daily

Children (less than 3 years of age)

1. Major burn
   - One children's multivitamin daily
   - 250 mg ascorbic acid twice daily*
   - 5000 IU vitamin A daily
   - 100 mg zinc sulfate daily*
   - 1600 IU vitamin D_3 daily
3. Minor burn (< 20%) or reconstructive patient
   - One multivitamin daily

*Delivery should be in suspension for tube feeding because oral vitamin C and zinc in large doses may precipitate nausea or vomiting.

Source: Reprinted with permission from Gottschlich, Michele M., Warden, Glenn D. Vitamin Supplementation in the Person with Burns. *Journal of Burn Care & Rehabilitation.* 11(3):275–279, May/June 1990.

organ failure, septicemia, mechanical ventilation, or any other presenting condition limits the ability to obtain vital nutrients.

Small Burn Area (Less Than 20%)

Small burns (less than 20% surface area) not complicated by facial injury, psychologic problems, inhalation injury, or preburn malnutrition can usually be supported by an oral high-protein, high-calorie diet. Between-meal snacks should be encouraged. Commercial meal-replacement beverages or the addition of nutrient modules to menu selections may be helpful in boosting a marginal intake of calories or protein.

Larger Surface Burns (More Than 20%)

Children with burns covering a larger surface area (20% or more) generally cannot meet their nutrient requirements by oral intake alone. In these cases, alternative forms of feeding must be implemented. Nutrients should be provided enterally to the burned youngster whenever possible. The enteral route is preferred over intravenous because it is safer, gastrointestinal function is preserved, and the integrity of the small intestinal mucosal surface is better maintained,[70,92,93] thus possibly minimizing bacterial translocation from the gastrointestinal tract.[92,94,95] In general, gastric feedings are not supported for a number of reasons, including the fact that postburn gastric ileus often inhibits the initial advancement and full-volume delivery of enteral feedings. In addition, the multiple position changes (for example, prone and neck hyperextension) that patients undergo for dressing changes, physical therapy, and operative procedures increase the aspiration risk when they are fed nasogastrically. Gastric feedings also potentiate limited oral intake because the patient minimally experiences hunger.

Enteral Feeding

Owing to the grave concern for possible aspiration, enteral alimentation that bypasses the stomach and uses the functional small intestine is desirable. Feeding tube placement into the third portion of the duodenum can be a safe means of enteral nutritional support, even during critical periods such as resuscitation, surgery, anesthesia for major dressing changes, or septic ileus.[95,96] Small bowel feedings permit minimal interruption of the nutrition regimen, thereby maximizing nutrient intake.

Determining the correct time for initiating a tube feeding program requires consideration. In general, enteral nutrition support should commence as soon as possible postburn. The obvious reasons include the fact that a significant nutrient deficit can develop when alimentation is delayed following thermal injury, which has a direct bearing on morbidity and mortality. In addition, aggressive enteral support has been associated with improved tube feeding tolerance and sustained bowel mucosal integrity.[70,93,97] Furthermore, when tube feeding is initiated within the first few hours postburn, the hypermetabolic response can be partially suppressed, as evidenced by decreased energy expenditure and improvements in measurements of nitrogen balance, visceral proteins, and catabolic hormones.[63,93,98,99]

Gottschlich and colleagues evaluated the effects of early versus delayed enteral feeding on various outcomes postburn.[100] Patients were randomized to receive enteral feedings within 24 hours (study group) or 48 hours (control group) of burn injury. Results indicate that early feeding reduces cumulative caloric deficits and potentially stimulates insulin secretion while conserving lean body mass. Feeding within 24 hours of injury did not limit postburn hypermetabolism, nor did it improve nutritional status, reduce infection, or decrease hospital stay. Some question the definition of early feeding (initiated within 24 hours) applied in this study. Perhaps benefit would have been increasingly apparent if nutrition support was initiated within a few hours of insult or if the control group delayed feeds for a greater period of time. Nevertheless, this is the only prospective clinical feeding trial of its nature in pediatric burns. Additional studies are recommended to establish feeding times that maximize clinical benefit and minimize morbid outcomes.

Fluids

Riegel and associates examined the effects of fluid resuscitation, inotrope use, and early feeding on the development of bowel necrosis.[101] Results indicated that patients with bowel necrosis had similar characteristics that divided them from those who did not infarct. Patients who sustained bowel necrosis required more fluid resuscitation during burn shock and tended to have prolonged (greater than 24 to 48 hours) burn shock. This subgroup of patients required higher doses of dopamine during burn shock and tended to receive dopamine more frequently during burn shock. Initiation of enteral feeds within 24 hours of insult did not increase the incidence of bowel necrosis in this study. As a result of this study, patients who are underresuscitated and require inotropic support greater than renal dose dopamine should be monitored for bowel necrosis during the postresuscitation phase. In addition, some recommend that trophic enteral feeds be employed for this subpopulation until fluid resuscitation is complete.

Because burn patients usually have unscathed digestive and absorptive capabilities, products containing intact nutrients should be used. Elemental or dipeptide formulations are unnecessary, unless dictated by concomitant disease or anatomic anomalies, and appear to yield less-favorable results in burns.[102] Most tube feedings can be started at full strength. The initial hourly infusion rate should begin at approximately half of the final desired volume and be increased by 5 mL/hour in the infant and toddler, 10 mL/hour in the school-age child, and 20 mL/hour in the teenager, as tolerated, until the final hourly rate is achieved.

As oral intake improves and nutrient needs decrease, the child can be gradually weaned from the tube feeding regimen. Initially, tube feedings can be held at mealtime to stimulate appetite. Once the patient demonstrates the ability to consume 25–50% of caloric needs by mouth, the tube feeding program may be necessary only at night. Eventually, when the patient is able to meet approximately 75% or greater of his or her caloric needs orally, tube feedings can be discontinued.

The composition of the enteral infusate should take into account the unique metabolic and age-related alterations in nutrient utilization that accompany an extensive burn injury. Suggested tube feeding regimens for pediatric burn patients can be divided into two major categories: (1) those appropriate for children younger than 6 months of age and (2) those for patients 6 months of age or older.

Enteral protocols for infants less than 6 months of age are generally conservative, relying on commercial infant formulas. The normal dilution of infant formula is 20 kcal/oz (0.66 kcal/mL). Gradually advancing the concentration to 24 kcal/oz is routinely safe. Further progression to 27–30 kcal/oz to meet the infant's energy needs must be monitored carefully, due to the resulting increased renal solute load.

The protein content of infant formulas ranges from 9% to 12% of total calories. This level is sometimes insufficient for those with large surface area burns. The addition of a protein module to the infant formula may be indicated in such cases if, once again, the patient is carefully monitored. Infant formulas derived from soy protein should not be used unless casein or whey intolerances have been confirmed, because the biologic value of soy protein is less than that of animal protein. Nutritional support regimens containing significantly reduced fat content are likewise not routinely recommended during infancy because fat is an extremely important nutrient during the period of central nervous system maturation.

Tube feeding products for children over 6 months of age can generally be selected from formularies established for adults. The coincident fluid needs and energy requirements normally result in utilizing a tube feeding concentration of 30 kcal/oz or 1 kcal/mL. If the tube feeding product selected is low in protein, according to the guidelines established for burn patients,[8,62,68,103] products should be enriched with protein modules to yield 20–23% of their energy content as protein.

To date, there are no commercially manufactured tube feeding formulas specifically designed for the burn patient. However, it is clear from recent studies that this patient population has atypical nutritional needs that transcend traditional recommendations for a high-calorie, high-protein solution. Modular tube feeding recipes have evolved that not only take into consideration energy and quantitative protein guidelines, but also currently offer the only means of incorporating findings regarding unique fat, amino acid, vitamin, and mineral requirements.[44,70,99,104] Employment of modular tube feeding prescriptions has been correlated with statistically significant reductions in infection rates and length of hospital stay.[44] However, because complex recipes are not feasible at many institutions, due to the laborious, complicated preparation procedures involved, protein enrichment of commercial substrates or careful scrutiny of the formulary for a high-protein, low-fat, low–linoleic acid, omega-3 fatty acid–enriched product is recommended as a practical alternative.

Parenteral Hyperalimentation

During the late 1960s, when intravenous feeding was shown to permit growth and development, it became possible to provide nutritional support to virtually any child.[98] Although the gastrointestinal tract is the preferred route of nutritional support, under certain circumstances intravenous feeding can become a necessary, and even lifesaving, part of burn management.

Appropriate indications for intravenous feeding in burns are listed in **Table 18-6**. There are two general categories of pediatric patients for whom parenteral nutrition is indicated. The first major category includes youngsters with protracted diarrhea or serious tube feeding intolerance, resulting in caloric insufficiency. If at all possible, however, at least some nutrients should be administered enterally via trophic feeds during episodes of diarrhea. Children with gastrointestinal disease or injury form a second group that frequently requires parenteral nutrition (PN).

In general, peripheral parenteral support does not provide adequate calories and nitrogen, and the delivery of intravenous nutrients via a central line is necessary to promote anabolism in the presence of burns.[105] Standard central venous regimens for the thermally injured patient usually consist of a final concentration of 25% dextrose and 5% crystalline amino acids, although individualized balancing is often warranted.

TABLE 18-6 Indications for Total Parenteral Nutrition in Burns

- Gastrointestinal trauma
- Curling's ulcer
- Severe pancreatitis
- Superior mesenteric artery syndrome
- Obstructions of the gastrointestinal tract
- Severe vomiting or abdominal distention
- Intractable diarrhea
- Adjunct to insufficient enteral support
- Necrotic bowel

If essential fatty acid requirements are being met in the trophic enteral feeds, then additional intravenous fat is not warranted. Patients receiving 100% of their energy needs via the parenteral route require the administration of modest amounts of intravenous fat. Five hundred milliliters of 10% lipid emulsion (or 250 mL of 20% lipid emulsion) infused two to three times weekly will suffice in meeting essential fatty acid requirements.

The metabolic and mechanical complications of parenteral hyperalimentation and the high incidence of septic morbidity in burns speak for reserving PN for those whose nutritional needs cannot be met by the enteral route. Adherence to strict protocols of infection control, along with continuous monitoring of tolerance, will most often promote a successful intravenous feeding program. Every attempt should be made to advance the enteral feeding rate with subsequent decrease in parenteral feeds to minimize the immunosuppression concomitant with the intravenous route.

Nutritional Assessment

Nutritional assessment is the process of identifying an individual's energy and nutrient requirements and evaluating the adequacy of enteral or parenteral nutrition support programs in meeting these needs. Clinical nutrition protocols for the care of burned children have been published; however, there is little specific information regarding their precise nutritional requirements.[106,107] Therefore, assessment and monitoring of patient response to diet therapy are especially important, so that the clinician can react to alterations in metabolism that occur over time and reduce the opportunity for complications. **Tables 18-7 and 18-8** summarize the nutrition assessment program successfully employed at the Cincinnati Shriners Hospital for Children.

Conclusion

Burn injury in pediatrics has important ramifications for nutrition. Decisions regarding what and how to feed patients continue to pose perplexing problems. Prompt provision of individually tailored diet therapy is of paramount importance in preventing malnutrition in burned children. This nutritional challenge is complicated by the fact that the knowledge of these patients' precise nutrient requirements remains incomplete. Burned infants and children represent separate and much more complex diet therapy problems, compared with their adult counterparts, because requirements for growth and development must be considered, as well as the increased nutrient needs imposed by burns. It is obvious that there is much to learn regarding optimal feeding practices in pediatric burn patients. Further research is needed to establish more definitive guidelines for nutritional intervention in burned children.

TABLE 18-7 Acute Burns: Guidelines for Initial Nutrition Assessment

Collect Objective Data	Obtain Appropriate Histories	Determine Preburn Nutritional Status	Calculate	Determine Appropriate Route of Feeding	Initiate Assessment Tool
Age Percent total body surface area burn Percent full thickness burn Body areas burned Inhalation injury Ventilatory status Gastric decompression initiated Anthropometrics: • Weight • Height/length • Body mass index • Head circumference (< 3 years)	Past medical history Social history Concomitant injuries Routine medications Referring hospital course as applicable	Diet history Food restrictions/ allergies Dentition Appetite Vitamin/mineral supplementation	Calorie and protein needs Vitamin/mineral supplementation recommendations Weight percentage: Percent ideal body weight (> 20 years) CDC growth chart percentile (≤ 20 years)	Oral Nasoenteral Parenteral	Obtain indirect calorimetry within 24 hours of admission. Begin 24-hour urinary urea collection for nitrogen balance determination. Obtain serum prealbumin. Begin monitoring calorie and protein intake.

*National Center for Health Statistics

Source: Reprinted from Mayes T, Gottschlich MM. Burns and wound healing. In: *The Science and Practice of Nutrition Support: A Case-Based Core Curriculum*. Silver Spring, MD: A.S.P.E.N.; 2001: 402. With permission from the American Society for Parenteral and Enteral Nutrition (A.S.P.E.N.). A.S.P.E.N. does not endorse the use of this material in any form other than its entirety.

TABLE 18-8 Acute Burns: Recommendations for Nutrition Reassessment

Daily	Weekly	Upon Discharge
Calorie and protein intake	Weight (once edema is resolved)	Percent preburn weight at discharge
Labs:	Prealbumin	Adequacy of oral intake
• BUN/creatinine	Nitrogen balance trend	Nutrition supplementation requirements
• Glucose	Wound healing (% open wound)	Need for nutrition follow-up in the outpatient setting
• Electrolytes	Indirect calorimetry:	
• Nitrogen balance	• REE	
Tolerance (nausea, vomiting, distention, diarrhea, constipation)	• RQ	
Clinical course (sepsis, infection, surgeries, fluid status, medications, respiratory status)		
Appropriateness of diet/enteral or parenteral nutrition order		

Abbreviations: BUN, blood urea nitrogen; REE, resting energy expenditure; RQ, respiratory quotient.

Source: Reprinted from Mayes T, Gottschlich MM. Burns and wound healing. In: *The Science and Practice of Nutrition Support: A Case-Based Core Curriculum*. Silver Spring, MD: A.S.P.E.N.; 2001: 402. With permission from the American Society for Parenteral and Enteral Nutrition (A.S.P.E.N.). A.S.P.E.N. does not endorse the use of this material in any form other than its entirety.

Case Study

Nutrition Assessment

TD is a previously healthy 11-month-old female admitted to the intensive care unit. She suffered 40% total body surface area (TBSA) burns, 35% full thickness, when she pulled on the electric cord of a frying pot, tipping the container. The hot liquid splattered over her face, head, neck, and right side of her upper body and thigh.

In anticipation of face and neck swelling over the course of the next few hours, TD is sedated and intubated to maintain oxygen and airway. A nasogastric tube is placed to low wall suction. Her abdomen is soft and nondistended. She is 9 kg in weight and 74 cm in length. Her intravenous resuscitative fluids are infusing to maintain a urine output of approximately 1.0 mL/kg/hour. Past medical history is noncontributory. Labs are initially monitored every 6 hours and electrolyte adjustment, glucose management, blood product replacement, and ventilator therapies are coordinated with respective panel results. A nutrition history from the mother indicated the baby is beginning to wean from the bottle and increasing her intake of baby foods and soft table foods. She accepts a pacifier at afternoon nap and bedtimes. The patient has no known food allergies or intolerances.

Nutrition Intervention

TD's initial goals for calorie, protein, and micronutrients were established. Within 6 hours of admission to the unit, feeding tube placement is confirmed in the upper portion of the duodenum. Given her adequate hydration status and hemodynamic stability (i.e., lack of vasopressor use), tube feeding (TF) rate is initiated at 5 mL per hour and advanced every 2 hours by 5 mL to a goal of 35 mL per hour. The goal TF rate provides 95% of kcal and 103% of protein goals.

TD undergoes surgery six times. Each excision procedure is followed by a 24-hour period of stabilization prior to donor site harvest and skin grafting over the burned areas. Enteral feeds are continued through surgery to ensure adequate nutritional support throughout the perioperative period.[96]

While on mechanical ventilatory support, oral stimulation is provided during physical therapy sessions. As TD progresses and sedation is weaned, a pacifier is provided for comfort as well as oral stimulation. Given her young age, she maintains a high risk for subsequent oral feeding coordination deficiencies due to prolonged NPO status. The pacifier supports skills necessary for eventual oral feeding coordination.

The patient's endotracheal tube is uncuffed so indirect calorimetry is not possible initially; however, once extubated, indirect calorimetry is performed biweekly. The tube feeding rate is adjusted based upon a 30% addition to the resting energy expenditure. This ensures sufficient calories to cover additional metabolic influences such as fever spikes, pain, anxiety, dressing changes, therapy sessions, and the like that are not an inherent component of the test.

Following extubation on postburn day 10, TD is permitted an oral diet. Clear liquids are provided via bottle and accepted well. Gastrointestinal tolerance is deemed appropriate and the diet therefore advanced to regular, age-appropriate provision. As wounds are increasingly covered, appetite improves and tube feedings are tapered. When TD is consuming 20% of the calorie goal consistently for a period of 2 days, feeds are tapered to be held 2 hours at meal times. When her wounds are 95% covered, and she is accepting 80% of her nutrition goal orally, the feeding tube is discontinued.

Monitoring and Evaluation

The enteral regimen is assessed daily for calorie and protein intake and gastrointestinal tolerance. TD's clinical course is evaluated daily for parameters related to nutritional status and regimen tolerance. These include surgery, labs including fluid and electrolytes, infection, antibiotic use, respiratory status, physical therapy gains (e.g., head control, sitting up independently in a high chair, feeding self), and wound status. BUN/creatinine levels are assessed daily to ensure proper balance of fluids/hydration status. Glucose levels and need for insulin supplementation are monitored daily; however, the enteral regimen is not changed when insulin needs are increased. The preference for carbohydrate versus fat calories for wound healing supersedes a regimen change to a higher fat formula in an effort to assist glucose management. As TD's clinical course progresses, the appropriateness of an enteral feeding taper is evaluated daily.

Discharge

On postburn day 39, TD is discharged to home. She has 98% wound coverage. TD is at 95% of her preburn weight. She is eating well, having improved to 90% of her estimated goal, and including a diet similar to that consumed prior to injury. TD does not require any nutritional supplementation at this time.

Questions for the Reader

1. What are the patient's energy, protein, and micronutrient supplementation needs upon admission to the burn unit (weight = 9 kg)?
2. What are TD's weight and height percentiles on the CDC growth chart upon admission?
3. Complete a PES statement for this patient.
4. What type of tube feeding product was recommended for TD?
5. What other weekly assessment parameters were closely monitored in TD?
6. What type of nutritional follow-up will TD receive in the outpatient clinic?

REFERENCES

1. Curreri PW, Luterman A, Braun DW, et al. Burn injury: analysis of survival and hospitalization time for 937 patients. *Ann Surg.* 1980;192:472–478.
2. Erickson EJ, Merrell SW, Saffle JR, Sullivan JJ. Differences in mortality from thermal injury between pediatric and adult patients. *J Pediatr Surg.* 1991;26:821–825.
3. Sheridan RL, Remensnyder JP, Schnitzer JJ, et al. Current expectations for survival in pediatric burns. *Arch Pediatr Adolesc Med.* 2000;154:245–249.
4. Klein GL, Herndon DN, Rutan TC, et al. Bone diseases in burn patients. *J Bone Miner Res.* 1993;8(3):337–345.
5. Rutan RL, Herndon DN. Growth delay in postburn pediatric patients. *Arch Surg.* 1990;125:392–395.
6. Grybowski JD. Gastrointestinal function in the infant and young child. *Clin Gastroenterol.* 1977;6:253–265.
7. Lebenthal E, Lee PC. Development of functional response in human exocrine pancreas. *Pediatrics.* 1980;66:556–560.
8. Spitzer A. The role of the kidney in sodium homeostasis during maturation. *Kidney Int.* 1982;21:539–545.
9. Gottschlich M, Alexander JW, Bower RH. Enteral nutrition in patients with burns or trauma. In: Rombeau JL, Caldwell MD, eds. *Enteral and Tube Feeding*, 2nd ed. Philadelphia: WB Saunders; 1990:306–324.
10. Cuthbertson DP, Zagreb H. The metabolic response to injury and its nutritional implications: retrospect and prospect. *J Parenter Enteral Nutr.* 1979;3:108–130.
11. Aikawa N, Caulfield JB, Thomas RJS, et al. Post burn hypermetabolism: relation to evaporative heat loss and catecholamine level. *Surg Forum.* 1975;26:74–76.
12. Wilmore DW, Long JM, Mason AD, et al. Catecholamines: mediators of the hypermetabolic response to thermal injury. *Ann Surg.* 1974;180:653–669.
13. Bane JW, McCaa RE, McCaa CS. The pattern of aldosterone and cortisone blood levels in thermal burn patients. *J Trauma.* 1974;14:605–611.
14. Jeshke MG, Chinkes D, Finnerty C, et al. Pathophysiologic response to severe burn injury. *Ann Surg.* 2008;248:387-401.
15. Vaughn GM, Becker RA, Allen JP, et al. Cortisol and corticotrophin in burned patients. *J Trauma.* 1982;22:263–273.
16. Wilmore DW, Lindsey CA, Moylan JA, et al. Hyperglucagonemia after burns. *Lancet.* 1974;1:73–75.
17. Johoor F, Herndon DH, Wolfe RR. Role of insulin and glucagon in the response of glucose and alanine kinetics in burn-injured patients. *J Clin Invest.* 1986;78:807–814.
18. Orton CI, Segal AW, Bloom SR, et al. Hypersecretion of glucagon and gastrin in severely burned patients. *Br Med J.* 1975;2:170–172.
19. Nygren J, Sammann M, Malm M, et al. Disturbed anabolic hormonal patterns in burned patients: the relation to glucagons. *Clin Endocrinol.* 2008;43:491–500.
20. Nair KS, Halliday D, Matthews DE, Welle SL. Hyperglucagonemia during insulin deficiency accelerates protein catabolism. *Am J Physiol Endocrinol Metab.* 1987;253:E208–E213.
21. Wilmore DW. Nutrition and metabolism following thermal injury. *Clin Plast Surg.* 1974;1:603–619.
22. Barrow RE, Jeschke MG, Herndon DN. Early fluid resuscitation improves outcomes in severely burned children. *Resuscitation.* 2000;45:91–96.

23. Baxter CR, Shires T. Physiological response to crystalloid resuscitation of severe burns. *Ann NY Acad Sci.* 1968;150:874–894.
24. Finnerty CC, Herndon DN, Przkora R, et al. Cytokine expression profile overtime in severely burned pediatric patients. *Shock.* 2006;26:13–19.
25. Tracey KJ. TNF and other cytokines in the metabolism of septic shock and cachexia. *Clin Nutr.* 1992;11:1–11.
26. Tredgett EE, Yu YM, Zhong S, et al. Role of interleukin-1 and tumor necrosis factor on energy metabolism in rabbits. *Am J Physiol.* 1988;255:E760–E768.
27. Dinarello CA. Overview: interleukin-1 and tumor necrosis factor in inflammatory disease and the effect of dietary fatty acids on their production. In: Kinney JM, Tucker HN, eds. *Organ Metabolism and Nutritional Ideas for Future Critical Care.* New York: Raven Press; 1994:181–195.
28. Warren RS, Starnes HF, Gabrilove JL. The acute metabolic effects of tumor necrosis factor administration. *Arch Surg.* 1987;122: 1396–1400.
29. Gottschlich MM, Jenkins ME, Mayes T, et al. A prospective clinical study of the polysomnographic stages of sleep following burn injury. *J Burn Care Rehabil.* 1994;15:486–492.
30. Copinschi, G. Metabolic and endocrine effects of sleep deprivation. *Essent Psychopharmacol.* 2005;6:341–347.
31. Van Cauter E, Homback U, Knutson K, et al. Impact of sleep and sleep loss on neuroendocrine and metabolic function. *Horm Res.* 2007;67(Suppl 1):2–9.
32. Gottschlich MM, Khoury J, Warden GD, Kagan RJ. An evaluation of the neuroendocrine response to sleep in pediatric burn patients. *J Parenter Enteral Nutr.* 2009;33:317–326.
33. Day T, Dean P, Adams MC, et al. Nutritional requirements of the burned child: the Curreri junior formula. *Proc Am Burn Assoc.* 1986;18:86.
34. Davies JWL, Liljedahl SL. Metabolic consequences of an extensive burn. In: Polk HC, Stone HH, eds. *Contemporary Burn Management.* Boston: Little Brown; 1971:151–169.
35. Hildreth M, Caravajal HF. Caloric requirements in burned children: a simple formula to estimate daily caloric requirements. *J Burn Care Rehabil.* 1982;3:78–80.
36. Hildreth MA, Herndon DN, Desai MH, Duke MA. Calorie needs of adolescent patients with burns. *J Burn Care Rehabil.* 1989;10:523–526.
37. Hildreth MA, Herndon DN, Parks DH, et al. Evaluation of a caloric requirement formula in burned children treated with early excision. *J Trauma.* 1987;27:188–189.
38. Hildreth MA, Herndon DN, Desai MH, Broemeling LD. Current treatment reduces calories required to maintain weight in pediatric patients with burns. *J Burn Care Rehabil.* 1990;11:405–409.
39. Mayes TM, Gottschlich MM, Khoury J, Warden GD. An evaluation of predicted and measured energy requirements in burned children. *J Am Diet Assoc.* 1996;96:24–29.
40. Klein CJ, Stanek GS, Wiles CE. Overfeeding macronutrients to critically ill adults. *Metab Complications.* 1998;98:795–806.
41. Aarsland A, Chinkes D, Wolfe RR. Hepatic and whole-body fat synthesis in humans during carbohydrate overfeeding. *Am J Clin Nutr.* 1997;65:1774–1782.
42. Klein S, Kinney J, Jeejeebhoy K, et al. Nutrition support in clinical practice: review of published data and recommendations for future research directions. *Am J Clin Nutr.* 1997;66:683–706.
43. da Rocha EE, Alves VG, da Fonseca RB. Indirect calorimetry: methodology, instruments and clinical application. *Curr Opin Clin Nutr Metab Care.* 2006;9:247–256.
44. Gottschlich MM, Jenkins M, Warden GD, et al. Differential effects of three enteral regimens on selected outcome parameters. *J Parenter Enteral Nutr.* 1990;14:225–236.
45. Kagan RJ, Gottschlilch MM, Mayes T, Warden GD. Estimation of calorie needs in the thermally injured child. *Proc Am Burn Assoc.* 1995;27:283.
46. Wilmore DW, Goodwin CW, Aulick LH, et al. Effect of injury and infection on visceral metabolism and circulation. *Ann Surg.* 1980;192:491–500.
47. Gauglitz GG, Herndon DN, Jeschke MG. Insulin resistance postburn: underlying mechanisms and current therapeutic strategies. *J Burn Care Res.* 2008;29:683–694.
48. McGowen KC, Malhotra A, Bistrian BR. Stress-induced hyperglycemia. *Crit Care Clin.* 2001;17:107–124.
49. Hart DW, Wolf SE, Zhang X-J, et al. Efficacy of a high-carbohydrate diet in catabolic illness. *Crit Care Med.* 2001;29:1318–1324.
50. Barrocas A, Tretola R, Alonso A. Nutrition and the critically ill pulmonary patient. *Respir Care.* 1983;28:50–61.
51. Askanazi J, Rosenbaum SH, Hyman AI, et al. Respiratory changes induced by large glucose loads of total parenteral nutrition. *JAMA.* 1980;243:1444–1447.
52. Young VR, Motil KJ, Burke JF. Energy and protein metabolism in relation to requirements of the burned pediatric patient. In: Suskind RM, ed. *Textbook of Pediatric Nutrition.* New York: Raven Press; 1981:309–340.
53. Van den Berghe G, Wouters P, Weekers F, et al. Intensive insulin therapy in critically ill patients. *N Engl J Med.* 2001;345:1359–1367.
54. Van den Berghe G, Wouters P, Bouillion R, et al. Outcomes benefit of intensive insulin therapy in the critically ill: insulin dose versus glycemic control. *Crit Care Med.* 2003;31:359–366.
55. Van den Berghe C, Wilmer A, Hermans G, et al. Intensive insulin therapy in the medical ICU. *N Engl J Med.* 2006;354:449–461.
56. Collier BC, Diaz J, Forbes R, et al. The impact of a normoglycemic management protocol on clinical outcomes in the trauma intensive care unit. *J Parenter Enteral Nutr.* 2005;29:353–359.
57. Cochran A, Davis L, Morris SE, Saffle JE. Safety and efficacy of an intensive insulin protocol in a burn-trauma intensive care unit. *J Burn Care Res.* 2008;29:187–191.
58. Hemmila MR, Taddonio MA, Arbabi S, et al. Intensive insulin therapy is associated with reduced infectious complications in burn patients. *Surg.* 2008;144:629–635.
59. Pham TN, Warren AJ, Phan HH, et al. Impact of tight glycemic control in severely burned children. *J Trauma.* 2005;59:1148–1154.
60. Thomas SJ, Morimoto K, Herndon DN, et al. The effect of prolonged euglycemic hyperinsulinemia on lean body mass after severe burn. *Surg.* 2002;132:341–347.
61. Jeschke MG, Klein D, Herndon DN. Insulin treatment improves the systemic inflammatory reaction to severe trauma. *Ann Surg.* 2004;239:553–560.
62. Alexander JW, MacMillan BG, Stinnett JD, et al. Beneficial effects of aggressive protein feeding in severely burned children. *Ann Surg.* 1980;192:505–517.
63. Dominioni L, Trocki O, Mochizuki H, et al. Prevention of severe postburn hypermetabolism and catabolism by immediate intragastric feeding. *J Burn Care Rehabil.* 1984;5:106–112.

64. Serog P, Baigts F, Apfelbaum M, et al. Energy and nitrogen balances in 24 severely burned patients receiving 4 isocaloric diets of about 10 MJ/m^2/day (2392 kcal/m^2/day). *Burns.* 1983;9:422–427.
65. Saito H, Trocki O, Wang S, et al. Metabolic and immune effects of dietary arginine supplementation after burn. *Arch Surg.* 1987;122:784–789.
66. Dominioni L, Trocki O, Fang CH, et al. Nitrogen balance and liver changes in burned guinea pigs undergoing prolonged high-protein enteral feeding. *Surg Forum.* 1983;34:99–101.
67. Dominioni L, Trocki O, Fang CH, et al. Enteral feeding in burn hypermetabolism: nutritional and metabolic effects of different levels of calorie and protein intake. *J Parenter Enteral Nutr.* 1985;9:269–279.
68. Gottschlich MM. Acute thermal injury. In: Lang CE, ed. *Nutritional Support in Critical Care.* Gaithersburg, MD: Aspen Publishers; 1987:159–181.
69. Gottschlich MM, Mayes T, Allgeier C, et al. Differential effects of three enteral regimens in burned infants and toddlers. *Proc Am Burn Assoc.* 2005;26:S105.
70. Gottschlich MM, Warden GD, Michel MA, et al. Diarrhea in tube-fed burn patients: incidence, etiology, nutritional impact and prevention. *J Parenter Enteral Nutr.* 1988;12:338–345.
71. Mochizuki H, Trocki O, Dominioni L, et al. Optimal lipid content for enteral diets following thermal injury. *J Parenter Enteral Nutr.* 1984;8:638–646.
72. Gottschlich MM, Alexander JW. Fat kinetics and recommended dietary intake in burns. *J Parenter Enteral Nutr.* 1987;11:85–89.
73. Long JM, Wilmore DW, Mason AD, et al. Effect of carbohydrate and fat intake on nitrogen excretion during total intravenous feeding. *Ann Surg.* 1977;185:417–422.
74. Souba WW, Long JM, Dudrick SJ. Energy intake and stress as determinants of nitrogen excretion in rats. *Surg Forum.* 1978;29:76–77.
75. Freund H, Yoshimura N, Fischer JE. Does intravenous fat spare nitrogen in the injured rat? *Am J Surg.* 1980;140:377–383.
76. Gottschlich MM, Warden GD. Vitamin supplementation in the burn patient. *J Burn Care Rehabil.* 1990;11:275–279.
77. Gamliel Z, DeBiasse MA, Demling RH. Essential microminerals and their response to burn injury. *J Burn Care Rehabil.* 1996;17:264–272.
78. Jenkins ME, Gottschlich MM, Kopcha R, et al. A prospective analysis of serum vitamin K and dietary intake in severely burned pediatric patients. *J Burn Care Rehabil.* 1998;19:75–81.
79. Gottschlich MM, Mayes T, Khoury J, Warden GD. Hypovitaminosis D in acutely injured pediatric burn patients. *J Am Diet Assoc.* 2004;104:931–941.
80. Pochon JP. Zinc and copper replacement therapy: a must in burns and scalds in children? *Prog Pediatr Surg.* 1981;14:151–172.
81. King N, Goodwin CW. Use of vitamin supplements for burned patients: a national survey. *J Am Diet Assoc.* 1984;84:923–925.
82. Council on Scientific Affairs. Vitamin preparations as dietary supplements and as therapeutic agents. *JAMA.* 1987;257:1929–1936.
83. Shippee RL, Wilson SW, King N. Trace mineral supplementation of burn patients: a national survey. *J Am Diet Assoc.* 1987;87:300–303.
84. Weinberg ED. Iron and susceptibility to infectious disease. *Science.* 1974;184:952–956.
85. Klein GL, Langman CB, Herndon DN. Vitamin D depletion following burn injury in children: a possible factor in post-burn osteopenia. *J Trauma.* 2002;52:346–350.
86. Klein GL, Herndon DN, Langman CB, et al. Long term reduction in bone mass after severe burn injury in children. *J Pediatr.* 1995;126:252–256.
87. Klein GL, Herndon DN, Rutan TC, et al. Bone disease in burn patients. *J Bone Miner Res.* 1993;8:337–345.
88. Mayes T, Gottschlich MM, Scanlon J, Warden GD. Four year review of burns as an etiologic factor in the development of long bone fractures in pediatric patients. *J Burn Care Rehabil.* 2003;24:279–284.
89. Gottschlich MM, Mayes T, Allgeier C, et al. Prospective randomized evaluation of vitamin D2 versus D3 supplementation in critically ill pediatric burn patients. Proceedings of the American Burn Association, *J Burn Care Res.* 2010;31:S151.
90. Klein GL. The interaction between burn injury and vitamin D metabolism and consequences for the patient. *Curr Clin Pharmacol.* 2008;3:204–210.
91. Klein GL, Chen TC, Holick MF, et al. Synthesis of vitamin D in skin after burns. *Lancet.* 2004;363:291–292.
92. Saito H, Trocki O, Alexander JW, et al. The effect of route of nutrient administration on the nutritional state, catabolic hormone secretion, and gut mucosal integrity after burn injury. *J Parenter Enteral Nutr.* 1987;11:1–7.
93. Saito H, Trocki O, Alexander JW. Comparison of immediate postburn enteral versus parenteral nutrition. *J Parenter Enteral Nutr.* 1985;9:115.
94. Herek O, Kara IG, Kaleli I. Effects of antibiotics and *Saccharomyces boulardii* on bacterial translocation in burn injury. *Surg Today.* 2004;34:256–260.
95. Gottschlich MM. Early and perioperative nutrition support. In: Matarese L, Gottschlich MM, eds. *Contemporary Nutrition Support Practice.* Philadelphia: WB Saunders; 1998:265–278.
96. Jenkins M, Gottschlich M, Baumer T, et al. Enteral feeding during operative procedures. *J Burn Care Rehabil.* 1994;15:199–205.
97. Mochizuki H, Trocki O, Dominioni L, et al. Mechanism of prevention of postburn hypermetabolism and catabolism by early enteral feeding. *Ann Surg.* 1984;200:297–310.
98. Jenkins M, Gottschlich M, Waymack JP, et al. An evaluation of the effect of immediate enteral feeding on the hypermetabolic response following severe burn injury. *Proc Am Burn Assoc.* 1988;112.
99. Jenkins M, Gottschlich MM, Alexander JW, et al. Enteral alimentation in the early postburn phase. In: Blackburn GL, Bell SJ, Mullen JL, eds. *Nutritional Medicine: A Case Management Approach.* Philadelphia: WB Saunders; 1989:1–5.
100. Gottschlich MM, Jenkins MJ, Mayes T, et al. An evaluation of the safety of early versus delayed enteral support and effects on clinical, nutritional and endocrine outcomes after severe burns. *J Burn Care Rehabil.* 2002;23:401–415.
101. Riegel T, Allgeier C, Gottschlich M, et al. Fluid resuscitation, inotropic agents and early feeding: is there a relationship to bowel necrosis? *J Burn Care Rehabil.* 2003;24:S61.
102. Trocki O, Mochizuki H, Dominioni L, et al. Intact protein versus free amino acids in the nutritional support of thermally injured animals. *J Parenter Enteral Nutr.* 1986;10:139–145.

103. Gottschlich MM, Alexander JW, Jenkins M, et al. Burns. In: Blackburn GL, Bell SJ, Mullen JL, eds. *Nutritional Medicine: A Case Management Approach.* Philadelphia: WB Saunders; 1989:6–9.
104. Bell SJ, Molnar JA, Carey M, et al. Adequacy of a modular tube feeding diet for burned patients. *J Am Diet Assoc.* 1986;86:1386–1391.
105. Gottschlich MM, Warden GD. Parenteral nutrition in the burned patient. In: Fischer JE, ed. *Total Parenteral Nutrition.* Boston: Little Brown & Co.; 1991:270–298.
106. Mayes T, Gottschlich MM, Warden GD. Clinical nutrition protocols for continuous quality improvements in the outcomes of patients with burns. *J Burn Care Rehabil.* 1997; 18:365–368.
107. Prelack K, Dylewski M, Sheridan RL. Practical guidelines for nutritional management of burn injury and recovery. *Burns.* 2007;33:14–24.
108. Mayes T, Gottschlich MM, Allgeier C, et al. Overweight and obesity: over-representation in the pediatric reconstructive burn population. *J Burn Care Res.* 2010:31(3):423–428.
109. Mayes T, Gottschlich M, Khoury J, et al. A comparison of polysomnographic and respiratory recordings between obese and non-obese burned children in the outpatient setting. *J Burn Care Res.* 2010;31:S67.

Enteral Nutrition

Lisa Simone Sharda

Introduction

Normal nutrition is received through the voluntary ingestion of a variety of foods both liquid and solid. Nutritional intake provides the required nutrients for the normal growth and development of infants and children. This process can be interrupted as a result of some acute or chronic conditions that affect an infant or child's ability to ingest, digest, or absorb nutrients. When infants and children are unable to obtain adequate nutrients from oral intake, supplemental feedings are warranted.

Enteral nutrition (EN) or enteral nutrition support (ENS) is the delivery of nutrition in the form of glucose, protein, and/or lipid directly into the gastrointestinal (GI) tract via a tube, catheter, or stoma. Indications for EN are a functioning GI tract of sufficient length and absorptive capacity. Infants and children meeting these criteria who possess the inability to consume adequate nutrition via the oral cavity are candidates for EN.[1,2]

Enteral nutrition is often preferred over parenteral nutrition because it is associated with fewer complications and is less expensive.[3–5] Advances in commercial formulas and equipment for the delivery of ENS have made enteral feeding safe and efficacious to administer to pediatric patients in either the hospital or home setting.

This chapter provides practical guidelines for:

- Selecting appropriate candidates for enteral nutrition, ranging in age from birth to 18 years
- Selecting specific products
- Administering and monitoring enteral feedings
- Considering specific factors of the pediatric population

Note that enteral feeding of the premature infant is addressed in Chapter 4 of this book.

Patient Selection

Patients can be treated with ENS in hospitals and rehabilitation facilities, as well as at home. The healthcare team should establish inpatient and outpatient criteria for consideration of EN. Nutrition screening should identify patients who are failing to thrive from either inorganic or organic sources or those who possess feeding disorders that affect their ability to ingest adequate nutrition. Factors to evaluate include:[3,5]

- Usual caloric intake of less than 80% of needs
- Weight maintenance or loss
- Weight-to-length or weight-to-height ratio under the 5th percentile
- Excessive feeding time
- Oral and/or texture aversion
- Mechanical problems with mastication, swallowing, or peristalsis

Pediatric patients with a variety of diseases who are at nutritional risk have been shown to benefit from ENS (**Exhibit 19-1**). Specific screens can be developed for a particular disease state or condition, as the need arises.[6–9]

When enteral nutrition is contraindicated due to severe intestinal dysfunction (**Exhibit 19-2**), parenteral nutrition constitutes the appropriate route for specific nutritional support (see Chapter 20).

Product Selection

Enteral formulas are classified by the U.S. Food and Drug Administration (FDA) under the heading of medical foods. Medical foods are described as "a food which is formulated to be consumed or administered enterally under the supervision of a physician."[1] Medical foods are not regulated as either conventional foods or drugs.[10] Infant formula must meet FDA assurance of nutrition quality, as well as labeling criteria, nutrient content, and manufacturers quality control procedures prior to marketing of the infant formula.

A wide variety of commercially prepared infant, pediatric, and adult enteral formulas can be utilized for pediatric patients requiring ENS. The proper product selection is

EXHIBIT 19-1 Indications for Enteral Nutrition in the Pediatric Patient

Functional

1. Neurologic disorders
2. Neuromuscular disorders
3. Prematurity
4. Inability to take in adequate nutrition
5. Genetic/metabolic disorders

Structural

1. Congenital anomalies
   a. Tracheoesophageal fistula
   b. Esophageal atresia
   c. Cleft palate
   d. Pierre Robin syndrome
2. Obstruction
   a. Cancer of head/neck
   b. Intubation
3. Injury
   a. Ingestions
   b. Trauma
   c. Sepsis
4. Surgery

EXHIBIT 19-2 Potential Complications for Enteral Nutrition in Pediatric Patients

- Acute pancreatitis
- Gastrointestinal obstruction
- Inflammatory bowel disease
- Intestinal atresia
- Limited or impaired absorptive surface
- Necrotizing enterocolitis
- Overwhelming sepsis
- Side effects of cancer therapy

contingent on a number of factors related to the specific medical and nutritional status of the patient. Patient-specific factors include:

- Age
- Gastrointestinal function
- History of feeding tolerance
- Nutrient requirements
- Feeding route

Several formula-specific factors must also be considered prior to choosing an enteral formula; these include:

- Osmolality
- Renal solute load
- Nutrient complexity
- Product availability
- Cost
- Caloric density

Infants Less than 1 Year of Age

Human milk and/or commercial infant formulas constitute the most appropriate feedings for infants who are less than 1 year of age. Human milk is the optimal choice when available. When human milk is not available, commercially prepared infant formulas are the next best choice.

Breast Milk Tube Feedings

Human milk provides the optimal food for infants and offers many immunologic and nutritional benefits.[3] Infants who are unable to nurse at the breast can receive pumped breast milk through a feeding tube; however, the delivery of breast milk by tube requires some unique considerations. First of all, the mother must be taught safe methods for the collection and storage of her milk.[11] Breast milk administration techniques also should be devised and implemented.

Continuous drip feedings of human milk have been associated with appreciable fat losses, which result in a significant reduction of energy delivered to the infant.[12] These losses occur because the fat in human milk separates and collects in the infusion system. A caloric loss of approximately 20% is typical. The delivery of essential fatty acids, phospholipids, cholesterol, and associated fat-soluble vitamins may also be diminished. It should be noted that when residual milk is flushed from the tubing, a large fat bolus may be delivered to the patient. Patients with impaired gastrointestinal function may not tolerate a fat bolus.

Short-term refrigeration of human milk has been shown to increase the delivery of fat during continuous feedings.[13] Therefore, when delivering a continuous feeding of breast milk, the use of refrigerated milk may be advantageous. Unfortunately, significant fat losses still occur. If continuous feedings of expressed breast milk are required, combining the expressed breast milk with a liquid fortifier or other liquid formulas can promote more efficient delivery of breast milk nutrients via tube.[11] Use of a syringe pump helps to decrease the adherence of fat to the feeding pump bag and tubing. It is also advantageous to invert the syringe pump to encourage any separation of fat to be pushed through the pump first.

Intermittent bolus feeding of human milk, in contrast, does not result in a significant loss of fat in the tubing or the terminal delivery of a large fat bolus. Therefore, intermittent bolus feeding is the preferred method of delivery for the tube feeding of human milk, whenever possible.

Infant Formula Feedings

Iron-fortified infant formulas are an appropriate substitute for infants who are not able to receive breast milk. The most common breast milk substitutes are manufactured as dried powders, which then require reconstitution using water. Several manufacturing companies also offer a concentrated liquid formula that still requires reconstitution with water. Ready-to-feed infant formulas, provided by a small number of manufacturers and in a limited number of products, are also available. It is not possible to sterilize powdered formulas. It is best to use sterile water when reconstituting powdered formulas.[10,14,15] When available, the use of a nutritionally appropriate sterile liquid infant formula is preferred, such as liquid concentrated formulas or ready-to-feed infant formulas.[1]

A broad range of tube feeding products are available with different characteristics. These products are suited for a variety of medical problems found in pediatrics, and are listed in **Table 19-1**. Most manufacturers' product guides have detailed information about the indicated use of formulas and absorption/utilization routes.[16–21] Infant formulas can be classified according to the protein source: cow's milk, soy, protein hydrolysate, or amino acid. The use of highly specialized formulas for infants and children with inborn errors of metabolism is addressed in Chapter 9.

The standard dilution for infant formulas is 20 kcal/oz; however, infants who have increased metabolic needs and/or a decreased fluid tolerance may not be able to consume an adequate volume of standard formulas to promote growth. In this instance, a more concentrated formula may be needed. Formulas with a caloric density greater than 20 kcal/oz are most commonly provided to infants with chronic lung disease and congenital heart disease or to those infants with chronic renal failure who require continuous ambulatory peritoneal dialysis. Concentrated infant formulas may also be useful for infants with nonorganic failure to thrive during periods of catch-up growth.

Infant formulas can be concentrated cautiously to a maximum of 30 kcal/oz (without modular additives) by adding less water to a concentrated liquid or powdered formula base.[22] If human milk is used in lieu of infant formulas, it can be "concentrated" with the addition of powdered infant formula. When this formula base (or human milk) is concentrated, the infant's water balance in relation to renal solute load should be monitored. Patients on formulas concentrated to more than 120% (24 kcal/oz)[23] should be monitored frequently for signs of dehydration as noted by irregular output of urine, stool, or emesis) or high urine specific gravity or nutrient imbalances.

To ensure adequate hydration for the initial fluid prescription, it is a general practice to use 100 mL/kg for the first 10 kg of body weight. For weight between 10 and 20 kg, use 1000 mL plus 50 mL/kg for each kg over 10 kg; for weight over 20 kg, use 1500 mL plus 20 mL/kg for each kg over 20 kg.[24,25] Fluid should be adjusted frequently based on weight gain changes. Insensible water loss should be factored, as well as additional needs caused by any medical condition.

If insensible water losses are high, it is advisable to concentrate the base formula (or human milk) to only 24 kcal/oz. The caloric density can be further increased by utilizing modular additives of carbohydrate (glucose polymers) or fat (vegetable oil or medium-chain triglycerides [MCT]). Carbohydrate and fat additives do not increase the renal solute load; however, carbohydrate additives can cause a moderate increase in osmolality. With the addition of a long-chain triglyceride, the gastric emptying time may be decreased. This effect may be clinically significant for those patients who are at risk for aspiration and already have delayed gastric emptying.

Increases in caloric density of the tube feeding are best tolerated by the patient when advanced gradually in increments of 2–4 kcal/oz/day.[22] Formulas that consist of a base concentration of 24–26 kcal/oz and also contain modular additives of fat (e.g., 0.25–0.50 g corn oil/oz, 2.5–5.0 kcal/oz, respectively) and/or carbohydrates (e.g., 0.5–1.0 g glucose polymer/oz, 2–4 kcal/oz, respectively) are generally tolerated by infants. The change in the percentage of calories from carbohydrate and fat and the ratio of protein/100 calories by the addition of modulars must be taken into account when offered to infants.

Table 19-2 contains three comparisons of nutrient percentages and the percentage change with modulars. Patients on concentrated formulas should be monitored closely and changed to a more appropriate distribution of macronutrients, as tolerated.

The distribution of calories in breast milk is approximately 6–7% calories from protein, 50–52% calories from fat, and 40–43% from carbohydrate. Infant formula's distribution of macronutrients is 8–12% calories from protein, 45–50% calories from fat and 40–45% calories from carbohydrate.[16,17,26–28]

Protein intakes accounting for more than 16% of calories could contribute to azotemia and negative water balance if associated fluid intakes are low. Established protein needs are 2.5 to 3.3 grams per 100 calories. A minimum of 2.2 g/kg is recommended for infants younger than 3 months and a minimum of 1.8 g/kg for infants older than 3 months.[29] Additionally, high carbohydrate intakes may contribute to osmotic diarrhea, and fat intakes that exceed 60% of the formula calories could lead to ketosis.

TABLE 19-1 Characteristics of Selected Enteral Formulas

Formula Classification	Product Classification	Possible Indications for Use	Infant Formula up to 12 Months	Pediatric Formula 1 to 10 Years	Adult Formula 10+ Years
Standard milk-based (SMB)	Intact protein Contains lactose Long-chain triglycerides Moderate residue Low to moderate osmolality	Normally functioning GI tract Lactose tolerance	Human milk Abbott Laboratories Similac Advanced Mead Johnson Enfamil Lipil Nestle Good Start Bright Beginnings Gentle		
Standard milk-based altered	Intact protein Electrolyte manipulation (low iron, altered calcium, phosphorous) Low renal solute load Lactose free Added starch	Renal, endocrine conditions Lactose intolerant Mild reflux	Abbott Laboratories PM 60/40 Mead Johnson Enfamil AR Abbott Labs Similac Sensitive RS	Abbott Laboratories Pediasure[‡] Nestle Compleat Pediatric[‡] Resource Boost Nutren Junior[‡] Kid Essentials	Abbott Laboratories Ensure Products Jevity[‡] Osmolite[‡] Nestle Compleat[‡] Boost Nutren[‡] Carnation Instant Breakfast Impact
Standard soy lactose free	Intact protein Low-moderate residue Low-moderate osmolality	Primary lactose deficiency Secondary lactose deficiency (intestinal injury or PEM) Galactosemia	Abbott Laboratories Isomil Products Mead Johnson Prosobee Nestle Good Start Soy Plus	Bright Beginnings Soy Pediatric Drink	
Standard added fiber	Intact protein Lactose free 4.3–14 g fiber/1000 mL Low-moderate osmolality	Constipation Diarrhea Normal digestive/absorptive capacity	Abbott Labs Isomil DF	Abbott Laboratories Pediasure with fiber[‡] Nestle Nutrition Compleat Pediatric[‡] Nutren Jr with fiber[‡] Bright Beginnings Soy drink with fiber	Abbott Laboratories Ensure with fiber Jevity[‡] Osmolite Nestle Nutrition Compleat[‡] Boost Nutren[‡] Impact with fiber
Lactose free/ modified fat	Intact protein Fat content 88% MCT 12% long-chain triglycerides	Chylothorax Intestinal lymphangiectasia, severe steatorrhea, cholestasis, liver disease	Nutricia North America Monogen[‡]	Mead Johnson Portagen[‡] Nestle Nutrition Vivonex Pediatric[‡]	Mead Johnson Portagen[‡]

Semi-elemental	Hydrolyzed protein Lactose free Low-moderate osmolality Partial MCT content	Steatorrhea Intestinal resection Cystic fibrosis Chronic liver disease Inflammatory bowel disease Diarrhea associated with hypoalbuminemia Allergy to cow's milk and soy proteins Not needed for jejunal feedings in patients with normal GI function	Abbott Laboratories Alimentum Advanced‡ Mead Johnson Pregestimil Lipil‡ Nutramigen Lipil	Abbott Laboratories Vital Junior‡ Nestle Nutritionals Peptamen Junior‡	Abbott Laboratories Vital HN‡ Nestle Nutritionals Peptamen‡
Elemental	Protein as free amino acids Lactose free High osmolality Low fat Carbohydrate in form of glucose oligosaccharides	Intestinal fistula Glycogen storage disease Chylothorax, intestinal lymphangiectasia not responsive to Monogen Short gut syndrome HIV + inflammatory bowel disease	Mead Johnson Nutramigen AA Nutricia Neocate Infant‡ Neocate Nutra‡ Abbott Laboratories Elecare‡	Nestle Nutrition Vivonex Pediatric‡ Nutricia Neocate One Plus‡ Neocate Junior‡ Pediatric E028‡ Pepdite Junior‡ Abbott Laboratories Elecare‡	Nestle Nutrition Vivonex Plus‡ Vivonex RTF‡ Vivonex TEN‡ Tolerex
Calorically dense	Intact protein Lactose free High renal solute load High osmolality 1.5–2.0 kcal/mL	Fluid restriction Increased metabolic needs Not recommended for transpyloric feeds		Nestle Nutrition Boost Kid Essentials	Abbott Laboratories Oxepa Pulmocare TwoCal HN Nestle Nutritionals Boost High Protein Fibersource HN Isosource HN Isosource 1.5 Nutren Replete‡ Nutren 1.5 ‡ Nutren 2.0‡ Resource 2.0‡ Impact 1.5

(continued)

TABLE 19-1 *(Continued)*

Formula Classification	Product Classification	Possible Indications for Use	Infant Formula up to 12 Months	Pediatric Formula 1 to 10 Years	Adult Formula 10+ Years
Premature	Increased calories Increased calcium, phosphorous, protein	Premature infants for first year of life	Abbott Laboratories Similac Neosure‡ Similac Special Care‡ Mead Johnson Enfamil Enfacare‡ Bright Beginnings NeoCare		
Follow-up	Over 1 year of age iron fortified Balanced nutrition with vitamins, minerals			Mead Johnson Enfamil Next Step Enfamil Next Step Soy Abbott Laboratories Similac Advanced-2 Bright Beginnings Follow-On formula Nestle Nutrition Good Start 2	

* Blenderized feedings contain 6 g dietary fiber per liter.

‡ Contains medium-chain triglycerides (MCT) as part of total fat.

Source: Mead Johnson, referenced on December 20, 2009, http://www.enfamil.com; Abbott Laboratories, referenced on December 20, 2009, http://www.abbott.com; Nestle Nutrition, referenced on December 20, 2009, http://www.nestle-nutrition.com; Bright Beginnings, referenced on December 20, 2009, http://www.brightbeginnings.com; Nutricia North America, referenced on December 20, 2009, http://www.nutricia.com.

TABLE 19-2 Nutrients in Different Concentrations and Formula Recipes

+ 4 kcal/oz Formula	24 kcal/oz from Standard Dilution	24 kcal/oz from Liquid Concentrates	20 kcal/oz Formula Powder or 20 kcal/oz Corn Oil
Oz per 100 calories	5	4.16	3.57
Cholesterol (g/oz)	2.4	2.5	2.5
% calories	43	43	36
Protein (g/oz)	0.43	0.51	0.51
% calories	9	9	7
Fat (g/oz)	1.08	1.3	1.82
% calories	48	48	57
Protein (g per 100 kcal)	2.14	2.14	1.82

Diluting formula to less than 20 kcal/oz should be done only with careful consideration and monitoring because of the risk of hyponatremia, diluted or insufficient nutrients, and/or excess fluid.[23,30]

It is important to ensure that caregivers clearly understand the instructions for mixing formulas correctly when counseling for either increased of decreased caloric density.

Children Older than 1 Year

Feedings for children between 1 and 10 years of age include a choice of pediatric follow-up formulas, pediatric enteral formulas, and/or various homemade blenderized feedings. The caloric density of feedings utilized for children in this age group can range from 30 kcal/oz to 60 kcal/oz. A change to a more calorically dense formula may not always be appropriate. Therefore, the caloric density of an enteral formula may need to be increased with the use of a modular if the patient has increased metabolic needs and/or decreased fluid tolerance.

Formulas designed for pediatric enteral feedings meet the daily recommended dietary allowances (RDAs) or the adequate intakes (AIs) in a volume of 900 to 1300 mL per day (see Appendix H).[26–28] These enteral products are isotonic and lactose free, with a partial MCT content to facilitate absorption.

Under specific conditions, infant formulas can be continued through 4 years of age. These formulas can be concentrated to provide higher levels of nutrients, but also have a higher osmolality. Additional vitamin or mineral supplementation may also be needed, depending on the specific volume provided. Altered formulas have not been tested in vitro or processed by the manufacturer to be absorbed or used by the body as the original product. Adding nutrient supplementation, such as calcium or phosphorus, to a formula does not guarantee that the patient will be able to utilize the extra nutrients.

Infant formulas have a lower renal solute load than do products designed for patients who are older than 1 year of age. These formulas may be more appropriate for malnourished toddlers who may actually be infant size.

Adolescents

Standard milk-based, lactose-free, elemental, fiber-containing, and calorically dense formulas are commercially available for children between the ages of 10 and 18 years. For these children, many factors require consideration, such as maturation level, physical ability or limitations, calorie requirements, and volume tolerance. Adolescent nutrient needs increase with the last growth phase. Their calorie and protein needs may be met in a pediatric formula but other nutrient needs, such as calcium, sodium, and iron, are not met. It is important to assess the adequacy of the micronutrients provided by the volume of formula, particularly when assessing the intake of a child who requires low volumes to promote growth. Micronutrient analysis is helpful in matching a formula or combination of pediatric and adult formulas to meet the unique needs of the teen.

A variety of computer nutrition assessment programs are available; when selecting one, pediatric parameters and pediatric formulas within the database should be considered in the selection criteria.

Blenderized Feedings

Blenderized feedings consist of a mixture of various meats, fruits, vegetables, milk (or formula), carbohydrates, fats, water, vitamins, and minerals that have been blenderized and strained. These blenderized feeding recipes can be made for use in an institution or in the home setting. Blenderized feedings are moderate in residue and moderate to high in osmolality and viscosity. Because their high viscosity hinders flow through small feeding tubes, these feedings are most often administered as gastrostomy tube feedings.

Other disadvantages of blenderized feedings include a potentially high bacteria count,[11–14] and the additional labor required for preparation. Homemade blenderized feedings:

- Provide a more variable nutrient content than do commercially manufactured products
- Are not emulsified
- Can be used only when enteral feeding is delivered into the stomach
- May not provide all essential nutrients in the level required by a pediatric patient

Blenderized feedings are considered for use today in the healthcare arena when third-party reimbursement or support is not provided. Although homemade formulas seem to be more economical in the home setting using food products, nutrient adequacy or variety is not taken into account. However,economics is particularly important to families of children with chronic diseases, so blenderized concoctions will continue to represent a viable feeding alternative when a pediatric-specific product is not covered by a third-party payor.

Because inappropriate homemade tube feedings can result in hypernatremic dehydration[22] and a number of nutrient deficiencies, it is important to perform a periodic analysis of the recipe, including verification of how the family is making the formula at home, the adequacy of the nutrients, and the associated fluids. It is equally important to monitor the intake of protein and electrolytes because excess may lead to a negative water balance in the patient.[25,31]

Commercial Adult Formulas

A large variety of adult enteral products are commercially available primarily through Abbott Laboratories or Nestlé. These products contain macronutrients in various forms and amounts. As with adolescent formulas, they can also be divided into several general categories: standard milk-based, lactose-free, elemental, fiber-containing, and calorically dense. General characteristics of selected adult enteral products with possible indications for use are covered in Table 19-1. This list is not inclusive of all products that are commercially available, but is intended to provide examples of products that are available in each general category. Information regarding the complete nutrient composition of commercial adult formulas is readily available from various manufacturers.

It should be noted that adult enteral products are not designed for use in children and have not been extensively tested in the pediatric population. Specific concerns regarding the use of these products in children are addressed in the following discussions of renal solute load and nutrient requirements.

Renal Solute Load and Fluid Balance

The renal solute load of a formula consists primarily of electrolytes and metabolic end products of protein metabolism that the kidneys must excrete in the urine.[23] These solutes require water for urinary excretion and therefore have a major effect on water balance. Infants have an immature renal system with limited concentrating ability, and they require more free water to excrete solutes than do older children and adults. Therefore, infants are at particular risk for negative water balance and subsequent dehydration. Potential renal solute load (PRSL) does not need to be calculated routinely, but is important to determine with patients who have medical problems or formula prescriptions that would influence renal metabolism. Equations for PRSL vary in the units of measurement for solute load.[3] An example equation is as follows:

$$\text{PRSL (mOsm/L)} = \text{mEq sodium/L} + \text{mEq potassium/L} + \text{mEq chloride/L} + [4 \times \text{protein g/L}]$$

The renal solute load and fluid balance should be closely monitored when infants have a low fluid intake, are receiving calorically dense feedings, or have increased extrarenal fluid losses (i.e., fever, diarrhea, sweating) and/or impaired renal concentrating ability.[23] Neurologically impaired infants and children who are unable to indicate thirst may also be at risk for dehydration.

Infant formulas at standard dilution contain approximately 90% free water[16–18,27] (preformed water plus water of oxidation). In contrast, standard pediatric and adult enteral formulas contain approximately 85% free water. Because adult formulas are also higher in protein and electrolytes, they possess a higher renal solute load. Therefore, when administering adult products to infants and toddlers, proper precautions should be taken; for example, additional water may be required and can usually be given while flushing the feeding tube.

Osmolality

Osmolality refers to the number of active particles in a kilogram of solution. The osmolality of a formula may affect the tolerance. Feeding intolerances associated with delivering a hyperosmolar formula may include delayed gastric emptying, abdominal distention, vomiting, or diarrhea.

Carbohydrates, electrolytes, and amino acids are the major factors that determine the gastrointestinal osmotic load of a formula. Smaller particles, such as glucose and free amino acids, contribute more to a higher osmolality than do larger particles, such as polysaccharides or intact protein molecules. Thus, formulas that contain hydrolyzed protein and monosaccharides will tend to have a higher osmolality than will formulas with intact protein and glucose polymers.

Recommendations for infant formulas are at osmolality less than 460 mOsm/kg.[23] Therefore, the osmolality in formulas for infants and children younger than 4 years should be less than 400 mOsm/kg and for older children under 600 mOsm/kg.[3] The osmolality of infant formulas at a caloric density of 20 kcal/oz generally falls below this suggested limit (range of 200–380 mOsm/kg); however, several pediatric and adult enteral products exceed this limit at a caloric density of 30 kcal/oz and may require a dilution to two-thirds strength prior to use in infants. Medications can also increase osmolality significantly and should be evaluated prior to selecting a formula.[25] The osmolality of Pregestimil, for example, concentrated to 27 kcal/oz is approximately 446 mOsm/kg, whereas a multivitamin with iron (Poly-Vi-Sol with Iron) at 10 mg/mL Fe is 10,683 mOsm/kg.[25]

Nutrient Requirements

When using DRIs (RDAs) as a standard for comparison, differences in the needs of nonambulatory, ill, or physically delayed children must be considered. Values for specific conditions such as spina bifida, Down syndrome, and bronchopulmonary dysplasia have been established.[33] Calorie levels are based on height in centimeters or percentage of RDAs.

The DRI and the RDA may both be lower than potential therapeutic needs dictated by specific disease or deficiency states. In specific circumstances, both infant and adult formulas may require vitamin and/or mineral supplementation.

Supplements may not be absorbed or utilized in the body as desired and should be evaluated frequently. Infant formulas generally provide adequate amounts of vitamins and minerals with a volume of 1 quart. However, infants who have restricted fluid intakes (e.g., infants with congenital heart disease) may require vitamin and mineral supplementation.

Adult enteral formulas are designed to provide the adult RDAs for vitamins and minerals when a volume of 1500–2000 mL/day is administered. However, when these adult enteral products are administered to children at lower volumes, some nutrients may not be adequate. A micronutrient analysis may be warranted.

Product Availability and Cost

The cost of commercial enteral formulas may exceed the financial resources of some families. Therefore, whenever medically possible, the least specialized enteral product should be considered. The more specialized the feedings are (e.g., hydrolyzed protein and MCT oil), the higher will be the cost.

Formula costs do not necessarily constitute a socioeconomic barrier. Infants and children who range in age from birth to 5 years may be enrolled in the Women, Infants, and Children (WIC) nutrition program if their family income falls below a certain level. A variety of infant and pediatric formulas are available through this program. The Medicaid program and private insurance companies may cover enteral formulas and needed supplies, such as tubes, bags, or pumps. Coverage varies, and the healthcare team should work closely with home care companies and insurers to ensure that the patient obtains the best coverage possible. Letters of medical necessity are sometimes helpful in obtaining coverage for a specific enteral feeding product.

Selection of Specific Feeding Routes

Common routes for enteral nutrition in pediatric patients include nasogastric, nasoduodenal, nasojejunal, gastrostomy, and jejunostomy feedings. The risk of aspiration becomes a major consideration when determining whether the tube should be placed in the stomach or small intestine. The evaluation process for gastroesophageal reflux (GER) may include upper gastrointestinal endoscopy (UGI), modified barium swallow, pH probe, occasional esophageal motility, or gastric emptying study. If the patient is determined to have a high risk of aspiration due to GER, a gastrostomy tube is placed surgically. Fundoplication (surgical repair for GER) can sometimes be beneficial in reducing GER; however, postoperative complications can range from retching to dumping syndrome, swallowing problems, impaired esophageal emptying, slow feeding, and abdominal distention. **Figure 19-1** gives criteria for making a decision as to whether to use a nasogastric or enterostomy feeding route.[33]

Gastric Feeding

A direct gastric feeding is preferable to an intestinal feeding because it allows for a more normal digestive process. This is generally true because the stomach serves as a reservoir and provides for a gradual release of nutrients into the small bowel. Gastric feedings are associated with a larger osmotic and volume tolerance, a more flexible feeding schedule, easier tube insertions, and a lower frequency of diarrhea and dumping syndrome. In addition, gastric acid has a bactericidal effect that may be an important factor in decreasing the patient's susceptibility to various infections. See **Table 19-3** for enteral feeding sites and routes.[32]

Nasogastric (NG) feeding tubes are used for the short term (4 to 6 weeks). Patients requiring long-term enteral nutrition are often evaluated after this time to determine the best enteral device to meet their needs (such as a gastrostomy [g] tube).

Nasogastric feeding is contraindicated in patients with severe esophagitis or who have an intestinal obstruction between the nose and stomach. In addition, nasogastric tubes may not be tolerated in neonates, who are obligate nose breathers. To prevent airway occlusion in this instance, orogastric tubes are often used when tube feeding is indicated.

Transpyloric Feedings

Nasoduodenal, nasojejunal, or gastrojejunal feeding is desirable for patients who are at risk of aspiration or who are unable to tolerate feedings into the stomach. Typically, this

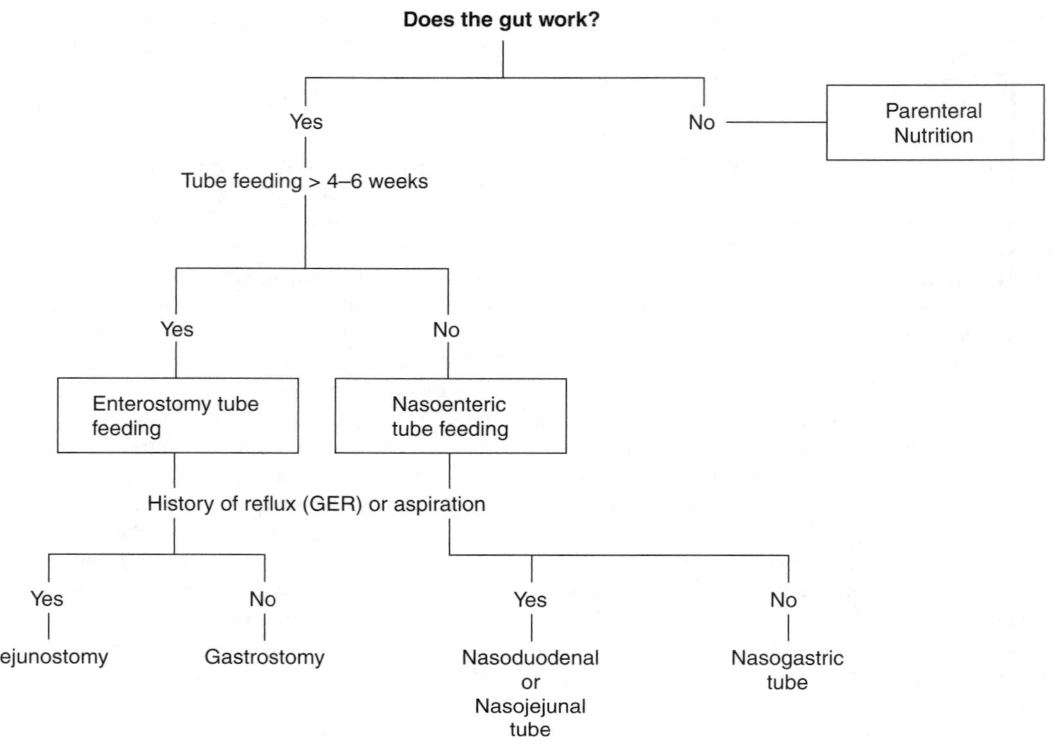

FIGURE 19-1 Decision Making for Selecting the Feeding Site

Source: Adapted with permission from Enteral and tube feedings, Figure 16-1, page 263. In: Rombeau JL, Caldwell MD, eds., *Clinical Nutrition*, vol. 1. © 1984, WB Saunders Co.

includes patients who have a diminished gag reflex, delayed gastric emptying, frequent vomiting, or severe GER. Nasoenteric tube placement is the most common route of enteral access. These tubes may fail secondary to tube occlusion or tube dislodgement and interrupt tube feeding and medication schedule.[34,35]

Nasojejunal feeding may be more efficacious than nasoduodenal feeding in preventing aspiration.[36] Gastric reflux of duodenally administered solutions can be a problem. Additionally, nasoduodenal tubes may fail to enter or stay in the duodenum, resulting in aspiration.[36] Nasojejunal tubes may also be less likely than nasoduodenal tubes to become dislodged in children with cystic fibrosis, who may experience severe coughing episodes. This is also true for children with cancer, who may have vomiting associated with chemotherapy. Specific procedures for nasoduodenal or nasojejunal intubation have been outlined by Wesley.[37] The enteric position of the tube requires radiographic verification before feeding is initiated. A potential complication of transpyloric feeding is intestinal perforation with use of stiff, large-bore tubes.[37] Use of small-bore tubes made of polyurethane or silicone might decrease the incidence of this complication; however, there may be an increase in tube clogging.

Jejunostomy Feeding

Endoscopically placed gastrostomies or jejunostomies (PEG/PEJ) are less invasive and require less time under anesthesia. In some cases the use of conscious sedation can be used.[38,39] Low-profile gastrostomy devices are frequently used as replacement devices after the stoma tract is well healed (usually 6 to 8 weeks). There are also low-profile devices that can be placed initially as a one-step procedure.[38,40] Enteral feedings, although safer than parenteral nutrition, are not without complications (see **Table 19-4**).[41]

Administration of Feeding

The methods of delivery and advancing the feeding rate and formula concentration are other key factors that the practitioner must consider in providing EN for patients.

Methods of Delivery

The specific method utilized for feeding delivery is contingent on the clinical condition of the patient and the

TABLE 19-3 Enteral Feeding Sites and Routes

Site	Route	Advantage	Disadvantages	Indications	Contraindication
Stomach		Anti-infective mechanism Allows for normal processes and hormonal responses Tolerances of larger osmotic loads Decreased incidence of dumping syndrome Greater mobility between feedings Greater flexibility in feeding schedule and formula choice		As the first consideration for enteral nutrition	Delayed gastric emptying Pulmonary aspiration GER Intractable vomiting Impaired or absent gag reflex
	Orogastric	Does not obstruct nasal passage	May increase salivary flow and make clearance more difficult	< 34-wk gestation with gag; doesn't obstruct nasal passage	> 34-wk gestation or when patient acquires a gag
	Nasogastric	Easy intubation Surgery not required	Nasal, esophageal, or tracheal irritation Local skin care required Easily dislodged by a toddler Easily dislodged by a forceful cough May stimulate gag Caretaker must be well-trained Limited long-term compliance in the home care setting	For short-term use	Same as for the stomach
	Gastrostomy	Allows patient greater mobility Feedings are generally well-tolerated Larger diameter feeding tube lessens chances of obstruction/clogged feeding tube Doesn't obstruct the airway	Requires a surgical procedure for placement May result in increased GER Occasional leakage around the insertion site Skin irritation and infection Difficulty hiding the external portion of the tube under clothing Risk of intra-abdominal leak with peritonitis	Prolonged enteral nutrition support	Same as for the stomach

(continued)

TABLE 19-3 *(Continued)*

Site	Route	Advantage	Disadvantages	Indications	Contraindication
Small Bowel		Can feed enterally despite poor gastric motility and persistent high gastric residuals Lessens the chances of gastric distention	Less mixing of formula with pancreatic enzymes Tube easily malpositioned Greater exposure to radiation when checking placement Greater risk of bacterial overgrowth Changes small bowel intestinal flora May limit choices of feeding schedule and formula selection	Congenital upper GI anomalies Inadequate gastric motility After upper GI surgery Patients with increased risk of aspiration	Nonfunctioning GI tract
	Nasojejunal		Requires radiographic proof of adequate placement Takes a long time to pass without radiographic placement Tube easily displaced during peristalsis	For short-term nutrition support	
	Jejunostomy		Technically difficult to place	Jejunal feedings for >6 mo For postop nutritional management of abdominal surgery while an ileus exists	Patient at operative risk

Source: Copyright © 1990, K. Hendricks and W. Walker.

TABLE 19-4 Complications of Enteral Feeding

Complication	Possible Causes	Management/Prevention
Gastrointestinal		
Aspiration pneumonia	Aspiration of feedings	Confirm placement of tube prior to administration of feeds.
	Emesis	
	Displacement or migration	
	Supine position during feeds	Elevate head 30–45 degrees.
	Gastrointestinal reflux	
	Presence of nasogastric tube preventing complete closure of esophagus	Tube placement into the duodenum.
	Delayed gastric emptying	Use prokinetics.
Bloating/cramps, gas	Air in tubing	Remove as much air as possible when setting up feed.
Diarrhea	Bacterial contamination of formula	Proper storage, preparation and administration of feeds.
		Change feeding bag daily.
		Limit hang time to 4 hours for commercially prepared formula.
		Undiluted "ready to feed" products minimize risk.
	Food allergies	Consider changing to a lactose-free formula.
	Hyperosmolar formula	Consider changing formula to an isotonic formula.
	Too rapid infusion	Decrease rate of infusion to previously tolerated rate.
	Low fiber intake	Consider using formula containing fiber.
	Fat malabsorption	Consider changing formula to a product with partial MCT content.
	Medications (antibiotics), antacids, sorbitol, magnesium, antineoplastic agents	
Dumping syndrome	Cold formula	Administer formula at room temperature.
	Rapid feeding	Decrease infusion rate.
Vomiting	Hyperosmolar formula	Consider changing formula to an isotonic product.
	Delayed gastric emptying	Consider transpyloric route.
		Consider continuous infusion.
		Elevate head of bed 45 degrees during feeding.
		Check for residuals prior to feedings.
	Obstruction	Consider utilizing prokinetics.
		Discontinue feedings.
	Too rapid advancement of volume/concentration	Return to previously tolerated strength/volume, and advance more slowly.
Mechanical		
Clogged tubing	Inadequate flushing	Flush tube before and after aspirating residuals, after bolus feedings, and every 4–8 hours during continuous feedings.
	Inadequate crushing of medications	Dissolve crushed tablets in warm water.
		Use liquid form of medications when available.
	Formula and medication residual	Flush tube before and after medication administration.
		Avoid mixing formula with medication.
	Kinking of tubing	Replace feeding tube.
	Highly viscous fiber rice formulas	

(continued)

TABLE 19-4 *(Continued)*

Complication	Possible Causes	Management/Prevention
Tube displacement	Coughing Vomiting Inadvertent dislodgment Removal of tube by patient	Replace feeding tube.
Metabolic		
Dehydration	Inadequate free water Hyperosmolar formulas	Monitor intake and output. Monitor hydration status routinely. Assess renal solute load of formula.
Overhydration	Excessive fluid administration Too rapid refeeding of patients with moderate to severe PEM	Advance feedings slowly. Allow a 5- to 7-day period to reach nutritional goals.
Electrolyte imbalance	Formula components Medical condition/diagnosis	Evaluate electrolyte adequacy of specific formula and appropriateness of formula dilution. Monitor electrolytes, phosphorus, BUN, creatinine, and glucose.
Failure to achieve appropriate weight gain	Inadequate nutrient intake	Evaluate adequacy of nutrient intake. Perform routine nutritional assessments.
Psychologic		
Fear of tube insertion	Psychologic trauma associated with insertion of nasogastric tube/gastrostomy	Utilize relaxation techniques. Medical play: allow child to handle tube and insert tube in doll. Comfort child after insertion. Consider sedation prior to replacement of tube.
Altered body image	Visible presence of nasogastric tube or gastrostomy tube	Consider nocturnal feedings and removal of tube during the day. Consider use of low-profile gastrostomy device.
Food refusal	Deprivation of normal oral feeding experiences	Initiate oral feedings when medically possible. Provide positive oral experience during tube feedings. Refer to speech therapist.

Source: Data from Grumow JE, Al-Hafidh AS, Tunell WP. Gastroesophageal reflux following percutaneous endoscopic gastrostomy in children. *J Pediatr Surg*. 1989;24:44–45.

anatomic location of the tube (gastric or transpyloric). Continuous drip and intermittent bolus administration are the two methods most often used for delivery of enteral feedings to infants and children. Intermittent bolus feedings are generally delivered to the stomach by gravity over 15 to 30 minutes on a schedule of every 2 to 4 hours or via pump over a 1-hour period several times during 24 hours. Bolus feeding more closely mimics a normal oral feeding pattern and is often preferred for this reason. Bolus feeds are typically used during the day as opposed to overnight because there is an increased likelihood of GER with bolus feeds.[34,42] Intermittent feedings better facilitate transition to a home setting and eventually the transition off enteral feeds.

In contrast, the continuous drip method provides an infusion of nutrients at a constant rate over several hours. Continuous drip feedings are beneficial for patients who cannot tolerate bolus feedings or those with altered gastrointestinal function, and are essential for those receiving enteral transpyloric or nocturnal feedings. Continuous feedings require the use of a feeding pump to deliver formula at a consistent rate over a period of time.

In practice, the individual patient's tolerance ultimately dictates the method of delivery. In many cases a combination of intermittent bolus feeds during the day and a continuous drip overnight is used. Each method of delivery provides a number of specific advantages and disadvantages (see **Exhibit 19-3**).

Pumps

Enteral feeding pumps are typically utilized to control the rate of delivery of continuous drip feedings and bolus feedings. A number of enteral feeding pumps are available for use in pediatric patients.[43] Portable enteral pumps or backpack pumps allow for greater patient mobility while receiving their enteral feeding.

Important features of enteral pumps for use in the pediatric population include the ability to provide low delivery rates (less than 5 mL/hour) and to advance in small increments (1–5 mL/hour). Other desirable features of pediatric pumps include tamper-proof controls, an occlusion alarm, and a low-battery indicator.[11] These features all contribute to the safe and efficient delivery of continuous tube feedings for the pediatric population.

Delivery of human milk via enteral feeding requires a different system than that for infant, pediatric, or adult formulas. The loss of fat and fat-soluble vitamins due to the adherence of the fat to the enteral pump bag and tubing poses a unique complication. Because the required volumes of human milk are often low, particularly with continuous infusions, a syringe pump is typically used to deliver human milk via an

EXHIBIT 19-3 Methods of Delivering Enteral Feedings

Continuous Drip Feedings

Advantages

1. Ability to increase volume of formula more rapidly
2. Improved absorption of major nutrients in infants with intestinal diseases
3. Reduced stool output in hypermetabolic patients
4. Associated with a reduced incidence of vomiting in infants with gastroesophageal reflux
5. Greater caloric intake when volume tolerance may be a problem

Disadvantages

1. More expensive feeding method because a pump is required for delivery
2. Restricts patient ambulation
3. Less physiologic

Intermittent Feedings

Advantages

1. More physiologic because a normal feeding schedule is mimicked
2. Less expensive because an enteral pump is not required
3. Greater flexibility in feeding schedule
4. Freedom from infusion equipment
5. Improved nitrogen retention with less fat and fluid accumulation

Disadvantages

1. Associated with a longer time to reach nutritional goals
2. Reduced weight gain and nutrient absorption in infants with malabsorption
3. Larger-bore tube may be required for gravity administration
4. More time required for administration than for pump-delivered feedings

enteral feeding system. The use of the syringe pump also helps to avoid the adherence of fat to the feeding bag.[1]

In cases where enteral feeding pumps are not used, enteral formula can be delivered by gravity infusions either as intermittent or continuous drip. The feeding bag is suspended on a bedside pole where the rate is dependant only on the height of the feeding bag. The delivery rate is not precise and often predisposes the patient to gastroesophageal reflux or aspiration.[44]

Initiation and Advancement of Feedings

There are published recommendations for advancing enteral nutrition in pediatric patients.[1,42] Many of these recommendations are based on institutional practices and modification of adult regimens. Generally, the rate of advancement of a feeding regimen (**Exhibit 19-4**) is contingent on the structure and function of the patient's gastrointestinal tract and should be guided by the patient's age, underlying disease, nutrition status, and nutritional requirements, as well as the enteral access device.[26,36]

Isotonic formulas should be used initially at a rate of 1–2 mL/kg/hour for children < 35 kg and at a rate of 1 mL/kg/hour for children > 35 kg. Changes in volume and concentration should never be made simultaneously. Stable and/or older patients may be able to tolerate a rapid increase in the enteral feedings rate, generally reaching the nutritional goal within a 24- to 48-hour time frame.[1,42]

Diluting enteral feedings in the initial stages is not necessary and may increase the risk of microbial contamination.[43,45] However, diluted formulas can be considered for patients with altered gastrointestinal function or when transitioning to enteral feeding from parenteral nutrition. For gut-sensitive patients, advancing from a diluted to full strength product over several days may be warranted.

Volume of the tube feeding should be increased before concentration when administering transpyloric feedings. Advance concentration before volume when delivering gastric feedings. If feeding intolerance develops, return to the previously tolerated concentration and volume, and advance at a slower rate with caution.

For intermittent feedings, determine the total volume of a full strength, isotonic formula needed to provide the nutritional goal. A volume of 2.5–5 mL/kg (or 25% of goal volume for day 1) can be given over five to eight bolus feedings

EXHIBIT 19-4 Initiation and Advancement of Feedings

*Continuous Drip Feeding**

Age	Weight Maximum Range (kg)	Volume Range (mL/kg/d)	Initial Rate (mL/h)	Advancement Rate (mL/h)	Rate (mL/h)
Infant	3–10	125–160	1	1.5–3	25–50
Toddler/preschool	10–20	110–130	1	5–10	60–70
School age	20–40	70–110	2	5–10	80–100
Teenage	> 40	60–80	2	20–100	100–150

*Intermittent Feedings***

Age	Weight (kg)	Suggested Advancement***		
		Kcal/kg	1st day (mL)	Advance to and Evaluate for Tolerance (mL)
Infant	3–10	98–108	250	1000
Toddler/preschool	10–20	70–100	450	1800
School age	20–40	60–90	675	2700
Teenage	> 40	40–55	700	2800

*Adjust per needs, tolerance, and medical condition

**Adjust to needs and intake by mouth

***Divided over number of feeds

Sources: Data from Texas Children's Hospital. *Pediatric Nutrition Reference Guide*, 8th ed. Houston, TX: McGraw-Hill Professional; 2008; and American Academy of Pediatrics. *Pediatric Nutrition Handbook*, 6th ed. Elk Grove, IL: American Academy of Pediatrics: 2009:552–554.

per day. Gradually advance by 25% per day to reach the desired goal volume. Bolus feeds may be further increased in volume to reduce the number of feedings per day. Feedings can be administered via pump over 1 hour or by gravity over 15 to 30 minutes.[11] Bolus feedings should be given during the same period of time as it would take the child to consume the same volume orally.

For continuous feedings, the total volume of a full strength, isotonic formula needed to meet nutritional needs must be determined. Feedings should be initiated at 1–2 mL/kg/hour and advance by 0.5–1 mL/kg/hour every 6–12 hours as tolerated until the goal volume is reached. Maximum volumes for continuous or bolus feeds are determined by the individual child's tolerance.

Infants and children who are being weaned from parenteral nutrition and/or who are malnourished generally require a more conservative feeding progression than what is typically administered to children who have normal gastrointestinal function. (See also Chapter 20 on parenteral nutrition.)

Prevention and Treatment of Complications

Potential complications are generally classified into gastrointestinal, mechanical (tube-related), metabolic, and psychologic categories. Some pediatric studies have reported complications that include various mechanical problems related to gastrostomy[45,46] and to nasogastric tubes,[47,48] metabolic disturbances, and feeding disorders that are related to the delayed introduction of oral feedings.[49] Additionally, gastrointestinal complications have been associated with low serum albumin levels in pediatric surgical patients,[50–52] delayed enteral support in pediatric burn patients,[53] and contaminated feedings. A summary of the most common complications and associated management suggestions is presented in Table 19-4.

Hang Time

Formulas that require reconstitution or manipulation (dilution or additives) are at the greatest risk for bacterial contamination.[54] In contrast, the use of sterile, undiluted, ready-to-feed products minimizes the risk of contamination (see **Exhibit 19-5**).[4,26,36,45]

Precautions to guard against the contamination of enteral feedings include frequently changing the feeding bag tubing, paying careful attention to clean technique during handling of the feedings, and limiting hang time of the formulas. Specific recommendations for preparation, administration, and monitoring of enteral feedings to maximize

EXHIBIT 19-5 Guidelines for Storage and Administration of Enteral Feedings (in hours)*

Product	Storage Time Room Temp	Storage Time in Refrigerator	Hang Time[1]	Bag Change	Tubing Change
EBM/EBM with fortifiers[2]	2	24	2/2–4[5]	4	4
Sterile formula,[3] nonsterile with additives, or powdered formula[4]	< 4	24	4	4	4
Infant, pediatric, and adult sterile, canned/bottled liquid products	8	48	4	8	Infant 8 Pediatric 24
Closed system formula	24	48	24	24	24

*See references for neonates and immune-compromised patients. Manufacturer's guidelines and/or hospital policy should be followed for any manipulation of enteral nutrition products. Equipment with ice packs may be used in overnight delivery, but temperatures must be checked routinely to ensure safety. All enteral nutrition products should be placed in food-grade containers.

1. Hang time includes all periods of time that the product is not refrigerated below 45°F (i.e., transport time; tubing or equipment setup).
2. For hospitalized infants.
3. Sterile feeds include industrially produced, prepacked liquid formulas that are "commercially sterile."
4. Nonsterile feedings are those that may contain live bacteria and include hospital- or home-prepared formulas, reconstituted powdered feedings, and commercial liquid formulas to which nutrients and/or other supplements have been added in the hospital kitchen, pharmacy, unit, school, or home. Powdered formula is not recommended for neonates or immune-compromised patients, unless there is no alternative available.
5. One manufacturer recommends 2 hours and other companies recommend 4 hours.

Sources: Data from Lavine M, Clark RM. The effect of short-term refrigeration of milk and addition of breast milk fortifier on the delivery of lipids during tube feeding. *J Pediatr Gastroenterol Nutr.* 1989;8:496–499; Texas Children's Hospital. *Pediatric Nutrition Reference Guide*, 8th ed. Houston, TX: McGraw-Hill Professional. 2008; and American Academy of Pediatrics. *Pediatric Nutrition Handbook*, 6th ed. Elk Grove, IL: American Academy of Pediatrics; 2009:552–554.

bacteriologic safety have been published.[54,55] Of note, disposable enteral feeding bags should not be reused.

When nutritionally appropriate, sterile liquid formulas are recommended for all enteral feedings. Breast milk and all formulas either decanted, with modular additives, reconstituted, or diluted should hang no longer than 4 hours.[1,14] Recent research has indicated that the use of an enteral formula in a closed system is safe for a 24-hour hang time.[44,45] Some pediatric and adult products are available in a closed system that can be hung for up to 48 hours as defined by the nursing policies of the hospital.

Transition to Oral Intake

Many factors must be considered before weaning the patient off a tube feeding. Typically, the transition is done slowly with the incorporation of oral feedings used to replace nutrition previously provided by the enteral feedings.

Weaning

When the patient's medical condition allows for normal oral feedings, weaning from tube feedings can be initiated. The management of the transition back to oral feedings is multifaceted and involves the medical team, the patient, and the caregivers.[56] A complete weaning from ENS should not be considered until the patient has achieved a satisfactory nutritional status, because the patient may stop gaining weight for a time during the transition.

The weaning time may vary from a few days to several months. Records of the patient's oral intake should be kept during this time because it is important to maintain an adequate intake. Tube feedings should be continued until the patient can demonstrate that nutrient requirements can be met consistently by oral intake. Some patients use enteral nutrition in combination with parenteral nutrition and/or oral intake.[57] The combination of enteral and cycled parenteral nutrition is controlled on the basis of patient tolerance. Monitoring for intolerance or complications would be completed similarly to any nutrition delivery that is provided and not patient initiated.

A combination of enteral and oral feedings is more difficult to project. Total daily requirements in fluid and calories are calculated, then enteral feedings are used to complete what the oral feedings lack. To stimulate hunger, the enteral feeds will need to be decreased. A guideline is to begin with a 25% decrease in the caloric intake by tube, then start to offer oral feeds. This transition will require frequent evaluation because of the risk of decrease in growth with a lower caloric intake or if the child has trouble or delay in progressing. If the oral intake varies from day to day, a sliding scale for supplemental enteral feeds should be created. To summarize the recommendations at the time of transition, Glass and Lucas[58] suggest normalizing the tube feeding schedule to approximate the timing of meals and snacks, altering the feeding schedule to promote hunger, reducing the calories from tube feedings, providing adequate fluids, and, as oral intake increases, adjusting the tube feedings accordingly.

Formula Change and Acceptance

When a change in formula is indicated as part of the treatment of a GI problem, there is concern about acceptance. As infant formulas become more elemental, the taste becomes less sweet and more bitter or sour. Partially hydrolyzed and elemental formulas often also have a less pleasant odor and an unpleasant aftertaste.[59] Amniotic fluid and breast milk are sweet and vary in flavor based on the mother's diet.[60] A difference has been noted by clinicians between an infant who is initially offered a hydrolysate formula (and accepts it well) versus an older infant who is changed to the formula. The rejection does not occur until after 4 months of age. An interesting study by Mennella and associates looked at acceptance of a protein-hydrolysate formula after initially being given either a hydrolysate or a milk-based formula. Infants who were given a hydrolysate throughout infancy continued to accept it at 7.5 months (and disliked the better tasting cow's milk–based formula) whereas an infant who is switched to a hydrolysate at 7.5 months rejects it.[59] Their research indicates that responses to olfactory components of flavor are influenced by the child's experience.[60] This is also shown in 4- to 5-year-old children who were fed hydrolysates as infants and had more positive responses to them years later.[61,62]

Adolescents with phenylketonuria who went off of their formula have been shown to be able to go back to the formula with some difficulty but with fewer problems than those who were not exposed as infants.[63] Infants will readily drink hydrolyzed formulas if introduced before 4 months of age. If required after this age, it should be mixed with a formula that is already accepted while gradually increasing the proportion of hydrolysate.[59] The parent needs to work closely with a dietitian to make this transition acceptable to the child.

Feeding Disorders

Infant and toddler feeding disorders constitute a tube-feeding complication that is unique to the pediatric population. Many times, when a chronically ill infant is medically ready to begin oral feedings, the infant or toddler may display no interest in eating or may respond with manifested oral aversion when food, liquid, or utensils are near the face. In this situation, the child typically refuses, cries, gags, or vomits when offered feedings. This oral aversion can occur in children with or without mechanical eating problems.

Due to the emotional component of eating/feeding, a dysfunctional or uninformed family may further the trauma of eating by force feeding. Children who have been given ENS often do not have normal hunger cycles, normal eating experiences at a table, or a mealtime routine. All of these points should be addressed when the transition to oral feeding occurs. Severe cases of oral aversion require intervention and behavior modification from pediatric psychologists, as well as other health professionals such as speech pathologists, dietitians, and occupational therapists.[64]

Illingsworth and Lister[65] suggest that resistant feeding behavior may be due to missing a "critical period" in the development of the child's feeding skills. They indicate that the critical period for the development of chewing skills is 6 to 7 months of age; if solids are not introduced during this time, the child typically will have difficulty accepting them later.

Other important oral experiences during the first year of life include the development of the rooting and sucking reflexes, the oral exploration of objects, and the association of hunger with feeding. When a child is deprived of these normal oral feeding experiences during the first year of life, he or she may subsequently experience feeding difficulties that last throughout the toddler and preschool years. These children may also demonstrate significant delays in gross motor and personality development.[49] Daily oral therapy or "mouth play" can help to eliminate or reduce the problems that typically occur in the patient with nonoral nutrition support. Most feeding problems can be resolved or improved through medical, oral motor, and behavioral therapy.[66,67]

Initiating oral feedings as soon as medically possible can minimize feeding disorders. Concomitant speech or feeding therapy with ENS can help to alleviate oral aversion.[68] Nonnutritive sucking during tube feedings in infancy can help to stimulate oral sucking and swallowing behavior. Pediatric occupational therapists or speech pathologists are the health professionals most qualified to assess an infant's feeding potential and to design an appropriate, ongoing oral motor stimulation program. Intervention should be considered during enteral feeding rather than at the termination of enteral feeding. Lastly, textured foods ideally should be offered, if medically feasible, when the infant is at a developmental age of 6 to 7 months. Positive caregiver–child mealtime interactions are critical for achieving feeding success.[69]

Swallowing Disorders

Eating/swallowing disorder therapy often includes recommendations to thicken liquids for therapy in the management of an infant or child who has been diagnosed with misswallowing by modified barium swallow studies using videofluoroscopy. This diagnosis means that, on regular fluid consistency, the patient is at risk for aspiration or actually aspirates. Several disease states or conditions contribute to misswallowing.[70]

Swallowing dysfunction is compounded in infants or young children who have not learned the act of swallowing. A behavioral eating plan is a complicated process because the family and/or medical team are often trying to avoid an alternative feeding delivery. Developmental progress, therapy, and nutrition all must be considered as the patient's plan is developed.[71]

Adding a thickening agent or food to the formula or liquid thickens the fluid so that the patient can swallow liquid with decreased risk of aspiration. If at all possible, a gel thickener should be considered. They are made from gum substances and contribute no calorie or carbohydrate value.[72] Powdered thickeners have nutritional consequences. The more thickener that is required, the more effect this will have on the nutrition content of the intake. Available powdered commercial thickening agents are carbohydrate based, with few or no other nutrients. Adding a carbohydrate product will skew the nutrients, add calories, and increase free water needs in a medically unstable patient or one who is at risk for dehydration. The recipe for thickened consistency is included with the package label, and the categories for thickening generally are nectar, honey, and pudding consistencies.

An example of a higher calorie formulation is given to illustrate how this can be done. A 4-month-old baby, EK was diagnosed with silent aspiration and a history of ventricular septal defect (VSD). The patient was 84% his ideal body weight, current weight of 5.2kg. Estimated energy needs were 120–130 kcal/kg. The patient required intake of 120 mL eight times per day of a standard 20 kcal/oz formula. EK was only able to consume orally 75 mL at each feed.

Speech recommendations following video fluoroscopy swallow study (VFSS) was for thin nectar liquid consistency for all oral feeds offered using medium flow nipple. Nectar thick consistency was accomplished by the addition of 1 teaspoon of crushed rice cereal per ounce of formula. The addition of rice cereal provides 5kcals/ teaspoon, increasing the caloric density of standard 20kcal/oz formula to 25kcal/oz.

Using a combination of nocturnal enteral feedings and oral feedings, the recommended feedings would be 75 mL of nectar thick formula three times during the day (225mL, 187.5 kcal) plus nocturnal feeds at 60 mL/hr run for 12 hours (720ml, 480kcal). Total nutrition provided 667.5kcal (128.4kcal/kg).

Baby rice cereal can be used a thickener, and it will provide some nutrients other than carbohydrate. Dehydrated baby cereal flakes are difficult to blend with the formula in a liquid form, do not thicken evenly, are not an exact measured substitute for thickener, and vary in the amount of time they take to thicken. Crushing the rice cereal prior to its addition to the formula creates a more uniform thickness and allows for easier passage through the opening of the nipple.[3]

In all situations, there may be an increased need for fluid or free water with no method of delivery unless ENS is considered as a means of alternative delivery. Because of these factors, judicious prescription and follow-up must be made. Time frames for trial therapy should be established. A well-developed behavioral and skill progression feeding plan is helpful and should include a multidisciplinary team familiar with pediatric dysphagia. Oral intake is important to encourage—as much as is medically safe. At the conclusion of the trial therapy, the patient should be evaluated for progress and/or level of rehabilitation. If there has been no change in ability, a different modality for fluid delivery should be established, with swallowing therapy to work with oral skills. Lefton-Grief has published a detailed skill list matched with nutrition modality recommendations that is helpful to use as an evaluation tool.[71]

For a growing infant, 3 to 4 weeks on an altered regimen would be the maximum for a trial period; for a toddler or older child 2 to 3 months would be the maximum.

In summary, the management plan for dysphagia should focus on the reduction or elimination of factors that potentially contribute to airway compromise, provide adequate nutrition and hydration, and facilitate a workable interaction between the caregiver and the child.[70]

Planning for Home Enteral Support

Whenever possible, ENS should be provided in the home rather than in the hospital. There are psychosocial benefits for the child and the family, and an economic benefit due to reduced hospital stay. Often, third-party payers are making the decision of when to provide home enteral support because of the much-reduced cost of home management. A patient who is a candidate for home enteral feedings should be evaluated based on the following criteria:[74]

- The patient must be medically stable and have demonstrated a tolerance to the feeding regimen in the hospital.
- A safe home environment is required, with available running water, electricity, refrigeration, and adequate storage space.
- The family (or patient) must be educated and capable of administering the feedings at home.
- A payment source is needed for the formula and tube-feeding equipment.
- A home care agency should be available to service the patient in his or her home locale. If an agency is not available, a hospital team that takes responsibility for home monitoring must be identified (pediatric nurse, dietitian, and pharmacist).
- A physician must be willing to assume responsibility for following the patient after discharge from the hospital.
- Supplies and equipment must be available.
- Patient/caregiver education must be arranged.
- A nutrition plan must be established.
- A social support system must be identified.
- Outpatient follow-up must be established.

Monitoring forms should be used for these patients to document data collected between medical evaluations (see **Exhibit 19-6**). Any forms used or developed should allow for quality improvement monitoring or the collection of data to measure outcomes.[75] Lastly, arrangements should be made for outpatient follow-up.

Successful ENS can be delivered in the medical or home environment to provide for a patient's nutritional needs. The improvement in products and supplies and the reduction in complications of ENS have enabled many ill children to improve nutrition and health outcomes in a more naturalized setting.

EXHIBIT 19-6 Pediatric Home Care Monitoring Form

Date ______

Patient ______ DOB ______ Primary Care Physician ______
Caregiver ______ Hospital RD ______
Address ______ Monitoring Comments ______

Phone no. ______ Nutrition Support Contact Person ______

Age ___ Last measurements ______ Last nutrition Rx: Date ______
Wt ___ Wt ___ Formula ______
Ht ___ Ht ___ Total Volume ______
OFC ___ OFC ___ Delivery Schedule ______

Procurement Enteral ☐ Parenteral ☐ Supporting Medical Equipment ______
Formula ___ Provider ___ Monitor ☐ provider ___
Equipment ___ Provider ___ Oxygen ☐ provider ___
Supplies ___ Provider ___ Other ☐ provider ___
Problems ___ Problems ___

Formula and Delivery ☐ Same ☐ Change to

Formula ______ Concentration ______
Vol/day ______ Substitute Formula ______

EXHIBIT 19-6 *(Continued)*

Infusion and Schedule
☐ By mouth (PO)—attach diet history
☐ PO in combination with—attach diet history
☐ Intermittent Infuse ________ mL over ________ minutes ________ times per day
☐ Continuous Infuse ________ mL/hr for ________ hours from ______ to ______
☐ Parenteral Infuse ________ mL/hr for ________ hours from ______ to ______
(See formula that follows)

Feeding Tube Type Size
☐ Nasogastric ☐ PEG ☐ Gastrostomy ☐ Jejunostomy ☐ Other

Water Flushes: Vol/day ________ mL ________ mL water per flush _____ flushes/day

Medications and Methods of Delivery: ________________________________

Monitoring Instructions (e.g., labs, anthropometrics, nutrition, specialists) ________________

Referral Recommendations ________________________________

Caregiver Issues ________________________________

Home Nutrition Support Information Given To ________________________________

Signature ________________________________

Home Care Staff ________________________________
Telephone ________________________________
Comments ________________________________
____
____

Problems: ☐ Vomiting ☐ Reflux ☐ Aspiration ☐ Gagging ☐ Diarrhea ☐ Illness ☐ Constipation
☐ Weight Loss ☐ Behavioral ☐ Sepsis ☐ Equip. Malfunction ☐ Other ____________

PLAN OF CARE

Signature ________________________

Parenteral Rx Date ______
Dextrose ______
Amino Acid ______
NaCl ______
KCl ______
Kphos ______
CaGlu ______
Mg ______
Na Acetate ______
Other ______
______
______
______
Calories Provided ______
Amt. Protein ______

Case Study

Nutrition Assessment

AP, a 21-month-old female, presented with failure to thrive. AP was born full term with an uncomplicated pregnancy and birth history.

Birth weight: 2.96 kg

Height: 50 cm

Patient has an unremarkable past medical history; family history is positive for diabetes in her paternal aunt.

No current medications or vitamins.

Parents report that AP eats a good variety of foods. Mom reports patient drinks three cans of Pediasure per 24-hour period. Meals are offered in a high chair at the table, without distractions. Mom reports meal times take 45 minutes to 1 hour. Mom reports occasional coughing with meals, but denies gagging during meals. AP has been evaluated for delayed speech; however, therapy has not yet started. Mom denies any swallow studies or oral motor assessments have been completed.

Anthropometric Measurements

Weight history:

15 months:	wt: 8 kg	ht: 73 cm
17 months:	wt: 8.2 kg	ht: 74.5 cm
18 months:	wt: 8.5 kg	ht: 75.2cm
19 months:	wt: 8.7 kg	ht: 76 cm

Pertinent labs: Hgb: 9 (L) Hct 12.5 (L), MCV 85.5, prealbumin 15 (L), albumin 3.2

Current weight: 8.97 kg, < 5th percentile

Height: 76 cm, 50th percentile

IBW: 11.6 kg

%IBW: 77%

Weight/height: < 5th percentile

Expected height for age: 83 cm

(Percentile, IBW, and weight/height determined using CDC growth charts.)

Typical intake:

Wakes at 6 am: patient drinks 6 oz Pediasure

Patient typically returns to sleep following bottle.

10 am: 3 tbsp tilapia, 2 strawberries, 3 oz water

12 pm: 4 oz Pediasure

Patient takes 1- to 2-hour afternoon nap.

5 pm: ¼ cup chicken soup, grapes, 2 oz juice

7 pm: 4 oz Pediasure

10 pm: 4 oz Pediasure

1 am: 6 oz Pediasure

Patient 77% IBW and 92% expected height for age. This places her in moderate chronic malnutrition and mild acute malnutrition based on the Waterloo Criteria.

Nutrition Diagnosis

Based on the above information, a nutrition diagnosis or problem is determined.

Nutrition Intervention

Plan: Patient is to be admitted to an inpatient hospital for nasogastric tube placement and teaching. The goal is for her to receive overnight feedings of currently tolerated formula.

Nocturnal feed of Pediasure should run at 60 mL/hour × 12 hours (run from 7 pm to 7 am). While on the inpatient unit, AP is assessed by a speech therapist for oral motor function and to rule out aspiration secondary to the reports of coughing during feeds as well as prolonged feeding time. Patient received clearance from the speech therapist to continue oral feeds of age-appropriate solids and nectar-thickened liquids.

Nutrition Education

1. Provide nutrition education on high-calorie and high-protein age-appropriate foods.
2. Limit oral feeds to 30 minutes.
3. Initiate nocturnal feed of Pediasure at 7 pm at 60 mL/hr × 12 hours.

Monitoring and Evaluation

It is recommended that the patient continue to follow nutrition services monthly for assessment of anthropometrics until catch-up growth has been established. A 10% increase in total calories provided by enteral nutrition is recommended to achieve adequate weight gain. As patient's oral ability improves, a shift may be likely from nocturnal NG feeds to oral daytime feeds of Pediasure. Once the patient has exhibited good catch-up growth, follow-up should be shifted to once every 3–4 months. Adjustments to nocturnal feeds will be made to maintain adequate weight gain and linear growth.

The patient should continue to receive regular speech therapy for continued monitoring of oral motor function.

Questions for the Reader

1. What is the patient's estimated energy and protein needs per kg?
2. What percentage of the total energy needs and protein needs are provided by the Pediasure?
3. Write one PES statement for this patient.

REFERENCES

1. ASPEN Board of Directors. Enteral nutrition practice recommendations. *J Parenter Enteral Nutr*. 2009;33(2):122–167.
2. Joffe,A, Anton, N, Lequier, L, et al., ed. *Nutritional Support for Critically Ill Children*. Hoboken, NJ: Wiley; 2009:1–29.
3. Klawitter BM. Pediatric enteral nutrition support. In: Nevin-Folino NL, ed. *Pediatric Manual of Clinical Dietetics*, 2nd ed. Chicago: American Dietetic Association; 2003.
4. ASPEN Board of Directors. Clinical Guidelines for the use of parenteral and enteral nutrition in adult and pediatric patients, 2009. *J Parenter Enteral Nutr*. 2009;26(1 Suppl):1SA–138SA.
5. Schwart DB. Enhanced enteral and parenteral nutrition practice and outcomes in an intensive care unit with a hospital-wide performance improvement process. *J Am Diet Assoc*. 1996;96:484–489.
6. Cox JH, ed. *Nutrition Manual for At-Risk Infants and Toddlers* Chicago: Precept Press; 1997:183–186.
7. Theriot L. Routine nutrition care during follow-up. In: Groh-Wargo S, Thompson M, Cox JH, eds. *Nutritional Care for the High Risk Newborn*, 3rd ed. Chicago: Precept Press; 2000:457–583.
8. Campbell MK, Kelsey KS. The PEACH survey: a nutrition screening tool for use in early intervention programs. *J Am Diet Assoc*. 1994;94(10):1156–1158.
9. Feldhausen J, Thomson C, Duncan B, Taren D. *Referral Criteria in Pediatric Nutrition Handbook*. New York: Chapman & Hall; 1996:65.
10. Food and Drug Administration. Regulation of infant formula. Available at: http://www.fda.gov/Food/GuidanceCompliance RegulatoryInformation/GuidanceDocuments/InfantFormula/ucm056524.htm. Accessed August 24, 2010.
11. Wessel JJ. Feeding methodologies. In: Groh-Wargo S, Thompson M, Cox JH, eds. *Nutritional Care for the High Risk Newborn*, 3rd ed. Chicago: Precept Press; 2000:321–339.
12. Greer FR, McCormick A, Loker J. Changes in fat concentration of human milk during delivery by intermittent bolus and continuous mechanical pump infusion. *J Pediatr*. 1984;105:745–749.
13. Lavine M, Clark RM. The effect of short-term refrigeration of milk and addition of breast milk fortifier on the delivery of lipids during tube feeding. *J Pediatr Gastroenterol Nutr*. 1989;8:496–499.
14. Robbins ST, Beker LT. *Infant Feedings: Guidelines for Preparation of Formula and Breastmilk in Health Care Facilities*. Chicago: American Dietetic Association; 2004.
15. Centers for Disease Control and Prevention. *Enterobacter sakazakii* infections associated with the use of powdered infant formula—Tennessee, 2001. *MMWR*. 2002;51:297–300.
16. Ross Products Division, Abbott Laboratories. Available at: http://www.rosspediatrics.com. Accessed November 4, 2009.
17. Mead Johnson & Company. Available at: http://www.meadjohnson.com. Accessed November 4, 2009.
18. Nestle Clinical Nutrition. Available at: http://www.nestle-nutrition.com/Public/Default.aspx. Accessed August 24, 2010.
19. Novartis Nutrition Corporation. Currently Nestle Clinical Nutrition. Available at: http://www.novartis.com/. Accessed August 24, 2010.
20. Scientific Hospital Supplies. Available at: http://www.shsna.com. Accessed November 4, 2009.
21. Wyeth-Ayerst Labs. Available at: http://www.parentschoiceformula.com. Accessed November 4, 2009.
22. Sapsford AB. Human milk and enteral nutrition products. In: Groh-Wargo S, Thompson M, Cox JH, eds. *Nutritional Care for the High Risk Newborn*, 3rd ed. Chicago: Precept Press; 2000:286–287.
23. Fomon SJ. *Nutrition of Normal Infants*. St. Louis, MO: Mosby-Year Book; 1993:100.
24. Cowen SL. Feeding gastrostomy: nutritional management of the infant or young child. *J Pediatr Perinat Nutr*. 1987;1:51.
25. Jew RK, Owen D, Kaufman D, Balmer D. Osmolality of commonly used medications and formulas in the neonatal intensive care unit. *Nutr Clin Pract*. 1997;12:158–163.
26. Texas Children's Hospital. *Pediatric Nutrition Reference Guide*, 8th ed. Huston, TX: McGraw-Hill Professional; 2008.
27. Gerber Good Start. Gerber Products. Available at: http://www.gerber.com/Products. Accessed December 2, 2009.
28. Joeckel RJ, Phillips SK. Overview of infant and pediatric formulas. *Nutr Clin Pract*. 2009;24:356–362.
29. Denne, SC. Protein requirements. In: Polin RA, Fox WW, eds. *Fetal and Neonatal Physiology*, 2nd ed. Philadelphia, PA: Sanders; 1998:315–325.
30. Fuentebella J, Kerner JA. Refeeding syndrome. *Pediatr Clin N Am*. 2009;56:1201–1210.
31. Santos VF, Morais TB. Nutritional quality and osmolality of home-made enteral diets, and follow-up growth of severely disabled children receiving home enteral nutrition therapy. *J Trop Pediatr*. 2010;56(2):127–128..
32. Warman KY. Enteral nutrition: support of the pediatric patient. In Walker WA, Hendricks KM, eds. In: *Manual of Pediatric Nutrition*. Philadelphia, PA: WB Saunders; 1990:70–76.
33. Rombeau JL, Jacobs DO. Nasoenteric tube feeding. In: Rombeau JL, Caldwell MD, eds. Clinical nutrition volume 1: Enteral and tube feeding. Philadelphia: Sanders; 1984:263.
34. American Academy of Pediatrics. *Pediatric Nutrition Handbook*, 6th ed. Elk Grove, IL: American Academy of Pediatrics. 2009:108–554.
35. Delegge, MH. Enteral access: the foundation of feeding. *J Parenter Enteral Nutr*. 2000;25:S8–S13.
36. Cone LC, Gilligan MF, Kagan RJ, et al. Enhancing patient safety: the effect of process improvement on bedside fluoroscopy time related to nasoduodenal feeding tube placement in pediatric burn patients. *J Burn Care Res*. 2009;30(4):606–611.
37. Wesley JR. Special access to the intestinal tract. In: Balistreri WF, Farrell MK, eds. *Enteral Feeding: Scientific Basis and Clinical Applications*. Report of the 94th Ross Conference on Pediatric Research. Columbus, OH: Ross Products; 1988:57–62.
38. Lord LM. Enteral access devices. *Nurs Clin North Am*. 1997; 32(4):685–702.
39. Meyer R, Harrison S, Ramnarayan P, et al. The impact of enteral feeding protocols on nutritional support in critically ill children. *J Hum Nutr Diet*.2009;22:428–436.
40. El-Marary W. Percutaneous endoscopic gastrostomy in children. *Can J Gastroenterol*. 2008;22(12):993–998
41. Grumow JE, Al-Hafidh AS, Tunell WP. Gastroesophageal reflux following percutaneous endoscopic gastrostomy in children. *J Pediatr Surg*. 1989;24:44–45.
42. American Society for Parenteral and Enteral Nutrition Board of Directors. Clinical guidelines for the use of parenteral and

enteral nutrition in adolescent and pediatric patients, 2009. *J Parenter Enteral Nutr.* 2009;33:255.
43. Walker WA, Hendricks KM, eds. Enteral nutrition support of the pediatric patient. In: *Manual of Pediatric Nutrition*. Philadelphia, PA: WB Saunders; 1985.
44. American Gastroenterological Association. American Gastroenterological Association Medical Position Statement: Guidelines for the Use of Enteral Nutrition. http://www3.us.elsevierhealth.com/gastro/policy/v108n4p1280.html. Accessed August 31, 2010.
45. Vanek VW. Closed versus open enteral delivery systems: a quality improvement study. *Nutr Clin Pract*. 2000;15:234–243.
46. Canal DF, Vane DW, Goto S, et al. Reduction of lower esophageal sphincter pressure with Stamm gastrostomy. *J Pediatr Surg*. 1987;22:54–57.
47. Kellie SJ, Fitch SJ, Kovnar EH, et al. A hazard of using adult-sized weighted-tip enteral feeding catheters in infants. *Am J Dis Child*. 1988;142:916–917.
48. Allen DB. Postprandial hypoglycemia resulting from nasogastric tube malposition. *Pediatrics*. 1988;81:582–584.
49. Rommel N, DeMeyer A, Feenstra L, Veereman-Wauters G. The complexity of feeding problems in 700 infants and young children presenting to a tertiary care institution. *J Pediatr Gastroenterol Nutr*. 2000;37:75–84.
50. Ford EG, Jennings M, Andrassy RJ. Serum albumin (oncotic pressure) correlates with enteral feeding tolerance in the pediatric surgical patient. *J Pediatr Surg*. 1987;22:597–599.
51. Skillman HE, Wischmeyer PE. Nutrition therapy in critically ill infants and children. *J Parenter Enteral Nutr*. 2008;32(5);520–534.
52. Huhmann MB, August DA. Nutrition support in surgical oncology. *Nutr Clin Pract*. 2009;24(4):520–526.
53. Gottschlich MM, Warden GD, Michel M, et al. Diarrhea in tube-fed burn patients: incidence, etiology, nutritional impact, and prevention. *J Parenter Enteral Nutr*. 1988;12:388–445.
54. Hutsler D. Delivery and bedside management of infant feedings. In: Robbins S, Beker L, eds. *Infant Feedings: Guidelines for Preparation of Formula and Breast Milk in Health Care Facilities*. Chicago: American Dietetic Association; 2003;1–10.
55. Arnold LDW. *Recommendations for Collection, Storage, and Handling of a Mother's Milk for Her Own Infant in the Hospital Setting*. Denver, CO: Human Milk Banking Association of North America; 1999.
56. Forchielli ML, Bines J. Enteral Nutrition. *Nutrition in Pediatrics*. 4th ed. Hamilton ON. 2008;765–775.
57. Issacs JS, Lucas BL, Feucht SA, Grieger LE. Nutritional care for the gastrostomy-fed child with neurological impairments. *Top Clin Nutr*. 1993;8(4):58–65
58. Glass RP, Lucas B. *Making the Transition from Tube Feeding to Oral Feeding. Nutrition Focus for Children with Special Health Care Needs*. Seattle, WA: Children's Development and Mental Retardation Center, University of Washington; 1990;5:1–4.
59. Mennella JA, Griffin CE, Beauchamp GK. Flavor programming during infancy. *Pediatrics*. 2004;113:840–845.
60. Mennella JA, Johnson A, Beauchamp GK. Garlic ingestion by pregnant women alters the odor of amniotic fluid. *Chem Senses*. 1995;20:207–209.
61. Mennella JA, Beauchamp GK. Flavor experiences during formula feeding are related to preferences during childhood. *Early Human Dev*. 2002;68:71–82.
62. Liem DG, Mennella JA. Sweet and sour preferences during childhood: role of early experiences. *Dev Psychobiol*. 2002;41:388–395.
63. Owada M, Anki K, Kitagawa T. Taste preferences and feeding behavior in children with phenylketonuria on a semisynthetic diet. *Eur J Pediatr*. 2000;159(11):846–850.
64. Stein, K. Children with feeding disorders: an emerging issue. *J Am Diet Assoc*. 2000;100(9):1000–1001.
65. Illingsworth RS, Lister J. The critical or sensitive period, with special reference to certain feeding problems in infants and children. *J Pediatr*. 1964;65:8.
66. Rudolph, CD, Link D. Feeding disorders in infants and children. *Pediatr Gastroenterol Nutr*. 2002;49:97–112.
67. Burklow KA, McGrath AM, Allred KE. Parent perceptions of mealtime behaviors in children fed enterally. *Nutr Clin Pract*. 2002;17:291–295.
68. Camp KM, Kalscheur MC. Nutritional approach to diagnosis and management of pediatric feeding and swallowing disorders. In: Tuchman DN, Walter RS, eds. *Disorders of Feeding and Swallowing in Infants and Children: Pathophysiology, Diagnosis, and Treatment*. San Diego, CA: Singular Publishing Group; 1994:153–185.
69. Manikam R, Perman JA. Pediatric feeding disorders. *J Clin Gastroenterol*. 2000;30:34–46.
70. American Academy of Pediatrics. *Pediatric Nutrition Handbook*, 6th ed. Elk Grove, IL: American Academy of Pediatrics. 2009;108–554.
71. Lefton-Grief MA. Diagnosis and management of pediatric feeding and swallowing disorders: role of the speech-language pathologist. In: Tuchman DN, Walter RS, eds. *Disorders of Feeding and Swallowing in Infants and Children: Pathophysiology, Diagnosis, and Treatment*. San Diego, CA: Singular Publishing Group; 1994:97–113.
72. Phagia-Gel Technologies. Available at: http://www.simplythick.com. Accessed May 29, 2004.
73. Feucht S. Guidelines for the use of thickeners in foods and liquids. In: *Nutrition Focus for Children with Special Health Care Needs*. Seattle, WA: Children's Developmental and Mental Retardation Center, University of Washington;1995:1–6.
74. Vanderhoff JA, Young RJ. Overview of considerations for the pediatric patient receiving home parenteral and enteral nutrition. *Nutr Clin Pract*. 2003;18:221–226.
75. Gallagher AL, Onda RM. Using quality assurance procedures to improve compliance with standards to nutrition care for patients receiving isotonic tube feeding. *J Am Diet Assoc*. 1993;93:678–679.

Parenteral Nutrition

Janice Hovasi Cox and Ingrida Mara Melbardis

Introduction

Parenteral nutrition (PN) is the intravenous delivery of nutrients, including water, carbohydrates, fat, protein, electrolytes, vitamins, minerals, and trace elements. The proportions of these nutrients are individualized, based on an assessment of the child's clinical and nutritional needs. The goal of PN is to support normal growth and development as well as to promote tissue repair and maintenance while oral/enteral feedings are precluded.

PN in pediatrics is commonly used for the treatment of a wide variety of conditions in both the hospital and home settings.[1–4] This chapter summarizes the complexities of pediatric PN as it is utilized in the hospital and in the home.

Clinical Indications

PN is needed when an infant or child is unable to meet ongoing nutrition needs with an oral diet and/or enteral feedings. In extremely premature infants, gastrointestinal tract immaturity may prevent sufficient enteral feedings for several weeks. Because premature infants have low nutritional stores, PN should be started within 24 hours of birth. Undernourished infants and children require nutrition support within 1 to 2 days if they will not be able to consume adequate feedings. Well-nourished infants and children are better able to tolerate longer periods without nutrition intervention, up to 3–5 and 5–7 days, respectively.[5,6] Intravenous solutions (dextrose/sodium chloride/potassium chloride) are usually provided during this time to meet fluid needs and prevent hypoglycemia.

It is important to ensure that PN is used appropriately and that the infants and children who receive PN are managed effectively to support the best outcome at the lowest cost. Policies and decision trees can help practitioners choose the most suitable form of nutrition support (see **Figure 20-1**).[6] Conditions that may require PN are listed in **Exhibit 20-1**. Some hospitals utilize interdisciplinary nutrition support teams (physicians, dietitians, nurses, and pharmacists)[7] and clinical pathways[8,9] to help evaluate and manage patients requiring enteral nutrition or PN.[10]

Gastrointestinal (GI) tract dysfunction can occur at any age due to disease, injury, or radiation/chemotherapy.[5,11] In GI conditions requiring surgical resection, the extent of macronutrient and micronutrient malabsorption depends on the amount of bowel resected, the presence or absence of the ileocecal valve, and the function of the remaining bowel. Often children with short gut syndrome are able to tolerate at least partial enteral feedings. When the ileocecal valve is not intact, the rapid transit time of enteral formulas through the bowel may require a greater dependence upon PN.[12] The extent of the resection, paired with the tolerance of enteral feedings, can help predict the duration of a neonate's dependence on PN.[13,14]

Although PN may help bring about disease remission in children with irritable bowel disease (IBD), ulcerative colitis, or Crohn's disease, relapse occurs soon after a normal diet is resumed.[15] Elemental enteral feedings may be more beneficial for inducing remission of IBD, improving nutrition status, and reversing growth failure.[16] PN should be reserved only for those children who are unable to tolerate enteral feedings. Gastrointestinal disorders requiring nutritional support are discussed in detail in Chapter 12.

Children with cancer are at increased risk for malnutrition. The causes for cancer cachexia seem to be multifaceted and include anorexia, anxiety, and increased metabolic needs.[11] Whether enteral feeding has been impeded by the side effects of radiation and chemotherapy or by surgical procedures, the child with cancer may have an improved quality of life with PN.[17–20] Helping children maintain optimal nutrition during therapy may promote improved growth and better tolerance of therapies.[21] Some children may be able to tolerate small gastric feedings along with PN to meet nutrition needs. Most practitioners agree that children receiving aggressive cancer therapy should also receive supportive nutrition therapy, but the benefits of PN

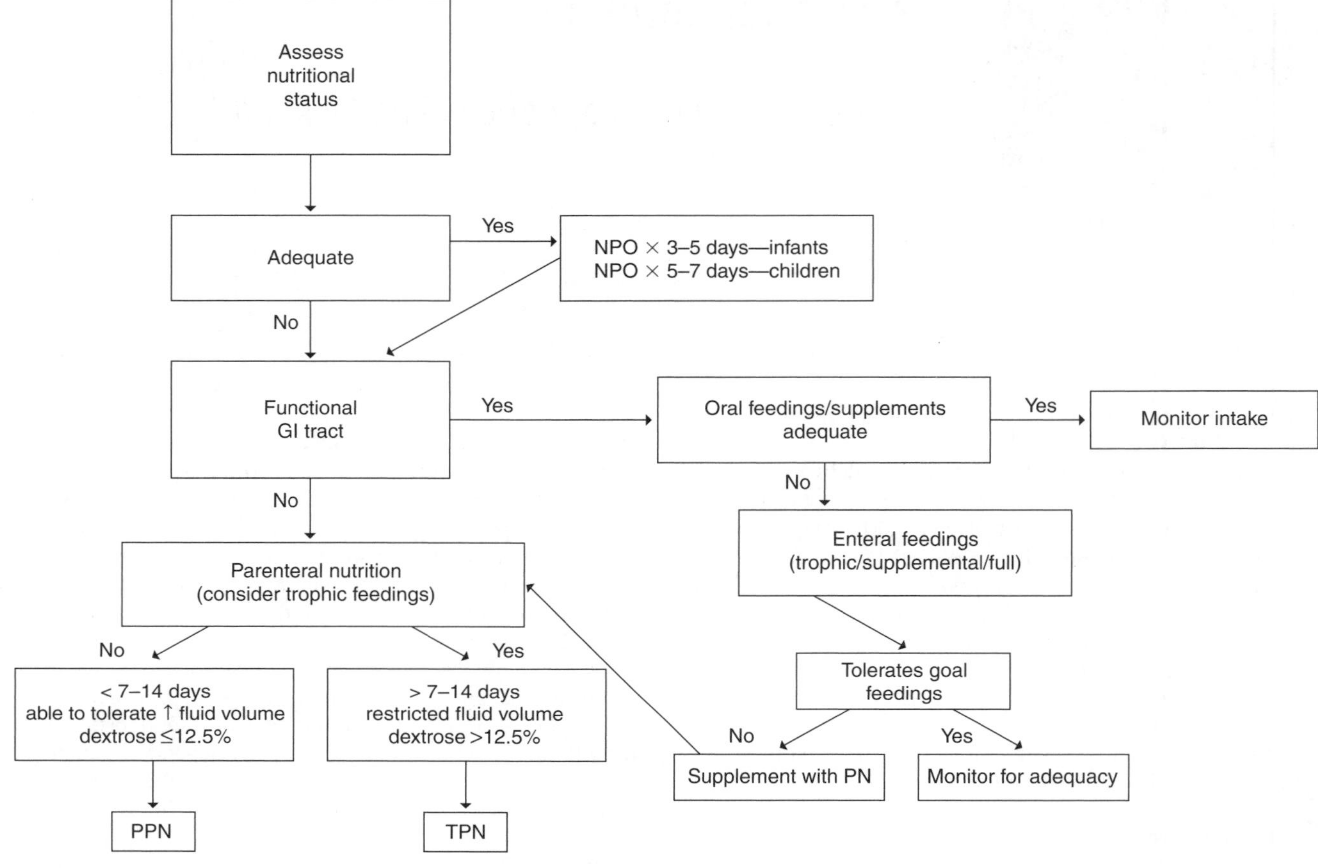

FIGURE 20-1 Pediatric Nutrition Support Algorithm

EXHIBIT 20-1 Conditions that May Require Parenteral Nutrition

GI Conditions

- Bowel obstruction
- Crohn's disease
- Diaphragmatic hernia
- Gastroschisis
- High-output fistulas
- Intestinal atresia
- Intractable diarrhea
- Intussusception
- Malrotation/volvulus
- Meconium ileus
- Necrotizing enterocolitis
- Neuromuscular intestinal disorders
- Omphalocele
- Radiation enteritis
- Severe Hirschsprung's disease
- Short bowel syndrome
- Ulcerative colitis

Other Circumstances

- Anorexia nervosa
- Bronchopulmonary dysplasia
- Cancer cachexia
- Chylothorax
- Low-birth-weight neonate (< 1500 g)

should be weighed against the potential risks of PN, which include increased infection rates and metabolic abnormalities.[22,23]

PN may be used in the refeeding process for children with anorexia nervosa simply because it has less resemblance to food than the enteral feeding. The use of PN in these patients depends on the severity of malnutrition and on the patient's tendency to interfere with the infusion apparatus.[24,25]

Vascular Access

Use of central versus peripheral venous access is an important factor to consider when providing parenteral nutrition to the patient.

Peripheral Venous Access

PN may be delivered through a peripheral or central venous catheter, depending on the anticipated length of therapy, nutrition needs, and fluid tolerance. Peripheral parenteral nutrition (PPN) is used when the anticipated length of therapy is less than 2 weeks, PN is needed to maintain rather than replete nutrition status, and fluid tolerance is ample. Because PPN solutions are not as calorie dense as total PN (TPN) solutions, greater fluid volumes are required to provide comparable nutrition. The major complications associated with PPN are soft tissue sloughs and phlebitis, which are more likely to occur if the infused solution has an osmolality greater than 900 mOsm/L. A final concentration of no more than 12.5% dextrose with a maximum solution osmolality less than 900 mOsm/L with lipids, or less than 600 mOsm/L without lipids, is recommended in the administration of PPN.[4] A simple equation can be used to estimate osmolality.[26] Using g/L for glucose and amino acids, mg/L for phosphorus and mEq/L for sodium, the equation is osmolality (mOsm/L) = (amino acids × 8) + (glucose × 7) + (sodium × 2) + (phosphorus × 2) − 50. Limiting calcium to a maximum of 8 mEq/L may also help decrease the risk of phlebitis.[4]

A negative aspect of the peripheral delivery route is that it may be more restrictive than central delivery to normal activity, depending on the site and stability of venous access.

Central Venous Access

Providing TPN through a central vein is indicated when an infant or child requires fluid restriction or long-term nutrition therapy, or when an infant or child is a candidate for home PN. Infusion of TPN into a central vein allows the high blood flow to rapidly dilute the hypertonic solution. Central venous catheters (CVCs) are also used to provide chemotherapy, prolonged antibiotic therapy, and blood components. Although blood sampling from a CVC site that is being used for PN administration is thought to increase the risk of contamination, risks may be diminished by strict use of aseptic technique.[5]

Central venous access can be temporary or permanent. In neonates, umbilical vessels may be used temporarily as a central route for TPN. Risk of thrombosis increases if umbilical artery catheters are used beyond 5 days or if umbilical venous catheters are used beyond 14 days.[5] To avoid complications associated with their use, many institutions restrict use of umbilical catheters to lab and blood pressure monitoring, and PN is administered through a peripherally inserted central catheter (PICC) if central access is required.[27]

A PICC line provides reliable central venous access and may be inserted at the bedside using strict sterile techniques.[28–30] Insertion-related complications inherent in the surgically placed CVC, such as pneumothorax and hemothorax, are virtually eliminated with the PICC line. Some studies have also found that sepsis rates tend to be lower in neonates and children with PICC lines versus surgically placed central catheters.[31,32] PICC lines are being used in increasing numbers in both neonates and older children because they provide central venous access less invasively, with lower risks, and at lower cost than surgically placed CVCs or multiple insertions of peripheral lines.[5,33–36]

Permanent catheters are indicated when long-term access (over 3 weeks) is needed.[33] The surgically placed right atrial catheter (e.g., Broviac, Hickman) is the most suitable CVC for pediatric patients who require long-term or home TPN. The catheter is placed in the external jugular or the facial vein and threaded through the internal jugular vein and down into the superior vena cava. Tip placement outside the pericardial sac avoids the risk of pericardial tamponade.[5] Location of the catheter tip should be verified every 6 to 12 months for children undergoing significant linear growth.[37] The distal end of the catheter is tunneled subcutaneously and exits mid-chest. The Dacron cuff affixed to the tunneled portion of the catheter helps secure the catheter because subcutaneous fibrous tissue adheres to the cuff. The major complications associated with CVC insertion and use include infection and thrombosis.[33,38]

Although a single-lumen CVC is the venous access device most often used for the pediatric PN patient, two- and three-lumen CVCs also have been used for the pediatric population. Double- and triple-lumen catheters are particularly useful in patients who require frequent infusions of blood products and medications in addition to the nutrition solution. Designating one port exclusively for PN or PN with compatible medications and using the other ports for blood drawing, blood product delivery, and central venous pressure measurements may help decrease the risk for sepsis associated with multiple lumen catheters.[5] Lumens not in use must be heparinized and capped. Multiple-lumen catheters may be more suitable for the larger child rather than the neonate because of total catheter size. Strict aseptic technique is critical when a multiple-lumen CVC is in place.[39,40]

In order to avoid some of the problems associated with the externalized CVC, a totally implantable vascular device consisting of a catheter connected to a chamber or port can be used.[41] The advantages of the implantable port are that it eliminates daily dressing changes when not in use and it is not as disruptive to body image.

For the child on home PN, the implanted CVC requires daily access. Daily percutaneous puncture or leaving a Huber needle in place with a dressing for days at a time may negate the overall benefits of the implanted device. Skin irritation and breakdown have been associated with frequent port access, and other CVC-related complications such as occlusion and infection remain risks with the implanted CVC.[30]

Solution Administration

Due to the wide range in nutrient needs, fluid requirements, and clinical conditions of infants and children who require PN, individualized solutions are generally preferred over standard solutions.[5] Standard solutions may be used for short periods of time, particularly during the neonatal period, provided that electrolyte adjustment is possible and laboratory monitoring is consistent.[5,42] For individualized solutions, nutrient doses are calculated based on the infant's or child's weight (per kg) or daily need and ordered per unit of volume, usually per liter, or per day in a specified volume. When prescribing individualized solutions, standardized order forms should be designed to help ensure the prescription of appropriate, safe, and nutritionally complete solutions.[43,44] (Recommendations are provided in **Exhibit 20-2**.) Computerized and Web-based programs also are available to simplify order entry for PN.[45–47]

Parenteral nutrient solutions may be prepared as 2-in-1 solutions, or as 3-in-1 or total nutrient admixtures (TNAs). In 2-in-1 solutions, dextrose and amino acids are combined with electrolytes, minerals, and trace elements. This solution is infused through one arm of a Y-connector, while lipids are infused in the other arm. Administering lipids separately allows for the visualization of potential calcium phosphate precipitates in the dextrose/amino acid solution, but increases the risk for increased bacterial growth in the lipid emulsion, especially if lipid is transferred from the original bottle into smaller syringes.[48] Vitamin stability may be greater if dosed in the lipid emulsion rather than the dextrose and amino acid solution. Administration tubing and extension sets for dextrose and amino acid solutions should be changed at least every 72 hours, or as recommended by the manufacturer. Tubing for lipids should be changed every 24 hours.[5,44]

A 3-in-1 or TNA combines the lipid emulsion, amino acid, and dextrose solutions in the same container. Although the TNA is more convenient to use, there has been concern about the stability and safety of these solutions. TNAs, unlike 2-in-1 solutions, are emulsions and, therefore, are more significantly influenced by pH and temperature.[49,50] Of concern also is the potential peroxidation of lipid emulsions by phototherapy lights.[51] Using aluminum foil to shield the

EXHIBIT 20-2 Recommendations for Writing Parenteral Nutrition Prescriptions

1. Use standard order forms specifically developed for infants and children.
2. Identify prescription with patient's name and date of birth.
3. Provide patient's current weight; provide dosing weight if different than current weight due to malnutrition, edema, or obesity.
4. Identify whether intravenous access route is peripheral or central because this determines dextrose concentration limitations.
5. Include fluid prescription, accommodating other fluids needed for administration of flushes, medications, other intravenous fluids, and/or enteral feedings.
6. Specify total daily volume, hourly rate of delivery, and number of hours of delivery.
7. Each nutrient should be clearly identified, including chloride and acetate.
8. Include guidelines for nutrient requirements for various ages and/or acceptable ranges of nutrient concentration in admixture, including mineral content compatibility.
9. The list of nutrients in the prescription should be in the same order and units as in the guidelines and on the label. For example, do not use "mEq" for calcium in the prescription list but "mg" of calcium in the guidelines or "mL" of calcium gluconate on the label.
10. Avoid using percent concentration. Use amount per volume, amount per kg, or amount per day.
11. Use one zero before the decimal to hold a place, but do not use trailing zeros. For example, use 0.5, but do not use .5; use 5, but do not use 5.0.
12. Complete the form for all subsequent orders, even if only one nutrient is changed.
13. If standard solutions are used, provide options for adjusting electrolytes; decreasing lipid, copper, and manganese; and other modifications that may be clinically indicated.
14. Establish standard guidelines for laboratory monitoring.

bag and the tubing from phototherapy lights can prevent this from happening. Opaque tubing is also available.[52] Infusion of a multivitamin (MVI) preparation along with shielding the tubing may fully protect the solution from peroxidation.[53] Tubing for TNA should be changed every 24 hours.[5,44]

Three main variables affect the overall stability of the final TNA:[44,54,55] (1) the final concentration of the macronutrients, (2) the amount of added cations (especially polyvalent cations such as iron, magnesium, calcium, and zinc), and (3) the compounding order. If parenteral medications are to be infused simultaneously via a Y-site, compatibility with the TNA solution should be verified.[56] Care must be taken to identify any precipitates or emulsion breakdown in the TNA before infusion occurs. The most commonly found precipitate is calcium phosphate. Emulsion breakdown or "creaming" (liberation of free oil) can result when higher amounts of cations are used in the mixture. The presence of yellow-brown oil droplets at or near the TNA surface is an indicator that the solution is unsafe for administration.[44] Various methods of in-process end-product testing are described in the American Society for Parenteral and Enteral Nutrition (ASPEN) guidelines to ensure and document the safety of the end TNAs.[44] Compounding PN solutions, either manually or using an automated compounding device, requires meticulous adherence to standards that ensure safety, sterility, accuracy, quality, and labeling. These standards are published and reviewed elsewhere.[57,58]

Of greatest concern with neonatal and pediatric PN solutions is the solubility of calcium and phosphorus.[53] Although the addition of lipids to the PN solution does not directly affect the solubility of calcium and phosphorus, the opacity of the admixture makes visual detection of precipitates difficult. Computer and Web-based programs are available to help maximize the amount of calcium and phosphorus that can be provided safely in PN solutions.[44,46]

For neonates and children receiving home PN, the stability of the PN needs to be assured for longer periods of time. Using dual-chamber bags to separate the lipid from the rest of the solution and adding vitamins and trace minerals just before infusion helps improve the shelf-life of TNAs used in this setting.[54,59] Use of an MCT/LCT-based TNA may also improve stability.[60,61] Caretakers administering PN in the home need to be trained on how to visually assess the stability of the emulsion.

The use of filters with PN provides additional safety.[5,44,62] Filters can prevent the infusion of particulate matter, air, and microorganisms. Different types of filters are used for 2-in-1 and 3-in-1 solutions. Positively charged filters and 0.22-micron filters can be used with 2-in-1 solutions. These filters remove microorganisms and pyrogens (gram-negative endotoxins) and reduce the risk of air embolism. For TNAs, larger 1.2-micron filters are used to allow administration of lipid droplets. These filter out particulate matter and larger organisms, such as *Candida albicans*, but are unable to filter out common smaller bacterial contaminants. Infusion sets for 2-in-1 solutions should be changed at least every 72 hours, or per manufacturer's instruction. Infusion sets for TNAs or lipids administered separately should be changed as soon as the infusion is delivered, or if a second infusion is given, at least every 24 hours.[5,44]

PN solutions should be initiated slowly and advanced gradually as the child's fluid and glucose tolerance permits. Infusion pumps are used to maintain a constant flow rate, thereby maintaining steady glucose delivery. If the PN infusion is interrupted or discontinued abruptly, a 10% dextrose solution may be infused to maintain euglycemia (or to prevent hypoglycemia) until the PN solution can be replaced.

Cycling

Administration of PN in cycles provides for planned interruption of the nutrient infusion. Cycling more closely simulates normal patterns of food ingestion and fasting and may help prevent PN-associated hepatic complications.[63] Whether at home or in the hospital, cyclic PN allows a more normal daytime routine, enhancing mobility and activity patterns and also leaving a window of time for lipid clearance.

The nutrition needs of the child, compared with the ability to tolerate oral/enteral feedings, should be taken into consideration when deciding on cyclic PN. Infants younger than 4 to 6 months of age who are receiving all of their nutrition parenterally may be able to tolerate breaks from PN up to only 4 hours in duration. Older infants and children may tolerate interruptions of up to 6 to 8 hours. Infants and children who are receiving enteral feedings or are eating in addition to their PN may receive adequate PN in shorter spans of time. Supplemental PN can usually be provided over 8 to 12 hours. Children who are more tolerant of the necessary fluid load can receive their total required nutrition and fluid loads condensed into 10- to 16-hour cycles.

Glucose infusion rate should not exceed 20 mg/kg/min (1.2 g/kg/hr) to prevent wide variations in serum glucose.[5] Gradually increasing the rate when starting the infusion and slowly weaning the rate at the end of the infusion may lessen the likelihood of hyper/hypoglycemia. The rate is adjusted over a period of 1 to 2 hours (i.e., run at half rate for the first hour and last hour) to maintain euglycemia. Infusion pumps that can be programmed to accomplish the gradual introduction and weaning of PN are available. A rate adjustment for cycling may not be necessary in children over 2 years of age.[64]

Weaning

Minimal enteral feedings should be given whenever possible to prevent bowel atrophy and improve adaptation for tolerance of feeding advancement.[5] When increasing enteral feedings, making one change at a time in substrate, volume, or rate makes it easier to assess tolerance. Newborn infants are best weaned to mother's milk, although fortification may be needed for preterm infants to adequately meet their nutrient needs. Older infants and children who recover gastrointestinal function quickly may be weaned to a diet that is age appropriate. When bowel function is expected to return gradually or remain somewhat compromised, mother's milk or hydrolyzed protein- or amino acid-based enteral products may be better tolerated.[5]

As an infant or child is able to make the transition to enteral/oral feedings, the volume of PN is gradually weaned by decreasing the hourly rate and/or decreasing the infusion time.[5] Total energy intake is adjusted as the percentage of enteral nutrition increases. Enteral energy needs are usually higher than PN needs because energy is required for digestion, and absorptive losses may be small or significant, depending on gastrointestinal function. When PN is cycled, providing PN at night offers supplemental nutrition with limited suppression of appetite during the day, which may better support a transition to oral feedings.

Fluid and Electrolytes

Guidelines for the administration of parenteral fluids to infants and children are based on normal maintenance estimates with adjustments for increased or decreased losses due to disease or environmental conditions (see **Table 20-1**). During the first week of life, infants experience three phases of fluid and electrolyte homeostasis.[5,44] During the first 12 to 36 hours of life, or the prediuretic phase, renal excretion of sodium, potassium, and fluid is minimal. Electrolytes may not be needed during the first 1–2 days, and fluid administration is conservative unless insensible water loss (IWL) is high. The onset of the diuretic phase usually occurs within the first 2 days and accounts for most of the weight, sodium, and potassium loss that occurs during the first week of life. The postdiuretic phase usually begins between 3 and 5 days of age and is characterized by improved homeostasis of fluid, sodium, and potassium.[65,67] This initial adjustment to extrauterine life usually results in up to 10% weight loss in term infants. Prematurely born infants may lose up to 20% of their body weight, due primarily to their greater percentage of total body water as extracellular water. Insensible water losses may be greater due to their greater body surface area to body mass ratio and their more permeable epidermis.[68] Weight loss greater than 15% to 20% of birth weight may represent some loss of lean tissue due to energy deficit.[69]

Fluid losses through urine and the gastrointestinal tract may be relatively easy to measure, although IWL through the respiratory tract and skin is more elusive and may be affected by environmental conditions. Radiant heat warmers and ultraviolet light therapy may increase IWL by 20% to 25%.[70] Use of double-walled isolettes may prevent this increase in water loss.[71] Use of mist tents and humidified air may decrease IWL. In older infants and children, hyperventilation and visible sweating often associated with fever may increase IWL by 20% to 25%.[72]

Low-birth-weight infants may require up to 200 mL/kg/day due to their renal immaturity and increased IWL. They may also be intolerant of excessive fluid intake. Patent ductus arteriosus, bronchopulmonary dysplasia, intraventricular hemorrhage, and necrotizing enterocolitis each has been linked with excessive fluid administration.[67,73–76] Frequent monitoring of fluid and electrolyte intake, serum and urine electrolyte levels, weight changes, and urine output may be needed to appropriately manage fluid and electrolyte balance during the neonatal period.

Beyond the first week of life and throughout childhood, maintenance fluid and electrolyte requirements are directly related to metabolic rate.[77] Infants and children generally

TABLE 20-1 Daily Maintenance Fluid Requirements

Clinical Condition	Fluids Required per Day
Sick newborn, day 1	40–80 mL/kg
Sick newborn, week 1	80–150 mL/kg
Newborn to 1 year, stable growth	140–160 mL/kg/day
Anuria, extreme oliguria	45 mL/kg
Diabetes insipidus	Up to 400 mL/100 kcal
1–10 kg body weight	100 mL/kg
11–20 kg body weight	1000 mL + 50 mL/kg above 10 kg
Body weight above 20 kg	1500 mL + 20 mL/kg above 20 kg
Body surface area	1500–1800 mL/m^2

Sources: Data from Koletzko B, Goulet O, Hunt J, Krohn K, Shamir R for the Parenteral Nutrition Guidelines Working Group. Guidelines on paediatric parenteral nutrition of the European Society of Paediatric Gastroenterology, Hepatology and Nutrition (ESPGHAN) and the European Society for Clinical Nutrition and Metabolism (ESPEN), supported by the European Society of Paediatric Research (ESPR). *J Pediatr Gastroenterol Nutr.* 2005;41:S1–S87; Mirtallo J, Canada T, Johnson D, et al., Task Force for the Revision of Safe Practices for Parenteral Nutrition. Safe practices for parenteral nutrition formulations. *J Parenter Enteral Nutr.* 2004;28:S39–S70; Kerner JA Jr, ed. *Manual of Pediatric Parenteral Nutrition*. New York: John Wiley and Sons; 1983; Nelson WE, Behrman RE, Vaughan VC, eds. *Nelson's Textbook of Pediatrics*, 12th ed. Philadelphia: WB Saunders; 1983:231; and Baumgart S, Costarino AT. Water and electrolyte metabolism of the micropremie. *Clin Perinatol.* 2000;27:131–146.

require at least 115 mL of fluid for every 100 kcal of energy provided[78] (see Table 20-1). The amount of fluid needed to maintain adequate hydration often does not provide adequate nutrition when using peripheral venous access, though administration of fluids 30–50% above maintenance levels are usually well tolerated. Changes in metabolic rate, respiratory rate, IWL, and water production from the oxidation of protein, carbohydrate, and fat also affect fluid needs. Older infants and children may initially require fluids and electrolytes in excess of maintenance requirements to establish normal hydration if they have had prolonged or excessive vomiting or diarrhea.

Losses of fluid and electrolytes through the GI tract in disease states may be measured directly for replacement or estimated by monitoring changes in body weight every 8 or 24 hours. GI losses may be due to vomiting, nasogastric suctioning, diarrhea, or ostomy drainage.[79] Due to the wide range in electrolyte composition of various GI fluids, direct measurement may be required to provide adequate replacement.

Urinary losses of fluid and electrolytes depend largely on intake and renal maturity. Infants less than 1 year of age can dilute urine to 50 mOsm/kg of water. Concentrating ability at birth is about 600 mOsm/kg of water and gradually increases to 1000 to 1200 mOsm/kg of water during the first year. During periods of growth, the renal solute load is lower, as nitrogen, phosphorus, sodium, potassium, and chloride are retained as constituents of body tissues. During periods of stress and tissue catabolism, the renal solute load is higher.

Various conditions may alter urinary losses of fluid and electrolytes. Preterm infants have an immature capacity to either excrete or retain electrolytes and maintain acid–base balance.[5,80,81] Excessive sodium losses are common and may require up to 12 mmol/kg/day of sodium. Inappropriate or excessive antidiuretic hormone (ADH) secretion, often associated with hypoxia, hemorrhage, central nervous system insult, hypotension, anesthesia, pneumothorax, or pain, requires fluid restriction and sodium supplementation to maintain normal extracellular fluid volumes and prevent hyponatremia.[80] However, hyperchloremic acidosis in preterm infants is associated with excessive chloride intake when sodium is provided solely as sodium chloride. Using sodium acetate (up to 14.2 mmol/kg/day) has been shown to reduce the incidence of metabolic acidosis and hyperchloremia.[81] If IWL (which is all free water) is high in prematurely born infants, particularly during the diuretic phase of initial fluid and electrolyte homeostasis, hypernatremia may develop.[68,82]

Fluid and electrolyte restriction may be necessary in some disease states such as congestive heart failure, head trauma, and renal insufficiency. Medications may be a significant source of fluid and/or electrolytes. Saline flushes used in routine care of intravenous lines may be a significant source of sodium and chloride.[83] Some medications may cause increased excretion or retention of various electrolytes. Direct measurement of urine volume and electrolytes may be necessary to provide appropriate replacement.

Energy

Parenteral energy needs are probably about 10% to 15% lower than estimated enteral needs for most infants and children due to reduced fecal losses and reduced energy required for digestion and absorption (see **Table 20-2**). Although meeting basal energy needs prevents catabolism and weight loss, the energy needed to support catch-up growth, or even normal growth and activity levels, may be nearly double basal energy needs.[92] Energy requirements for postoperative infants and children increase immediately after surgery, but return to normal within 12 to 24 hours, possibly due to administration of sedative medications and temporary interruption of growth. Subsequent energy needs are more related to growth and the underlying illness.[5,93] Energy needs during the acute phase of critical illness, sedation, or paralysis may be lower than normal.

Various equations have been developed that include length, specific age, body temperature, and heart rate to estimate individual energy needs.[5,47] When considering preexisting malnutrition or obesity, fluctuations in clinical condition, activity levels, growth spurts, and so forth, these methods may be cumbersome and perhaps no more accurate than simpler methods based on estimated lean weight and general age category[5] (see Table 20-2). However, underfeeding may result in poor growth or decline in nutritional status. Overfeeding may result in hepatic steatosis, hyperglycemia, increased risk of infection, or obesity.

Numerous reports describe the comparison of established equations to indirect calorimetry for estimating individual energy needs.[1,5,94–98] Technical constraints and limited resources are the most often cited barriers to routine use of indirect calorimetry in the pediatric population. Energy expenditure can also be estimated using bicarbonate dilution kinetics.[99] Whatever method is used to estimate energy needs, frequent monitoring of anthropometric, clinical, and laboratory parameters allows adjustment of energy delivery to meet individual energy needs.

The percentage contribution of protein, carbohydrate, and fat to total energy intake varies with individual tolerance to fluid, carbohydrate, lipid infusion, clinical condition, and the route of delivery. General guidelines for energy distribution are 8–15% protein, 45–60% carbohydrate, and 25–40% fat.[65] Positive nitrogen balance is best achieved when the nonprotein calorie to nitrogen ratio is 150–300:1.[89,100]

TABLE 20-2 Recommendations for Daily Parenteral Administration of Macronutrients, Electrolytes, and Minerals

	Dose Unit	Premature Infants	Term Infants	1–3 Years	4–6 Years	7–10 Years	11–18 Years	Maximum Dose
Fluid	mL/kg	140–160	120–150	80–120	80–100	60–80	50–70	
Basal energy[1]	kcal/kg	46–55	55	40–55	38–40	25–38	23–25	
Total energy[2]	kcal/kg	90–120	80–105	75–90	65–80	55–70	30–55	
Dextrose[3]	mg/kg/min	5–15	5–15	5–12	5–11	6–10	4–7	See text
Carbohydrate	g/kg	8–21	8–21	8–18	8–16	8–14	6–10	See text
Protein[4]	g/kg	2.5–4	2–3	1–2	1–2	1–2	0.8–1.5	4
Fat[5]	g/kg	0.6–3	0.6–3	0.6–2.5	0.5–2.5	0.5–2.5	0.4–1.8	4
Sodium	mEq/kg	2–5	2–3	1–5	1–5	1–5	60–150 mEq/d	150 mEq/d
Potassium	mEq/kg	2–4	2–3	2–4	2–4	2–4	70–180 mEq/d	180 mEq/d
Chloride	mEq/kg	2–5	2–3	2–4	2–4	2–4	60–150 mEq/d	150 mEq/d
Calcium[6]	mEq/kg	2.5–3	1–2	0.5–1	0.5–1	0.5–1	10–20 mEq/d	See text
Phosphorus[7]	mmol/kg	1–1.5	1–1.5	0.5–1.3	0.5–1.3	0.5–1.3	10–40 mEq/d	See text
Magnesium[8]	mEq/kg	0.5–1	0.25–1	0.25–0.5	0.25–0.5	0.25–0.5	10–30 mEq/d	See text
Zinc[9]	µg/kg	325–400	100–250	100	100	50	2000–5000 µg/d	5000 µg/d
Copper[9]	µg/kg	20	20	20	20	5–20	200–300 µg/d	300 µg/d
Chromium[9]	µg/kg	0.05–0.2	0.14–0.2	0.14–0.2	0.14–0.2	0.14–0.2	5–15 µg/d	15 µg/d
Manganese[9]	µg/kg	1	1	1	1	1	40–50 µg/d	50 µg/d
Selenium[9]	µg/kg	2–3	2	2	2	1–2 µg/d	40–60 µg/d	60 µg/d
Molybdenum[9]	µg/kg	0.25–1	0.25	0.25	0.25	0.25	5 µg/d	5 µg/d
Iron[10]	mg/kg	See text	0.1/See text	See text	See text	See text	See text	See text

[1]Basal energy needs increase: 12% for every degree of fever, 15–25% in cardiac failure, 20–30% in traumatic injury or major surgery, 25–30% in severe respiratory distress or bronchopulmonary dysplasia, 40–50% in severe sepsis, 6 kcal/g weight gain for catch-up growth.

[2]Total parenteral energy needs include basal energy needs, activity, and growth but do not include energy required for digestion or energy losses in stool that occur with enteral feeding. Adjust energy intake if activity or growth needs are higher or lower than normal. Although surgery may increase basal needs temporarily, total energy needs may not increase due to inactivity and temporary interruption of growth.

[3]Peripheral venous access limits dextrose concentration to 12% solutions due to high osmolality and increased risk of tissue damage. Central venous access allows up to 25% dextrose solutions.

[4]Protein needs may vary with diagnoses: 0.8–2 g/kg/day for renal failure; 3 g/kg/day for necrotizing enterocolitis, major surgery, traumatic injury, or sepsis; 4–8 g/kg/day for thermal injury. Most efficient protein utilization occurs when nonprotein/calorie ratio is 150–250:1 (100–150:1 in burns and multiple trauma).

[5]Minimum fat dose to meet essential fatty acid requirements varies depending upon fat source and total energy needs. See text.

[6]Calcium conversions: 1 mEq = 0.5 mmol = 20 mg elemental calcium; 1 mL calcium gluconate 10% contains 100 mg calcium gluconate = 9.3 mg elemental calcium = 0.47 mEq = 0.25 mmol calcium.

[7]Phosphorus conversions: 1 mmol = 31 mg elemental phosphorus; 1 mL sodium phosphate contains 3 mmol or 93 mg elemental phosphorus (and 4 mEq sodium); 1 mL potassium phosphate contains 3 mmol or 93 mg elemental phosphorus (and 4.4 mEq potassium).

[8]Magnesium conversions: 1 mEq = 0.5 mmol = 12.5 mg elemental magnesium; magnesium sulfate 50% contains 500 mg magnesium sulfate heptahydrate or 4.1 mEq (or 51.3 mg) elemental magnesium.

[9]Trace mineral additives are currently available individually and in various combinations/concentrations for various ages. Doses vary. Copper and manganese needs may be lower with cholestasis.

[10]Many institutions do not routinely include iron in parenteral admixtures due to incompatibility with other nutrients, contraindication during sepsis, and risks associated with overdose with multiple blood transfusions.

Sources: Data from Koletzko B, Goulet O, Hunt J, Krohn K, Shamir R for the Parenteral Nutrition Guidelines Working Group. Guidelines on paediatric parenteral nutrition of the European Society of Paediatric Gastroenterology, Hepatology and Nutrition (ESPGHAN) and the European Society for Clinical Nutrition and Metabolism (ESPEN), supported by the European Society of Paediatric Research (ESPR). *J Pediatr Gastroenterol Nutr.* 2005;41:S1–S87; American Society for Parenteral and Enteral Nutrition. Guidelines for the use of parenteral and enteral nutrition in adult and pediatric patients. *J Parenter Enteral Nutr.* 1993;17(Suppl):27SA–52SA; Mirtallo J, Canada T, Johnson D, et al., Task Force for the Revision of Safe Practices for Parenteral Nutrition. Safe practices for parenteral nutrition formulations. *J Parenter Enteral Nutr.* 2004;28:S39–S70; Kerner JA Jr, ed. *Manual of Pediatric Parenteral Nutrition.* New York: John Wiley and Sons; 1983; Heimler R, Doumas BT, Jendrzejcak BM, et al. Relationship between nutrition, weight change, and fluid compartments in preterm infants during the first week of life. *J Pediatr.* 1993;122:110–114; Tilden SJ, Watkins S, Tong TK, Jeevanandam M. Measured energy expenditure in pediatric intensive care patients. *Am J Dis Child.* 1989;143:490–492; Lowery GH. *Growth and Development of Children*, 6th ed. Chicago: Year Book Medical Publishers; 1973:331–332; Heird WC, Kashyap S, Gomez MR. Parenteral alimentation of the neonate. *Semin Perinatol.* 1991;15:493–502; Greene HL, Hambidge KM, Schanler R, et al. Guidelines for the use of vitamins, trace elements, calcium, magnesium, and phosphorus in infants and children receiving total parenteral nutrition: report of the Subcommittee on Pediatric Parenteral Nutrient Requirements from the Committee on Clinical Practice Issues of the American Society for Clinical Nutrition. *Am J Clin Nutr.* 1988;48:1324. (Revised in 1990.); Kleinman RE, ed. *Pediatric Nutrition Handbook.* Elk Grove Village, IL: American Academy of Pediatrics, Committee on Nutrition; 1998:285–305; Khaldi N, Coran AG, Wesley JR. Guidelines for parenteral nutrition in children. *Nutr Supp Serv.* 1984;4:27; Sunehag AL, Haymond MW. Glucose extremes in newborn infants. *Clin Perinatol.* 2002;29:245–260; Prelack K, Sheridan RL. Micronutrient supplementation in the critically ill patient: strategies for clinical practice. *J Trauma.* 2001;51:601–620; and Illingworth RS, Lister J. The critical or sensitive period, with special reference to certain feeding problems in infants and children. *J Pediatr.* 1964;65:839–848.

Carbohydrate

Glucose (dextrose monohydrate, 3.4 kcal/g) is the primary source of parenterally administered carbohydrate, and generally provides 60–75% of nonprotein calories. Glycerol, found in parenterally administered fat emulsions, is also a source of carbohydrate. Glucose dose recommendations for infants and children are found in Table 20-2. Glucose infusions of less than 2 mg/kg/min (3 g/kg/day) may be insufficient to prevent ketosis caused by mobilization of fat stores as a source of energy. Glucose utilization by infants (6–8 mg/kg/min or 8.6–11.5 g/kg/day) is significantly different from adults (2 mg/kg/min or 3 g/kg/day) primarily due to brain metabolism. The brain requires glucose as the primary source of energy, and the brain to body weight ratio in infants is 12% compared to 2% in adults.[90,101] Brain utilization of glucose may account for as much as 90% of basal glucose needs. In addition, infants and children require glucose to support normal growth. Prematurely born infants may require as much as 16 mg/kg/min (24 g/kg/day) of glucose if fat is poorly tolerated as a source of energy.[90,100]

Maximum glucose tolerance varies with age, total energy expenditure, and clinical condition.[47,90,101] Net fat synthesis is shown to occur in infants when glucose intake exceeds 12.5 mg/kg/min (18 g/kg/day) or 6 mg/kg/min (8.6 g/kg/day) in older children. Prematurely born infants or severely malnourished children often require lipogenesis because they may lack adequate fat stores.[5] Glucose intake for full term infants and children up to 2 years of age should not exceed 13 mg/kg/min (18 g/kg/day). Glucose given in excess of need may be associated with hyperglycemia, hepatic steatosis, and/or increased carbon dioxide production and minute ventilation.[1,89,92] During periods of critical illness, glucose tolerance may be limited to 5 mg/kg/min (7.2 g/kg/day).[5]

Generally, insulin is not added to parenteral nutrient admixtures because dose response varies widely, particularly in the low-birth-weight infant. Insulin, when needed, may be given in a separate infusion starting at 0.1 U/kg/hour and increased or decreased as needed to maintain euglycemia.[102,103] Small glycogen stores in low-birth-weight infants and undernourished infants and children place them at a greater risk of developing hypoglycemia following abrupt cessation of parenteral glucose. Gradual weaning from parenteral glucose and adequate enteral feeding help prevent the development of hypoglycemia.

The recommended dose of carbohydrate may be delivered while meeting normal fluid requirements by using a 10% to 12.5% dextrose solution. This concentration is compatible with peripheral intravenous infusion. Greater concentrations of carbohydrate are given by central venous infusion, generally up to a maximum concentration of 25%.[104] These may be needed when caloric needs are greater than normal, when parenterally administered fat is poorly tolerated, or when fluid restriction is necessary.

Protein

Studies attempting to define parenteral protein needs are more abundant for preterm infants than for older infants and children. Parenteral administration of 1.1 to 2.5 g/kg/day along with 30 to 60 kcal/kg/day supports neutral or positive nitrogen balance in very-low-birth-weight (VLBW) infants during the first 24 hours of life. Subsequently, 3.0 to 3.5 g/kg/day (3.5 to 4.0 g/kg/day in infants less than 1000 g) is needed to support normal tissue accretion.[105–111] Early amino acid delivery may improve glucose tolerance by enhancing endogenous insulin secretion.[92,110] Insulin-like growth factor I (IGF-1) is lower in prematurely born infants and may be further reduced by inadequate protein intake. Low levels of IGF-1 are associated with increased risk of retinopathy of prematurity, bronchopulmonary dysplasia, intraventricular hemorrhage, and necrotizing enterocolitis.[112] Recommendations beyond infancy are more empirical or disease related.[89,111,113] General recommendations for protein administration for infants and children are given in Table 20-2. Protein usually comprises about 10–15% of total energy intake. Individual protein needs can be determined from nitrogen balance studies.

Unlike energy needs, protein needs do not decrease during periods of acute stress.[113] The administration of amino acids during periods of acute stress does not completely prevent endogenous protein catabolism, but, in conjunction with enough energy to meet basal requirements, helps maintain normal plasma amino acid concentrations, increases nitrogen retention, and may stimulate endogenous insulin secretion to improve glucose tolerance.[5,92,110] Although evidence is insufficient to make clear recommendations for protein intake, suggestions for reasonable and safe intake during critical illness are 3 g/kg/day for infants and children and up to 2 g/kg/day for adolescents.[5,44] Protein status is generally evaluated by monitoring serum total protein and albumin levels, although changes in serum prealbumin, transferrin, retinol binding protein, or blood urea nitrogen (BUN) levels may identify changes in protein status more quickly. Monitoring acid–base balance and BUN or ammonia levels helps identify excess protein intake. Recommendations concerning monitoring and complications of protein administration are found in **Tables 20-3 and 20-4**.

Crystalline amino acid (CAA) products have been developed for infants reflecting the amino acid composition of human milk or plasma aminograms of healthy term infants fed mature human milk. Metabolic immaturity has also been considered, because cystine, taurine, tyrosine, and histidine may be essential amino acids for neonates and young children.[114–118] Methionine, phenylalanine, and glycine concentrations have been decreased in these solutions, while histidine, tyrosine, taurine, arginine, glutamic acid, and aspartic acid may be added or their concentrations increased.[118] Although cystine may be a conditionally essential amino acid, it is not included in CAA solutions because it is unstable in solution for prolonged periods of time.[119] It is available as L-cystine hydrochloride to be added separately at the time of administration. Cystathionase activity matures to 70% of adult activity by 9 days of age in preterm infants and by 3 days of age in term infants. Cystine supplementation does not increase overall nitrogen retention or improve growth in neonates when 120 mg methionine per kilogram per day is provided, suggesting that cystine may not be needed beyond the neonatal period.[120,121] However, children 1 to 7 years of age with short bowel syndrome receiving home parenteral nutrition demonstrate low serum taurine levels that are increased to within normal reference range by the addition of cystine to their pediatric amino acid preparation, even though the preparation itself contains taurine.[122] The most commonly recommended dose for cystine is 30 to 40 mg/g of protein for pediatric CAA products, although cystine may not be needed for standard solutions due to higher methionine content.[121–124] Adding

TABLE 20-3 Suggested Laboratory Monitoring During Pediatric Parenteral Nutrition

Laboratory Index	Initial	Stable	Home Monitoring
Blood glucose	Daily	Daily to 3×/week	Daily to 3×/week
Acid–base status	Daily to weekly	Every other week	Monthly < 6 months Every 3 months < 1 year Every 6 months > 1 year
Electrolytes Na, K, Cl, CO_2	Daily	Weekly or every other week	
Chemistry profile: total protein albumin BUN, creatinine Ca, P, Mg triglyceride	Weekly	Weekly or every other week	Monthly < 6 months Every 3 months < 1 year Every 6 months > 1 year
Liver profile: total bilirubin alkaline phosphatase LDH, ALT, AST PTT	Weekly	Monthly	Monthly < 6 months Every 3 months < 1 year Every 6 months > 1 year
Hematology profile: HBG/HCT platelet count	Baseline	Weekly	Monthly < 6 months Every 3 months < 1 year Every 6 months > 1 year
CBC w/diff	Weekly	Monthly or as indicated*	As above or as indicated*
iron/TIBC/ferritin	As indicated*	As indicated*	As indicated*
Other: trace minerals vitamins carnitine	As indicated*	As indicated*	As indicated*
Urine glucose specific gravity pH	2–4 times a day	Daily to weekly	As indicated*

*As indicated by clinical condition or symptoms indicating deficiency, imbalance, or abnormality

Abbreviations: BUN, blood urea nitrogen; LDH, lactic dehydrogenase; ALT, alanine amino transferase; AST, aspartate amino transferase; PTT, prothrombin time; HGB, hemoglobin; HCT, hematocrit; CBC, complete blood count; TIBC, total iron binding capacity.

TABLE 20-4 Metabolic Complications of Pediatric Parenteral Nutrition

Complication	Cause	Treatment
Hyperglycemia, glycosuria, osmotic diuresis, hyperosmolar nonketotic dehydration, coma	Excessive dose or rate of glucose infusion	Decrease rate and concentration of glucose; use insulin with caution; results are often erratic in the very-low-birth-weight infant.
Hypoglycemia	Abrupt discontinuation of glucose infusion; excess insulin	Maintain constant glucose infusion; decrease glucose infusion rates slowly; decrease insulin.
Metabolic acidosis, hyperammonemia, prerenal azotemia	Excessive amino acid infusion, inappropriate protein/calorie ratio	Decrease amino acids, increase nonprotein calories.
Hyperchloremic metabolic acidosis	Excessive chloride administration causing cation gap	Provide equal amount of sodium and chloride in infusate; neutralize cation gap with lactate or acetate if respiratory status allows.
Hypokalemia	Inadequate potassium infusion relative to increased requirements for protein anabolism	If potassium needs are greater than the potassium provided by potassium phosphate, potassium acetate is generally recommended.
Hyperkalemia	Excessive potassium administration, especially in metabolic acidosis	Decrease potassium in infusate.
Volume overload, congestive heart failure	Excessive rate of fluid administration	Monitor weight daily; monitor intake and output daily to prevent volume overload; do not attempt to "catch up" by increasing rate of infusion; to treat, decrease rate of infusion.
Hypocalcemia	Inadequate calcium administration or phosphorus administration without simultaneous calcium infusion; hypomagnesemia or hypoalbuminemia	Increase calcium infusion, maintaining appropriate phosphorus and magnesium infusion.
Hypophosphatemia	Inadequate phosphorus administration especially relative to increased needs of protein anabolism	Increase phosphorus infusion, maintaining appropriate calcium/phosphorus precipitation.
Hypomagnesemia	Inadequate magnesium infusion relative to increased gastrointestinal losses in chronic diarrhea or increased needs for protein anabolism	Increase magnesium infusion.
Essential fatty acid deficiency	Inadequate linoleic acid infusion	Provide at least 4–8% of total calories as intravenous fat emulsion to provide 1–4% of total calories as linoleic acid.
Hypertriglyceridemia, hypercholesterolemia	Lipids infused at a rate greater than the capacity to metabolize	Decrease or interrupt lipid infusion; add heparin to infusate.
Anemia	Deficiency of iron, folic acid, vitamin B_{12}, or copper	Administer appropriate nutrient.
Cholestatic jaundice	Sepsis, prematurity, starvation, essential fatty acid deficiency, lipid infusion, amino acid deficiency, amino acid excess, carbohydrate excess, decreased bile flow, bowel obstruction, lack of enteral feedings	Begin enteral feedings as soon as possible, maintain adequate but not excessive intake; liver function generally returns to normal within 6–9 months after cessation of therapy, but may progress to chronic liver disease; consider enteral fish oil; parenteral fish oil is currently for compassionate use only in the United States.

Source: Adapted with permission from Hendricks KM, Walker WA. *Manual of Pediatric Nutrition*, 3rd ed. Philadelphia: Decker, 2000:265–277.

L-cystine hydrochloride decreases the solution's pH, which increases calcium and phosphorus solubility, thus increasing mineral delivery.[125,126]

Although glutamine is not routinely added to parenteral nutrition solutions due to solubility problems, this amino acid may be conditionally essential during periods of sepsis, trauma, surgery, or shock when circulating levels decrease and needs, particularly in maintaining GI mucosal cell integrity, are increased.[127,128] For extremely low-birth-weight infants, glutamine added to parenteral nutrition in amounts of 0.3 to 0.5 g/kg/day (or 20% of amino acid intake) appears safe and may support lower occurrence rates of GI dysfunction and severe neurological sequelae and earlier achievement of full enteral feedings.[129,130]

Most of the studies comparing or evaluating the efficacy of pediatric and standard CAA products have been done in small numbers of patients over relatively short duration (5 to 21 days).[102,114–116,126] Although greater weight gain and nitrogen balance with pediatric products may be statistically significant, these differences may not be clinically significant. The greatest advantage seems to be that plasma amino acid patterns are similar to those of healthy breastfed neonates. Implications for use with older infants or children have not been clearly identified. Although the data are inconclusive, there may be a decreased incidence of cholestatic liver disease during specific pediatric CAA product administration.[124,131–134]

In practice, based on current literature, pediatric CAA products may be of benefit to the prematurely born infant or the infant who requires long-term parenteral nutrition. Pediatric CAA products may require cystine supplementation with 55 to 77 mg/kg/day for infants less than 4 months of age due to inadequate cystathionase activity. All other infants and children may need 3 to 22 mg cystine per gram of total amino acid content due to reduced methionine content.[102,119,121–124]

Special solutions of L-isomer CAA formulated for adults with severe hepatic or renal failure appear to also be efficacious in children with severe hepatic or chronic renal failure, though standard CAA solutions may better meet the amino acid needs of children with acute renal failure.[135–139] Older children with sepsis or traumatic injury may benefit from using formulations with increased amounts of branched-chain amino acids.[140]

Fat

Fat is included in PN regimens for infants and children as a source of essential fatty acids (EFA) and to provide 25–40% of nonprotein energy intake. Linoleic acid (LA) deficiency is clinically manifested as dry, flaky skin; dry hair; poor growth; decreased platelets; and impaired wound healing. Biochemical deficiency of LA precedes these clinical manifestations. Plasma levels of LA and arachidonic acid (AA) decline, and the ratio of plasma eicosatrienoic acid to AA (triene:tetraene) becomes elevated. Numbness, paresthesia, weakness, inability to walk, and blurring of vision may occur if linolenic acid (LNA) deficiency is present, and docosapentaenoic acid (DPA) levels increase while docosahexaenoic acid (DHA) levels decrease.[5,141,142] Long-chain polyunsaturated acids AA and DHA are involved in the structure and function of cell membranes, specifically retinal and central nervous system structures, and dietary intake of these fatty acids may be essential during infancy.[143] Very-low-birth-weight infants or infants and children with depleted body stores of fat or with a chronic history of fat malabsorption are at greatest risk of developing EFA deficiencies.[144]

Providing as little as 2% to 4% of the total daily caloric intake as LA (0.25 g/kg/day for infants and 0.1 g/kg/day in older children) and 0.25% to 0.5% of the total daily caloric intake as LNA can prevent deficiency in most infants and children.[5,11,44,65,145] Parenteral lipids currently available in the United States contain soy oil (Intralipid and Liposyn III) or safflower oil and soy oil (Liposyn II). Soy oil preparations provide 0.5 g LA and 0.09 g LNA per gram of fat. Safflower oil and soy oil mixtures contain 0.65 g LA and 0.04 g LNA per gram of fat. Usual recommendations for prevention of EFA deficiency using these emulsions are 0.5–1 g/kg/day or 2.5–5 mL of 20% lipid emulsion/kg/day. Children over 4 years of age require 0.5 g/kg/day and adolescents require 0.4 g/kg/day to meet estimated essential fatty acid needs.

In Europe and South America, other parenteral lipid preparations are available that contain medium-chain triglycerides (MCT), olive oil, and/or fish oil, but the experience and research with these preparations in pediatric patients is somewhat limited. Products containing MCT oil may provide advantages of more rapid hydrolyzation and oxidation with improved tolerance and better energy delivery, but they also contain lower amounts of essential fatty acids.[146] Products made with olive oil may have fewer immunologic effects and reduced lipid peroxidation.[92,147,148] The most promising advance in PN therapy is the use of fish-oil-based lipid emulsions to prevent or reverse PN-associated liver disease.[149–151] Each of these emulsions contains lower amounts of essentially fatty acids. The fatty acid compositions of parenteral lipid emulsions are listed elsewhere.[118,149]

Limitations of glucose or fluid tolerance and high energy needs usually dictate a greater intake of lipid than that which prevents deficiency. Fifty percent of energy intake is derived from fat in the breastfed infant. Parenteral lipid doses of 2.5 to 3.0 g/kg/day provide infants with only 25–35% of total energy intake as fat, but higher doses may be poorly tolerated, especially in prematurely born or small for gestational age infants.[65,89,152,153] In children over 2 years of age, it may be advisable to limit fat to 30% of total calories (generally 1.0 to 2.5 g/kg/day), as recommended by the

American Academy of Pediatrics.[154] Fat should not provide more than 60% of total calories in any patient, because ketotic acidosis may occur.[155]

The rate of administration may be just as significant a factor in lipid tolerance as daily dose. Adverse effects of intravenous fat when given in boluses or in doses exceeding 0.15 g/kg/hour or 3.6 g/kg/day have been reported, including altered pulmonary function, impaired neutrophil function, and an increased risk of kernicterus in infants with elevated serum bilirubin level.[156–158] Preterm or malnourished infants and children may be at greater risk for impaired fat tolerance due to decreased adipose tissue mass, reduced lipoprotein lipase activity, hepatic immaturity, or carnitine deficiency. Although heparin stimulates the release of lipoprotein lipase, it may not significantly affect lipid clearance over time and is not routinely recommended for that purpose.[5]

Parenteral lipid emulsions contain egg phospholipid as an emulsifying agent. Because phospholipids interfere with enzymes that help metabolize and clear plasma lipids, 20% emulsions are recommended over 10% emulsions due to lower phospholipid-to-lipid ratio. Parenteral lipid emulsions also contain glycerol and are relatively isotonic and pH neutral, providing a favorable environment for the proliferation of several common pathogens. When infused separately, lipid emulsions are associated with an increased incidence of coagulase-negative staphylococcal bacteremia, particularly when hang times exceed 12 hours. When administered as a component of a TNA, this association is no longer apparent, likely due to the hypertonic and relatively acidic environment provided by the presence of other nutrients.[158] Both of these factors may decrease the stability of the lipid emulsion, causing separation, particularly when higher amounts of amino acids and minerals are used, as for low-birth-weight infants. The opacity of TNAs may also mask the presence of incompatibilities and precipitates, resulting in adverse outcomes, although use of a 1.2-micron filter can remove larger organisms, particles, precipitates, and fat globules.[159]

Intravenous fat may be safely given if:

- The initial dose is 0.5 g/kg/day and it is gradually increased by 0.25 or 0.5 g/kg/day.
- The highest dose is under 0.12 to 0.15 g/kg/hour (3 to 3.6 g/kg/day) or less than 0.08 g/kg/hour (2 g/kg/day) during periods of acute sepsis.
- Serum triglycerides are monitored and kept within the normal range, although various recommendations are given in the literature for the acceptable upper limit of normal, ranging from 100 to 200 mg/dL.[145,156,157]
- Whenever possible, lipids are administered as a component of a TNA over 24 hours using a 1.2-micron filter to best maintain physiochemical stability and minimize infectious risk.[159,160]

When lipids must be infused separately due to higher protein and mineral needs, such as for low-birth-weight infants, recommendations for reducing risk of nosocomial bacteremia include: (1) aseptic transfer of lipid emulsion from the original container directly to infusion devices by pharmacy personnel under a class A laminar air flow hood, and (2) hang times limited to 12 hours whenever possible.[161] Limiting hang times to 12 hours ultimately limits total lipid dose to 1.8 g/kg/day or 17–20% of total energy intake. When energy needs exceed 95 kcal/kg/day and fluid tolerance is limited to 120–150 mL/kg/day, dextrose solutions of 15–18% given through centrally placed catheters may be required. Because this may exceed glucose tolerance, particularly in extremely low-birth-weight infants, using administration sets up to 24 hours to accommodate a second lipid infusion has been suggested.[160]

If serum bilirubin levels are greater than 8–10 mg/dL (while the serum albumin level is 2.5 to 3 g/dL), lipids should be given only in amounts adequate to prevent EFA deficiency.[158] If intravenous fat is given in greater amounts or given in bolus doses, the free fatty acid to serum albumin molar ratio should be maintained at less than 6 while bilirubin levels remain elevated.[65] (See Chapter 4 for further discussion on this issue.)

Carnitine facilitates transport of long- and medium-chain fatty acids across mitochondrial membranes. Carnitine is normally synthesized by the liver from methionine and lysine. Pediatric amino acid solutions are lower in methionine than in standard solutions, and patients at risk for carnitine deficiency demonstrate lower plasma concentrations of carnitine when receiving carnitine-free parenteral products as their single source of nutrition.[162] Patients at highest risk for carnitine depletion include those who are less than 30 weeks' gestation, have a birth weight under 1500 g or a history of fetal malnutrition, or have hepatic or renal dysfunction, infection, or medium-chain acetyl-dehydrogenase deficiency.[163]

Studies are somewhat conflicting as to whether routine carnitine supplementation is needed, even in high-risk individuals, or if carnitine supplementation significantly affects parenteral lipid utilization.[164–169] Carnitine supplementation may be considered in patients identified at high risk if parenteral nutrition is expected to be the single source of nutrition for longer than 2 weeks, or if hypertriglyceridemia, hypoglycemia, and low serum carnitine are present.[5,163,165] Dose recommendations for oral or intravenous supplementation of carnitine vary from 50 to 100 mmol/kg/day (approximately 10–20 mg/kg/day).[164–168] Doses of 300 mmol/kg/day (50 mg/kg/day) or greater are not recommended, because these doses are associated with increased metabolic rate, decreased protein deposition, and impaired growth.[163,168] Although carnitine is not routinely added to parenteral nutrition solutions in all institutions at this time, it is available for parenteral use.

Vitamins

Recommendations for term infants and children up to 11 years of age were established by the Nutrition Advisory Group of the American Medical Association in 1975.[170] They are based on the 1974 recommended dietary allowances (RDAs), which are guidelines for enteral nutrient intake. Recommendations for adolescents are based on guidelines for adults. Vitamin requirements of prematurely born infants may vary from those of term infants due to the immaturity of vitamin absorption, excretion, enterohepatic recirculation, and renal tubular reabsorption mechanisms. Current estimates of need are based on numerous studies and extrapolations from term infant data.[87] Two different vitamin dose regimens for infants who weigh less than 2500 g have been suggested. Doses based on broad weight categories are more likely to underdose larger infants and/or overdose smaller infants, particularly with vitamins E and K and B-complex vitamins.[171–173] Either dose regimen is likely to underdose vitamin A, particularly for smaller infants, though vitamin A is often dosed separately for these infants and given intramuscularly.[171,174]

Studies have shown the Food and Drug Administration's current dose recommendations produce serum levels at or above the reference range for a-tocopherol, 25-hydroxycholecalciferol, thiamin, riboflavin, niacin, pyridoxine, folate, pantothenic acid, cyanocobalamin, and biotin.[175,176] There are no reports of toxic vitamin levels using these recommended doses. Thiamin deficiency has been reported in infants and children during shortages of parenteral multivitamin (MVI) products. Oral or enteral administration of thiamin, and perhaps other vitamins, may not be sufficient in patients who require total or partial delivery of nutrition parenterally. Thiamin should be given as a separate intravenous additive during MVI shortages.[177] The vitamin content of MVI Pediatric for Infusion and MVI-12 Multivitamin Infusion (Astra USA, Inc.) are compared to the current vitamin dose recommendations in **Table 20-5**.

Levels of several vitamins may decrease over time in parenteral nutrient admixtures due to light degradation, decomposition in the presence of bisulfite (an antioxidant additive) or varying pH, and adsorbance to plastic or glass. For these reasons, multivitamins should be added to TNA solutions immediately prior to administration, excessive light exposure (direct sunlight or phototherapy light) should be avoided, and administration of these admixtures completed within 24 hours. If lipids are given separately, adding both fat-soluble and water-soluble vitamins to the lipid emulsion may increase vitamin stability and delivery.[5]

Minerals

It is important to monitor key minerals such as magnesium, calcium, and phosphorus as well as trace minerals, and adjust the intake of these minerals as needed while on parenteral nutrition.

Magnesium

Magnesium deficiency is identified by decreased serum levels. Hypomagnesemia can occur in many conditions such as protein-calorie malnutrition, chronic malabsorption, proximal jejunal resection, ileostomy, cystic fibrosis, neonatal hepatitis, congenital biliary atresia, DiGeorge's syndrome, or hypokalemia; in infants born to diabetic mothers; or during chronic diuretic therapy, aminoglycoside therapy, or chemotherapy.[13] If serum levels are below 1.4 mg/dL or if seizures occur, repletion dose is 0.2 mEq/kg given intramuscularly or intravenously every 6 hours until symptoms subside. Older children may require 0.8–1 mEq/kg/day for repletion or during critical illness.[91] Blood pressure should be monitored when providing intravenous magnesium repletion, because hypotension may occur.[65]

Parenteral doses of 0.5–1 mEq/kg/day may be needed to allow adequate retention for prematurely born infants, though general dose recommendations for all other infants and children are 0.25 to 0.5 mEq/kg/day of magnesium with a maximum allowable dose of 24 mEq/day.[65,100,153] Upper-range doses may be needed during rapid growth phases, diuretic therapy, or chronic malabsorption. Lower range doses may be indicated if renal function is impaired. Magnesium is added to parenteral admixtures as magnesium sulfate (50% $MgSO_4$), which contains 4.1 mEq (49.3 mg) of magnesium per milliliter. Excessive doses may cause central nervous system depression and hypotonia.[87] Serum magnesium levels may be transiently elevated in preterm infants whose mothers received significant amounts of magnesium sulfate to prevent premature labor or treat preeclampsia. Magnesium may be withheld from PN solutions for these infants until serum levels are within normal limits.

Calcium

Calcium deficiency is not usually identified by low serum levels because serum calcium is usually maintained at the expense of bone stores.[87] Hypocalcemia is most common during the neonatal period, particularly in infants born prematurely, due to their relatively low calcium stores and inappropriately low parathyroid hormone levels. This initial hypocalcemia usually resolves within the first few days of life when treated with intravenous administration of calcium 1 to 2 mEq/kg/day.[114]

Nutrition recommendations for parenteral calcium administration to prematurely born infants range from 50 to 80 mg/kg/day (which is 1.3–2 mmol/kg/day or 2.5–3 mEq/kg/day).[87,157,178,179] Most published sources empirically recommend 10–50 mg/kg/day (which is 0.25 to 1.3 mmol/kg/day or 0.5 to 2 mEq/kg/day) for all other ages[50] (see Table 20-2). Calcium should be administered over 24 hours because parenteral calcium administered chronically as bolus doses over 20 minutes to 1 hour has been associated with hypercalcemia and hypercalciuria.[180,181] Nephrolithiasis and

TABLE 20-5 Recommendations for Pediatric Parenteral Daily Vitamin Dosage

	A IU	D IU	E mg	K μg	C mg	B_1 mg	B_2 mg	B_3 mg	B_6 mg	B_{12} μg	FA μg	PA mg	Biotin μg
Recommended amount/kg/day													
Preterm infant (≤ 2.5 kg)	500–1700	32–160	2.8–3.5	10–80	15–25	0.35–0.5	0.15–0.2	4–6.8	0.15–0.2	0.3	56	1–2	5–8
MVI Pediatric** doses													
30% dose/day (0.5–1 kg)	700–1400	120–240	2.1–4.2	60–120	24–48	0.4–0.7	0.3–0.6	5–10	0.3–0.6	0.3–0.6	42–84	1.5–3	6–12
65% dose/day (1–2.5 kg)	600–1500	100–260	1.8–4.5	50–130	21–52	0.3–0.8	0.4–0.9	4–11	0.3–0.6	0.3–0.6	36–90	1.5–3	5–13
40% dose/kg/day (≤ 2.5 kg)*	920	160	2.8	80	32	0.48	0.56	6.8	0.4	0.4	56	2	8
Recommended amount/day													
Preterm infant (> 2.5 kg)	700–1500	40–160	2–4	6–10	35–50	0.3–0.8	0.4–0.9	5–12	0.3–0.7	0.3–0.7	40–90	2–5	6–13
Term infant/child (age 1–11 yrs)	2300	400	5–7	200	80	1.2	1.4	17	1	1	140	5	20
MVI Pediatric,** 1 dose/day	2300	400	7	200	80	1.2	1.4	17	1	1	140	5	20
Recommended amount/day													
Adolescents (11–18 yrs)	3300	200	10	150–700	100	3	3.6	40	4	5	400	15	60
MVI–12,** 1 dose/day	3300	200	10	150	100	3	3.6	40	4	5	400	15	60

* Maximum dose not to exceed 1 full dose per day.

** Pediatric MVI (pediatric parenteral multivitamin) and MVI-12 Injection or Unit Vial, Astra USA, Inc., Westboro, MA.

Abbreviations: A, retinol; D, cholecalciferol; E, alpha-tocopherol; K, phytonadione; B1, thiamin; B2, riboflavin; B3, niacin; B6, pyridoxine; B12, cyanocobalamin; FA, folic acid; PA, pantothenic acid.

Sources: Data from Koletzko B, Goulet O, Hunt J, Krohn K, Shamir R for the Parenteral Nutrition Guidelines Working Group. Guidelines on paediatric parenteral nutrition of the European Society of Paediatric Gastroenterology, Hepatology and Nutrition (ESPGHAN) and the European Society for Clinical Nutrition and Metabolism (ESPEN), supported by the European Society of Paediatric Research (ESPR). *J Pediatr Gastroenterol Nutr.* 2005;41:S1–S87; Storm HM, Young SL, Sandler RH. Development of pediatric and neonatal parenteral nutrition order forms. *Nutr Clin Pract.* 1995;10:54–59; John E, Klavdianou M, Vidyasagar D. Electrolyte problems in neonatal surgical patients. *Clin Perinatol.* 1989;16:219–232; Greene HL, Hambidge KM, Schanler R, et al. Guidelines for the use of vitamins, trace elements, calcium, magnesium, and phosphorus in infants and children receiving total parenteral nutrition: report of the Subcommittee on Pediatric Parenteral Nutrient Requirements from the Committee on Clinical Practice Issues of the American Society for Clinical Nutrition. *Am J Clin Nutr.* 1988;48:1324. (Revised in 1990.); Friedman Z, Danon A, Stahlman MT, et al. Rapid onset of essential fatty acid deficiency in the newborn. *Pediatrics.* 1976;58:640–649; Magnusson G, Boberg M, Cederblad G, et al. Plasma and tissue levels of lipids, fatty acids, and plasma carnitine in neonates receiving a new fat emulsion. *Acta Paediatr.* 1997;86:638–644; and McDonald CM, MacKay MW, Curtis J, et al. Carnitine and cholestasis: nutritional dilemmas for the parenterally nourished newborn. *Support Line.* 2003;25:10.

hypercalciuria have been associated with furosemide therapy and inadequate phosphorus intake.[178,182] Older children receiving cyclic parenteral nutrition may have greater urinary losses of calcium due to higher rates of infusion.[183]

Calcium gluconate is generally the additive of choice, though there is some concern about aluminum contamination, especially at higher doses.[184] Solutions that deliver 15 to 30 μg aluminum/kg/day may result in tissue loading and are considered unsafe.[87,185] Calcium gluconate 10% contains 100 mg of calcium gluconate per 1 mL, providing 0.5 mEq, 0.25 mmol, or 10 mg of elemental calcium per 1 mL.

Phosphorus

Phosphorus depletion has been reported in infants and children; it may be more pronounced when calcium is given without phosphorus, or may occur during chronic aminoglycoside or vancomycin therapy.[186] Phosphorus depletion is characterized by hypercalciuria (at least 4 mg calcium/kg/day), hypophosphatemia (serum levels less than 4 mg/dL), and undetectable levels of urinary phosphorus excretion.[87,178,188] Parenteral repletion of phosphorus may be accomplished by an initial one to two doses of 5 to 11 mg/kg (0.15 to 0.36 mmol/kg), each given over 6 hours. When refeeding malnourished individuals, the initial 7 to 10 days of the anabolic phase is accompanied by increased needs for phosphorus, and, to a lesser extent, potassium and magnesium, because these electrolytes are incorporated into cells of lean tissue. Phosphorus needs may be twice the normal recommended allowance during this time, though consistent monitoring is recommended to prevent excessive phosphorus administration that may cause hyperphosphatemia, hypocalcemia, and secondary hyperparathyroidism.[87]

Recommendations for parenteral administration of phosphorus to infants and children are given in Table 20-2. Doses for phosphorus are often given in proportion to calcium as 1–1.3:1 molar ratio or 1.3–1.7:1 calcium/phosphorus ratio by weight.[87] Phosphorus is added to parenteral nutrient solutions as potassium phosphate or sodium phosphate salts. Potassium phosphate contains 93 mg (3 mmol) of phosphorus and 4.4 mEq of potassium per mL. Sodium phosphate contains 93 mg (3 mmol) of phosphorus and 4 mEq of sodium per mL.

The greatest difficulty in providing adequate calcium and phosphorus parenterally is their relative insolubility in the same admixture, limited further by increasing pH and temperature. Alternating calcium and phosphorus administration is not recommended due to adverse effects including alternating elevations of serum mineral levels, increased mineral losses due to urinary excretion, and altered mineral homeostasis.[189–191] Recommendations for compounding to minimize precipitation usually include adding phosphate salts early in the process and calcium salts late (but before the lipid emulsion in 3-in-1 admixtures).[191,192] Adherence to compounding protocol is particularly important when lipid is present, because precipitates are more difficult to identify due to the opacity of the admixture. The addition of L-cysteine increases mineral solubility; the use of calcium glycerophosphate or monobasic phosphate formulations may also improve solubility.[53] Solubility studies and guidelines for simultaneous administration of calcium and phosphorus have been published for various amino acid products.[189,192–194] Filters are recommended to prevent precipitate delivery: a 1.2-micron air-eliminating filter for lipid-containing admixtures and a 0.22-micron air-eliminating filter for non-lipid-containing admixtures.[192] The higher doses of minerals needed for young infants are given through central intravenous access to prevent vascular damage and tissue sloughs. Separate administration of lipid may be needed to allow higher concentrations of calcium and phosphorus for prematurely born infants.

Trace Minerals

Recommendations for daily parenteral doses of trace minerals are given in Table 20-2.[87,195] Zinc, copper, chromium, manganese, selenium, and iodine are available singly or in combination for use in PN admixtures. Product concentrations and dose recommendations are given in **Table 20-6**. Neither clinical nor biochemical deficiency of molybdenum or iodine with parenteral nutrition has been reported in the literature, and they are generally not included in parenteral nutrition admixtures. Transdermal absorption of iodine from cleansing or disinfecting solutions or ointments may be an adequate source of iodine.[182] Fluorine is not added, because its role in human nutrition is limited primarily to dental health and may be of greater benefit when administered topically once teeth have erupted around 6 months of age.[88]

Very-low-birth-weight infants and infants and children with protein-calorie malnutrition, thermal injury, neoplasms, chronic diarrhea, enterocutaneous fistulas, or bile salt malabsorption are at greatest risk for developing trace element deficiency.[195–198] Zinc supplementation without copper supplementation may interfere with copper metabolism.[196] Copper doses are reduced or eliminated and manganese is often withheld for infants and children who develop cholestatic jaundice, because these minerals are excreted primarily through bile and their accumulation is potentially hepatotoxic and, in the case of magnesium, neurotoxic.[65,199–201] However, serum copper and manganese levels may not correlate with serum direct bilirubin levels.[202] Hepatic copper content has been shown to decrease as evidence of cholestasis increases, and copper deficiency has been reported when omitted from parenteral nutrition due to presence of cholestasis.[203–205] Serum manganese levels may become markedly elevated after several months of PN. A contributory role of manganese in the development

TABLE 20-6 Dose Concentrations and Recommendations for Combined Trace Mineral Products

Product Category	Dose mL	Zinc μg	Copper μg	Chromium μg	Manganese μg	Selenium[1] μg
Neonatal[2]	1	1500	100	0.85	25	—
	0.2/kg	300/kg[3]	20/kg	0.17/kg	5/kg[4]	—
Pediatric	1	500 or 1000	100	0.85 or 1	25	0 or 15
	0.1/kg	50 or 100/kg	10/kg	~ 0.1/kg	2.5/kg	0 or 1.5/kg
	0.2/kg	100 or 200/kg	20/kg	~ 0.2/kg	5/kg[4]	0 or 2/kg
	2[5]	2000	200	2	50	30
	5[5]	2500 or 5000	500	4.25 or 5	125	0
Adult[6,7] (standard)	1	1000	400	4	100	0 or 20
	0.05/kg	50/kg	20/kg	0.2/kg	5/kg[4]	0 or 1/kg
Adult[6] (concentrate)	1	5000	1000	10	500	0 or 60
	0.01/kg	50/kg	10/kg	0.1/kg	5/kg[4]	0 or 0.6/kg

[1]Neonatal and select pediatric and adult products do not contain selenium or molybdenum. These may be added separately when total parenteral nutrition is required for longer than 4 weeks.

[2]Neonatal products are generally recommended for preterm infants until term age. Maximum dose is 3 mL/day.

[3]Additional zinc is needed to meet recommendations for preterm neonates.

[4]Manganese dose may be excessive in cholestatic jaundice.

[5]Maximum dose of pediatric product with selenium is limited by the amount of selenium. Maximum dose of pediatric product without selenium is limited by cwopper content.

[6]Adult products are generally used for adolescents, or children over 10 years of age.

[7]Iodine is included in one standard and one concentrated adult product in concentrations of 25 and 75 mcg/mL respectively; molybdenum is included in one standard adult product in a concentration of 25 μg/mL.

Sources: Data from product literature; Intravenous nutritional therapy. Trace metals. In: Killion KH, Kastrup EK, eds. *Drug Facts and Comparisons,* 57th ed. St. Louis, MO: Wolters Kluwer Health; 2003:125.

of PN-related cholestasis has been considered, particularly in individuals receiving PN for longer than 30 days.[206] The literature suggests monitoring levels of both copper and manganese, and adjusting parenteral supplementation as needed to maintain serum levels within the normal range.[64] Selenium and molybdenum are not generally used when parenteral nutrition is required for only a short period of time. Selenium is present as a contaminant in parenteral dextrose solutions, providing up to 0.9 mg/dL. Parenteral selenium toxicity has not been reported, though lower doses may be indicated when renal function is impaired.[87]

Iron deficiency is probably the most common trace mineral deficiency. It manifests as microcytic hypochromic anemia and is characterized by low serum hemoglobin and ferritin levels, low hematocrit, and low percent transferrin saturation. Infants and children at risk for iron deficiency include those who are prematurely born, chronically ill, protein-calorie malnourished, have significant unreplaced blood loss, or who receive unsupplemented parenteral nutrition for long periods of time.

There is some controversy over whether iron should be routinely included in parenteral nutrition therapy. Intramuscular injections of iron may not be the best choice in the small prematurely born infant or the protein-calorie malnourished patient due to small muscle mass and increased risk of sarcoma at the site of injection.[208] Anaphylaxis has been reported in some patients with administration of iron dextran.[208] Several authors report that iron may be safely given daily in parenteral nutrition admixtures or in bolus doses given intravenously over 2 to 3 hours weekly or monthly.[207–210] Often, iron is given parenterally only in treatment of iron deficiency anemia.

Although standard dose recommendations for prematurely born infants are 0.1 to 0.2 mg/kg/day,[87,211] trials of recombinant erythropoietin have used iron supplements of 1 mg/kg/day without evidence of harmful side effects, though these are short-term studies.[212,213] Iron toxicity may be difficult to ascertain because iron is quickly stored in hepatic tissue and serum iron levels may not reflect overload. Excess iron may also increase risk of gram-negative septicemia and increase antioxidant requirements. These risks do not preclude use of standard doses of parenteral iron, but higher doses must be used with caution beyond 4 weeks duration.[87] Very-low-birth-weight infants who have received blood transfusion of at least 180 mL of packed cells may not need additional iron supplementation.[214] Doses of 0.1 mg/kg/day up to 1 mg/day are recommended for all other infants and children. Iron dextran is available as the source of iron for parenteral use. Guidelines for dosage and administration of iron dextran in treatment of iron deficiency are given in the manufacturer's package insert.

Patient Monitoring

A comprehensive monitoring program for infants and children receiving PN includes evaluation of laboratory measurements of metabolic and electrolyte status (see Table 20-3), anthropometric measurements (see **Table 20-7**), intake and output measurements, and physical examination (see **Table 20-8**). Baseline and regularly scheduled laboratory measurements allow timely identification of metabolic complications and assessment of nutritional adequacy. Metabolic complications that may occur during pediatric nutrition support are summarized in Table 20-4. Laboratory monitoring protocols may vary from one setting to another, but should take into consideration smaller blood volumes in pediatric patients, using microtechniques whenever possible and avoiding unnecessary bloodwork. For patients on long-term PN, the need and frequency for some tests can be reevaluated once a stable regimen has been established. See also Chapter 3 on nutrition assessment and Appendix G for biochemical evaluation of nutritional status.

Temperature instability, apnea and bradycardia, and increased respiration rate and pulse may be early signs of sepsis in the pediatric patient. Records of intake provide documentation that actual administration equals planned intake. Documentation of output establishes a basis for evaluation of fluid balance, as does evaluation of skin turgor and the presence of edema. Insertion sites are monitored for redness, swelling, leaking, or other signs of infection or infiltration. Changes in behavior and/or mental status may precede other signs of sepsis or fluid and electrolyte balance.

TABLE 20-7 Growth Parameters Monitored During Pediatric Parenteral Nutrition

Parameter	Frequency
Weight	Daily (neonates up to 1 month corrected age) Weekly (1–6 months corrected age) Monthly (infants, 6 months corrected age; children)
Length or height	Weekly (infants, 6 months corrected age) Monthly (infants, 6 months corrected age) Every 3 months (ages 1–3) Every 6 months (ages 4–18)
Head circumference	Weekly (infants, 6 months corrected age) Monthly (infants, 6 months corrected age) Every 3 months (ages 1–3)
Body composition triceps skinfold arm muscle area	As clinically indicated; comparison against established norms is more useful in children over 3 years than in younger children

TABLE 20-8 Clinical Monitoring During Pediatric Parenteral Nutrition

Clinical Parameter	Initial	Stable
Temperature Pulse/respirations	Hourly, then every 4–8 hr	Daily or as indicated
Intake	Hourly, then every 4–8 hr	Daily
Output	Hourly, then every 4–8 hr	As indicated
Administration system	Hourly, then every 4–8 hr	Daily
Infusion site/dressing	Hourly, then every 4–8 hr	Daily
Mental status, behavioral status, edema, skin turgor	Every 4–8 hr	Daily or as indicated

Psychosocial Issues

Eating is basic to life. Parents feed their infants and children. When normal feeding is replaced with PN, parents may feel helpless or useless. An infant or child of any age may feel frustrated at not being able to eat. Older children may have fears or insecurities about body function or body image. The ability of an infant or child and their family to accept and adapt to PN depends on the presenting diagnosis, the acuity or chronic nature of the disease or condition, the duration and complexity of the hospitalization, the duration of nutrition support therapy, and the physical and emotional development of the infant or child.[215-217] Eighty to 90% of children requiring home TPN will likely continue to receive this support 1 year after initiation.[218] When long-term or home PN is needed, the stability of the family unit and its financial, physical, and emotional resources are important factors as well.

Keeping the family informed; providing consistent support through a social worker, care manager, and/or primary nurse; and involving the family and child (appropriately for age and level of understanding) in the actual care activities can empower the family and child to meet some of their own needs and lessen their feelings of helplessness. Family involvement is crucial in preparing a family for successful home PN.

Members of the hospital-based multi-disciplinary team, including the physician, nurse, dietitian, pharmacist, social worker, and developmental specialist, must plan a program of home PN that is feasible, given the resources of the family and the community. Resources that support success of home PN are listed in **Table 20-9**. Education of family members must take into account their readiness and ability to learn. Assessment of learning includes measuring the family's ability to accurately repeat instructions or demonstrate techniques. Communication with home healthcare providers is essential for continuity of care.

The technical nature of PN must not overshadow the infant or child and his or her developmental progress. Occupational and physical therapists, speech pathologists, and child life and/or developmental specialists ensure that the hospital setting is modified as much as possible to support the normal development of the child on PN.

For the neonate whose feedings are limited or who is unable to take oral feedings, pleasant oral stimulation, non-nutritive sucking, and other sensory stimulation is needed to support normal oral development. Prolonged, early oral deprivation can lead to increased oral sensitivity and abnormal tongue movements that can adversely influence the development of future speech patterns.[219] Eating is a basic, essential function and many parents, particularly mothers, may feel responsible for their infant's problems and may suffer loss of self-esteem or have feelings of inadequacy at being unable to perform the simple caregiving task of feeding. Healthcare professionals can enhance the parents' involvement in "feeding" the PN-dependent infant by encouraging them to hold, cuddle, and offer other forms of oral stimulation during "normal" feeding times. When possible, the infant on PN should be offered some type of oral feeding, if only in very small amounts. If totally deprived of oral sustenance, the introduction of oral feedings may be met with gagging, vomiting, swallowing difficulties, or other signs of feeding aversion.

Infants use their mouths to explore much of their environment. Sucking on fingers or toys can be encouraged to help infants experience and develop trust in their environment. Other types of tactile and visual stimulation can be provided to distract infants from manipulating or chewing on tubes and equipment. Creative ways to protect equipment and maintain safety should be used rather than physical restraint. Clothing that covers the catheter insertion site and tubing helps prevent pulling and manipulation of equipment and allows more limited exploration of the environment.

Toddlers present many challenges to the safe delivery of PN. These challenges may include temperament, mobility,

TABLE 20-9 Resources that Support Successful Home Parenteral Nutrition

Environment	Grounded electrical outlets. Backup electricity, either battery, generator, or power company priority for loss of power. Lack of physical barriers to maneuvering equipment or storing supplies. Refrigeration to store adequate supplies of solutions. Reliable telephone service. Convenient and safe water supply and hand-washing facilities.
Medical support	Convenient and reliable home healthcare agency for nursing care. Ongoing nutritional assessment, supplies, laboratory assessment. Local physician experienced and amenable to home parenteral nutrition. Responsive local community emergency care, both ambulance and local emergency room.
Family characteristics	At least two responsible adults are competent to provide all care associated with home parenteral nutrition; extended family support. All children (both the patient and siblings, particularly small children) are protected from harm associated with home parenteral nutrition, such as needle sticks; damage to catheter, tubing, or other equipment; removal of catheter; etc.
Financial	Adequate medical insurance coverage with certified medical necessity for home parenteral nutrition.
Attitude	Family and patient must see home parenteral nutrition as having a positive influence on the life of the child. Respect for risks and safety issues associated with parenteral nutrition. Ability and willingness to comply with medical plan and techniques.

and the development of other normal milestones such as toileting. Creative strategies to allow toddlers some control and independence in their environment can promote autonomy and lessen the negative impact of hospitalization or home PN on normal development. Providing clothes, toys, and photographs from home, sibling visits, and a high level of parent involvement can help the young child deal with the fear of painful procedures, the strange hospital environment, separation from loved ones, and feelings that the illness is a punishment for being naughty. A backpack that contains solution, pump, and tubing in fastened compartments can allow mobility and prevent toddlers from handling equipment, but it allows parents easy access for managing PN. Nocturnal cyclic PN may reduce interference with developmental needs.

The school-age child who is frequently hospitalized and requires PN needs to maintain involvement in school and with friends, to have some conformity with peers in appearance, and to have as much control over personal issues as possible. In-hospital teachers or private tutors may be needed to maintain educational progress. Choices for the child are offered whenever possible, including selection of the type and placement of the CVC and assisting with dressing changes. An established routine that allows the child to accomplish as many aspects of care as possible is important to avoid feelings of inferiority and prevent excessive dependency. During home PN, children are encouraged to resume as many normal school and play activities as their clinical condition allows.

Although the technical aspects of PN in the adolescent may be easier to manage, other issues may present greater challenges. With greater intellectual and social sophistication, the adolescent may have concerns, fears, and/or anxiety regarding many issues such as loss of control; altered body image or appearance; peer acceptance or isolation; dependence on technology, technical failures, or malfunctions; health and life expectancy; ability to participate in sports and other peer group activities; financial issues; and the effects on other family members. Sleep disturbances may occur due to anxiety or frequent urination that occurs with nocturnal fluid administration. Many of these issues may cause anger or depression and lead to poor compliance with the therapeutic regimen.

Backpacks or vests designed to hold PN solutions and equipment may be used to maximize mobility and minimize changes in physical appearance. Nocturnal cyclic PN circumvents changes in appearance during the day and places less limitation on activities with peers. Other strategies to improve compliance with the PN regimen include:

- Providing information using appropriate terminology for age and educational level
- Encouraging active participation in decision making and management of PN
- Providing psychological counseling when needed

Reimbursement

In response to rapidly escalating healthcare costs starting in the mid-1970s, reimbursement strategies have been changing dramatically. PN is a complex and expensive therapy. Costs include nutrient solutions; technical equipment such as catheters, tubing, and automated pumps; laboratory monitoring; and healthcare providers such as physicians, nurses, dietitians, pharmacists, and developmental therapists. Though PN administered at home may generate fewer costs, it is still expensive.

In efforts to contain healthcare costs, many third-party payers have developed regulations that restrict who can be reimbursed and what is reimbursed, and place a capitation on reimbursement for PN.[220] PN provided in the hospital may be considered part of "room and board," because nutrition/feeding is considered a basic need. Because PN is not a directly reimbursed service, reimbursement often depends on the assigned primary diagnosis or specific diagnosis-related group (DRG) or co-morbid condition (CC). DRGs or CCs that include the presence of malnutrition or nonfunctioning gastrointestinal tract with malabsorption are often required, particularly in the home setting. Medical necessity for PN must be justified by the prescribing physician at the initiation of therapy and periodically throughout the course of therapy. Even then, reimbursement is usually less than 100%, which leaves the family (or supplemental insurance) with the remaining costs.

Healthcare providers who prescribe and/or monitor PN need to keep abreast of changes in regulations governing reimbursement. Documentation is needed regarding effectiveness and outcomes with PN in terms of costs and benefits from length of hospital stay and complication rates to quality of life and functional status. If PN yields no perceived benefit, it is not needed and those who provide it will not be reimbursed. Constant efforts must be employed to control costs through exploring effective but less expensive modalities of care or designing clinical pathways or standardized policies that maximize the effectiveness of PN.

Case Study

Nutrition Assessment

HC, an 8-year, 4-month-old male, is admitted to the hospital with a medical history of blunt abdominal trauma 4 years ago with ruptured duodenum and gastro-jejunostomy with pyloric exclusion. Current radiologic findings indicate possible partial bowel obstruction.

Anthropometric Measurements

- **Weight:** 22.2 kg, 10th percentile, gaining only 0.3 kg over the past year when weight was 21.9 kg, 25th percentile. Normal gain over this time at this age is 2.1–2.4 kg, which would maintain the 25th percentile.
- **Height:** 125 cm, 25th percentile
- **Body mass index:** 14.2 kg/m^2, 7th percentile
- Ideal weight for height and age, given previous growth, is likely 24 kg.

Lab work: All within normal limits for age

Diet order: Clear liquids. Physician has recommended parenteral nutrition and peripheral IV placement. RD consulted for TPN recommendations.

Intake: Oral intake provides less than 200 kcal/day and is not adequate to meet estimated needs at this time. Patient experiences severe abdominal cramps with food and beverage intake at this time. No known food allergies.

Nutrition Diagnosis

Based on the data obtained above, a nutrition diagnosis or problem is made. Inadequate oral intake related to pain associated with eating, as evidenced by low weight gain and intake records.

Nutrition Intervention/Recommendations

Nutritional needs at this time can be met by the following parenteral nutrient delivery:

- Start parenteral nutrition at 55 mL/hour to meet minimum fluid requirements and gradually increase over the next 2–3 days to 92 mL/hour to meet estimated nutritional needs.
- Goal volume: 2208 mL, providing approximately 100 mL/kg/day at a rate of 92 mL/hour.
- Providing 10% dextrose, 1.5% protein with standard amino acids, 2% liposyn at goal volume supplies: 60 kcal/kg/day, 1.5 g protein/kg/day, 2 g fat/kg/day; energy source: 57% cholesterol, 10% protein, 33% fat.
- 30 mEq/L sodium chloride with sodium phosphate provides 3.8 mEq/kg/day sodium (normal level is 1-5).
- 6 mmol/L sodium phosphate provides 0.6 mmol/kg/day phosphorus (normal level is 0.5–1.3).
- 10 mEq/L potassium chloride with sodium chloride provides a total chloride dose of 4 mEq/kg/day (normal level is 2–4).
- 10 mEq/L potassium acetate with potassium chloride provides a total potassium dose of 2 mEq/kg/day (normal level is 2–4).
- 3 mEq/L magnesium sulfate provides 0.3 mEq/kg/day magnesium (normal level is 0.25–0.5).
- 6 mEq/L calcium gluconate provides 0.6 mEq/kg/day calcium (normal level is 0.5–1).

Provide a dose of pediatric multivitamins and 0.2 mL pediatric trace mineral package/kg/day.

This provides 100% of needs peripherally. If oral intake provides a significant amount of nutrients, the rate can be reduced, although a clear liquid diet does not meet many nutritional needs and the patient's weight is lower than expected for growth history and current height.

Monitoring and Evaluation

- Although the patient should not experience refeeding syndrome because he does not appear to be in a malnourished state, standard laboratory assessment for parenteral nutrition will be monitored as well as changes in weight (normal weight gain is 0.24 kg/month).
- Follow up in 3–5 days.

Questions for the Reader

1. Lab work on day 3 includes a serum phosphorus level of 3.4 g/dL (normal level is 3.6–5.6 mg/dL). What is one possible nutrition diagnosis or problem?
2. What changes would you make in this patient's parenteral nutrition prescription to address his current nutrition diagnosis?
3. On day 5, the patient is taken to surgery and laparoscopic surgical findings are significant. A large colon mesenteric rent was found with rotation of cecum through the defect. Rotation was corrected and venous congestion was relieved. Lysis of adhesions and reconstruction of the previous gastrojejunostomy was performed. After surgery, what adjustments might be necessary in this patient's TPN?
4. Lab work on day 7 includes a serum triglyceride level of 250 mg/dL (normal level $<$ 150 mg/dL). What adjustment would you recommend in this patient's parenteral nutrition prescription?

Resources

The Marvin MediSoft TPN 2000 computerized neonatal and pediatric TPN ordering program can be accessed at http://tpn2000.com; email: info@tpn2000.com; or call (877) TPN-EASY.

REFERENCES

1. Steinhorn DM. Nutrition in the PICU: who needs it?! Guidelines for nutritional support of critically ill children. In: Green TP, Zucher AR, eds. *Current Concepts in Pediatric Critical Care*. Chicago: Society of Critical Care Medicine; 1996:77–86.
2. Archer S, Burnett R, Fischer J. Current uses and abuses of total parenteral nutrition. In: *Advances in Surgery*. Chicago: Mosby-Year Book; 1996;29:165–189.
3. Chellis MJ, Sanders SV, Webster H, et al. Early enteral feeding in the pediatric intensive care unit. *J Parenter Enteral Nutr*. 1996;20:71–73.
4. Acra S, Rollins C. Principles and guidelines for parenteral nutrition in children. *Pediatr Ann*. 1999;28:113–120.
5. Koletzko B, Goulet O, Hunt J, Krohn K, Shamir R for the Parenteral Nutrition Guidelines Working Group. Guidelines on paediatric parenteral nutrition of the European Society of Paediatric Gastroenterology, Hepatology and Nutrition (ESPGHAN) and the European Society for Clinical Nutrition and Metabolism (ESPEN), supported by the European Society of Paediatric Research (ESPR). *J Pediatr Gastroenterol Nutr*. 2005;41:S1–S87.
6. Davis A. Pediatrics. In: Matarese LE, Gottschlich MM, eds. *Contemporary Nutrition Support Practice*. Philadelphia: WB Saunders; 1998:349–351.
7. Fisher G, Opper F. An interdisciplinary nutrition support team improves quality of care in a teaching hospital. *J Am Diet Assoc*. 1996;96:176–178.
8. Fisher A, Poole R, Machie R, et al. Clinical pathway for pediatric parenteral nutrition. *Nutr Clin Pract*. 1997;12:76–80.
9. Phillips S. Pediatric parenteral nutrition clinical pathway. *Building Block Life*. Winter 2003:1.
10. Trujillo EB, Young LS. Metabolic and monetary costs of avoidable parenteral nutrition use. *J Parenter Enteral Nutr*. 1999;23:109–113.
11. American Society for Parenteral and Enteral Nutrition. Guidelines for the use of parenteral and enteral nutrition in adult and pediatric patients. *J Parenter Enteral Nutr*. 1993;17(Suppl):27SA–52SA.
12. Okada A. Clinical indications of parenteral and enteral nutrition support in pediatric patients. *Nutrition*. 1988;14:116–118.
13. Sondheimer JM, Cadnapaphornchai M, Sontag M, et al. Predicting the duration of dependence on parenteral nutrition after neonatal intestinal resection. *J Pediatr*. 1998;132:80–84.
14. Vantini I, Benini L, et al. Survival rate and prognostic factors in patients with intestinal failure. *Dig Liver Dis*. 2004;36:46–55.
15. Sitrin MD. Nutrition support in inflammatory bowel disease. *Nutr Clin Pract*. 1992;7:53–60.
16. Polk DB, Hattner JA, Kerner JA Jr. Improved growth and disease activity after intermittent administration of a defined formula diet in children with Crohn's disease. *J Parenter Enteral Nutr*. 1992;16:499–504.
17. Rickard KA, Grosfield JL, Kirksey A, et al. Reversal of protein-energy malnutrition in children during treatment of advanced neoplastic disease. *Ann Surg*. 1979;190:771–781.
18. Filler RM, Dietz W, Suskind RM, et al. Parenteral feeding in management of children with cancer. *Cancer*. 1979;43(Suppl):2117–2120.
19. Copeland EM, MacFadgen BV, Dudrick SJ. Effect of intravenous hyperalimentation on established delayed hypersensitivity in the cancer patient. *Ann Surg*. 1976;184:60–64.
20. Copeland EM, Daly JM, Ota DM, et al. Nutrition, cancer, and intravenous hyperalimentation. *Cancer*. 1979;43:2108–2116.
21. Andrassay RJ, Chwals WJ. Nutritional support of the pediatric oncology patient. *Nutrition*. 1998;14:124–129.
22. Christensen ML, Hancock ML, Gattuso J, et al. Parenteral nutrition associated with increased infection rate in children with cancer. *Cancer*. 1993;72:2732–2738.
23. Copeman MC. Use of total parenteral nutrition in children with cancer: a review and some recommendations. *Pediatr Hematol Oncol*. 1994;11:463–470.
24. Perl M. TPN and the anorexia nervosa patient. *Nutr Supp Serv*. 1981;1:13.
25. Pertschuk MJ, Forster J, Buzby G, et al. The treatment of anorexia nervosa with total parenteral nutrition. *Biol Psychiatr*. 1981;16:539–550.
26. Pereira-da-Silva L, Virella D, Henriques G, et al. A simple equation to estimate the osmolarity of neonatal parenteral nutrition solutions. *J Parenter Enteral Nutr*. 2004;28:34–37.
27. Kanarek KS, Kuznicki MB, Blair RC. Infusion of total parenteral nutrition via the umbilical artery. *J Parenter Enteral Nutr*. 1991;15:71–74.
28. Chathas MK. Percutaneous central venous catheters in neonates. *J Obstet Gynecol Neonatal Nurs*. 1986;15:324–332.
29. Goodwin ML. The Seldinger method of PICC insertion. *J Intraven Nurs*. 1989;12:238–243.
30. Brown JM. Peripherally inserted central catheters: use in home care. *J Intraven Nurs*. 1989;12:144–147.
31. Yeung CY, Lee HC, Huang FY, Wang CS. Sepsis during total parenteral nutrition: exploration of risk factors and determination of the effectiveness of peripherally inserted central venous catheters. *Pediatr Infect Dis J*. 1998;17:135–142.
32. Chathas MK, Paton JB. Sepsis outcomes in infants and children with central venous catheters: percutaneous versus surgical insertion. *J Obstet Gynecol Neonatal Nurs*. 1996;25:500–506.
33. Chung D, Ziegler M. Central venous catheter access. *Nutrition*. 1988;14:119–123.
34. Dubois J, Garel L, Tapiero B, et al. Peripherally inserted central catheters in infants and children. *Radiology*. 1997;204:622–626.
35. Pettit J. Assessment of infants with peripherally inserted central catheters: part 1. Detecting the most frequently occurring complications. *Adv Neonatal Care*. 2002;2:304–315.
36. Liossis G, Bardin C, Papageorgiou A, et al. Comparison of risks from percutaneous central venous catheter and peripheral lines in infants of extremely low birth weight: a cohort controlled study of infants, 1000 g. *J Matern Fetal Neonatal Med*. 2003;13:171–174.
37. Reed T, Phillips S. Management of central venous catheter occlusions and repairs. *J Intraven Nurs*. 1996;19:289–294.
38. Kakzanov V, Monagle P, Chan AKC. Thromboembolism in infants and children with gastrointestinal failure receiving long-term parenteral nutrition. *J Parenter Enteral Nutr*. 2008;32:88–93.

39. Pemberton LB, Lyman B, Lander V, et al. Sepsis from triple versus single lumen catheters during total parenteral nutrition in surgical or chronically ill patients. *Arch Surg.* 1986;121:591.
40. Yeung C, May J, Hughes R. Infection rate for single lumen versus triple lumen subclavian catheters. *Inf Control Hosp Epidemiol.* 1988;9:154.
41. Hughes CB. A totally implantable central venous system for chemotherapy administration. *NITA.* 1985;8:523–527.
42. Valentine CJ, Puthoff TD. Enhancing parenteral nutrition therapy for the neonate. *Nutr Clin Pract.* 2007;22:183–193.
43. Storm HM, Young SL, Sandler RH. Development of pediatric and neonatal parenteral nutrition order forms. *Nutr Clin Pract.* 1995;10:54–59.
44. Mirtallo J, Canada T, Johnson D, et al., Task Force for the Revision of Safe Practices for Parenteral Nutrition. Safe practices for parenteral nutrition formulations. *J Parenter Enteral Nutr.* 2004;28:S39–S70.
45. Puangco M, Nguyen H, Sheridan M. Computerized PN ordering optimizes timely nutrition therapy in a neonatal intensive care unit. *J Am Diet Assoc.* 1997;97:258–261.
46. Schloerb PR. Electronic parenteral and enteral nutrition. *J Parenter Enteral Nutr.* 2000;24:23–29.
47. Lehmann CU, Conner KG. Preventing provider errors: online total parenteral nutrition calculator. *Pediatrics.* 2004;113:748–753.
48. Hardy G, Puzovic M. Formulation, stability, and administration of parenteral nutrition with new lipid emulsions. *Nutr Clin Pract.* 2009;24:616–625.
49. Mirtallo J. Should the use of total nutrient admixtures be limited? *Am J Hosp Pharm.* 1994;51:2831–2836.
50. Lee MD, Yoon JE, Kim, SI, et al. Stability of total nutrient admixtures in reference to ambient temperatures. *Nutrition.* 2003;19:886–890.
51. Neuzil J, Darlow BA, Inder TE, et al. Oxidation of parenteral lipid emulsion by ambient and phototherapy lights: potential toxicity of routine parenteral feeding. *J Pediatr.* 1995;126:785–790.
52. Laborie S, Lavoie JC. Protecting solutions of parenteral nutrition from peroxidation. *J Parenter Enteral Nutr.* 1999;23:104–108.
53. Silvers KM, Sluis KB. Limiting light-induced lipid peroxidation and vitamin loss in infant parenteral nutrition by adding multivitamin preparations to Intralipid. *Acta Paediatr.* 2001;90:242–249.
54. Alwood M, Driscoll D, Sizer T, Ball P. Physicochemical assessment of total nutrient admixture stability and safety: quantifying the risk. *Nutrition.* 1998;14:166–167.
55. Skouroliakou M, Matthaiou C, Chiou A, et al. Physicochemical stability of parenteral nutrition supplied as all-in-one for neonates. *J Parenter Enteral Nutr.* 2008;32:201–209.
56. Trissel LA, Gilbert DL. Compatibility of medications with 3-in-1 parenteral nutrition admixtures. *J Parenter Enteral Nutr.* 1999; 23:67–74.
57. Pharmaceutical compounding—sterile preparations. In: *Revision Bulletin, The United States Pharmacopeia.* Rockville, MD: United States Pharmacopeial Convention; 2008:1–61.
58. Curtis C, Sacks GS. Compounding parenteral nutrition: reducing the risks. *Nutr Clin Pract.* 2009;24:441–446.
59. Steger PJ, Muhlebach SF. Lipid peroxidation of intravenous lipid emulsions and all-in-one admixtures in total parenteral nutrition bags: the influence of trace elements. *J Parenter Enteral Nutr.* 2000;24:37–41.
60. Driscoll DF, Bacon MN. Physicochemical stability of two types of intravenous lipid emulsion as total nutrient admixtures. *J Parenter Enteral Nutr.* 2000;24:15–22.
61. Driscoll DF, Nehne J, Peterss H, et al. Physicochemical stability of intravenous lipid emulsions as all-in-one admixtures intended for the very young. *Clin Nutr.* 2003;22:489–495.
62. Driscoll D, Bacon M, Bistrian B. Effects of in-line filtration on lipid particle size distribution in total nutrient admixtures. *J Parenter Enteral Nutr.* 1996;20:296–301.
63. Muller MJ. Hepatic complications in parenteral nutrition. *Z Gastroenterol.* 1996;34:36–40.
64. Slicker J, Vermilyea S. Pediatric parenteral nutrition: putting the microscope on macronutrients and micronutrients. *Nutr Clin Pract.* 2009;24:481–486.
65. Kerner JA Jr, ed. *Manual of Pediatric Parenteral Nutrition.* New York: John Wiley and Sons; 1983.
66. Nelson WE, Behrman RE, Vaughan VC, eds. *Nelson's Textbook of Pediatrics*, 12th ed. Philadelphia: WB Saunders; 1983:231.
67. Baumgart S, Costarino AT. Water and electrolyte metabolism of the micropremie. *Clin Perinatol.* 2000;27:131–146.
68. Lorenz JM, Kleinman LI, Ahmed G, et al. Phases of fluid and electrolyte homeostasis in the extremely low birth weight infant. *Pediatrics.* 1995;96:484–489.
69. Heimler R, Doumas BT, Jendrzejcak BM, et al. Relationship between nutrition, weight change, and fluid compartments in preterm infants during the first week of life. *J Pediatr.* 1993;122:110–114.
70. Oh W, Karechi H. Phototherapy and insensible water loss in the newborn infant. *Am J Dis Child.* 1972;124:230–232.
71. Yeh TF, Voora S, Lillien J. Oxygen consumption and insensible water loss in premature infants in single versus double walled incubators. *J Pediatr.* 1980;97:967–971.
72. Gruskin AB. Fluid therapy in children. *Urol Clin North Am.* 1976;3:277–291.
73. Stevenson JG. Fluid administration in the association of patent ductus arteriosus complicating respiratory distress syndrome. *J Pediatr.* 1977;90:257–261.
74. Bell EF, Acarregui MJ. Restricted versus liberal water intake for preventing morbidity and mortality in preterm infants. *Cochrane Database Syst Rev.* 2001;3:CD000503.
75. Goldman HI. Feeding and necrotizing enterocolitis. *Am J Dis Child.* 1980;134:553.
76. Goldberg RN, Chung D, Goldman SL, et al. The association of rapid volume expansion and intraventricular hemorrhage in the preterm infant. *J Pediatr.* 1980;96:1060–1063.
77. Rao M, Koenig E, Li S, et al. Estimation of insensible water loss in low birth weight infants by direct calorimetric measurement of metabolic heat release. *Pediatr Res.* 1989;25:295A.
78. Ford EG. Nutrition support of pediatric patients. *Nutr Clin Pract.* 1996;11:183–191.
79. Carlson S. Acid/base balance in special care nurseries. *Support Line.* 2002;24:17.
80. Aperia A, Broberger O, Elinder G, Herin P, Zetterstrom R. Postnatal development of renal function in pre-term and full-term infants. *Acta Paediatr Scand.* 1981;70:183–187.
81. Peters O, Ryan S, Matthew L, et al. Randomised controlled trial of acetate in preterm neonates receiving parenteral nutrition. *Arch Dis Child.* 1997;77:F12–F15.

82. John E, Klavdianou M, Vidyasagar D. Electrolyte problems in neonatal surgical patients. *Clin Perinatol.* 1989;16:219–232.
83. Groh-Wargo S, Ciaccia A, Moore J. Neonatal metabolic acidosis: effect of chloride from normal saline flushes. *J Parenter Enteral Nutr.* 1988;12:159–161.
84. Tilden SJ, Watkins S, Tong TK, Jeevanandam M. Measured energy expenditure in pediatric intensive care patients. *Am J Dis Child.* 1989;143:490–492.
85. Lowery GH. *Growth and Development of Children*, 6th ed. Chicago: Year Book Medical Publishers; 1973:331–332.
86. Heird WC, Kashyap S, Gomez MR. Parenteral alimentation of the neonate. *Semin Perinatol.* 1991;15:493–502.
87. Greene HL, Hambidge KM, Schanler R, et al. Guidelines for the use of vitamins, trace elements, calcium, magnesium, and phosphorus in infants and children receiving total parenteral nutrition: report of the Subcommittee on Pediatric Parenteral Nutrient Requirements from the Committee on Clinical Practice Issues of the American Society for Clinical Nutrition. *Am J Clin Nutr.* 1988;48:1324. (Revised in 1990.)
88. Kleinman RE, ed. *Pediatric Nutrition Handbook*. Elk Grove Village, IL: American Academy of Pediatrics, Committee on Nutrition; 1998:285–305.
89. Khaldi N, Coran AG, Wesley JR. Guidelines for parenteral nutrition in children. *Nutr Supp Serv.* 1984;4:27.
90. Sunehag AL, Haymond MW. Glucose extremes in newborn infants. *Clin Perinatol.* 2002;29:245–260.
91. Prelack K, Sheridan RL. Micronutrient supplementation in the critically ill patient: strategies for clinical practice. *J Trauma.* 2001;51:601–620.
92. Adamkin DH. Total parenteral nutrition. *Neonatal Intensive Care.* Sept/Oct 1997:24.
93. Pierro A, Eaton S. Metabolism and nutrition in the surgical neonate. *Semin Pediatr Surg.* 2008;17:276–284.
94. Mehta NM, Compher C. A.S.P.E.N. clinical guidelines support of the critically ill child. *J Parenter Enteral Nutr.* 2009;33:260–276.
95. Coss-Bu JA, Klish WJ, Walding D, et al. Energy metabolism, nitrogen balance, and substrate utilization in critically ill children. *Am J Clin Nutr.* 2001;74:664–669.
96. Mehta NM, Bechard LJ, Leavitt K, et al. Cumulative energy imbalance in the pediatric intensive care unit: role of targeted indirect calorimetry. *J Parenter Enteral Nutr.* 2009;33:336–344.
97. Mellecker RR, McManus AM. Measurement of resting energy expenditure in healthy children. *J Parenter Enteral Nutr.* 2009;33:640–645.
98. Soares FVM, Moreira MEL, Abranches AD, et al. Indirect calorimetry: a tool to adjust energy expenditure in very low birth weight infants. *J Pediatr (Rio J).* 2007;83:567–570.
99. Sy J, Gourishankar A, Gordon WE, et al. Bicarbonate kinetics and predicted energy expenditure in critically ill children. *Am J Clin Nutr.* 2008;88:340–347.
100. Zlotkin SH, Bryan MH, Anderson GH. Intravenous nitrogen and energy intakes required to duplicate in utero nitrogen accretion in prematurely born human infants. *J Pediatr.* 1981;99:115–120.
101. Kalhan SC, Kilic I. Carbohydrate as nutrient in the infant and child: range of acceptable intake. *Eur J Clin Nutr.* 1999;53:S94–S100.
102. Cochran EB, Phelps SJ, Helms RA. Parenteral nutrition in pediatric patients. *Clin Pharm.* 1988;7:351–366.
103. Sajbel TA, Dutro MP, Radway PR. Use of separate insulin infusions with total parenteral nutrition. *J Parenter Enteral Nutr.* 1987;11:97–99.
104. Groh-Wargo S. Prematurity/low birth weight. In: Lang C, ed. *Nutritional Support in Critical Care*. Gaithersburg, MD: Aspen Publishers; 1987:287.
105. Rubecz I, Mestyan J, Varga P, Klujber L. Energy metabolism, substrate utilization, and nitrogen balance in parenterally fed postoperative neonates and infants. *J Pediatr.* 1981;98:42–46.
106. Thureen PJ, Anderson AH, Baron KA, et al. Protein balance in the first week of life in ventilated neonates receiving parenteral nutrition. *Am J Clin Nutr.* 1998;68:1128–1135.
107. Poindexter BB, Denne SC. Protein needs of the preterm infant. *NeoReviews.* 2003;4:E52.
108. Thureen PJ, Hay WW Jr. Intravenous nutrition and postnatal growth of the micropremie. *Clin Perinatol.* 2000;27:197–219.
109. Kalhan SC, Iben S. Protein metabolism in the extremely low-birth-weight infant. *Clin Perinatol.* 2000;27:23–56.
110. Micheli J-L, Schultz Y, Junod S, et al. Early postnatal intravenous amino acid administration to extremely-low-birth-weight infants. In: Hay WW Jr, ed. *Seminars in Neonatal Nutrition and Metabolism*, vol 2. Columbus, OH: Ross Products Division; 1994:1–3.
111. Zlotkin SH, Stallings VA, Pencharz PB. Total parenteral nutrition in children. *Pediatr Clin North Am.* 1985;32:381–400.
112. Hellstrom A, Engstrom E, Hard A-L, et al. Postnatal serum insulin-like growth factor I deficiency is associated with retinopathy of prematurity and other complications of premature birth. *Pediatr.* 2003;112:1016–1020.
113. Adan D, LaGamma EF, Browne LE. Nutritional management and the multisystem organ failure/systemic inflammatory response syndrome in critically ill preterm neonates. *Crit Care Clin.* 1995;11:751–784.
114. Coran AG, Drongowski RA. Studies on the toxicity and efficacy of new amino acid solution in pediatric parenteral nutrition. *J Parenter Enteral Nutr.* 1987;11:368–377.
115. Helms RA, Christensen ML, Mauer EC, Storm MC. Comparison of a pediatric versus standard amino acid formulation in preterm neonates requiring parenteral nutrition. *J Pediatr.* 1987;110:466–470.
116. Chessex P, Zebiche H, Pineault M, Lepage D, Dallaire L. Effect of amino acid composition of parenteral solutions on nitrogen retention and metabolic response in very-low-birth weight infants. *J Pediatr.* 1985;106:111–117.
117. Heird WC, Dell RB, Helms RA, et al. Amino acid mixture designed to maintain normal plasma amino acid patterns in infants and children requiring parenteral nutrition. *Pediatrics.* 1987;80:401–408.
118. Intravenous nutritional therapy. Crystalline amino acid infusions. *Drug Facts and Comparisons*. St. Louis, MO: Drug Facts & Comparisons; 2010;96–97.
119. Heird WC. Essentiality of cyst(e)ine for neonates. Clinical and biochemical effects of parenteral cysteine supplementation. In: Kinney JM, Borum PR, eds. *Perspectives in Clinical Nutrition*. Munich, Germany: Urban Schwarzenberg; 1989:275–282.
120. Gaull GE, Sturman JA, Raiha NCR, Sturman JA. Development of mammalian sulfur metabolism. Absence of cystathionase in human fetal tissues. *Pediatr Res.* 1972;6:538–547.

121. Zlotkin SH, Bryan H, Anderson H. Cysteine supplementation to cysteine-free intravenous feeding regimens in newborn infants. *Am J Clin Nutr.* 1981;34:914–923.
122. Helms RA, Storm MC, Christensen ML, et al. Cysteine supplementation results in normalization of plasma taurine concentrations in children receiving home parenteral nutrition. *J Pediatr.* 1999;134:358–361.
123. Heird WC, Hay W, Helms RA, Storm MC, Kashyap S, Dell RB. Pediatric parenteral amino acid mixture in low birth weight infants. *Pediatrics.* 1988;81:41–50.
124. Heird WC, Dell RB, Helms RA, et al. Amino acid mixture designed to maintain normal plasma amino acid patterns in infants and children requiring parenteral nutrition. *Pediatrics.* 1987;80:401–408.
125. Eggert LD, Rusho WJ, MacKay MW, Chan GM. Calcium and phosphorus compatibility in parenteral nutrition solutions for neonates. *Am J Hosp Pharm.* 1982;39:49.
126. Battista MA, Price PT, Kalhan SC. Effect of parenteral amino acids on leucine and urea kinetics in preterm infants. *J Pediatr.* 1996;128:130–134.
127. Lowe DK, Benfell K, Smith RJ, et al. Safety of glutamine-enriched parenteral nutrient solutions in humans. *Am J Clin Nutr.* 1990; 52:1101–1106.
128. Wischmeyer PE. Clinical applications of L-glutamine: past, present, and future. *Nutr Clin Pract.* 2003;18:377.
129. Lacey JM, Crouch JB, Benfell K, et al. The effects of glutamine-supplemented nutrition in premature infants. *J Parenter Enteral Nutr.* 1996;20:74–80.
130. Vaughn P, Thomas P, Clark R, et al. Enteral glutamine supplementation and morbidity in low birth weight infants. *J Pediatr.* 2003;142:662–668.
131. Adamkin DH, McClead RE, Desai NS, et al. Comparison of two neonatal amino acid formulations in preterm infants in a multicenter study. *J Perinatol.* 1991;11:375–382.
132. Forchielli ML, Gura KM, Sandler R, et al. Aminosyn PF or Trophamine: which provides more protection from cholestasis associated with total parenteral nutrition? *J Pediatr Gastroenterol Nutr.* 1995;21:374–382.
133. Wright K, Ernst KD, Gaylord MS, et al. Increased incidence of parenteral nutrition-associated cholestasis with Aminosyn PF compared to Trophamine. *J Perinatol.* 2003;23:444–450.
134. Adamkin DH. Total parenteral nutrition-associated cholestasis: prematurity or amino acids? *J Perinatol.* 2003;23:437–438.
135. Abitbol CL, Holliday MA. Total parenteral nutrition in anuric children. *Clin Nephrol.* 1976;5:153–158.
136. Holliday MA, Wassner S, Ramirez J. Intravenous nutrition in uremic children with protein-energy malnutrition. *Am J Clin Nutr.* 1978;31:1854–1860.
137. Motil KJ, Harmon WE, Grupe WE. Complications of essential amino acid hyperalimentation in children with acute renal failure. *J Parenter Enteral Nutr.* 1980;4:32–35.
138. Takala J. Total parenteral nutrition in experimental uremia: studies of acute and chronic renal failure in the growing rat. *J Parenter Enteral Nutr.* 1984;8:427–432.
139. Helms RA, Phelps SJ, Mauer EC, Christensen ML, Storm MC. Parenteral protein use in liver disease. *Pediatr Res.* 1989;25:115A.
140. Maldonato J, Gil A, Faus MJ, Periago JL, Loscertales M, Molina JA. Differences in the serum amino acid pattern of injured and infected children promoted by two parenteral nutrition solutions. *J Parenter Enteral Nutr.* 1989;13:41–46.
141. Holman RT, Johnson SB, Hatch TF. A case of human linolenic acid deficiency involving neurologic abnormalities. *Am J Clin Nutr.* 1982;35:617–623.
142. Uauy R, Mena P, Rojas C. Essential fatty acid metabolism in the micropremie. *Clin Perinatol.* 2000;27:71–93.
143. Jensen CL, Heird WC. Lipids with an emphasis on long-chain polyunsaturated fatty acids. *Clin Perinatol.* 2002;29:261–281.
144. Friedman Z, Danon A, Stahlman MT, et al. Rapid onset of essential fatty acid deficiency in the newborn. *Pediatrics.* 1976;58: 640–649.
145. Baugh N, Recupero MA, Kerner JA Jr. Nutritional requirements for pediatric patients. In: Merritt RJ, ed. *The ASPEN Nutrition Support Practice Manual.* Silver Spring, MD: American Society for Parenteral and Enteral Nutrition; 1998:1–13.
146. Waitzberg DL, Torrinhas RS, Jacintho TM. New parenteral lipid emulsions for clinical use. *J Parenter Enteral Nutr.* 2006;30:351–367.
147. Putet G. Lipid metabolism of the micropremie. *Clin Perinatol.* 2000;27:57–69.
148. Driscoll DF, Nehne J, Peterss H, et al. Physicochemical stability of intravenous lipid emulsions as all-in-one admixtures intended for the very young. *Clin Nutr.* 2003;22:489–495.
149. deMeijer VE, Gura KM, Le HD, et al. Fish oil–based lipid emulsions prevent and reverse parenteral nutrition-associated liver disease: the Boston experience. *J Parenter Enteral Nutr.* 2009;33:541–547.
150. Gura KM, Lee S, Valim C, et al. Safety and efficacy of a fish-oil-based fat emulsion in the treatment of parenteral nutrition-associated liver disease. *Pediatrics.* 2008;121:e678–e686.
151. Diamond IR, Pencharz PB, Wales PW. Omega-3 lipids for intestinal failure associated liver disease. *Semin Pediatr Surg.* 2009;18:239–245.
152. American Academy of Pediatrics, Committee on Nutrition. Commentary on parenteral nutrition. *Pediatrics.* 1983;71:547–552.
153. Levy JS, Winters RW, Heird WC. Total parenteral nutrition in pediatric patients. *Pediatr Rev.* 1980;2:99.
154. American Academy of Pediatrics, Committee on Nutrition. Prudent life-style for children: dietary fat and cholesterol. *Pediatrics.* 1986;78:521–525.
155. Sapsford A. Energy, carbohydrate, protein, and fat. In: Groh-Wargo S, Thompson M, Cox JH, eds. *Nutritional Care for High-Risk Newborns.* Chicago: Precept Press; 1994:83.
156. Mitton SG. Amino acids and lipid in the total parenteral nutrition for the newborn. *J Pediatr Gastroenterol Nutr.* 1994;18:25–31.
157. Pereira GR. Nutritional care of the extremely premature infant. *Clin Perinatol.* 1995;22:61–75.
158. American Academy of Pediatrics, Committee on Nutrition. Use of intravenous fat emulsions in pediatric patients. *Pediatrics.* 1981;68:738–743.
159. Driscoll DF, Bacon MN, Bistrian BR. Effects of in-line filtration on lipid particle size distribution in total nutrient admixtures. *J Parenter Enteral Nutr.* 1996;20:296–301.
160. Sacks GS, Driscoll DF. Does lipid hang time make a difference? Time is of the essence. *Nutr Clin Prac.* 2002;17:284–290.

161. Pearson ML, Hospital Infection Control Practices Advisory Committee. Guideline for prevention of intravascular-device-related infections. *Infect Control Hosp Epidemiol.* 1996;17:438–479.
162. Magnusson G, Boberg M, Cederblad G, et al. Plasma and tissue levels of lipids, fatty acids, and plasma carnitine in neonates receiving a new fat emulsion. *Acta Paediatr.* 1997;86:638–644.
163. McDonald CM, MacKay MW, Curtis J, et al. Carnitine and cholestasis: nutritional dilemmas for the parenterally nourished newborn. *Support Line.* 2003;25:10.
164. Helms RA, Mauer EC, Hay WW Jr, et al. Effect of intravenous L-carnitine on growth parameters and fat metabolism during parenteral nutrition in neonates. *J Parenter Enteral Nutr.* 1990;14:448–453.
165. Borum P. Carnitine in neonatal nutrition. *J Child Neurol.* 1995;10(Suppl 2):S25–S31.
166. Winter SC, Szabo-Aczel S, Curry CJR, et al. Plasma carnitine deficiency: clinical observations in 51 pediatric patients. *Am J Dis Child.* 1987;141:660–665.
167. Coran AG, Drongowshi RA, Baker PJ. The metabolic effects of oral L-carnitine administration in infants receiving total parenteral nutrition with fat. *J Pediatr Surg.* 1985;20:758–764.
168. Crill CM, Wang B, Storm MC, et al. Carnitine: a conditionally essential nutrient in the neonatal population? *J Pediatr Pharmacol Ther.* 2001;6:225.
169. Cairns PA, Stalker DJ. Carnitine supplementation of parenterally fed neonates. *Cochrane Database Syst Rev.* 2000;4:CD000950.
170. American Medical Association, Nutrition Advisory Group. Multivitamin preparations for parenteral use. *J Parenter Enteral Nutr.* 1979;3:258–262.
171. Greer FR. Vitamin metabolism and requirements in the micropremie. *Clin Perinatol.* 2000;27:95–118.
172. Kumar D, Greer FR, Super DM, et al. Vitamin K status of premature infants: implications for current recommendations. *Pediatrics.* 2001;108:1117–1122.
173. Brion LP, Bell EF, Raghuveer TS, et al. What is the appropriate intravenous dose of vitamin E for very-low-birth-weight infants? *J Perinatol.* 2004;24:205–207.
174. Darlow BA, Graham PJ. Vitamin A supplementation for preventing morbidity and mortality in very low birthweight infants. *Cochrane Database Syst Rev.* 2002;4:CD000501.
175. Moore MC, Greene HL, Phillips B, et al. Evaluation of a pediatric multiple vitamin preparation for total parenteral nutrition in infants and children. I. Blood levels of water-soluble vitamins. *Pediatrics.* 1986;77:530–538.
176. Greene HL, Moore MC, Phillips B, et al. Evaluation of a pediatric multivitamin preparation for total parenteral nutrition. II. Blood levels of vitamins A, D, and E. *Pediatrics.* 1986;77:539.
177. Hahn JS, Berquist W, Alcorn DM, et al. Wernicke encephalopathy and beriberi during total parenteral nutrition attributable to multivitamin infusion shortage. *Pediatrics.* 1998;101:E10.
178. Greer FR, Tsang RC. Calcium and vitamin D metabolism in term and low-birth-weight infants. *Perinatol Neonatol.* 1986:14.
179. Koo WWK, Tsang RC. Mineral requirements for low-birth-weight infants. *J Amer Coll Nutr.* 1991;10:474–486.
180. Changaris DG, Purohit DM, Balentine JD, et al. Brain calcification in severely stressed neonates receiving parenteral calcium. *J Pediatr.* 1984;104:941–946.
181. Goldsmith MA, Bhatia SS, Kanto AP, et al. Gluconate calcium therapy and neonatal hypercalciuria. *Am J Dis Child.* 1981;135:538–543.
182. Hufnagle KF, Khan SN, Penn D, et al. Renal calcifications: a complication of long-term furosemide therapy in preterm infants. *Pediatrics.* 1982;70:360–363.
183. Wood RJ, Bengoa JM, Sitrin MD, Rosenberg IH. Calciuretic effect of cyclic versus continuous total parenteral nutrition. *Am J Clin Nutr.* 1985;41:614–619.
184. Koo WWK, Kaplan LA, Horn J, Tsang RC, Steichen JJ. Aluminum in parenteral nutrition solution—sources and possible alternatives. *J Parenter Enteral Nutr.* 1986;10:591–595.
185. Moreno A, Dominguez C, Ballabriga A. Aluminum in the neonate related to parenteral nutrition. *Acta Paediatr.* 1994;83:25–29.
186. Giapros VI, Papdimitriou FK, Andronikou SK. Tubular disorders in low birth weight neonates after prolonged antibiotic treatment. *Neonatology.* 2007;91:140–144.
187. Vileisis RA. Effect of phosphorus intake in total parenteral nutrition infusates in premature neonates. *J Pediatr.* 1987;110:586–590.
188. Aladjem M, Lotan D, Biochis H, et al. Changes in the electrolyte content of serum and urine during total parenteral nutrition. *J Pediatr.* 1980;97:437–439.
189. Kimura S, Nose O, Seino Y, et al. Effects of alternate and simultaneous administrations of calcium and phosphorus on calcium metabolism in children receiving total parenteral nutrition. *J Parenter Enteral Nutr.* 1986;10:513–516.
190. Pelegano JF, Rowe JC, Carey DE, et al. Effect of calcium/phosphorus ratio on mineral retention in parenterally fed premature infants. *J Pediatr Gastroenterol Nutr.* 1991;12:351–355.
191. Hoehn GJ, Carey DE, Rowe JC, et al. Alternate day infusion of calcium and phosphate in very low birth weight infants: wasting of the infused mineral. *J Pediatr Gastroenterol Nutr.* 1987;5:752–757
192. U.S. Department of Health and Human Services. *FDA Safety Alert: Hazards of Precipitation Associated with Parenteral Nutrition.* Rockville, MD: Food and Drug Administration; 1994.
193. Fitzgerald KA, MacKay MW. Calcium and phosphate solubility in neonatal parenteral nutrient solutions containing Trophamine. *Am J Hosp Pharm.* 1986;43:88.
194. Fitzgerald KA, MacKay MW. Calcium and phosphate solubility in neonatal parenteral nutrient solutions containing Aminosyn PF. *Am J Hosp Pharm.* 1987;44:1396.
195. Shils ME, Burke AW, Greene HL, et al. Guidelines for essential trace element preparations for parenteral use: a statement by an expert panel. *JAMA.* 1979;241:2051–2054.
196. Pyati SP, Ramamurthy RS, Krauss MT, Pildes RS. Absorption of iodine in the neonate following topical use of povidone iodine. *J Pediatr.* 1977;91:825–828.
197. Shaw JC. Trace elements in the fetus and young infant II. Copper, manganese, selenium and chromium. *Am J Dis Child.* 1980;134:74–81.
198. Triplett WC. Clinical aspects of zinc, copper, manganese, chromium and selenium metabolism. *Nutr Int.* 1985;1:60.
199. American Academy of Pediatrics, Committee on Nutrition. Zinc. *Pediatrics.* 1978;62:408–412.
200. Reynolds AP, Keily E, Meadows N. Manganese in long term paediatric parenteral nutrition. *Arch Dis Child.* 1994;71:527–528.

201. Hardy G. Manganese in parenteral nutrition: who, when and why should we supplement? *Gastroenterology.* 2009;137:S29–S35.
202. McMillan NB, Mulroy C, MacKay MW, et al. Correlation of cholestasis with serum copper and whole-blood manganese levels in pediatric patients. *Nutr Clin Pract.* 2008;23:161–165.
203. Hurwitz M, Garcia MG, Poole RL et al. Copper deficiency during parenteral nutrition: a report of four pediatric cases. *Nutr Clin Pract.* 2004;19:305–308.
204. Fuhrman MP, Herrmann V, Masidonski P, et al. Pancytopoenia after removal of copper from total parenteral nutrition. *J Parenter Enteral Nutr.* 2000;24:361–366.
205. Zambrano E, El-Hennawy M, Ehrenkranz RA, Zelterman D, Reyes-Mugica M. Total parenteral nutrition induced liver pathology: an autopsy series of 24 newborn cases. *Pediatr Dev Pathol.* 2004;7:425–432.
206. Fok TF, Chui KK, Cheung R, et al. Manganese intake and cholestatic jaundice in neonates receiving parenteral nutrition: a randomized controlled study. *Acta Paediatr.* 2001;90:1009–1115.
207. Reed MD, Bertino JS, Halpin TC. Use of intravenous iron dextran injection in children receiving total parenteral nutrition. *Am J Dis Child.* 1981;135:829–831.
208. Seashore JH. Metabolic complications of parenteral nutrition in infants and children. *Surg Clin North Am.* 1980;60:1239.
209. Wan KK, Tsallas G. Dilute iron dextran formulation for addition to parenteral nutrient solutions. *Am J Hosp Pharm.* 1980;37:206.
210. Halpin T, Reed M, Bertino J. Use of intravenous iron dextran in children receiving TPN for nutritional support of inflammatory bowel disease. *J Parenter Enteral Nutr.* 1980;4:600.
211. Ehrenkranz RA. Iron requirements of preterm infants. *Nutrition.* 1994;10:77.
212. Ohls RK, Harcum J, Schibler KR, et al. The effect of erythropoietin on the transfusion requirements of preterm infants weighing 750 grams or less: a randomized, double-blind, placebo-controlled study. *J Pediatr.* 1995;126:421–426.
213. Meyer MP, Haworth C, Meyer JH, et al. A comparison of oral and intravenous iron supplementation in preterm infants receiving recombinant erythropoietin. *J Pediatr.* 1996;129:258–263.
214. Ng PC, Lam CWK, Lee CH, et al. Hepatic iron storage in very low birthweight infants after multiple blood transfusions. *Arch Dis Child Fetal Neonatal Ed.* 2001;84:F101–F105.
215. Bastian C, Driscoll R. Enteral tube feeding at home. In: Rombeau JL, Caldwell MD, eds. *Enteral and Tube Feeding.* Philadelphia: WB Saunders; 1984:494–512.
216. Beghin L, Michaud L. Total energy expenditure and physical activity in children treated with home parenteral nutrition. *Pediatr Res.* 2003;53:684–690.
217. Johnson T, Sexton E. Managing children and adolescents on parenteral nutrition: challenges for the nutritional support team. *Proc Nutr Soc.* 2006;65:217–221.
218. Puntis JW. Nutritional support at home and in the community. *Arch Dis Child.* 2001;84:295–298.
219. Illingworth RS, Lister J. The critical or sensitive period, with special reference to certain feeding problems in infants and children. *J Pediatr.* 1964;65:839–848.
220. Nelson JK. Economics of nutrition support. In: Matarese LE, Gottschlich MM, eds. *Contemporary Nutrition Support Practice.* Philadelphia: WB Saunders; 1998:643.

Botanicals in Pediatrics

John Westerdahl

Introduction

Since the beginning of time, botanicals have played an important part in the diet and well-being of every major culture. The people of the ancient world relied heavily on various herbs for their medicines. Used by both adults and children, many of these plants were their chief therapy, offering comfort and healing during illness and disease. Botanicals were once the conventional medicines used in treating common health problems such as colds, flu, nausea, heart disease, depression, and most other conditions, including childhood illnesses. Many medicinal plants are listed in early *materia medica* from ancient China, Babylon, Egypt, India, Greece, and other parts of the world. The ancient Egyptian medical text *Papyrus Ebers*, written in 1550 BC, lists over 800 medicinal formulas using herbs. The Greek physician Hippocrates (ca. 468–ca. 377 BC), known as the father of medicine, used herbs extensively with his patients and wrote about their healing benefits. In the first century, another Greek physician, Dioscorides, listed 500 plant medicines in his classic herbal guide, *De Materia Medica*. Many of the currently popular medicinal herbs were once listed in official monographs in the United States Pharmacopoeia (USP) and the National Formulary (NF) and were used extensively by physicians. Today, some 25% of prescription drugs marketed in the United States are derived from plants.[1,2] From a global perspective, the World Health Organization (WHO) estimates that 80% of the world's population currently relies mainly on traditional medicines, most of which utilize medicinal plants.[3]

Table 21-1 lists the botanicals that are currently approved by the U.S. Food and Drug Administration (FDA) as effective over-the-counter (OTC) drug ingredients. However, the FDA does not regulate herbal supplements.

During the past three decades, the use of herbs and phytomedicines has increased as consumers have become more aware of their uses. This can be attributed both to increased published scientific research documenting the therapeutic efficacy of many medicinal herbs and to the passing of the Dietary Supplement Health and Education Act of 1994 (DSHEA), which created a regulatory framework for dietary supplement products. It allows herbal manufacturers to make truthful, nonmisleading claims about the herb's effect on the structure and function of the body. These claims are required to be accompanied by a disclaimer that states, "This statement has not been evaluated by the Food and Drug Administration. This product is not intended to diagnose, treat, cure, or prevent any disease."[4]

When using commercial herbal products, it is wise to look for standardized versions with measured amounts of active ingredients as much as possible. Consumers interested in using herbs should seek reputable manufacturers' products and call companies to ascertain the source of their herbs and manufacturing procedures. Pregnant or nursing women should not use herbal supplements without first consulting a knowledgeable physician.

Growth of the Herbal Market

Consumers have shown a growing interest in trying natural alternatives to synthetic drugs that address their health concerns.[5] As a result, the herbal market has experienced steady growth. In 2008, the botanical medicine market had grown to an estimated annual retail sales figure of $4.8 billion. **Table 21-2** identifies the best-selling herbal products sold in the United States in 2008.[6] This marketing information is helpful to the health professional to identify the types of herbs that many patients are using today.

With the growing interest in herbs, an increasing number of parents use botanical medicines with their children. Several herbal product companies now market phytomedicines especially formulated for children. More and more parents perceive herbal remedies as effective and having actions that are "gentler," with fewer side effects than those of most conventional drugs. In the United States, the majority of doctors and pharmacists recognize that there is a

TABLE 21-1 Botanicals Approved as OTC Drug Ingredients

Herb	Approved Use
Capsicum (*Capsicum* spp.)	Counterirritant
Ipecac root (*Cephaelis ipecacuanha*)	Emetic
Peppermint oil (*Mentha piperita*)	Antitussive
Psyllium (*Plantago psyllium*)	Bulk laxative
Senna (*Senna alexandrina; Cassia senna*)	Stimulant laxative
Slippery elm (*Ulmus fulva*)	Demulcent
Witch hazel (*Hamamelis virginiana*)	Astringent

Source: Food and Drug Administration. *OTC Drug Review Ingredient Status Report.* Rockville, MD: Food and Drug Administration; July 2003.

TABLE 21-2 20 Top-Selling Herbal Dietary Supplements in the Food, Drug, and Mass Market Channel in the United States, 2008

Rank	Herb	Rank	Herb
1.	Cranberry	11.	Green tea
2.	Soy	12.	Evening primrose
3.	Garlic	13.	Valerian
4.	Saw palmetto	14.	Horny goat weed
5.	Ginkgo	15.	Grape seed
6.	Echinacea	16.	Elderberry
7.	Milk thistle	17.	Bilberry
8.	St. John's wort	18.	Ginger
9.	Ginseng	19.	Horse chestnut seed
10.	Black cohosh	20.	Yohimbe

Source: Information Resources, Inc. Available at: http://www.us.infores.com. Accessed August 23, 2010.

growing consumer interest in herbal medicine, but most of them have little or no knowledge and absolutely no training in this area. Doctors, pharmacists, registered dietitians, and other healthcare practitioners need to increase their knowledge about herbal products to better assist their patients who use them.

Definitions

In the world of herbs and phytomedicines, the health professional should be familiar with some basic nomenclature when working with patients who use these preparations. This starts with adequately defining the word *herb*. Depending on the context, the term *herb* can be defined in a few different ways.

An herb is defined botanically as a seed-producing, nonwoody plant that dies down to its roots at the end of its growing season. Others have described an herb simply as a useful plant. In the culinary arts field, the term *herb* is described as a vegetable product that is used in cooking to add flavor and/or aroma to foods.[1] However, in the field of herbal medicine, the term *herb* takes on a more medical meaning. Perhaps the most precise and accurate definition of the term *herb* as it pertains to medicinal values is the definition offered by the late Dr. Varro E. Tyler, former dean and distinguished professor emeritus of the School of Pharmacy and Pharmacal Sciences at Purdue University. In his book, *Tyler's Herbs of Choice: The Therapeutic Use of Phytomedicinals*, 3rd edition, Dr. Tyler defines medicinal herbs as "crude drugs of vegetable origin utilized for the treatment of disease states, often of a chronic nature, or to attain or maintain a condition of improved health."[7]

Commercial herbal and phytomedicine preparations are available in several different forms. Some of the key forms are defined as follows:[1]

- *Extract:* An herbal concentrate that contains the phytochemical constituents found in the herb. Extracts are made when the plant constituents are extracted from the plant by physical and/or chemical means.
- *Standardized extract:* An herbal extract that is guaranteed to provide a standardized level of a particular phytochemical constituent. In many cases, this phytochemical constituent is considered to be the key active compound.
- *Infusion:* An herbal tea. An herbal extract is prepared by steeping dried plant parts in hot water.
- *Decoction:* An herbal extract prepared by putting the plant material (usually hard or woody parts) in water and boiling the water, then allowing it to simmer gently for extended periods of time. The liquid is then cooled and strained for use.
- *Tincture:* An herbal extract prepared by mixing the herb with a solvent (usually an alcohol and water mixture) for a specified period of time (hours to days). The solvent extracts phytochemical constituents from the herb. Any remaining solids are removed, and the solution that results is used medicinally.
- *Glycerite:* An herbal extract that is similar to a tincture; however, glycerol is used as the solvent in preparation instead of alcohol. Because they are alcohol-free, glycerites have recently become very popular for use with children.
- *Fluid extract:* Liquid preparations that usually contain a ratio of one part solvent to one part herb. They are much more concentrated than tinctures, and their alcohol content can vary.
- *Solid extract:* Made by evaporating all the residual solvent or liquid used during the extraction process. (Also called powdered extract.)

- *Powder:* A preparation in the form of finely divided, sieved herbal particles made from dried and finely milled herbs for use in herbal preparations such as tablets and capsules.
- *Syrup:* A water and sugar solution to which flavoring and an herbal extract may be added. Syrups are often used to relieve coughs or to mask the unpleasant flavor of a tincture. Syrups are a popular form of herbal medicine in pediatrics.

The Use of Herbs and Phytomedicines in Pediatrics

Although herbs have been used for centuries, most controlled clinical trials using herbs have included only adults. The scientific data examining the use of herbs with children are limited. As a result, herbal medicine experts do not have a consensus of opinion as to the appropriate use of botanicals for children, particularly the very young. Although more conservative experts feel strongly that botanicals should not be used by children under the age of 12 until there is more research in the pediatric population to confirm their safety, other experts have less concern and recommend their use for young children and even infants. Nevertheless, there are growing numbers of parents who are using many herbal products to treat minor illnesses in small children. The concern among many health professionals, however, is the potential hazards of the inappropriate use of herbal preparations by parents treating their children for serious health conditions without the consultation of a pediatrician.

In general, the safety of most responsibly formulated commercial herb products has been well established. However, there are situations in which specific herbs should not be used. If a child has an allergy to a specific herb, it must be avoided. Certain plants in the *Asteraceae*, *Apiaceae*, and other plant families possess a high degree of allergenicity with some children. It is advised to observe caution in the consumption of plants classified as ragweeds, especially flowers found in the *Asteraceae* family, such as chamomile.

Parents should observe the child who takes an herbal preparation for the first time for several hours for any adverse reactions. Watery, itchy eyes; sneezing; wheezing; coughing; or hives could be signs of allergy. Pediatricians who utilize herbal remedies in their practice recommend to concerned parents of allergy-prone children that they introduce an herb in the same way they would introduce new foods to an infant. The pediatrician's advice is to try only one herb at a time, administered in very small doses.

Herbs should not be given by the parent to a child who is currently taking a medication without first consulting a doctor. The interaction of an herb with medicinal substances should always be considered. Although there is little data available today on herb–drug interactions, some important information in this area is known by the medical profession such as the risks of using St. John's Wort with other antidepressants or garlic while taking other anticoagulants.

There is debate among herbal medicine experts as to which herbal remedies are safe and appropriate for use by children. In Germany, Commission E, an interdisciplinary expert committee on herbal medicines consisting of physicians, pharmacists, pharmacologists, toxicologists, representatives of the pharmaceutical industry, and laypersons, is responsible for evaluating the scientific data on the safety and efficacy of phytomedicines. Commission E members are appointed by the Federal Institute for Drugs and Medical Devices (formerly the German Federal Health Agency) and are assigned the task of preparing monographs on medicinal plants. Most experts regard these monographs as the most accurate scientific information available in the world on the safety and efficacy of herbs and phytomedicines. Although the monographs describe the medicinal use of herbs primarily for adults, they also identify herbs that are contraindicated for children (**Exhibit 21-1**).[8] **Table 21-3** gives an overview of several of the internal and external uses of many of the medicinal herbs commonly used in pediatrics.

EXHIBIT 21-1 Herbs and Herbal Products Contraindicated for Children According to the German Commission E Monographs

Aloe
Buckthorn bark and berry
Camphor
Cajeput oil
Cascara sagrada bark
Eucalyptus leaf
Eucalyptus oil
Fennel oil
Horseradish
Mint oil (external)
Nasturtium
Peppermint oil (external)
Rhubarb root
Senna leaf and pod
Watercress

Source: Blumenthal M, et al., eds., Klein S, Rister RS, trans., *The Complete German Commission E Monographs: Therapeutic Guide to Herbal Medicines.* © 1998 American Botanical Council and Integrative Medicine Communications.

TABLE 21-3 Common Herbal Remedies Used in Pediatrics

Common and Latin Names	Internal and External Uses	Contraindications/Precautions
Aloe (*Aloe vera*)	External use: wound healing, minor skin irritation, burns	Not recommended internally for pediatrics.
Anise (*Pimpinella anisum*)	Internal use: common colds, coughs, bronchitis, indigestion	Rare allergic reactions to anise and its constituent anethole.
Bilberry (*Vaccinium myrtillus*)	Internal use: diarrhea	None known.
Calendula flowers (*Calendula officinalis*)	Internal use: inflammation of mouth and pharynx External use: wounds and burns	Rare allergic reactions through frequent skin contact.
Catnip (*Nepeta cataria*)	Internal use: nervous disorders, sleep aid, common colds, colic	None known.
Chamomile flowers (*Matricaria chamomilla*)	Internal use: carminative, sleep aid External use: inflammation and irritations of the skin, wounds, burns	Rare allergic reactions.
Cherry bark (*Prunus sp.*)	Internal use: coughs, common colds	None known.
Comfrey leaf (*Symphytum officinale*)	External use: minor wounds, ulcers, inflammations, bruises, and sprains; used as poultice for skin disorder	Not to be taken internally. Internal use promotes hepatotoxic effects.
Echinacea (*Echinacea angustifolia*) (*Echinacea purpurea*)	Internal use: common colds, flu, coughs, bronchitis, fever, immune stimulant External use: wounds, burns	Allergic reactions may occur with some individuals. Not recommended for individuals with autoimmune diseases.
Elder flowers (*Sambucus nigra*)	Internal use: common colds, antiviral, diaphoretic	None known.
Eucalyptus (*Eucalyptus globulus*)	Internal use: expectorant, coughs, congestion of the respiratory tract	Nausea, vomiting, and diarrhea may occur after ingestion in rare cases. Eucalyptus preparations should not be applied to the face or nose of infants and very young children.
Fennel seed (*Foeniculum vulgare*)	Internal use: carminative, indigestion, coughs, bronchitis, gastrointestinal afflictions	Allergic reactions may occur with some individuals.
Garlic (*Allium sativum*)	Internal use: common colds, bronchitis, fever External use: antibacterial, antifungal, ear infections	Intake of large quantities can lead to stomach complaints. Rare allergic reactions.
Ginger (*Zingiber officinale*)	Internal use: carminative, antinausea, indigestion	None known.
Goldenseal (*Hydrastis canadensis*)	Internal use: common colds, flu, inflammation of mucous membranes External use: antiseptic, antimicrobial, cuts, wounds, ear infections	Internal use can cause nausea, vomiting, and diarrhea, and may disrupt intestinal flora. Internal use is not recommended for young children by many experts due to the herb's alkaloid (berberine and hydrastine) content.
Hops (*Humulus lupulus*)	Internal use: nervous disorders, sleep aid	Rare allergic reactions.
Horehound (*Marrubium vulgare*)	Internal use: coughs, bronchitis	None known.
Hyssop (*Hyssopus officinalis*)	Internal use: coughs, common colds	None known.

TABLE 21-3 *(Continued)*

Common and Latin Names	Internal and External Uses	Contraindications/Precautions
Lemon balm (*Melissa officinalis*)	Internal use: nervous disorders, sleep aid	None known.
Licorice root (*Glycyrrhiza glabra*)	Internal use: coughs, bronchitis	Prolonged use with high doses may promote hypertension, edema, and hypokalemia.
Marshmallow root (*Althaea officinalis*)	Internal use: coughs, bronchitis, sore throat	None known.
Mullein leaf (*Verbascum thapsus*)	Internal use: coughs, bronchitis, common colds, flu	None known.
Oat straw (*Avena sativa*)	External use: inflammation of the skin, itching	None known.
Passion flower (*Passiflora incarnata*)	Internal use: nervous disorders, sleep aid	None known.
Peppermint leaf (*Mentha piperita*)	Internal use: carminative, indigestion, nausea, gastrointestinal disorders, common colds, cough, bronchitis	Preparations containing peppermint oil should not be applied to the face or nose of infants or very young children.
Pleurisy root (*Asclepias tuberosa*)	Internal use: coughs, pleurisy	Excessive amounts can be toxic due to the herb's cardioactive steroid content that can lead to digitalis-like poisonings. High doses can promote vomiting.
St. John's wort (*Hypericum perforatum*)	Internal use: emotional upsets, including anxiety and depressive moods. External use: cuts and abrasions	Safety of internal use with children has not been established. The safety and ethics of the use of herbal antidepressants with children without the consultation of a doctor is questionable. Should not be taken by children already taking prescription medications for depression without first consulting a doctor. May cause sun sensitivity in some individuals.
Thyme (*Thymus vulgarus*)	Internal use: cough, bronchitis, common colds	None known.
Valerian root (*Valeriana officinalis*)	Internal use: nervous disorders, sleep aid	The safety and ethics of the use of herbal sedatives with children without the consultation of a doctor is questionable.

Note: Clinical efficacy for each of these herbs has not necessarily been established.

Laxatives and Stimulants

Most herbal medicine experts caution against the use of herbal stimulant laxatives by children under the age of 12. Herbal stimulant laxatives include aloe (*Aloe ferox*), buckthorn bark (*Rhamnus frangula*), cascara sagrada bark (*Rhamnus purshiana*), and senna leaf or pod (*Cassia senna*). Stimulants such as caffeine-containing herbs are also generally contraindicated for young children.[8,9]

Herbs that are classified as stimulants include not only coffee and black and green tea (*Camellia sinensis*), but also cola nut (also called kola nut; *Cola nitida*), guarana (*Paullinia cupana*), and maté (*Ilex paraguariensis*). Ma huang (also known as ephedra herb) is also a potent stimulant and is contraindicated for young children. It has been taken off the U.S. market. Asian ginseng (*Panax ginseng*) and American ginseng (*Panax quinquefolium*), traditionally regarded as herbal stimulants, are also not recommended for young children by many herbal medicine authorities.[1,9]

Sedatives and Antidepressants

Many plants have traditionally been used for their sedative properties. There is controversy as to whether it is proper or even ethical to administer any sedative to young children without the consultation of a physician. Definitely, this is quite clear in regard to prescription drugs, but naturally derived herbal sedatives have not always been looked at in the same light. Most health authorities would agree that any sedative, herbal or otherwise, should be given to a child only under medical direction. Many herbal medicine experts would agree that strong sedative herbs such as valerian (*Valeriana officinalis*) should not be given to young children. There is no consensus of opinion on the use of some of the other popular traditional sedative herbs for children, despite the fact that many of them have been used with children for centuries. These herbs include catnip (*Nepeta cataria*), German chamomile (*Matricaria recutita*), hops (*Humulus lupulus*), lemon balm (*Melissa officinalis*), and passion flower (*Passiflora incarnata*). St. John's wort (*Hypericum perforatum*), an herb that has proven efficacy in treating mild and moderate depression in adults, has not been adequately studied for use by children.

Herbs Containing Alkaloids

Many herbal experts have concerns about children's use of herbs that contain powerful alkaloids. One of the alkaloids of concern is berberine. Berberine is a key principal phytochemical constituent found in several of the currently popular herbal products found in natural food and drug stores. Herbs containing berberine include goldenseal root (*Hydrastis canadensis*), Oregon grape root (*Mahonia aquifolium*), and barberry root (*Berberis vulgaris*). Berberine has antibacterial properties. Overuse of herbs containing this and other alkaloids could disrupt the normal flora in a child's gastrointestinal tract.[9]

Alkaloids that affect the central nervous system (caffeine, ephedrine, pseudoephedrine, and others) are generally not recommended for young children except under a doctor's direction.[9]

Traditional Herbal Remedies Used with Infants and Children

For centuries, medicinal herbs have been used with children worldwide with an apparently good record of safety. Clinical research has shown that many traditional herbal remedies appear to be effective;[9] however, more research is needed to confirm the safety and efficacy of the use of medicinal herbs in pediatric medicine.

Few studies have been done with infants using herbal preparations. Unfortunately, in recent years pediatric herbal medicine studies have not been made a priority. In 1993, a prospective, randomized, double-blind, placebo-controlled study published in the *Journal of Pediatrics* examined the effects of an herbal tea in treating infantile colic.[10] The tea was made from herbs known to have antispasmodic activity and traditionally used to treat indigestion and colic in infants. The tea contained chamomile (*Matricaria chamomilla*), vervain (*Verbena officinalis*), licorice root (*Glycyrrhiza glabra*), fennel (*Foeniculum vulgare*), and lemon balm (*Melissa officinalis*). The use of the herbal tea eliminated the colic in 19 (57%) of the 33 infants, whereas the placebo was helpful in only 9 (26%) of 35 ($p < 0.01$). The mean colic score was significantly improved in the infants treated with herbal tea. None of the infants in the study experienced any adverse effects from the herbal tea.[10]

Additional studies demonstrating the effectiveness of herbal remedies with children have been published in the scientific literature. Standardized ginger root has been shown to be effective in treating motion sickness in children ages 4 to 8 years of age.[11] Enteric-coated peppermint oil capsules have been demonstrated to be safe and effective as a treatment for pain associated with the acute phases of irritable bowel syndrome (IBS) in older children and adolescents.[12] A study conducted on 171 children (ages 5 to 18 years) using herbal ear drops containing a combination of mullein, marigold (calendula), St. John's wort, lavender, and garlic in an olive oil base reduced ear pain associated with acute otitis media (AOM) as effectively as standard anesthetic eardrops.[13] A review of randomized controlled trials indicates that ivy leaf extract (*Hedra helix*) preparations show effects respective to improving the respiratory functions of children with chronic asthma.[14]

Heinz Schilcher, an expert in pharmacognosy at the Institute of Pharmaceutical Biology at Berlin's Independent University and a member of the German Commission E, points out the value of herbal remedies in pediatrics in his book *Phytotherapy in Paediatrics: Handbook for Physicians and Pharmacists*.[15] He notes that the benefits of many phytomedicines outweigh the risks because they have a relatively good benefit/risk ratio. In European studies, the actions of many combinations of naturally occurring compounds in herbs have been experimentally established and/or clinically confirmed, with minimal or negligible side effects. Other advantages of herbal remedies mentioned by Schilcher are that herbs have gentle medicinal actions, and their common methods of administration (inhalation, baths, ointments, syrups) are particularly appropriate for children. As a result, this can provide for good compliance. He points out that herbal medicines in pediatrics may be used at a preventive level, not just for treating symptoms. Schilcher also notes that, as a general rule, phytomedicines are less expensive than conventional medicines.[15]

Determining Proper Pediatric Dosage for Medicinal Herbs

There is little scientific or even traditional information available on the proper dosage of herbs and phytomedicines in pediatrics. Because most clinical trials using herbs have been with adults, official dosages have been established for only the adult population. The posology in the German Commission E monographs refers to adults. A general pediatric guide used for determining the dosage of phytotherapeutic drugs is one third of the adult dose (as established in the Commission E monographs) for very young and young children and one half the adult dose for school-age children.[15] Two classic pharmacy rules that are traditionally used in determining the dosages for drugs for children are sometimes used by herbal medicine experts as well. These rules are known as *Clark's Rule* and *Young's Rule*. **Exhibit 21-2** illustrates how they are calculated. Because children have lower body weight than adults and do not have the sufficient development of liver enzymes necessary to metabolize many medications, their dosages of conventional as well as herbal medicines must be reduced. The proper pediatric dosage is best determined by an experienced and trained health professional. In recent years, some herbal product manufacturers have formulated their preparations for dosage levels appropriate for children.

EXHIBIT 21-2 How to Calculate a Child's Dosage for Herbal Medicines

The following are two classic rules used to calculate the approximate dosage for a child.

Clark's Rule: Divide the child's weight by 150. The example given is for a 50-pound child:

$$\frac{50}{150}=\frac{1}{3}\text{ adult dosage}$$

Young's Rule: Divide the child's age by the child's age + 12. The example given is for a 4-year-old child:

$$\frac{4}{4+12}=\frac{4}{16}=\frac{1}{4}\text{ adult dosage}$$

Conclusion

Medicinal herbs have been used in pediatrics since ancient times. There is a growing trend among parents to use botanical and other natural medicines with their children as alternatives to conventional medicines. Increased public awareness of the therapeutic value of certain herbs and an increasing amount of scientific research in this area have led to an explosion in the marketplace of herbal medicine preparations and products. Several leading pharmaceutical companies are now adding herbal medicines to their product lines. Herbal medicine preparations specifically formulated for children are being sold in natural food stores. Based on current trends, herbal medicine will undoubtedly play a more prominent role in the pediatric medicine of the 21st century. Increased medical expenses associated with the cost of pharmaceuticals has contributed to the high cost of today's healthcare. Lower cost, safe, and effective alternative herbal medicines can play an important role in reducing overall healthcare costs. Pediatricians and other health professionals who work with pediatric patients need to gain more knowledge about herbal medicine and its potential role in the health care of infants and children. More clinical research is needed to evaluate the safety and efficacy of medicinal herbs in the pediatric population.

Case Study

Nutrition Assessment

Patient history: A 7-year-old female visited her pediatrician for digestive problems including feelings of nausea. The pediatrician diagnosed the patient with having a mild case of dyspepsia (indigestion, upset stomach). The patient has a history of remarkable good health throughout her childhood. On one previous occasion, about 7 months ago, the patient had a similar episode of mild dyspepsia associated with eating a rich meal. The patient's parents are interested in complementary and alternative medicine approaches to treating their child's dyspepsia without the use of conventional medicines.

Family history: There is no family history of any serious digestive problems.

Medical/lab tests: No medical or lab tests were performed.

Anthropometric Measurements

Height: 122.0 cm

Weight: 23.0 kg

BMI: 15.5 kg/m^2

Nutrition History

No known food allergies.

Typical day's intake: Patient and her family typically follow a very healthy, low-fat vegetarian diet: three vegetarian meals with healthy vegetarian snacks throughout the day. This typical diet is routinely followed with the exception of occasional holidays, parties, and special social events when the vegetarian diet is not always followed.

Diet on day of dyspepsia:

- Breakfast: Granola cereal with blueberries and soy milk, whole wheat toast with whole fruit strawberry jam, and small glass of fresh squeezed orange juice.
- Lunch: Birthday party lunch: Vanilla milkshake, cheeseburger, French fries, nachos, candy, birthday cake, and chocolate ice cream cone.
- Dinner: Could not eat dinner that evening due to indigestion and stomachache.

Children's multivitamin taken with breakfast.

Nutrition Diagnosis

Based on the above information, a nutrition diagnosis or problem is determined.

Nutrition and Botanical Medicine Interventions

Goal: To alleviate patient's dyspepsia and offer plan to avoid future episodes.

Food/nutrient delivery: Patient will temporarily avoid solid foods. Tolerable clear liquids will be advised and recommended, starting with an appropriate warm herbal tea/beverage.

Nutrition education: Educate parents and patient about a recommended clear liquid diet and how to begin using an appropriate warm herbal tea/beverage to help alleviate symptoms of dyspepsia.

Nutrition counseling: Patient to remain on appropriate clear liquid diet and warm herbal tea/beverage until symptoms of dyspepsia have resolved. Then reinstitute the healthy diet plan the family regularly follows. Counsel parents and patient to be moderate in consumption of rich foods at parties and celebrations to avoid future episodes of dyspepsia.

Monitoring and Evaluation

Should symptoms persist or later reoccur, follow up with patient with appropriate diet plan and nutrition counseling in conjunction with recommendations from patient's pediatrician.

Questions for the Reader

1. What percentiles on the NCHS growth chart are the patient's height and weight?
2. Based on the list of herbs in Table 21-3, what appropriate herbs (herbal remedies) can be used in the preparation of a warm herbal tea or beverage for the treatment of symptoms of dyspepsia (indigestion, upset stomach)?

Resources

Associations

American Botanical Council, P.O. Box 144345 Austin, TX 78714, Phone: (800) 373-7105, http://www.herbalgram.org

Herb Research Foundation, 4140 15th Street, Suite 200, Boulder, CO 80304, Phone: (303) 449-2265, http://www.herbs.org

Books and Periodicals

Awang DVC. *Tyler's Herbs of Choice: The Therapeutic Use of Phytomedicinals*, 3rd ed. Boca Raton, FL: CRC Press; 2009.

Blumenthal M. *The ABC Clinical Guide to Herbs*. Austin, TX: American Botanical Council; 2003.

Blumenthal M, Busse WR, Goldberg A, et al. *The Complete German Commission E Monographs: Therapeutic Guide to Herbal Medicines*. Austin, TX: American Botanical Council; 1998.

HerbalGram. Austin, TX, Journal of the American Botanical Council.

Gruenwalk J, Brendler T, Jaenicke C, eds. *PDR for Herbal Medicines*, 4th ed. Montvale, NJ: Thomson Healthcare; 2007.

The Review of Natural Products. St. Louis, MO: Facts and Comparisons.

REFERENCES

1. Westerdahl J. *Medicinal Herbs: A Vital Reference Guide*. Dallas, TX: Bruce Miller Enterprises; 1998.
2. Principe PP. The economic significance of plants and their constituents as drugs. *Econ Med Plant Res*. 1989;3:1–17.
3. Farnsworth NR, Akerele O, Bingel AS, Soejarto DD, Guo Z. Medicinal plants in therapy. *Bull World Health Org*. 1985;63:965–981.
4. Dietary Supplement Health and Education Act of 1994 (DHEA), Pub.L No. 103-417, 108 Stat, 1994. U.S. Food and Drug Administration, Center for Food Safety and Applied Nutrition. Available at: http://www.vm.cfsan.fda.gov/ndMS/dietsupp.html. Accessed August 23, 2010.
5. Eisenberg DM, Kessler RC, Foster C, et al. Unconventional medicine in the United States. *N Engl J Med*. 1993;328:246–252.
6. Cavaliere C, Rea P, Lynch ME, Blumenthal M. Herbal supplement sales experience slight increase in 2008. *HerbalGram*. 2009;82:58–61.
7. Awang DVE. *Tyler's Herbs of Choice: The Therapeutic Use of Phytomedicinals*, 3rd ed. Boca Raton, FL: CRC Press; 2009:1.
8. Blumenthal M, Busse WR, Goldberg A, et al., eds. Klein S, Rister RS, trans. *The Complete German Commission E Monographs: Therapeutic Guide to Herbal Medicines*. Austin, TX: American Botanical Council; 1998.
9. Gruenwalk J, Brendler T, Jaenicke C, eds. *PDR for Herbal Medicines*, 4th ed. Montvale, NJ: Thomson Healthcare; 2007.
10. Weizman Z, Alkrinawi S, Goldfarb D, Bitran C. Efficacy of herbal tea preparation in infantile cholic. *J Pediatr*. 1993;122:650–652.
11. Careddu P. Motion sickness in children: results of a double-blind study with ginger (*Zintona*) and dimenhydrinate. *European Phytotherapy*. 1999;2:102–107.
12. Kline RM, Kline JJ, Di Palma J, Barbero GJ. Enteric-coated, pH-dependent peppermint oil capsules for the treatment of irritable bowel syndrome in children. *J Pediatr*. 2001;138:125–128.
13. Sarrel FM, Cohen HA, Kahan E. Naturopathic treatment for ear pain in children. *Pediatrics*. 2003;111:574–579.
14. Hofmann D, Hecker M, Volp A. Efficacy of dry extract of ivy leaves in children with bronchial asthma—a review of randomized controlled trials. *Phytomedicine*. 2003;10:213–220.
15. Schilcher H. *Phytotherapy in Pediatrics: Handbook for Physicians and Pharmacists*. Stuttgart, Germany: MedPharm Scientific Publishers; 1997.

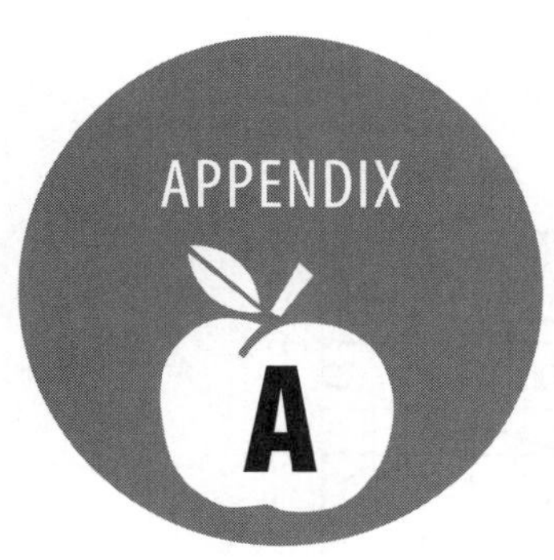

Premature Infant Growth Charts

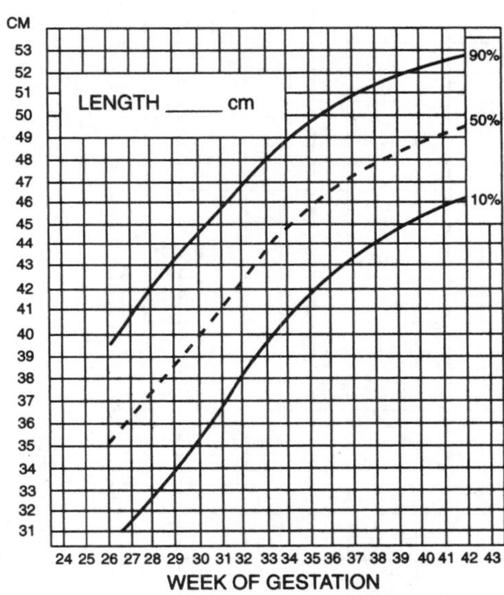

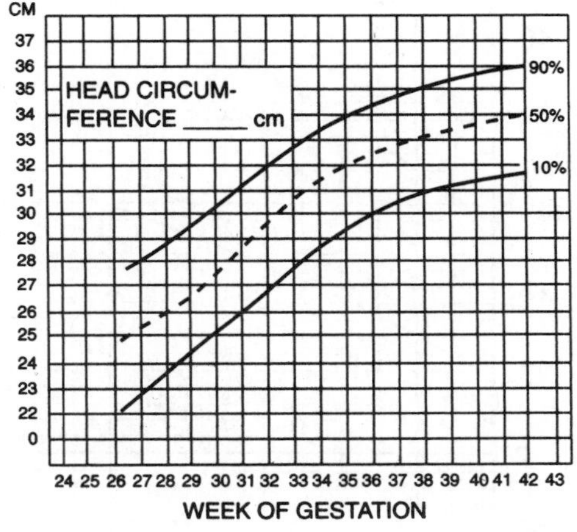

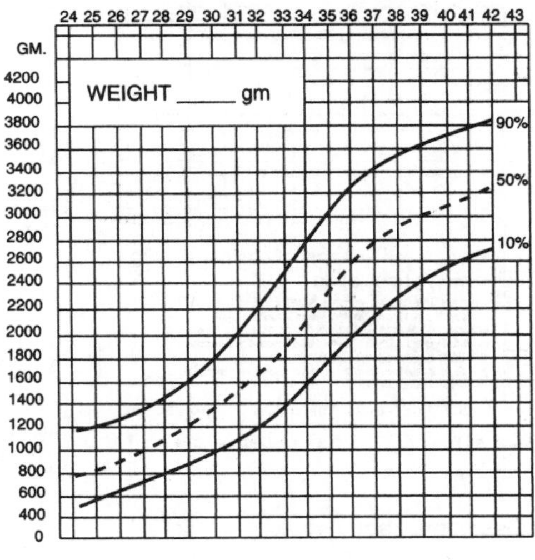

FIGURE A-1 Intrauterine growth charts.

Source: Data from Mead Johnson and Co., Classification of newborns based on maturity and intrauterine growth, 1978; Lubchenco LC, Hansman C, Boyd E. *Pediatrics* 1966;37:403; and Battaglia FC, Lubchenco LC. *J Ped.* 1967;71:159.

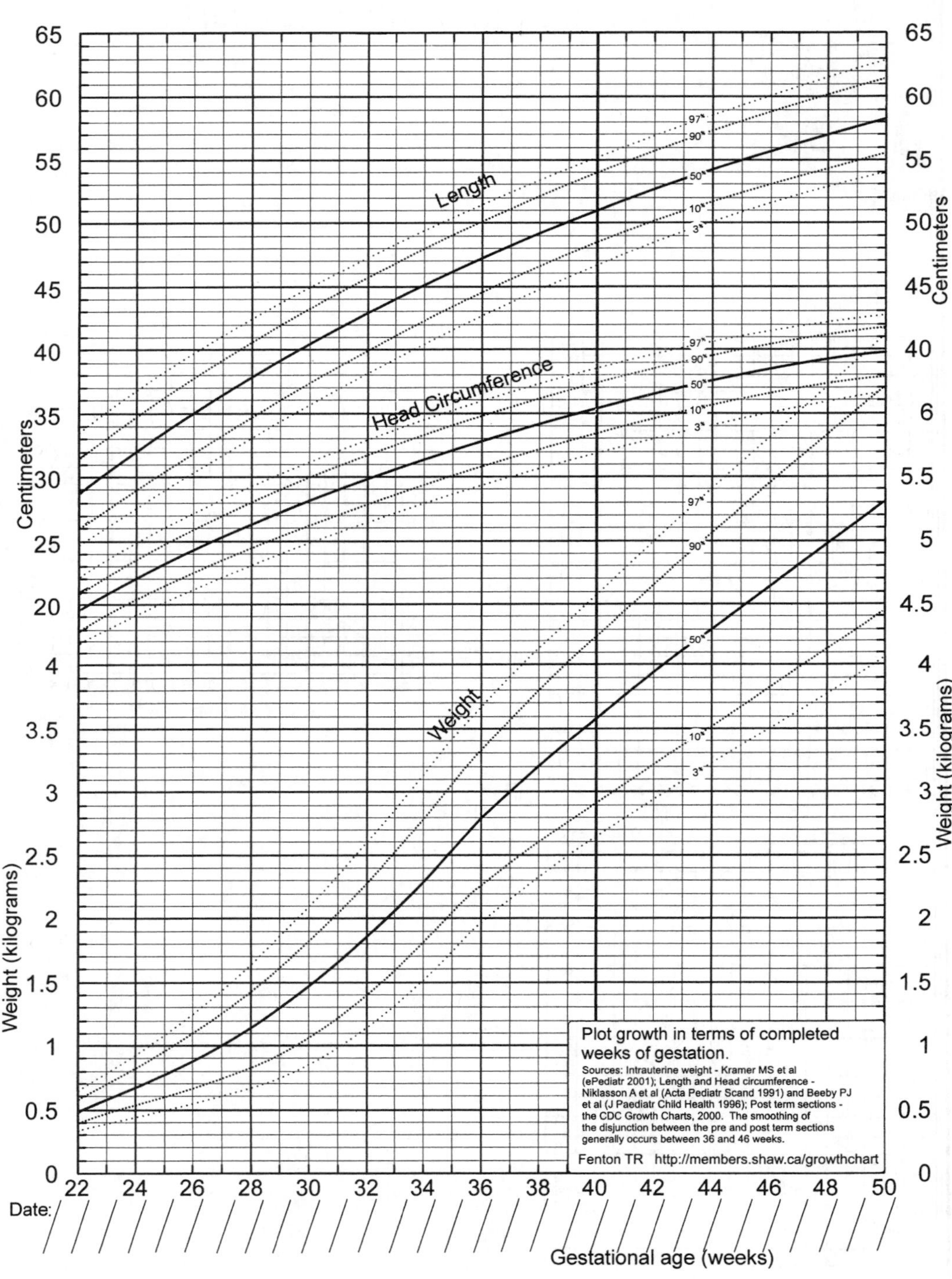

FIGURE A-2 Babson and Benda's growth chart for preterm babies.

Source: Fenton TR, *BMC Peds* 2003;3:13. Available at: www.members.shaw.ca/growthchart.

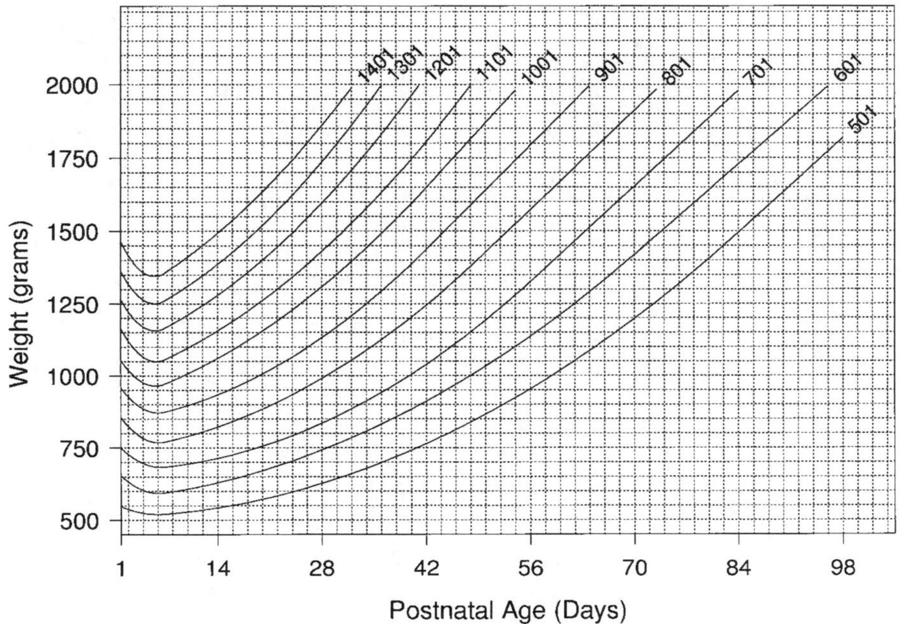

FIGURE A-3 Average daily body weight versus postnatal age in days for infants stratified by 100-g birth weight intervals.

Source: Ehrenkranz RA, Younes N, Lemons JA, et al. Longitudinal growth of hospitalized very low birth weight infants. *Pediatrics.* 1999;104:280–289.

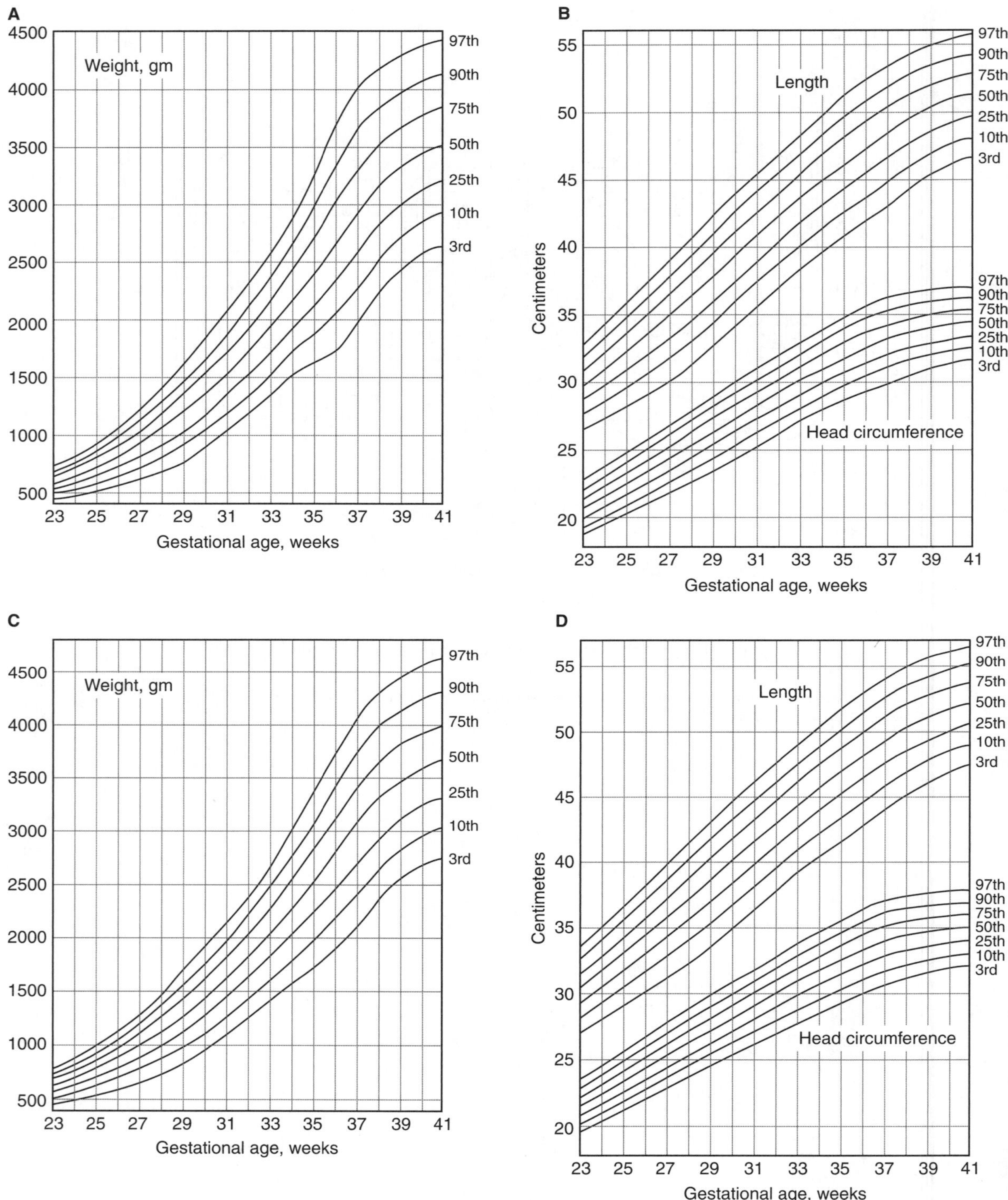

FIGURE A-4 New gender-specific intrauterine growth curves for girls' weight-for-age (A), girls' length- and HC-for-age (B), boys' weight-for-age (C), and boys' length- and HC-for-age (D). Of note, 3rd and 97th percentiles on all curves for 23 weeks should be interpreted cautiously given the small sample size; for boys' HC curve at 24 weeks, all percentiles should be interpreted cautiously because the distribution of data is skewed left.

Source: Adapted from Olsen IE, Groveman SA, Lawson ML, Reese HC, Zemel BS. New intrauterine growth curves based on United States data. *Pediatrics*. 2010;125:e214–e224. Available at: http://www.pediatrics.org. Accessed February 24, 2010.

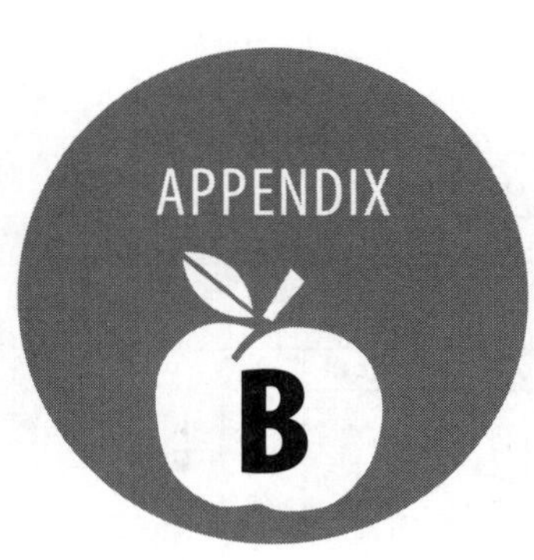

CDC and WHO Growth Charts

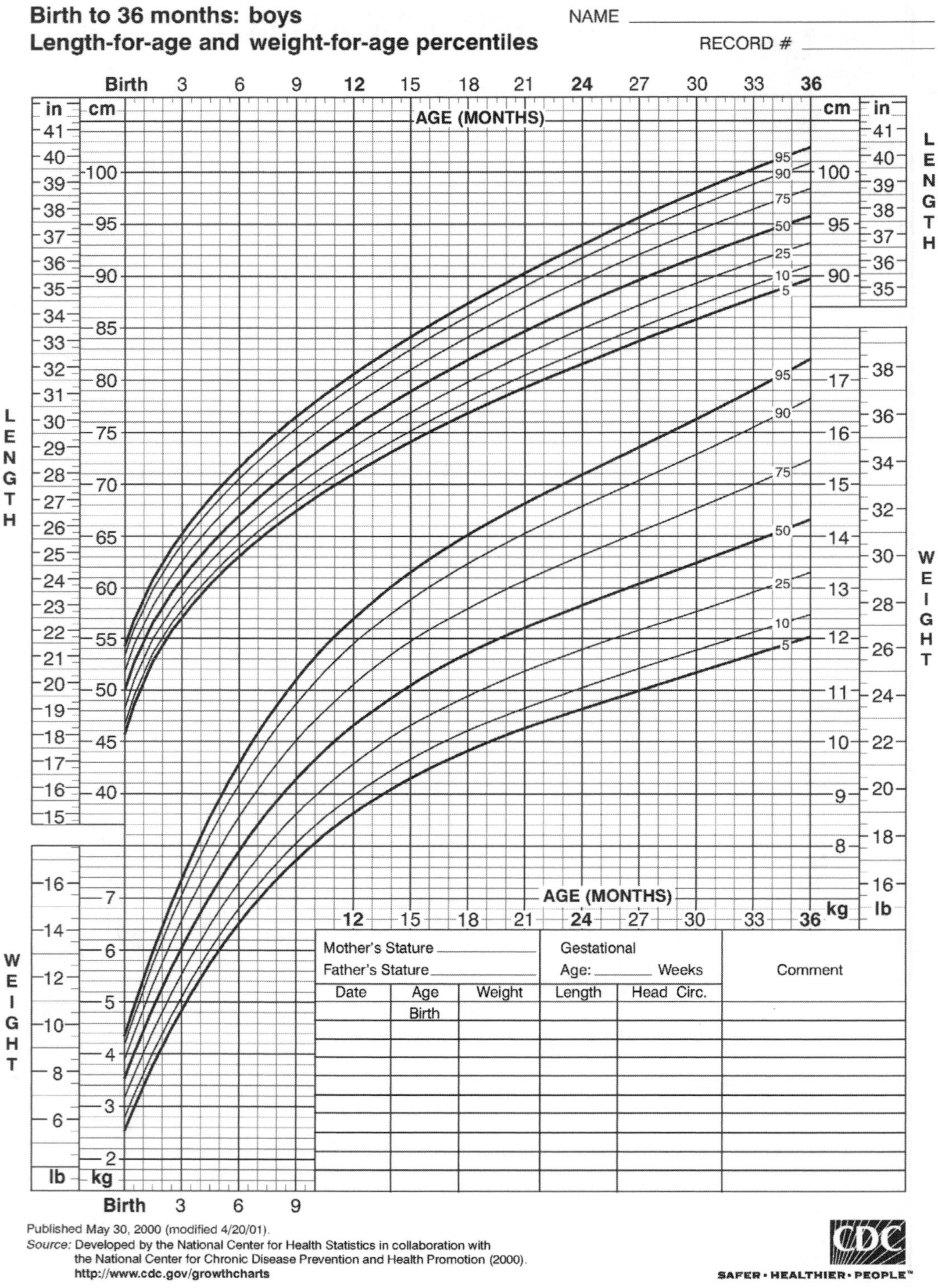

Birth to 36 months: boys
Length-for-age and weight-for-age percentiles

NAME ______________________

RECORD # ____________

Mother's Stature ____________ Gestational Age: ________ Weeks

Father's Stature ____________

Comment

Date	Age	Weight	Length	Head Circ.	Comment
	Birth				

Published May 30, 2000 (modified 4/20/01).
Source: Developed by the National Center for Health Statistics in collaboration with the National Center for Chronic Disease Prevention and Health Promotion (2000).
http://www.cdc.gov/growthcharts

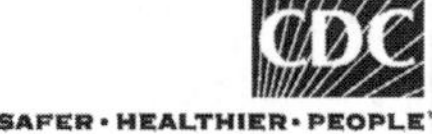

FIGURE B-1 Birth to 36 months: boys. Length-for-age and weight-for-age percentiles.

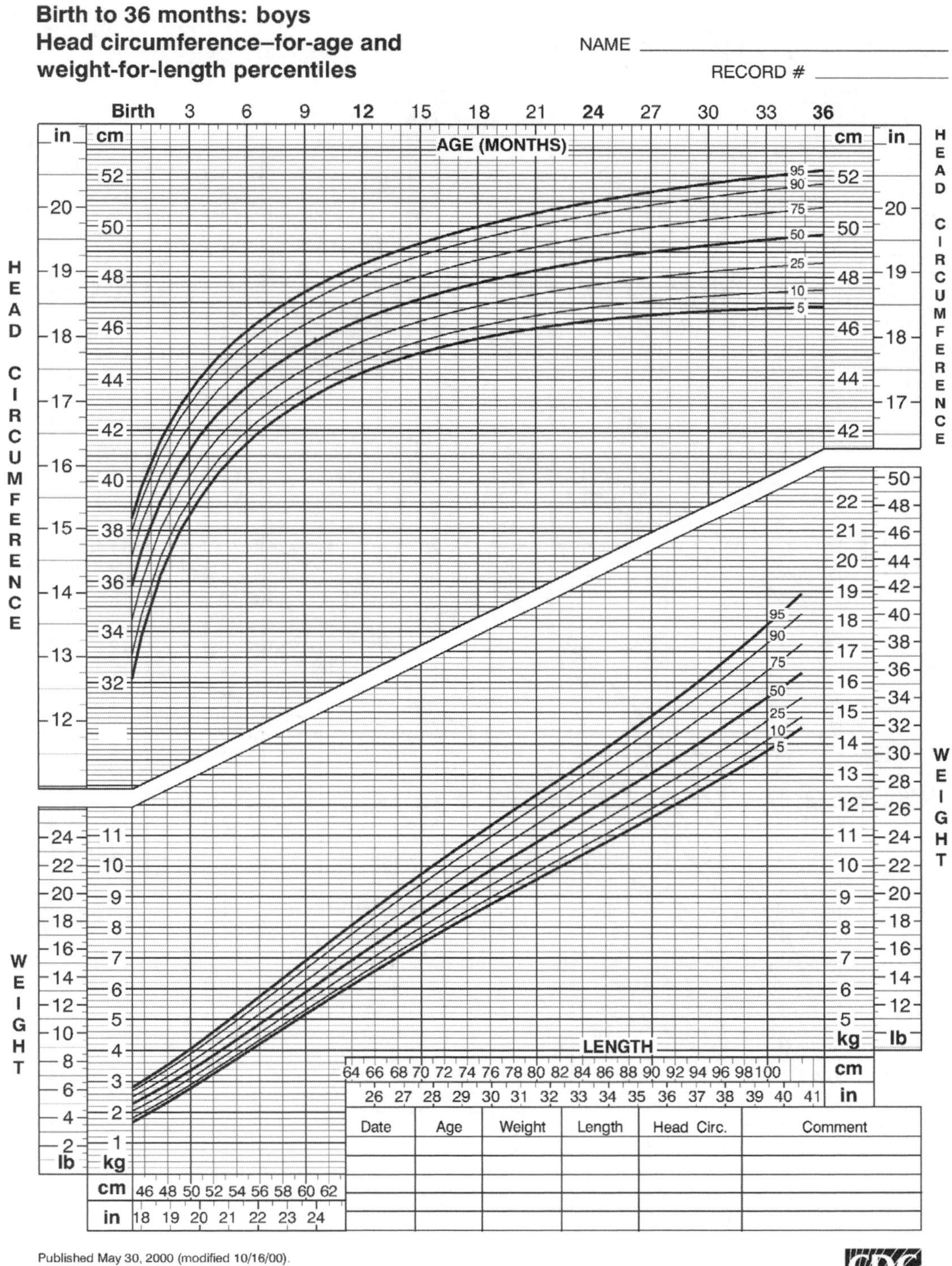

FIGURE B-2 Birth to 36 months: boys. Head circumference–for-age and weight-for-length percentiles.

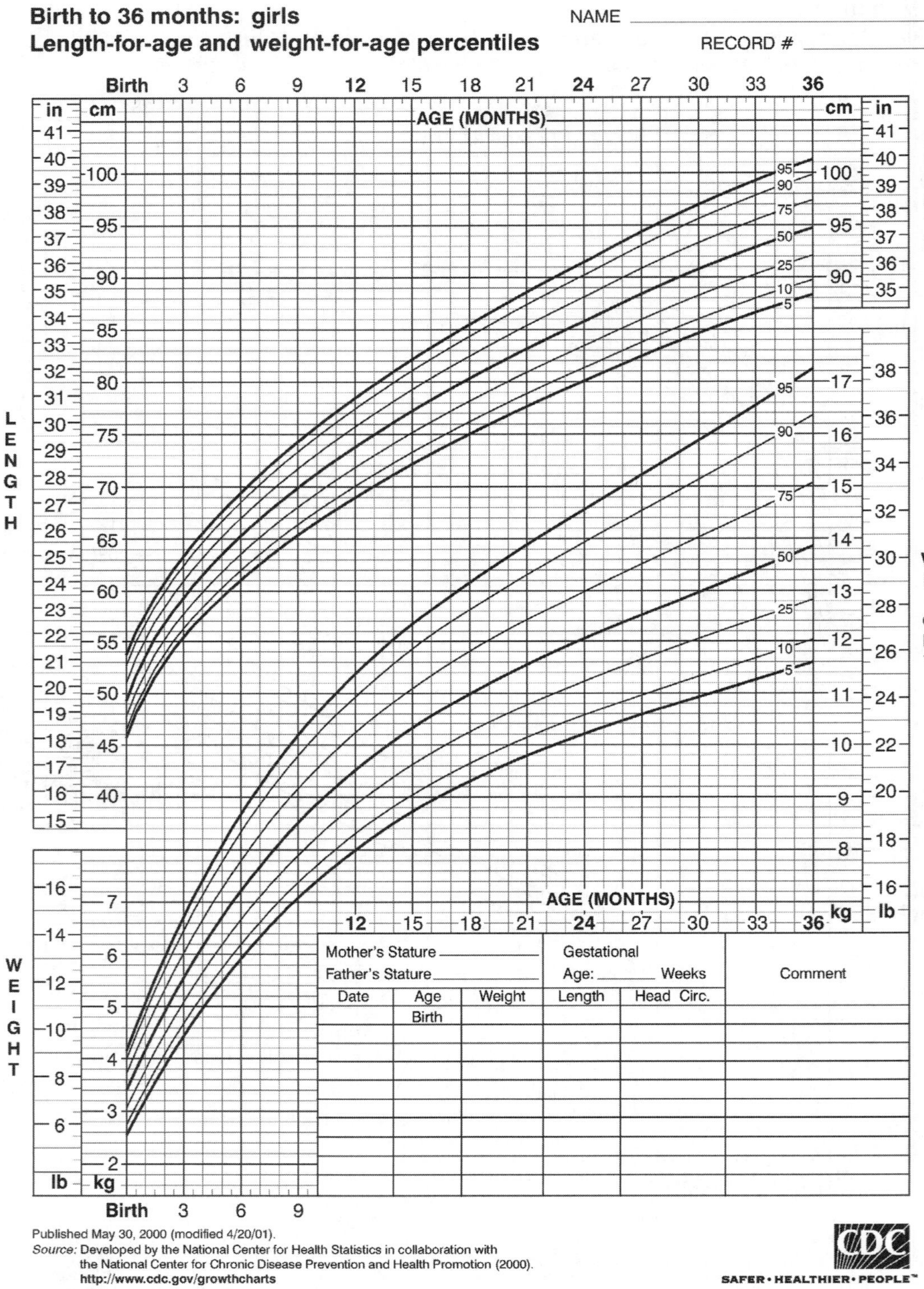

Birth to 36 months: girls
Length-for-age and weight-for-age percentiles
NAME
RECORD #
Birth 3 6 9 12 15 18 21 24 27 30 33 36
AGE (MONTHS)
in
cm
LENGTH
WEIGHT
95
90
75
50
25
10
5
kg
lb
Mother's Stature
Father's Stature
Gestational Age: Weeks
Comment
Date
Age
Weight
Length
Head Circ.
Birth
Published May 30, 2000 (modified 4/20/01).
Source: Developed by the National Center for Health Statistics in collaboration with the National Center for Chronic Disease Prevention and Health Promotion (2000).
http://www.cdc.gov/growthcharts
CDC
SAFER • HEALTHIER • PEOPLE

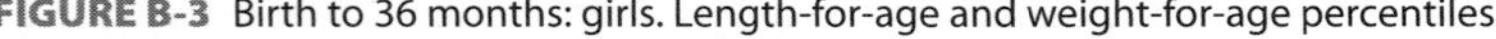

FIGURE B-3 Birth to 36 months: girls. Length-for-age and weight-for-age percentiles.

Birth to 36 months: girls
Head circumference–for-age and weight-for-length percentiles

NAME ____________________

RECORD # ____________

Birth 3 6 9 12 15 18 21 24 27 30 33 36

AGE (MONTHS)

HEAD CIRCUMFERENCE

in: 12 13 14 15 16 17 18 19 20

cm: 32 34 36 38 40 42 44 46 48 50 52

95 90 75 50 25 10 5

WEIGHT

kg: 1 2 3 4 5 6 7 8 9 10 11 12 13 14 15 16 17 18 19 20 21 22

lb: 2 4 6 8 10 12 14 16 18 20 22 24 26 28 30 32 34 36 38 40 42 44 46 48 50

LENGTH

cm: 46 48 50 52 54 56 58 60 62 64 66 68 70 72 74 76 78 80 82 84 86 88 90 92 94 96 98 100

in: 18 19 20 21 22 23 24 25 26 27 28 29 30 31 32 33 34 35 36 37 38 39 40 41

Date	Age	Weight	Length	Head Circ.	Comment

Published May 30, 2000 (modified 10/16/00).
Source: Developed by the National Center for Health Statistics in collaboration with the National Center for Chronic Disease Prevention and Health Promotion (2000).
http://www.cdc.gov/growthcharts

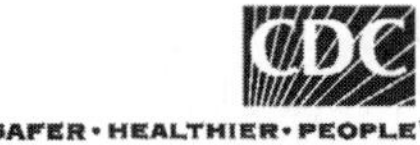

FIGURE B-4 Birth to 36 months: girls. Head circumference–for-age and weight-for-length percentiles.

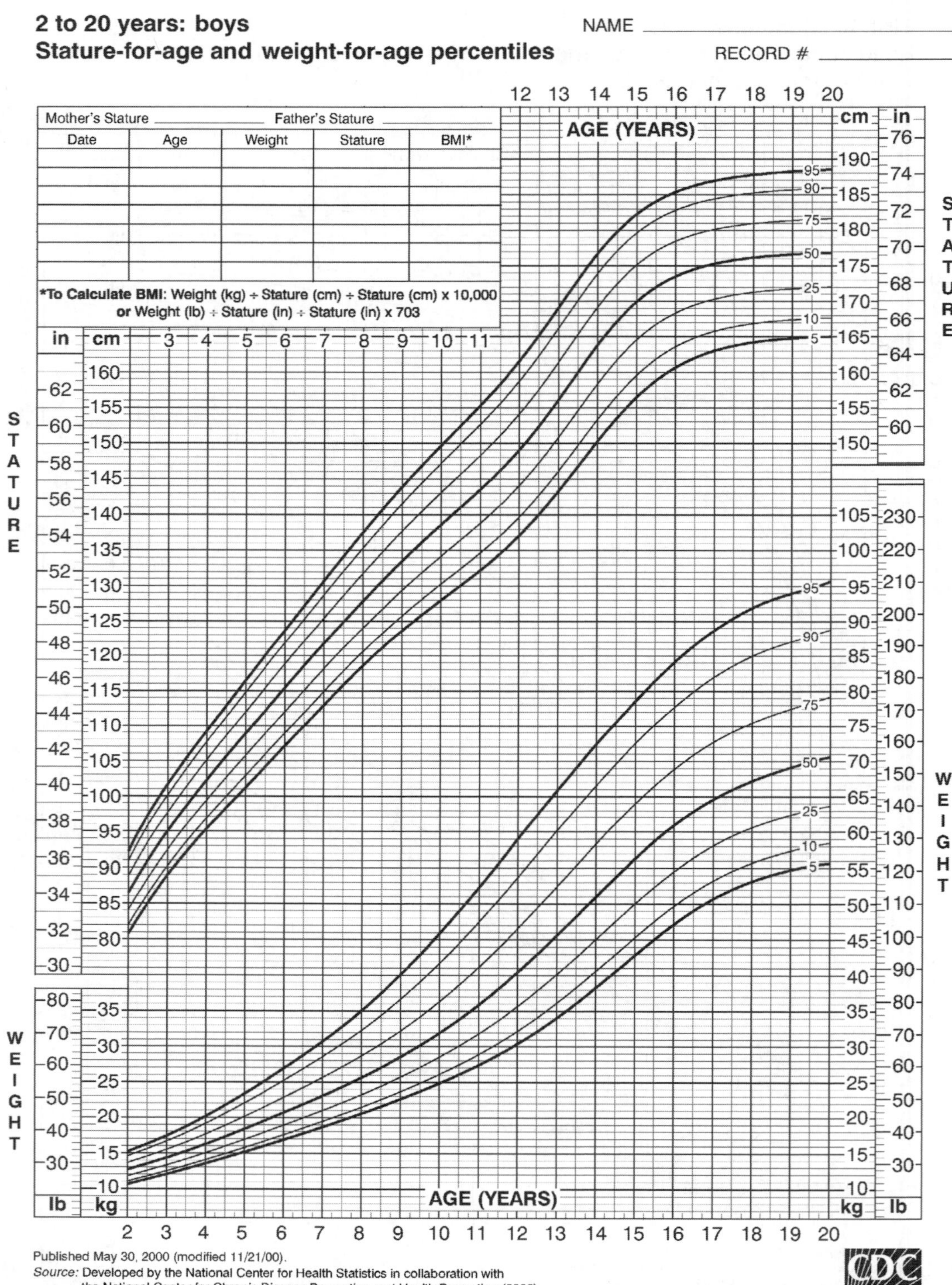

FIGURE B-5 2 to 20 years: boys. Stature-for-age and weight-for-age percentiles.

2 to 20 years: boys
Body mass index–for-age percentiles

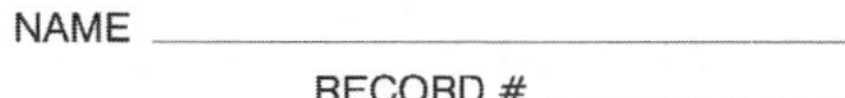

Date	Age	Weight	Stature	BMI*	Comments

***To Calculate BMI:** Weight (kg) ÷ Stature (cm) ÷ Stature (cm) x 10,000
or Weight (lb) ÷ Stature (in) ÷ Stature (in) x 703

BMI

35
34
33
32
31
30
29
28
27
26
25
24
23
22
21
20
19
18
17
16
15
14
13
12

kg/m²

95
90
85
75
50
25
10
5

AGE (YEARS)

2 3 4 5 6 7 8 9 10 11 12 13 14 15 16 17 18 19 20

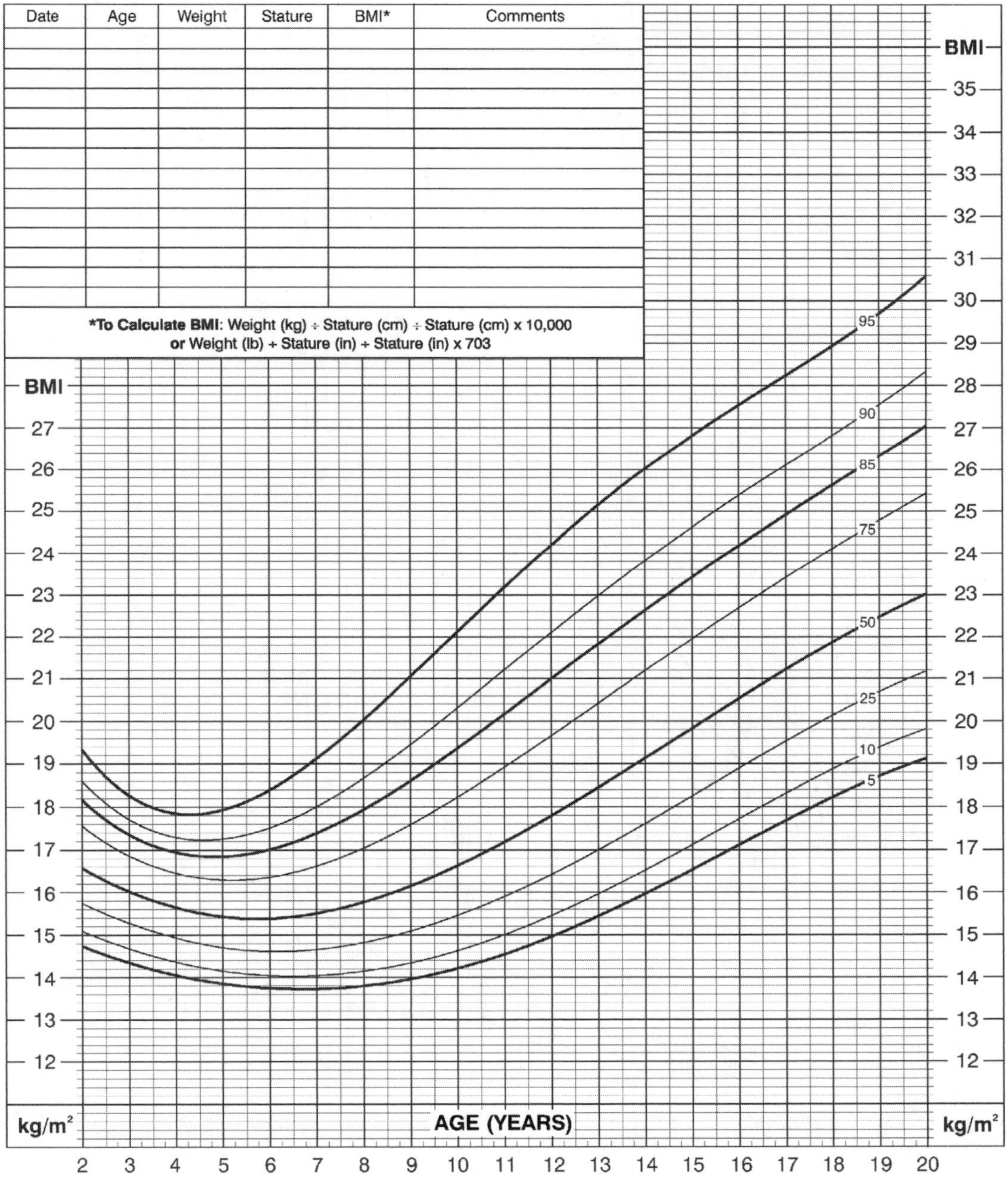

Published May 30, 2000 (modified 10/16/00).
Source: Developed by the National Center for Health Statistics in collaboration with the National Center for Chronic Disease Prevention and Health Promotion (2000).
http://www.cdc.gov/growthcharts

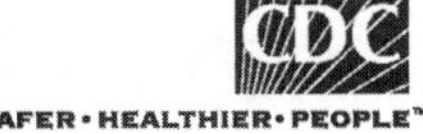

FIGURE B-6 2 to 20 years: boys. Body mass index–for-age percentiles.

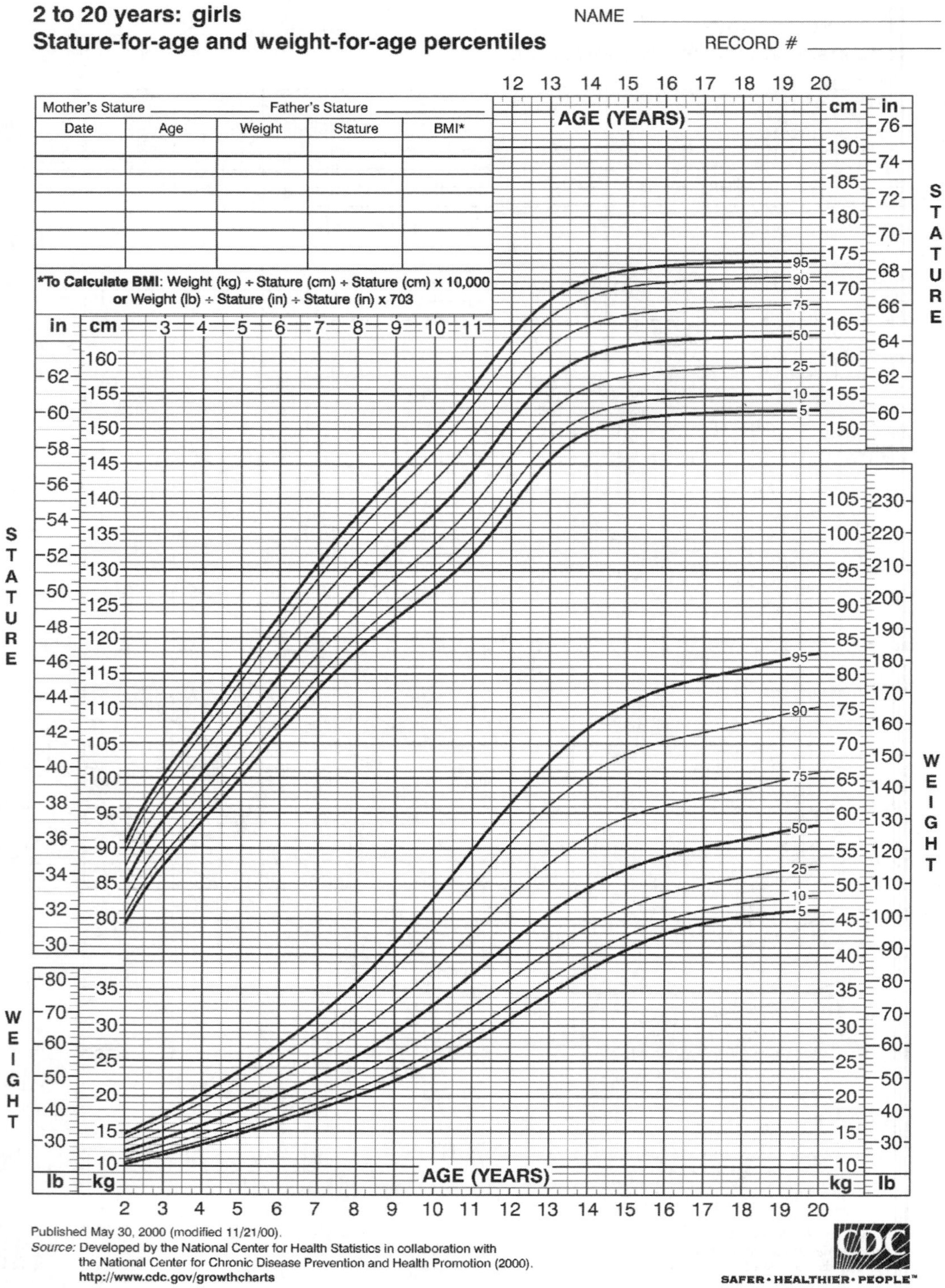

2 to 20 years: girls
Stature-for-age and weight-for-age percentiles
NAME
RECORD #
Mother's Stature
Father's Stature
Date
Age
Weight
Stature
BMI*
*To Calculate BMI: Weight (kg) ÷ Stature (cm) ÷ Stature (cm) x 10,000
or Weight (lb) ÷ Stature (in) ÷ Stature (in) x 703
AGE (YEARS)
STATURE
WEIGHT
cm
in
kg
lb
Published May 30, 2000 (modified 11/21/00).
Source: Developed by the National Center for Health Statistics in collaboration with the National Center for Chronic Disease Prevention and Health Promotion (2000).
http://www.cdc.gov/growthcharts
CDC
SAFER • HEALTHIER • PEOPLE™

FIGURE B-7 2 to 20 years: girls. Stature-for-age and weight-for-age percentiles.

2 to 20 years: girls
Body mass index–for-age percentiles

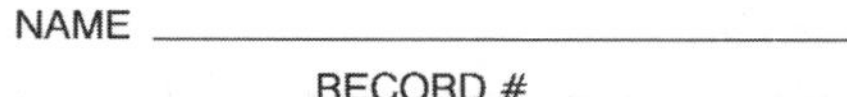

Date	Age	Weight	Stature	BMI*	Comments

***To Calculate BMI:** Weight (kg) ÷ Stature (cm) ÷ Stature (cm) x 10,000
or Weight (lb) ÷ Stature (in) ÷ Stature (in) x 703

BMI

35 34 33 32 31 30 29 28 27 26 25 24 23 22 21 20 19 18 17 16 15 14 13 12

95 90 85 75 50 25 10 5

kg/m²

AGE (YEARS)

2 3 4 5 6 7 8 9 10 11 12 13 14 15 16 17 18 19 20

Published May 30, 2000 (modified 10/16/00).
Source: Developed by the National Center for Health Statistics in collaboration with the National Center for Chronic Disease Prevention and Health Promotion (2000).
http://www.cdc.gov/growthcharts

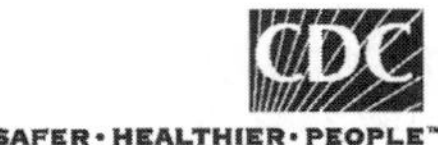

FIGURE B-8 2 to 20 years: girls. Body mass index–for-age percentiles.

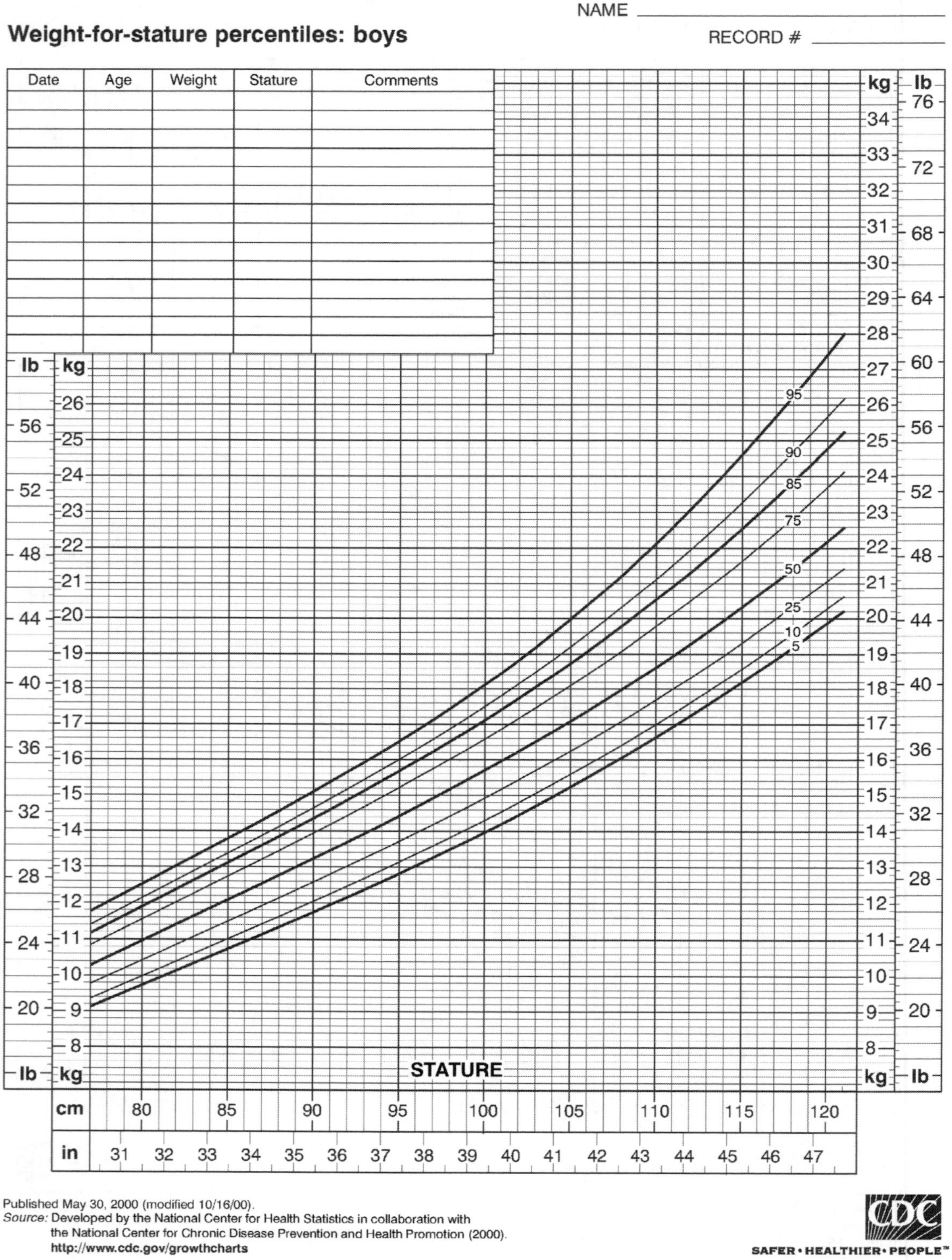
NAME
Weight-for-stature percentiles: boys
RECORD #
Date
Age
Weight
Stature
Comments
kg
lb
STATURE
cm
in
95
90
85
75
50
25
10
5
Published May 30, 2000 (modified 10/16/00).
Source: Developed by the National Center for Health Statistics in collaboration with the National Center for Chronic Disease Prevention and Health Promotion (2000).
http://www.cdc.gov/growthcharts
CDC
SAFER • HEALTHIER • PEOPLE™

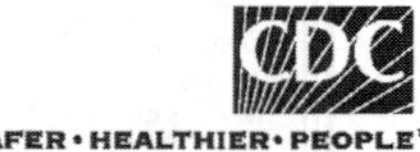

FIGURE B-9 Weight-for-stature percentiles: boys.

NAME ______________________

RECORD # ____________

Weight-for-stature percentiles: girls

Date	Age	Weight	Stature	Comments

Published May 30, 2000 (modified 10/16/00).
Source: Developed by the National Center for Health Statistics in collaboration with the National Center for Chronic Disease Prevention and Health Promotion (2000).
http://www.cdc.gov/growthcharts

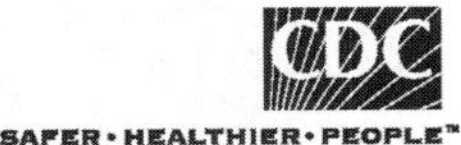

FIGURE B-10 Weight-for-stature percentiles: girls.

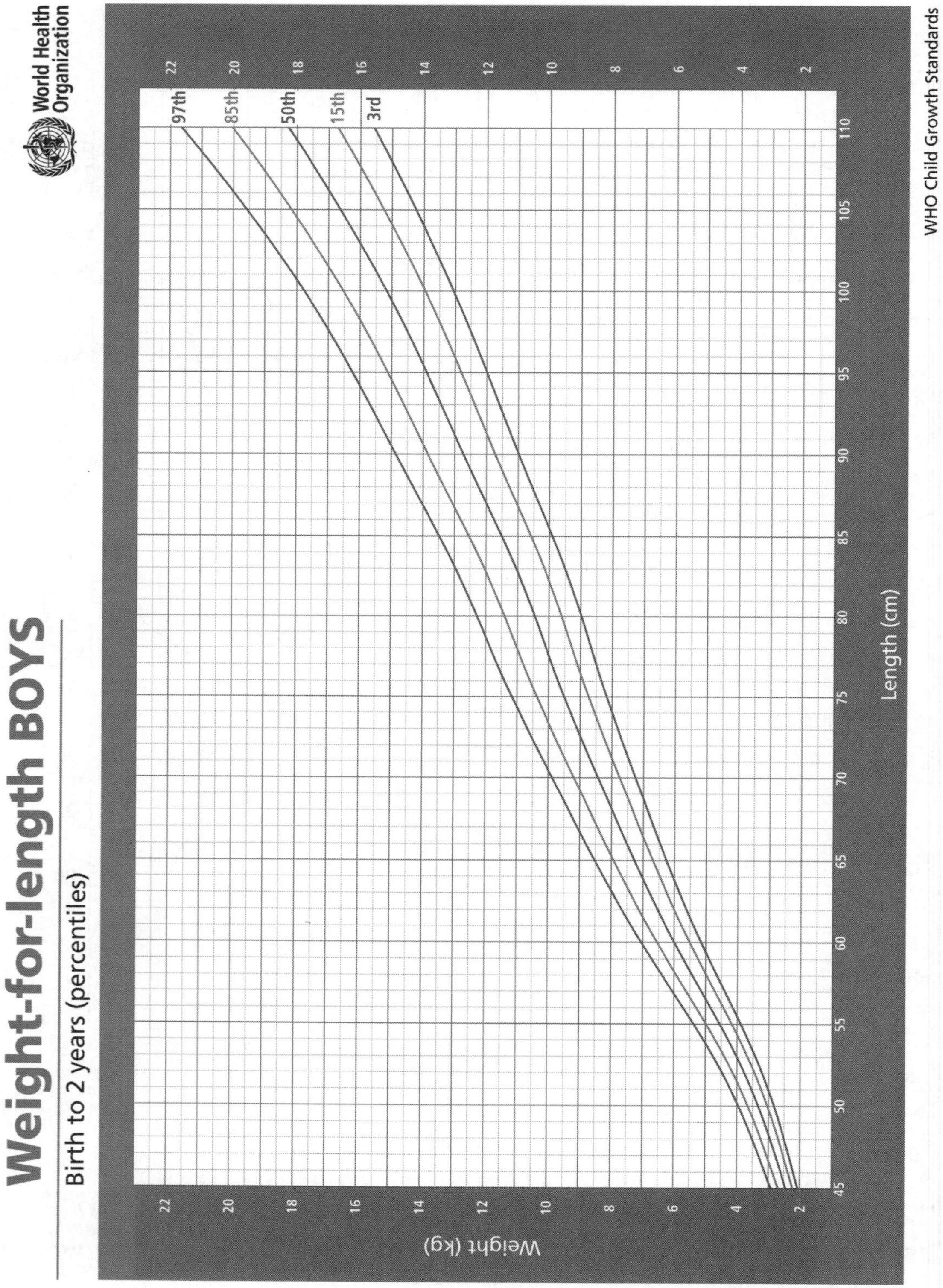
Weight-for-length BOYS
Birth to 2 years (percentiles)
World Health Organization
97th
85th
50th
15th
3rd
Weight (kg)
Length (cm)
45 50 55 60 65 70 75 80 85 90 95 100 105 110
2 4 6 8 10 12 14 16 18 20 22
WHO Child Growth Standards

FIGURE B-11 Weight-for-length: percentile boys.

Source: World Health Organization.

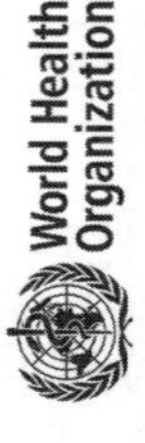

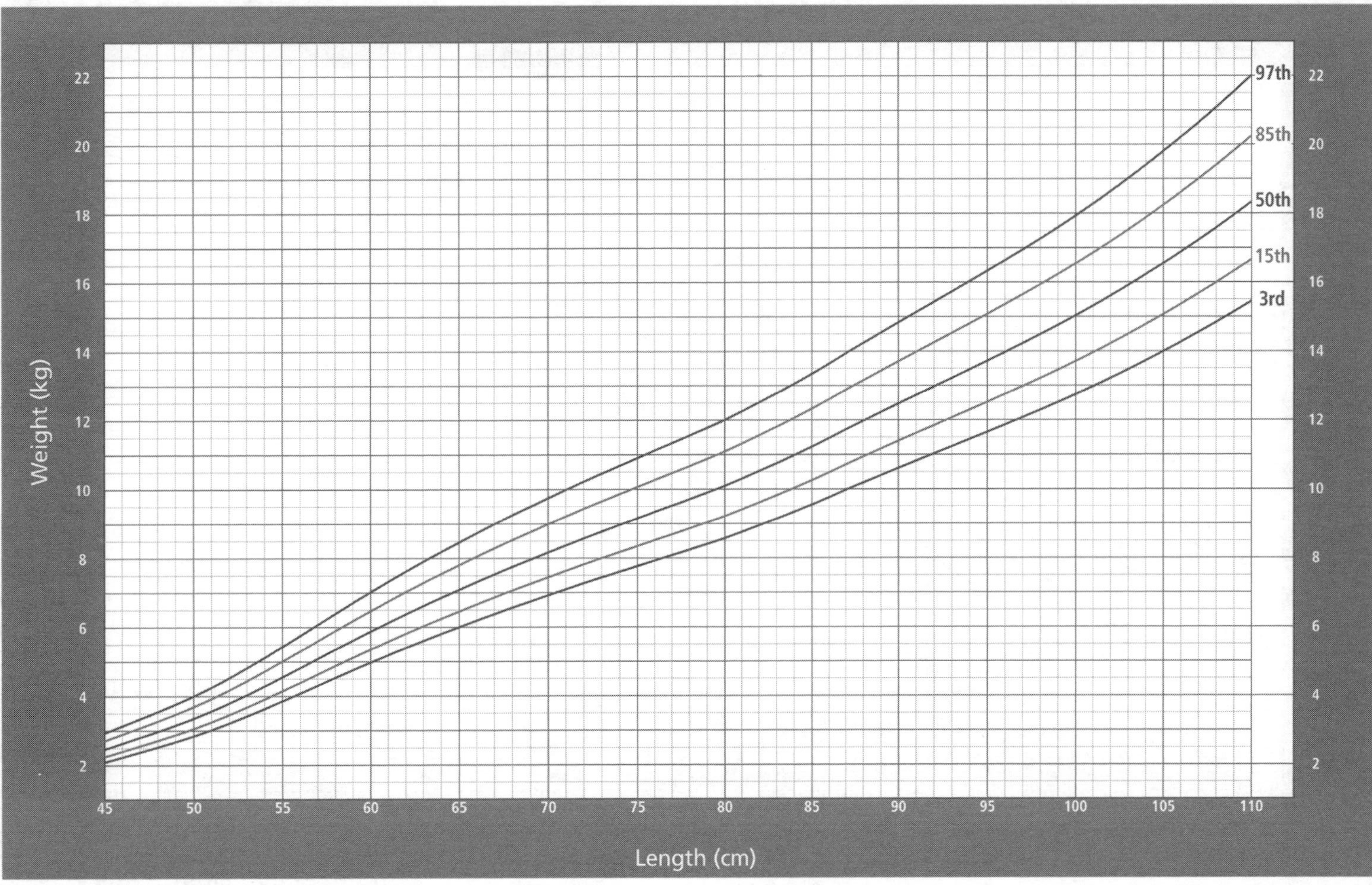

FIGURE B-12 Weight-for-length: percentile girls.

Source: World Health Organization.

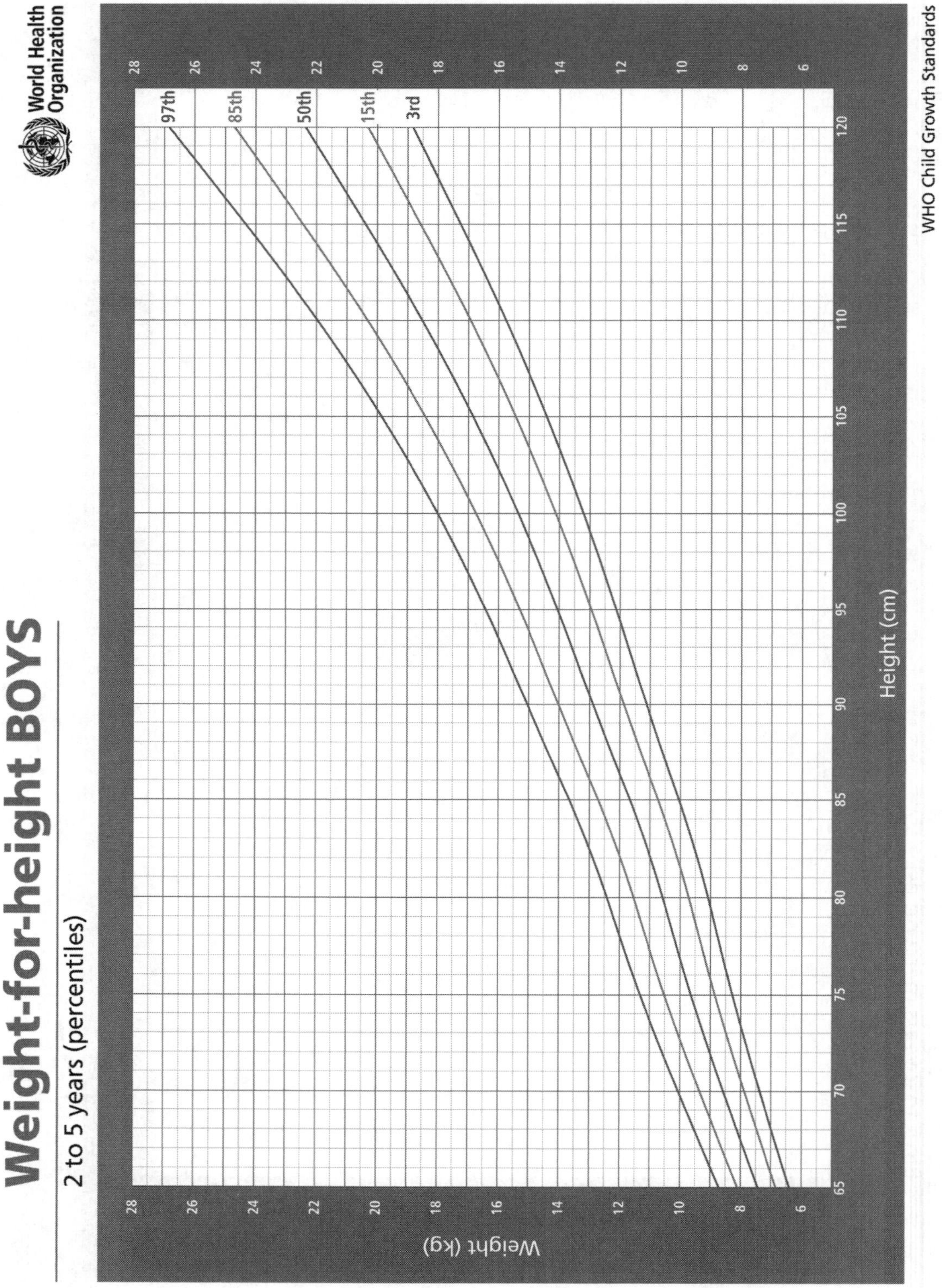
Weight-for-height BOYS
2 to 5 years (percentiles)
World Health Organization
97th
85th
50th
15th
3rd
Weight (kg)
Height (cm)
6
8
10
12
14
16
18
20
22
24
26
28
65
70
75
80
85
90
95
100
105
110
115
120
WHO Child Growth Standards

FIGURE B-13 Weight-for-height: boys.

Source: World Health Organization.

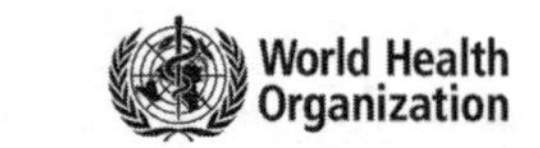

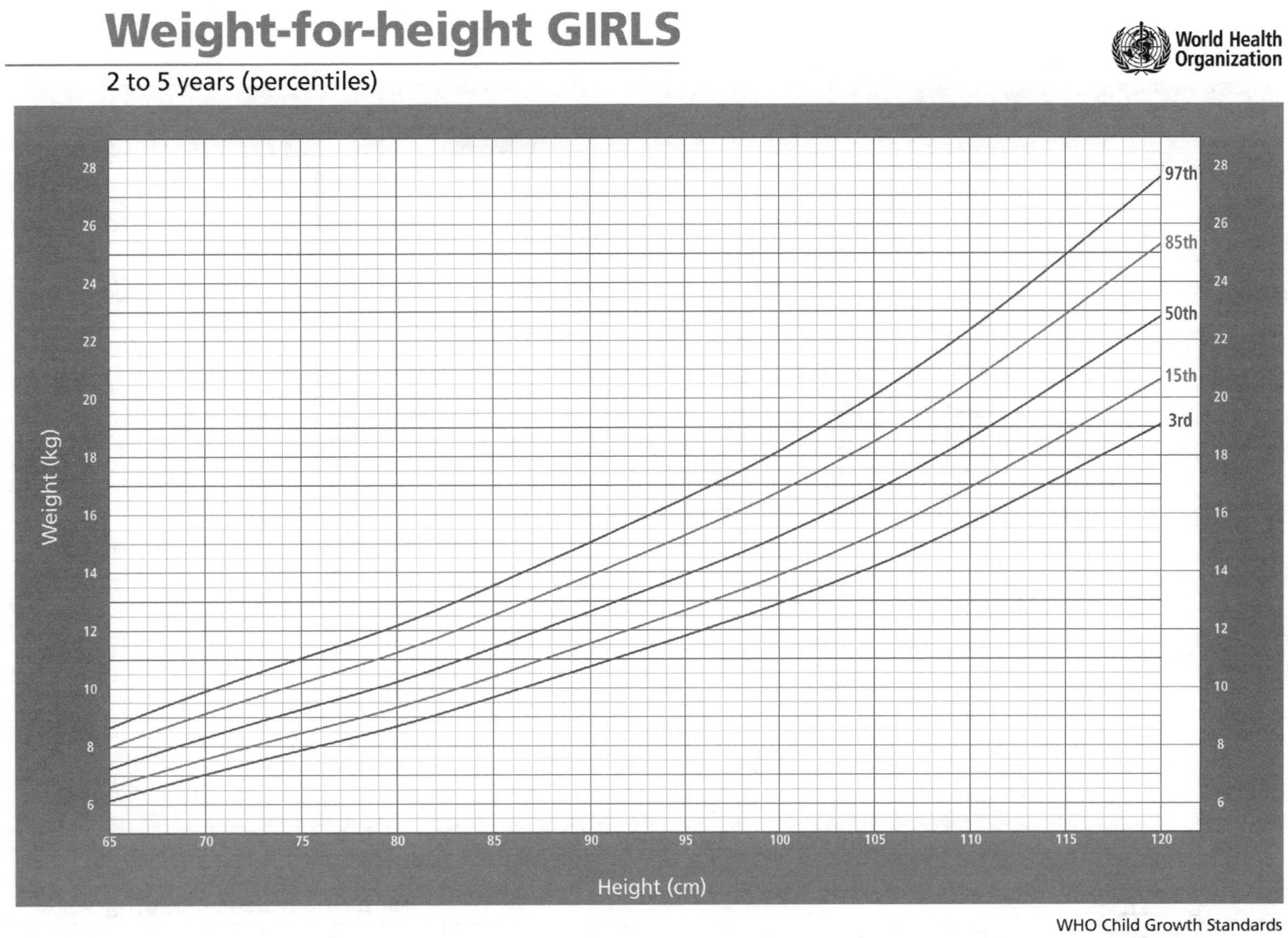

Weight-for-height GIRLS

2 to 5 years (percentiles)

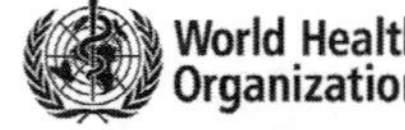

FIGURE B-14 Weight-for-height: girls.

Source: World Health Organization.

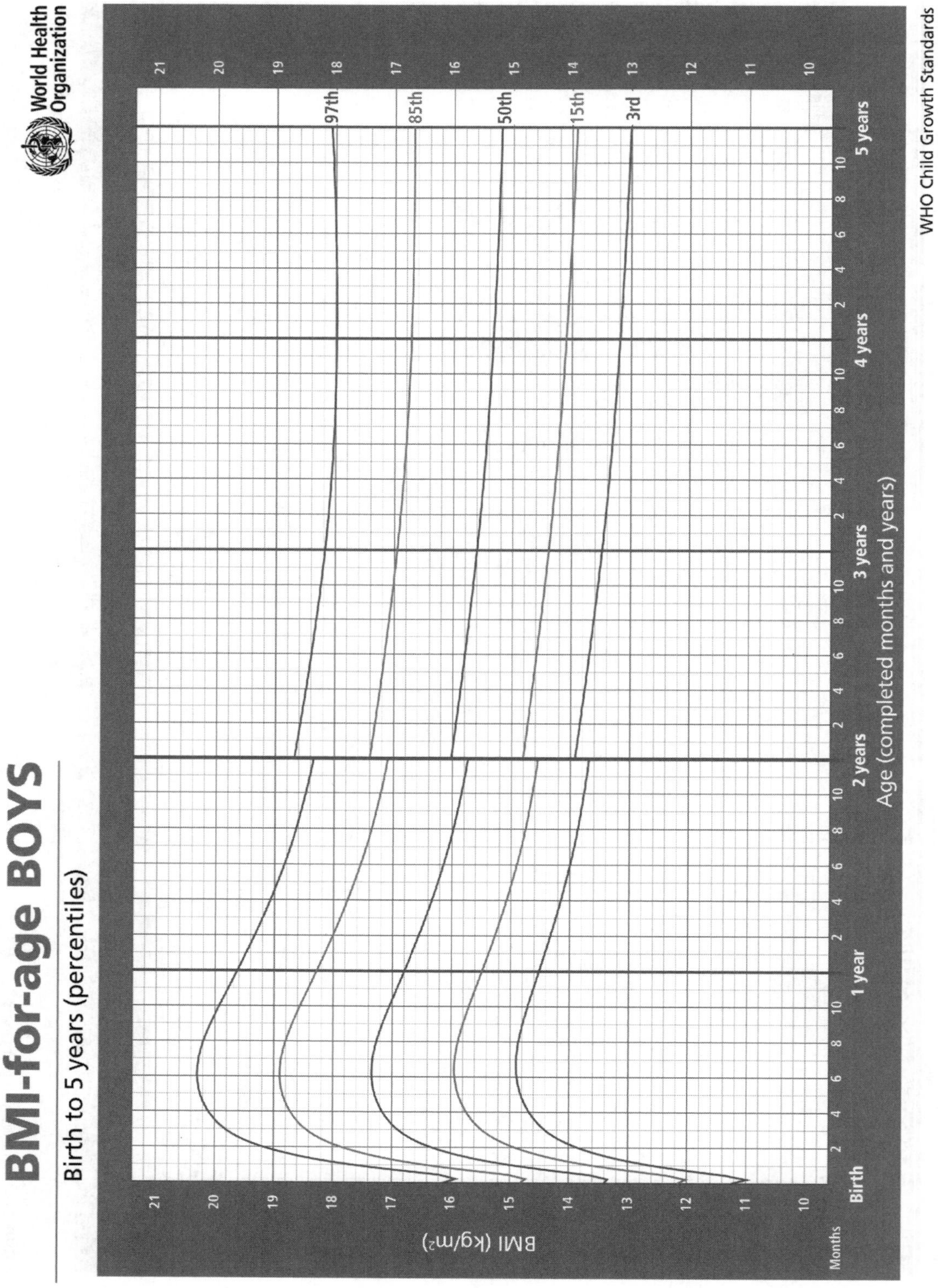

BMI-for-age BOYS

Birth to 5 years (percentiles)

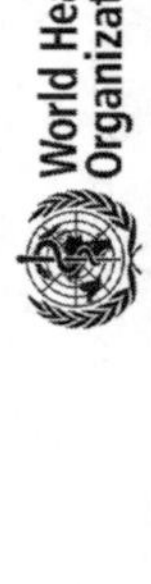

BMI (kg/m²)

21 20 19 18 17 16 15 14 13 12 11 10

97th 85th 50th 15th 3rd

Months Birth 2 4 6 8 10 1 year 2 4 6 8 10 2 years 2 4 6 8 10 3 years 2 4 6 8 10 4 years 2 4 6 8 10 5 years

Age (completed months and years)

WHO Child Growth Standards

FIGURE B-15 Body mass index: boys.

Source: World Health Organization.

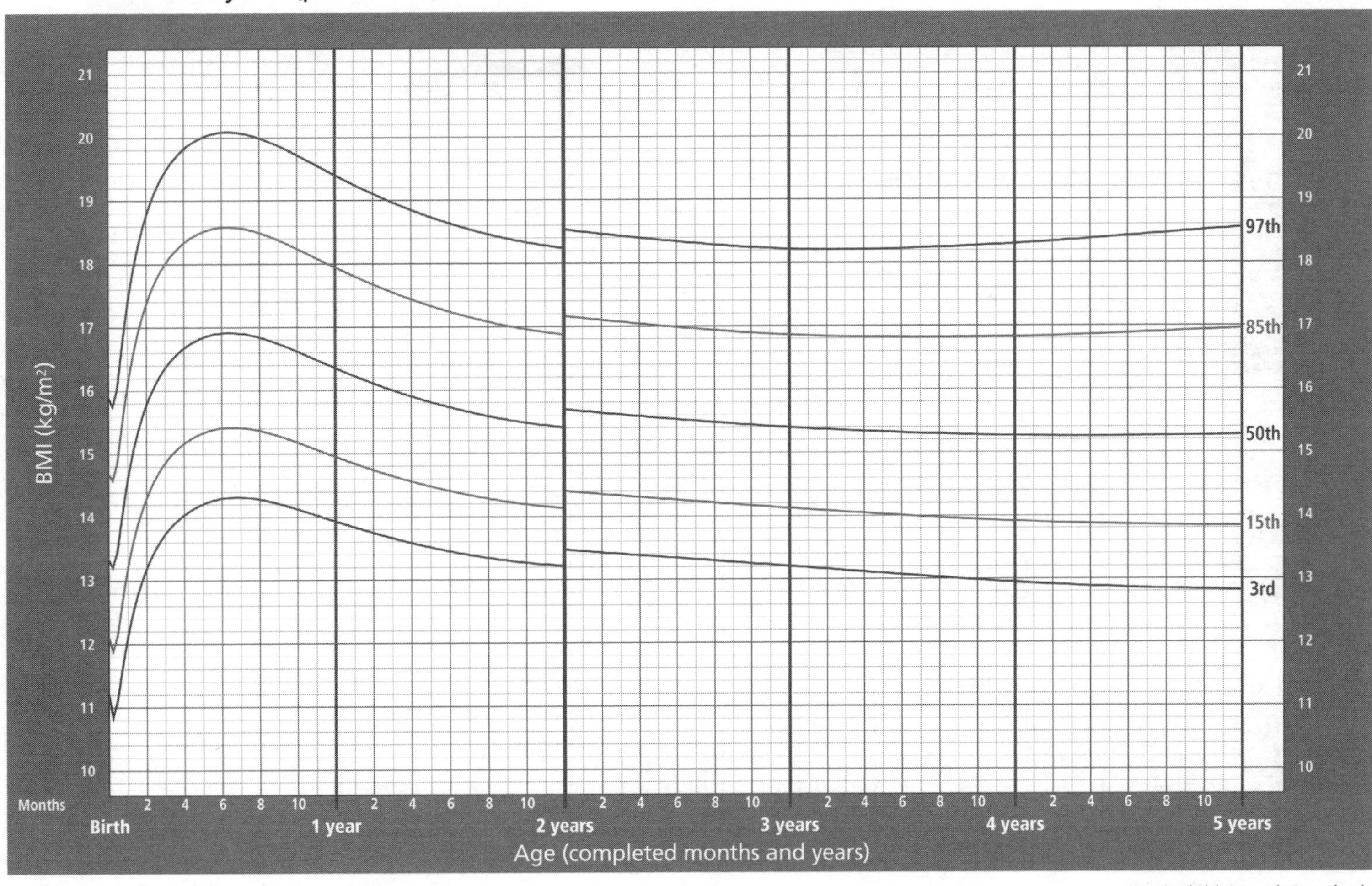

FIGURE B-16 Body mass index: girls.

Source: World Health Organization.

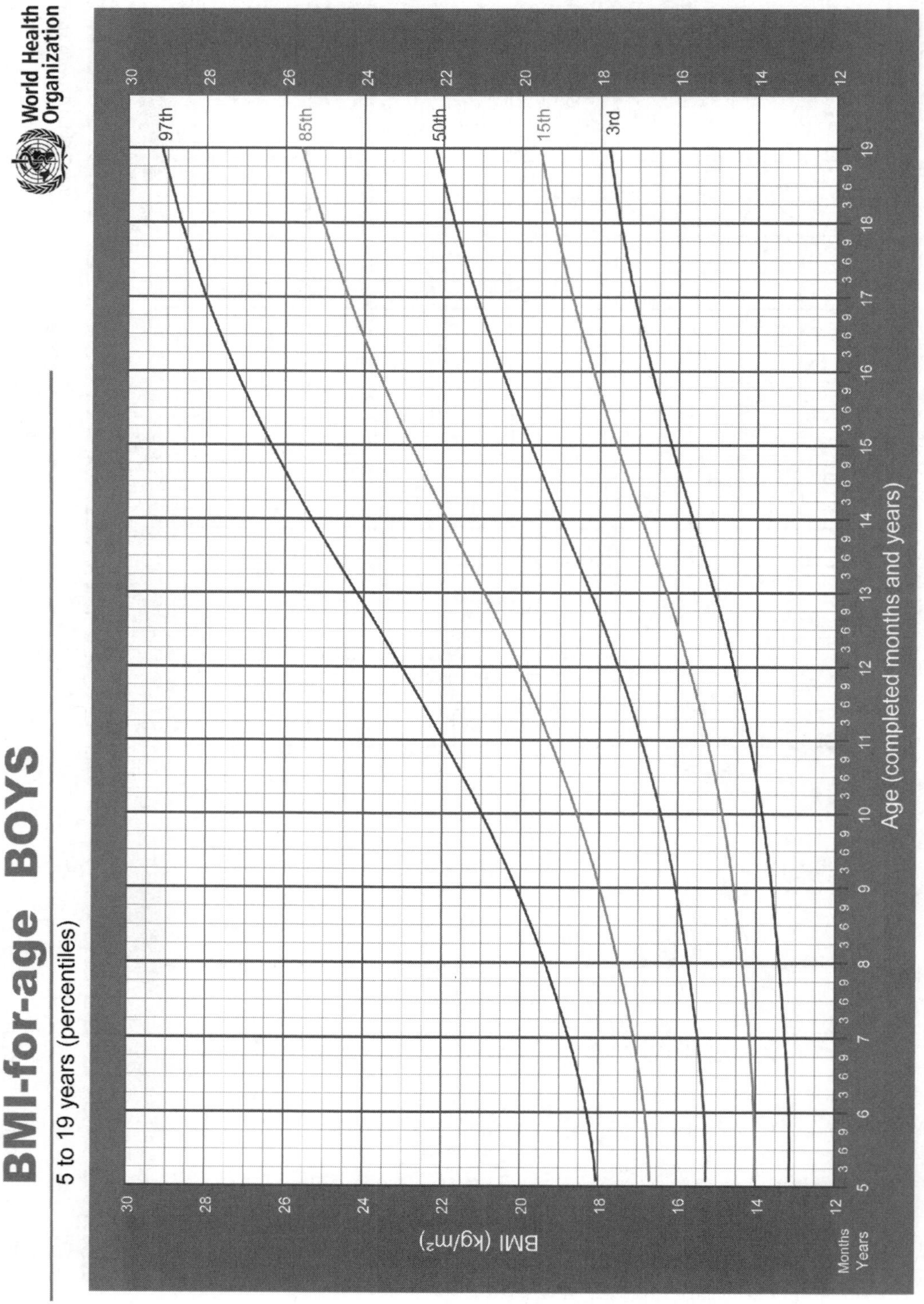

BMI-for-age BOYS
5 to 19 years (percentiles)
World Health Organization
97th
85th
50th
15th
3rd
BMI (kg/m²)
Age (completed months and years)
Months
Years
2007 WHO Reference

FIGURE B-17 Body mass index: boys.

Source: World Health Organization.

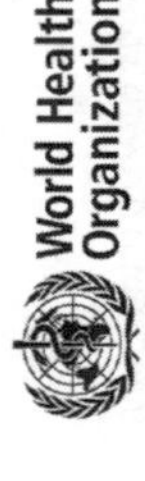

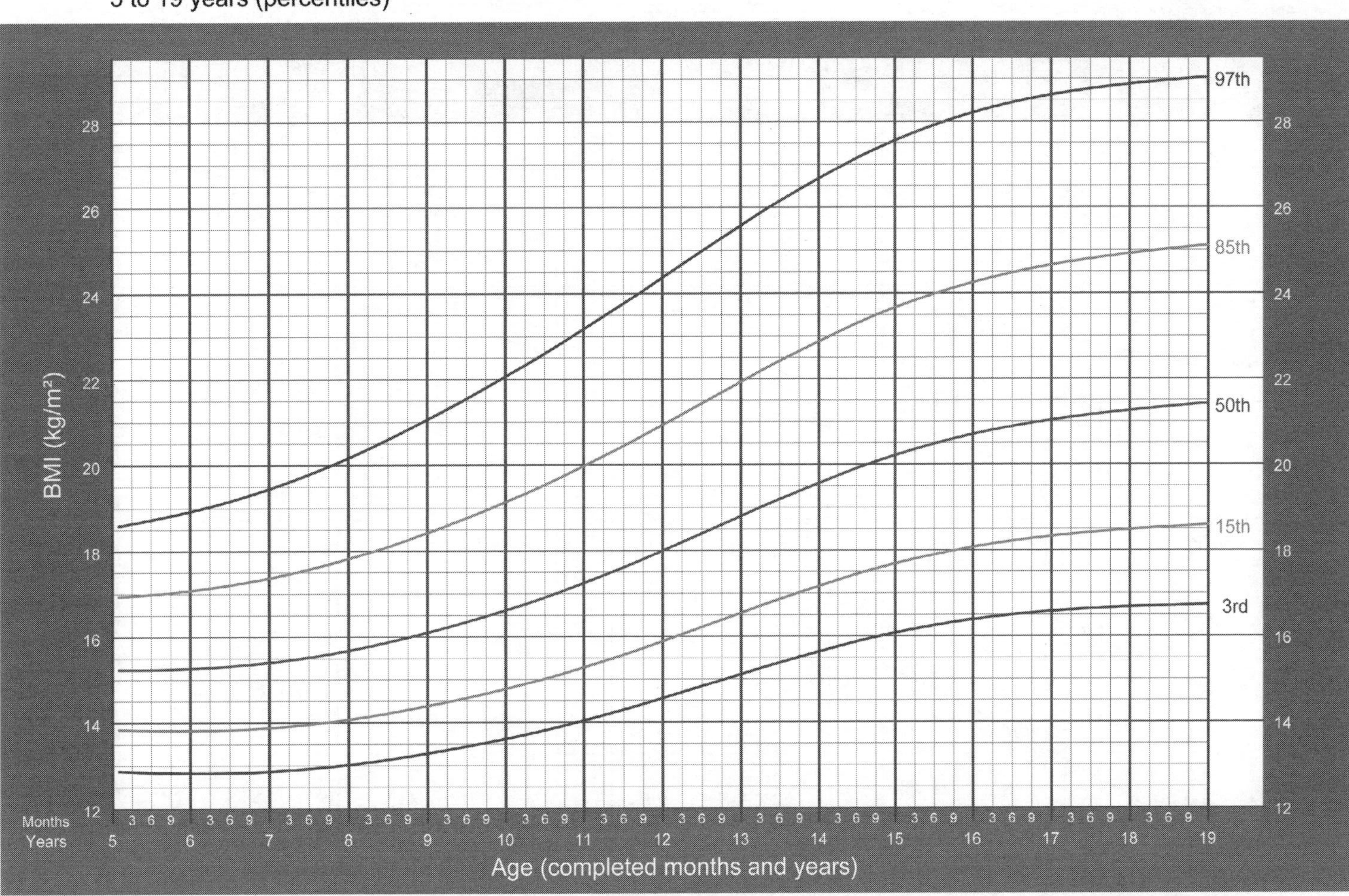

FIGURE B-18 Body mass index: girls.

Source: World Health Organization.

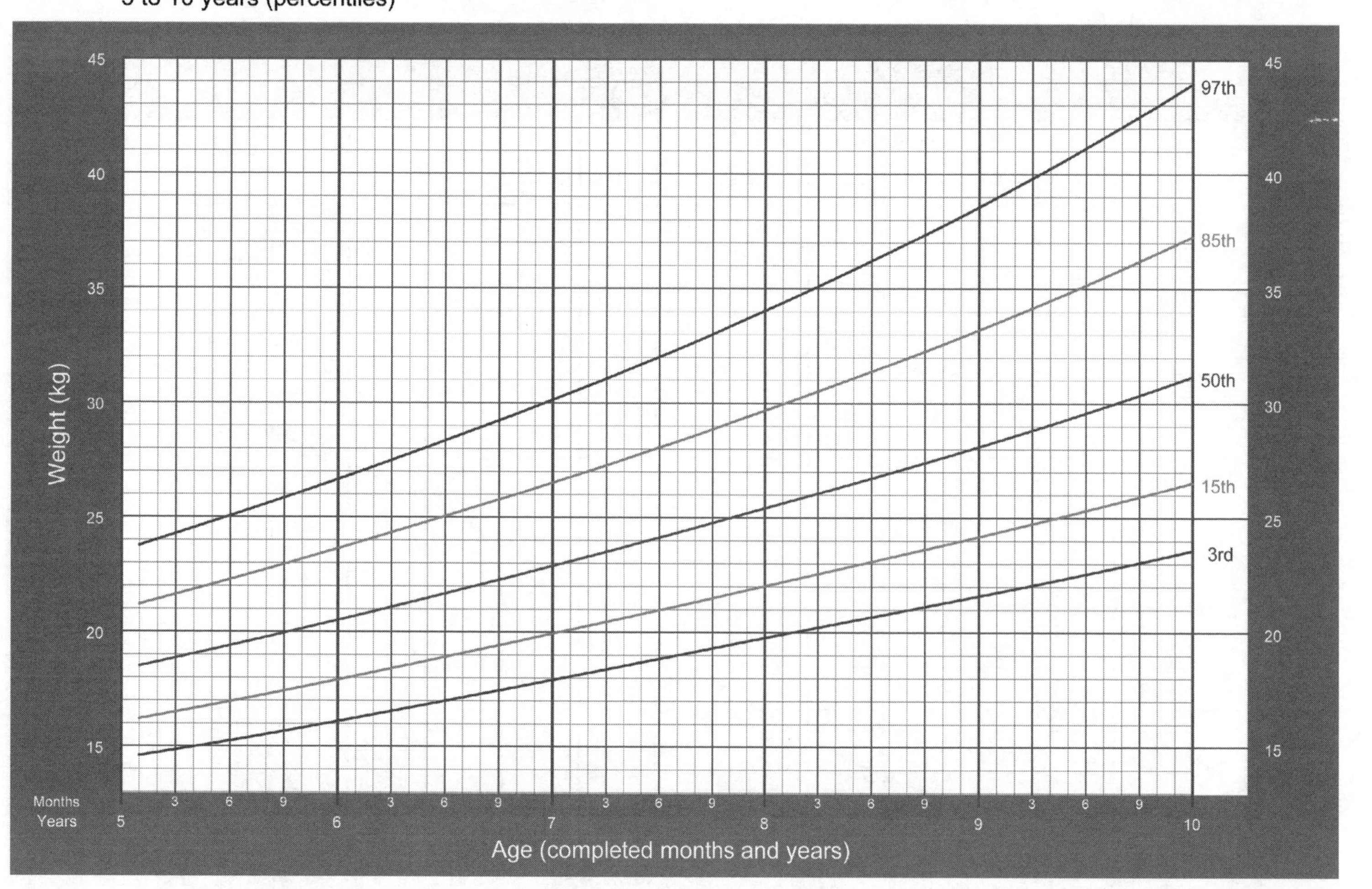

FIGURE B-19 Weight-for-age: boys.

Source: World Health Organization.

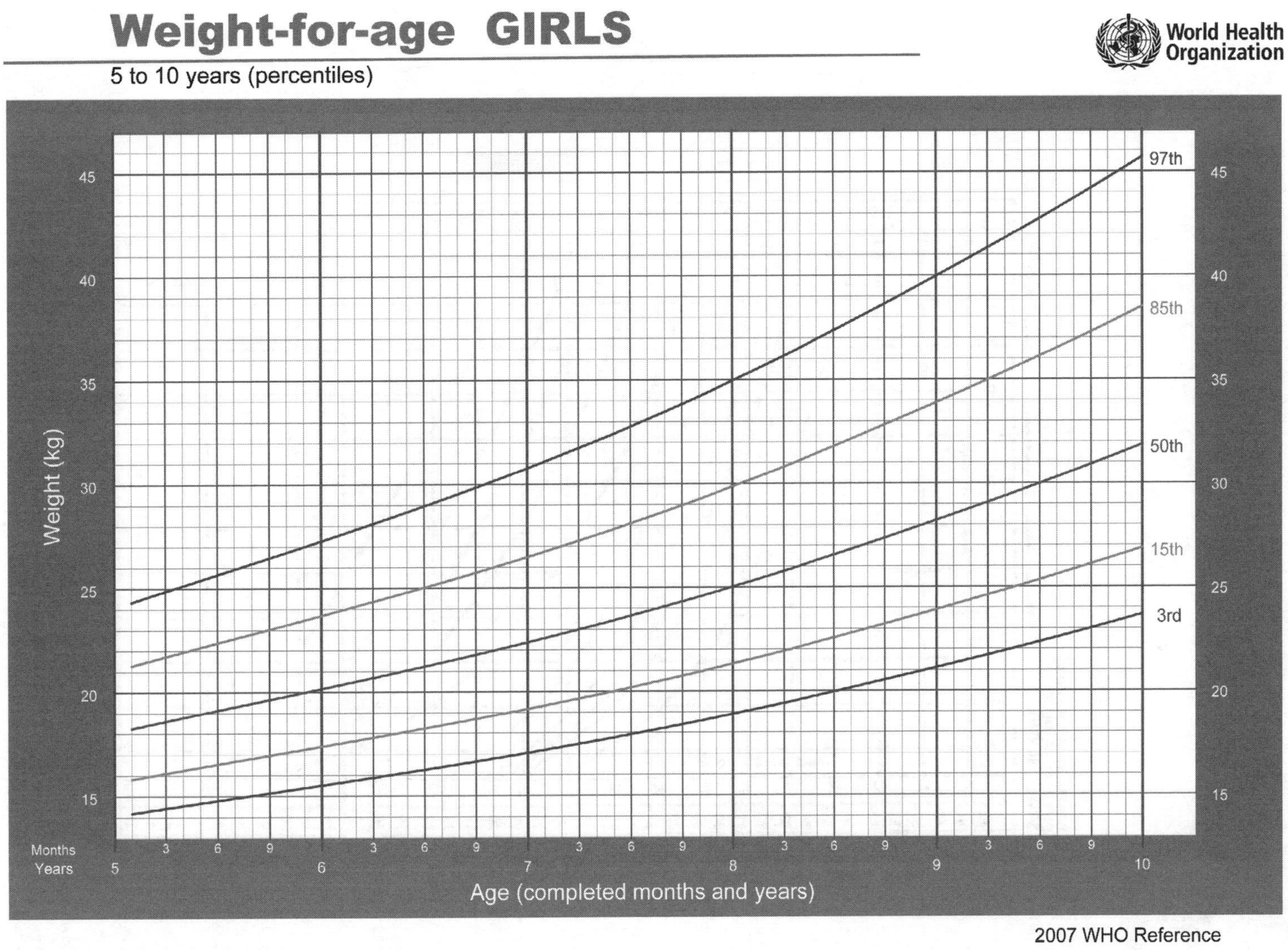
Weight-for-age GIRLS
5 to 10 years (percentiles)
World Health Organization
Weight (kg)
45
40
35
30
25
20
15
97th
85th
50th
15th
3rd
Months
Years
5
3
6
9
6
7
8
9
10
Age (completed months and years)
2007 WHO Reference

FIGURE B-20 Weight-for-age: girls.

Source: World Health Organization.

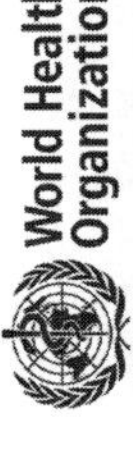

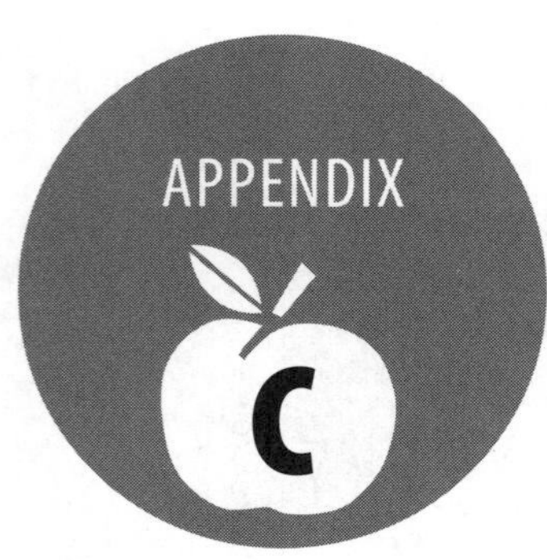

Down Syndrome Growth Charts

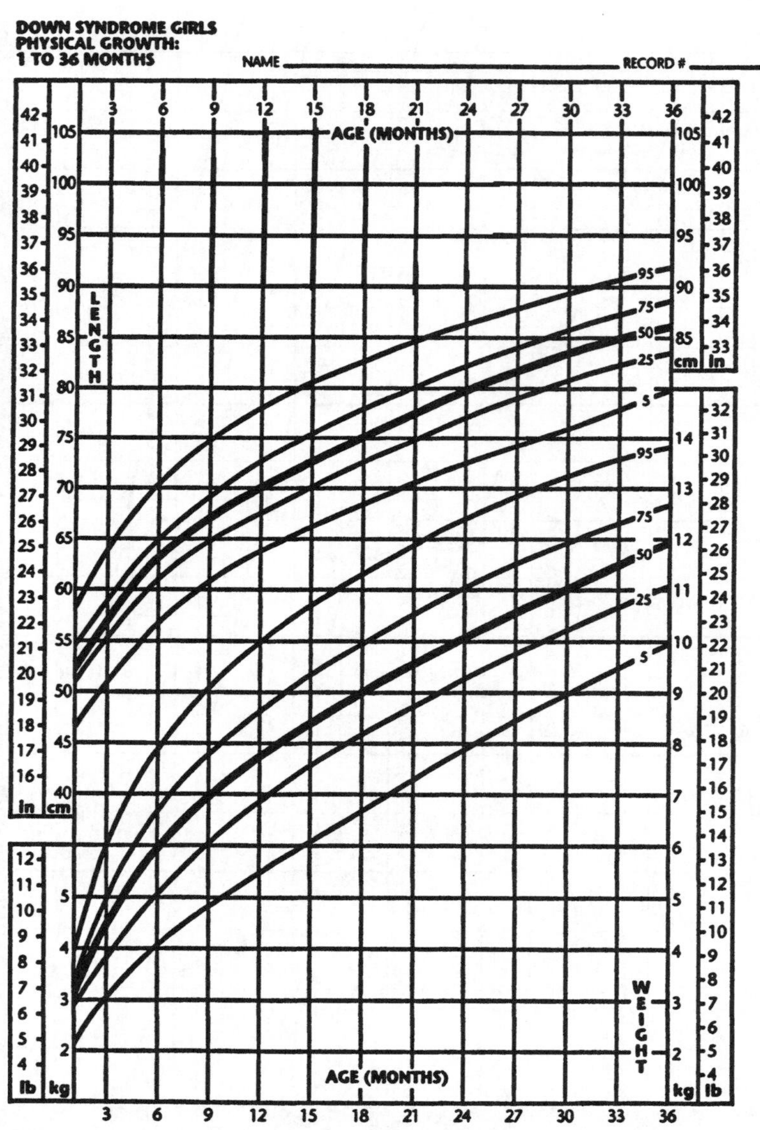

FIGURE C-1 Down syndrome, length and weight for girls, 1 to 36 months.

Source: Reprinted with permission from Crocker CC et al., Growth Charts for Children with Down Syndrome: 1 Month to 18 Years of Age, *Pediatrics*, Vol. 81, pp. 102–110; © 1988, American Academy of Pediatrics.

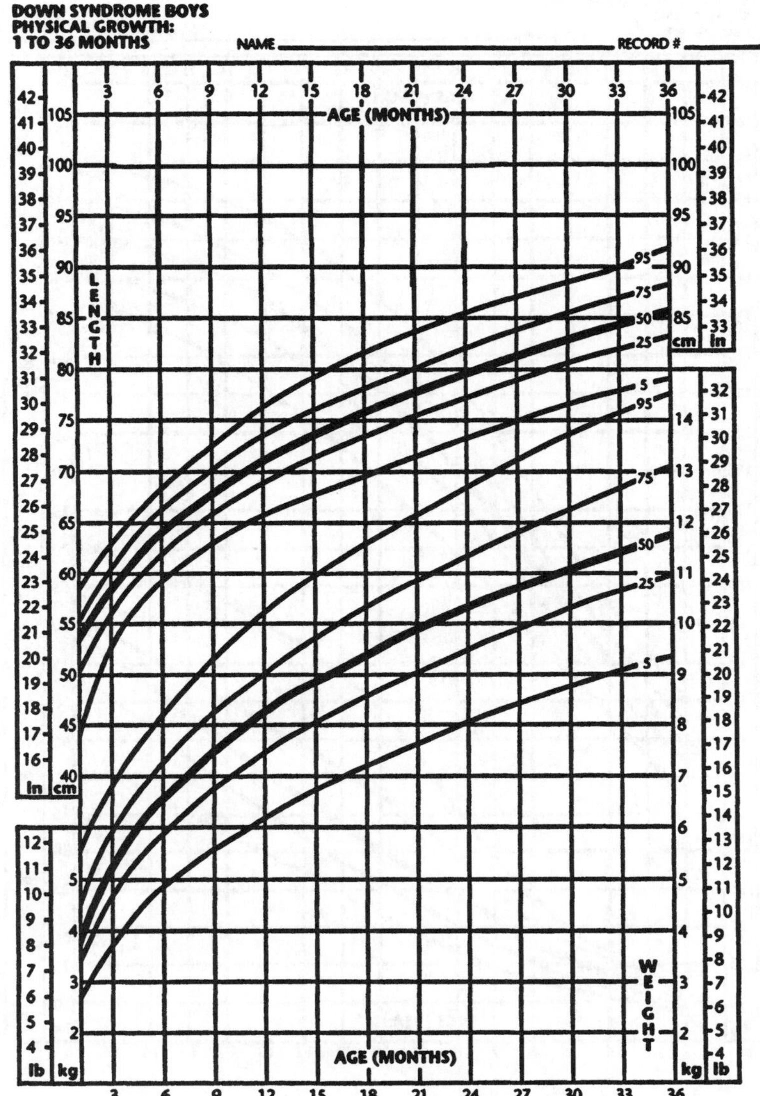

FIGURE C-2 Down syndrome, length and weight for boys, 1 to 36 months.

Source: Reprinted with permission from Crocker CC et al., Growth Charts for Children with Down Syndrome: 1 Month to 18 Years of Age, *Pediatrics*, Vol. 81, pp. 102–110; © 1988, American Academy of Pediatrics.

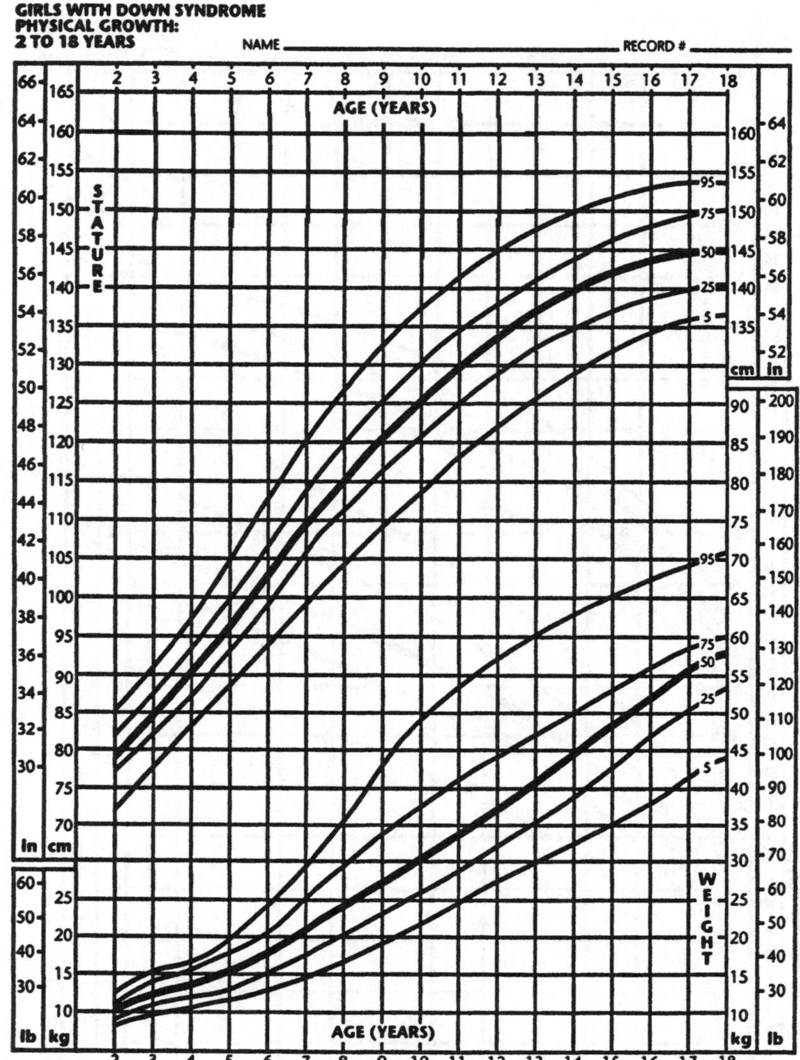

FIGURE C-3 Down syndrome, height and weight for girls, 2 to 18 years.

Source: Reprinted with permission from Crocker CC et al., Growth Charts for Children with Down Syndrome: 1 Month to 18 Years of Age, *Pediatrics*, Vol. 81, pp. 102–110; © 1988, American Academy of Pediatrics.

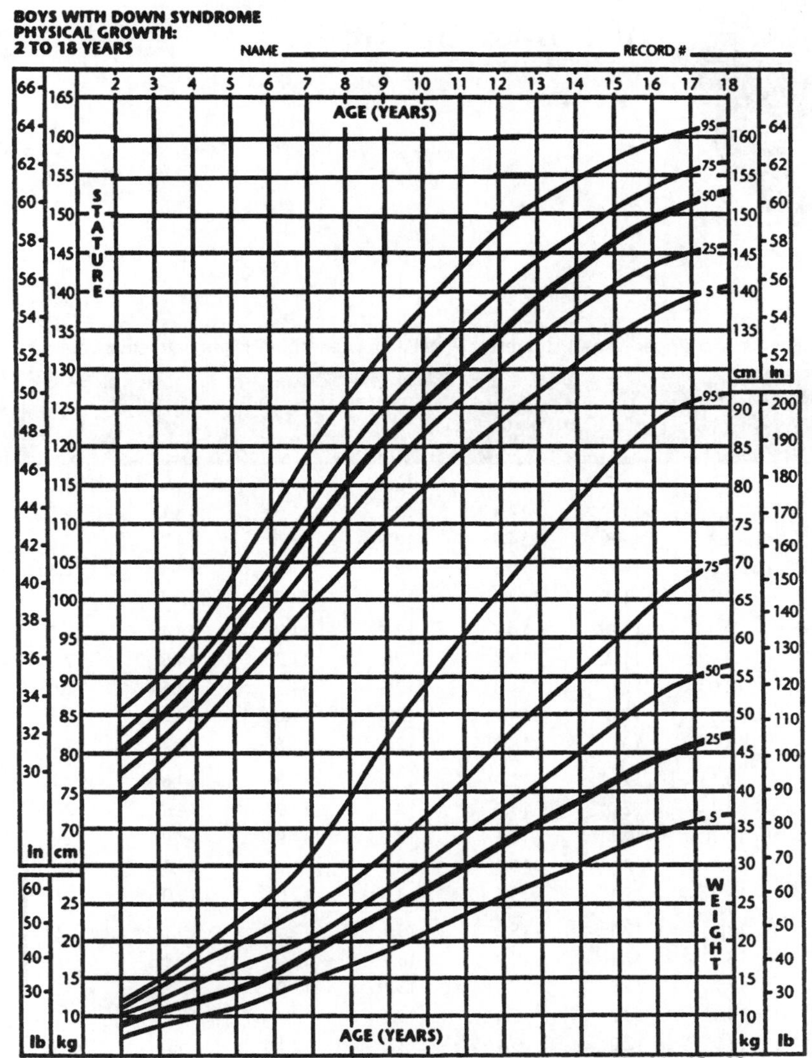

FIGURE C-4 Down syndrome, height and weight for boys, 2 to 18 years.

Source: Reprinted with permission from Crocker CC et al., Growth Charts for Children with Down Syndrome: 1 Month to 18 Years of Age, *Pediatrics*, Vol. 81, pp. 102–110; © 1988, American Academy of Pediatrics.

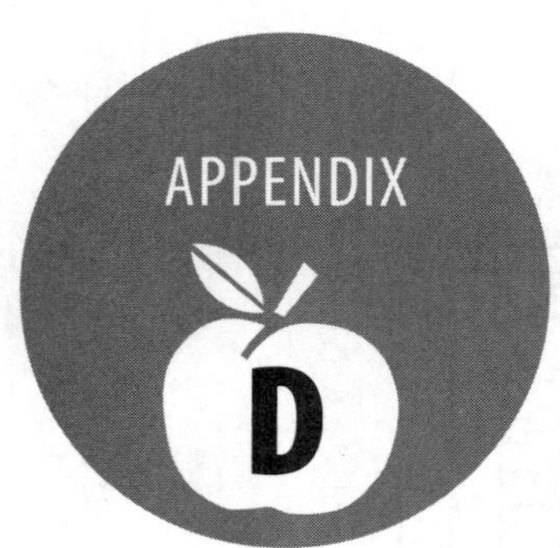

Arm Measurements

TABLE D-1 Arm Measurements: Mid-Upper-Arm-Circumference (MUAC) for Length or Height Reference Data

Length/ Height* (cm)	Boys			Combined Sexes			Girls			Length/ Height* (cm)
	Median	−2 SD	−3 SD	Median	−2 SD	−3 SD	Median	−2 SD	−3 SD	
65.0	14.6	12.7	11.7	14.3	12.4	11.5	14.0	12.1	11.2	65.0
65.5	14.7	12.7	11.8	14.4	12.5	11.5	14.1	12.2	11.2	65.5
66.0	14.7	12.8	11.8	14.5	12.5	11.6	14.2	12.3	11.3	66.0
66.5	14.8	12.8	11.8	14.5	12.6	11.6	14.3	12.3	11.3	66.5
67.0	14.9	12.9	11.9	14.6	12.6	11.6	14.4	12.4	11.4	67.0
67.5	14.9	12.9	11.9	14.7	12.7	11.7	14.4	12.4	11.4	67.5
68.0	15.0	12.9	11.9	14.7	12.7	11.7	14.5	12.5	11.5	68.0
68.5	15.0	13.0	12.0	14.8	12.8	11.7	14.6	12.6	11.5	68.5
69.0	15.1	13.0	12.0	14.9	12.8	11.8	14.7	12.6	11.6	69.0
69.5	15.1	13.0	12.0	14.9	12.8	11.8	14.7	12.7	11.6	69.5
70.0	15.1	13.1	12.0	15.0	12.9	11.8	14.8	12.7	11.7	70.0
70.5	15.2	13.1	12.0	15.0	12.9	11.9	14.8	12.8	11.7	70.5
71.0	15.2	13.1	12.1	15.1	13.0	11.9	14.9	12.8	11.7	71.0
71.5	15.3	13.1	12.1	15.1	13.0	11.9	15.0	12.8	11.8	71.5
72.0	15.3	13.2	12.1	15.2	13.0	12.0	15.0	12.9	11.8	72.0
72.5	15.3	13.2	12.1	15.2	13.1	12.0	15.1	12.9	11.8	72.5
73.0	15.4	13.2	12.1	15.2	13.1	12.0	15.1	13.0	11.9	73.0
73.5	15.4	13.2	12.2	15.3	13.1	12.0	15.2	13.0	11.9	73.5
74.0	15.4	13.3	12.2	15.3	13.1	12.1	15.2	13.0	11.9	74.0
74.5	15.5	13.3	12.2	15.4	13.2	12.1	15.2	13.1	12.0	74.5
75.0	15.5	13.3	12.2	15.4	13.2	12.1	15.3	13.1	12.0	75.0
75.5	15.5	13.3	12.2	15.4	13.2	12.1	15.3	13.1	12.0	75.5
76.0	15.6	13.4	12.2	15.5	13.3	12.2	15.4	13.2	12.1	76.0
76.5	15.6	13.4	12.3	15.5	13.3	12.2	15.4	13.2	12.1	76.5
77.0	15.6	13.4	12.3	15.5	13.3	12.2	15.4	13.2	12.1	77.0
77.5	15.6	13.4	12.3	15.6	13.3	12.2	15.5	13.3	12.1	77.5
78.0	15.7	13.4	12.3	15.6	13.4	12.2	15.5	13.3	12.2	78.0
78.5	15.7	13.4	12.3	15.6	13.4	12.3	15.6	13.3	12.2	78.5
79.0	15.7	13.5	12.3	15.6	13.4	12.3	15.6	13.3	12.2	79.0
79.5	15.7	13.5	12.4	15.7	13.4	12.3	15.6	13.4	12.2	79.5
80.0	15.8	13.5	12.4	15.7	13.4	12.3	15.6	13.4	12.3	80.0
80.5	15.8	13.5	12.4	15.7	13.5	12.3	15.7	13.4	12.3	80.5
81.0	15.8	13.5	12.4	15.8	13.5	12.4	15.7	13.4	12.3	81.0
81.5	15.8	13.6	12.4	15.8	13.5	12.4	15.7	13.5	12.3	81.5
82.0	15.9	13.6	12.4	15.8	13.5	12.4	15.8	13.5	12.3	82.0

TABLE D-1 *(Continued)*

Length/ Height* (cm)	Boys			Combined Sexes			Girls			Length/ Height* (cm)
	Median	−2 SD	−3 SD	Median	−2 SD	−3 SD	Median	−2 SD	−3 SD	
82.5	15.9	13.6	12.5	15.8	13.6	12.4	15.8	13.5	12.4	82.5
83.0	15.9	13.6	12.5	15.9	13.6	12.4	15.8	13.5	12.4	83.0
83.5	15.9	13.6	12.5	15.9	13.6	12.5	15.8	13.6	12.4	83.5
84.0	15.9	13.7	12.5	15.9	13.6	12.5	15.9	13.6	12.4	84.0
84.5	16.0	13.7	12.5	15.9	13.6	12.5	15.9	13.6	12.5	84.5
85.0	16.0	13.7	12.5	15.9	13.6	12.5	15.9	13.6	12.5	85.0
85.5	16.0	13.7	12.6	16.0	13.7	12.5	15.9	13.6	12.5	85.5
86.0	16.0	13.7	12.6	16.0	13.7	12.5	15.9	13.7	12.5	86.0
86.5	16.0	13.7	12.6	16.0	13.7	12.6	16.0	13.7	12.5	86.5
87.0	16.1	13.8	12.6	16.0	13.7	12.6	16.0	13.7	12.5	87.0
87.5	16.1	13.8	12.6	16.0	13.7	12.6	16.0	13.7	12.6	87.5
88.0	16.1	13.8	12.6	16.1	13.8	12.6	16.0	13.7	12.6	88.0
88.5	16.1	13.8	12.7	16.1	13.8	12.6	16.1	13.8	12.6	88.5
89.0	16.1	13.8	12.7	16.1	13.8	12.7	16.1	13.8	12.6	89.0
89.5	16.2	13.9	12.7	16.1	13.8	12.7	16.1	13.8	12.7	89.5
90.0	16.2	13.9	12.7	16.2	13.9	12.7	16.1	13.8	12.7	90.0
90.5	16.2	13.9	12.8	16.2	13.9	12.7	16.2	13.8	12.7	90.5
91.0	16.2	13.9	12.8	16.2	13.9	12.7	16.2	13.9	12.7	91.0
91.5	16.3	14.0	12.8	16.2	13.9	12.8	16.2	13.9	12.7	91.5
92.0	16.3	14.0	12.8	16.3	13.9	12.8	16.2	13.9	12.8	92.0
92.5	16.3	14.0	12.9	16.3	14.0	12.8	16.2	13.9	12.8	92.5
93.0	16.3	14.0	12.9	16.3	14.0	12.8	16.3	14.0	12.8	93.0
93.5	16.4	14.1	12.9	16.3	14.0	12.9	16.3	14.0	12.8	93.5
94.0	16.4	14.1	12.9	16.4	14.0	12.9	16.3	14.0	12.8	94.0
94.5	16.4	14.1	13.0	16.4	14.1	12.9	16.3	14.0	12.9	94.5
95.0	16.4	14.1	13.0	16.4	14.1	12.9	16.4	14.1	12.9	95.0
95.5	16.5	14.2	13.0	16.4	14.1	13.0	16.4	14.1	12.9	95.5
96.0	16.5	14.2	13.0	16.5	14.1	13.0	16.4	14.1	12.9	96.0
96.5	16.5	14.2	13.1	16.5	14.2	13.0	16.4	14.1	13.0	96.5
97.0	16.6	14.2	13.1	16.5	14.2	13.0	16.5	14.1	13.0	97.0
97.5	16.6	14.3	13.1	16.5	14.2	13.1	16.5	14.2	13.0	97.5
98.0	16.6	14.3	13.1	16.6	14.2	13.1	16.5	14.2	13.0	98.0
98.5	16.6	14.3	13.2	16.6	14.3	13.1	16.5	14.2	13.1	98.5
99.0	16.7	14.3	13.2	16.6	14.3	13.1	16.6	14.3	13.1	99.0
99.5	16.7	14.4	13.2	16.6	14.3	13.2	16.6	14.3	13.1	99.5
100.0	16.7	14.4	13.2	16.7	14.4	13.2	16.6	14.3	13.1	100.0
100.5	16.8	14.4	13.3	16.7	14.4	13.2	16.7	14.3	13.2	100.5
101.0	16.8	14.5	13.3	16.7	14.4	13.2	16.7	14.4	13.2	101.0
101.5	16.8	14.5	13.3	16.8	14.4	13.3	16.7	14.4	13.2	101.5
102.0	16.9	14.5	13.4	16.8	14.5	13.3	16.7	14.4	13.2	102.0
102.5	16.9	14.6	13.4	16.8	14.5	13.3	16.8	14.4	13.3	102.5
103.0	16.9	14.6	13.4	16.9	14.5	13.4	16.8	14.5	13.3	103.0
103.5	16.9	14.6	13.4	16.9	14.6	13.4	16.8	14.5	13.3	103.5
104.0	17.0	14.6	13.5	16.9	14.6	13.4	16.9	14.5	13.4	104.0
104.5	17.0	14.7	13.5	17.0	14.6	13.4	16.9	14.6	13.4	104.5

(continued)

TABLE D-1 *(Continued)*

Length/ Height* (cm)	Boys			Combined Sexes			Girls			Length/ Height* (cm)
	Median	–2 SD	–3 SD	Median	–2 SD	–3 SD	Median	–2 SD	–3 SD	
105.0	17.0	14.7	13.5	17.0	14.6	13.5	16.9	14.6	13.4	105.0
105.5	17.1	14.7	13.6	17.0	14.7	13.5	17.0	14.6	13.4	105.5
106.0	17.1	14.8	13.6	17.1	14.7	13.5	17.0	14.6	13.5	106.0
106.5	17.1	14.8	13.6	17.1	14.7	13.6	17.0	14.7	13.5	106.5
107.0	17.2	14.8	13.6	17.1	14.8	13.6	17.1	14.7	13.5	107.0
107.5	17.2	14.8	13.7	17.2	14.8	13.6	17.1	14.7	13.6	107.5
108.0	17.3	14.9	13.7	17.2	14.8	13.6	17.1	14.8	13.6	108.0
108.5	17.3	14.9	13.7	17.2	14.9	13.7	17.2	14.8	13.6	108.5
109.0	17.3	14.9	13.7	17.3	14.9	13.7	17.2	14.8	13.6	109.0
109.5	17.4	15.0	13.8	17.3	14.9	13.7	17.3	14.9	13.7	109.5
110.0	17.4	15.0	13.8	17.4	15.0	13.8	17.3	14.9	13.7	110.0
110.5	17.4	15.0	13.8	17.4	15.0	13.8	17.3	14.9	13.7	110.5
111.0	17.5	15.1	13.9	17.4	15.0	13.8	17.4	15.0	13.8	111.0
111.5	17.5	15.1	13.9	17.5	15.0	13.8	17.4	15.0	13.8	111.5
112.0	17.5	15.1	13.9	17.5	15.1	13.9	17.5	15.0	13.8	112.0
112.5	17.6	15.1	13.9	17.6	15.1	13.9	17.5	15.1	13.9	112.5
113.0	17.6	15.2	14.0	17.6	15.1	13.9	17.6	15.1	13.9	113.0
113.5	17.7	15.2	14.0	17.6	15.2	14.0	17.6	15.2	13.9	113.5
114.0	17.7	15.2	14.0	17.7	15.2	14.0	17.7	15.2	14.0	114.0
114.5	17.7	15.3	14.0	17.7	15.2	14.0	17.7	15.2	14.0	114.5
115.0	17.8	15.3	14.0	17.8	15.3	14.0	17.8	15.3	14.0	115.0
115.5	17.8	15.3	14.1	17.8	15.3	14.1	17.8	15.3	14.1	115.5
116.0	17.9	15.4	14.1	17.9	15.3	14.1	17.9	15.3	14.1	116.0
116.5	17.9	15.4	14.1	17.9	15.4	14.1	17.9	15.4	14.1	116.5
117.0	18.0	15.4	14.1	18.0	15.4	14.1	18.0	15.4	14.1	117.0
117.5	18.0	15.4	14.2	18.0	15.4	14.2	18.0	15.5	14.2	117.5
118.0	18.0	15.5	14.2	18.1	15.5	14.2	18.1	15.5	14.2	118.0
118.5	18.1	15.5	14.2	18.1	15.5	14.2	18.1	15.5	14.2	118.5
119.0	18.1	15.5	14.2	18.2	15.6	14.3	18.2	15.6	14.3	119.0
119.5	18.2	15.6	14.2	18.2	15.6	14.3	18.2	15.6	14.3	119.5
120.0	18.2	15.6	14.3	18.3	15.6	14.3	18.3	15.7	14.3	120.0
120.5	18.3	15.6	14.3	18.3	15.7	14.3	18.4	15.7	14.4	120.5
121.0	18.3	15.6	14.3	18.4	15.7	14.4	18.4	15.7	14.4	121.0
121.5	18.4	15.7	14.3	18.4	15.7	14.4	18.5	15.8	14.4	121.5
122.0	18.4	15.7	14.3	18.5	15.8	14.4	18.5	15.8	14.5	122.0
122.5	18.5	15.7	14.4	18.5	15.8	14.4	18.6	15.9	14.5	122.5
123.0	18.5	15.8	14.4	18.6	15.8	14.5	18.7	15.9	14.5	123.0
123.5	18.6	15.8	14.4	18.6	15.9	14.5	18.7	16.0	14.6	123.5
124.0	18.6	15.8	14.4	18.7	15.9	14.5	18.8	16.0	14.6	124.0
124.5	18.7	15.8	14.4	18.8	15.9	14.5	18.9	16.1	14.6	124.5
125.0	18.7	15.9	14.5	18.8	16.0	14.6	18.9	16.1	14.7	125.0
125.5	18.8	15.9	14.5	18.9	16.0	14.6	19.0	16.1	14.7	125.5
126.0	18.8	15.9	14.5	19.0	16.1	14.6	19.1	16.2	14.7	126.0
126.5	18.9	16.0	14.5	19.0	16.1	14.6	19.2	16.2	14.8	126.5
127.0	18.9	16.0	14.5	19.1	16.1	14.7	19.2	16.3	14.8	127.0

TABLE D-1 *(Continued)*

Length/ Height* (cm)	Boys			Combined Sexes			Girls			Length/ Height* (cm)
	Median	-2 SD	-3 SD	Median	-2 SD	-3 SD	Median	-2 SD	-3 SD	
127.5	19.0	16.0	14.5	19.2	16.2	14.7	19.3	16.3	14.8	127.5
128.0	19.1	16.1	14.6	19.2	16.2	14.7	19.4	16.4	14.9	128.0
128.5	19.1	16.1	14.6	19.3	16.3	14.7	19.5	16.4	14.9	128.5
129.0	19.2	16.1	14.6	19.4	16.3	14.8	19.5	16.5	14.9	129.0
129.5	19.3	16.2	14.6	19.4	16.3	14.8	19.6	16.5	15.0	129.5
130.0	19.3	16.2	14.6	19.5	16.4	14.8	19.7	16.6	15.0	130.0
130.5	19.4	16.2	14.6	19.6	16.4	14.9	19.8	16.6	15.1	130.5
131.0	19.5	16.3	14.7	19.7	16.5	14.9	19.9	16.7	15.1	131.0
131.5	19.5	16.3	14.7	19.8	16.5	14.9	20.0	16.7	15.1	131.5
132.0	19.6	16.3	14.7	19.8	16.6	14.9	20.1	16.8	15.2	132.0
132.5	19.7	16.4	14.7	19.9	16.6	15.0	20.2	16.8	15.2	132.5
133.0	19.8	16.4	14.7	20.0	16.7	15.0	20.2	16.9	15.2	133.0
133.5	19.8	16.5	14.8	20.1	16.7	15.0	20.3	17.0	15.3	133.5
134.0	19.9	16.5	14.8	20.2	16.8	15.0	20.4	17.0	15.3	134.0
134.5	20.0	16.5	14.8	20.3	16.8	15.1	20.5	17.1	15.3	134.5
135.0	20.1	16.6	14.8	20.4	16.9	15.1	20.6	17.1	15.4	135.0
135.5	20.2	16.6	14.9	20.5	16.9	15.1	20.7	17.2	15.4	135.5
136.0	20.3	16.7	14.9	20.6	17.0	15.2	20.8	17.2	15.5	136.0
136.5	20.4	16.7	14.9	20.7	17.0	15.2	20.9	17.3	15.5	136.5
137.0	20.5	16.8	14.9	20.8	17.1	15.2	21.1	17.4	15.5	137.0
137.5	20.5	16.8	15.0	20.9	17.1	15.3	21.2	17.4	15.6	137.5
138.0	20.7	16.9	15.0	21.0	17.2	15.3	21.3	17.5	15.6	138.0
138.5	20.8	16.9	15.0	21.1	17.2	15.3	21.4	17.6	15.7	138.5
139.0	20.9	17.0	15.0	21.2	17.3	15.4	21.5	17.6	15.7	139.0
139.5	21.0	17.0	15.1	21.3	17.4	15.4	21.6	17.7	15.7	139.5
140.0	21.1	17.1	15.1	21.4	17.4	15.4	21.7	17.8	15.8	140.0
140.5	21.2	17.2	15.2	21.5	17.5	15.5	21.9	17.8	15.8	140.5
141.0	21.3	17.2	15.2	21.7	17.6	15.5	22.0	17.9	15.9	141.0
141.5	21.5	17.3	15.2	21.8	17.6	15.6	22.1	18.0	15.9	141.5
142.0	21.6	17.4	15.3	21.9	17.7	15.6	22.2	18.0	15.9	142.0
142.5	21.7	17.5	15.3	22.0	17.8	15.7	22.4	18.1	16.0	142.5
143.0	21.9	17.5	15.4	22.2	17.9	15.7	22.5	18.2	16.0	143.0
143.5	22.0	17.6	15.4	22.3	17.9	15.8	22.7	18.3	16.1	143.5
144.0	22.1	17.7	15.5	22.5	18.0	15.8	22.8	18.4	16.1	144.0
144.5	22.3	17.8	15.5	22.6	18.1	15.9	22.9	18.4	16.2	144.5
145.0	22.4	17.9	15.6	22.8	18.2	15.9	23.1	18.5	16.2	145.0

*Length below 85 cm, height ≥ 85 cm.

Source: Reprinted with permission from: Mei Z, et al. The development of a MUAC-for-height reference, including a comparison to other nutritional status screening indicators. *WHO Bull.* 1997;75:333–341.

TABLE D-2 Arm Measurements: MUAC-for-Age Reference Data for Boys Ages 6–59 Months*

Age (Months)	−4 SD	−3 SD	−2 SD	−1 SD	Mean	+1 SD	+2 SD	+3 SD
6	10.3	11.5	12.6	13.8	14.9	16.1	17.3	18.4
7	10.4	11.6	12.7	13.9	15.1	16.3	17.5	18.6
8	10.5	11.7	12.8	14.0	15.2	16.4	17.6	18.8
9	10.5	11.7	12.9	14.2	15.4	16.6	17.8	19.0
10	10.6	11.8	13.0	14.2	15.5	16.7	17.9	19.1
11	10.6	11.9	13.1	14.3	15.6	16.8	18.0	19.3
12	10.7	11.9	13.2	14.4	15.7	16.9	18.1	19.4
13	10.7	12.0	13.2	14.5	15.7	17.0	18.2	19.5
14	10.8	12.0	13.3	14.5	15.8	17.1	18.3	19.6
15	10.8	12.1	13.3	14.6	15.9	17.1	18.4	19.7
16	10.8	12.1	13.4	14.6	15.9	17.2	18.5	19.8
17	10.8	12.1	13.4	14.7	16.0	17.3	18.6	19.8
18	10.8	12.1	13.4	14.7	16.0	17.3	18.6	19.9
19	10.9	12.2	13.5	14.8	16.1	17.4	18.7	20.0
20	10.9	12.2	13.5	14.8	16.1	17.4	18.7	20.0
21	10.9	12.2	13.5	14.8	16.1	17.5	18.8	20.1
22	10.9	12.2	13.5	14.9	16.2	17.5	18.8	20.1
23	10.9	12.2	13.5	14.9	16.2	17.5	18.9	20.2
24	10.9	12.2	13.6	14.9	16.2	17.6	18.9	20.2
25	10.9	12.2	13.6	14.9	16.3	17.6	18.9	20.3
26	10.9	12.3	13.6	14.9	16.3	17.6	19.0	20.3
27	10.9	12.3	13.6	15.0	16.3	17.7	19.0	20.4
28	10.9	12.3	13.6	15.0	16.3	17.7	19.1	20.4
29	10.9	12.3	13.7	15.0	16.4	17.7	19.1	20.4
30	10.9	12.3	13.7	15.0	16.4	17.8	19.1	20.5
31	11.0	12.3	13.7	15.1	16.4	17.8	19.2	20.5
32	11.0	12.3	13.7	15.1	16.5	17.8	19.2	20.6
33	11.0	12.4	13.7	15.1	16.5	17.9	19.2	20.6
34	11.0	12.4	13.8	15.1	16.5	17.9	19.3	20.6
35	11.0	12.4	13.8	15.2	16.5	17.9	19.3	20.7
36	11.0	12.4	13.8	15.2	16.6	18.0	19.3	20.7
37	11.0	12.4	13.8	15.2	16.6	18.0	19.4	20.8
38	11.0	12.4	13.8	15.2	16.6	18.0	19.4	20.8
39	11.1	12.5	13.9	15.3	16.7	18.1	19.5	20.9
40	11.1	12.5	13.9	15.3	16.7	18.1	19.5	20.9
41	11.1	12.5	13.9	15.3	16.7	18.1	19.6	21.0
42	11.1	12.5	13.9	15.4	16.8	18.2	19.6	21.0
43	11.1	12.5	14.0	15.4	16.8	18.2	19.7	21.1
44	11.1	12.5	14.0	15.4	16.8	18.3	19.7	21.1
45	11.1	12.6	14.0	15.4	16.9	18.3	19.8	21.2
46	11.1	12.6	14.0	15.5	16.9	18.4	19.8	21.3
47	11.1	12.6	14.0	15.5	17.0	18.4	19.9	21.3
48	11.1	12.6	14.1	15.5	17.0	18.4	19.9	21.4
49	11.1	12.6	14.1	15.6	17.0	18.5	20.0	21.4
50	11.1	12.6	14.1	15.6	17.1	18.5	20.0	21.5
51	11.1	12.6	14.1	15.6	17.1	18.6	20.1	21.6
52	11.1	12.6	14.1	15.6	17.1	18.6	20.1	21.6
53	11.1	12.6	14.1	15.7	17.2	18.7	20.2	21.7
54	11.1	12.6	14.2	15.7	17.2	18.7	20.2	21.8
55	11.1	12.6	14.2	15.7	17.2	18.8	20.3	21.8
56	11.1	12.6	14.2	15.7	17.3	18.8	20.4	21.9
57	11.1	12.6	14.2	15.8	17.3	18.9	20.4	22.0
58	11.1	12.6	14.2	15.8	17.3	18.9	20.5	22.1
59	11.1	12.6	14.2	15.8	17.4	19.0	20.6	22.2

*Reprinted with permission from: de Onis M, et al. The development of MUAC-for-age reference data recommended by a WHO expert committee. *WHO Bull.* 1997;75:11–18.

TABLE D-3 Arm Measurements: MUAC-for-Age Reference Data for Girls Ages 6–59 Months*

Age (Months)	−4 SD	−3 SD	−2 SD	−1 SD	Mean	+1 SD	+2 SD	+3 SD
6	9.2	10.4	11.5	12.7	13.9	15.0	16.2	17.4
7	9.4	10.6	11.8	13.0	14.1	15.3	16.5	17.7
8	9.6	10.8	12.0	13.2	14.4	15.6	16.8	18.0
9	9.8	11.0	12.2	13.4	14.6	15.8	17.0	18.2
10	9.9	11.1	12.3	13.6	14.8	16.0	17.2	18.4
11	10.0	11.3	12.5	13.7	15.0	16.2	17.4	18.6
12	10.1	11.4	12.6	13.9	15.1	16.4	17.6	18.8
13	10.2	11.5	12.7	14.0	15.2	16.5	17.7	19.0
14	10.3	11.6	12.8	14.1	15.4	16.6	17.9	19.2
15	10.4	11.7	12.9	14.2	15.5	16.7	18.0	19.3
16	10.4	11.7	13.0	14.3	15.6	16.8	18.1	19.4
17	10.5	11.8	13.1	14.4	15.7	16.9	18.2	19.5
18	10.5	11.8	13.1	14.4	15.7	17.0	18.3	19.6
19	10.6	11.9	13.2	14.5	15.8	17.1	18.4	19.7
20	10.6	11.9	13.2	14.5	15.8	17.2	18.5	19.8
21	10.6	11.9	13.3	14.6	15.9	17.2	18.5	19.8
22	10.7	12.0	13.3	14.6	15.9	17.3	18.6	19.9
23	10.7	12.0	13.3	14.7	16.0	17.3	18.6	20.0
24	10.7	12.0	13.4	14.7	16.0	17.4	18.7	20.0
25	10.7	12.0	13.4	14.7	16.1	17.4	18.7	20.1
26	10.7	12.1	13.4	14.7	16.1	17.4	18.8	20.1
27	10.7	12.1	13.4	14.8	16.1	17.5	18.8	20.2
28	10.7	12.1	13.4	14.8	16.1	17.5	18.9	20.2
29	10.7	12.1	13.5	14.8	16.2	17.5	18.9	20.3
30	10.8	12.1	13.5	14.8	16.2	17.6	18.9	20.3
31	10.8	12.1	13.5	14.9	16.2	17.6	19.0	20.3
32	10.8	12.1	13.5	14.9	16.3	17.6	19.0	20.4
33	10.8	12.2	13.5	14.9	16.3	17.7	19.0	20.4
34	10.8	12.2	13.6	14.9	16.3	17.7	19.1	20.5
35	10.8	12.2	13.6	15.0	16.3	17.7	19.1	20.5
36	10.8	12.2	13.6	15.0	16.4	17.8	19.2	20.5
37	10.8	12.2	13.6	15.0	16.4	17.8	19.2	20.6
38	10.9	12.2	13.6	15.0	16.4	17.8	19.2	20.6
39	10.9	12.3	13.7	15.1	16.5	17.9	19.3	20.7
40	10.9	12.3	13.7	15.1	16.5	17.9	19.3	20.7
41	10.9	12.3	13.7	15.1	16.6	18.0	19.4	20.8
42	10.9	12.3	13.8	15.2	16.6	18.0	19.4	20.8
43	10.9	12.4	13.8	15.2	16.6	18.1	19.5	20.9
44	10.9	12.4	13.8	15.2	16.7	18.1	19.5	21.0
45	11.0	12.4	13.8	15.3	16.7	18.1	19.6	21.0
46	11.0	12.4	13.9	15.3	16.7	18.2	19.6	21.1
47	11.0	12.4	13.9	15.3	16.8	18.2	19.7	21.2
48	11.0	12.4	13.9	15.4	16.8	18.3	19.8	21.2
49	11.0	12.5	13.9	15.4	16.9	18.3	19.8	21.3
50	11.0	12.5	14.0	15.4	16.9	18.4	19.9	21.4
51	11.0	12.5	14.0	15.5	17.0	18.4	19.9	21.4
52	11.0	12.5	14.0	15.5	17.0	18.5	20.0	21.5
53	11.0	12.5	14.0	15.5	17.0	18.6	20.1	21.6
54	11.0	12.5	14.0	15.6	17.1	18.6	20.1	21.7
55	11.0	12.5	14.1	15.6	17.1	18.7	20.2	21.7
56	11.0	12.5	14.1	15.6	17.2	18.7	20.3	21.8
57	11.0	12.5	14.1	15.7	17.2	18.8	20.3	21.9
58	11.0	12.5	14.1	15.7	17.3	18.8	20.4	22.0
59	11.0	12.5	14.1	15.7	17.3	18.9	20.5	22.1

*Reprinted with permission from: de Onis M, et al. The development of MUAC-for-age reference data recommended by a WHO expert committee. *WHO Bull.* 1997;75:11–18.

TABLE D-4 Percentiles for Triceps Skinfold for Whites of the U.S. Health and Nutrition Examination Survey I of 1971–1974

Age Group	Triceps Skinfold Percentiles (mm^2)															
	n	*5*	*10*	*25*	*50*	*75*	*90*	*95*	*n*	*5*	*10*	*25*	*50*	*75*	*90*	*95*
	Males								Females							
1–1.9	228	6	7	8	10	12	14	16	204	6	7	8	10	12	14	16
2–2.9	223	6	7	8	10	12	14	15	208	6	8	9	10	12	15	16
3–3.9	220	6	7	8	10	11	14	15	208	7	8	9	11	12	14	15
4–4.9	230	6	6	8	9	11	12	14	208	7	8	8	10	12	14	16
5–5.9	214	6	6	8	9	11	14	15	219	6	7	8	10	12	15	18
6–6.9	117	5	6	7	8	10	13	16	118	6	6	8	10	12	14	16
7–7.9	122	5	6	7	9	12	15	17	126	6	7	9	11	13	16	18
8–8.9	117	5	6	7	8	10	13	16	118	6	8	9	12	15	18	24
9–9.9	121	6	6	7	10	13	17	18	125	8	8	10	13	16	20	22
10–10.9	146	6	6	8	10	14	18	21	152	7	8	10	12	17	23	27
11–11.9	122	6	6	8	11	16	20	24	117	7	8	10	13	18	24	28
12–12.9	153	6	6	8	11	14	22	28	129	8	9	11	14	18	23	27
13–13.9	134	5	5	7	10	14	22	26	151	8	8	12	15	21	26	30
14–14.9	131	4	5	7	9	14	21	24	141	9	10	13	16	21	26	28
15–15.9	128	4	5	6	8	11	18	24	117	8	10	12	17	21	25	32
16–16.9	131	4	5	6	8	12	16	22	142	10	12	15	18	22	26	31
17–17.9	133	5	5	6	8	12	16	19	114	10	12	13	19	24	30	37
18–18.9	91	4	5	6	9	13	20	24	109	10	12	15	18	22	26	30
19–24.9	531	4	5	7	10	15	20	22	1060	10	11	14	18	24	30	34
25–34.9	971	5	6	8	12	16	20	24	1987	10	12	16	21	27	34	37
35–44.9	806	5	6	8	12	16	20	23	1614	12	14	18	23	29	35	38
45–54.9	898	6	6	8	12	15	20	25	1047	12	16	20	25	30	36	40
55–64.9	734	5	6	8	11	14	19	22	809	12	16	20	25	31	36	38
65–74.9	1503	4	6	8	11	15	19	22	1670	12	14	18	24	29	34	36

Source: Reprinted with permission from Frisancho AR, New norms of upper limb fat and muscle areas for assessment of nutritional status, in *American Journal of Clinical Nutrition* (1981;34:2540–2545).

TABLE D-5 Percentiles of Upper Arm Circumference and Estimated Upper Arm Muscle Circumference for Whites of the U.S. Health and Nutrition Examination Survey I of 1971–1974

Males

Age Group	Arm Circumference (mm)							Arm Muscle Circumference (mm)						
	5	10	25	50	75	90	95	5	10	25	50	75	90	95
1–1.9	142	146	150	159	170	176	183	110	113	119	127	135	144	147
2–2.9	141	145	153	162	170	178	185	111	114	122	130	140	146	150
3–3.9	150	153	160	167	175	184	190	117	123	131	137	143	148	153
4–4.9	149	154	162	171	180	186	192	123	126	133	141	148	156	159
5–5.9	153	160	167	175	185	195	204	128	133	140	147	154	162	169
6–6.9	155	159	167	179	188	209	228	131	135	142	151	161	170	177
7–7.9	162	167	177	187	201	223	230	137	139	151	160	168	177	190
8–8.9	162	170	177	190	202	220	245	140	145	154	162	170	182	187
9–9.9	175	178	187	200	217	249	257	151	154	161	170	183	196	202
10–10.9	181	184	196	210	231	262	274	156	160	166	180	191	209	221
11–11.9	186	190	202	223	244	261	280	159	165	173	183	195	205	230
12–12.9	193	200	214	232	254	282	303	167	171	182	195	210	223	241
13–13.9	194	211	228	247	263	286	301	172	179	196	211	226	238	245
14–14.9	220	226	237	253	283	303	322	189	199	212	223	240	260	264
15–15.9	222	229	244	264	284	311	320	199	204	218	237	254	266	272
16–16.9	244	248	262	278	303	324	343	213	225	234	249	269	287	296
17–17.9	246	253	267	285	308	336	347	224	231	245	258	273	294	312
18–18.9	245	260	276	297	321	353	379	226	237	252	264	283	298	324
19–24.9	262	272	288	308	331	355	372	238	245	257	273	289	309	321
25–34.9	271	282	300	319	342	362	375	243	250	264	279	298	314	326
35–44.9	278	287	305	326	345	363	374	247	255	269	286	302	318	327
45–54.9	267	281	301	322	342	362	376	239	249	265	281	300	315	326
55–64.9	258	273	296	317	336	355	369	236	245	260	278	295	310	320
65–74.9	248	263	285	307	325	344	355	223	235	251	268	284	298	306

(continued)

TABLE D-5 *(Continued)*

	Females													
	Arm Circumference (mm)							*Arm Muscle Circumference (mm)*						
Age Group	*5*	*10*	*25*	*50*	*75*	*90*	*95*	*5*	*10*	*25*	*50*	*75*	*90*	*95*
1–1.9	138	142	148	156	164	172	177	105	111	117	124	132	139	143
2–2.9	142	145	152	160	167	176	184	111	114	119	126	133	142	147
3–3.9	143	150	158	167	175	183	189	113	119	124	132	140	146	152
4–4.9	149	154	160	169	177	184	191	115	121	128	136	144	152	157
5–5.9	153	157	165	175	185	203	211	125	128	134	142	151	159	165
6–6.9	156	162	170	176	187	204	211	130	133	138	145	154	166	171
7–7.9	164	167	174	183	199	216	231	129	135	142	151	160	171	176
8–8.9	168	172	183	195	214	247	261	138	140	151	160	171	183	194
9–9.9	178	182	194	211	224	251	260	147	150	158	167	180	194	198
10–10.9	174	182	193	210	228	251	265	148	150	159	170	180	190	197
11–11.9	185	194	208	224	248	276	303	150	158	171	181	196	217	223
12–12.9	194	203	216	237	256	282	294	162	166	180	191	201	214	220
13–13.9	202	211	223	243	271	301	338	169	175	183	198	211	226	240
14–14.9	214	223	237	252	272	304	322	174	179	190	201	216	232	247
15–15.9	208	221	239	254	279	300	322	175	178	189	202	215	228	244
16–16.9	218	224	241	258	283	318	334	170	180	190	202	216	234	249
17–17.9	220	227	241	264	295	324	350	175	183	194	205	221	239	257
18–18.9	222	227	241	258	281	312	325	174	179	191	202	215	237	245
19–24.9	221	230	247	265	290	319	345	179	185	195	207	221	236	249
25–34.9	233	240	256	277	304	342	368	183	188	199	212	228	246	264
35–44.9	241	251	267	290	317	356	378	186	192	205	218	236	257	272
45–54.9	242	256	274	299	328	362	384	187	193	206	220	238	260	274
55–64.9	243	257	280	303	335	367	385	187	196	209	225	244	266	280
65–74.9	240	252	274	299	326	356	373	185	195	208	225	244	264	279

Source: Reprinted with permission from Frisancho AR, New norms of upper limb fat and muscle areas for assessment of nutritional status, in *American Journal of Clinical Nutrition* (1981;34:2540–2545).

TABLE D-6 Percentiles for Estimates of Upper Arm Fat Area and Upper Arm Muscle Area for Whites of the U.S. Health and Nutrition Examination Survey I of 1971–1974

	Males													
	Arm Muscle Area Percentiles (mm^2)							Arm Fat Area Percentiles (mm^2)						
Age Group	5	10	25	50	75	90	95	5	10	25	50	75	90	95
1–1.9	956	1014	1133	1278	1447	1644	1720	452	486	590	741	895	1036	1176
2–2.9	973	1040	1190	1345	1557	1690	1787	434	504	578	737	871	1044	1148
3–3.9	1095	1201	1357	1484	1618	1750	1853	464	519	590	736	868	1071	1151
4–4.9	1207	1264	1408	1579	1747	1926	2008	428	494	598	722	859	989	1085
5–5.9	1298	1411	1550	1720	1884	2089	2285	446	488	582	713	914	1176	1299
6–6.9	1360	1447	1605	1815	2056	2297	2493	371	446	539	678	896	1115	1519
7–7.9	1497	1548	1808	2027	2246	2494	2886	423	473	574	758	1011	1393	1511
8–8.9	1550	1664	1895	2089	2296	2628	2788	410	460	588	725	1003	1248	1558
9–9.9	1811	1884	2067	2288	2657	3053	3257	485	527	635	859	1252	1864	2081
10–10.9	1930	2027	2182	2575	2903	3486	3882	523	543	738	982	1376	1906	2609
11–11.9	2016	2156	2382	2670	3022	3359	4226	536	595	754	1148	1710	2348	2574
12–12.9	2216	2339	2649	3022	3496	3968	4640	554	650	874	1172	1558	2536	3580
13–13.9	2363	2546	3044	3553	4081	4502	4794	475	570	812	1096	1702	2744	3322
14–14.9	2830	3147	3586	3963	4575	5368	5530	453	563	786	1082	1608	2746	3508
15–15.9	3138	3317	3788	4481	5134	5631	5900	521	595	690	931	1423	2434	3100
16–16.9	3625	4044	4352	4951	5753	6576	6980	542	593	844	1078	1746	2280	3041
17–17.9	3998	4252	4777	5286	5950	6886	7726	598	698	827	1096	1636	2407	2888
18–18.9	4070	4481	5066	5552	6374	7067	8355	560	665	860	1264	1947	3302	3928
19–24.9	4508	4777	5274	5913	6660	7606	8200	594	743	963	1406	2231	3098	3652
25–34.9	4694	4963	5541	6214	7067	7847	8436	675	831	1174	1752	2459	3246	3786
35–44.9	4844	5181	5740	6490	7265	8034	8488	703	851	1310	1792	2463	3098	3624
45–54.9	4546	4946	5589	6297	7142	7918	8458	749	922	1254	1741	2359	3245	3928
55–64.9	4422	4783	5381	6144	6919	7670	8149	658	839	1166	1645	2236	2976	3466
65–74.9	3973	4411	5031	5716	6432	7074	7453	573	753	1122	1621	2199	2876	3327

(continued)

TABLE D-6 *(Continued)*

	Females													
	Arm Muscle Area Percentiles (mm²)							*Arm Fat Area Percentiles (mm²)*						
Age Group	*5*	*10*	*25*	*50*	*75*	*90*	*95*	*5*	*10*	*25*	*50*	*75*	*90*	*95*
1–1.9	885	973	1084	1221	1378	1535	1621	401	466	578	706	847	1022	1140
2–2.9	973	1029	1119	1269	1405	1595	1727	469	526	642	747	894	1061	1173
3–3.9	1014	1133	1227	1396	1563	1690	1846	473	529	656	822	967	1106	1158
4–4.9	1058	1171	1313	1475	1644	1832	1958	490	541	654	766	907	1109	1236
5–5.9	1238	1301	1432	1598	1825	2012	2159	470	529	647	812	991	1330	1536
6–6.9	1354	1414	1513	1683	1877	2182	2323	464	508	638	827	1009	1263	1436
7–7.9	1330	1441	1602	1815	2045	2332	2469	491	560	706	920	1135	1407	1644
8–8.9	1513	1566	1808	2034	2327	2657	2996	527	634	769	1042	1383	1872	2482
9–9.9	1723	1788	1976	2227	2571	2987	3112	642	690	933	1219	1584	2171	2524
10–10.9	1740	1784	2019	2296	2583	2873	3093	616	702	842	1141	1608	2500	3005
11–11.9	1784	1987	2316	2612	3071	3739	3953	707	802	1015	1301	1942	2730	3690
12–12.9	2092	2182	2579	2904	3225	3655	3847	782	854	1090	1511	2056	2666	3369
13–13.9	2269	2426	2657	3130	3529	4081	4568	726	838	1219	1625	2374	3272	4150
14–14.9	2418	2562	2874	3220	3704	4294	4850	981	1043	1423	1818	2403	3250	3765
15–15.9	2426	2518	2847	3248	3689	4123	4756	839	1126	1396	1886	2544	3093	4195
16–16.9	2308	2567	2865	3248	3718	4353	4946	1126	1351	1663	2006	2598	3374	4236
17–17.9	2442	2674	2996	3336	3883	4552	5251	1042	1267	1463	2104	2977	3864	5159
18–18.9	2398	2538	2917	3243	3694	4461	4767	1003	1230	1616	2104	2617	3508	3733
19–24.9	2538	2728	3026	3406	3877	4439	4940	1046	1198	1596	2166	2959	4050	4896
25–34.9	2661	2826	3148	3573	4138	4806	5541	1173	1399	1841	2548	3512	4690	5560
35–44.9	2750	2948	3359	3783	4428	5240	5877	1336	1619	2158	2898	3932	5093	5847
45–54.9	2784	2956	3378	3858	4520	5375	5964	1459	1803	2447	3244	4229	5416	6140
55–64.9	2784	3063	3477	4045	4750	5632	6247	1345	1879	2520	3369	4360	5276	6152
65–74.9	2737	3018	3444	4019	4739	5566	6214	1363	1681	2266	3063	3943	4914	5530

Source: Reprinted with permission from Frisancho AR, New norms of upper limb fat and muscle areas for assessment of nutritional status, in *American Journal of Clinical Nutrition* (1981;34:2540–2545).

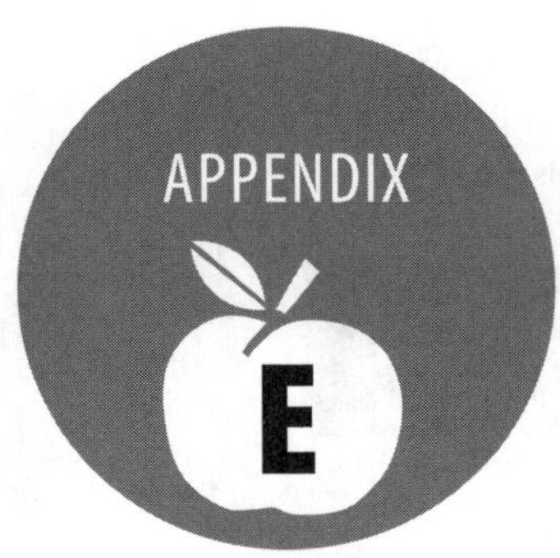

Progression of Sexual Development

TABLE E-1 Median Ages at Entry into Each Maturity Stage and Fiducial Limits* in Years for Pubic Hair and Breast Development in Girls by Race

Stage	Age at Entry for Girls					
	Non-Hispanic White		Non-Hispanic Black		Mexican American	
	Median	FL	Median	FL	Median	FL
Pubic hair						
PH2	10.57†	10.29–10.85	9.43†	9.05–9.74	10.39	—
PH3	1180†	11.54–12.07	10.57†	10.30–10.83	11.70†	11.14–12.27
PH4	13.00†	12.71–13.30	11.90†	11.38–12.42	13.19†	12.88–13.52
PH5	16.33†	15.86–16.88	14.70†	14.32–15.11	16.30†	15.90–16.76
Breast development						
B2	10.38†	10.11–10.65	9.48†	9.41–9.76	9.80	0–11.78
B3	11.75†	11.49–12.02	10.79†	10.50–11.08	11.43	8.64–14.50
B4	13.29†	12.97–13.61	12.24†	11.87–12.61	13.07†	12.79–13.36
B5	15.47†	15.04–15.94	13.92†	13.57–14.29	14.70†	14.37–15.04

FL indicates fiducial limit.

*Calculated 98.3% FLs to adjust for multiple comparisons between races for an overall of 0.05.

† Significant pair-wise racial difference, $P < 0.05$.

Source: Reprinted with permission from *Pediatrics,* Vol 110, pp. 911–918. Copyright 2002. Sun SS, Schuber CM, Chumlea WC, Roche AE, et al. National estimates of the timing of sexual maturation and racial differences among US children. *Pediatrics*. 2002;110:911–918.

Tanner Stage, or sexual maturity rating: 1. Prepubertal; 2. First visible signs of pubertal change appear; 3. Pubic hair increases and becomes darker and coarser, breast enlarge; 4. Pubic hair becomes more abundant and coarse, breasts increase in size; 5. Adult characteristics visible for breasts and pubic hair.

TABLE E-2 Mean Ages in Years and Standard Errors for Being in a Stage for Pubic Hair and Breast Development in Girls by Race

Stage	Age in a Stage for Girls								
	Non-Hispanic White			Non-Hispanic Black			Mexican American		
	N	Mean	SE	*N*	Mean	SE	*N*	Mean	SE
Pubic hair									
PH2	67	10.96*	0.23	85	10.25*	0.15	105	11.17*	0.21
PH3	61	12.41*	0.19	98	11.37*	0.23	108	12.84*	0.18
PH4	154	15.11*	0.18	184	13.69*	0.31	177	14.61*	0.26
PH5	133	16.53*	0.17	282	16.05*	0.14	161	16.61*	0.12
Breast development									
B2	82	11.05*	0.18	99	10.25*	0.20	129	10.70	0.21
B3	80	12.80*	0.19	106	11.94*	0.22	131	12.61*	0.20
B4	110	15.16*	0.32	112	13.61*	0.34	97	14.03*	0.27
B5	173	16.25*	0.18	338	15.78*	0.14	254	16.21*	0.12

SE indicates standard error.
*Significant pair-wise racial difference, $P < 0.05$.
Source: Reprinted with permission from *Pediatrics*, Vol. 110, pp. 911–918, Copyright 2002. Sun SS, Schuber CM, Chumlea WC, Roche AF, et al. National estimates of the timing of sexual maturation and racial differences among US children. *Pediatrics.* 2002;110:911–918.
Tanner Stage, or sexual maturity rating: 1. Prepubertal; 2. First visible signs of pubertal change appear; 3. Pubic hair increases and becomes darker and coarser, breasts enlarge; 4. Pubic hair becomes more abundant and coarse, breasts increase in size; 5. Adult characteristics visible for breasts and pubic hair.

TABLE E-3 Median Ages of Entry into Each Stage and FLs* in Years for Pubic Hair and Genitalia Development in Boys by Race

Stage	Age at Entry for Boys					
	Non-Hispanic White		Non-Hispanic Black		Mexican American	
	Median	FL	Median	FL	Median	FL
Pubic hair						
PH2	11.98†	11.69–12.29	11.16†	10.89–11.43	12.30†	12.06–12.56
PH3	12.65	12.37–12.95	12.51†	12.26–12.77	13.06†	12.79–13.36
PH4	13.56	13.27–13.86	13.73	13.49–13.99	14.08	13.83–14.32
PH5	15.67	15.30–16.05	15.32	14.99–15.67	15.75	15.46–16.03
Genitalia development						
G2	10.03	9.61–10.40	9.20†	8.62–9.64	10.29†	9.94–10.60
G3	12.32	12.00–12.67	11.78†	11.50–12.08	12.53†	12.29–12.79
G4	13.52	13.22–13.83	13.40	13.15–13.66	13.77	13.51–14.03
G5	16.01†	15.57–16.50	15.00†	14.70–15.32	15.76†	15.39–16.14

FL indicates fiducial limit.
*Calculated 98.3% FLs to adjust for multiple comparisons between races for an overall of 0.05.
† Significant pair-wise racial difference, $P < 0.05$.
Source: Reprinted with permission from *Pediatrics*, Vol. 110, pp. 911–918, Copyright 2002. Sun SS, Schuber CM, Chumlea WC, Roche AF, et al. National estimates of the timing of sexual maturation and racial differences among US children. *Pediatrics.* 2002;110:911–918.
Tanner Stage, or sexual maturity rating: 1. Prepubertal; 2. First visible signs of pubertal change appear; 3. Pubic hair increases and becomes darker and coarser, and genitalia lengthen and enlarge; 4. Pubic hair becomes more abundant and coarse, genitalia increase in size; 5. Adult characteristics visible for pubic hair and genitalia.

TABLE E-4 Mean Ages in Years and SEs for Being in a Stage for Pubic Hair and Genitalia Development in Boys by Race

Stage	Age in a Stage for Boys								
	Non-Hispanic White			Non-Hispanic Black			Mexican American		
	N	Mean	SE	*N*	Mean	SE	*N*	Mean	SE
Pubic hair									
PH2	42	11.81	0.16	106	11.48*	0.13	50	12.20*	0.24
PH3	39	13.03	0.27	86	12.79*	0.19	55	13.44*	0.26
PH4	75	14.89	0.18	94	15.21	0.26	93	15.25	0.16
PH5	133	16.84	0.13	238	16.67*	0.08	211	17.14*	0.10
Genitalia development									
G2	136	11.08	0.18	181	10.79	0.13	183	11.09	0.17
G3	63	12.55	0.29	113	12.03*	0.28	80	12.97*	0.28
G4	91	15.29	0.19	98	15.07	0.33	104	15.38	0.19
G5	120	16.64	0.15	253	16.42*	0.09	219	16.85*	0.13

*Significant pair-wise racial difference, $P < 0.05$.

Source: Reprinted with permission from *Pediatrics*, Vol. 110, pp 911–918, Copyright 2002. Sun SS, Schuber CM, Chumlea WC, Roche AF, et al. National estimates of the timing of sexual maturation and racial differences among US children. *Pediatrics.* 2002;110:911–918.

Tanner Stage, or sexual maturity rating: 1. Prepubertal; 2. First visible signs of pubertal change appear; 3. Pubic hair increases and becomes darker and coarser, and genitalia lengthen and enlarge; 4. Pubic hair becomes more abundant and coarse, genitalia increase in size; 5. Adult characteristics visible for pubic hair and genitalia.

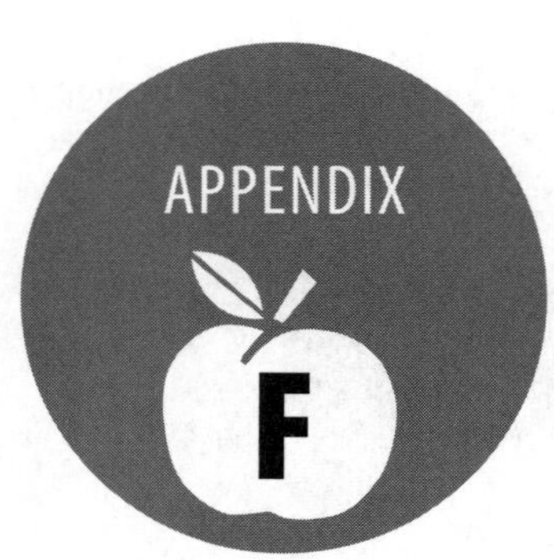

Nomograms

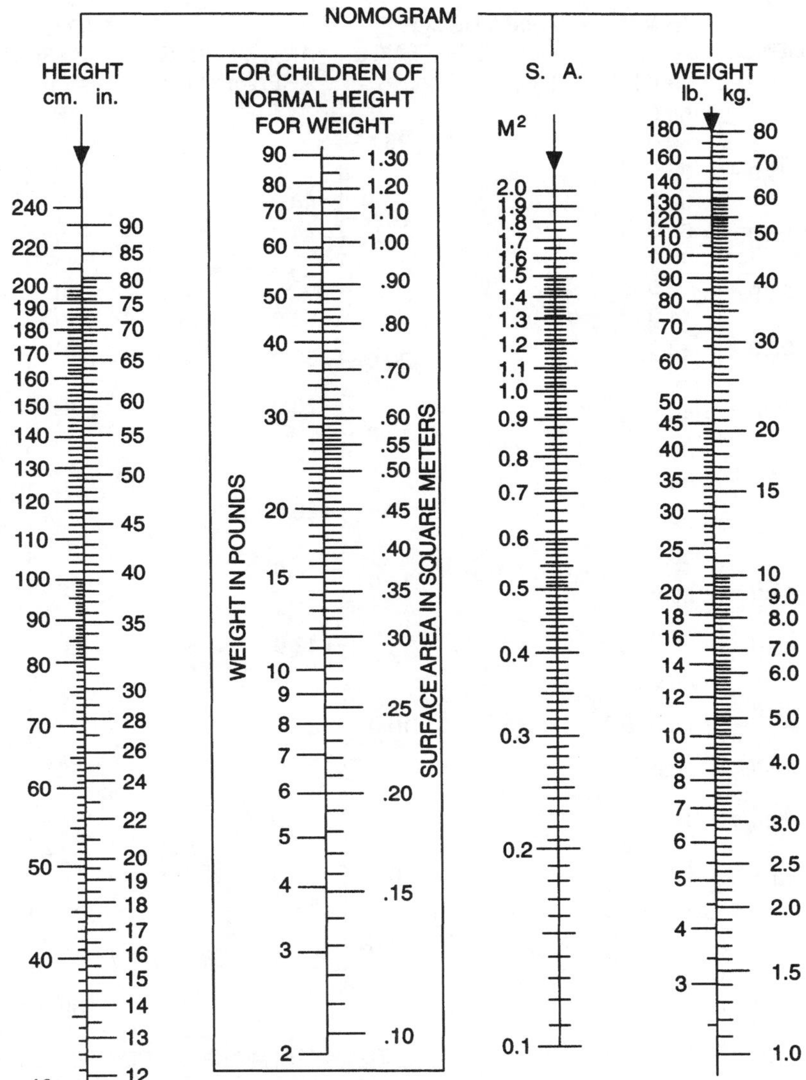

NOMOGRAM FOR ESTIMATION OF SURFACE AREA. THE SURFACE AREA IS INDICATED WHEN A STRAIGHT LINE THAT CONNECTS THE HEIGHT AND WEIGHT LEVELS INTERSECTS THE SURFACE AREA COLUMN, OR IF THE PATIENT IS ROUGHLY OF AVERAGE SIZE, FROM THE WEIGHT ALONE (ENCLOSED AREA). (NOMOGRAM MODIFIED FROM DATA OF E. BOYD BY C.D. WEST.)

FIGURE F-1 Nomogram for estimation of surface area.

Source: Reprinted from *Nelson's Textbook of Medicine,* ed 17 (p 2396) by Behrman RE and Vaughn VC (eds) with permission of WB Saunders © 2003.

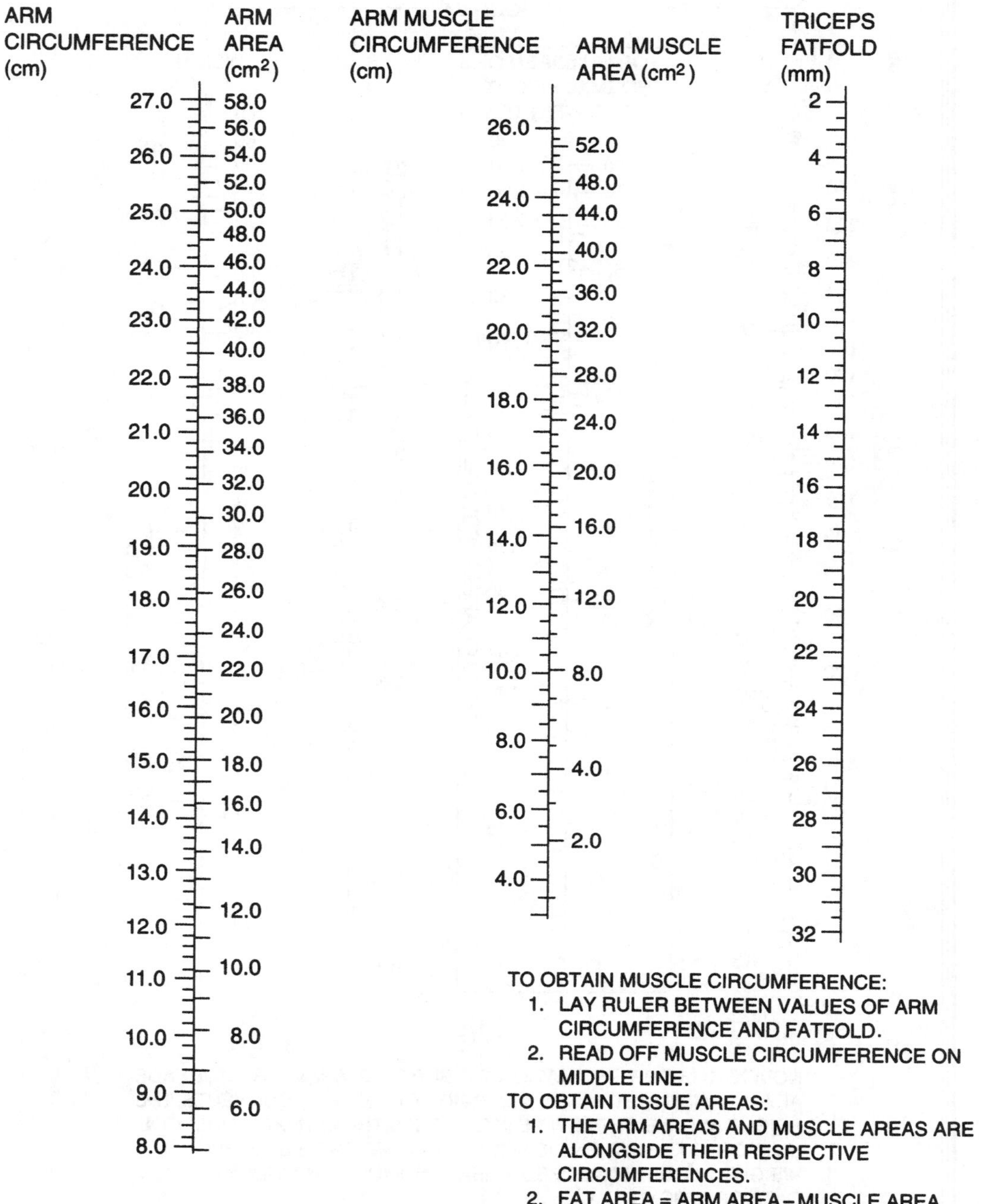

FIGURE F-2 Arm antropometry nomogram for children.

Source: Reprinted with permission from Gurney JM and Jeliffe DB, Arm anthropometry in nutritional assessment: nomogram for rapid calculation of muscle circumference and cross-sectional muscle and fat areas, in *American Journal of Clinical Nutrition* (1973;26:912–915). Copyright © 1973, American Society for Clinical Nutrition.

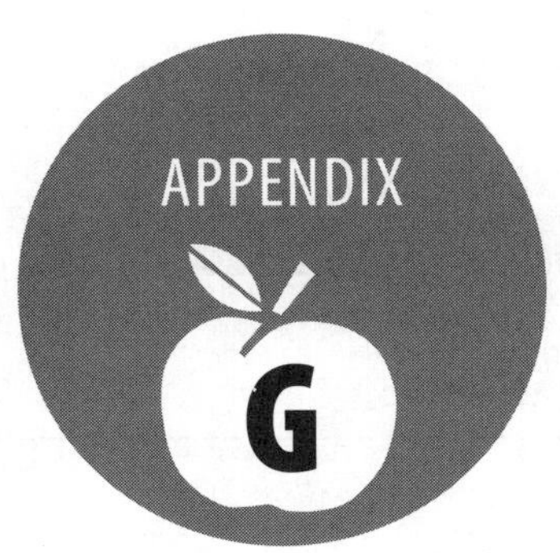

Biochemical Evaluation of Nutritional Status

TABLE G-1 Normal Values: Biochemical Measurement of Specific Nutritional Parameters

Test	Normal Value	Exceptions
Protein, Blood		
Serum albumin, g/dL	3.7–5.5	Infant 2.9–5.5
Retinol binding protein, mg/dL	1.3–9.9	Children $<$ 9 y, 1–7.8
Blood urea nitrogen, mg/dL	7–22	
Thyroxine binding protein, mg/dL	20–50	
Transferrin, mg/dL	170–440	
Fibronectin, mg/dL	30–40	
Prealbumin, mg/dL	17–42	Preterm infant, 4–14; term infant, 4–20; 6- to 12-mo-old child, 8–24; 1- to 6-y-old child, 17–30
Protein, Urine		
Creatinine/height index	$>$ 0.9	
3-methyl histidine, μmol/kg	3.2 $\pm$ 0.6 male, 2.1 $\pm$ 0.4 female, 4.2 $\pm$ 1.3 neonate	
3-methyl histidine, μmol/g	126 $\pm$ 32 male, 92 $\pm$ 23 female	
Creatinine	253 $\pm$ 78 neonate	
Hydroxyproline index	$>$ 2	
Vitamin A		
Plasma retinol, μg/dL	20–72	Infant, 13–50
Vitamin D		
25-OH-D_3, μg/L	2–30	. . .
1-25-OH-D_3, μg/L	15–60	
Riboflavin		
Red blood cell glutathione reductase stimulation, %	$<$ 20	. . .
Vitamin B_6		
Red blood cell transaminases, plasma pyridoxal phosphate, xanthurenic acid excretion	Feasible and useful in all age groups, but not readily available and not practical in children $<$ 9 y	. . .

(continued)

TABLE G-1 *(Continued)*

Test	Normal Value	Exceptions
Folic Acid		
Serum folate, ng/mL	> 6	. . .
Red blood cell folate, ng/mL	> 160	
Vitamin K		
Prothrombin time, sec	11–15	11–15
Vitamin E		
Plasma alphatocopherol, mg/dL	0.7–10	Preterm infant, 0.5–3.5
Red blood cell hemolysis test, %	10	
Vitamin C		
Plasma level, mg/dL	0.2–2.0	. . .
Leukocyte level, mg/100 cells	Difficult to perform on children because of sample requirements	
Thiamine		
Red blood cell transketolase stimulation, %	< 15	. . .
Vitamin B_{12}		
Serum vitamin B_{12}, pg/mL	200–900	. . .
Absorption test	Excretion of more than 7.5% of ingested labeled vitamin B_{12}	
Iron		
Hematocrit, %	39	Neonate, 31; infant, 33; child and menstruating females, 36
Hemoglobin, g/dL	14	Neonate, 11; infant, 12; child and menstruating females, 13
Serum ferritin, ng/mL	> 15	Neonate, < 60
Serum iron, µg/dL	> 60	Neonate, > 30; infant, > 40; child < 4 y, > 50
Serum total iron binding capacity, µg/dL	350–400	
Serum transferrin saturation, %	> 16	Infant, > 12; child, 9 y, > 14–15
Serum transferrin, mg/dL	170–250	Neonate, < 80; infant < 75
Erythrocyte protoporphyrin, µg/dL red blood cells	< 70	
Zinc		
Serum level, µg/dL	60–120	. . .
Erythrocyte level	Erythrocytes contain approximately 10 times more zinc than does plasma	
Phosphorus		
Serum phosphate, mg/dL	2.9–5.6	Newborn, 4.0–8.0; 1-y-old child, 3.8–6.2; 2- to 5-y-old child, 3.5–6.8
Calcium		
Serum total calcium, mg/dL	8.5–10.5	Preterm infant, 6–10; term infant, 7–12; child, 8–10.5
Serum ionized calcium, mg/dL	4.48–4.92	
Magnesium		
Serum magnesium, mEq/L	1.5–2.0	. . .

Source: Adapted with permission from *Nelson's Texbook of Pediatrics*, 13th ed., pp. 1535–1558, © 1989, W.B. Saunders Company.

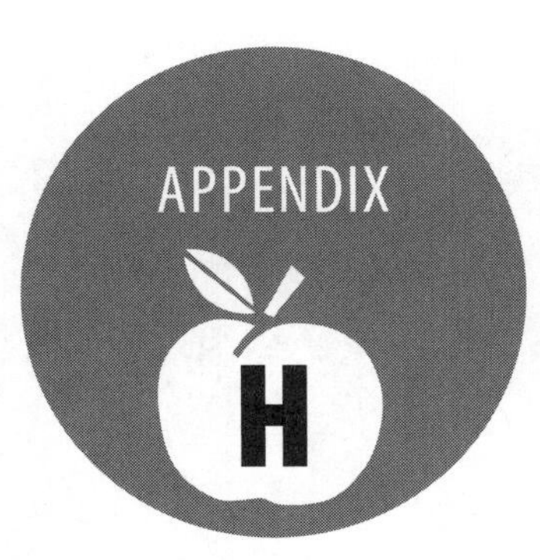

Recommended Dietary Allowances/Dietary Reference Intakes

TABLE H-1 Dietary Reference Intakes: Recommended Intakes for Individuals, Food and Nutrition Board, National Academy of Sciences

	Infants 0–6 mo	Infants 7–12 mo	Children 1–2 y	Children 3–8 y	Males 9–13 y	Males 14–18 y	Females 9–13 y	Females 14–18 y	Pregnancy 14–18 y	Lactation 14–18 y
Active PAL[k] EER (kcal/day)	Male 570 Female 520 (3 mo)	Male 743 Female 676 (9 mo)	Male 1046 Female 992 (24 mo)	Male 1742 Female 1642 (6 y)	2279 (11 y)	3152 (16 y)	2071 (11 y)	2368 (16 y)	1st trimester 2368 2nd trimester 2708 3rd trimester 2820 (16 y)	1st 6 mo 2698 2nd 6 mo 2768
Carbohydrates			130	130	130	130	130	130	175	210
Total Fiber	ND[n]	ND	19	25	31	48	26	26	28	29
AI (g/day)[m] Fat	31	30	ND	ND	ND	ND	ND	ND	ND	ND
ω-6 Polyunsaturated Fatty Acids (g/day) (Linoleic Acid)	4.4	4.6	7	10	12	16	10	11	13	13
ω-3 Polyunsaturated Fatty Acids (g/day) (α-Linoleic Acid)	0.5	0.5	0.7	0.9	1.2	1.6	1.0	1.1	1.4	1.3
Protein (g/kg/day)		1.5	1.10	0.95	0.95	0.85	0.95	.085		
Vitamin A (μg/day)[a]	400*	500*	**300**	**400**	**600**	**900**	**600**	**700**	**750**	**1200**
Vitamin C (mg/day)	40*	50*	**15**	**25**	**45**	**75**	**45**	**65**	**80**	**115**
Vitamin D (μg/day)[b,c]	5*	5*	5*	5*	5*	5*	5*	5*	5*	5*
Vitamin E (mg/day)[d]	4*	5*	6	7	**11**	**15**	**11**	**15**	**15**	**19**
Vitamin K (μg/day)	2.0*	2.5*	30*	55*	60*	75*	60*	75*	75*	75*
Thiamin (mg/day)	0.2*	0.3*	**0.5**	**0.6**	**0.9**	**1.2**	**0.9**	**1.0**	**1.4**	**1.4**
Riboflavin (mg/day)	0.3*	0.4*	**0.5**	**0.6**	**0.9**	**1.3**	**0.9**	**1.0**	**1.4**	**1.6**
Niacin (mg/day)[e]	2*	4*	**6**	**8**	**12**	**16**	**12**	**14**	**18**	**17**
Vitamin B_6 (mg/day)	0.1*	0.3*	**0.5**	**0.6**	**1.0**	**1.3**	**1.0**	**1.2**	**1.9**	**2.0**
Folate (μg/day)[f]	65*	80*	**150**	**200**	**300**	**400**	**300**	**400**[g]	**600**[h]	500
Vitamin B_{12} (mg/day)	0.4*	0.5*	0.9	1.2	1.8	2.4	1.8	2.4	2.6	2.8
Pantothenic Acid (mg/day)	1.7*	1.8*	2*	3*	4*	5*	4*	5*	6*	7*
Biotin (μg/day)	5*	6*	8*	12*	20*	25*	20*	25*	30*	35*
Choline[j] (mg/day)	125*	125*	200*	250*	375*	550*	375*	400*	450*	550*
Calcium (mg/day)	210*	270*	500*	800*	1300*	1300*	1300*	1300*	1300*	1300*
Chromium (μg/day)	0.2*	5.5*	11*	15*	25*	35*	21*	24*	29*	44
Copper (μg/day)	200*	220*	**340**	**440**	**700**	**890**	**700**	**890**	**1000**	**1300**

Fluoride (mg/day)	0.01*	0.5*	0.7*	1*	2*	3*	2*	2*	3*	3*
Iodine (μg/day)	110*	130*	**90**	**90**	**120**	**150**	**120**	**150**	**220**	**290**
Iron (mg/day)	0.27*	**11**	**7**	**10**	**8**	**11**	**8**	**15**	**27**	**10**
Magnesium (mg/day)	30*	75*	**80**	**130**	**240**	**410**	**240**	**360**	**400**	**360**
Manganese (mg/day)	0.003*	0.6*	1.2*	1.5*	1.9*	2.2*	1.6*	1.6*	2.0*	2.6*
Molybdenum (μg/day)	2*	3*	**17**	**22**	**34**	**43**	**34**	**43**	**50**	**50**
Phosphorus (mg/day)	100*	275*	**460**	**500**	**1250**	**1250**	**1250**	**1250**	**1250**	**1250**
Selenium (μg/day)	15*	20*	**20**	**30**	**40**	**55**	**40**	**55**	**60**	**70**
Zinc (mg/day)	2*	**3**	**3**	**5**	**8**	**11**	**8**	**9**	**13**	**14**

Note: This table (taken from the DRI reports, see http://www.nap.edu) presents Recommended Dietary Allowances (RDAs) in **bold type** and Adequate Intakes (AIs) in ordinary type followed by an asterisk (*). RDAs and AIs may both be used as goals for individual intake. RDAs are set to meet the needs of almost all individuals in a group. For healthy breastfed infants, the AI is the mean intake. The AI for other life stage and gender groups is believed to cover needs of all individuals in the group, but lack of data or uncertainty in the data prevent being able to specify with confidence the percentage of individuals covered by this intake.

[a] As retinol activity equivalents (RAEs). 1 RAE = 1 μg retinol, 12 μg β-carotene, 24 μg α-carotene, or 24 μg β-cryptoxanthin in foods. To calculate RAEs from retinol equivalents (REs) of provitamin A carotenoids in foods, divide the REs by 2. For preformed vitamin A in foods or supplements and for provitamin A carotenoids in supplements, 1 RE = 1 RAE.

[b] Cholecalciferol, 1 mg cholecalciferol = 40 IU vitamin D.

[c] In the absence of adequate exposure to sunlight.

[d] As α-tocopherol. α-Tocopherol includes *RRR*-α-tocopherol, the only form of α-tocopherol that occurs naturally in foods, and the 2R-stereoisomeric forms of α-tocopherol (*RRR-*, *RSR-*, *RRS-*, and *RSS-* α-tocopherol) that occur in fortified foods and supplements. It does not include the 2S-stereoisomeric forms of α-tocopherol (*SRR-*, *SSR-*, *SRS-*, and *SSS*-α-tocopherol), also found in fortified foods and supplements.

[e] As niacin equivalents (NE). 1 mg niacin = 60 mg tryptophan; 0–6 months = preformed niacin (not NE).

[f] As dietary folate equivalents (DFE). 1 DFE = 1 μg food folate = 0.6 μg folic acid from fortified food or as a supplement consumed with food = 0.5 μg of a supplement taken on an empty stomach.

[g] In view of evidence linking folate intake with neural tube defects in the fetus, it is recommended that all women capable of becoming pregnant consume 400 μg from supplements or fortified foods in addition to intake of food folate from the diet.

[h] It is assumed that women will continue consuming 400 μg from supplements or fortified food until their pregnancy is confirmed and they enter prenatal care, which ordinarily occurs after the end of the preconceptional period—the critical time for formation of the neural tube.

[i] Although AIs have been set for choline, there are few data to assess whether a dietary supply of choline is needed at all stages of the life cycle, and it may be that the choline requirement can be met by endogenous synthesis at some of these stages.

[j] For healthy moderately active Americans and Canadians.

[k] PAL = physical activity level, EER = estimated energy requirement, TEE = total energy expenditure. The intake that meets the average energy expenditure of individuals at the reference height, weight, and age.

[l] RDA = Recommended Dietary Allowance. The intake that meets the nutrient need of almost all (97–98 percent) individuals in a group.

[m] AI = Adequate Intake. The observed average or experimentally determined intake by a defined population or subgroup that appears to sustain a defined nutritional status, such as growth rate, normal circulating nutrient values, or other functional indicators of health. The AI is used if sufficient scientific evidence is not available to derive an Estimated Average Requirement (EAR). For healthy infants receiving human milk, the AI is the mean intake. The AI is not equivalent to an RDA. Based on 14 g/1000 kcal of required energy.

[n] ND = not determined. The observed average of experimentally determined intake by a defined population or subgroup that appears to sustain a defined nutritional status, such as growth rate, normal circulating nutrient values, or other functional indicators of health. The AI is used if sufficient scientific evidence is not available to derive an EAR. For healthy infants receiving human milk, the AI is the mean intake. The AI is not equivalent to an RDA.

No determined biological function in humans has been identified for the nutrients silicon and vanadium.

TABLE H-2 Dietary Reference Intakes (DRIs): Tolerable Upper Intake Levels (UL[a]), Food and Nutrition Board, National Academy of Sciences

	Infants 0–6 mo	Infants 7–12 mo	Children 1–3 y	Children 4–8 y	Males/ Females 9–13 y	Males/ Females 14–18 y	Pregnancy ≤18 y	Lactation ≤18 y
Vitamin A (μg/day)[b]	600	600	600	900	1700	2800	2800	2800
Vitamin C (mg/day)	ND[f]	ND	400	650	1200	1800	1800	1800
Vitamin D (μg/day)	25	25	50	50	50	50	50	50
Vitamin E (mg/day)[c,d]	ND	ND	200	300	600	800	800	800
Vitamin K (μg/day)	ND	ND	ND	ND	ND	ND	ND	ND
Thiamin (mg/day)	ND	ND	ND	ND	ND	ND	ND	ND
Riboflavin (mg/day)	ND	ND	ND	ND	ND	ND	ND	ND
Niacin (mg/day)[d]	ND	ND	10	15	20	30	30	30
Vitamin B_6 (mg/day)	ND	ND	30	40	60	80	80	80
Folate (μg/day)[d]	ND	ND	300	400	600	800	800	800
Vitamin B_{12} (mg/day)	ND	ND	ND	ND	ND	ND	ND	ND
Pantothenic Acid (mg/day)	ND	ND	ND	ND	ND	ND	ND	ND
Biotin (μg/day)	ND	ND	ND	ND	ND	ND	ND	ND
Choline (mg/day)	ND	ND	1.0	1.0	2.0	3.0	3.0	3.0
Carotenoids[e]	ND	ND	ND	ND	ND	ND	ND	ND
Arsenic	ND	ND	ND	ND	ND	ND	ND	ND
Boron (mg/day)	ND	ND	3	6	11	17	17	17
Calcium (mg/day)	ND	ND	2.5	2.5	2.5	2.5	2.5	2.5
Chromium (μg/day)	ND	ND	ND	ND	ND	ND	ND	ND
Copper (μg/day)	ND	ND	1000	3000	5000	8000	8000	8000
Fluoride (mg/day)	.07	.09	1.3	2.2	10	10	10	10
Iodine (μg/day)	ND	ND	200	300	600	900	900	900
Iron (mg/day)	40	40	40	40	40	45	45	45
Magnesium (mg/day)[c]	ND	ND	65	110	350	350	350	350
Manganese (mg/day)	ND	ND	2	3	6	9	9	9
Molybdenum (μg/day)	ND	ND	300	600	1100	1700	1700	1700
Nickel (mg/day)	ND	ND	0.2	0.3	0.6	1.0	1.0	1.0
Phosphorus (mg/day)	ND	ND	3	3	4	4	3.5	4
Selenium (μg/day)	45	60	90	150	280	400	400	400
Silicon[d]	ND	ND	ND	ND	ND	ND	ND	ND
Vanadium (mg/day)[e]	ND	ND	ND	ND	ND	ND	ND	ND
Zinc (mg/day)	4	5	7	12	23	34	34	34

[a]UL = The maximum level of daily nutrient intake that is likely to pose no risk of adverse effects. Unless otherwise specified, the UL represents total intake from food, water, and supplements. Due to lack of suitable data, ULs could not be established for vitamin K, thiamin, riboflavin, vitamin B_{12}, pantothenic acid, biotin, or carotenoids. In the absences of ULs, extra caution may be warranted in consuming levels above recommended intakes.

[b]As preformed vitamin A only.

[c]As α-tocopherol; applies to any form of supplemental α-tocopherol.

[d]The ULs for vitamin E, niacin, and folate apply to synthetic forms obtained from supplements, fortified foods, or a combination of the two.

[e]β-Carotene supplements are advised only to serve as a provitamin A source for individuals at risk of vitamin A deficiency.

[f]ND = Not determinable due to lack of data of adverse effects in this age group and concern with regard to lack of ability to handle excess amounts.

Source: This table is taken from the DRI report; see http://www.nap.edu.

TABLE H-3 Dietary Reference Intakes (DRIs) During Pregnancy[1]

	Females			Pregnancy		
Life Stage Group	**14–18 y**	**19–30 y**	**31–50 y**	**≤18y**	**19–30 y**	**31–50 y**
Calcium (mg/day)	1300*	1000*	1000*	1300*	1000*	1000*
Phosphorus (mg/day)	1250	700	700	1250	700	700
Magnesium (mg/day)	360	310	320	400	350	360
Vitamin A (μg/day)	700	700	700	750	770	770
Vitamin D (μg/day)[a,b]	5*	5*	5*	5*	5*	5*
Fluoride (mg/day)	3*	3*	3*	3*	3*	3*
Thiamin (mg/day)	1.0	1.1	1.1	1.4	1.4	1.4
Riboflavin (mg/day)	1.0	1.1	1.1	1.4	1.4	1.4
Niacin (mg/day)[c]	14	14	14	18	18	18
Vitamin B_6 (mg/day)	1.2	1.3	1.3	1.9	1.9	1.9
Folate (μg/day)[d]	400[g]	400[g]	400[g]	600[h]	600[h]	600[h]
Vitamin B_{12} (μg/day)	2.4	2.4	2.4	2.6	2.6	2.6
Pantothenic acid (mg/day)	5*	5*	5*	6*	6*	6*
Biotin (μg/day)	25*	30*	30*	30*	30*	30*
Choline[e] (mg/day)	400*	425*	425*	450*	450*	450*
Vitamin C (mg/day)	65	75	75	80	85	85
Vitamin E[f] (mg/day)	15	15	15	15	15	15
Iron (mg/day)	15	18	18	27	27	27
Zinc (mg/day)	9	8	8	13	11	11
Copper (μg/day)	890	900	900	1000	1000	1000
Selenium (μg/day)	55	55	55	60	60	60
Iodine (μg/day)	150	150	150	220	220	220

[1]Institute of Medicine.
*Adequate Intakes (AI).
[a]As cholecalciferol. 1 μg cholecalciferol = 40 IU vitamin D.
[b]In the absence of adequate exposure to sunlight.
[c]As niacin equivalents (NE). 1 mg niacin = 60 mg tryptophan.
[d]As dietary folate equivalents (DFE). 1 DFE = 1 μg food folate = 0.6 μg folic acid from fortified food or as a supplement consumed with food = 0.5 μg of a supplement taken on an empty stomach.
[e]Although AIs have been set for choline, there are few data to assess whether a dietary supply of choline is needed at all stages of the life cycle, and it may be that the choline requirement can be met by endogenous synthesis at some of these stages.
[f]As α-tocopherol. α-Tocopherol includes *RRR*-α-tocopherol, the only form of α-tocopherol that occurs naturally in foods, and the 2*R*-stereoisomeric forms of α-tocopherol (*SRR-*, *SSR-*, *SRS-*, and *SSS*-α-tocopherol), also found in fortified foods and supplements.
[g]In view of evidence linking folate intake with neural tube defects in the fetus, it is recommended that all women capable of becoming pregnant consume 400 μg from supplements or fortified foods in addition to intake of food folate from a varied diet.
[h]It is assumed that women will continue consuming 400 μg from supplements or fortified food until their pregnancy is confirmed and they enter prenatal care, which ordinarily occurs after the end of the periconceptional period—the critical time for formation of the neural tube.

1a. Institute of Medicine. Vitamin A. In: *Dietary Intakes for Vitamin A, Vitamin K, Arsenic, Boron, Chromium, Copper, Iodine, Iron, Manganese, Molybdenum, Nickel, Silicon, Vanadium, and Zinc*. Washington, DC: National Academies Press; 2001:65–126.
1b. Institute of Medicine FNB. *Dietary Reference Intakes for Calcium, Phosporus, Magnesium, Vitamin D, and Fluoride*. Washington, DC: Institute of Medicine; 1997.
1c. Institute of Medicine FNB. *Dietary Reference Intakes for Thiamin, Riboflavin, Niacin, Vitamin B_6, Folate, Vitamin B_{12}, Pantothenic Acid, Biotin, and Choline*. Washington, DC: Institute of Medicine; 1998.
1d. Institute of Medicine FNB. *Dietary Reference Intakes for Vitamin C, Vitamin E, Selenium, and Carotenoids*. Washington, DC: Institute of Medicine; 2000.

Source: This table is taken from the DRI report; see http://www.nap.edu.

Table H-4 Equations to Estimate Energy Requirement

Infants and Young Children Estimated Energy Requirement (kcal/day) = Total Energy Expenditure + Energy Deposition	
0–3 months	EER[a] = (89 × weight [kg] − 100) + 175
4–6 months	EER = (89 × weight [kg] − 100) + 56
7–12 months	EER = (89 × weight [kg] − 100) + 22
13–35 months	EER = (89 × weight [kg] − 100) + 20
Children and Adolescents 3–18 Years Estimated Energy Requirement (kcal/day) = Total Energy Expenditure + Energy Deposition	
Boys	
3–8 yrs	EER = 88.5 − (61.9 × age [y]) + PA[b] × [(26.7 × weight [kg]) + (903 × height [m])] + 20
9–18 yrs	EER = 88.5 − (61.9 × age [y]) + PA × [(26.7 × weight [kg]) + (903 × height [m])] + 25
Girls	
3–8 yrs	EER = 135.3 − (30.8 × age [y] + PA × [(10.0 × weight [kg]) + (934 × height [m])] + 20
9–18 yrs	EER = 135.3 − (30.8 × age [y] + PA × [(10.0 × weight [kg]) + (934 × height [m])] + 25
Adults 19 Years and Older Estimated Energy Requirement (kcal/day) = Total Energy Expenditures	
Men	EER = 662 − (9.53 × age [y]) + PA × [(15.91 × weight [kg]) + (539.6 × height [m])]
Women	EER = 354 − (6.91 × age [y]) + PA × [(9.36 × weight [kg]) + (726 × height [m])]
Pregnancy Estimated Energy Requirement (kcal/day) = Nonpregnant EER + Pregnancy Energy Deposition	
1st trimester	EER = Nonpregnant EER + 0
2nd trimester	EER = Nonpregnant EER + 340
3rd trimester	EER = Nonpregnant EER + 452
Lactation Estimated Energy Requirement (kcal/day) = Nonpregnant EER + Milk Energy Output − Weight Loss	
0–6 months postpartum	EER = Nonpregnant EER + 500 − 170
7–12 months postpartum	EER = Nonpregnant EER + 400 − 0

Note: These equations provide an estimate of energy requirement. Relative body weight (i.e., loss, stable, gain) is the preferred indicator of energy adequacy.

[a]EER = Estimated Energy Requirement.

[b]PA = Physical Activity Coefficient (see Table H-5).

Source: Otten JJ, Hellwig JP, Meyers LD. *DRIs: The Essential Guide to Nutrient Requirements*. Washington, DC: Institute of Medicine, The National Academies Press; 2006. Reprinted with permission.

TABLE H-5 Physical Activity Coefficients (PA Values) for Use in EER Equations

	Sedentary (PAL* 1.0–1.39)	Low Active (PAL 1.4–1.59)	Active (PAL 1.6–1.89)	Very Active (PAL 1.9–2.5)
	Typical daily living activities (e.g., household tasks, walking to the bus)	Typical daily living activities PLUS 30–60 minutes of daily moderate activity (e.g., walking at 5–7 km/h)	Typical daily living activities PLUS at least 60 minutes of daily moderate activity	Typical daily living activities PLUS at least 60 minutes of daily moderate activity PLUS an additional 60 minutes of vigorous activity or 120 minutes of moderate activity
Boys 3–18 y	1.00	1.13	1.26	1.42
Girls 3–18 y	1.00	1.16	1.31	1.56
Men 19 y +	1.00	1.11	1.25	1.48
Women 19 y +	1.00	1.12	1.27	1.45

*PAL = Physical Activity Level.

Source: Otten JJ, Hellwig JP, Meyers LD. *DRIs: The Essential Guide to Nutrient Requirements*. Washington, DC: Institute of Medicine, The National Academies Press; 2006. Reprinted with permission.

TABLE H-6 Estimated Energy Requirement (EER) for Boys 0 Through 2 Years of Age

Age (mo)	Reference Weight (kg [lb])	Total Energy Expenditure (kcal/day)	Energy Deposition (kcal/day)	EER (kcal/day)
1	4.4 (9.7)	292	180	472
2	5.3 (11.7)	372	195	567
3	6.0 (13.2)	434	138	572
4	6.7 (14.8)	496	52	548
5	7.3 (16.1)	550	46	596
6	7.9 (17.4)	603	42	645
7	8.4 (18.5)	648	20	668
8	8.9 (19.6)	692	18	710
9	9.3 (20.5)	728	18	746
10	9.7 (21.4)	763	30	793
11	10.0 (22.0)	790	27	817
12	10.3 (22.7)	817	27	844
15	11.1 (24.4)	888	20	908
18	11.7 (25.8)	941	20	961
21	12.2 (26.9)	986	20	1006
24	12.7 (28.0)	1030	20	1050
27	13.1 (28.9)	1066	20	1086
30	13.5 (29.7)	1101	20	1121
33	13.9 (30.6)	1137	20	1157
35	14.2 (31.3)	1164	20	1184

Source: Otten JJ, Hellwig JP, Meyers LD. *DRIs: The Essential Guide to Nutrient Requirements*. Washington, DC: Institute of Medicine, The National Academies Press; 2006. Reprinted with permission.

TABLE H-7 Estimated Energy Requirement (EER) for Girls 0 Through 2 Years of Age

Age (mo)	Reference Weight (kg [lb])	Total Energy Expenditure (kcal/day)	Energy Deposition (kcal/day)	EER (kcal/day)
1	4.2 (9.3)	274	164	438
2	4.9 (10.8)	336	164	500
3	5.5 (12.1)	389	132	521
4	6.1 (13.4)	443	65	508
5	6.7 (14.8)	496	57	553
6	7.2 (15.9)	541	52	593
7	7.7 (17.0)	585	23	608
8	8.1 (17.8)	621	22	643
9	8.5 (18.7)	656	22	678
10	8.9 (19.6)	692	25	717
11	9.2 (20.3)	719	23	742
12	9.5 (20.9)	745	23	768
15	10.3 (22.7)	817	20	837
18	11.0 (24.2)	879	20	899
21	11.6 (25.6)	932	20	952
24	12.1 (26.7)	977	20	997
27	12.5 (27.5)	1013	20	1033
30	13.0 (28.6)	1057	20	1077
33	13.4 (29.5)	1093	20	1113
35	13.7 (30.2)	1119	20	1139

Source: Otten JJ, Hellwig JP, Meyers LD. *DRIs: The Essential Guide to Nutrient Requirements*. Washington, DC: Institute of Medicine, The National Academies Press; 2006. Reprinted with permission.

TABLE H-8 Estimated Energy Requirements (EER; kcal/day) for Boys 3 Through 18 Years of Age

Age (years)	Reference Weight (kg [lbs])	Reference Height (m [in])	Sedentary PAL*	Low Active PAL*	Active PAL*	Very Active PAL*
3	14.3 (31.5)	0.95 (37.4)	1162	1324	1485	1683
4	16.2 (35.7)	1.02 (40.2)	1215	1390	1566	1783
5	18.4 (40.5)	1.09 (42.9)	1275	1466	1658	1894
6	20.7 (45.6)	1.15 (45.3)	1328	1535	1742	1997
7	23.1 (50.9)	1.22 (48.0)	1393	1617	1840	2115
8	25.6 (56.4)	1.28 (50.4)	1453	1692	1931	2225
9	28.6 (63.0)	1.34 (52.8)	1530	1787	2043	2359
10	31.9 (70.3)	1.39 (54.7)	1601	1875	2149	2486
11	35.9 (79.1)	1.44 (56.7)	1691	1985	2279	2640
12	40.5 (89.2)	1.49 (58.7)	1798	2113	2428	2817
13	45.6 (100.4)	1.56 (61.4)	1935	2276	2618	3038
14	51.0 (112.3)	1.64 (64.6)	2090	2459	2829	3283
15	56.3 (124.0)	1.70 (66.9)	2223	2618	3013	3499
16	60.9 (134.1)	1.74 (68.5)	2320	2736	3152	3663
17	64.6 (142.3)	1.75 (68.9)	2366	2796	3226	3754
18	67.2 (148.0)	1.76 (69.3)	2383	2823	3263	3804

*PAL = physical activity level
Source: Otten JJ, Hellwig JP, Meyers LD. *DRIs: The Essential Guide to Nutrient Requirements*. Washington, DC: Institute of Medicine, The National Academies Press; 2006. Reprinted with permission.

TABLE H-9 Estimated Energy Requirements (EER; kcal/day) for Girls 3 Through 18 Years of Age

Age (years)	Reference Weight (kg [lbs])	Reference Height (m [in])	Sedentary PAL*	Low Active PAL*	Active PAL*	Very Active PAL*
3	13.9 (30.6)	0.94 (37.0)	1080	1243	1395	1649
4	15.8 (34.8)	1.01 (39.8)	1133	1310	1475	1750
5	17.9 (39.4)	1.08 (42.5)	1189	1379	1557	1854
6	20.2 (44.5)	1.15 (45.3)	1247	1451	1642	1961
7	22.8 (50.2)	1.21 (47.6)	1298	1515	1719	2058
8	25.6 (56.4)	1.28 (50.4)	1360	1593	1810	2173
9	29.0 (63.9)	1.33 (52.4)	1415	1660	1890	2273
10	32.9 (72.5)	1.38 (54.3)	1470	1729	1972	2376
11	37.2 (81.9)	1.44 (56.7)	1538	1813	2071	2500
12	41.6 (91.6)	1.51 (59.4)	1617	1909	2183	2640
13	45.8 (100.9)	1.57 (61.8)	1684	1992	2281	2762
14	49.4 (108.8)	1.60 (63.0)	1718	2036	2334	2831
15	52.0 (114.5)	1.62 (63.8)	1731	2057	2362	2870
16	53.9 (118.7)	1.63 (64.2)	1729	2059	2368	2883
17	55.1 (121.4)	1.63 (64.2)	1710	2042	2353	2871
18	56.2 (123.8)	1.63 (64.2)	1690	2024	2336	2858

*PAL = physical activity level
Source: Otten JJ, Hellwig JP, Meyers LD. *DRIs: The Essential Guide to Nutrient Requirements*. Washington, DC: Institute of Medicine, The National Academies Press; 2006. Reprinted with permission.

TABLE H-10 Dietary Reference Intakes for Total Protein by Life Stage Group

	DRI Values (g/kg/day)				
	EAR[a]		RDA[b]		AI[c]
	Males	Females	Males	Females	
Life stage group					
0 through 6 mo					1.52 (9.1)
7 through 12 mo	1.0	1.0	1.2 (11)[d]	1.2 (11)	
1 through 3 y	0.87	0.87	1.05 (13)	1.05 (13)	
4 through 8 y	0.76	0.76	0.95 (19)	0.95 (19)	
9 through 13 y	0.76	0.76	0.95 (34)	0.95 (34)	
14 through 18 y	0.73	0.71	0.85 (52)	0.85 (46)	
19 through 30 y	0.66	0.66	0.80 (56)	0.80 (46)	
31 through 50 y	0.66	0.66	0.80 (56)	0.80 (46)	
51 through 70 y	0.66	0.66	0.80 (56)	0.80 (46)	
> 70 y	0.66	0.66	0.80 (56)	0.80 (46)	
Pregnancy		0.88[e]		1.1 (71)[e]	
Lactation		1.05		1.3 (71)	

[a]EAR = Estimated Average Requirement. An EAR is the average daily nutrient intake level estimated to meet the requirements of half of the healthy individuals in a group.

[b]RDA = Recommended Dietary Allowance. An RDA is the average daily dietary intake level sufficient to meet the nutrient requirements of nearly all (97–98 percent) healthy individuals in a group.

[c]AI = Adequate Intake. If sufficient scientific evidence is not available to establish an EAR, and thus calculate an RDA, an AI is usually developed. For healthy breastfed infants, the AI is the mean intake. The AI for other life stage and gender groups is believed to cover the needs of all healthy individuals in the group, but a lack of data or uncertainty in the data prevents being able to specify with confidence the percentage of individuals covered by this intake.

[d]Values in parentheses ( ) are examples of the total g/day of protein calculated from g/kg/day times the reference weights.

[e]The EAR and RDA for pregnancy are only for the second half of pregnancy. For the first half of pregnancy, the protein requirements are the same as those of nonpregnant women.

Source: This table is taken from the DRI report: see http://www.nap.edu.

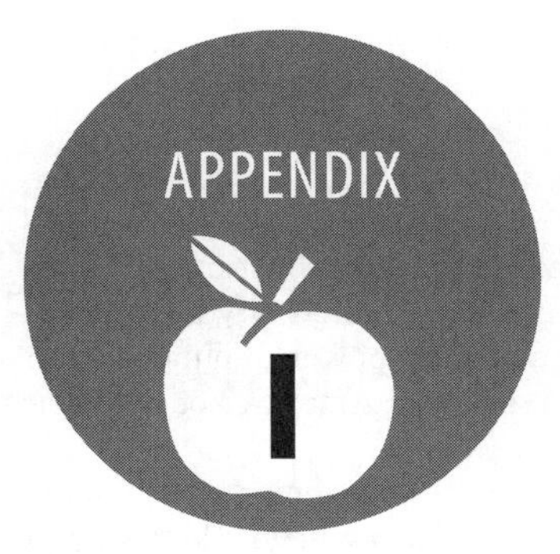

2010 Dietary Guidelines

Part A: Executive Summary

The 2010 Dietary Guidelines Advisory Committee (DGAC) was established jointly by the Secretaries of the U.S. Department of Agriculture (USDA) and the U.S. Department of Health and Human Services (HHS). The Committee's task was to advise the Secretaries of USDA and HHS on whether revisions to the 2005 Dietary Guidelines were warranted, and if so, to recommend updates to the Guidelines. The DGAC immediately recognized that, on the basis of the vast amount of published research and emerging science on numerous relevant topics, an updated report was indeed needed.

The 2010 DGAC Report is distinctly different from previous reports in several ways. First, it addresses an American public of whom the majority are overweight or obese and yet undernourished in several key nutrients. Second, the Committee used a newly developed, state-of-the-art, Web-based electronic system and methodology, known as the Nutrition Evidence Library (NEL), to answer the majority of the scientific questions it posed. The remaining questions were answered by data analyses, food pattern modeling analyses, and consideration of other evidence-based reviews or existing reports, including the 2008 *Physical Activity Guidelines for Americans*. The 2005 Dietary Guidelines for Americans were the starting place for most reviews. If little or no scientific literature had been published on a specific topic since the 2005 Report was presented, the DGAC indicated this and established the conclusions accordingly.

A third distinctive feature of this Report is the introduction of two newly developed chapters. The first of these chapters considers the total diet and how to integrate all of the Report's nutrient and energy recommendations into practical terms that encourage personal choice but result in an eating pattern that is nutrient dense and calorie balanced. The second chapter complements this total diet approach by integrating and translating the scientific conclusions reached at the individual level to encompass the broader environmental and societal aspects that are crucial to full adoption and successful implementation of these recommendations.

The remainder of this Executive Summary provides brief synopses of these and all of the other chapters, which reviewed current evidence related to specific topics and presents the resulting highlights that comprise the fundamental essence of this report.

Major Cross-Cutting Findings and Recommendations

Total Diet: Combining Nutrients, Consuming Foods

The 2010 DGAC report concludes that good health and optimal functionality across the life span are achievable goals but require a lifestyle approach including a total diet that is energy balanced and nutrient dense. Now, as in the past, a disconnect exists between dietary recommendations and what Americans actually consume. On average, Americans of all ages consume too few vegetables, fruits, high-fiber whole grains, low-fat milk and milk products, and seafood and they eat too much added sugars, solid fats, refined grains, and sodium. SoFAS (added sugars and solid fats) contribute approximately 35 percent of calories to the American diet. This is true for children, adolescents, adults, and older adults and for both males and females. Reducing the intake of SoFAS can lead to a badly needed reduction in energy intake and inclusion of more healthful foods into the total diet.

The diet recommended in this Report is not a rigid prescription. Rather, it is a flexible approach that incorporates a wide range of individual tastes and food preferences. Accumulating evidence documents that certain dietary patterns consumed around the world are associated with beneficial health outcomes. Patterns of eating that have been shown to be healthful include the Dietary Approaches to Stop Hypertension (DASH)-style dietary patterns and certain Mediterranean-style dietary patterns. Similarly, the USDA Food Patterns illustrate that both nutrient adequacy and moderation goals can be met in a variety of ways. The daunting

The 2010 Dietary Guidelines Advisory Committee (DGAC) report is available online at http://www.dietaryguidelines.gov. This report is very detailed and 800 pages long, so the executive summary is listed here.

public health challenge is to accomplish population-wide adoption of healthful dietary patterns within the context of powerful influences that currently promote unhealthy consumer choices, behaviors, and lifestyles.

Translating and Integrating the Evidence: A Call to Action

Complementing the Total Diet chapter, this chapter describes the four major findings that emerged from the DGAC's review of the scientific evidence and articulates steps that can be taken to help all Americans adopt health-promoting nutrition and physical activity guidelines:

- Reduce the incidence and prevalence of overweight and obesity of the U.S. population by reducing overall calorie intake and increasing physical activity.
- Shift food intake patterns to a more plant-based diet that emphasizes vegetables, cooked dry beans and peas, fruits, whole grains, nuts, and seeds. In addition, increase the intake of seafood and fat-free and low-fat milk and milk products and consume only moderate amounts of lean meats, poultry, and eggs.
- Significantly reduce intake of foods containing added sugars and solid fats because these dietary components contribute excess calories and few, if any, nutrients. In addition, reduce sodium intake and lower intake of refined grains, especially refined grains that are coupled with added sugar, solid fat, and sodium.
- Meet the 2008 Physical Activity Guidelines for Americans.

The 2010 DGAC recognizes that substantial barriers make it difficult for Americans to accomplish these goals. Ensuring that all Americans consume a health-promoting dietary pattern and achieve and maintain energy balance requires far more than individual behavior change. A multisectoral strategy is imperative. For this reason, the 2010 DGAC strongly recommends that USDA and HHS convene appropriate committees, potentially through the Institute of Medicine (IOM), to develop strategic plans focusing on the actions needed to successfully implement key 2010 DGAC recommendations. Separate committees may be necessary because the actions needed to implement key recommendations likely differ by goal.

A coordinated strategic plan that includes all sectors of society, including individuals, families, educators, communities, physicians and allied health professionals, public health advocates, policy makers, scientists, and small and large businesses (e.g., farmers, agricultural producers, food scientists, food manufacturers, and food retailers of all kinds), should be engaged in the development and ultimate implementation of a plan to help all Americans eat well, be physically active, and maintain good health and function. It is important that any strategic plan is evidence informed, action oriented, and focused on changes in systems in these sectors.

Any and all systems-based strategies must include a focus on children. Primary prevention of obesity must begin in childhood. This is the single most powerful public health approach to combating and reversing America's obesity epidemic over the long term.

Strategies to help Americans change their dietary intake patterns and be physically active also will go a long way to ameliorating the disparities in health among racial and ethnic minorities and among different socioeconomic groups, which have been recognized as a significant concern for decades. While the reasons for these differences are complex and multifactorial, this Report addresses research indicating that certain dietary changes can provide a means to reduce health disparities.

Change is needed in the overall food environment to support the efforts of all Americans to meet the key recommendations of the 2010 DGAC. To meet these challenges, the following sustainable changes must occur:

- Improve nutrition literacy and cooking skills, including safe food handling skills, and empower and motivate the population, especially families with children, to prepare and consume healthy foods at home.
- Increase comprehensive health, nutrition, and physical education programs and curricula in U.S. schools and preschools, including food preparation, food safety, cooking, and physical education classes and improved quality of recess.
- For all Americans, especially those with low income, create greater financial incentives to purchase, prepare, and consume vegetables and fruit, whole grains, seafood, fat-free and low-fat milk and milk products, lean meats, and other healthy foods.
- Improve the availability of affordable fresh produce through greater access to grocery stores, produce trucks, and farmers' markets.
- Increase environmentally sustainable production of vegetables, fruits, and fiber-rich whole grains.
- Ensure household food security through measures that provide access to adequate amounts of foods that are nutritious and safe to eat.
- Develop safe, effective, and sustainable practices to expand aquaculture and increase the availability of seafood to all segments of the population Enhance access to publicly available, user-friendly benefit/risk information that helps consumers make informed seafood choices.
- Encourage restaurants and the food industry to offer health-promoting foods that are low in sodium; limited in added sugars, refined grains, and solid fats; and served in smaller portions.

- Implement the U.S. National Physical Activity Plan, a private-public sector collaborative promoting local, state, and national programs and policies to increase physical activity and reduce sedentary activity (http://www.physicalactivityplan.org/index.htm). Through the Plan and other initiatives, develop efforts across all sectors of society, including health care and public health; education; business and industry; mass media; parks, recreation, fitness, and sports; transportation, land use and community design; and volunteer and non-profit. Reducing screen time, especially television, for all Americans also will be important.

Topic-Specific Findings and Conclusions

Energy Balance and Weight Management

The prevalence of overweight and obesity in the United States has increased dramatically in the past three decades. This is true of children, adolescents, and adults and it is more severe in minority groups. The American environment is conducive to this epidemic, presenting temptation to the populace in the form of tasty, energy-dense, micronutrient-poor foods and beverages. The macronutrient distribution of a person's diet is not the driving force behind the current obesity epidemic. Rather, it is the over-consumption of total calories coupled with very low physical activity and too much sedentary time. The energy density of foods eaten is an important factor in overeating. Americans eat too many calories from foods high in solid fats and added sugars (SoFAS) that offer few or no other nutrients besides calories. This is true not only for adults but also for children, who consume energy-dense SoFAS, especially in the form of sugar-sweetened beverages, at levels substantially higher than required to maintain themselves at a normal weight as they grow.

With regard to special subgroups, maternal obesity before pregnancy and excessive weight gain during pregnancy are deleterious for the mother and the fetus. One-fifth of American women are obese when they become pregnant, often put on much more weight than is healthy during pregnancy, and have trouble losing it after delivery, placing their offspring at increased risk of obesity and type 2 diabetes (T2D) later in life. Breastfeeding has no sustained impact on maternal weight gain or loss, but has numerous benefits for mother and infant and should be encouraged.

Older overweight or obese adults can derive as much benefit from losing weight and keeping it off as do younger persons, with resulting improvements in quality of life, including diminished disabilities and lower risks of chronic diseases.

Selected behaviors that lead to a greater propensity to gain weight include too much TV watching, too little physical activity, eating out frequently (especially at Quick Service Restaurants [i.e. fast food restaurants]), snacking on energy-dense food and drinks, skipping breakfast, and consuming large portions. Self-monitoring, including knowing one's own calorie requirement and the calorie content of foods, helps make individuals conscious of what, when, and how much they eat. Mindful, or conscious, eating is an important lifestyle habit that can help to prevent inappropriate weight gain, enhance weight loss in those who should lose weight, and assist others in maintaining a healthy weight.

Nutrient Adequacy

Americans are encouraged to lower overall energy intakes to match their energy needs. Energy-dense forms of foods, especially foods high in SoFAS, should be replaced with nutrient-dense forms of vegetables, fruits, whole grains, and fluid milk and milk products to increase intakes of shortfall nutrients and nutrients of concern—vitamin D, calcium, potassium, and dietary fiber. Women of reproductive capacity should consume foods rich in folate and iron, and older individuals should consume fortified foods rich in vitamin B_{12} or B_{12} supplements, if needs cannot be met through whole foods. Nutritious breakfast consumption and in some cases nutrient-dense snacking may assist in meeting nutrient recommendations, especially in certain subgroups.

A daily multivitamin/mineral supplement does not offer health benefits to healthy Americans. Individual mineral/vitamin supplements can benefit some population groups with known deficiencies, such as calcium and vitamin D supplements to reduce risk of osteoporosis or iron supplements among those with deficient iron intakes. However, in some settings, mineral/vitamin supplements have been associated with harmful effects and should be pursued cautiously.

Fatty Acids and Cholesterol

Intakes of dietary fatty acids and cholesterol are major determinants of cardiovascular disease (CVD) and T2D, two major causes of morbidity and mortality in Americans. Fats contribute 9 calories per gram. The health impacts of dietary fats and cholesterol are mediated through levels of serum lipids, lipoproteins, and other intermediate markers. The U.S. consumption of harmful types and amounts of fatty acids and cholesterol has not changed appreciably since 1990.

In order to reduce the population's burden from CVD and T2D and their risk factors, the preponderance of the evidence indicates beneficial health effects are associated with several changes in consumption of dietary fats and cholesterol. These include limiting saturated fatty acid intake to less than 7 percent of total calories and substituting instead food sources of mono- or polyunsaturated fatty acids. As an interim step toward achieving this goal, individuals should first aim to consume less than 10 percent of energy as saturated fats and gradually reduce intake over time, while increasing polyunsaturated and monounsaturated sources. Other beneficial changes include limiting dietary cholesterol to less than 300 mg per day, but aiming at further reductions of dietary cholesterol to less than 200 mg per day in persons with or at high risk for CVD or T2D, and limiting cholesterol-raising fats (saturated fats exclusive of stearic acid and *trans* fatty acids) to less than 5 to 7 percent of energy.

Beneficial changes also include avoiding *trans* fatty acids from industrial sources in the American diet, leaving small amounts (<0.5% of calories) from *trans* fatty acids from natural (ruminant) sources, and consuming two servings of seafood per week (4 oz. cooked, edible seafood per serving) that provide an average of 250 mg/day of *n*-3 fatty acids from marine sources (i.e., docosahexaenoic acid [DHA] and eicosapentaenoic acid [EPA]). Ensuring maternal dietary intake of long chain n-3 fatty acids, in particular DHA, during pregnancy and lactation through two or more servings of seafood per week also has benefits for the infant, especially when women emphasize types of seafood high in *n*-3 fatty acids and with low methyl mercury content.

Protein

Proteins are unique because they provide both essential amino acids to build body proteins and are a calorie source. Protein contributes 4 calories per gram. Because protein requirements are based on ideal body weight (0.8 g protein/kg body weight/day for ages 19 years and older), lower-calorie diets result in a higher percentage of protein intake. Animal sources of protein, including meat, poultry, seafood, milk, and eggs, are the highest quality proteins. Plant proteins can be combined to form complete proteins if combinations of legumes and grains are consumed. Plant-based diets are able to meet protein requirements for essential amino acids through planning and offer other potential benefits, such as sources of fiber and nutrients important in a health-promoting diet.

Carbohydrates

Carbohydrates contribute 4 calories per gram and are the primary energy source for active people. Sedentary people, including most Americans, should decrease consumption of energy-dense carbohydrates, especially refined, sugar-dense sources, to balance energy needs and attain and maintain ideal weight. Americans should choose fiber-rich carbohydrate foods such as whole grains, vegetables, fruits, and cooked dry beans and peas as staples in the diet. Low-fat and fat-free milk and milk products are also nutrient-dense sources of carbohydrates in the diet and provide high-quality protein, vitamins, and minerals. High-energy, non-nutrient-dense carbohydrate sources that should be reduced to aid in calorie control include sugar-sweetened beverages; desserts, including grain-based desserts; and grain products and other carbohydrate foods and drinks that are low in nutrients.

Sodium, Potassium, and Water

At present, Americans consume excessive amounts of sodium and insufficient amounts of potassium. The health consequences of excessive sodium and insufficient potassium are substantial and include increased levels of blood pressure and its consequences (heart disease and stroke). In 2005, the DGAC recommended a daily sodium intake of less than 2,300 mg for the general adult population and stated that hypertensive individuals, Blacks, and middle-aged and older adults would benefit from reducing their sodium intake even further to 1,500 mg per day. Because these latter groups together now comprise nearly 70 percent of U.S. adults, the goal should be 1,500 mg per day for the general population. Given the current U.S. marketplace and the resulting excessively high sodium intake, it will be challenging to achieve the lower level. In addition, time is required to adjust taste perception in the general population. Thus, the reduction from 2,300 mg to 1,500 mg per day should occur gradually over time. Because early stages of blood pressure-related atherosclerotic disease begin during childhood, both children and adults should reduce their sodium intake.

Individuals also should increase their consumption of dietary potassium because increased potassium intakes helps to attenuate the effects of sodium on blood pressure. Water is needed to sustain life. However, there is no evidence, except under unusual circumstances, that water intake among Americans is either excessive or insufficient.

Alcohol

An average daily intake of one to two alcoholic beverages is associated with the lowest all-cause mortality and a low risk of diabetes and coronary heart disease among middle-aged and older adults. Despite this overall benefit of moderate alcohol consumption, the DGAC recommends that if alcohol is consumed, it should be consumed in moderation, and only by adults. Moderate alcohol consumption is defined as average daily consumption of up to one drink per day for women and up to two drinks per day for men, with no more than three drinks in any single day for women and no more than four drinks in any single day for men. One drink is defined as 12 fl. oz. of regular beer, 5 fl. oz. of wine, or 1.5 fl. oz. of distilled spirits.

The DGAC found strong evidence that heavy consumption of four or more drinks a day for women and five or more drinks a day for men has harmful health effects. A number of situations and conditions call for the complete avoidance of alcoholic beverages.

Food Safety and Technology

Since the release of the 2005 Dietary Guidelines, food safety concerns have escalated, with the apparent increase in voluntary recalls of foods contaminated with disease-causing bacteria and adulterated with non-food substances. These food safety issues affect commercial food products and food preparations in the home.

The basic four food safety principles identified to reduce the risk of foodborne illnesses remain unchanged. These principles are Clean, Separate, Cook, and Chill. Consumers must take more responsibility for carrying out these essential food safety practices. These actions, in tandem with sound government policies and responsible food industry practices, can help prevent foodborne illness. Even with current and future introductions of food safety technologies, food safety fundamentals in the home remain foundational.

The health benefits from consuming a variety of cooked seafood outweigh the risks associated with exposure to methyl mercury and persistent organic pollutants, provided that the types and sources of seafood to be avoided by some consumers are clearly communicated to consumers. Overall, consumers can safely eat at least 12 oz. of a variety of cooked seafood per week provided they pay attention to local seafood advisories and limit their intake of large, predatory fish. Women who may become or who are pregnant, nursing mothers, and children ages 12 and younger can safely consume a variety of cooked seafood in amounts recommended by this Committee while following Federal and local advisories.

Conclusion

The 2010 DGAC recognizes the significant challenges involved in implementing the goals outlined in this Report. The challenges go beyond cost, economic interests, technological and societal changes, and agricultural limitations, but together, stakeholders and the public can make a difference. We must value preparing and enjoying healthy food and the practices of good nutrition, physical activity, and a healthy lifestyle. The DGAC encourages all stakeholders to take actions to make every choice available to Americans a healthy choice. To move toward this vision, all segments of society—from parents to policy makers and everyone else in between—must now take responsibility and play a leadership role in creating gradual and steady change to help current and future generations live healthy and productive lives. A measure of success will be evidence that meaningful change has occurred when the 2015 DGAC convenes.

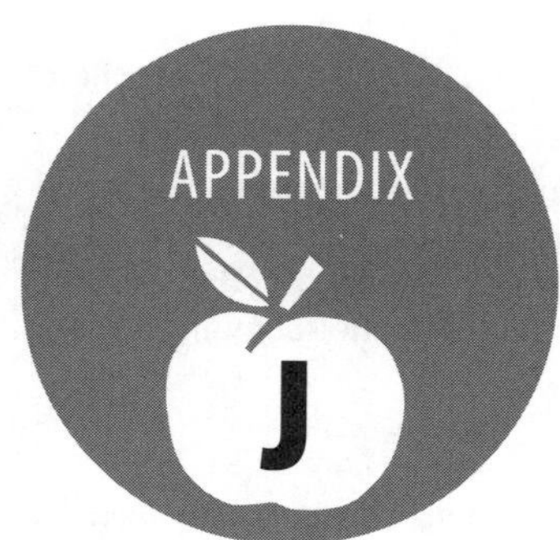

Conversion Tables

EXHIBIT J-1 Conversion Tables

Volume

1 t	= 1/3 T	= 1/6 fl oz	= 4.9 mL
3 t	= 1 T	= 1/2 fl oz	= 14.8 mL
2 T	= 1/8 cup	= 1 fl oz	= 29.6 mL
4 T	= 1/4 cup	= 2 fl oz	= 59.1 mL
5 1/3 T	= 1/3 cup	= 2 2/3 fl oz	= 78.9 mL
8 T	= 1/2 cup	= 4 fl oz	= 118.3 mL
10 2/3 T	= 2/3 cup	= 5 1/3 fl oz	= 157.7 mL
12 T	= 3/4 cup	= 6 fl oz	= 177.4 mL
14 T	= 7/8 cup	= 7 fl oz	= 207.0 mL
16 T	= 1 cup	= 8 fl oz	= 236.6 mL
1 mL	= 0.034 fl oz	= 1 mL	= 0.001 liter
1 liter	= 34 fl oz	= 1000 mL	
1 pint (pt)	= 2 cups	= 0.473 liter	= 473 mL
1 quart (qt)	= 2 pt	= 0.946 liter	= 946 mL
1 gallon	= 4 qts	= 3.785 liter	= 3785 mL
1 liter	= 1.057 qts	= 0.264 gallon	= 1000 mL

To convert mLs to oz divide by 30.
To convert oz to mLs multipy by 30.

Weight

1 gram (g) = 0.035 oz = 0.001 kg = 1000 mg = 1,000,000 mcg
1 mg = 0.001 g = 1000 mcg
1 oz = 28.35 g (often rounded to 28 g)
1 lb = 16 oz = 453.59 g = 0.454 kg
1 kg = 2.21 lb = 1000 g

Length

1 inch = 2.54 centimeters
1 foot = 30.5 centimeters
1 yard = 0.91 meters
1 mile = 1.61 kilometers
1 centimeter = 0.4 inches
1 meter = 3.3 feet
1 meter = 1.1 yards
1 kilometer = 0.6 miles

(continued)

EXHIBIT J-1 *(Continued)*

To convert inches to centimeters, multiply by 2.54; centimeters to inches, multiply by 0.4.

Area
1 square inch = 6.5 square centimeters
1 square foot = 9.29 square meters
1 square yard = 0.84 square meters
1 square centimeter = 0.16 square inches
1 square meter = 1.2 square yards

Heat Measures
1 kilojoule = 0.239 kilocalories
1 kilocalorie = 4.184 kilojoules

Temperatures

Water freezes	0°C	32°F
Room temperature	27°C	72°F
Body temperature	37°C	98.6°F
Water boils	100°C	212°F

To convert Fahrenheit to Celsius (centigrade), subtract 32, multiply by 5, divide by 9; Celsius (centigrade) to Fahrenheit, multiply by 9, divide by 5, and add 32.

Milliequivalent-milligram conversion table

Mineral element	Chemical symbol	Atomic weight	Valence
Calcium	Ca	40	2
Choline	Cl	35.4	1
Magnesium	Mg	24.3	2
Phosphorus	P	31	2
Potassium	K	39	1
Sodium	Na	23	1
Sulfate	SO_4	96	2
Sulfur	S	32	2
Zinc	Zn	65.4	2

$$\text{Milliequivalents} = \frac{\text{milligrams}}{\text{atomic weight}} \times \text{valence}$$

Example: convert 1000 mg sodium to MEq of sodium

1 g NaCl = 0.4 g Na
(Na+ = 40% of weight of NaCl)
1 g Na+ = 2.5g NaCl

$$\frac{1000}{23} \times 1 = 43 \text{ MEq sodium}$$

To change milliequivalents back to milligrams, multiply the milliequivalents by the atomic weight and divide by the valence.

Example: convert 10 MEq sodium to mg sodium

$$\frac{10 \times 23}{1} = 230 \text{ mg sodium}$$

EXHIBIT J-2 Pound to Kilogram Conversion Chart

lb	kg	lb	kg	lb	kg	lb	kg	lb	kg
85.0	38.6	108.0	49.1	131.0	59.5	154.0	70.0	177.0	80.5
85.5	38.9	108.5	49.3	131.5	59.8	154.5	70.2	177.5	80.7
86.0	39.1	109.0	49.5	132.0	60.0	155.0	70.5	178.0	80.9
86.5	39.3	109.5	49.8	132.5	60.2	155.5	70.7	178.5	81.1
87.0	39.5	110.0	50.0	133.0	60.5	156.0	70.9	179.0	81.4
87.5	39.8	110.5	50.2	133.5	60.7	156.5	71.1	179.5	81.6
88.0	40.0	111.0	50.5	134.0	60.9	157.0	71.4	180.0	81.8
88.5	40.2	111.5	50.7	134.5	61.1	157.5	71.6	180.5	82.0
89.0	40.5	112.0	50.9	135.0	61.4	158.0	71.8	181.0	82.3
89.5	40.7	112.5	51.1	135.5	61.6	158.5	72.0	181.5	82.5
90.0	40.9	113.0	51.4	136.0	61.8	159.0	72.3	182.0	82.7
90.5	41.1	113.5	51.6	136.5	62.0	159.5	72.5	182.5	83.0
91.0	41.4	114.0	51.8	137.0	62.3	160.0	72.7	183.0	83.2
91.5	41.6	114.5	52.0	137.5	62.5	160.5	73.0	183.5	83.4
92.0	41.8	115.0	52.3	138.0	62.7	161.0	73.2	184.0	83.6
92.5	42.0	115.5	52.5	138.5	63.0	161.5	73.4	184.5	83.9
93.0	42.3	116.0	52.7	139.0	63.2	162.0	73.6	185.0	84.1
93.5	42.5	116.5	53.0	139.5	63.4	162.5	73.9	185.5	84.3
94.0	42.7	117.0	53.2	140.0	63.6	163.0	74.1	186.0	84.5
94.5	43.0	117.5	53.4	140.5	63.9	163.5	74.3	186.5	84.8
95.0	43.2	118.0	53.6	141.0	64.1	164.0	74.5	187.0	85.0
95.5	43.4	118.5	53.9	141.5	64.3	164.5	74.8	187.5	85.2
96.0	43.6	119.0	54.1	142.0	64.5	165.0	75.0	188.0	85.5
96.5	43.9	119.5	54.3	142.5	64.8	165.5	75.2	188.5	85.7
97.0	44.1	120.0	54.5	143.0	65.0	166.0	75.5	189.0	85.9
97.5	44.3	120.5	54.8	143.5	65.2	166.5	75.7	189.5	86.1
98.0	44.5	121.0	55.0	144.0	65.5	167.0	75.9	190.0	86.4
98.5	44.8	121.5	55.2	144.5	65.7	167.5	76.1	190.5	86.6
99.0	45.0	122.0	55.5	145.0	65.9	168.0	76.4	191.0	86.8
99.5	45.2	122.5	55.7	145.5	66.1	168.5	76.6	191.5	87.0
100.0	45.5	123.0	55.9	146.0	66.5	169.0	76.8	192.0	87.3
100.5	45.7	123.5	56.1	146.5	66.6	169.5	77.0	192.5	87.5
101.0	45.9	124.0	56.4	147.0	66.8	170.0	77.3	193.0	87.7
101.5	46.1	124.5	56.6	147.5	67.0	170.5	77.5	193.5	88.0
102.0	46.4	125.0	56.8	148.0	67.3	171.0	77.7	194.0	88.2
102.5	46.6	125.5	57.0	148.5	67.5	171.5	78.0	194.5	88.4
103.0	46.8	126.0	57.3	149.0	67.7	172.0	78.2	195.0	88.6
103.5	47.0	126.5	57.5	149.5	68.0	172.5	78.4	195.5	88.9
104.0	47.3	127.0	57.7	150.0	68.2	173.0	78.6	196.0	89.1
104.5	47.5	127.5	58.0	150.5	68.4	173.5	78.9	196.5	89.3
105.0	47.7	128.0	58.2	151.0	68.6	174.0	79.1	197.0	89.5
105.5	48.0	128.5	58.4	151.5	68.9	174.5	79.3	197.5	89.8
106.0	48.2	129.0	58.6	152.0	69.1	175.0	79.5	198.0	90.0
106.5	48.4	129.5	58.9	152.5	69.3	175.5	79.8	198.5	90.2
107.0	48.6	130.0	59.1	153.0	69.5	176.0	80.0	199.0	90.5
107.5	48.9	130.5	59.3	153.5	69.8	176.5	80.2	199.5	90.7

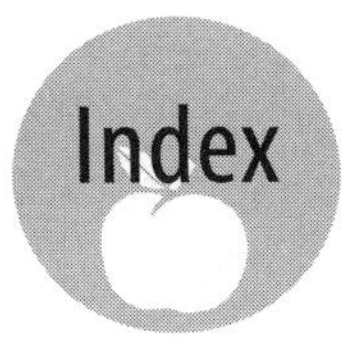

Index

Note: Page numbers followed by *f* indicate figures; page numbers followed by *t* indicate tables; page numbers followed by *e* indicate exhibits.